THE SCIENCE OF PHARMACOLOGY

THE SCIENCE OF PHARMACOLOGY

JAHANGIR MOINI, MD, MPH
Professor of Science and Health (retired)
Eastern Florida State College, Palm Bay, FL.

MANDANA NADERI, PHARMD, MPH, BCIDP
Medical Science Director in the pharmaceutical industry
Former Assistant Professor of Practice
R. Ken Coit College of Pharmacy at the University of Arizona
Los Angeles, CA

JENNIFER G. SCHNELLMANN, PH.D.
Associate Professor
University of Arizona, Colleges of Medicine and Pharmacy

ANTHONY SCOTT, PHARMD, MBA, FASHP
Director, Pharmacy Operations and Account Management
Cardinal Health, Atlanta, GA

ELSEVIER

ACADEMIC PRESS
An imprint of Elsevier

Academic Press is an imprint of Elsevier
125 London Wall, London EC2Y 5AS, United Kingdom
50 Hampshire Street, 5th Floor, Cambridge, MA 02139, United States

ISBN: 978-0-443-29038-1

For information on all Academic Press publications visit our website at
https://www.elsevier.com/books-and-journals

Publisher: Peter Linsley
Acquisitions Editor: Emma Sykes
Editorial Project Manager: Bhaviya Koul
Publishing Services Manager: Deepthi Unni
Production Project Manager: Surya Narayanan Jayachandran

Typeset by TNQ Tech
Printed in Great Britain by CPI Group (UK) Ltd,
Croydon, CR0 4YY

Last digit is the print number: 10 9 8 7 6 5 4 3 2 1

Contents

VIII

Respiratory drugs

IX

Chemotherapeutic drugs

X

Special topics

This is the link to the companion site of the book
https://shop.elsevier.com/books/book-companion/9780443290381

Dedication

Dr. Moini:

To my precious grandchildren, Artemis, Anastasia, Anabelle, and Laila; to my wonderful wife, Hengameh, and my beautiful daughters, Mahkameh and Morvarid

Dr. Naderi:

To the younger me, whose perseverance made dreams become reality, and to my family, who made it all possible.

Dr. Schnellmann:

To RGS, my favorite pharmacologist.

Dr. Scott:

My father, Kenneth, my aunt Simone, and my grandmothers, Aileen and Isme, continue to motivate and support me in all my personal and professional endeavors. This is only possible with your ongoing help and guidance day in and day out.

About the authors

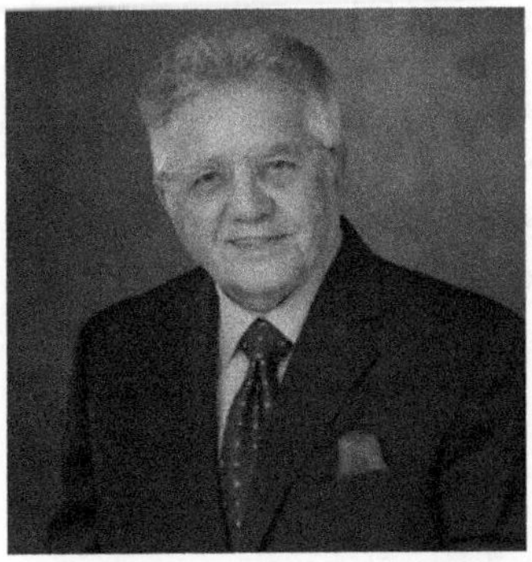

Dr. Moini served as an assistant professor in the Department of Epidemiology and Preventive Medicine at Tehran University Medical School for 9 years. He served as Director of Epidemiology for the Brevard County Health Department for 15 years. He served as Director of Science and Health at Everest University in Melbourne, FL, for 15 years. He also served as Professor of Science and Health at Everest for 24 years. He served as Professor of Science and Health at Eastern Florida State College for 6 years and is now retired. Dr. Moini has authored 60 books published internationally. His "Anatomy & Physiology for Healthcare Professionals" was translated and released in Japan and South Korea in 2020. His "Complication of Diabetes Mellitus" was translated into Spanish and released in 2023.

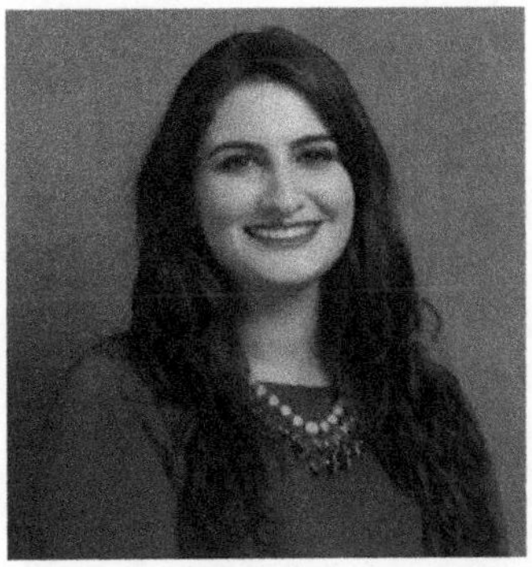

Dr. Mandana Naderi is an infectious diseases pharmacist and Medical Science Director at Paratek Pharmaceuticals. She previously served as an Assistant Professor at the University of Arizona College of Pharmacy. In that role, she served as the Lead Antimicrobial Stewardship Expert and Co-chair of the Antimicrobial Stewardship Subcommittee at the Arizona Department of Health Services (ADHS) in Phoenix, Arizona. Her ADHS responsibilities also included serving as a Clinical Therapeutics Lead during the COVID-19 and Mpox public health emergency response efforts. She earned her Bachelor of Science in Public Health from the University of Washington, her Doctor of Pharmacy degree from Washington State University, and her Master of Public Health degree from the University of Arizona. She completed a postgraduate pharmacy residency at Geisinger Wyoming Valley Medical Center in Wilkes-Barre, Pennsylvania, and a specialized infectious diseases residency at the University of Arizona/Banner University Medical Center in Tucson, Arizona.

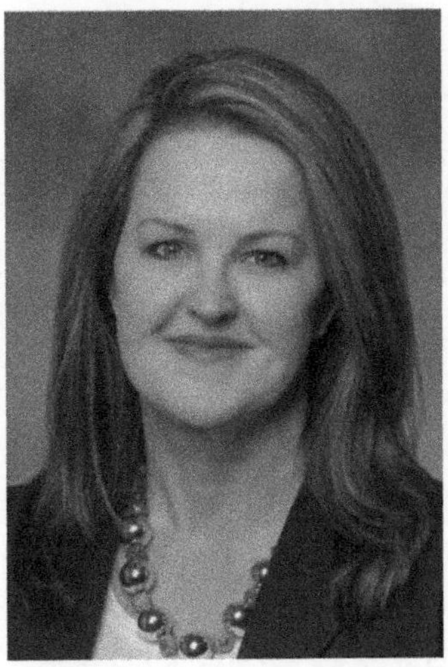

Dr. Jennifer G. Schnellmann is an Associate Professor in the Colleges of Medicine (Department of Medical Pharmacology) and Pharmacy (Department of Pharmacology and Toxicology) at the University of Arizona. She co-directs the Bachelor of Science in Pharmaceutical Sciences within the College of Pharmacy.

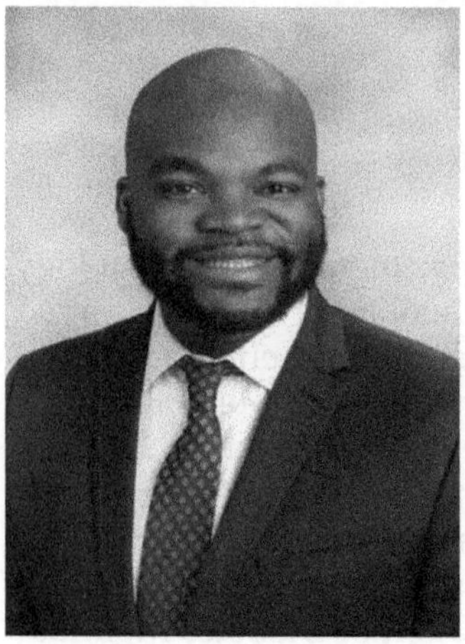

Dr. Anthony (Tony) Scott earned his PharmD from the University of Georgia and his MBA in Healthcare Management from New England College. He completed a PGY-1 Pharmacy Practice Residency at Piedmont Hospital in Atlanta, GA, followed by a PGY-2 Health-System Pharmacy Administration Residency at North Florida. He is also a diplomat of the ASHP Foundation Pharmacy Leadership Academy. Dr. Scott is the Director of Pharmacy Services at Emory University Hospital. Before joining Emory, he served as Assistant Director of Pharmacy Operations at The University of Chicago Medicine. Dr. Scott has been an active member of the American Society of Health-System Pharmacists (ASHP) and was recently elected Director-at-Large of the Sections of Pharmacy Practice Leaders Executive Committee. He has also been active with the Georgia Society of ASHP since returning to Georgia.

Preface

The authors welcome you to the first edition of "*The Science of Pharmacology*." We aim to provide thorough, up-to-date information on general principles of pharmacology and drug effects on various body systems. This book also includes discussions of special topics. It is intended for all medical students, nurses, nurse practitioners, and physician assistants. It can be translated into many languages and remains a valuable resource worldwide.

This book is organized into nine units. The first eight chapters discuss general principles of pharmacology. Unit 2 focuses on the effects of drugs on the central nervous system and spans more than eight chapters. Unit 3 covers drug effects on the autonomic nervous system—neurotransmitters, adrenergic and cholinergic agonists, and antagonists.

Unit 4 focuses on mental and behavioral health drugs, including anxiolytics and hypnotics, antidepressants, antipsychotics, schizophrenia drugs, and attention-deficit/hyperactivity disorder drugs. Unit 5 focuses on cardiovascular drugs, including antihyperlipidemics, drugs for angina pectoris and myocardial conditions, antihypertensives, antiarrhythmics, anti-anemia drugs, drugs for coagulation disorders, drugs for heart failure, diuretics, and drugs affecting the renin-angiotensin-aldosterone system.

Unit 6 focuses on endocrine drugs, and Unit 7 focuses on gastrointestinal medications, including peptic ulcers, bowel disease treatments, and vitamins. Unit 8 reviews respiratory drugs, while Unit 9 focuses on chemotherapeutic drugs. Unit 10 features special topics, including immunizations, NSAIDs and acetaminophen, medications for osteoporosis, rheumatoid arthritis, and gout, and a chapter on toxicology.

The book's three appendices cover dosage calculations, the ISMP list of high-alert medications, and the answers to the case study's critical-thinking questions. The book also includes a glossary and an index.

The features and content most beneficial to readers include real-world case studies with critical-thinking questions. Four-color printing helps illustrate non-text components and makes the e-book version more engaging. Each chapter's figures, graphs, and tables help illuminate the text material, engage readers, and provide additional insights and understanding—clinical case studies with critical-thinking questions and answers.

Acknowledgments

The authors appreciate the contributions of everyone who helped create this book, particularly the publisher, Peter Linsley; the acquisition editor, Emma Sykes; the editorial project manager, Bhaviya Koul; the production project manager, Surya Narayanan Jayachandran; and the cover designers, Greg Harris and Greg Vadimsky.

UNIT I

General principals

CHAPTER

1

Introduction

OUTLINE

LEARNING OUTCOMES

After study of the chapter, readers should be able to:

1. Identify the most critical events in the history of pharmacology.
2. Differentiate between therapeutic and pharmacologic drug classifications.
3. Define the term "prototype drug."
4. Explain the various types of drug names and give examples.
5. Describe the differences between prescription and over-the-counter drugs.
6. Explain the period of exclusivity of a drug.
7. List examples of prototype drugs in various classes.
8. Name three examples of statins.

Overview

Pharmacology studies how a drug affects a biological system and how the body responds to the medication. The discipline encompasses the sources, chemical properties, physical effects, and therapeutic uses of drugs. These effects can be therapeutic or toxic, depending on many factors. Pharmacology, a term derived from the Greek word *pharmakon* ("poison" in classic Greek, "drug" in modern Greek), is a branch of biology and medicine that is concerned with the study of drug action. Specifically, pharmacology examines the interactions between a living organism and chemicals that affect normal or abnormal biochemical functions. This includes drug composition, synthesis and design, molecular and cellular communication, molecular diagnostics, interactions, toxicology, chemical biology, therapy, medical applications, and antipathogenic capabilities. Furthermore, pharmacology is experimental and does not necessarily have therapeutic purposes. Even though they are not synonymous, both terms are often used interchangeably.

The Science of Pharmacology
https://doi.org/10.1016/B978-0-443-29038-1.00001-4

Brief history of pharmacology

The history of pharmacology began when herbs were first used to treat various disease symptoms. In about 2700 BCE, the *Great Herbal* was recorded by the Chinese, containing many different plant remedies for disease. In 1500 BCE, the Egyptians recorded treatments on *Eber's papyrus*, which included more than 700 formulas for treating illness. Much later, the Greek physician named Galen recorded more than 1000 treatments that used plant products in approximately 200 CE. During the Dark Ages, pharmacology continued with little documentation of any advancement. In 1693, Samuel Dale made the first recorded reference to *pharmacology*.

Modern pharmacology is believed to have evolved in the early 1800s. Chemists learned how to separate substances from complex mixtures and activate agents isolated from plants. These included colchicine, morphine, cocaine, and curare. Animal and human studies were conducted to understand the effects of these new substances. In 1847, the first ever department of pharmacology was established in Estonia. The father of American pharmacology, John Jacob Abel, founded the first pharmacy in the United States at the University of Michigan in 1890.

Experimental medicine, including significant advances in pharmacology, flourished during the 20th century. For the first time, drugs could be synthesized in the laboratory and tested over shorter periods. Researchers began to understand the molecular mechanisms of action for many drug products. The central purpose of pharmacology has never changed—to improve the quality of patients' lives.

Today, the area of **psychopharmacology** has dramatically evolved, with one in every six people taking some psychotropic drug. Modern psychopharmacology began in 1950 when the drug called *chlorpromazine* was synthesized. Over the next 50 years, the understanding and treatment of mental illness changed radically. Psychotropic drugs played a significant role; as state hospitals closed, psychotherapy became common, and the prescription of psychotropic medications increased. The earliest drugs included opiates, barbiturates, and lithium. Rapidly after that, tricyclic antidepressants, monoamine oxidase inhibitors and benzodiazepines were developed. The early 1960s saw Julius Axelrod describe nerve signals and synaptic transmission in a revolutionary way, followed by a dramatic increase in biochemical brain research related to psychotropic agents and brain chemistry.

You should remember

Pharmacology developed in the 19th century as a biomedical science that applied the principles of scientific experimentation to therapeutic contexts. The advancement of research techniques propelled pharmacological research and understanding.

Drug classification

There are thousands of different drugs, both legal and illegal. Because of this variety, it is often necessary to classify drugs into several types for legal, medical, and treatment purposes. There are several ways to organize medicines, including chemical similarities, effects on the mind and body, and legal definitions. Most countries have a legal classification system for drugs. These systems determine the circumstances, if any, under which that drug is legal, various requirements for that drug, and any legal penalties associated with its possession, distribution, or manufacture. Legal classifications are generally based on a drug's perceived medical value, risk, and danger. According to the *Approved Drug Products with Therapeutic Equivalence Evaluations*, known as the "**Orange Book**," the US Food and Drug Administration (FDA) lists more than 11,000 approved drugs. Similar agents are grouped for better understanding. The two primary classifications of drugs are therapeutic, describing the condition being treated, and pharmacologic, describing the drug's actions. Restorative classes are created based on a drug's value in treating a particular disease. For example, cardiovascular drugs are organized by their therapeutic classifications in Table 1.1.

Cardiovascular drugs may treat **heart failure**, hypertension, **arrhythmia**, cardiogenic shock, **angina pectoris,** and myocardial infarction. This means that cardiovascular medicines, as just one example, may be within a few different therapeutic classes. For therapeutic classification, it is essential to state which condition is being treated by each drug. A pharmacologic type focuses on a drug's mechanism of action or how it produces its effects. Tables 1.1 and 1.2 use hypertension as an example to summarize medications related to this condition.

TABLE 1.1 Cardiovascular drugs organized by therapeutic classification.

Therapeutic classification	Indication
Antianginals	Angina
Anticoagulants	Blood clotting regulation
Antidysrhythmics	Restoring normal heart rhythm
Antihyperlipidemics	Lowering blood cholesterol
Antihypertensives	Lowering blood pressure

In each example, Table 1.2 shows how hypertension may be controlled. Pharmacologic classifications are more specific than therapeutic classifications. Biochemistry and physiology must be understood; these classifications often use the chemical names of drugs. However, most drugs have multiple categories, and therapeutic and pharmacologic varieties may be mixed. For example, *epinephrine* has many different types of actions, as follows:

- Adrenergic agonist: to stimulate adrenergic receptors
- Anaphylactic agent: to prevent life-threatening hypersensitivity
- Antiglaucoma agent: to prevent glaucoma
- Autonomic nervous system agent: to affect the function of the heart, respiratory system, gastrointestinal tract, bladder, eyes, and glands
- Bronchodilator: to dilate the vessels of the airways
- Ocular mydriatic: to dilate the pupils and relax eye muscles
- Sympathomimetic: to increase systemic and pulmonary vascular resistance, increase blood pressure, and increase myocardial contractility and heart rate while relaxing smooth muscles in the skeletal muscle vascular bed and bronchi
- Topical hemostatic: to reduce bleeding
- Vasoconstrictor: to constrict the blood vessels

The specific classification chosen is mainly based on the condition being treated. It is essential to understand all the different types of each drug. Classifying drugs by their chemical similarities is useful because those that are chemically similar often have similar impacts and risks.

TABLE 1.2 Antihypertensive drugs organized by pharmacologic classification.

Pharmacologic classification	Indication
Adrenergic agonists or blockers	Blocking physiologic reactions to stress
Angiotensin-converting enzyme inhibitors	Blocking hormonal activity
Calcium channel blockers	Blocking heart calcium channels
Diuretics	Lowering plasma volume
Vasodilators	Dilating peripheral blood vessels

Prototype drugs

In pharmacology and pharmaceutics, a **prototype drug** is an individual drug that represents a drug class: a group of medications having similar chemical structures, mechanisms of action, and **adverse effects** of other drugs of the same type can be better predicted. An example is *penicillin V.* Understanding how penicillin V works and the outcomes it produces allows us to understand all of the other penicillins. There is some disagreement between healthcare providers about which drugs are the ideal prototypes. Usually, the oldest and most widely understood drug in any given glass is the prototype drug. Morphine is the prototype of opioid analgesics, diazepam is the prototype of benzodiazepine, propranolol is the prototype of beta blockers, and chlorpromazine is the prototypical phenothiazine antipsychotic.

In some cases, newer drugs are developed in a specific drug class with increased effects or a better safety profile. As time passes, some older drugs are not prescribed as often as they previously were, and therefore the prototype drug chosen for the class may be changed to a newer and more helpful drug. The following is a list of prototype drugs that are generally agreed upon, with their classes:

- Acyclovir: antiviral agent
- Aspirin: nonsteroidal antiinflammatory agent
- Chloroquine: antimalarial agent
- Chlorpromazine: phenothiazine antipsychotic
- Diazepam: benzodiazepine
- Diphenhydramine: ethanolamine antihistamine
- Imipramine: tricyclic antidepressant
- Morphine: opioid analgesic
- Nifedipine: dihydropyridine calcium channel blocker
- Propranolol: beta blocker

Drug names

Drugs may have three different names: chemical, generic, and trade. Chemical names are derived using standards established by the *International Union of Pure and Applied Chemistry.* There is only one chemical name for each drug, which helps predict the drug's chemical and physical properties. However, **chemical names** are often complicated to pronounce or remember.

Chemical names such as calcium gluconate or sodium chloride are generally used only when short and easy to remember. Sometimes, drugs are named and classified by part of their chemical structure, known as the *chemical group name*. Drug classes include benzodiazepines, aminoglycosides, fluoroquinolones, phenothiazines, and thiazides. Understanding common chemical group names helps to remember the actions of major drug classes.

The **generic name** of a drug is usually much less complicated and more accessible to remember. The United Nations Adopted Names Council (NANC) assigns it. Organizations such as the FDA and World Health Organization (WHO) regularly use generic names to describe drugs. Each drug also has only one generic name. Healthcare providers usually prefer generic names and must learn and remember many. To simplify it, parts of generic names help students recognize other drugs of the same class. Examples include the following:

- Antiasthma medications: albuterol, formoterol, salmeterol
- Antibiotics: amoxicillin, ampicillin, penicillin
- Antidepressants: duloxetine, fluoxetine, paroxetine
- Antihistamines: fexofenadine, loratadine, terfenadine
- Antiulcer medications: lansoprazole, omeprazole, pantoprazole
- Beta blockers: acebutolol, atenolol, metoprolol
- Narcotic analgesics: buprenorphine, morphine, nalbuphine
- Nonsteroidal antiinflammatory drugs: fenoprofen, ibuprofen, ketoprofen
- Statins: lovastatin, rosuvastatin, simvastatin
- Thiazide diuretics: chlorothiazide, hydrochlorothiazide, methychlothiazide

A **trade name** is also called a brand name, proprietary ("owned") name, or product name. It is assigned by the pharmaceutical company that markets the drug. Therefore each generic drug may have multiple trade names created by a unique manufacturer. Trade names are short and easy to remember, so patients can quickly become familiar with them. In the United States, the FDA grants a pharmaceutical company exclusive rights to a new generic drug, which the company can market under its chosen trade name for several years after its new drug application is approved. This is known as the **exclusivity** period, during which competitors cannot market generic versions of the same drug. This allows the company that developed the drug to recover the millions of dollars spent on research, development, design, and testing. Each manufacturer would not find developing new, unique drugs worthwhile without exclusivity.

Once exclusivity expires, competing companies can sell generically equivalent drug versions using different trade names. The FDA must approve each alternate version of the drug. Usually, exclusivity for a new drug lasts for 5 years, but this can be extended for 3 more years if the drug has a further indication or different route of administration or if it is manufactured in another dosage form. If a manufacturer tests the drug in children and determines its dosage and safety level in this age group, the FDA will grant the company 6 more months of exclusivity. **Orphan drugs**, however, have 7 years of exclusivity. Because extended exclusivity can result in millions of additional dollars in profit, pharmaceutical companies usually do everything they can to receive FDA extensions.

Trade names may be difficult to remember due to the potential for applying many different terms to the same generic drug. Drugs that have more than one active generic ingredient are called **combination drugs**. This creates difficulty when trying to match generic and product names. The generic drug *diphenhydramine* is popularly known as *Benadryl*, along with many other trade names. Diphenhydramine is sold over the counter in low doses, but higher doses require a prescription. The drug is often combined with many different drugs and sold under even more unique trade names, as follows:

- Benadryl Cold: acetaminophen/diphenhydramine/pseudoephedrine
- Theraflu Nighttime Severe Cold & Cough: acetaminophen/diphenhydramine/phenylephrine
- Contac Day and Night Cold and Flu: acetaminophen/dextromethorphan/diphenhydramine/pseudoephedrine
- Tylenol PM: acetaminophen/diphenhydramine
- Mucinex Fast-Max Day Time Severe Cold and Night Time Cold & Flu Maximum Strength

To avoid confusion, generic names should be used when naming active **ingredients** in a combination drug. It is conventional always to write generic names in lowercase letters first, followed by the trade name in parentheses, with the first letter *capitalized*. Examples of this include the following:

- atorvastatin (Lipitor)
- clopidogrel (Plavix)
- lansoprazole (Prevacid)
- esomeprazole (Nexium)
- montelukast (Singulair)
- levothyroxine (Synthroid)
- fluticasone/salmeterol (Advair Diskus)
- venlafaxine (Effexor XR)
- escitalopram (Lexapro)
- valsartan (Diovan)

Table 1.3 gives even more examples of generic drugs in various trade name products.

You should remember

Sometimes a drug's trade name comes from rather strange factors. For example, diazepam's best-known trade name is "Valium." This term comes from the Latin word vale, meaning "farewell" or "goodnight." The drug is used to reduce anxiety, muscle spasms, and even seizures and often results in the patient relaxing comfortably overnight or for an intended number of hours, as needed.

TABLE 1.3 Generic drugs found in many trade name products.

Generic name	Trade names
aspirin	Acetylsalicylic Acid, Acuprin, Anacin, Aspergum, Bayer, Bufferin, Ecotrin, Empirin, Excedrin, Maprin, Norgesic, Salatin, Salocol, Salsprin, Supac, Talwin, Traphen-10, Vanquish, Verin, Zorprin
buprenorphine	Belbuca, Buprenex, Butrans, Probuphine, Sixmo, Sublocade, Subutex
diphenhydramine	Allerdryl, Benadryl, Benahist, Bendylate, Caladryl, Compoz, Diahist, Diphenadril, Eldadryl, Fenylhist, Fynex, Hydramine, Hydril, Insomnal, Noradryl, Nordryl, Nytol, Tusstat, Wehdryl
ibuprofen	Advil, Amersol, Apsifen, Brufen, Haltran, Medipren, Midol 200, Motrin, Nuprin, Pamprin-IB, Rufen, Trendar
levothyroxine	Levothroid, Levoxyl, Synthroid, Tirosint, Unithroid

Key Terms

Adverse effects
Angina pectoris
Arrhythmia
Chemical names
Combination drugs
Exclusivity
Generic name
Heart failure
Ingredients
Orange Book
Orphan drugs
Prototype drug
Psychopharmacology
Trade name

Further Reading

[1] American Pharmacists Association, Drug Information Handbook with International Trade Names Index: Adapted from the Drug Information Handbook, 26th Edition, Lexi-Comp Inc, 2017.
[2] American Society of Health-System Pharmacists, D.A. Holdford, Introduction to Acute & Ambulatory Care Pharmacy Practice, second ed., ASHP Publications, 2017.
[3] I. Ebenezer, Neuropsychopharmacology and Therapeutics, Wiley-Blackwell, 2015.
[4] S. Jansen, OTC Pocket Guide: OTC Pocket Guide: Quick Nonprescription Drug Reference, CreateSpace Independent Publishing Platform, 2016.
[5] B. Levin, A. Hanson, P.D. Hurd, Introduction to Public Health in Pharmacy, second ed., Oxford University Press, 2018.
[6] J.J. Li, Top Drugs: Their History, Pharmacology, and Syntheses, Oxford University Press, 2015.
[7] A.W. Lovett, S.K. Peasah, H. Xiao, G.J. Ryan, Introduction to the Pharmacy Profession, Jones & Bartlett Learning, 2013.
[8] N.K. Pandit, R.P. Soltis, Introduction to the Pharmaceutical Sciences: An Integrated Approach, second ed., Lippincott, Williams, and Wilkins, 2011.
[9] G. Patrick, An Introduction to Medicinal Chemistry, sixth ed., Oxford University Press, 2017.
[10] L.M. Posey, The pharmacy technician's introduction to pharmacy: APhA pharmacy technician training series, Amer. Pharm. Assoc. (2009).
[11] K.D. Tripathi, Pharmacological Classification of Drugs with Doses and Preparations, fifth ed., Jaypee Brothers Medical Publishers Ltd, 2016.

[12] C.J. Watkins, Pharmacology Clear and Simple: A Guide to Drug Classifications and Dosage Calculations, third ed., F.A. Davis Company, 2018.
[13] B. Levin, A. Hanson, P.D. Hurd, Introduction to Public Health in Pharmacy, second ed., Oxford University Press, 2018.
[14] J.J. Li, Top Drugs: Their History, Pharmacology, and Syntheses, Oxford University Press, 2015.
[15] S. Marie, The Art and Science of Psychopharmacology: Essential Tools for Treating Anxiety, Depression, Bipolar Disorder & Psychosis, PESI Publishing & Media, 2020.
[16] N.K. Pandit, R.P. Soltis, Introduction to the Pharmaceutical Sciences: An Integrated Approach, second ed., Lippincott, Williams, and Wilkins, 2011.
[17] L.M. Posey, The pharmacy technician's introduction to pharmacy: APhA pharmacy technician training series, Amer. Pharm. Assoc. (2009).
[18] S.M. Stahl, Prescriber's Guide: Stahl's Essential Psychopharmacology, sixth ed., Cambridge University Press, 2017.
[19] K.D. Tripathi, Pharmacological Classification of Drugs with Doses and Preparations, fifth ed., Jaypee Brothers Medical Publishers Ltd, 2016.
[20] C.J. Watkins, Pharmacology Clear and Simple: A Guide to Drug Classifications and Dosage Calculations third ed., 20, F.A. Davis Company, 2018.

CHAPTER

2

Pharmacodynamics

OUTLINE

LEARNING OUTCOMES

After study of the chapter, readers should be able to:

1. Describe drug receptors and the mechanisms of drug action.
2. Explain the terms therapeutic index and therapeutic window.
3. Describe a drug's duration of action.
4. Describe the dose-response relationship.
5. Compare the differences between potency and efficacy.
6. Discuss agonists and an antagonist.
7. Describe the various factors that cause the side effects of a drug.
8. Explain pharmacodynamics.
9. Describe downregulation and upregulation.
10. Explain pharmacogenetics.

Overview

Pharmacodynamics studies drugs' biochemical, physiologic, and molecular effects on the body. It involves receptor binding, postreceptor effects, and chemical interactions. Pharmacodynamics and pharmacokinetics explain the relationship between drug doses and patient responses. Pharmacologic responses are based on how drugs bind with their targets. Drug effects are influenced by the drug concentration at the receptor site. Pharmacodynamics can be affected by physiologic changes from disorders or diseases, aging, and the consequences of other medications. Conditions that affect pharmacodynamics include genetic mutations, malnutrition, thyrotoxicosis, myasthenia gravis, Parkinson disease, and insulin-resistant diabetes mellitus, to name only a few.

https://doi.org/10.1016/B978-0-443-29038-1.00002-6

Drug receptors

Most drugs produce their effects by activating or inhibiting specific cellular receptors, which are particular target molecules to which drugs bind. Drugs enhance or inhibit physiological and biochemical processes by interacting with body chemicals. Receptor theory predicts that responses to a drug are proportional to the number of receptors bound or occupied by the drug. This theory explains how most drugs produce their effects. Receptors typically bind endogenous molecules, including hormones, growth factors, and **neurotransmitters**. Drugs use existing targets to have their impact. A drug that attaches to a receptor will enhance or inhibit normal cellular functions. Binding is usually reversible. Drug actions end once the drug leaves the receptor. However, less often, binding is irreversible. Medicines that can bind to a receptor and produce an intense action have high intrinsic activity related to efficacy. Drugs with high **intrinsic activity** also have high efficacy. The three receptor families (see Fig. 2.1) are as follows:

- *Cell membrane–embedded enzymes*: The ligand-binding domain for drug binding is on the cell surface. A drug activates an enzyme inside the cell, and a response occurs.
- *Ligand-gated ion channels*: The channel crosses the cell membrane. When the channel opens, ions flow in and out of cells. This primarily affects sodium and calcium ions.
- *G protein–coupled receptor systems*: Proteins located in the cell membrane that bind extracellular substances and transmit signals from these substances to an intracellular molecule called a G protein (guanine nucleotide–binding protein).
- *Transcription factors are located in the cell nucleus on DNA, not* the cell surface. When activated, receptors regulate protein synthesis and last quite a while. This differs from the other receptor families, in which receptor activation is fast.

Drug receptors are usually proteins but can be any molecule. An extracellular receptor component often contains subunits arranged in a specific shape that will bind a drug or ligand. The receptor can form a membrane channel, which regulates substances that leave and enter cells. Drugs selectively bind to receptors. When a receptor is occupied, second messenger events are triggered in a cell. These include converting adenosine triphosphate into cyclic adenosine monophosphate, releasing intracellular calcium, and activating specific G proteins and their related enzymes. These biochemical events start drug actions by stimulating or inhibiting normal cellular activities. If small changes occur to the structure of the drug or its receptor, they may reduce or eliminate binding, and the drug becomes ineffective. Other receptors are intracellular molecules such as cytoplasmic DNA or enzymes. Interactions with these receptors allow drugs to inhibit protein synthesis or regulate cell division or metabolism. Agents that bind intracellular components include specific vitamins and steroid hormones.

Pharmacotherapy has improved over time as more was learned about receptor subtypes. When the *alpha* and *beta* subtypes were discovered, drugs that were selective for only one of them could be developed. This allowed for more specific therapy and fewer adverse effects. Medications became more specifically effective when the additional alpha-1, alpha-2, beta-1, and beta-2 subtypes were discovered. Research continues to find other drug receptor subtypes, further improving our abilities to give specific, accurate, and individualized treatments. Also, some drugs act independently of cellular receptors. Instead, they utilize altered cellular membrane permeability, inhibition of membrane excitability, or changing activities of cellular pumps.

Osmotic diuretics, ethyl alcohol, and general anesthetics use these nonspecific cellular responses. *Cholinergic receptors* are affected by these drugs, and there are multiple sites of cholinergic receptors, which include the eyes, heart,

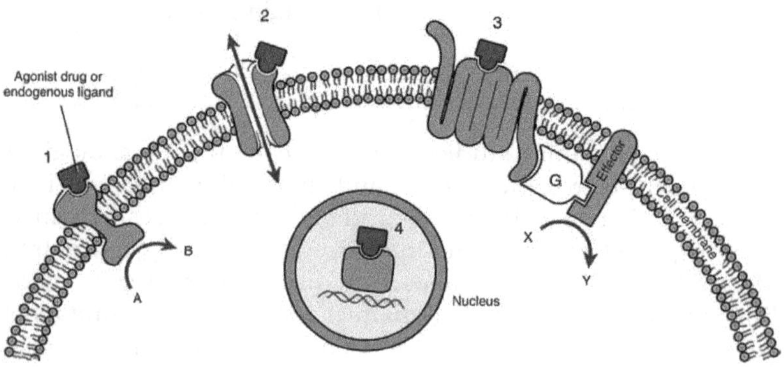

FIG. 2.1 The four receptor families: (1) cell membrane-embedded enzymes, (2) ligand-gated ion channels, (3) G protein-coupled receptor systems, and (4) transcription factors.

blood vessels, stomach, bronchus, and bladder (see Fig. 2.2). The example drug used in this figure is *bethanechol*, used for postoperative urinary retention—it stimulates bladder contraction so that the patient can urinate but also decreases the heart rate and BP, increases gastric acid secretion, and constricts the bronchioles as well as the pupils of the eyes. Other nonselective drugs, such as epinephrine, affect multiple receptors to treat anaphylaxis or severe asthma.

The mechanisms of drug action include stimulation, inhibition, irritation, replacement, cytotoxic action, antimicrobial action, and changes in immune status. These can be further explained as follows:

- *Stimulation*: enhancement of intrinsic activity, such as when adrenergic drugs increase heart rate, respiratory rate, and sweating during the fight-or-flight response
- *Inhibition*: decreasing of neural activity and bodily functions, such as by barbiturates and opiates
- *Irritation*: having harmful effects, such as astringents
- *Replacement*: being able to replace needed body compounds—examples include some hormones such as insulins and thyroid drugs
- *Cytotoxic action*: being able to kill cancers or invading parasites selectively
- *Antimicrobial action*: being able to inhibit, kill, or prevent infectious organisms from causing disease
- *Changes in immune status*: being able to depress, enhance, or modify the immune system; examples include interferons and methotrexate

Some drugs may have side and secondary effects even with correct drug doses. They are often predictable, but they range from minor to severe and can even be life-threatening. Side effects are affected by age, chronic illness, gender, weight, and ethnicity. Desirable side effects include drowsiness caused by some drugs taken at bedtime. Side effects are one of the main reasons patients stop taking the medications. Teaching patients about potential side effects and how to report them is essential. Dose adjustments can often manage side effects, though sometimes changing the drug to a different one within the same class or trying other treatment methods may be needed.

Tolerance is the decreased responsiveness to a drug over time, resulting in a patient needing more drugs to achieve the same therapeutic response. **Tachyphylaxis** is an acute decrease in drug responsiveness following an initial or several doses. It is most common with centrally acting analgesics, nitroglycerin, and ranitidine. It is essential to understand that tolerance and tachyphylaxis may result in patients not responding well to drug administration and failing to achieve adequate therapeutic outcomes. The placebo effect is a response to a drug unrelated to its chemical properties. Responses can be positive or negative, affected by the patient's attitudes, beliefs, and expectations concerning the drug. The placebo effect is of psychological origin, though physiologic responses include alterations in blood pressure, heart rate, and pain sensation.

A drug interaction is a changed action or effect of a drug because of an interaction with one or several drugs. It is not the same as an adverse drug reaction or *incompatibility*, a chemical or physical reaction between two or more drugs *in vitro*. The reaction may occur between drugs within some artificial environment outside the body, such as a syringe or IV bag. Drug interactions are still a significant feature of drug therapy, especially because 70% of Americans take one or more prescription drugs. Drug-nutrient, drug-disease, and drug-laboratory reactions must also be considered in which a drug interacts with food, alcohol, herbal supplements, specific conditions, and

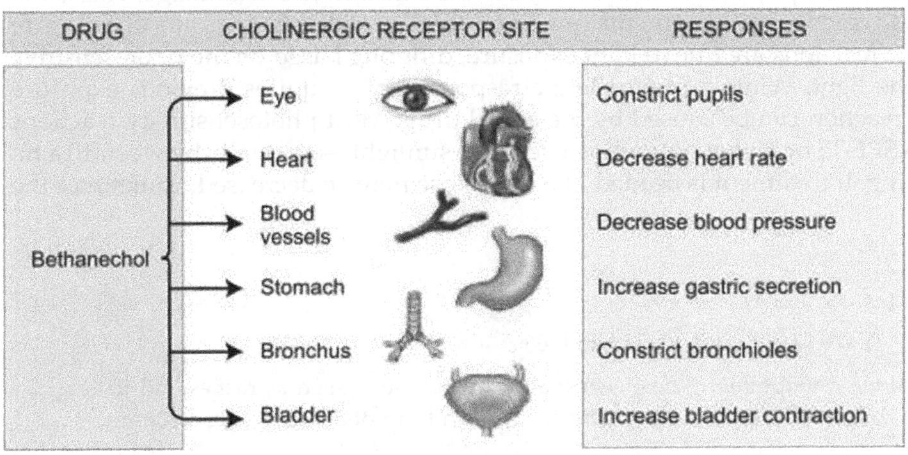

FIG. 2.2 The locations of cholinergic receptors.

laboratory tests, respectively. Patients should always be closely monitored for reactions between the drugs they are given and all these factors. Those at higher risk for drug interactions include patients taking multiple medications, having chronic health disorders, seeing more than one healthcare provider, and using more than one pharmacy. Older adults are at exceptionally high risk.

An **additive effect** occurs when two drugs are given in combination, and the response is increased to an impact more significant than either drug could produce alone ($1 + 1 = 2$). A desirable additive effect occurs if a diuretic and a beta-blocker are offered to treat hypertension, which results in a more potent blood pressure–lowering effect. An undesirable additive effect is when hydralazine for hypertension is given with nitroglycerin for angina and a severe hypotensive response occurs.

A **synergistic effect** also occurs when two drugs are given together. The clinical outcome has a much more significant impact than when either drug is given alone ($1 + 1 = 3$). A desirable synergistic effect occurs when two cytotoxic drugs are administered, reducing individual drug dosing and decreasing side effects. An undesirable synergistic effect occurs if a sedative hypnotic drug is taken with alcohol, increasing CNS depression. An antagonistic effect occurs if two medications are administered that reduce or block each other's products. A desirable negative result occurs when naloxone is given to secure the narcotic effects of morphine.

Most drug-drug interactions cause symptoms such as heartburn, nausea, headache, and lightheadedness. The most serious interactions cause severe hypotension and arrhythmias. Some drug interactions cause organ-specific toxicity, such as damage to the heart, liver, kidney, and other vital organs. Fortunately, most drug interactions are not severe or life-threatening. It is essential to understand that besides prescription drugs, OTC and herbal supplements can also cause drug interactions. Severe adverse reactions are indicated inside *boxed warnings* in the paperwork accompanying drug products.

Drug-nutrient interactions may involve increases, decreases, or delays in the body's response to a drug. One example is tyramine-rich foods consumed along with a monoamine oxidase inhibitor (MAOI) antidepressant. These foods include cheese, organic meats, wine, beer, sour cream, bananas, and yogurt. Because tyramine is a potent vasoconstrictor when taken with an MAOI antidepressant, a hypertensive crisis could occur. Therefore these foods must be avoided with MAOI antidepressants. Grapefruit affects the metabolism of more than 44 drugs, so it must be avoided when indicated to prevent severe drug reactions. Protein energy malnutrition and other nutritional deficiencies can also affect drug responses and metabolic processes, causing toxicity. The two forms of protein energy malnutrition are **kwashiorkor** and **marasmus**. With either form, there can be reduced drug absorption and protein binding, altered biotransformation and volume of distribution, and decreased elimination. Therefore anyone with these forms of malnutrition must be monitored because the risk for toxicity is high.

Drugs may also interfere with laboratory tests. They can cross react with antibodies, alter chemical reactions, and interfere with enzyme reactions. As a result, there can be test results that need to be validated or misinterpreted. This can lead to additional testing requirements or unneeded repeats of tests. Drug-laboratory reactions can also result in incorrect or missed diagnoses. Another factor to consider is drug-induced **photosensitivity** (see Fig. 2.3). This is a skin reaction from exposure to sunlight, usually caused by a drug interacting with exposure to ultraviolet A light, which may result in cellular damage to the epidermis. Photosensitivity reactions can also involve ultraviolet B light. There are two forms of these reactions. A *photoallergic reaction* occurs if a drug such as sulfonamide is activated within the skin by ultraviolet light, becoming a highly allergenic compound.

Over time, as antibodies develop, this type of skin reaction is a form of delayed hypersensitivity. A *phototoxic reaction* occurs if a photosensitive drug experiences photochemical reactions in the skin and causes damage. This is not immune mediated. The onset of phototoxic reaction with erythema can occur quickly, within 2 to 6 hours of exposure to sunlight. Both types of photosensitivity reactions are due to light exposure, differing based on the photosensitive drug involved and the wavelength of the light. While a photoallergic response only requires previous exposure (sensitization) to the drug, a phototoxic reaction can be caused by the actual drug. Most photosensitivity reactions can be avoided by using sunscreen (with SPF-15 or higher), avoiding excessive sunlight—especially between 10 a.m. and 4 p.m., and wearing protective clothing. If treatment is needed, the drug dose may be decreased. Sometimes the drug must be discontinued entirely.

You should remember

The potential to cause allergic reactions. Symptoms include cough, nausea, vomiting, diarrhea, and headaches, but skin reactions such as rashes and itching are the most common form of allergic drug reactions.

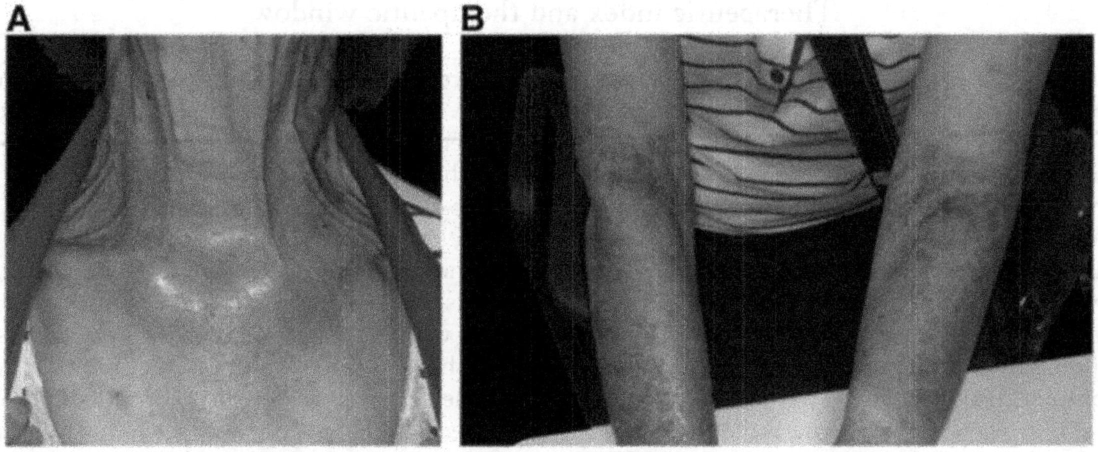

FIG. 2.3 Drug-induced photosensitivity on (A) the neck and upper chest and (B) the arms.

Receptor regulation

Receptors are extensively regulated in terms of amount, location, and sensitivity. Changes may occur over as short a period as a minute to as long as several days. When frequently or continuously exposed to an *agonist*, there is often a short-term reduction of the receptor response, sometimes referred to as tachyphylaxis. There are three mechanisms of action for this, as follows:

- *Intracellular molecules block access of a G protein to the activated receptor molecule*: such as when the *β-arrestin* molecule binds to an intracellular loop of the *β adrenoceptor* when the receptor is continually activated; *β-arrestin* stops access to the *G_s-coupling protein*, desensitizing tissues to more *β-agonist* activation, within minutes. Removal of the *β-agonist* causes a reduction of *β-arrestin*, and the complete response is restored over a few minutes to hours.
- *Agonist-bound receptors are internalized by endocytosis*: this removes them from additional exposure to extracellular molecules. The receptor molecule is then reinserted into the membrane (such as with morphine receptors) or degraded (such as with *β adrenoceptors* and *epidermal growth factor receptors*). The internalization/reinsertion process may sometimes be needed for the receptor-effector system to function normally.
- *Continuous activation of the receptor-effector system* may result in the depletion of some essential substrates needed for downstream effects. Depletion of *thiol cofactors* may be the reason for developing a tolerance to *nitroglycerin*. Sometimes repletion of a missing substrate, such as by administering *glutathione*, reverses the tolerance.

Downregulation can occur as a response to continual exposure to agonists. Oppositely, **upregulation** may occur when receptor activation is blocked for several days or prolonged, either from pharmacologic antagonists or by denervation. Continuous exposure of receptors to agonists often results in decreased receptors in the cell membrane, known as downregulation, due to increased internalization or degradation. Oppositely, continual exposure of receptors to antagonists often results in increased receptors in the cell membrane, known as upregulation, due to increased receptor synthesis (see Fig. 2.4).

You should remember

The regulation of drug receptors is the homeostatic increase or decrease in receptor activity or number as a response to activation or blockage. Regulation mechanisms are related to upregulation, downregulation, decreased activity by uncoupling of second messenger receptors, decreased activity by depletion of second messengers, tolerance, and tachyphylaxis.

Therapeutic index and therapeutic window

The study of how drugs affect the body is known as **pharmacodynamics**, and the most common mechanism is drug interaction with tissue receptors in the cell membranes or intracellular fluid. A drug's therapeutic index is its margin of safety. Several important factors must be considered. First, the correct therapeutic response for each patient must be achieved. Second, the dosage must be safe for the patient. The toxic *dose* of a drug is abbreviated as TD_{50}. The therapeutic index, comparing therapeutic and toxic effects, is shown in Fig. 2.5.

Frequency distribution curves can be used to visualize the safety of a drug. In preclinical experiments using laboratory animals, the median lethal dose (LD_{50}) is often determined as part of the drug development process. The drug dose will kill 50% of a theoretical population of test animals. However, the dose in the middle of a frequency distribution curve is known as the **median effective dose (ED_{50})**, which is the dose that will produce a specific therapeutic response in 50% of patients. Laboratory test animals will show a wide variance in median effective and lethal doses. A nontoxic drug for one animal can be fatally toxic to another. A drug's safety is determined by comparing the LD_{50} and the ED_{50}. If 10 mg of a drug is the average effective dose and 40 mg is the average lethal dose, for example, the drug's therapeutic index—the ratio between these two amounts—is calculated as follows:

FIG. 2.4 Regulation of receptor density by agonists and antagonists.

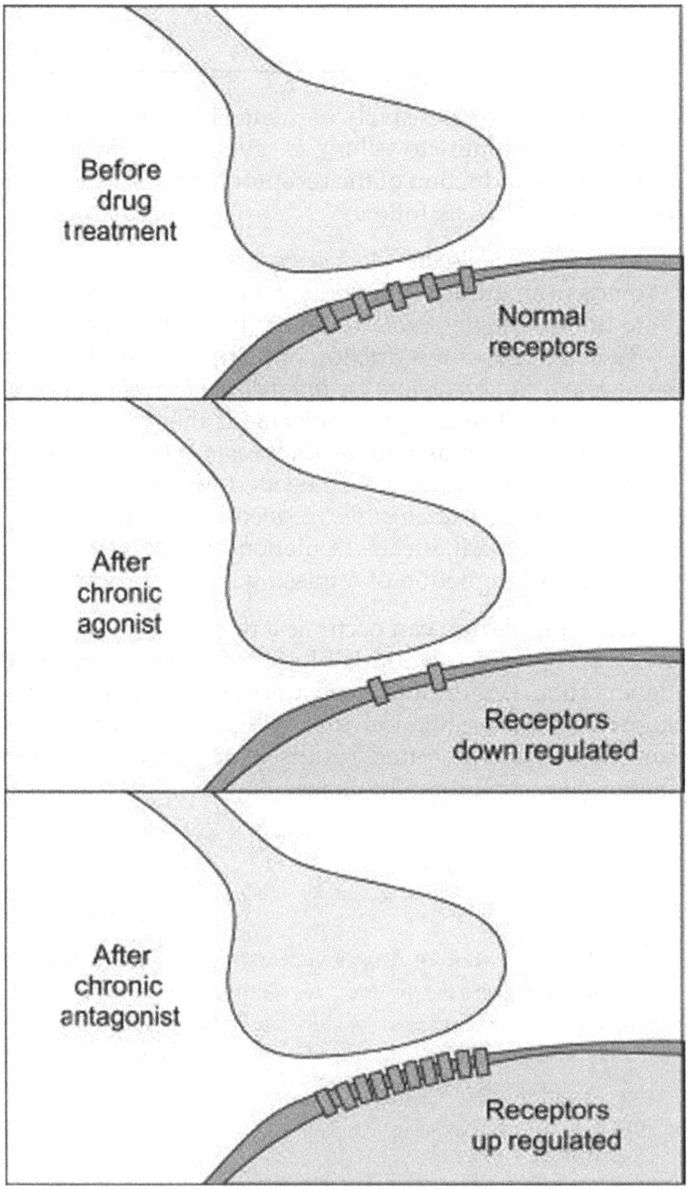

$$\text{Therapeutic index} = \frac{LD_{50}}{ED_{50}}$$

So, using the sample amounts described:

$$\text{Therapeutic index} = \frac{40 \text{ mg}}{10 \text{ mg}}$$

This means that the therapeutic index is equal to 4. A dosage, to be lethal to a patient, would have to be four times larger than the effective dose. This is a relatively safe margin, and any slight medication errors or changes in the bioavailability of the drug would not be dangerous. The therapeutic index is demonstrated to be a measurement of the safety margin of a drug. The higher this value is, the safer the medication is. Drugs have a large variability in their therapeutic indices, from as low as 1 to 2 to as much as 100.

The danger is much higher for a fatal outcome for a drug with a low therapeutic index such as 2. The difference between an effective and lethal dose is small, and the safety margin is narrow. Slight medication errors or changes in the metabolism or excretion of the drug could be deadly. Careful assessment of each patient's renal and hepatic function is needed before a drug with a narrow safety margin is administered. The lowest dose possible is given and only increased when careful monitoring is done.

Other measurements are used to determine drug safety. The median toxic dose (TD_{50}) is a dose that will cause specific toxicity in 50% of a theoretical group of animals or subjects. This value may be determined from animal studies or based on adverse effects that occur in human clinical trials. The **margin of safety** also helps assess a drug's safety and effectiveness. It is the amount of medicine that is lethal to 1% of test animals (LD_1) divided by the amount that produces a therapeutic effect in 99% of the animals (ED_{99}). Generally, the higher the margin of safety value, the safer the drug. It would be best to understand that only the drug's potential to be lethal is considered, and severe but nonlethal adverse effects that can occur from lower drug doses are not a consideration.

The **therapeutic window** describes the dose range between a minimum effective therapeutic concentration and the minimum toxic concentration. If a drug's average minimum therapeutic plasma concentration is 10 mg/L and its poisonous effects occur at 20 mg/L, the therapeutic window would be 10 to 20 mg/L. A drug's therapeutic index and window are based on the specific toxic effects. An example of a drug with a narrow therapeutic window is warfarin. It must be given great care to achieve the desired anticoagulation without excess risk of bleeding—the difficulties associated with warfarin lead to developing new oral anticoagulants, such as *dabigatran* and *rivaroxaban*.

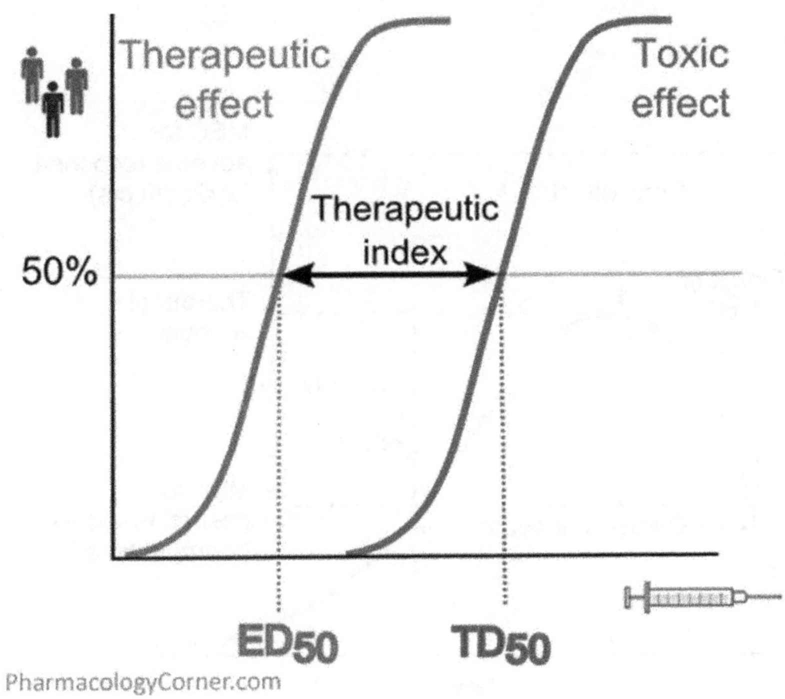

FIG. 2.5 The therapeutic index is the ratio between a drug's toxic and therapeutic doses.

You should remember

Drugs with a narrow therapeutic index must be used cautiously because they differ slightly between their therapeutic and toxic doses. Therapeutic drug monitoring is essential to determine the amount at which the drug will be safe and effective. Drug metabolism varies between individual people. The key to avoiding drug-related problems is to consider the therapeutic index to ensure safety.

Duration of action

The time it takes for a drug to reach its minimal effective concentration is the drug's onset of action. The drug's peak concentration occurs when it comes to its highest bloodstream concentration. The length of time that the drug provides therapeutic effects is known as the duration of action (see Fig. 2.6). This information is essential for administering medications. Some drugs are effective in only minutes, while others require hours or days. When the drug plasma concentration decreases below the minimal effective concentration, adequate dosing is not achieved. Also, an excessively high drug concentration can cause toxicity. If a drug is given IV, the peak time is usually 30–60 minutes. The peak time for a drug given orally may be within 2–3 hours. The *trough drug level* is the lowest plasma concentration of a drug and can be used to measure the elimination rate. Trough levels are drawn just before the next drug dose, regardless of how it is administered.

You should remember

The duration of drug action depends on several factors. These include the absolute amount of drug given, the pharmaceutical preparation, the reversibility of drug action, the drug's half-life, the slope of the concentration-response curve, the activity of metabolites, and the influence of disease upon drug elimination.

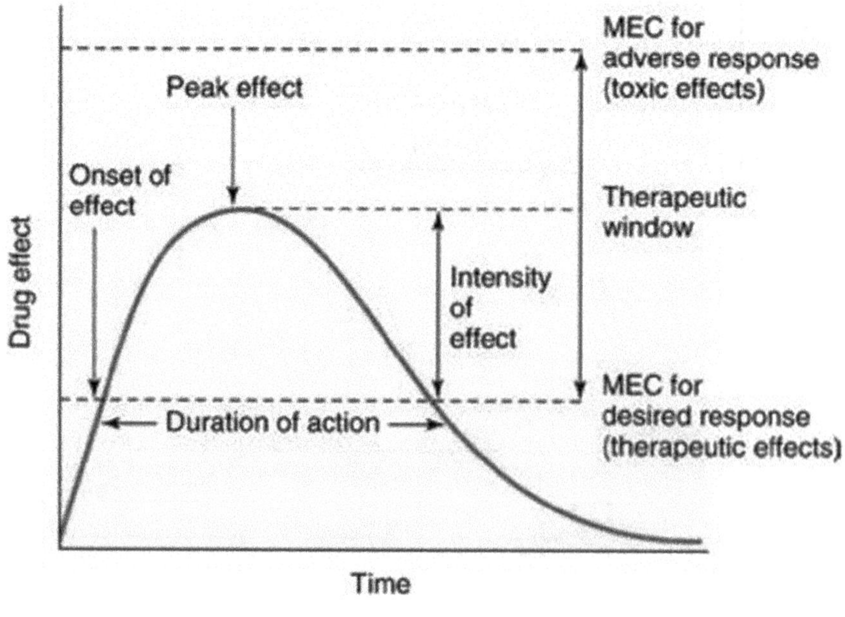

FIG. 2.6 A drug's duration of action, showing its onset and peak.

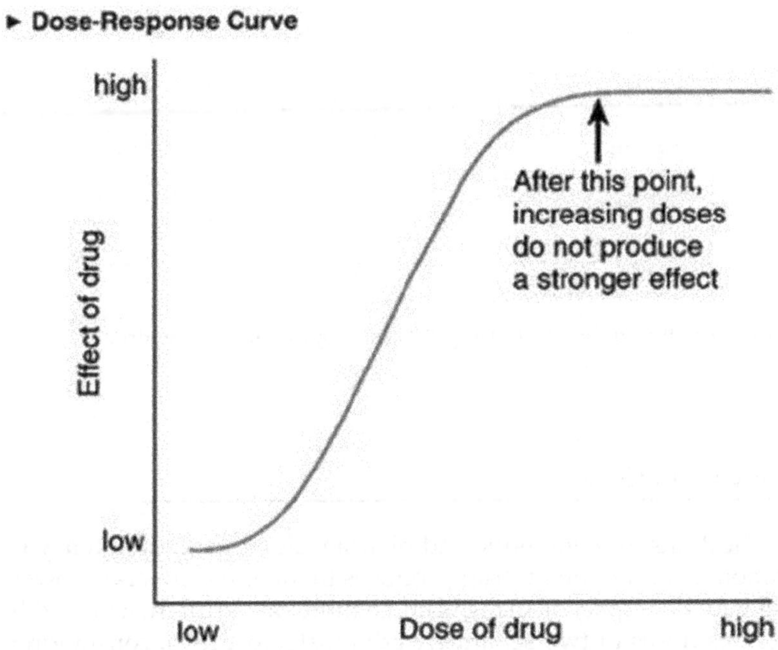

FIG. 2.7 The dose-response relationship.

Dose-response relationship

The **dose-response relationship** explains how drug actions change with different doses. Thus small amounts of a drug would produce modest effects, and more drugs would produce more visible results. The dose-response relationship is a straightforward concept shown in Fig. 2.7. Dose-response curves, which plot a drug dose given to a patient and its intensity or degree of response, can provide an extensive collection of drug information.

In a dose-response curve, there are three distinct phases. Phase 1 is when the lowest doses of a drug are administered. The curve at this point is relatively flat, showing that only a few target cells are reacting to the drug. Insufficient drug amounts do not produce any therapeutic effect. Phase 2, however, rises upward dramatically, nearly as a straight vertical line. There is a linear relationship between the amount of drug given and the amount of response in the patient. If a dose is doubled, twice as much drug response occurs. This is the most desirable dose range because giving more of the drug causes a proportionately increasing effect, and lower doses give less effect. In phase 3, a plateau is reached, and increased quantities provide no additional therapeutic effect. This may occur because all of the target receptors for the drug are now occupied, or it can mean that the drug has been 100% effective in treating the patient. No additional relief can be obtained from higher doses. However, the practitioner must know that increased amounts can potentially cause more adverse effects.

Because the dose-response curve is continuous and smooth, it is sometimes called a *graded one*. By adjusting doses in small increments, nearly any amount of therapeutic response, from 0% to 100%, can be obtained within the linear drug dose range. This is most true when the intravenous route of administration is used and infusion rates can be changed in tiny increments. Understanding that many adverse effects follow a graded dose-response relationship is critical. Higher drug doses cause more intense adverse effects. The negative effects may be reduced if the amount is adjusted lower but is still in the therapeutic range. However, anaphylaxis is an example of an adverse effect independent of the dose amount, and tiny doses may trigger serious adverse events.

You should remember

The dose-response relationship is the most basic and essential fundamental toxicological concept. Many health, economic, and regulatory decisions depend upon the integrity of this relationship. Some drugs are absorbed quickly and distributed to many body tissues, but many only affect one or a few specific tissues. Other medicines have similar or identical properties but affect many more cells and tissues throughout the body.

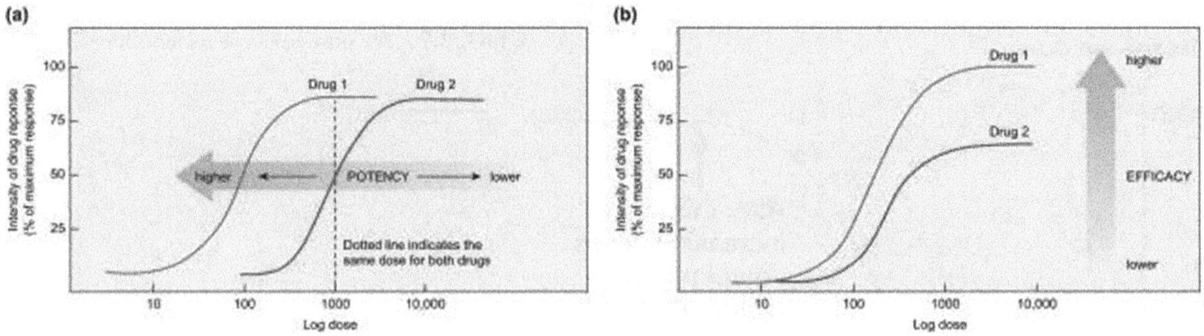

FIG. 2.8 Potency and efficacy. (A) Drug "1" has a higher potency than drug "2". (B) Drug "1" has a higher efficacy than drug "2".

Potency and efficacy

Two concepts must be understood to compare medications in therapeutic and pharmacologic classes. **Potency** is the strength of a drug at a specific dose or concentration. A more potent drug produces therapeutic effects in lower doses than other drugs within the same class. A drug with an impact of 10 mg is much more powerful than one with the same results at 100 mg. Therefore potency compares doses of two separately administered drugs, considering how much is needed for a specific response. Dose-response curves help to understand the concept of potency. Another method is called **efficacy**, which is the most excellent maximal response a drug produces. The ideas of potency and efficacy are illustrated in Fig. 2.8.

Pharmacotherapeutic experts agree that efficacy is nearly always more important than potency. Relief of a patient's condition is essential, so the most *effective* drug is of more significant concern. However, higher doses produce more intense adverse effects again, but this is only true when comparing doses of the same drug. Comparing two different medications used for the same condition gives a different result due to differences in their potency. However, we should never assume that when two other drugs are compared, the drug with the lower dose has fewer adverse effects. Then *potency* is sometimes misused to indicate a more "effective" drug.

Agonists

Actual biochemical mechanisms of therapeutic effects can be very complicated, with mechanisms of action not always understood. A drug binding to its receptor may produce a response that resembles the development of an endogenous regulatory molecule. Activity that occurs when there is no **ligand** is called **constitutive activity**. An **agonist** is a drug that activates a receptor, producing the same type of response as an endogenous substance. An agonist sometimes causes a more excellent maximal response than an endogenous chemical. A **full agonist** can activate the effector system when binding to a receptor. A **partial agonist** is a medication that produces a less productive or weaker response than an agonist. A partial agonist acts as an inhibitor when a full agonist is present. For example, *buprenorphine* is a mixed partial agonist used to treat opioid addiction. When administered with an opioid such as morphine, oxycodone, or heroin, the effects of the opioid are reduced to the level caused by buprenorphine alone (see Fig. 2.9).

Neutral antagonists bind with *equal affinity* to the most active and inactive receptors. This prevents binding by an agonist and deviations from levels of constitutive activity. Conversely, inverse agonists have a much higher affinity for passive receptors than active receptors. They decrease or stop constitutive activities. Drugs form a chemical bond with specific receptor sites, similar to a key and lock. The better they fit, the better the response. Fig. 2.10 shows the ways that agonists, as well as antagonists, attach to receptor sites and the resulting reactions. An example of an inverse agonist is *diphenhydramine*, which acts at the H1 receptor, reversing the effects of histamine on capillaries to reduce allergic reaction symptoms.

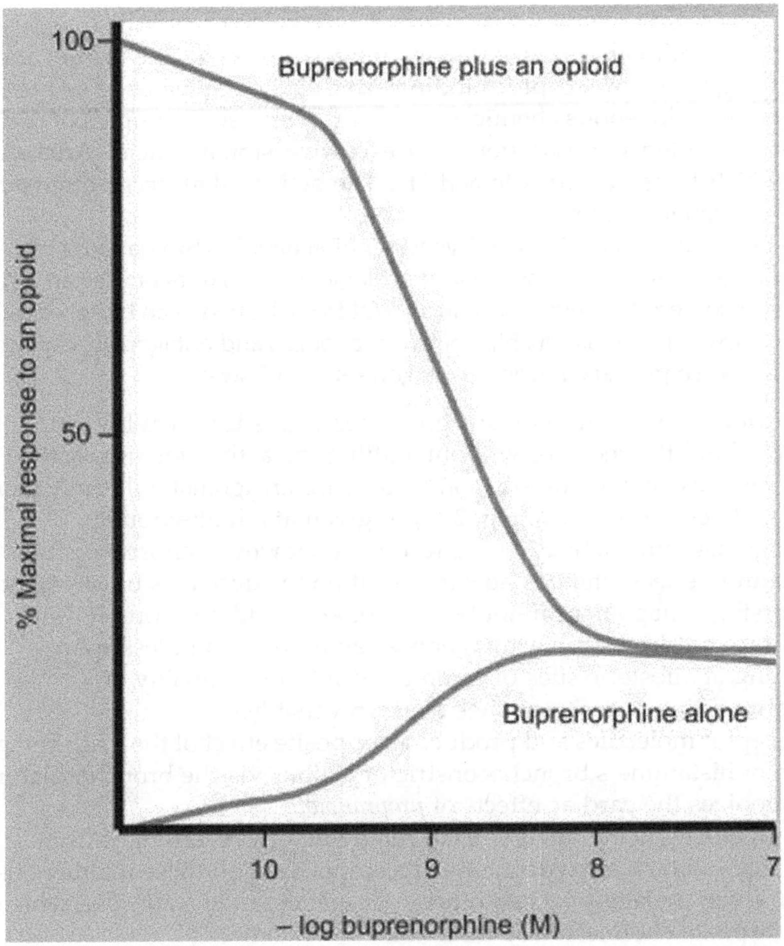

FIG. 2.9 The effect of a partial agonist on a response to a full agonist, using buprenorphine for reference.

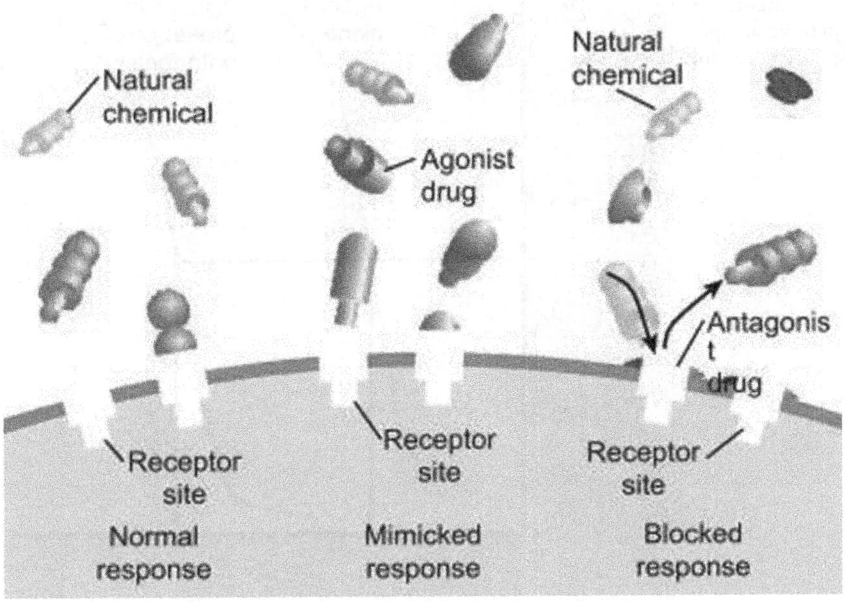

FIG. 2.10 Drugs act by forming a chemical bond with specific receptor sites, similar to a lock and key. The better they "fit," the better the response. Drugs with complete attachment and response are called agonists. Drugs that attach but do not elicit a reaction are called antagonists.

Antagonists

An **antagonist** is a drug that occupies a receptor, preventing the endogenous chemical from being able to bind and produce its action. Antagonists often compete with agonists for receptor-binding sites. They may be used as medications if the body has an excessive response from an endogenous chemical or a drug overdose. Examples of conditions that antagonists treat include tachycardia, hypertension, sedation, and excessive stomach acid. Adverse effects are often reversed by using antagonists, which have no intrinsic activity. The actions that occur after the administration of an antagonist are due to a lack of agonist actions.

However, antagonists are not always associated with receptors. *Functional antagonists* inhibit agonists by changing pharmacokinetic factors. They can slow the absorption of agonists to reduce their pharmacologic effects. Antagonists can also alter fluids' pH and neutralize agonists before they are absorbed. The removal of an agonist from the body can be enhanced by antagonists that increase the speed of metabolism or excretion. Relationships between agonists and antagonists explain many drug-drug and drug-food interactions. There are three primary forms of antagonists, as follows:

- *Competitive and irreversible*: These drugs bind to (or extremely close to) an agonist receptor site reversibly without activating its effector system. Neutral antagonists bind the receptor without shifting the active versus inactive receptor equilibrium. If a competitive antagonist is present, the dose-response curve for an agonist will show that higher doses are required for the same maximal effect to occur (see Fig. 2.11). If given at a high-enough concentration, the agonist can displace the antagonist, fully activating the receptors. However, an irreversible antagonist causes a downward shift of the maximum effect. There is no curve shift on the dose axis unless spare receptors are available. The impact of an irreversible antagonist cannot be overcome by adding more of the agonist. Competitive antagonists increase the ED_{50}, but irreversible antagonists cannot do this unless spare receptors exist. Noncompetitive antagonists acting at allosteric sites of receptors can bind reversibly or irreversibly. However, noncompetitive antagonists acting at receptor sites bind irreversibly.
- *Physiologic*: These antagonists bind to *different* receptor molecules and produce an opposite effect of the drug being antagonized. Examples include the antagonism of histamine's bronchoconstrictor actions via the bronchodilator actions of epinephrine and how glucagon antagonizes the cardiac effects of *propranolol.*
- *Chemical*: These antagonists directly interact with a drug being antagonized, removing or preventing it from binding to its target. These antagonists do not need interactions with agonist receptors, though these interactions sometimes occur. Examples include *dimercaprol*, which chelates lead and other toxic metals, and *pralidoxime*, which avidly combines with phosphorus in organophosphate cholinesterase inhibitors.

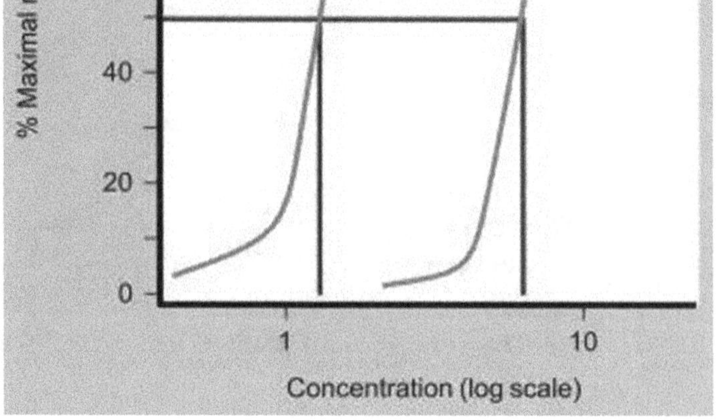

FIG. 2.11 An agonist response, modified by the administration of a competitive antagonist. Both the agonist and antagonist compete for and bind reversibly to the same receptor site. The competitive antagonist causes a parallel right shift of the concentration-response curve for the agonist.

You should remember

The critical difference between agonists and antagonists is their counteractive mechanism of action. Agonists produce actions, while antagonists inhibit actions. Examples of agonists include morphine and methadone. Examples of antagonists include naltrexone and naloxone.

Pharmacogenetics

Pharmacogenetics usually refers to how variation in one gene influences the patient's response to a single drug. Some people have excessive adverse effects with some medications or do not respond to them. Current advances point toward drugs becoming "customized" for patients with specific genetic similarities. In the past, pharmacologists often had to deal with distinctive **idiosyncratic responses**, which were unpredictable and unexplained drug reactions. These responses may be prevented by analyzing a patient's DNA before prescribing a specific drug. *Pharmacogenetics* is an aspect of pharmacology that reveals how genetics are related to drug responses. Significant advancements include identifying slight genetic differences in the drug-metabolizing enzymes of individuals. These genetic differences cause many drug-induced toxicities. In the future, pharmacogenetic information may allow drug therapies to be more customized to the individual molecules of each patient. Over time, this may become more cost effective and significantly improve pharmacotherapy. The term **pharmacogenomics** is broader and refers to studies of the genome.

Key Terms

Additive effect
Agonist
Antagonist
Constitutive activity
Dose-response relationship
Downregulation
Drug interaction
Efficacy
Frequency distribution curves
Full agonist
Idiosyncratic responses
Intrinsic activity
Inverse agonists
Kwashiorkor
Ligand
Marasmus
Margin of safety
Median effective dose
Median lethal dose
Neurotransmitters
Neutral antagonists
Partial agonist
Pharmacogenetics
Pharmacogenomics
Photosensitivity
Placebo
Potency
Side effects
Synergistic effect
Tachyphylaxis
Therapeutic index
Therapeutic window
Tolerance
Upregulation

Clinical Case Studies

Clinical Case Study 1

An 80-year-old male was taken to the hospital after vomiting large quantities of blood. He felt tired and was lightheaded. The patient stated that he had been prescribed warfarin for paroxysmal atrial fibrillation. The patient also had type 2 diabetes, hypertension, dyslipidemia, and Parkinson disease. His other medications included amiodarone, esomeprazole, carbidopa/levodopa, and clonidine. Examination revealed bradycardia, hypotension, and anemia, so he was transferred to the intensive care unit and transfused with packed red blood cells and fresh frozen plasma. His prothrombin time test was unremarkable at admission, so the warfarin was withheld. Tests revealed sinus bradycardia and mild fatty liver. Over 7 days, the patient's warfarin was slowly reinstated. A cardiologist reviewed his condition within 1 week, and the patient was discharged.

Critical Thinking Questions

1. What is the potential danger linked to the use of warfarin?
2. Which disorders affect pharmacodynamics?
3. What are the signs and symptoms of most drug-drug interactions?

Clinical Case Study 2

A 45-year-old male was brought to the emergency department with altered consciousness. He had previously told his family that he might have taken too much diphenhydramine—generally a safe medication. In the emergency department, he suffered a cardiac arrest, determined to be from an overdose of diphenhydramine. The patient was oxygenated. His arterial blood gases showed acidosis. The electrocardiogram showed an entirely right bundle branch block. His blood pressure slowly decreased, and he died on the third day of his hospitalization. After death, his serum diphenhydramine concentration was still excessively high. This drug can cause dose-dependent toxicity.

Critical Thinking Questions

1. How is a drug's safety determined?
2. What are the differences between a drug's potency and its efficacy?
3. What is diphenhydramine classified as, and how does it work?

Further Reading

[1] P.L. Bonate, Pharmacokinetic-Pharmacodynamic Modeling and Simulation, second ed., Springer, 2011.
[2] A.D. Bush, Laboratory Manual of Pharmacology, Including Materia Medica, Pharmacopedics, and Pharmacodynamics, Alpha Edition, 2020.
[3] M.H.H. Ensom, T.K.L. Kiang, K.J. Wilby, Pharmacokinetic and Pharmacodynamic Drug Interactions Associated with Antiretroviral Drugs, Adis, 2016.
[4] M.W. Jann, S.R. Penzak, L.J. Cohen, Applied clinical pharmacokinetics and pharmacodynamics of psychopharmacological agents, Adis (2016).
[5] Y. Kwon, Handbook of Essential Pharmacokinetics, Pharmacodynamics, and Drug Metabolism for Industrial Scientists, Springer, 2013.
[6] D.E. Mager, H.H.C. Kimko, Systems Pharmacology and Pharmacodynamics (AAPS Advances in the Pharmaceutical Sciences Series 23), Springer, 2016.
[7] C.H. Nightingale, P.G. Ambrose, G.L. Drusano, T. Murakawa, Antimicrobial Pharmacodynamics in Theory and Clinical Practice (Infectious Disease and Therapy), second ed., CRC Press, 2019.
[8] J.S. Owen, J. Fiedler-Kelly, Introduction to Population Pharmacokinetic / Pharmacodynamic Analysis with Nonlinear Mixed Effects Models, Wiley, 2014.
[9] M.A. Rudek, C.H. Chau, W.D. Figg, H.W. McLeod, Handbook of Anticancer Pharmacokinetics and Pharmacodynamics (Cancer Drug Discovery and Development), second ed., Humana Press, 2014.
[10] J. Schuttler, H. Schwilden, Modern Anesthetics (Handbook of Experimental Pharmacology 182), Springer, 2008.
[11] T.N. Tozer, M. Rowland, Essentials of Pharmacokinetics and Pharmacodynamics, second ed., Lippincott, Williams, and Wilkins, 2015.
[12] A.A. Udy, J.A. Roberts, J. Lipman, Antibiotic pharmacokinetic / pharmacodynamic considerations in the critically ill, Adis (2018).
[13] A.A. Vinks, H. Derendorf, J.W. Mouton, Fundamentals of Antimicrobial Pharmacokinetics and Pharmacodynamics, Springer, 2014.

CHAPTER

3

Pharmacokinetics

OUTLINE

LEARNING OUTCOMES

After study of the chapter, readers should be able to:

1. Identify the primary pharmacokinetic processes.
2. Describe the barriers that prevent drugs from crossing plasma membranes.
3. Discuss factors that affect drug absorption.
4. Discuss first-pass metabolism.
5. Describe the blood-brain barrier.
6. Explain drug binding to plasma proteins.
7. Describe blood barriers to drug distribution.
8. Explain fecal and biliary excretion.
9. Describe the significant processes of drug excretion.
10. Explain the minimum effective concentration of a drug.

The Science of Pharmacology
https://doi.org/10.1016/B978-0-443-29038-1.00003-8

Overview

Pharmacokinetics describes how body systems biologically affect medications. To prevent, control, and cure diseases, accurate drug doses must reach target tissues to obtain therapeutic—but not toxic—levels. The derivation of the word "pharmacokinetics" comes from "pharmaco," meaning *medicines*, and "kinetics," meaning *motion* or *movement. Many obstacles can* stop a drug from reaching its target cells. Medications' pharmacological and toxicological actions are mostly related to their plasma concentrations. Recognizing how fast drug actions occur, medication strengths, and drug action durations is vital. These factors are based on drug absorption, bioavailability, distribution, metabolism, and elimination. Drug absorption from the site of administration allows entry into the plasma. The drug may reversibly leave the bloodstream to be distributed into the interstitial and intracellular fluids and then metabolized by the liver. Eventually, the drug and its metabolites are removed via the urine, bile, or feces. Knowledge of pharmacokinetics helps to determine the correct routes of administration of medications.

The passage of drugs through plasma membranes

Most drugs cross plasma membranes, entering cells and producing specific effects. A plasma membrane comprises a lipid bilayer (see Fig. 3.1). Throughout the membrane, there are scattered lipoproteins and other molecules. Like other chemicals, drugs utilize *diffusion (passive transport)* and **active transport** as their primary methods of crossing plasma membranes. Distribution requires a therapeutic agent to be able to cross plasma membranes freely. This works well for lipid-soluble drug molecules but does not facilitate the movement of ionized molecules. Some drug molecules can enter via open channels in the plasma membrane. This requires them to be minimal-molecular-weight substances such as alcohol, urea, and water. Larger drug molecules, those that are water soluble, and those that are ionized require **facilitated diffusion** via a carrier protein to cross plasma membranes. Carrier proteins select only certain molecules with specific structures to transport through a plasma membrane. Active transport is a method that requires energy expenditure from a cell and a carrier protein to allow drug molecules to cross plasma membranes against their gradient from low to high concentrations. The carrier proteins are sometimes referred to as *pumps*.

Drug absorption

Pharmacokinetics begins with *drug absorption*, which is determined by the physiochemical properties, formulation, and route of administration of each drug. The two primary routes of drug administration are the *enteral* and *parenteral* routes. Enteral administration occurs through the mouth. It is the most common and simplest method of drug administration. The two common subtypes of enteral administration are the oral (swallowed) and sublingual (dissolved under the tongue) routes. The **parenteral route** of drug administration involves using injections,

FIG. 3.1 Structure of the cell membrane.

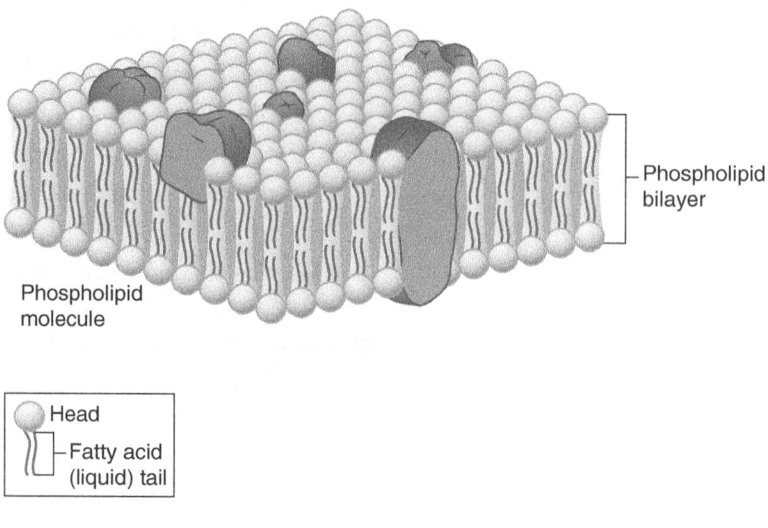

which are most often intramuscular (IM), subcutaneous (SC), or intravenous (IV). Additional routes of administration include inhalation, intranasal, intrathecal, topical, transdermal, and rectal routes. Regardless of the method of drug administration, absorption involves the drug being transferred from the administration site into the bloodstream. The drug is completely absorbed in parenteral administration, reaching the systemic blood circulation.

Barriers prevent some drugs from crossing plasma membranes. For oral medications, the plasma membranes of the GI tract and the capillary endothelial cells must be crossed to reach the bloodstream. When a drug leaves the bloodstream, it again strikes capillary cells, moves through the interstitial fluid, and may have to pass through the plasma membranes of target cells. The list of various membranes a drug may encounter includes the stomach, portal vein, liver, systemic circulation, target tissue, and target cell (see Fig. 3.2).

Routes of drug administration

Drug absorption is highly affected by the route of administration. Some drugs are formulated to be administered by several routes, and some are designed for one specific route. The **enteral route** is orally or through nasogastric or **gastrostomy** tubes. It is the most common route of all. Most enteral medications utilize the porous surfaces of the oral mucosa, the stomach, and the small intestine. Few enteral drugs are given for local effects, which include GI tract

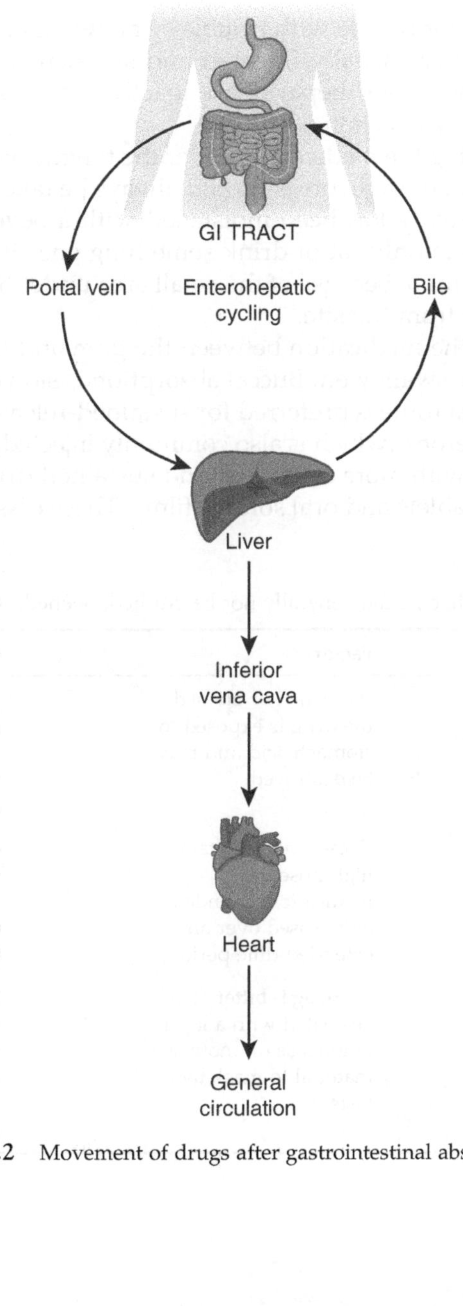

FIG. 3.2 Movement of drugs after gastrointestinal absorption.

infections. The most common oral drug forms are *tablets* and *capsules*, which are relatively easy to take. Tablets are sometimes *scored*, so they can be broken into two halves or four quarters for smaller doses. The oral route is very safe because the skin barrier does not have to be compromised. If an overdose of an oral drug occurs, vomiting can be induced, or the stomach contents can be suctioned. Because tablets and capsules must be dissolved before absorption, they have a relatively slow onset. The dissolution rate may be the slowest part of oral drug absorption. Oral liquids are absorbed faster because they do not require dissolution.

Solid acids destroy some enteral medications within the stomach. To avoid this, tablets may be coated with a hard, waxy substance that resists acidity. Known as **enteric-coated** tablets, they dissolve in the small intestine, which has an alkaline environment. Some enteric-coated drugs are so coated because they would otherwise irritate the stomach mucosa if dissolved there. Then, the need to take multiple daily doses often results in patients taking medications improperly. Therefore extended-release tablets or capsules are available for some drugs. Their labels contain notations for this particular release characteristic, which is often abbreviated as "XR" or "XL" for extended release, "LA" for *long-acting* drugs, and "SR" for slow and sustained release, and these dissolve slowly to provide a longer duration of action. These drugs are used only once or twice daily.

Children and older adults may have difficulty swallowing tablets and capsules. If the drug manufacturer intends to do so, some tablets can be crushed, and some capsules can be opened. The powder can then be sprinkled over food or mixed into juice for easier swallowing. This should only be done if the manufacturer indicates the practice is approved. Generally, drugs that should not be crushed, opened, or chewed (instead of swallowed) are summarized in Table 3.1.

Some drugs are available as liquids for people with trouble swallowing tablets or capsules. Liquid forms include elixirs, suspensions, and syrups. They are usually flavored and sweetened extensively, so their bitter taste is not experienced. Some drugs, such as insulin and heparin, are inactivated by stomach and small intestine enzymes. Therefore they must be administered by injection.

The **sublingual route** involves placing the medication under the tongue, where it slowly dissolves. This provides a rapid onset of drug action. Sublingual dosage forms should always be taken after oral medicines have been swallowed. They are taken after the oral cavity has been moistened with a beverage. The patient must not move the mixture around with the tongue and can only eat or drink something once it is dissolved. Extended-release formulations are not used via the sublingual route because of the small area under the tongue and the constant presence of saliva, which would remove the drug from the site.

The **buccal route** involves placing the medication between the gum and the cheek. The drug must stay in place and not reach the sublingual area or be swallowed. Buccal absorption is slower than the sublingual route. Due to its greater mucosal surface area, the buccal route is preferred for sustained-release delivery of medications. An example of a drug given via this route is testosterone (which is also commonly injected) because buccal administration allows the release of the drug over 12 hours, with more consistent and sustained drug levels. Newer options for oral medications include orally disintegrating tablets and oral soluble films. These dissolve in the mouth in under 30 seconds

TABLE 3.1 Drugs that should generally not be crushed, opened, or chewed

Type of drug	Factor	Comments
Enteric coated	If crushed or opened, the drug is exposed to stomach acid and may be destroyed.	Also, the drug may irritate the stomach mucosa, causing nausea, vomiting, or gastritis.
Extended release	These drugs contain a high dose of medication, intended to be released over an extended time period.	Opening or crushing will release all of the drug immediately, which can result in toxicity.
Undesired effects	If a drug is bitter, it may be coated with a layer of glucose or another material to mask the taste.	If crushed or opened, the bitterness is tasted; others stain teeth, irritate oral mucosa, or cause an anesthetic effect upon the tongue.

and do not require the patient to drink water. These forms are perfect for patients who have problems chewing or swallowing or are uncooperative, mentally impaired, or nauseated. The buccal and sublingual routes are illustrated in Fig. 3.3.

Medications applied to the skin or mucous membranes are topical. Topical drugs may also be used on the mucous membranes of the eyes, ears, nose, respiratory tract, urinary tract, vagina, and rectum. Some are absorbed quickly because the thin membranes contain a rich blood supply. Many topical drugs produce localized effects, such as antibiotics for skin infections. Antineoplastic drugs can be instilled into the urinary bladder through a catheter for localized bladder cancers. Corticosteroids can be sprayed into the nostrils and reduce inflammation of the nasal mucosa caused by allergic rhinitis.

Topical formulations of drugs cause fewer adverse effects than oral or parenteral forms because of slower absorption. The amount of the drug that reaches the general circulation is only minimal. Topical drugs' most common adverse effects are transient redness, stinging, or burning. Some topical medicines provide a slow release and absorption into the general circulation and are given for systemic effects. One example is a nitroglycerin patch applied to the skin to treat coronary artery disease.

Some medications are very well delivered by using **transdermal patches**. Examples include nitroglycerin (for angina pectoris), scopolamine (for motion sickness), and testosterone (for hypogonadism). A transdermal patch contains a specific amount of medication; the delivery rate and actual dose received may differ. Patches are changed regularly, often daily or weekly, based on the type of medication within.

The ophthalmic route is used for local conditions of the eye and its surrounding structures. This route can be perfect for treating eye infections, excessive dryness, glaucoma, and dilating the pupils for eye examinations. Ophthalmic drugs are absorbed systemically as the drug drains into the nasolacrimal ducts, nasopharynx, and,

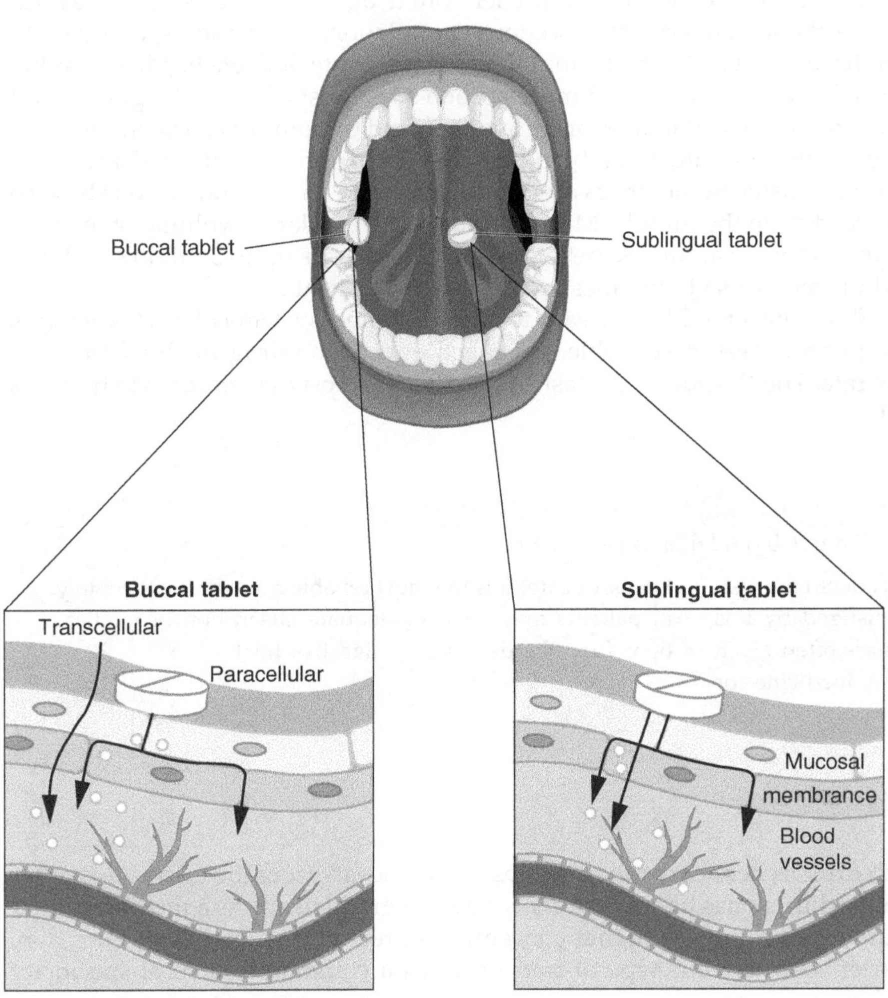

FIG. 3.3 The buccal and sublingual routes.

eventually, the GI tract. This is a slow process in most cases, and only a small amount reaches the general circulation. There are very few systemic adverse effects except in infants with greater circulating systemic drug concentration than adults, causing more risk for adverse effects.

The otic route is used for local ear conditions, including accumulations of earwax and infections. Otic medications must always be at room temperature before use because if they are cold, they can cause nausea or dizziness. Systemic adverse effects do not occur unless an otic drug is applied to injured or abrased areas, such as a ruptured tympanic membrane.

The intranasal route is used to attain localized effects upon the nasal mucosa or for systemic absorption. This route is convenient and provides a rapid onset of action. It is used to apply drops or sprays, shrink swollen nasal mucous membranes, or loosen sections and allow for drainage. Decongestant nasal sprays immediately relieve nasal congestion from the common cold. Intranasal corticosteroids are highly safe and effective for allergic rhinitis.

The vaginal route allows for the treatment of infections, itching, and pain because a rich blood supply allows for widespread absorption and systemic effects. Vaginal creams containing estrogen can produce localized vaginal impact and significantly increase estrogen in the bloodstream. The rectal route is also used for local and systemic drug delivery. It is a safe route for comatose patients or patients with nausea or vomiting who cannot take oral medications. Typically, rectal medications are suppositories, laxatives, and diagnostic substances that may be given via an enema.

The *parenteral route* requires using a needle to inject medications into the skin, SC tissue, muscles, or veins. Parenteral administration is more invasive to the body and can introduce pathogens into the tissues or blood. The primary difference between intradermal (ID) and SC injections is the depth that the needle reaches. Both methods are alternatives when a patient cannot take oral drugs. The digestive system is avoided, but small drug volumes can be administered parenterally.

Injections may cause pain and swelling at the site where they are given. The ID route brings medications into the skin's dermis, which has more blood vessels than the deeper SC layer. Therefore drugs are absorbed more readily, and the ID route is usually used for local anesthetic delivery before venous cannulation, allergy shots, and tests to screen for disease. Only 0.1 to 0.2 mL of medication is used in an ID injection. The SC route delivers heparin, insulin, vitamins, and certain vaccines. SC doses usually range from 0.5 to 1 mL. Injection sites must be rotated regularly and documented so that absorption can be maintained, tissue damage can be avoided, and discomfort can be minimized.

The IM route delivers medications to large muscles with a rich blood supply. The drug molecules quickly move into the blood vessels, and the onset of action is faster. Some drugs are formulated with an oily and viscous base so that they are slowly and continuously absorbed from the muscle. Muscle tissue receives a larger volume of medications than the SC region. Therefore an adult with normal muscle development can tolerate up to 3 mL injected into the gluteus medius muscles. If the deltoid muscle is used, volumes are usually 0.5 to 1 mL.

The IV route directly delivers drugs or fluids into the bloodstream to be distributed systemically. This route is used when a swift onset is needed. Absorption is very predictable. An exact level of the drug in circulation can be achieved by finely adjusting the IV flow rate. The IV route is the fastest but also the most dangerous. Medications cannot be retrieved after they are injected.

You should remember

The IV drug administration route is considered the fastest of all. Injections and infusions administered by this route have 100% bioavailability. IV drugs are often given in acute situations such as emergency medicine or intensive care. It is the most reliable route because acutely ill patients may have inadequate absorption of medications from the tissues and digestive tract.

Transport from the GI tract

As introduced previously, based on each drug's chemical properties, absorption occurs from the GI tract by either **passive diffusion** or active transport. Passive diffusion is based on a concentration gradient across a membrane that separates two body compartments. The drug moves from a higher concentration region to a lower concentration. Passive diffusion does not require a "carrier" because this type of transport has a common structural specificity

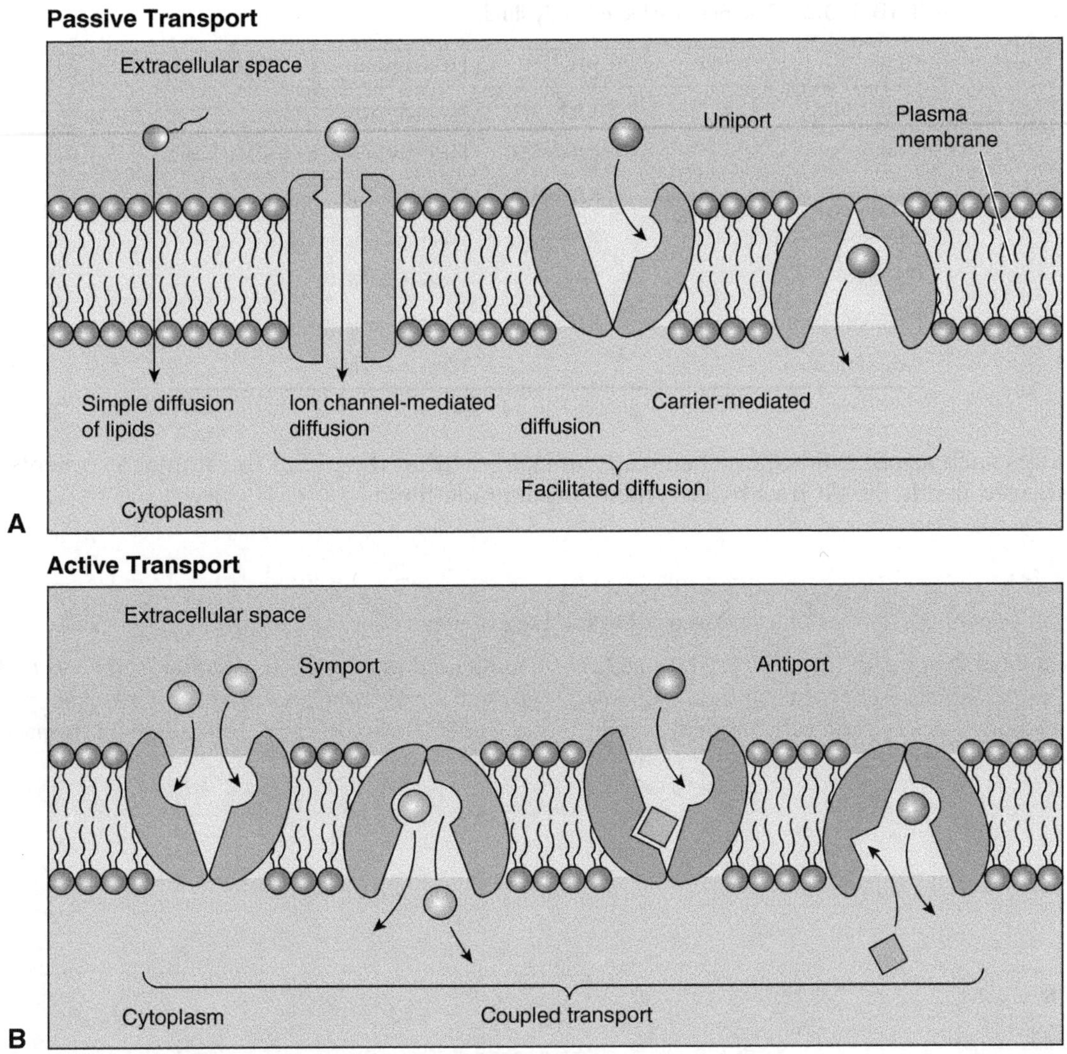

FIG. 3.4 Passive and active transport with adenosine triphosphate *(ATP). From Gartner, L.P. [2017]. Textbook of histology [4th ed.]. St. Louis: Elsevier.*

and is not saturable. Most drugs exert their effects via passive diffusion. Lipid-soluble drugs move quickly across most body membranes because of their solubility within the membrane bilayers. Water-soluble drugs penetrate cell membranes via aqueous channels or pores.

Other agents enter cells via specialized transmembrane carrier proteins that allow the passage of large molecules. The carrier proteins change structure to allow drugs or endogenous molecules to pass into cells from areas of high to low concentrations. This facilitated diffusion does not need energy and may be saturated or inhibited.

Active transport also involves specific carrier proteins over cell membranes. A few drugs that appear structurally similar to natural metabolites are transported over cell membranes via these carrier proteins. Active transport requires energy via the hydrolysis of adenosine triphosphate. Drugs are moved against a concentration gradient but from low- to high-concentration areas. This abides by saturation kinetics for the carriers, similar to how enzyme-catalyzed reactions have a maximal velocity at high substrate levels, and all active sites are filled with substrate (see Fig. 3.4).

Effects of pH

Drug absorption is affected by pH because most drugs are either weak acids or weak bases. They are ionized in some pH ranges and nonionized in others. An acid can dissociate and release a hydrogen ion with a pH lower than 7.0. A base can take up a hydrogen ion with a pH greater than 7.0. The pH of selected body fluids is shown

TABLE 3.2 The pH of selected body fluids.

Fluid	pH	Description
Gastric juice	1.0 to 3.0	Strongly acidic
Urine	4.0 to 8.0	Strongly acidic to weakly basic
Duodenum of small intestine	5.0 to 6.0	Weakly acidic
Cerebrospinal fluid	7.3	Weakly basic
Plasma	7.4	Weakly basic
Ileum of small intestine	8.0	Weakly basic
Large intestine	8.0	Weakly basic

in Table 3.2. Drugs such as *penicillin G* are chemically unstable within the pH of the stomach contents. *Insulin* and *heparin* are destroyed inside the GI tract by enzymes that degrade them.

You should remember

Weakly essential drugs with low solubility at high pH could have impaired absorption in patients with high gastric pH, leading to reduced and variable bioavailability. It is necessary to understand the behavior of the compound as a function of stomach pH and to develop a potent formulation that may provide enough exposure in patients who do not produce enough stomach acid.

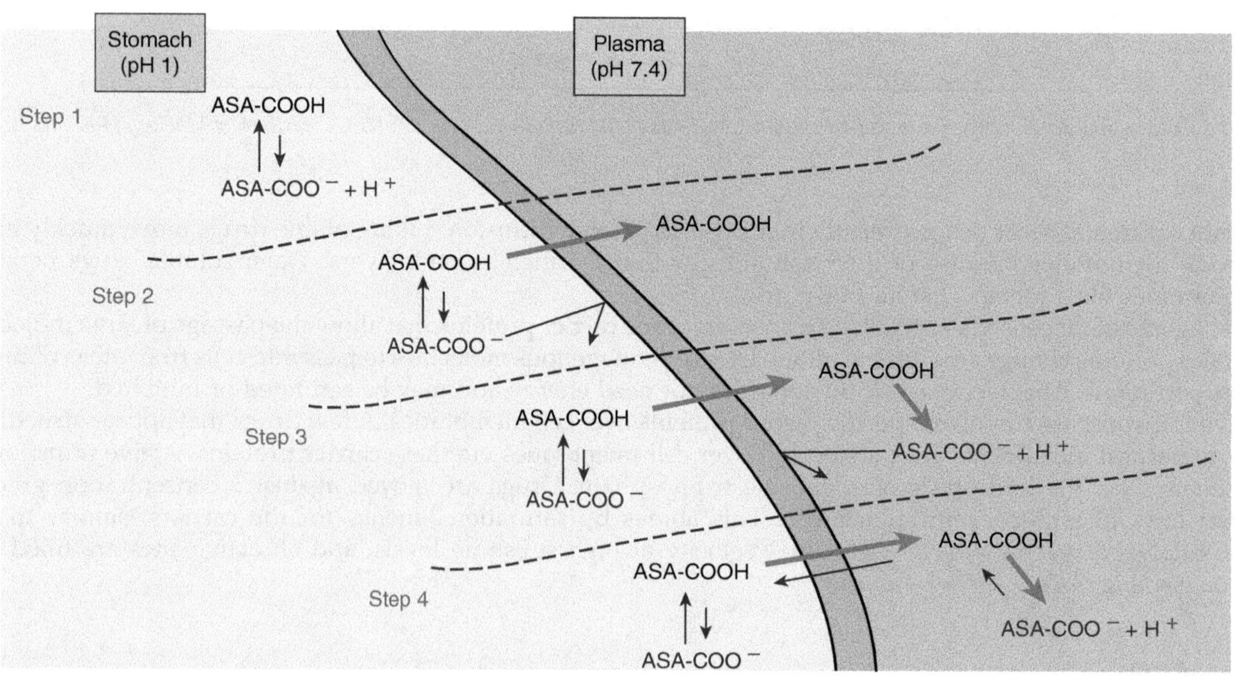

FIG. 3.5 Ion trapping of drugs. (Step 1: aspirin dissolves, and some molecules become ionized after losing a proton. Step 2: Because most molecules are still nonionized, they easily cross membranes of the stomach lumen into the plasma. Step 3: Most of the molecules lose a proton (H^+) and become negatively charged ions. Step 4: As the molecules become ionized, more of them pass from the stomach to the plasma to replace them.)

Blood flow to the site of absorption

A drug's administration site must have sufficient blood flow to be absorbed. Drugs are absorbed more quickly in areas with higher blood flow. An IM injection is inserted into larger muscles because their increased blood flow provides the best absorption. If a patient is experiencing shock or a myocardial infarction, blood flow to specific tissues is reduced. Absorption from the IM sites or GI tract may also be diminished. Topical drugs may be slowly absorbed because of the poor blood supply to the upper skin layers. Sometimes blood flow can be controlled to cause slower drug absorption because local anesthetics can be toxic with quick absorption, so a vasoconstrictor such as epinephrine can be added to the local anesthetic to reduce blood flow in the area of treatment. Another example is the application of ice packs to slow absorption to the site. Adding heat would speed up absorption.

Drug ionization

Ionized molecules carry positive or negative charges. Based on the pH of surrounding fluids, most drugs are in a charged or uncharged state. Drug ionization affects the drug's ability to cross plasma membranes and be excreted. Aspirin is an example of the effects of ionization upon absorption (see Fig. 3.5). Unlike aspirin, weakly basic medications are nonionized in an alkaline environment. Essential drugs are much more likely to be absorbed in alkaline environments such as the small intestine. The simplest way to understand drug ionization is as follows:

- Acids are absorbed in acids because they are nonionized.
- Bases are absorbed in bases because they are nonionized.

Drug distribution

Drug distribution is transferring a drug from the bloodstream to the body tissues. The drug's delivery from the plasma to the extracellular fluid, known as the *interstitial tissues*, is mainly based on blood flow, capillary permeability, drug binding to plasma and tissue proteins, and relative hydrophobicity. The circulatory system is the primary pathway for the delivery of a drug to its site of action. Fig. 3.6 illustrates possible entry routes and places of distribution and disposition.

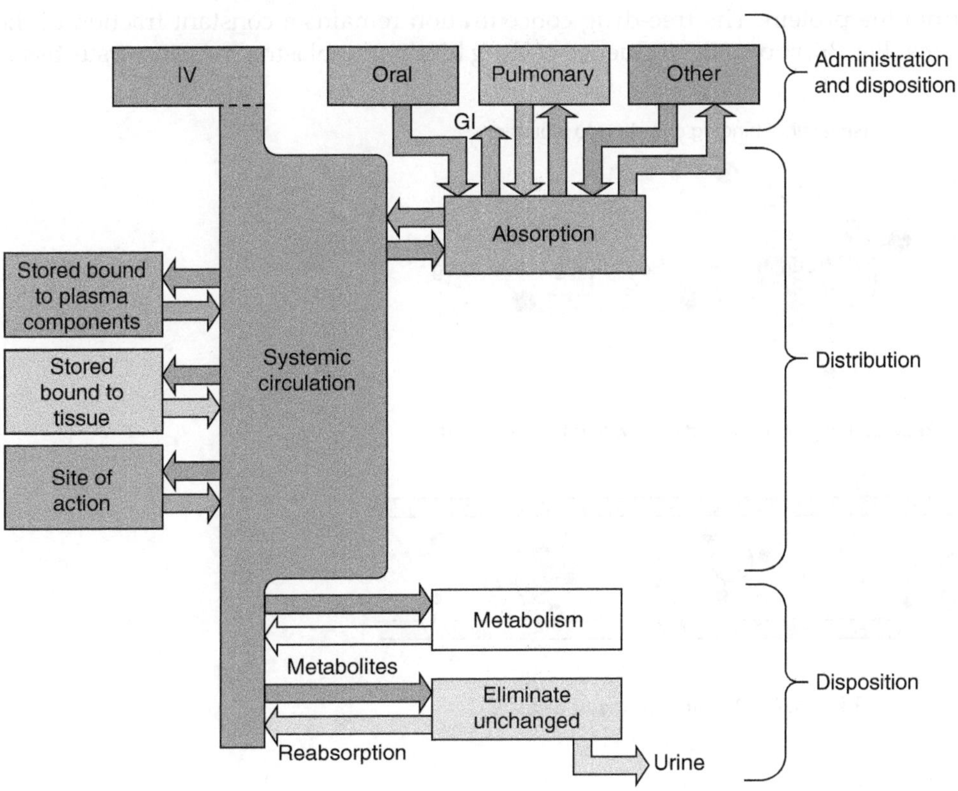

FIG. 3.6 Factors influencing drug concentration at the site of action and at different times after administration. This figure includes absorption, transport via the systemic circulation, storage areas, and metabolism.

Blood flow to tissues

Because of the unequal distribution of cardiac output to various body organs, blood flow rates to tissue capillaries are incredibly different. For example, blood flow is more significant to the brain, heart, kidneys, and liver than other organs. Fat tissues have decreased perfusion, resulting in lower amounts of drug distribution. Blood flow must be considered locally as well. After a traumatic injury, the blood supply to a fractured bone may be much less because of damaged blood vessels. Perfusion can also be blocked by cellular debris related to inflammation. Antibiotics may be unable to reach the area of injury until blood flow is restored. Delivery of large concentrations of drugs to injured, necrotic, or abscessed areas with insufficient perfusion is always tricky.

Drug solubility

A drug's physical properties greatly determine how it will move through the body. Lipid solubility determines how quickly the medicine is absorbed and how it will mix in the bloodstream, cross membranes, and become localized in body tissues. Lipid-soluble drugs are not stopped by barriers that usually prevent water-soluble drugs. Therefore lipid-soluble drugs are more wholly distributed to the body tissues.

Tissue storage

Some body tissues can accumulate and store medications in higher concentrations than other tissues. There is a high **affinity** for some medicines in the eyes, teeth, bone marrow, and adipose tissue. Agents stored in adipose tissue include diazepam, lipid-soluble vitamins, and tetracycline (which also binds to calcium salts, accumulating in the bones and teeth). After a drug is stored in the tissues, it can remain for months and be released extremely slowly into circulation. One example is the osteoporosis drug *alendronate*, which remains present for 4 to 7 months after administration stops.

Drug binding to plasma proteins

Drugs remain nondiffusible because of reversible binding to plasma proteins, which slows their transfer out of the vascular compartment. Binding is nonselective for chemical structure. It occurs at protein sites where bilirubin and other endogenous compounds usually attach. The major drug-binding protein is **plasma albumin**, which may function as a drug reservoir. A free drug's concentration is decreased due to elimination via **excretion** or metabolism. The bound drug becomes dissociated from the protein. The free-drug concentration remains a constant fraction of the total amount of medicine in the plasma. Fig. 3.7 shows the influence of drug binding to plasma protein versus tissue

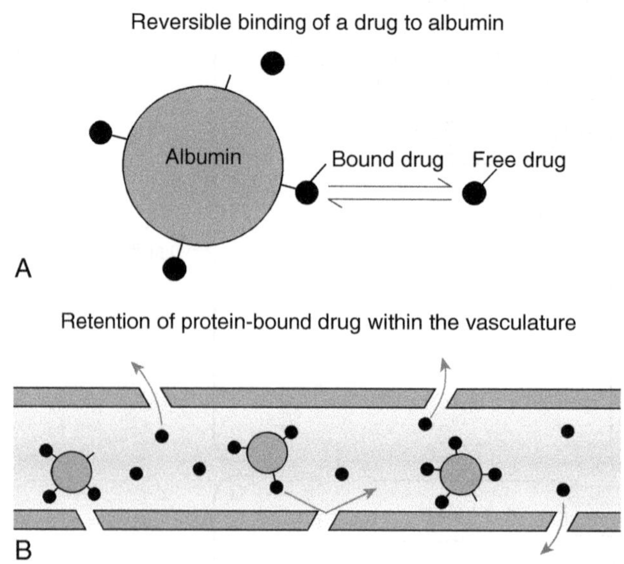

FIG. 3.7 Protein binding of drugs.

sites on volume of distribution, showing numbers that represent the relative quantity of a drug in 1 mL of plasma compared with adjacent tissue. Only the plasma is sampled, and the albumin-bound drug is included in this sample.

Volume of distribution

The *volume of distribution* is an imagined fluid volume into which a drug is dispersed. A drug, regardless of route of administration, can enter one of three distinct body water compartments or remain in a cellular location. When an anesthetic has a substantial molecular weight or binds well to plasma proteins, it is too large to move through endothelial **slit junctions** of capillaries. It becomes trapped in the vascular (plasma) compartment. Therefore the drug is distributed in a volume of about 6% of body weight. In a 154-pound (70-kg) person, this is about 4.2 quarts (4 L). An example of such a drug is *heparin.*

When a drug has a low molecular weight and is hydrophilic, it can move through endothelial slit junctions of capillaries into the interstitial fluid. Even so, hydrophilic drugs cannot cross lipid cell membranes to enter the water component inside of cells. Instead, these drugs are distributed into a volume consisting of the total of the interstitial fluid and plasma water. Together, these components comprise the extracellular fluid, about 20% of body weight, or about 14.8 quarts (14 L) in a 154-pound (70-kg) person. The *aminoglycoside antibiotics* are examples of such drugs.

When a drug has a low molecular weight but is hydrophobic, it can move into the interstitium through slit junctions and cell membranes into the intracellular fluid. These drugs are distributed into a volume of about 60% of body weight. In a 154-pound (70-kg) person, this is about 44.3 quarts (42 L). An example of such a drug is *ethanol* (ethyl alcohol). There are also other sites where drugs can be distributed. In a pregnant female, the fetus can take up drugs, increasing the volume of distribution.

You should remember

The distribution volume measures the relative affinity of a drug for plasma and tissue components. It may be altered in critically ill patients, with either an increase or decrease in total body fluid and intravascular volume. Remember, the volume of distribution is not a physical space but an "apparent" space.

Barriers to drug distribution

Because of spaces between endothelial cells, most capillaries are relatively porous. Many drugs exit the blood circulation by moving through these spaces to enter the interstitial fluid quickly. The brain and placenta have anatomic barriers that stop many chemicals and drugs from leaving the blood. These include the blood-brain barrier and the **fetal-placental barrier**. Brain capillaries have endothelial cells sealed by tight junctions and a thick basement membrane (see Fig. 3.8). Astrocytes in the brain are firmly pressed against the basement membrane and secrete chemicals

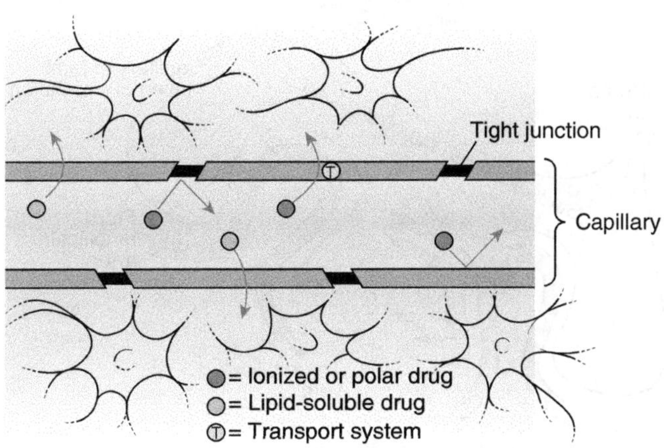

FIG. 3.8 Drug movement across the blood-brain barrier.

that regulate capillary permeability. The blood-brain barrier protects the brain from pathogens and toxic substances. Highly lipid-soluble agents, including antianxiety drugs, general anesthetics, sedatives, and anticonvulsant drugs, easily cross the blood-brain barrier to affect the central nervous system.

Conversely, many antibiotics and antitumor drugs cannot easily cross the barrier, so brain cancers and infections are difficult to treat. When a condition such as meningitis inflames the blood-brain barrier, it becomes more permeable. The blood-brain barrier is not entirely developed in neonates; many drugs can easily cross into the infant brain.

The fetal-placental barrier stops harmful substances from passing from the mother's bloodstream to the fetus (see Fig. 3.9). This barrier is relatively inefficient because alcohol, caffeine, cocaine, and some prescription medications easily cross, resulting in potential fetal harm. Therefore a pregnant female should take no prescription medication, over-the-counter drug, or herbal supplement if the physician disapproves.

You should remember

Barriers to drug distribution include plasma or tissue protein binding, body weight, body composition, and fluid spaces. The significant determinants of drug distribution include total body weight, muscle mass, and fat composition. Females and males are different regarding these factors.

Drug metabolism

Drug metabolism (**biotransformation**) involves chemical modifications of the drug by the body. The drug enters the hepatic portal and systemic circulation after absorption across the GI tract. Biotransformation utilizes **first-pass elimination** by the liver, the primary organ for drug metabolism (see Fig. 3.10), as part of **first-pass metabolism**. The hepatic microsomal enzyme system metabolizes the majority of drugs. Cytochrome 450 (CYP450) is a family of critical enzymes for metabolizing medications. This enzyme comprises families of **isozymes** that contain heme in the liver. An Arabic number indicates the specific family and is followed by a capital letter to designate the subfamily, such as CYP3A. Then another number is added, indicating distinct isozymes, such as CYP3A4. Many different genes and enzymes exist, as do various types of P450 or **isoforms**. However, an individual drug can be a substrate for multiple isozyme types. These enzymes have extreme genetic variability, affecting personal dosing regimens and determining therapeutic responses and risks of adverse events. Drugs such as *carbamazepine, phenobarbital*, and *rifampin* can increase synthesis of several CYP isozymes. **Induction** is a process in which a molecule, such as a drug, induces the expression of an enzyme, enhancing its activity. This causes increased drug biotransformation and may result in significant decreases in plasma concentrations of metabolized medicines and a loss of pharmacologic effects. In the example of rifampin, the drug decreases the plasma concentration of human immunodeficiency virus protease inhibitors, reducing their ability to suppress its virion maturation.

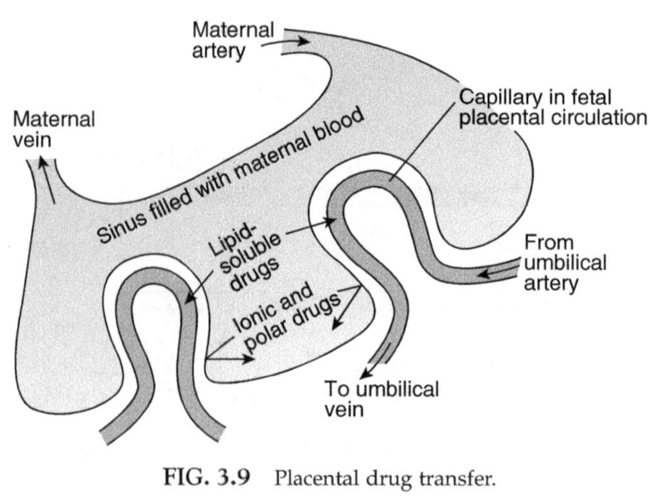

FIG. 3.9 Placental drug transfer.

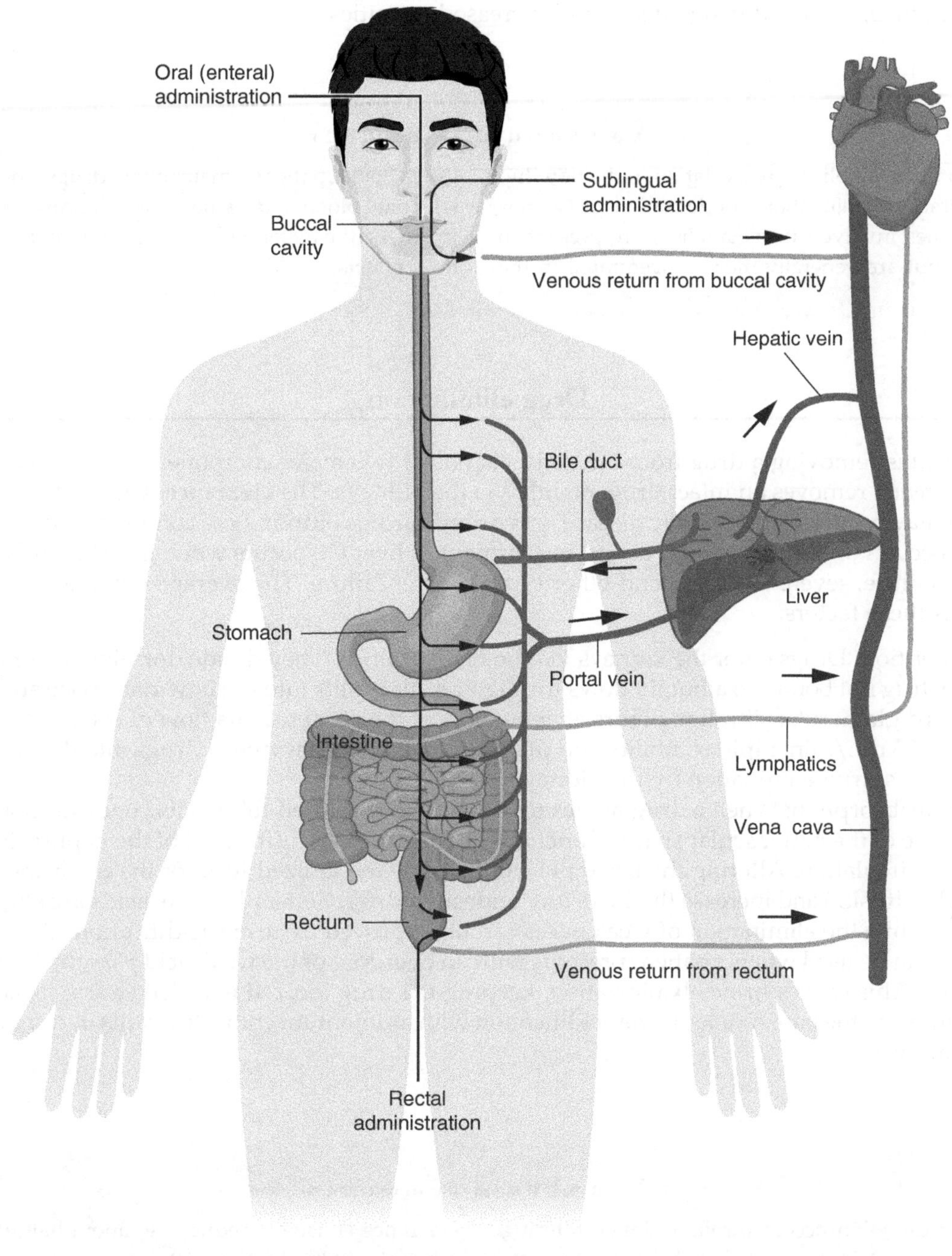

FIG. 3.10 First-pass metabolism.

Inhibition of isozyme activity is an essential source of drug interactions, leading to serious adverse effects. Usually, inhibition occurs through competition for the same isozyme. However, some drugs, such as *ketoconazole*, can inhibit reactions for which they are not substrates. Many drugs, including *omeprazole*, inhibit several CYP-dependent biotransformation pathways of *warfarin*. If these two drugs are coadministered, plasma concentrations of *warfarin* increase, leading to more coagulation inhibition and risks for severe bleeding. Important CYP inhibitors include *erythromycin*, *ketoconazole*, and *ritonavir* because they inhibit multiple CYP isozymes. The cimetidine drug blocks the metabolism of clozapine, theophylline, and warfarin. Natural substances, such as grapefruit juice, can also inhibit drug metabolism, which inhibits CYP3A4 and therefore medicines such as *amlodipine*, *clarithromycin*, and *indinavir*. This system metabolizes these drugs and is then found in more significant amounts in the blood, likely being able to increase their therapeutic or toxic effects. Inhibited drug metabolism can increase plasma concentrations with long-term medications, extended drug effects, and increased toxicities.

You should remember

Drugs can be metabolized by oxidation, reduction, hydrolysis, hydration, conjugation, condensation, or isomerization. Enzymes involved in metabolism are present in many tissues but are generally more concentrated in the liver. Some patients metabolize drugs so quickly that adequate blood and tissue concentrations are not reached. In others, the metabolism is so slow that usual doses have toxic effects.

Drug elimination

Drug *elimination* is removing a drug from the body via one of two major components: excretion and biotransformation. Drug *excretion* removes an intact drug, mainly via the kidneys. The **clearance** (CL) of drugs that depend on kidney function may be affected by kidney disease or reduced cardiac output. Less commonly, alterations of consent by the liver can occur. For high-extraction drugs, impairment of liver CL occurs when liver blood flow is decreased, such as in heart failure, severe cirrhosis, and other types of liver failure. The average elimination of a drug by the kidneys involves these factors:

- Glomerular filtration: Drugs enter the kidneys via the renal arteries. They divide, forming a glomerular capillary plexus. A free drug not bound to albumin flows through capillary slits into the Bowman space and the glomerular filtrate. Standard glomerular filtration occurs at about 20% of the renal plasma flow of 600 mL/min, meaning the average rate is 125 mL/min. Lipid solubility and pH do not affect the passage of drugs into the glomerular filtrate. Fig. 3.11 illustrates drug elimination by the kidneys.
- Distal tubular reabsorption: When a drug moves to the distal convoluted tubule, its concentrations increase to be higher than those of the perivascular space. If uncharged, the drug can diffuse out of the nephric lumen, returning to the systemic circulation. Altering the urine pH can increase the ionized form of the medicine in the lumen to minimize back diffusion and increase the CL of any undesired drug. Generally, weak acids are eliminated by urine alkalinization, while the elimination of weak bases can be improved by urine acidification. This is known as ion trapping. This can be used when a patient presents with an overdose of the weak acid *phenobarbital* and *bicarbonate* is administered. This causes urine alkalinization, keeping the drug ionized and decreasing its absorption. If a patient overdoses on the base *cocaine*, urine acidification with ammonium chloride results in drug protonation and increased clearance.

You should remember

Most drug excretion occurs through kidney filtering. As people age, renal drug excretion decreases. At age 80, clearance is usually reduced to about half of what it was when the individual was 30.

Clearance

CL explains a drug's elimination rate to its plasma concentration, expressed in units equaling the volume per unit of time. The formula is as follows:

$$CL = \frac{\text{Rate of drug elimination}}{\text{Plasma drug concentration}}$$

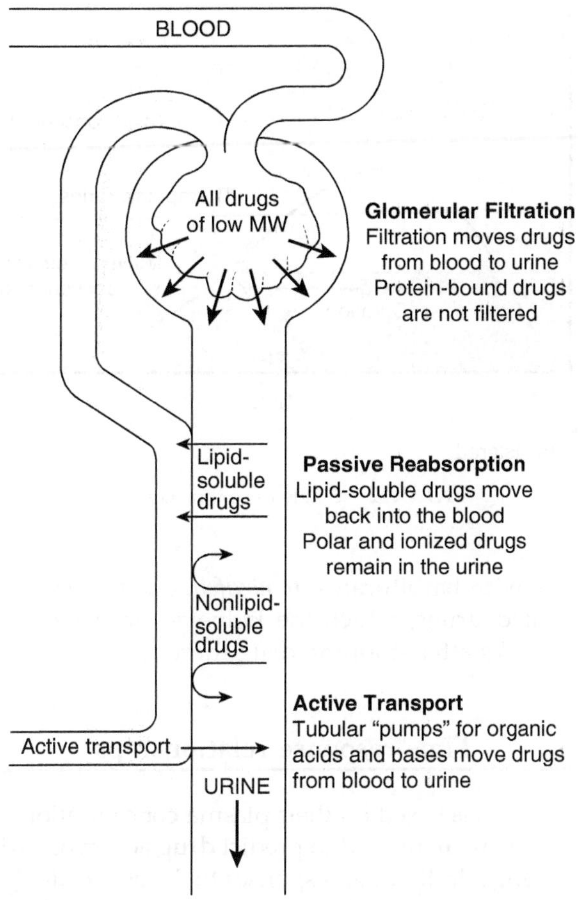

FIG. 3.11 Renal drug excretion. *MW*, Molecular weight.

Clearance is constant for any drug eliminated with **first-order kinetics**. The ratio of the elimination rate compared to plasma concentration is the same, no matter the plasma concentration. Clearance for various drugs can range widely, from a small percentage of blood flow to a maximum of total blood flow in the liver and kidneys. Drug choice is based on the drug, the individual's blood flow, and the condition of the liver and kidneys. Most medications used today (about 95%) are eliminated via first-order kinetics rather than zero-order kinetics. However, examples of drugs eliminated via zero-order kinetics include aspirin, ethanol, and phenytoin. Zero-order kinetics is described when a constant amount of drug is eliminated per unit of time, but the rate is independent of the concentration of the drug.

Pulmonary excretion

Drugs that are part of a gas or **volatile liquid** are well suited for excretion by the respiratory system. Rates of respiratory excretion are based on factors concerning gas exchange. These include diffusion, gas solubility, and blood flow to the lungs. Respiratory activity is the prime eliminator of gaseous and volatile anesthetics. The quicker the breathing rate, the faster the excretion. However, respiratory removal of water-soluble agents such as alcohol depends more on blood flow to the lungs. The quicker the blood flows through the lung capillaries, the more pulmonary excretion will occur. The lungs excrete most drugs in their original, unmetabolized form, unlike other forms of excretion.

Fecal and biliary excretion

Some oral drugs move through the GI tract without absorption and are excreted in the feces, such as *mebendazole* to treat intestinal worms and *barium sulfate*, used as a contrast agent in radiology. With **biliary excretion,** a drug is excreted in the bile. These drugs enter the duodenum and exit the body in the feces. Some bile substances are reabsorbed and returned to the liver via enterohepatic recirculation, which saves and reuses beneficial substances. Drugs and their metabolites may recirculate multiple times in the bile. This extends their half-lives and can prolong their

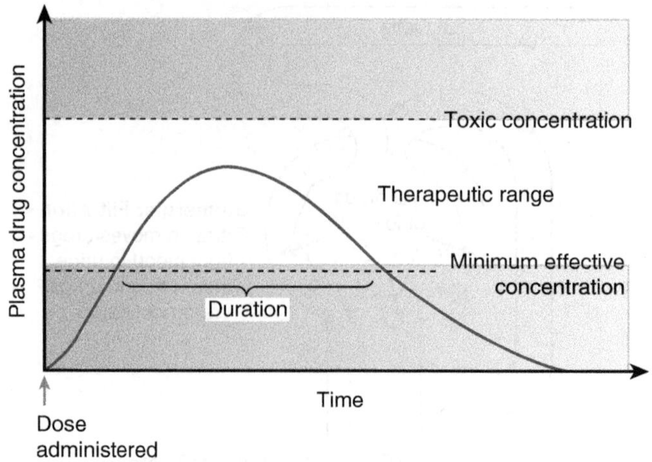

FIG. 3.12 Single-dose time course.

action. This type of excretion occurs with barbiturates, *tamoxifen*, *carbamazepine*, oral contraceptives, and *rifampin*. The liver later metabolizes recirculated drugs, which the kidneys can excrete. Recirculation and elimination via biliary excretion may continue for weeks after stopping drug therapy.

Time-response relationships

The therapeutic response of most drugs is based on their plasma concentrations. Therefore plasma drug concentrations for drugs with a low safety margin are monitored to predict drug action or toxicity. **Therapeutic drug monitoring** helps keep doses in a predetermined range. Individual responses to drugs are highly varied. Patients may have no toxic effects, which can occur even if the serum concentration remains in the normal range. To understand, imagine that a plasma drug concentration slowly increases and 2 hours pass before the **minimum effective concentration** is reached, which is needed to produce a therapeutic effect. The drug is at a therapeutic range where the desired therapeutic action is made. After peaking, the drug plasma concentration falls slowly out of the therapeutic range because of excretive processes (see Fig. 3.12). A higher dose could have caused the drug plasma concentration to be toxic, causing severe adverse effects. Pharmacotherapy attempts to reach and maintain levels within the therapeutic range while avoiding the toxic concentration. For some drugs, the therapeutic range is extensive, but for others, it is very narrow. The difference between a minimum effective dose and a toxic dose can be dangerously slight.

Half-life

A drug's duration of action is often described by its plasma half-life, abbreviated as $t_{1/2}$. It is the time needed for the plasma concentration to decrease the drug amount by one-half after administration. A **half-life** may be only a few minutes or as long as several hours or days. In rare cases such as *amiodarone*, the half-life is 40 to 55 days. Drugs with short half-lives are perfect if a condition or procedure lasts briefly, such as a dental procedure. If a drug with a long duration of action is given, there could be long-lasting adverse effects after the process is complete. Short-acting drugs are quickly excreted, reducing the risks of long-term adverse effects. Fig. 3.13 shows scales that assess the elimination of half-lives of two different formulations of the drug *topiramate*. In the figure, TPM-IR is the immediate-release formulation of the drug, and USL255 is the extended-release formulation.

Long-duration drugs are suitable for chronic conditions such as hypertension or heart failure and to prevent diseases such as seizures or migraine headaches. It is essential to understand that the longer a drug stays in the body, the higher the risk for long-term adverse effects. Patients with extreme renal or hepatic impairment must be carefully evaluated so that a drug does not remain in the body for too long, and doses may need to be adjusted. Generally, about four half-lives must pass when a drug is stopped before the drug is functionally eliminated. About 94% of the drug is eliminated after four half-lives. However, this rule does not apply to all medicines or medications for renal or hepatic impairment patients.

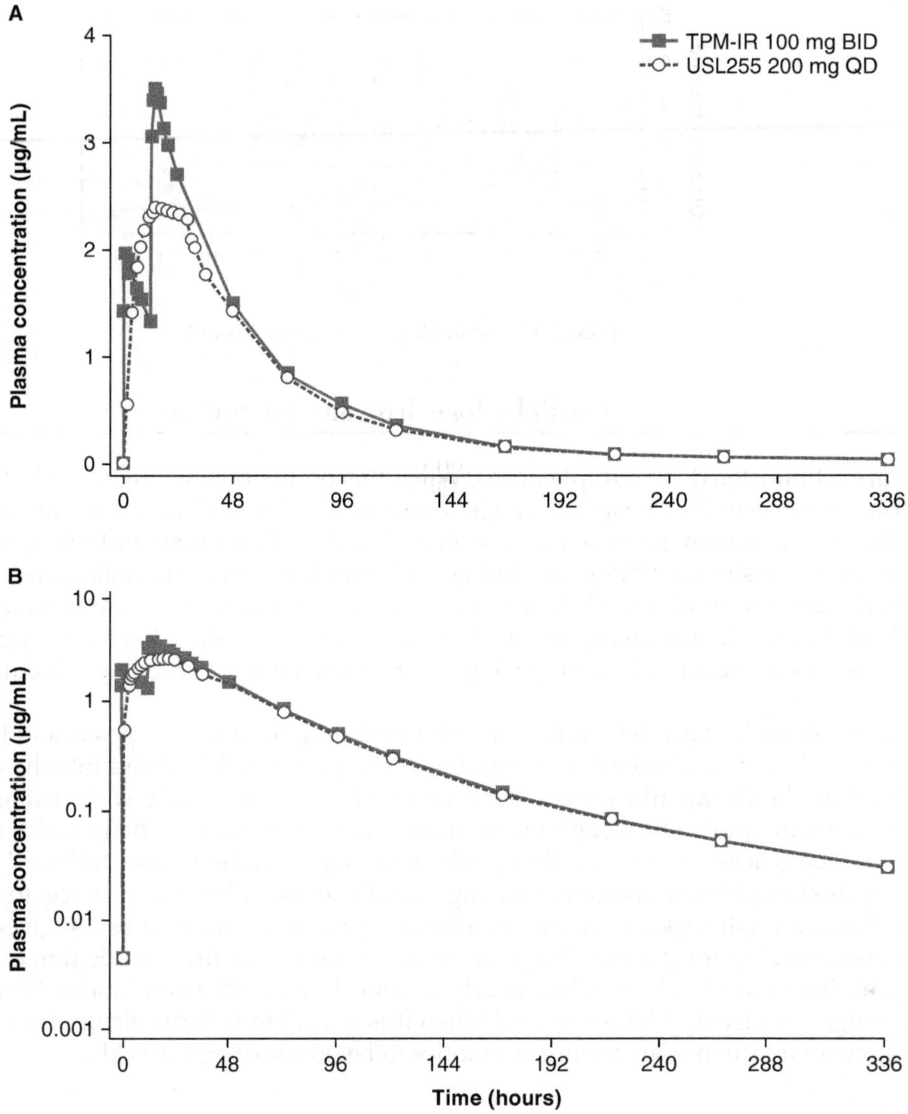

		48 h	72 h	168 h	264 h	336 h
$t_{1/2z_1}$	USL255 200 mg QD	35.6 (16.9)	31.3 (7.2)	40.4 (9.2)	58.8 (15.9)	80.2 (14.2)
mean (SD)	TPM-IR 100 mg BID	28.8 (7.0)	28.4 (5.6)	34.4 (5.1)	61.5 (16.5)	82.8 (14.4)

FIG. 3.13 The elimination half-lives of immediate-release topiramate *(TPM-IR)* and extended-release topiramate *(USL255)*, with (A) showing the linear scale and (B) showing the logarithmic scale. The linear scale has consistent measurements between points, and the logarithmic scale has progress measurements between points.

You should remember

While each drug has its elimination half-life, they all follow the same rule. After one half-life, 50% of the initial drug amount is removed from the body. Most clinically essential drugs follow first-order pharmacokinetics—their drug elimination rates are proportional to plasma concentrations.

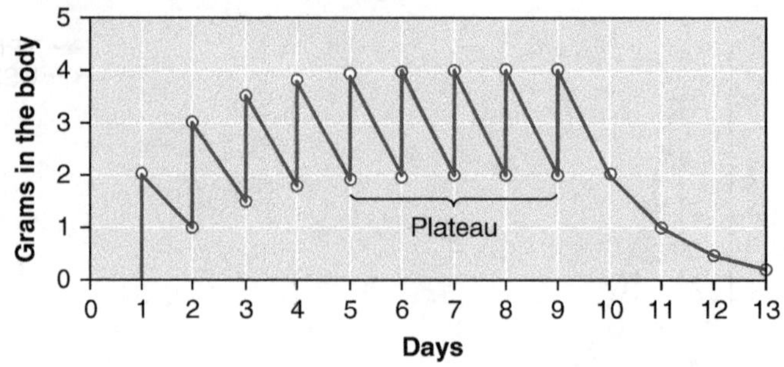

FIG. 3.14 Multiple-dose drug administration.

Multiple-dose drug administration

Most drugs are administered in multiple doses. When this occurs over a long period, the goal is to maintain the drug plasma concentration in the therapeutic range continuously. The next dose is administered before drug concentrations fall below the minimum effective concentration. Fig. 3.14 shows how multiple quantities result in the drug accumulating in the bloodstream. With good timing, a plateau is reached and maintained in the therapeutic range. At the plateau, the amount of absorbed drug equals the amount excreted. There is a steady therapeutic amount distributed to body tissues. It takes about four half-lives to reach this state. When a medication is given as a continuous infusion, the plateau can be achieved quickly and maintained with little or no fluctuation in the drug plasma concentration.

Plasma drug concentrations are sometimes smooth or continuous and have peaks and troughs. With oral drugs, there are fluctuations in peak and trough concentrations. The peak should not rise into the toxic range, and the track should not fall below the therapeutic range. The drug will be released slowly with sustained- or extended-release formulations, minimizing peak and trough fluctuations. An altered dosing schedule also reduces changes.

The plateau can be reached more quickly by administering a loading dose, followed by regular maintenance doses. A **loading dose** is a higher amount of a drug, usually given only once or twice, to "ready" the bloodstream with sufficient drugs for a therapeutic response. Intermittent maintenance doses are given before drug concentrations return to zero, keeping the plasma drug concentration within the therapeutic range. Though there are fluctuations, the equilibrium state can be reached nearly as quickly as with a continuous infusion. Loading doses are significant for drugs with lengthy half-lives and when it is critical to increase drug plasma concentrations rapidly. For example, a severe infection may require antibiotics to be administered quickly.

Key Terms

Active transport
Affinity
Biliary excretion
Bioavailability
Biotransformation
Blood-brain barrier
Buccal route
Clearance
Enteral route
Excretion
Extended release
Facilitated diffusion
Fetal-placental barrier
First-order kinetics
First-pass elimination
First-pass metabolism
Gastrostomy
Half-life
Hepatic portal circulation
Induction
Ion trapping
Isoforms

Isozymes
Loading dose
Maintenance doses
Microsomal enzyme system
Minimum effective concentration
Parenteral route
Passive diffusion
pH
Pharmacokinetics
Plasma albumin
Saturation kinetics
Slit junctions
Sublingual route
Therapeutic drug monitoring
Therapeutic range
Topical route
Transdermal patches
Volatile liquid
Zero-order kinetics

Clinical Case Studies

Clinical Case Study 1

A 44-year-old female is evaluated because of strep throat. She is currently taking celecoxib for arthritis and nizatidine for heartburn. The decision is made to start the patient on oral cefuroxime for 10 days, but after 5 days, the patient calls her physician to tell him that the sore throat is just as bad as it has been. The physician evaluates the cefuroxime, which requires a lower stomach pH to be adequately absorbed. In this case, nizatidine has probably caused the stomach pH to increase, impairing the absorption of cefuroxime. There is evidence that acid-suppressing drugs can lower the bioavailability of cefuroxime by as much as 60%. Because the patient needed nizatidine for her heartburn, it would have been better to prescribe a macrolide antibiotic or a cephalosporin such as cephalexin because these drugs do not require lower stomach pH to be effective.

Critical Thinking Questions

1. Because strong stomach acids destroy some enteral medications, what form of drugs can be used?
2. How do extended-release tablets or capsules work?
3. What are other enteral methods of administering medications?

Clinical Case Study 2

A 71-year-old male was hospitalized because of his altered mental status, confusion, and visual hallucinations. He had a 10-year history of type 2 diabetes, symptomatic peripheral vascular insufficiency, and chronic kidney disease because of diabetic nephropathy. He was required to have hemodialysis three times per week. His medications included aspirin, atorvastatin, insulin, gabapentin, and vancomycin. The patient underwent dialysis while in the hospital, and his symptoms improved, though they recurred between dialysis sessions. It was determined that because gabapentin is excreted, the patient's reduced kidney capacity had elevated gabapentin, triggering his neurologic symptoms.

Critical Thinking Questions

1. Where does most drug excretion occur, and what factors affect clearance?
2. What factors are involved in the regular elimination of a drug by the kidneys?
3. How much clearance is reduced in humans by the age of 80?

Further Reading

[1] American Society of Health-System Pharmacists, Clinical Pharmacokinetics, sixth ed., American Society of Health-System Pharmacists, 2017.
[2] S. Baxter, Medicine, Metaphors, and Metaphysics: An Interdisciplinary Analysis and Critique of Therapeutic Equivalence as a Health Policy, Scholars' Press, 2014.
[3] S.C. Chow, J.P. Liu, Design and Analysis of Bioavailability and Bioequivalence Studies (Chapman & Hall/CRC Biostatistics Series Book 27), third ed., Chapman and Hall/CRC Press, 2008.
[4] M.D. Coleman, Human Drug Metabolism, third ed., Wiley-Blackwell, 2020.
[5] J.W. Fisher, J.M. Gearhart, Z. Lin, Physiologically Based Pharmacokinetic (PBPK) Modeling: Methods and Applications in Toxicology and Risk Assessment, Academic Press, 2020.

[6] S. Ma, S. Chowdhury, Identification and Quantification of Drugs, Metabolites, Drug Metabolizing Enzymes, and Transporters: Concepts, Methods, and Translational Sciences, second ed., Elsevier Science, 2020.
[7] S.A. Peters, Physiologically-Based Pharmacokinetic (PBPK) Modeling and Simulations: Principles, Methods, and Applications in the Pharmaceutical Industry, Wiley, 2012.
[8] S.E. Rosenbaum, Basic Pharmacokinetics and Pharmacodynamics: An Integrated Textbook and Computer Simulations, second ed., Wiley, 2016.
[9] M. Rowland, T.N. Tozer, Clinical Pharmacokinetics and Pharmacodynamics: Concepts and Applications, fourth ed., Lippincott, Williams, & Wilkins, 2010.
[10] M.A. Rudek, C.H. Chau, W.D. Figg, H.L. McLeod, Handbook of Anticancer Pharmacokinetics and Pharmacodynamics: Cancer Drug Discovery and Development, second ed., Humana Press, 2016.
[11] L. Shargel, A. Yu, Applied Biopharmaceutics & Pharmacokinetics, seventh ed., McGraw-Hill Education/Medical, 2015.
[12] D.A. Smith, D. Fox, Metabolism, Pharmacokinetics and Toxicity of Functional Groups: Impact of Chemical Building Blocks on ADMET (Drug Discovery, Volume 1), Royal Society of Chemistry, 2010.
[13] R. Southwood, V.H. Fleming, Huckaby, Concepts in Clinical Pharmacokinetics, seventh ed., American Society of Health Systems, 2018.
[14] T.N. Tozer, M. Rowland, Essentials of Pharmacokinetics and Pharmacodynamics, second ed., Lippincott, Williams, & Wilkins, 2015.
[15] J.G. Wagner, Pharmacokinetics for the Pharmaceutical Scientist, CRC Press, 2019.
[16] B. Wu, D. Lu, D. Dong, Circadian Pharmacokinetics, Springer, 2020.

CHAPTER

4

Pharmacogenomics and drug toxicity

OUTLINE

LEARNING OUTCOMES

After study of the chapter, readers should be able to:

1. Describe pharmacogenomics and genome variations.
2. Explain idiosyncratic drug reactions.
3. Identify factors determining drug toxicity.
4. Explain adverse drug reactions.
5. Discuss teratogens and some examples.
6. Describe drug-drug interactions.
7. Explain anaphylactic shock and its treatment.
8. Discuss hepatotoxic drugs and list 10 medications that may damage the liver.
9. Explain how certain medicines may cause ototoxicity.
10. List some examples of antidotes.

Overview

Pharmacogenomics is the study of genetic variations that affect individual responses to drugs. Some drug therapies can be individualized if a genetic variation that affects drug disposition is known. This may improve the drug efficacy and reduce adverse effects. Pharmacogenomics merges biochemistry and other traditional pharmaceutical sciences with knowledge about common human genome DNA variations. Drug toxicity involves the accumulation

https://doi.org/10.1016/B978-0-443-29038-1.00004-X

of an excessive amount of any medication in the bloodstream. The medication's effects are more intense at toxic levels, and adverse effects may be severe or lethal. Drug toxicity can occur when a dose is too high or when drug clearance via the liver or kidneys is insufficient to remove the drug from the bloodstream.

Pharmacogenomics

Pharmacogenomics is the study of genetic factors that influence variations in drug responses. Pharmacogenomics emerged as severe adverse reactions were documented in patients who had drug-metabolizing enzymes with *genomic* variations. A **genome** contains all of the hereditary information belonging to an individual organism. After human genome sequencing was completed in 2003, this field has overgrown. Changes in genomes are considered **polymorphisms**, and these occur in genes that encode cytokines, human leukocyte antigen loci, and transporter proteins, among other gene products.

Polymorphisms help to predict variations in therapeutic and adverse drug responses, and more than 335 million different single-nucleotide polymorphisms exist in humans across many populations. Polymorphisms are linked to individual reactions to a drug. Susceptibility to certain diseases is also related to common single-nucleotide DNA variations. As a result, pharmacogenomics is currently focused on genes that encode metabolic enzymes to alter drug activity and defects in structural proteins that increase disease susceptibility. Fig. 4.1 shows different patient responses to certain medications.

Genomic medicine, also called *tailored or personalized medicine*, has evolved using genetic information to choose medications and doses for individual patients. Guidelines from the Clinical Pharmacogenetics Implementation Consortium (CPIC) have resulted in drugs being prescribed more effectively. Genomic medicine can also drive new therapeutics. For instance, *genome replication* about viruses requires specific triphosphates: *ribonucleoside triphosphates* for RNA viruses or *deoxyribonucleoside triphosphates* for DNA viruses.

A viral or cellular polymerase incorporates triphosphates into new viral genomes. This understanding has allowed scientists to develop new antivirals that are safer and more effective than ever before. This is explained by the differences between viral kinases and polymerases, which are unique compared to the kinases and polymerases of normal body cells. Therefore genomic medicine has allowed the development of drugs targeting two different steps in the viral replication pathway.

You should remember

Pharmacogenomics allows for individualized drug therapy based on genetic variations related to drug effects and adverse effects. Advances include more powerful medicines, more efficacious, safer drugs, and more accurate drug doses.

Drug toxicity

Drug toxicity can occur if a drug's concentration exceeds a therapeutic range. This may occur secondary to an unintentional or intentional overdose or because of drug accumulation. *Toxicity* is the state of being noxious or is described as a drug's ability to poison the body. Examples include severe hypoglycemia and death due to an overdose of insulin, excessive sedation to coma, or death from an overdose of morphine. Toxic, well-documented events are referred to as poisonous effects or side effects. They are peripheral or secondary effects beyond the therapeutic effect. Some side effects develop quickly after drug use begins, while others do not appear until the drug has been taken for weeks or more. Side effects are usually predictable, and their intensity is based on dosage amount. Adverse events are typically unpredictable and genetically determined.

Factors determining drug toxicity include patient age, preexisting conditions, genetics, and the drug dosage and drugs being used concurrently. Young or old patients are often more susceptible to toxicities due to immature or altered pharmacokinetics or drug-metabolizing enzymes. Disease states that influence drug toxicity include kidney or liver disease and allergies. Drug-drug, drug-supplement, and drug-food interactions can contribute to toxicity as well. The top 15 drugs or drug classifications that are involved in toxicity include acetaminophen, alcohol,

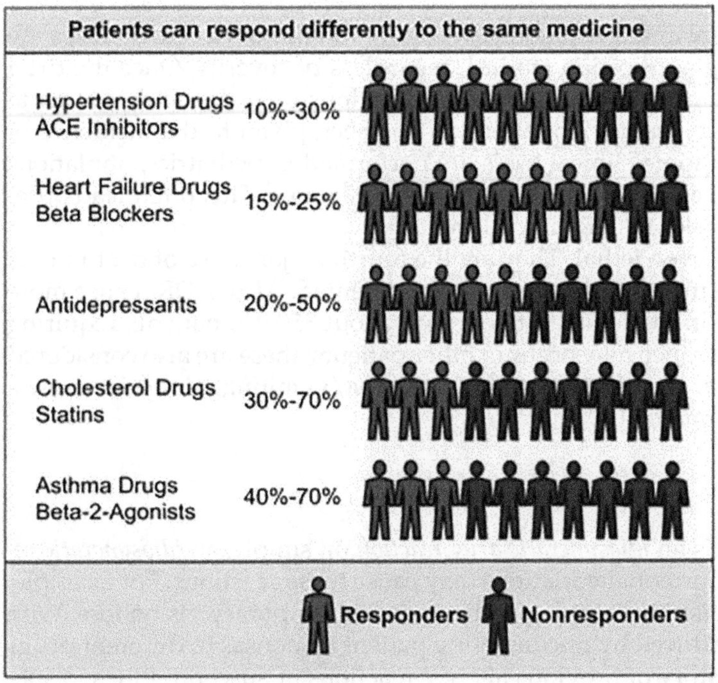

FIG. 4.1 Variable responses to drugs. *From Pharmacogenomics Laboratory, Indiana University School of Medicine. [2016]. Pharmacogenetics Brochure.* Ignite. *Https://gmkb.org/?utm_source-ignite-genomics.org&utm_medium-referral.*

benzodiazepines, anticoagulants, antidepressants, antihypertensives, bromocriptine (an anti-Parkinson medication), clarithromycin (an antibiotic), clozapine (an antipsychotic), cocaine, colchicine (an antiinflammatory), cough medicines, digoxin, heroin, and semisynthetic opioids.

Toxicity occurs when cellular defenses become overwhelmed. Repeated damage can harm the function of affected organs over time. Two outcomes may occur based on the severity of the injury. **Apoptosis** is programmed cell death. It allows cells to self-destruct via the activation of specific proteins. This is helpful when the process kills damaged cells but does not harm nearby tissue. In cancer cells, apoptosis is often inhibited. The second outcome is **necrosis**, the death of cells and tissues. This usually occurs in a localized area, where apoptosis cannot happen because toxicity is exceedingly severe. Enzymes digest the contents of the cells. Proteins experience changes in their structure, and membranes are disrupted. Necrotic cells may damage normal cells when they attract inflammatory cells. This occurs as apoptosis progresses, with only slight inflammation and disruption of adjacent tissues. **Antidotes** may exist for some drug toxicities, but discontinuing the offending drug is often the best approach.

Adverse effects

The **adverse effects** are unique from a side effect and may be genetically determined and largely unanticipated. When a negative impact occurs due to drug binding at the intended receptor but the result is altered, this is referred to as an "on target" adverse effect or event. Factors affecting drug binding include incorrect doses, pharmacokinetic changes, or administration into the wrong tissues. These factors are also known as *drug class effects*. When a drug binding to a false target or receptor causes an adverse effect, it is "off target." The immune system may also mediate adverse effects.

Sometimes, from medication errors, poor judgment, or attempted suicide, a patient may have a drug overdose. Any drug can theoretically be overdosed depending on the drug's *margin of safety* or *therapeutic window*. This refers to the difference between effective and toxic drugs. Margins of protection apply to all drugs, prescribed or OTC. Factors related to the margin of safety include gene characteristics, polymorphisms, enzymes, **comorbidities**, and reduced organ function. Comorbidities are disorders or diseases present in addition to a primary condition or illness. They can also be effects that are caused by additional disorders or diseases. An overdose often occurs with drugs with large margins of safety, while adverse effects can occur from therapeutic doses or when the margin of safety is small or nonexistent.

Adverse drug reactions

Adverse drug reactions (ADRs) are unexpected and unplanned reactions to drugs, even though average doses are used. All adverse events are reported during new drug application studies, regardless of severity. Once the drug reaches the market, all adverse events must still be reported. The FDA requires serious or unexpected events to be reported within 15 days of occurrence. Unfortunately, insufficient attention has been given to the incidence of ADRs in children of all ages. This may be because only some clinical trials are performed in pediatric populations due to myriad issues that include ethics, responsibility, cost, and drug approval regulations. This often leads prescribers to estimate doses and dosages, increasing the risk of ADRs in children.

ADRs can occur at any age and be minor, severe, and even lethal. They are the fourth major cause of death in the United States, especially among elderly patients, so they must be reported and documented. Also, ADRs cause more than 1.3 million emergency department visits annually in the United States, with about 350,000 patients requiring hospitalization for further treatment. Allergies and intolerance may occur in other patients; these are also considered reportable ADRs. The most common ADRs are diarrhea, constipation, fatigue, nausea/vomiting, **alopecia**, drowsiness, myelosuppression, skin reactions, **anorexia**, and **mucositis**.

Idiosyncratic drug reactions

A unique, strange, or unpredicted reaction to a drug is an *idiosyncratic drug reaction* or, simply, an *idiosyncratic reaction*. Underlying enzyme deficiencies from genetic or hormonal variations may cause these reactions. For example, carisoprodol may cause personal reactions such as transient quadriplegia, dizziness, or temporary vision loss. With continuing study, idiosyncratic drug reactions may be reduced by documenting patient responses to different drugs related to genetic and other mechanisms of action. A history of previous allergic reactions or susceptibilities to specific medications, vaccines, serum, or blood transfusions must be obtained from patients before treatment. This can prevent or help prepare for serious idiosyncratic drug reaction hazards. Patients predisposed to allergic reactions should wear an alert bracelet or necklace.

Teratogenic effects

A **teratogen** is any substance, agent, or process that interferes with normal prenatal development, causing the formation of one or more developmental abnormalities in the fetus. Examples of teratogens include alcohol, cigarette smoke, medications (thalidomide, some antibiotics, and antidepressants), illegal drugs (cocaine and heroin), certain vaccines, some viral infections (the rubella virus and cytomegalovirus), X-ray radiation, and environmental factors. A *teratogenic effect* is a drug-induced congenital disability such as enlargement of specific organs (such as the liver or spleen), congenital absence of any part of a limb, abnormal limb size, abnormal smallness of the eyes, and blindness. There are many causes of congenital malformations. They include genetic, environmental, and combinations of both. Genetic factors include chromosomal abnormalities and single-gene defects. Ecological factors include maternal metabolic disorders, chemicals, intrauterine infections, ionizing radiation, drugs, and medications.

You should remember

Regarding teratogens, major brain malformations are more common in early embryos than in newborns. The most severely affected embryos are spontaneously aborted during the first 6–8 weeks of gestation. During organogenesis (between days 15 to 60), teratogenic agents are more likely to cause severe congenital malformations.

Carcinogenic effects

A drug's *carcinogenic effect* is its ability to cause cancer. While only a few therapeutic agents can cause cancer, some include agents used to treat cancer. It is difficult to determine a substance's carcinogenic effects because cancer may not appear until 20 or more years after initial exposure to the substance. As a result, preclinical and clinical trials usually do not illuminate carcinogenic effects. Therefore new drugs are often released to the public without fully understanding their potential cancer-causing effects. An example of such delayed toxicity is *diethylstilbestrol*, a synthetic hormone with estrogen-like effects. The drug was previously used to prevent spontaneous abortion for women with high-risk pregnancies. Later, it was discovered that female fetuses exposed to the drug *in utero* developed vaginal and uterine cancers later in life.

Drug-drug interactions

Drug-drug interactions have become more common because of growing populations, longer lifespans, and polypharmacy. These interactions may have pharmacokinetic as well as pharmacodynamic implications. A pharmacokinetic drug-drug interaction occurs when a drug affects another drug's absorption, distribution, metabolism, or excretion. These interactions can change concentrations of either active drug in the body. If the same P450 enzyme metabolizes two medicines, there may be competitive or irreversible inhibition of the enzyme, affecting drug concentrations. Also, drug metabolism may be induced, causing toxicities or faster clearance and fewer therapeutic effects.

Next, particular drugs may affect the transport of other drugs in and out of body tissues. Pharmacokinetic interactions may be desired, such as when one drug is given with another to increase efficacy or therapeutic outcomes. Also, some medications can displace others by utilizing the same proteins, increasing the bioavailability of the other drug to body tissues. Examples of drug-drug interactions include clozapine, erythromycin, and some antifungal interactions with oral contraceptives.

Drug-drug interactions also occur when a drug changes how tissues respond, or do not respond, to another drug. These interactions can be toxic when the two drugs activate *complementary pathways*, increasing the effects of both drugs. Significant examples are *nitroglycerin,* used for angina pectoris, and *sildenafil*, a phosphodiesterase inhibitor for erectile dysfunction.

Drugs can also interact with herbs, herbal supplements, foods, and beverages. This occurs because many supplements contain biologically active compounds that have yet to be thoroughly studied or may be significantly toxic. Therefore physicians must always ask patients about all nondrug substances they consume when prescribing medications that could interact. An example of a supplement that interacts with NSAIDs is *ginkgo biloba*. Because both substances inhibit platelet aggregation, simultaneous use may increase the risk of bleeding.

You should remember

All patients must be questioned about any history of allergies, such as hay fever, rashes, or asthma, or if they have had unusual reactions to drugs taken orally or by injection.

Allergic drug reactions

Drugs also cause allergic and autoimmune reactions. Allergic or hypersensitivity reactions require the host's presensitized (immune) state. Such reactions may be uncomfortable and treatable or sudden and fatal. Autoimmune reactions arise from abnormal immune responses against substances and tissues usually present in the body. These drug responses are not simply intolerant to a drug. Thus practitioners must determine whether the patient is experiencing an actual allergic reaction or drug intolerance. For example, the administration of penicillin by injection may result in a severe allergic reaction that can be life-threatening. However, when a patient takes penicillin orally, an allergy may cause nausea and vomiting. The four types of allergic reactions include:

Type I hypersensitivity is described as immediate hypersensitivity or **anaphylaxis** resulting from IgE production after exposure to an antigen. This may be a foreign or endogenous protein modified by a **hapten**, which becomes immunogenic. For example, when fragments of penicillin act as haptens, they activate the immune system. Recurrent exposure to the antigen causes degranulation of **mast cells** and then the release of histamine, leukotrienes, or other inflammatory mediators. Type I reactions develop in the skin as *wheal-and-flare reactions.*

Anaphylactic shock is a life-threatening emergency that develops from anaphylaxis. The blood pressure drops suddenly, and the airways narrow, resulting in wheezing or difficulty breathing. Signs and symptoms include tachycardia, hives, flushed skin, pallor, a sensation of warmth, swollen tongue or lips, difficulty swallowing, nausea, vomiting, and abdominal pain. Treatment must begin immediately. To treat such an outcome, epinephrine is injected intradermally. Glucocorticoids and antihistamines are then injected intravenously, and oxygen is administered.

Type II hypersensitivity: antibody-dependent cytotoxic hypersensitivity responses resulting from a drug that binds to red blood cells, which IgG or other antibodies recognize. Cell lysis is triggered via **complement fixation**, cytolysis by cytotoxic T cells, or phagocytosis by macrophages.

Type III hypersensitivity: immune complex-mediated responses that require the formation of antibodies (usually IgG or IgM) against soluble antigens. Complexes of antigens and antibodies are deposited in tissues, mainly the joints, kidneys, and lung vascular endothelium. Damage is caused by *serum sickness* involving inflammation because of the activation of complement and leukocytes inside the tissues. Examples of agents that cause type III hypersensitivity include bupropion, cefaclor, and antivenins.

Type IV hypersensitivity: delayed-type hypersensitivity responses caused by activation of cytotoxic T cells and T helper cells. As a hapten binds to host proteins, contact dermatitis is common. This often occurs after subsequent exposures, not the first exposure to a causative agent. Langerhans cells are activated and migrate to nearby lymph nodes. T cells are activated and return to the skin, causing an immune response. Relatively common examples of type IV responses include reactions to latex and poison ivy. Severe allergies may arise when the exposure to a foreign agent is repeated. Such a painful outcome may be a **cytokine storm**, which may cause fever, hypotension, and organ failure.

When the immune system attacks its cells, *autoimmunity* develops. Drugs that can trigger autoimmunity include the antihypertensives *hydralazine* and *methyldopa*, isoniazid, and the antiarrhythmic *procainamide*. **Red man syndrome** is a rare condition caused by amphotericin B, ciprofloxacin, rifampin, teicoplanin, and vancomycin. The syndrome involves degranulation of mast cells, which occurs independently of preformed complement or IgE. Usually, wheals and **urticaria** develop on the neck, arms, and upper trunk (see Fig. 4.2). The syndrome usually resolves after the drug's infusion rate is reduced or discontinued.

Other drug-related reactions include skin rashes, known as **erythema multiforme**. Drugs such as antiepileptics, barbiturates, NSAIDs, and sulfonamides have caused severe skin rashes such as *Stevens-Johnson syndrome* and the more powerful and potentially fatal toxic *epidermal necrolysis*. Indeed, many drugs have been linked to Stevens-Johnson syndrome. Injury to the immune system is called *immunotoxicity* and may be related to drug therapy or an intended outcome of specific drug therapies. An example of the latter situation would be the use of cytotoxic agents to kill specific neoplastic cells. Immune system targeting is needed when normal immune responses worsen a disease. However, this therapy is rigidly controlled due to the possibility of other negative results, including dangerous infections.

You should remember

Anaphylaxis is a severe allergic reaction that is rapid in its onset and may be fatal. It is fatal in about 0.7% to 2% of cases. The peak severity of anaphylaxis is usually within 5 to 30 minutes, but in rare cases, it can last several days. It is an immediate medical emergency, and recovery is based on how quickly medical treatment is given to the patient.

Drug toxicity of specific organs

Drugs are primarily toxic to specific organs but not every organ system. The most critical toxicities occur in the liver, nervous system, kidneys, heart, and skeletal muscles. These toxicities are discussed below.

Nephrotoxicity

The kidneys are affected by many medications because they receive approximately 25% of all cardiac output and metabolize many drugs excreted in the urine. The kidneys also reabsorb or secrete some drugs, meaning the renal tubule cells are exposed to significant concentrations. A few medications obstruct the urinary system by causing

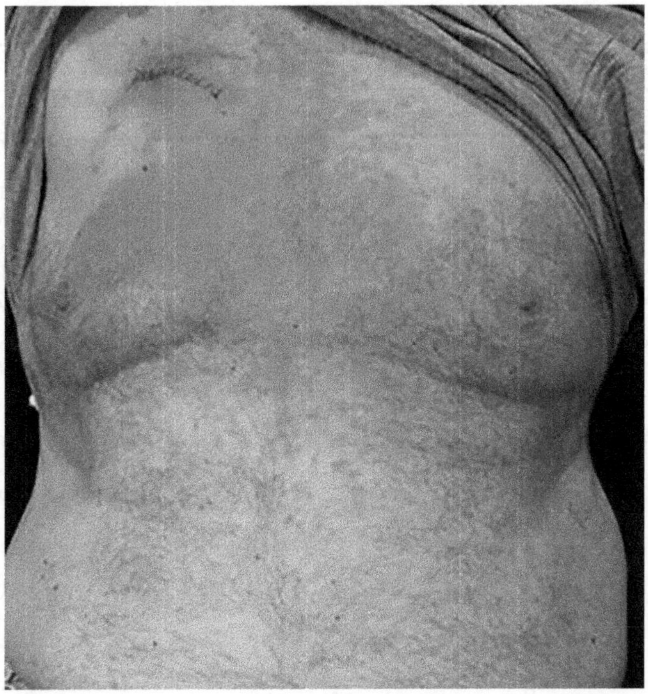

FIG. 4.2 Red man syndrome.

crystalluria to occur in the urinary tract. Nephrotoxic drugs can cause acute symptoms after one or more doses or can cause chronic effects, appearing after several months. Healthcare providers must identify any patient who is at risk for **nephrotoxicity**. Prevention of nephrotoxicity involves monitoring urinary lab values, proper hydration, and dosage adjustments for patients with impaired kidney function. If there is severe kidney impairment, the patient should not receive nephrotoxic drugs unless other therapies have failed.

Hepatotoxicity

Hepatotoxic drugs destroy the liver. These drugs are the leading cause of acute liver failure, which can be quickly fatal. Most medicines withdrawn from the United States drug market have hepatotoxic effects. More than 100 drugs are known to be hepatotoxic, examples of which are listed in Table 4.1. Because the liver is the leading site of drug metabolism, many drugs are biotransformed into toxic products that harm liver cells. Combinations of hepatotoxic medications with other substances, such as alcohol, can cause severe liver injury.

A prime example is the regular combination of acetaminophen with alcohol. Chronic drinkers can have liver toxicity with therapeutic doses of acetaminophen, so a black box warning was placed on OTC packages several decades ago. Specifically, toxic *N-acetyl-p-benzoquinone imine* is abundant and outpaces the liver's detoxification ability, causing centrilobular hepatic necrosis. Once the liver is severely damaged, death from fulminant liver failure can result within only several days after an acetaminophen overdose.

Any patient taking a hepatotoxic drug should undergo liver function tests, which assess the enzymes **aspartate aminotransferase** and **alanine aminotransferase**. Although these enzymes are released from the heart when damaged, they may point to liver damage when considered along with bilirubin, albumin, and alkaline phosphatase. Life-threatening liver damage can develop very quickly, so early detection of elevations in these enzymes is essential. Patients must be informed about the signs of liver damage, including **jaundice**, light-colored stools, dark urine, nausea, vomiting, abdominal discomfort, malaise, and loss of appetite.

Neurotoxicity

Even with the protective effect of the blood-brain barrier, some classifications of drugs regularly cause **neurotoxicity** because the brain receives an ample blood supply and is very sensitive to only small amounts of toxicants. Differences between therapeutic doses and those that produce adverse effects can be minimal, especially for

TABLE 4.1 Drugs that are toxic to the liver.

Drug classification	Examples
Statins and other lipid-lowering drugs	atorvastatin (Lipitor) fenofibrate (Tricor) fluvastatin (Lescol) gemfibrozil (Lopid) lovastatin (Mevacor) niacin (Niaspan) pravastatin (Pravachol) simvastatin (Zocor)
Oral antidiabetic drugs	acarbose (Precose) pioglitazone (Actos) rosiglitazone (Avandia)
Antiseizure drugs	carbamazepine (Tegretol) divalproex sodium (Depakote) felbamate (Felbatol)
Antifungal drugs	itraconazole (Sporanox) ketoconazole (Nizoral) terbinafine (Lamisil)
Antituberculosis drugs	isoniazid (generic) pyrazinamide (generic) rifampin (Rifadin)
Immunosuppressants	azathioprine (Imuran) methotrexate (Rheumatrex)
Antiretroviral drugs	nevirapine (Viramune) ritonavir (Norvir)
Miscellaneous drugs	acetaminophen (Tylenol) (when taken with alcohol) amiodarone (Cordarone) diclofenac (Voltaren) duloxetine (Cymbalta) leflunomide (Arava) methyldopa (Aldomet) nefazodone (Serzone) nitrofurantoin (Macrodantin) tamoxifen (Nolvadex) zileuton (Zyflo)

antidepressants, sedatives, anticonvulsants, antipsychotics, and antianxiety drugs. Most patients taking these medications experience drowsiness at the beginning of therapy. Signs and symptoms of CNS toxicity include depression, behavioral changes, sedation, hallucinations, suicidal thoughts, and seizures. In addition, there can be hearing impairment, visual changes, and loss of balance.

Patient education is essential when any drug is started that has neurotoxic potential. Until the patient becomes familiar with the drug's effects, they must avoid driving vehicles or doing anything hazardous. Family members or caregivers should monitor the patient for behavioral changes because they may not be aware of them. Neurotoxic drugs can make any preexisting mental health disorder much worse. Any healthcare practitioner who prescribes a neurotoxic medication should be alerted if a patient has severe symptoms. These include delirium, significant hearing or visual impairment, suicidal thoughts, or seizures.

Ototoxicity

Ototoxicity can occur because of damage to the eighth cranial nerve. Ototoxic medications known to cause permanent damage include certain aminoglycoside antibiotics such as gentamicin, tobramycin, streptomycin, neomycin, kanamycin, and vancomycin. Chemotherapeutic medicines, particularly those containing platinum (cisplatin and carboplatin), can cause **tinnitus** and hearing loss. Hearing loss can be profound and permanent, occurring immediately after the first dose, or it can be delayed until several months after the completion of treatment. Salicylates in high doses (more than 325-mg tablets of aspirin a day) cause temporary hearing loss and tinnitus. Ethacrynic acid and furosemide given IV have caused profound, permanent hearing loss in patients with renal failure receiving aminoglycoside antibiotics.

Cardiotoxicity

A few medications damage cardiac muscle cells and affect the heart. These include cardiac glycosides such as digoxin and digitalis and the anthracyclines, which are used to treat cancer. Digoxin (and less so, digitalis) is used clinically for heart failure due to systolic dysfunction and for certain supraventricular tachyarrhythmias. Digoxin has a narrow therapeutic window or margin, with the therapeutic range being 0.5–2 ng/mL and the toxic content being 2.5 ng/mL or more. Examples of anthracyclines include *daunorubicin (Cerubidine), doxorubicin (Adriamycin), epirubicin (Ellence), idarubicin (Adriamycin),* and *mitoxantrone (Novantrone)*. Their cardiotoxicity can be severe, causing dysrhythmia and heart failure.

Skeletal muscle toxicity

Even though the skeletal muscles have a large blood supply, they are primarily resistant to drug effects. The incidence of drug-induced **myopathy** is severe but rare, with the most extreme example being **rhabdomyolysis** (see Fig. 4.3). *Statins*, used to reduce hyperlipidemia, may cause rhabdomyolysis. Also, some fluoroquinolone antibiotics cause damage to cartilage and tendons, mostly in adults older than 65 years of age, and they most often rupture the **Achilles tendon**. These medications can also interfere with cartilage growth, so they should not be taken by patients younger than 18. During therapy with toxic drugs to the musculoskeletal system, unexplained muscle or joint pain or soreness must be assessed. Laboratory tests such as creatinine kinase are regularly done during treatment.

Antidotes

Antidotes are drugs or substances that oppose the actions of specific poisons. There are mechanical, chemical, or physiologic antidotes. A mechanical antidote is *activated charcoal*, which absorbs poisons in the GI tract and prevents

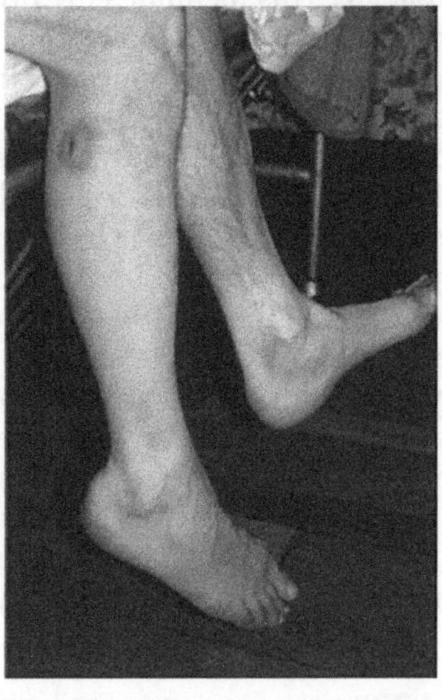

FIG. 4.3 Rhabdomyolysis of the leg.

TABLE 4.2 Poisons and their specific antidotes.

Poison	Name of antidote	Classification of antidote
Acetaminophen	*N*-Acetylcysteine	Mucolytic agent
Benzodiazepines	Flumazenil	Benzodiazepine antagonist
Carbon monoxide	Oxygen	Nonmetallic element
Cyanide	Amyl nitrate	Nitrate inhalant
Iron	Deferoxamine	Heavy metal antagonist
Methanol	Ethanol	Organic chemical
Opiates	Naloxone	Opioid antagonist
Organophosphates	Atropine or pralidoxime	(Atropine): anticholinergic or antiparasympathetic (parasympatholytic) drug, (Pralidoxime): oxime drug

them from being absorbed. Chemical antidotes neutralize toxins. Physiologic antidotes directly oppose the actions of a poison. Specific antidotes are available for just a few poisons (see Table 4.2). Specific systemic antidotes reduce concentrations of toxic substances by combining with them or increasing their excretion rate. Other systemic antidotes compete with poisons for their receptor sites. Antidotes have different mechanisms of action, described as follows:

- **Antagonizing toxic actions:** For example, atropine, a muscarinic receptor antagonist, is an antidote for anticholinesterase intoxication. It blocks the access of excessive acetylcholine to muscarinic receptors. Atropine and pralidoxime antagonize the actions of organophosphates, carbonates, and nerve gases.
- **Accelerating detoxification:** For example, *N-acetylcysteine* accelerates the detoxification of high doses of *acetaminophen*, which can otherwise cause liver necrosis due to metabolic activation by the cytochrome P450 enzymes. *N*-acetylcysteine donates cysteine, binds to, and facilitates excretion of the reactive metabolite, *N*-acetyl benzoquinone imine, and must be given as early as possible—within 8 to 10 hours after ingesting acetaminophen.
- **Providing an alternative target:** For example, two steps are used to treat *cyanide* poisoning. First, *sodium nitrite* is given to oxidize hemoglobin to methemoglobin, which has a high binding affinity for cyanide, producing *cyanmethemoglobin.* Amyl nitrite can also be used for the same purpose. The second step accelerates the detoxification of cyanide with *sodium thiosulfate.* This facilitates the production of *thiocyanate*, which is not nearly as toxic as cyanide, which is excreted. For a patient with smoke inhalation and cyanide toxicity, induction of methemoglobin is avoided unless the carboxyhemoglobin concentration is lower than 10%. Otherwise, the blood's oxygen-carrying capacity will become too low.
- **Reduction of metabolic activation:** For methanol, toxicity may be mediated by *formic acid*, produced when alcohol dehydrogenase metabolizes methanol to formaldehyde. Aldehyde dehydrogenase creates formic acid. *Fomepizole* inhibits alcohol dehydrogenase and decreases formic acid production.
- **Restoring an altered target**: When phosphorylation caused by organophosphorus compounds has inhibited acetylcholinesterase, it may be reactivated by using the pralidoxime antidote unless the offending agent has aged or covalently bound to the enzyme. After aging, the enzyme must be restored over time.
- **Chelation therapy**: Drugs that covalently bind with cationic metals can create a chelator-metal complex that can then be excreted. Because chelators are not specific to heavy metals, essential metals such as zinc may also be chelated. Also, some chelators have serious adverse effects, so they are used only when the benefits exceed metal toxicity risks. Examples of chelators include *dimercaprol, succimer (dimercaptosuccinic acid)*, and *edetate calcium disodium.* Dimercaprol is used to chelate mercury, arsenic, and lead. Succimer is used to chelate lead but may be effective for other metals. Edetate calcium disodium is used primarily to chelate lead but also can be used for different metals.

You should remember

While there may be no official "universal antidote," activated charcoal has been used for decades to combat most poisons. It can prevent the absorption of most toxic agents from the gastrointestinal tract and increase the elimination rate of some already absorbed agents.

Key Terms

Achilles tendon
Adverse effect
Alanine aminotransferase
Alopecia
Anaphylaxis
Anorexia
Antidotes
Apoptosis
Aspartate aminotransferase
Comorbidities
Complement fixation
Creatinine kinase
Crystalluria
Cytokine storm
Erythema multiforme
Genome
Hapten
Jaundice
Mast cells
Mucositis
Myopathy
Necrosis
Nephrotoxicity
Neurotoxicity
Ototoxicity
Pharmacogenomics
Polymorphisms
Red man syndrome
Rhabdomyolysis
Teratogen
Tinnitus
Urticaria

Clinical Case Studies

Clinical Case Study 1

A 10-year-old male went to his pediatrician's office with body aches, fever, severe sore throat, and nausea. A blood test was performed, and he was diagnosed with strep throat. His physician ordered a penicillin IM injection in the office and prescribed amoxicillin for 10 days. When the medical assistant questioned the child's mother about her child having any allergies to penicillin, the mother said he had never had any allergies. The inexperienced medical assistant administered penicillin G procaine without first performing an allergy test. Fifteen minutes later, the child went into anaphylactic shock. The pediatrician immediately began to treat the boy's reaction to the injection.

Critical Thinking Questions

1. **What is anaphylactic shock?**
2. **Explain the signs and symptoms of anaphylactic shock.**
3. **How is anaphylactic shock treated?**

Clinical Case Study 2

A 33-year-old female with acute psychosis was admitted to the hospital. She denied smoking and was taking long-term oral contraceptives. The patient was treated with antipsychotics. For one week, she received fluconazole gel after diagnosis of oral candidiasis. On day 24, clozapine was started with a resolution of her psychotic symptoms. After 3 weeks, the clozapine plasma levels had significantly increased, and eosinophilia was observed. The patient complained of nausea, vomiting, and palpitations. Echocardiography revealed heart abnormalities and pericardial effusion. The oral contraceptives were discontinued, and the clozapine was also interrupted. After 1 week, there was a complete resolution of adverse effects and pericardial effusion.

Critical Thinking Questions

1. How does a pharmacokinetic drug-drug interaction occur?
2. How can a drug-drug interaction be toxic?
3. Are there known interactions between clozapine and other drugs?

Further Reading

[1] R.B. Altman, D. Flockhart, D.B. Goldstein, Principles of Pharmacogenetics and Pharmacogenomics, Cambridge University Press, 2012.
[2] American Society of Health-System Pharmacists, Concepts in Pharmacogenomics, second ed., American Society of Health-System Pharmacists, 2017.
[3] D.G. Barceloux, Medical Toxicology of Drug Abuse: Synthesized Chemicals and Psychoactive Plants, Wiley, 2012.
[4] E. Benfenati, In Silico Methods for Predicting Drug Toxicity (Methods in Molecular Biology 1425), Humana Press, 2016.
[5] J. Bertino, A. Kashuba, J. Ma, U. Fuhr, C.L. DeVane, Pharmacogenomics: An Introduction and Clinical Perspective, McGraw-Hill Education/Medical, 2012.
[6] J. Carter, M. Slack, Pharmacy in Public Health: Basics and Beyond, ASHP, 2009.
[7] M.D. Coleman, Human Drug Metabolism, third ed., Wiley-Blackwell, 2020.
[8] S. Cox Gad, Drug Safety Evaluation (Pharmaceutical Development Series), third ed., Wiley, 2016.
[9] A. Dasgupta, C.A. Hammett-Stabler, Herbal Supplements: Efficacy, Toxicity, Interactions with Western Drugs, and Effects on Clinical Laboratory Tests, Wiley, 2011.
[10] A. Dasgupta, L.J. Langman, Pharmacogenomics of Alcohol and Drugs of Abuse, CRC Press, 2019.
[11] L. Di, E.H. Kerns, Drug-Like Properties: Concepts, Structure Design and Methods—From ADME to Toxicity Optimization, second ed., Academic Press, 2016.
[12] D.B. Durham, R. Thirumaran, C. Fluxman, Psychiatric Pharmacogenetics, Book 1: From Concepts to Cases, Fortis Caliga Academic Press, 2017.
[13] P. Frank, M.A. Ottoboni, The Dose Makes the Poison: A Plain-Language Guide to Toxicology, third ed., John Wiley and Sons, 2011.
[14] P. Greaves, Histopathology of Preclinical Toxicity Studies: Interpretation and Relevance in Drug Safety Evaluation, fourth ed., Academic Press, 2011.
[15] P.K. Gupta, Illustrated Toxicology: With Study Questions, Academic Press, 2018.
[16] M.J. Klepper, B. Cobert, Drug Safety Data: How to Analyze and Summarize Safety Data to Determine Risk, Jones & Bartlett Learning, 2010.
[17] D.A. Smith, D. Fox, Metabolism, Pharmacokinetics and Toxicity of Functional Groups: Impact of Chemical Building Blocks on ADMET (Drug Discovery, Volume 1), Royal Society of Chemistry, 2010.

CHAPTER

5

Medication errors

OUTLINE

LEARNING OUTCOMES

After study of the chapter, readers should be able to:

1. Identify the three stages of the medication process in which errors can occur.
2. Describe high-alert medications that are associated with an increased risk of patient harm.
3. Discuss the MedWatch program related to medication errors.
4. Explain the role of The Joint Commission regarding medication errors.
5. Describe the guidelines for risk reduction of medication errors.
6. Explain the strategies for handling medication errors.
7. Describe polypharmacy with medication errors.
8. Explain medication cartridges.

Overview

Medication errors frequently occur in the United States; the most vulnerable populations for medical mistakes are children and older adults. Medication errors include prescribing, dispensing, administration, and patient compliance. To avoid medication errors, patients and healthcare providers should ensure that all medications used by the patient are well understood. Then medication reconciliation, a safety strategy that involves comparing lists of

https://doi.org/10.1016/B978-0-443-29038-1.00005-1

medications taken by the patient with lists maintained by healthcare providers treating the patient, can be used to reduce drug-drug interactions and unnecessary drug use. The seven "rights" of drug administration must always be followed. Accurate documentation is always required, and medical staff members are legally and ethically responsible for reporting all medication errors. These strategies are only a few ways to reduce or prevent medication errors and improve patient morbidity and mortality.

Medication errors

A **medication error** is an inappropriate or incorrect drug administration and can occur in many ways. Sometimes, medication errors occur because of manufacturing mistakes. According to My Medical Score, over $40 billion was spent in 2020 to care for patients who experienced medication errors in the United States alone. Between 7000 and 9000 patients die from medication errors annually in the United States, with mistakes often occurring in three stages:

- *Prescribing or ordering medication.* In this stage, physicians or prescribing providers may need to be more focused and, as a result, provide complete orders. This dramatically increases the risk of errors. Medication errors mainly occur when choosing a medication, its dose, and the dosing schedule or dosage.
- *Dispensing the medication to patients or consumers.* Dispensing errors can occur due to insufficient or inexperienced pharmacy staffing and time constraints for patient counseling. This can lead to patient confusion about how to take the medication. All dispensed drugs should be double checked against the **medication administration record** (MAR). This stops errors before medications are dispensed.
- *Administering the medication and monitoring side effects.* At this stage, errors are most commonly attributed to those legally allowed to handle administration. They may be accountable for poor communication or misreading prescriptions, orders, or drug labels. Other factors include similar labeling and packaging of products and medications with lookalike names. After administering medications, healthcare professionals must ensure that the patient does not adversely react to the drug.

The most common medication error involves the dose or the entire dosing regimen, especially with antibiotics or analgesics. Medication errors may occur with outpatients due to the increasing number of prescriptions dispensed yearly and because pharmacists often need help adequately counseling patients. The current shortage of pharmacists and pharmacy technicians may also contribute to medication errors. Then, increased use of OTC drugs, various supplements such as "herbals," and the availability of medicines over the internet can cause medication errors.

A medication error must be reported as soon as it is noticed. Then, the patient must be monitored for undesirable effects or injury. Medication errors must be documented in the medical record with the signature of the individual who made the error, if possible. If health professionals involved with prescribing, dispensing, or administering medication follow the seven "rights" of medication administration and adhere to dispensing guidelines, medication errors should not occur. The seven rights of medication administration are described as follows.

You should remember

Medication errors harm an estimated 1.5 million people annually and cost more than $3.5 billion annually. Adverse drug events affect about 2 million hospitalized patients annually and increase the length of stay by 1.7 to 4.6 days. The most common cause of medication errors is poor communication among physicians, other staff members, and patients.

High-alert medications

High-alert medications are associated with an increased risk of patient harm if administered incorrectly. Though errors with these medications are uncommon, patient outcomes can be severe because of the drug's strength. Some high-alert drugs, defined by the Institute for Safe Medication Practices (ISMP), are shown in Table 5.1.

TABLE 5.1 High-alert medications by drug class and name.

Drug classes with examples	Drug names
Adrenergic agonists, IV (epinephrine, norepinephrine, phenylephrine)	Epoprostenol, IV
Adrenergic antagonists, IV (labetalol, metoprolol, propranolol)	Insulin, subcutaneous, and IV
General anesthetics, inhaled and IV (ketamine, propofol)	Methotrexate, oral for nonchemotherapy uses
Antiarrhythmics, IV (amiodarone, lidocaine)	Opium tincture
Antithrombotic agents (enoxaparin, dalteparin, heparin, fondaparinux, argatroban, lepirudin, bivalirudin, alteplase, reteplase, tenecteplase, eptifibatide, and warfarin)	Oxytocin, IV
Cardioplegic solutions	Nitroprusside injection
Chemotherapy medications, oral and IV	Potassium chloride concentrate injection
Hypertonic (20%+) dextrose solutions	Potassium phosphate injection
Hemodialysis and peritoneal solutions	Promethazine, IV
Medications given via epidural or intrathecal routes	Hypertonic (0.9%+) sodium chloride injection
Oral antidiabetic agents	Sterile water for injection, inhalation, and irrigation (containers of 100 mL+)
Inotropic medications, IV (digoxin, milrinone)	
Moderate sedatives, IV (midazolam)	
Pediatric moderate sedatives, oral (chloral hydrate)	
Narcotics, IV, oral, transdermal	
Neuromuscular blocking agents (succinylcholine, rocuronium, vecuronium)	
Radiocontrast agents, IV	
Total parenteral nutrition solutions	

The five medication classes most commonly involved in severe adverse events include insulin, IV heparin, IV narcotics, IV potassium concentrates, and IV hypertonic sodium chloride solutions. Most of these are available as floor stock in nursing areas, and a system of double checking their use may need to be implemented. Then, their IV administration increases the risk of errors due to inappropriate concentrations and infusion rates.

In addition, confusing abbreviations, acronyms, and symbols are often used. These include "U" for "unit," "IU" for "International Unit," trailing zeros such as X.0 mg, and the lack of a leading zero such as .X mg, the > sign for "greater than," the < signal for "less than," and abbreviated drug names. Writing out words, phrases, and drug names is always best.

You should remember

Factors that may cause medication errors include handwriting misinterpretation, verbal or phone order misunderstandings, inaccurate administration, and miscalculations.

Causes

Medication errors can happen anywhere at any time. Medication errors are the most common cause of morbidities and preventable hospital deaths. These errors affect patients, their families, and those healthcare professionals responsible for the error. Medication errors may cause extended stays in the hospital, higher costs, and patient separation from family and everyday activities. Every healthcare professional involved in a medication error may experience severe emotional trauma because of responsibility for the patient's welfare. High error rates can damage the reputations of healthcare staff and their facilities. Financial penalties and lawsuits may also result.

All healthcare facilities should reduce medication errors to the lowest possible. Each mistake should be closely investigated and documented to prevent future errors. Investigations should encourage the correct reporting of what occurred without the threat of penalties. After identifying error patterns, steps can be taken to stop activities that lead to errors. Several factors cause medication errors, including:

- *Use of incorrect abbreviations:* many abbreviations can be mistaken for different units and different doses
- *Miscommunication:* poor handwriting, similar drug names, and dosing unit confusion
- *Missing information:* lack of patient information (such as allergies, diseases, drug history, laboratory information, and drug information or warnings)
- *Lack of appropriate labeling:* by the manufacturer or the pharmacist
- *Environmental factors:* noise, lighting, stress, and fatigue that affect healthcare providers
- *Poor management:* unhealthy healthcare facility environments

Medication errors may occur in inpatient settings such as hospitals and nursing homes or outpatient settings such as physicians' offices or clinics. Errors, including formulation, packaging, labeling, and distribution errors, can also happen during drug manufacturing. Mistakes may also be the result of undiscovered toxicities. Medication errors are largely preventable and are the single largest source of all medical errors. Then, medication errors may occur due to the following, or the seven "rights" of drug administration:

- Wrong patient
- Incorrect route
- Incorrect drug
- Incorrect dose
- Incorrect time
- Incorrect technique
- False information on the patient chart

You should remember

The most common prescribing errors include dosing errors, prescribing medications to which the patient has had an allergic response, and errors involving prescribing inappropriate dosage forms.

Documentation

Documentation of medication errors must be clear and factual, following the facility's policy and procedure guidelines. Blame and judgment should be put aside. The goal is to determine the causes of the error so that future errors can be eradicated. Documentation of medication errors must include interventions undertaken to counteract them. The patient's medical record must be updated with complete information about the error. The MAR should also be fully updated if the patient is hospitalized.

After updating the records about a medication error, the person who made the error or observed its occurrence should create a separate written report (incident report or occurrence report). A factual, objective document containing the specific details of the error should be assembled. These reports are used by *risk management personnel* for quality improvement and assurance.

Accurate documentation in medical records and error reports is required for legal reasons. These documents help improve medication administration processes and verify that patient safety is protected. If there is an attempt to delay corrective action or hide a mistake, legal ramifications may be much more severe. This is also true if interventions are not documented in the patient's chart.

Healthcare facilities use quality and improvement programs to monitor medication errors. These alert practitioners to medication error trends and help create specific solutions. Many facilities use **root cause analysis** to prevent future mistakes, asking precisely what happened, why, and what can be done to avoid recurrence. It may also be used to determine whether recurrence risks have been reduced.

Reporting

Staff members are legally and ethically responsible for the reporting of all occurrences of medication errors. Patients sometimes undergo lifesaving interventions and may need follow-up supervision and treatments. At the federal level, the FDA coordinates the reporting of medication errors via its **MedWatch program** or the *FDA Safety Information and Adverse Event Reporting Program*. This program provides timely and clinically significant information about medical products, which includes data regarding safety issues for prescription and OTC drugs, biologics, medical devices, radiation-emitting devices, and unique nutritional products. Healthcare professionals should use the MedWatch database to report medication errors and situations that may lead to mistakes. Reporting may be anonymous, directly to the FDA, by the internet, or by telephone. MedWatch may be contacted at www.fda.gov/Safety/MedWatch/default.htm or (800) 332-1088.

The National Coordinating Council for Medication Error Reporting and Prevention (NCC MERP) assists with medication errors. This organization has helped to standardize the medication error reporting system. The NCC MERP coordinates medication error information and provides preventive education. They may be contacted at http://www.nccmerp.org/ or 800-233-7767. The ISMP publishes "Safe Medicine," a consumer newsletter on medication errors. The ISMP accepts consumer and healthcare professional reports related to medication safety. The ISMP may be contacted at www.ismp.org/newsletters/consumer/default.aspx.

The Joint Commission (TJC) has established standards that address many significant patient safety issues. These include patient safety programs, management practices focusing on safety, and continued analysis of medication ordering, preparation, and dispensing. TJC requires hospitals to inform patients when errors have harmed them. TJC has established National Patient Safety Goals. Because of this, barcoding for medication administration is now standard in all hospitals. TJC's website is https://www.jointcommission.org.

Prevention

Preventing medication errors begins with a system that encourages them to be reported positively and without blame. This requires cooperation among all team members. Patients should be educated about taking their medications correctly and urged to monitor prescription accuracy from pharmacies. They should report unexpected side effects from their medications. Patient education should occur during every interaction with healthcare providers, including pharmacists, to facilitate error reduction.

Newer technologies that aid in the prevention of medication errors include **computerized physician order entry**, automated dispensing machinery, **barcoding**, computerized MARs (CMARs), and **smart infusion pumps** (see Fig. 5.1). The primary advantage of computerized physician order entry was the reduction of illegible prescriptions. Automated dispensing machinery has also decreased medication errors, although incorrectly loading **medication cartridges** into this machinery has caused adverse outcomes.

Barcoding technology ensures that the medication and its dose match what has been prescribed, the drug is given to the correct patient, and all dispensing and administration processes are accurate and timely. CMARs reduce medication errors by providing consistent documentation, brief drug administration records, appropriate drug information, and integrating databases that improve patient care. These include purchasing, distribution, and patient information. Each CMAR documents the medication prescribed, the prescription date, doses, dose frequency, and medication discontinuation. Smart infusion pumps reduce IV drug administration errors because they contain "safety software" that can be adjusted based on parameters specific to the medical facility.

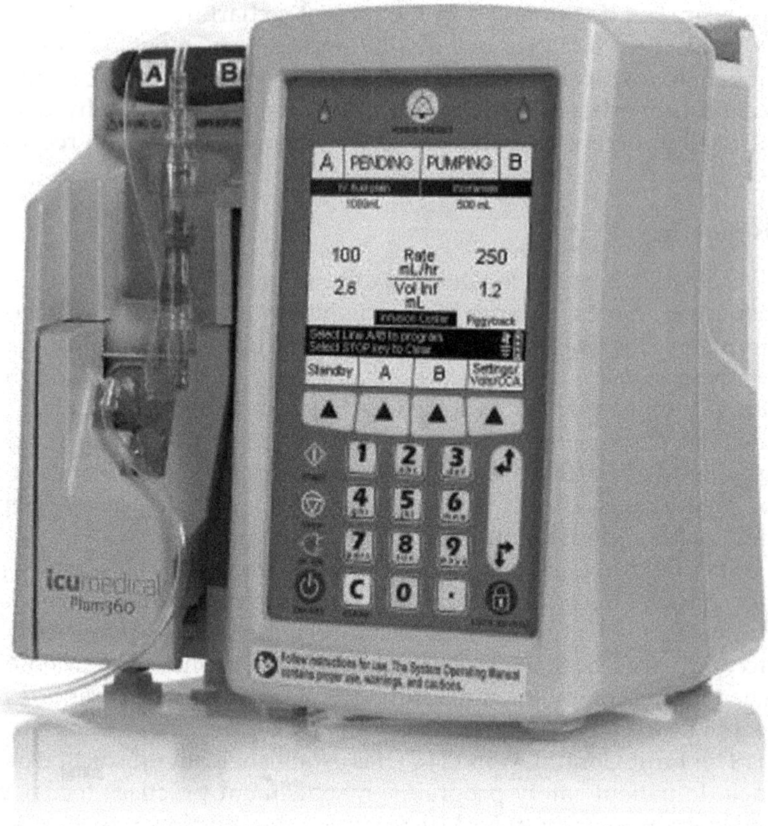

FIG. 5.1 Smart infusion pump, a device that significantly helps reduce medication errors.

You should remember

Systems that help decrease hospital medication errors are varied. They include electronic medical records, barcoding systems, standardized units of measure, avoiding confusing units of measure, weight-based dosing, and having a pharmacist available to assist in calculating correct doses.

Sentinel events

Sentinel events are unexpected occurrences involving death, serious physical or psychological injury, or risk thereof. They are recognized by TJC and are investigated so that interventions may be used to ensure zero recurrence. Root cause analysis is used to identify causes and the needed type of intervention. The most often reported sentinel events include patient suicide, operative or postoperative complications, wrong-site surgery, medication errors, delayed treatment, falling, patient death or injury while in restraints, and assaults.

You should remember

Use of OTC drugs and supplements by patients without any medical supervision may cause adverse reactions and medication errors. Potential risks include infrequent but severe adverse reactions, dangerous drug interactions, incorrect administration or dosages, incorrect choosing of the OTC drug or drugs, and possible overdoses if the dosing regimen is not followed carefully.

Reducing errors in healthcare facilities

Most healthcare facilities store medications in locked, automated, and computerized cabinets. A specific code is needed to access these cabinets. Automation allows for an accurate inventory of medication supplies to be maintained. In more extensive facilities, **risk management departments** minimize medication errors and examine risks for them. Risk management specialists track information, investigate incidents, find problems, and provide recommendations to improve the accuracy of patient care. Collaboration between staff members and risk management specialists helps modify policies and procedures. Errors can be reduced by correctly storing medications, keeping reference materials updated, and avoiding the following:

- Use of expired medications
- Transfer of medications between containers
- Overstocking
- Use of dangerous abbreviations

Medication errors may be related to professional practice, healthcare products, procedures, and systems. Guidelines for risk reduction include:

- Using an adequate number of health staff members who are trained to prepare, dispense, and administer medications to patients
- Using standardized measurement systems for inpatients and outpatients
- Using error-tracking systems that consistently target and monitor common patient errors
- Defining a strategy for drug ordering, dispensing, and administration that includes reviews of original drug orders
- Compiling medication profiles for all patients with updated allergy histories after each encounter
- Providing excellent work environments for safe, adequate drug preparation
- Using electronic medical records and e-prescribing so that automatic surveillance measures can find potential medication errors, especially if the information is lacking or conflicting with other information

You should remember

Preventable medical errors contribute significantly to healthcare costs, including higher health insurance costs. Health professionals working more closely together can only reduce or avoid medical mistakes. This can achieve success by reducing patient injury and related expenses.

Strategies for handling medication errors

Medication errors arise from treating children or older adults within certain healthcare facilities. Administering a wrong dose or an incorrect drug and using the wrong route of administration are typical examples of sources of medication errors. Because children receive amounts based on weight, they are more likely to experience medication errors than adults because of miscalculations. Also, older adults are at increased risk of errors due to using several drugs simultaneously (**polypharmacy**), age-related physiological changes, and multiple physicians. The following steps can help to avoid medication errors and promote safe administration of medications:

1. *Assessment:* Ask patients about allergies, health conditions, and the use of medications and herbal supplements in the correct doses, routes, and times for administration; educate patients about all needed medications; and assess bodily functions to determine if pharmacotherapy impairments exist.
2. *Planning:* Avoid abbreviations that may be misunderstood, unclear question orders, refusal of verbal orders, and strict compliance with all policies and procedures. Patients should restate dosing directions, dose amounts, administration routes, and drug dosing times. They should also repeat the goals of the medication therapy.

3. *Implementation:* Eliminate distractions during medication administration (noise, talking, and other events); ensure everything: the right patient, time, frequency, dose, route, and drug; verify identity, procedures and techniques, dose calculations, correct and timely opening of medications, proper documentation of processes, confirmation that the patient has wholly swallowed an oral dose of medicine, and double checking for long-acting oral dosage forms.
4. *Evaluation:* assess the patient for correct outcomes and determine any adverse effects.

There are nine categories of medication errors, and healthcare professionals should be familiar with them. These categories are:

- **Category A:** circumstances or events that can cause errors
- **Category B:** errors that occurred but did not affect the patient
- **Category C:** errors that affected the patient but did not cause any harm
- **Category D:** errors that occurred, affected the patient, and required monitoring to ensure that no harm occurred or that needed intervention to prevent patient harm
- **Category E:** errors that occurred and may have contributed to or resulted in temporary harm to the patient (and required intervention)
- **Category F:** errors that occurred that might have contributed to or resulted in temporary harm to the patient (and required initial or prolonged hospitalization)
- **Category G:** errors that occurred that might have contributed to or resulted in permanent patient harm
- **Category H:** errors that occurred that required intervention necessary to sustain life
- **Category I:** errors that occurred that might have contributed to or resulted in the patient's death

Most medication errors involve the administration of an incorrect dose (41%). Nearly 50% of fatal medication errors occur in patients older than 60. Up-to-date drug information must be available so healthcare practitioners can verify correct data for the medications they are administering.

You should remember

Physiologic changes associated with aging include altered memory, poorer vision, decreased kidney function; less complete and slower absorption from the GI tract; and reduced liver function. These changes can increase the chances for cumulative and toxic effects of medications.

Reconciling medications

Polypharmacy uses multiple medications, sometimes for the same condition, with often conflicting pharmacologic actions. Polypharmacy is most prevalent in older adults but may occur in patients of all ages. Keeping track of multiple medications and healthcare providers is difficult for many older adults. This is complicated further by poor medication information, documentation, and reporting. Keeping track of a patient's medications as they change healthcare providers is **medication reconciliation**. This requires accurately listing all medications a patient takes to reduce duplications, dosing errors, omissions, and drug interactions. For hospitalized patients, nurses document all medications previously taken at home, including the dose, frequency, and route. This list is used whenever the patient is admitted to other facilities or transferred to different hospital units. The list is rechecked when a patient is discharged from a hospital. Many possible medication errors have been revealed during medication reconciliation procedures. Medications a patient takes must be considered part of medication reconciliation, including prescription medications, OTC medications, herbal supplements, and even vitamins.

TJC has identified many severe medication errors related to medication reconciliation and developed recommendations for their prevention. TJC encourages hospitals to thoroughly document all medications used by every patient during the admission process. Prescription medications, OTC medications, vitamins, and herbal supplements are all recorded. Patient medication lists must be shared with all service providers inside and outside the hospital. After a patient is discharged, they must receive a complete list of medications to be taken and instructions on using any newly prescribed medications.

You should remember

The five steps of medication reconciliation include developing a list of current medications, developing a list of drugs to be prescribed, comparing the pills on the two lists, making clinical decisions based on the comparison, and communicating the new list to caregivers and the patient.

Patient education about medications

Educating patients about their medications is crucial. They must have a basic understanding of medication risks and benefits and how to administer medications safely and correctly. Patients must receive counseling to understand the information concerning this subject thoroughly. Studies have shown that most patients prefer to receive this information from their physicians. When patients do not receive adequate and direct education, they often rely on printed information on drug labels or package inserts, which they may need help understanding.

It is best to provide detailed, spoken instructions to each patient, which can then be followed up by giving complete written information. Poor health literacy is a barrier to adequate care. A typical example of a lack of understanding occurs in elderly patients, who may not know why certain medications must be taken at specific times during the day. When a physician communicates this information directly to them or their caregivers, the reasons behind specific dosing times are better understood. This results in greater compliance.

Regarding medications, patients must be provided with age-appropriate written information, audiovisual teaching aids if available, and the professionals' contact information to be notified in case of an adverse reaction. Patients should know the names of every medication they take, the correct uses and dosages, and when and how they should be taken. They must understand potential adverse effects that need to be reported immediately. Patients should always use specified medication devices to administer medications, not *household utensils* such as spoons, which may need to be more accurate. They should carry a list of all their prescription and OTC medications (plus vitamins and herbal supplements) with them at all times and should use one pharmacy for all their drugs. They must be encouraged to ask questions when working with healthcare providers to maintain safe medication principles.

Key Terms

Barcoding
Computerized physician order entry
Herbals
High-alert medications
Medication administration record
Medication cartridges
Medication error
Medication reconciliation
MedWatch program
Polypharmacy
Root cause analysis
Sentinel events
Smart infusion pumps
The Joint Commission

Clinical Case Studies

Clinical Case Study 1

A surgeon prescribed morphine ".4 mg IV" for postoperative pain for a 5-month-old infant. A secretary recorded the order in the MAR as "4 mg." An inexperienced nurse followed the directions on the MAR without question and gave the infant 4 mg of IV morphine initially and another 4 mg dose 4 hours later. About 50 minutes after the second dose, the infant stopped breathing and experienced respiratory and cardiac arrest. If the surgeon had written "0.4 mg," the unit secretary would probably not have misunderstood the intended amount, and the nurse would have administered the correct dose.

Critical Thinking Questions

1. Whose error prompted the medication error described in this case study?
2. When do medication errors mainly occur?

Clinical Case Study 2

A 75-year-old male took multiple medications for hypertension, prostate enlargement, and rheumatoid arthritis. Four drugs would be taken before bed, and three would be taken in the morning. One night, the male realized he had forgotten to take one of his medications. He got out of bed, went into the kitchen, and mistakenly took one of the medications he had already taken earlier in the dimly lit room. After 2 hours, he woke up to go to the bathroom, felt chest pain and dizziness, and almost collapsed, awakening his wife.

Critical Thinking Questions

1. What is the definition of polypharmacy?
2. How can polypharmacy complicate medication management?
3. Which medications a patient takes must be considered as part of medication reconciliation?

Further Reading

[1] K.R. Baker, Medication Safety: Dispensing Drugs Without Error, Cengage Learning, 2012.
[2] M.R. Cohen, Medication Errors, second ed., American Pharmacists Association, 2006.
[3] M. Courtenay, M. Griffiths, Medication Safety: An Essential Guide, Cambridge University Press, 2009.
[4] A.M. Curren, M.H. Witt, Curren's Math for Meds: Dosages and Solutions, eleventh ed., Cengage Learning, 2014.
[5] D. Farb, Medication Errors, University of Health Care, 2004.
[6] T. Guerra, How to Pronounce Drug Names: A Visual Approach to Preventing Medication Errors, Lulu.com, 2017.
[7] S. Haroutounian, Preventing Medication Errors at Home, Oxford University Press, 2019.
[8] J.B. Hart, R. Barrows, W. Schaller, D. Lidel, Dosage and Clinical Calculations: With Focus on Preventing Medication Errors, fourth ed., Kendall Hunt Publishing, 2009.
[9] Institute of Medicine, Board on Health Care Services, Committee on Identifying and Preventing Medication Errors, L.R. Cronenwett, J. L. Bootman, J. Wolcott, P. Aspden, Preventing Medication Errors (Quality Chasm Series), National Academies Press, 2007.
[10] W.N. Kelly, Prescribed Medications and the Public Health: Laying the Foundation for Risk Reduction, CRC Press, 2006.
[11] G. Kukhet, Your License is on the Line: Medication Errors – Dispensing Without Error Dietary Supplements, OTC Products, being an Active Member, and Medical Abbreviations, CreateSpace Independent Publishing Platform, 2017.
[12] C.M. Larson, D. Saine, The Medication Safety Officer's Handbook, American Society of Health-System Pharmacists, 2013.
[13] M.S. McAslan, Read the Prescription Label: And Other Tips to Prevent Deadly and Costly Medication Errors, Balboa Press, 2012.
[14] R. Persaud, R. Tabanao, Medication Administration: A Guide for Unregulated Healthcare Providers, Tellwell Talent, 2019.
[15] Z.M. Pronsky, D. Elbe, K. Ayoob, J.P. Crowe, S. Epstein, W.H. Roberts, Food Medication Interactions, eighteenth ed., FMI, 2015.
[16] N. Solanki, C. Shah, Study of Medication Errors in Western Population of India: Root Cause Analysis of Medication Errors at Multispecialty Hospital, Lap Lambert Academic Publishing, 2014.
[17] P.L. Spath, Error Reduction in Health Care: A Systems Approach to Improving Patient Safety, second ed., Jossey-Bass, 2011.
[18] United States Congress House Committee, Issues Relating to Medication Errors: Hearing Before the Subcommittee on Health of the Committee on Ways and Means, House of Representatives, Palala Press, 2015.
[19] T. Warholak, D. Nau, Quality and Safety in Pharmacy Practice, McGraw-Hill Education / Medical, 2010.
[20] M.L. Workman, L.A. LaCharity, Understanding Pharmacology: Essentials for Medication Safety, second ed., Saunders, 2015.
[21] B.J. Youngberg, Principles of Risk Management and Patient Safety, Jones & Bartlett Learning, 2010.

CHAPTER

6

Complementary and alternative dietary therapies

OUTLINE

LEARNING OBJECTIVES

After studying this chapter, the reader should be able to:

1. Define terms used to describe alternative and herbal treatments.
2. Identify informational resources/websites providing evidence-based information for herbal remedies.
3. Discuss the implications of the Dietary Supplement Health and Education Act of 1994.
4. Discuss safety concerns related to herbal preparations, including regulation and standardization.
5. Identify the indications of saw palmetto and goldenseal.
6. Describe the adverse effects of black cohosh.

https://doi.org/10.1016/B978-0-443-29038-1.00006-3

7. Explain the primary uses of ginkgo and ginseng.
8. Identify the adverse effects of echinacea.
9. Describe the numerous safety concerns with ephedra.
10 Discuss meaningful herbal-herbal and herbal-drug interactions.

Overview

Complementary and alternative dietary are increasingly common in the United States and worldwide. A recent National Health Interview Survey study found that 76% of patients reported taking dietary supplements. It is estimated that more than 170 million Americans take nutritional supplements, an increase from 38 million in 2002. Approximately one out of four individuals taking prescription medication also uses some dietary supplement. Around the world, about 80% of individuals routinely use nutritional supplements and alternative remedies to treat and prevent ailments. Individuals frequently see dietary supplement products as harmless or benign, although their use can be helpful. However, because the FDA does not regulate them, there can be contaminants and variances in quality that consumers may not be aware of. In some cases, these preparations can cause significant toxicity and side effects. Therefore drug interactions and drug toxicity must always be considered.

Popularity of dietary supplements

Because the FDA does not regulate or monitor the purity of supplement products, there can be contaminants in the products and fluctuations in the quality of the product due to variations in climate and soil where an herb was grown, along with manufacturing processes used. Healthcare providers should be aware of dietary supplements' potential benefits and risks. Given the number of products patients use, it is essential to determine when patients are taking these products while obtaining a drug history. As a patient develops more severe and complicated medical ailments, the temptation to try dietary supplements or herbal remedies for relief of symptoms and disease treatment is understandably strong.

When patients transition from one healthcare setting to another (from home to the hospital or from home to the outpatient surgery setting), identifying dietary supplement use is particularly important to minimize dangerous drug interactions and toxicity. Many patients do not recognize these supplements as "medications" and thus may not tell healthcare providers about these products. Of the 50.6 million individuals reporting the use of dietary supplements in the prior 12 months, only one-third reported this information to their healthcare providers. Patients less likely to report dietary supplement use include ethnic and racial minorities, males, and young adults. Unlike traditional medications, solid scientific evidence substantiating product claims and safety has been difficult to collect for many reasons. Along the same lines, it may be challenging to determine a strong relationship between dietary supplement use and side effects and whether the side effect was related to the active compound in the active ingredient or other substances in the product.

Some preparations may be manufactured using different plant parts (such as the root, seed, leaves, flower, or bark) and come in various formulations (tea, tincture, dried, or extract) that can have differing potency, effects, and toxicity. Clinical trials are frequently sponsored by pharmaceutical companies hoping to create, patent, and market a drug for economic profits. Because the products are not patent protected, manufacturers' financial gains tend to be less substantial. Thus the impetus to conduct extensive clinical trials investigating supplement claims is low (although some, notably glucosamine sulfate, had over $240 million in global sales in 2020).

National Center for Complementary and Alternative Medicine

The US National Center for Complementary and Alternative Medicine (NCCAM) was created partially in response to the need to compile more robust evidence on the effects of dietary supplement products. The NCCAM has been conducting well-designed clinical trials related to alternative medicine to answer important questions about safety and efficacy. Because patients may not identify these medications as drugs and healthcare providers may not even know that the patient is taking them, reporting supplement-drug interactions is limited. It is also challenging to determine if specific substances in herbs provide health benefits or if the whole plant and all its ingredients are helpful. Because data on herbals and their safety can be challenging to collect and interpret, caution should be exercised with pregnant females and children using supplements, for whom data regarding safety and long-term effects are scant.

Like other drugs, concerns with supplement-drug interactions are related to interference with liver metabolism pathways, such as the CYP450 family of hepatic metabolizing enzymes. Other problems associated with drugs and supplements are linked to altered drug absorption with these preparations or side effects that are more devastating in specific patient populations, such as those with cardiac or hepatic disease.

Dietary Supplement Health and Education Act of 1994

Although dietary supplements are not regulated the same as drugs, federal regulations are in place to promote the safety of these substances. The Dietary Supplement Health and Education Act (DSHEA) 1994 created supplement guidelines and definitions. Whereas drug manufacturers can claim that a drug can diagnose, cure, mitigate, or prevent a disease, supplements are considered foods. They thus can only assert a health claim (by reducing risk for an illness), a nutrient/supplement claim (describing the amount of the nutrient in the product), or a structure/function claim (explaining how a supplement may alter the function of an organ or body system).

The DSHEA mandates that all herbals contain the following labeling: "This product is not intended to diagnose, treat, or prevent any disease." Herbal preparations marketed before 1994 are assumed to be safe, given that humans have already used them with no adverse effects. New supplements sold after 1994 must inform the FDA of plans to sell the supplement and provide evidence that the product is safe for humans.

Common herbal remedies

Here, we discuss some of the most commonly used herbal remedies, providing information on their common uses, available evidence about the product benefits, contraindications, and safety and drug interaction concerns.

Garlic

Garlic is an herbal product from a perennial bulb grown worldwide (see Fig. 6.1). It is commonly used to prevent and treat vascular diseases, significantly reducing LDL, elevated triglycerides, and hypertension. Other uses for garlic have included treatment for **alopecia**, breast disease, and upper respiratory infection. A garlic-rich diet seems to confer a lower risk of developing colon, prostate, stomach, and breast cancer.

Many different garlic preparations include raw garlic, garlic powder tablets, garlic oil, and aged garlic extract. Thus the evidence on garlic includes trials that have used varying preparations. Recommended daily dosing for all these preparations varies greatly. These preparations may not have the same active ingredients; thus trial results cannot be generalized to other garlic preparations.

Side effects of using garlic may include garlicky breath, body odor, nausea, vomiting, flatulence, flushing, tachycardia, and insomnia. Garlic should not be used in large amounts during pregnancy because it may be fatal to the fetus or stimulate labor. Large quantities also should not be given directly or via breast milk because it may cause colic in infants or be deadly to children through uncharacterized mechanisms. It is contraindicated in those with known hypersensitivity or gastritis. Garlic should not be used in people before or after surgery due to the increased risk of bleeding.

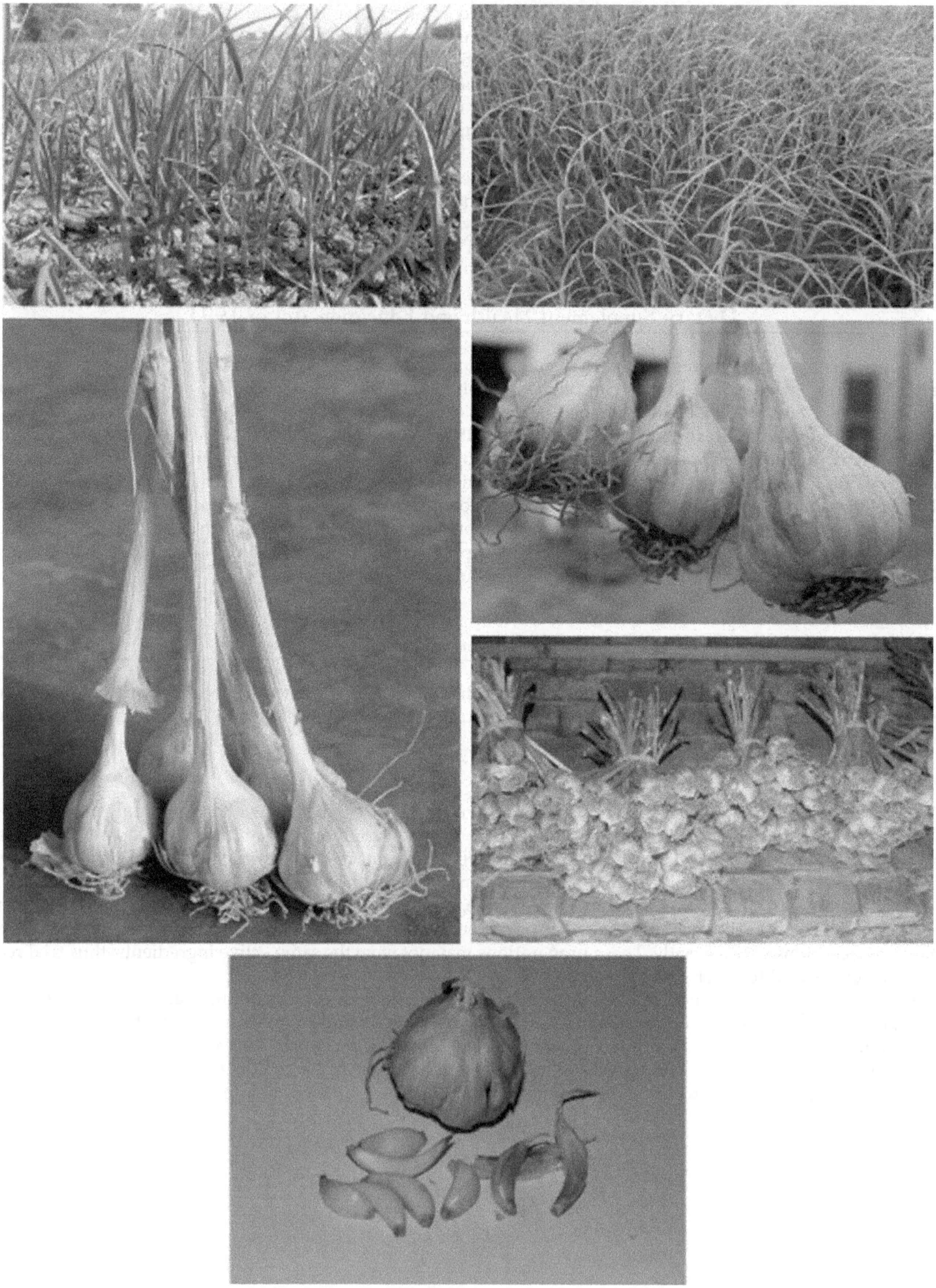

FIG. 6.1 Garlic.

You should remember

Garlic was one of the first herbs to be cultivated, beginning more than 4000 years ago. It has been used throughout history for culinary and medicinal purposes. Garlic's many health properties include anticoagulation, antioxidant, antiviral, and antimicrobial properties, lowering cholesterol, and even anticancer properties. It also helps regulate blood pressure.

St. John's wort

St. John's wort is a native plant with yellow, star-shaped flowers. It is found commonly in Europe, the United States, Africa, and Asia. The leaves are dried, made into tea, or prepared as a dried extract in pills/capsules. It is a favored treatment for depression, anxiety, premenstrual symptoms, and neuropathic pain. St. John's wort is likely safe when used in doses of up to 900 mg daily for 12 weeks. It can cause side effects such as diarrhea, nausea, dizziness, trouble sleeping, allergic reactions, restlessness, **xerostomia**, erectile dysfunction, and orgasm dysfunction. St. John's wort is possibly unsafe when taken by mouth during pregnancy. It might cause congenital disabilities in infants.

The herb has the potential for numerous drug interactions, as it induces hepatic enzyme CYP3A4 and thus can reduce drug concentrations and the effect of cyclosporine, theophylline, nifedipine, and other drugs metabolized by CYP3A4. St John's wort can also affect P-glycoprotein function in the GI tract, impairing absorption of certain drugs and resulting in lower serum concentrations. This is true with the protease inhibitor drugs used to treat HIV (ritonavir and atazanavir), and St. John's wort is contraindicated with patients taking this class of drugs.

You should remember

Pregnant or breastfeeding females must avoid St. John's wort. The supplement can also interfere with medications used in organ transplant patients, heart medications, and drugs used for HIV and cancer. It can also reduce the effectiveness of anxiety medications. Taking St. John's wort with antidepressants can cause a dangerous increase in serotonin, resulting in serotonin syndrome.

Ginger

Ginger (*Zingiber officinale*) is commonly used as an antiemetic to treat nausea associated with pregnancy, chemotherapy, motion sickness, and other causes (see Fig. 6.2). Ginger is also used to promote blood flow to the gallbladder and for antiinflammatory action and antiplatelet activity. The root is formulated into several forms: tablets, capsules, fresh or dried root, topical cream, tea, and liquid extract. Several components of the root have pharmacologic activity, including *gingerol and shogaol*. Ginger exhibits antihistamine and anticholinergic activity to reduce salivary output and improve peristalsis. It also inhibits **prostaglandin** and **leukotriene** synthesis, providing antiinflammatory and antiplatelet function.

Ginger has few side effects when taken at recommended doses. There have been reports of dyspepsia, diarrhea, heartburn at recommended doses, and some rashes from the topical cream. Because ginger has some antiplatelet activity, it should be used cautiously in patients taking other antiplatelet drugs such as aspirin, warfarin, and other nonsteroidal antiinflammatory drugs. Ginger does not appear to be metabolized via the CYP450 enzyme pathway.

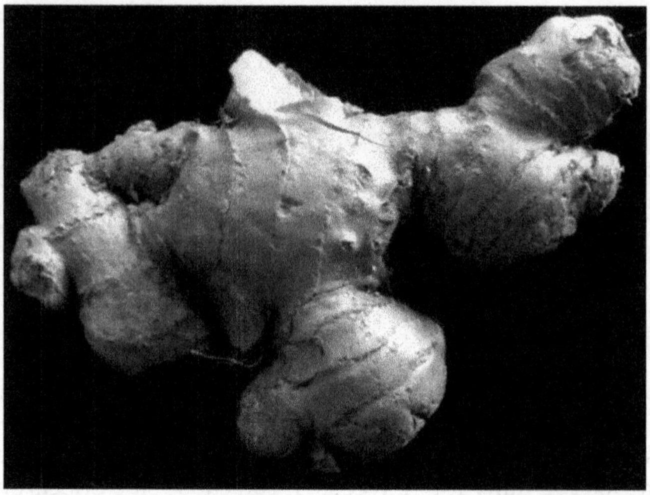

FIG. 6.2 Ginger.

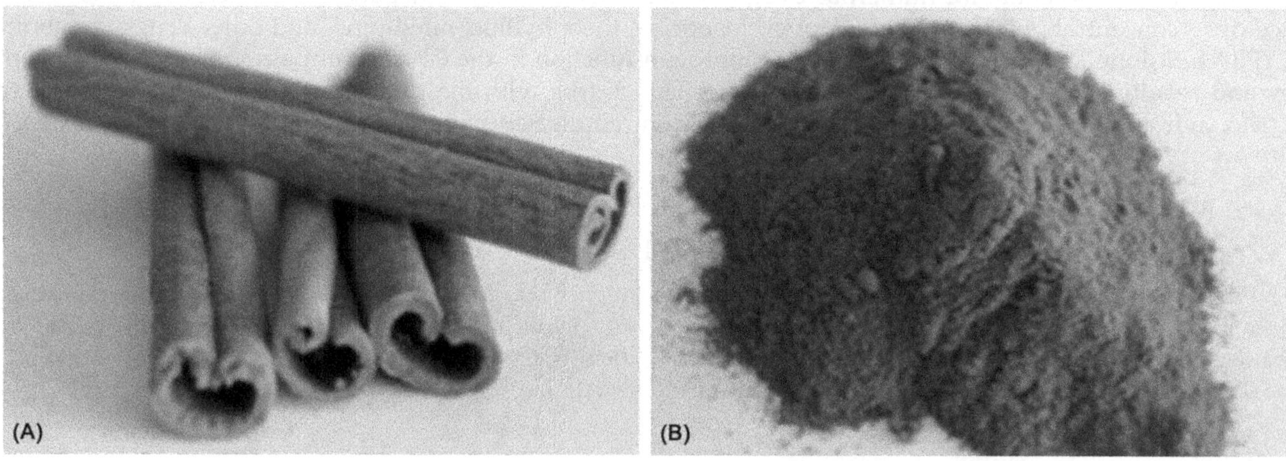

FIG. 6.3 (A) Raw and (B) ground cinnamon.

You should remember

Ginger, like garlic, has been used as a flavoring agent and medicinal plant for thousands of years. It has antiinflammatory properties and is considered a "carrier" herb because it enables other herbs to be more effective in the body. Ginger contains many essential vitamins and minerals as well as gingerol, a component with potent antioxidant and antiinflammatory properties. It can reduce hypertension, breakage of DNA, nausea, migraines, and the buildup of amyloid, which is implicated in Alzheimer disease.

Cinnamon

Cinnamon is a spice obtained from the inner bark of trees in the genus *Cinnamomum* (see Fig. 6.3). It reduces blood glucose levels, increases natural insulin production, and lowers blood cholesterol. Cinnamon enhances the odor and taste of many foods, including breakfast cereals and snacks. The distinctive qualities of cinnamon come from its

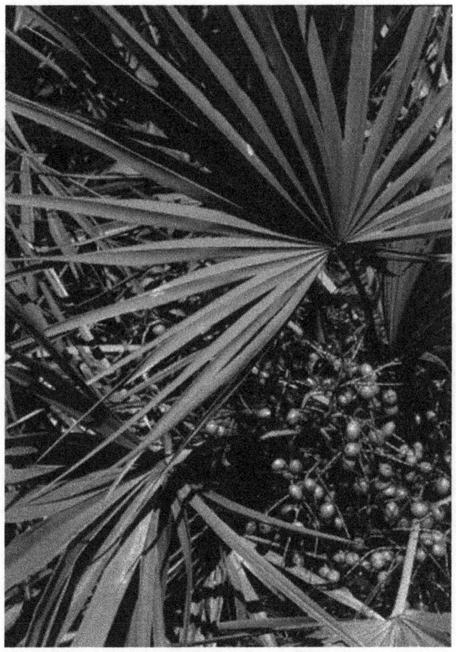

FIG. 6.4 Saw palmetto.

essential oil and primary component, *cinnamaldehyde*. Most of the world's cinnamon is grown in Sri Lanka, China, Indonesia, Vietnam, and other Southeast Asian countries. The many indications (though disputed) for the use of cinnamon include toothache, bad breath, memory problems, acne, coagulation, indigestion, nausea, vomiting, diarrhea, flatulence, excessive stomach acid, morning sickness, the common cold, influenza, sore throat, menstrual cramps, hemorrhoids, amenorrhea, amoebiasis, heart disease, fever, coughing, headache, diuresis, increased **libido**, lactation, and to relieve oxidative stress.

Adverse effects of excessive cinnamon include liver damage and increased risk of cancer, mouth sores, hypoglycemia, and breathing abnormalities. Cinnamon can also interact with medications for diabetes mellitus, heart disease, and liver disease, resulting in intensified effects of these medications. One reason is that cinnamon contains relatively high amounts of coumarin, which can cause liver toxicity and damage.

You should remember

The *Cassia* variety of cinnamon, from Indonesia and China, is the most common variety of cinnamon sold in America. It contains much more natural coumarin than the Ceylon variety. This toxic chemical compound can be dangerous if cinnamon is consumed in large quantities and must be avoided by pregnant females. Even with these dangers, cinnamon in small amounts helps lower lipids, including LDL cholesterol and triglycerides.

Saw palmetto

Saw palmetto is extracted from dried berries of *Serenoa repens* and is used to treat benign prostatic hypertrophy (BPH) in males (see Fig. 6.4). More than 2 million males in the United States have used saw palmetto to treat BPH, and it is commonly used as a first-line treatment for BPH in Germany, Austria, and Italy. Standard doses used for BPH are 160 mg twice daily. It is thought to work by inhibiting 5-α reductase activity and thus stops the conversion of testosterone to dihydrotestosterone along the androgen synthesis pathway. Saw palmetto may also inhibit dihydrotestosterone through competition at the androgen receptor site. Saw palmetto may have similar clinical effects to finasteride, prescribed for BPH, and can improve urinary flow and reduce nocturia. However, it is unclear if saw

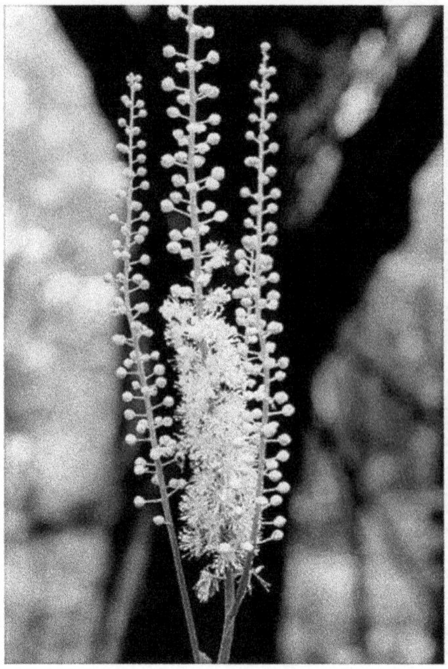

FIG. 6.5 Black cohosh.

palmetto can reduce prostate size in BPH. The supplement has also been used for male pattern hair loss, although the evidence is not strong.

Adverse effects of saw palmetto include increased bleeding risk for those with bleeding disorders or who take anticoagulants. Because saw palmetto affects androgen activity, it should be avoided in pregnancy due to adverse reproductive effects on the developing fetus. Likewise, saw palmetto can inhibit the action of androgen drugs such as testosterone and methyltestosterone and potentiate the effects of antiandrogen medications.

Saw palmetto has no known metabolism along the CYP450 pathway that would increase risks for drug interaction. Gastrointestinal side effects are common with saw palmetto, including nausea, vomiting, diarrhea, and abdominal pain. Other side effects include rhinitis, headache, decreased libido, and fatigue. This drug has had rare hypertension reports, palpitations, angina, and arrhythmias. However, determining strong causality between the use of saw palmetto and these side effects has been complex. One of the biggest concerns about the use of saw palmetto is that patients with developing prostate cancer can have symptoms similar to BPH, and the use of this remedy to treat symptoms of nocturia and poor urine stream could lead to delay in recognition or diagnosis of prostate cancer or prostatitis.

You should remember

Saw palmetto is not recommended for everyone. Those who are pregnant or nursing should avoid this supplement because of a lack of research on its safety and long-term effects. Because it can alter hormones, saw palmetto may be unsuitable for people taking hormone replacement therapy or hormonal contraceptives. It may also interfere with warfarin or heparin and increase bleeding risks.

Black cohosh

Black cohosh is found in the eastern United States, with a small plume of star-shaped white flowers (see Fig. 6.5). It contains chemicals known as phytoestrogens that have properties similar to estrogens. The herb is used very commonly to treat menopausal symptoms in females such as hot flashes, night sweats, vaginal dryness and

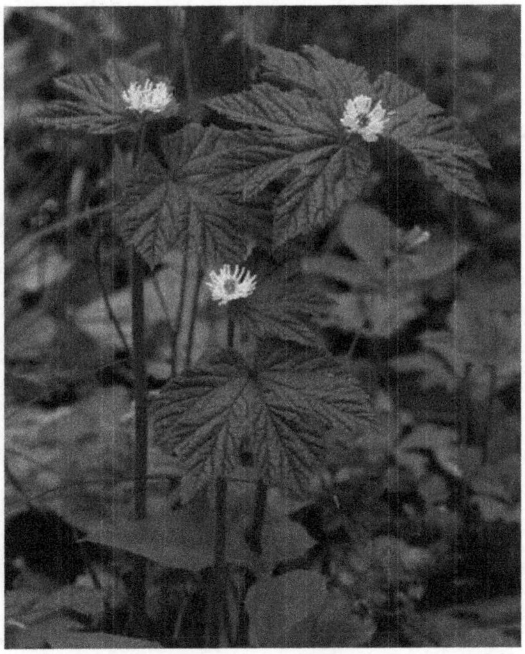

FIG. 6.6 Goldenseal.

irritation, and palpitations. Other uses include the treatment of dysmenorrhea, arthritis pain, menstrual migraines, breast cancer, and infertility.

Because black cohosh may affect estrogen receptors, it is unclear if this herbal product is safe for females with estrogen-dependent cancers (such as breast or endometrial). Black cohosh may precipitate premature labor in pregnant females, and one case report of liver failure occurred after a patient took black cohosh for several weeks. Side effects include headache, hypertension, palpitations, nausea, vomiting, and rash. Black cohosh may contain small amounts of salicylic acid, so those with aspirin allergies should not take this herb.

Goldenseal

Goldenseal is a perennial herb found in the Ohio River Valley (see Fig. 6.6). The plant bears fruit similar to a raspberry. Still, the root is used in herbal medicine to treat hypertension, poor appetite, menstrual problems, minor sciatic pain, muscle spasms, and infections, especially in the eyes and skin. Berberine salts constitute a significant component of goldenseal and are the source of some benefits. Common adverse effects include headache, hypotension, nausea, vomiting, leukopenia, and bradycardia. Goldenseal is probably unsafe when used at high doses or in the long term. The active constituent berberine can cause significant toxicity.

Goldenseal is contraindicated in females who are pregnant or breastfeeding and in infants because it has the potential to cause brain damage. It may also increase the risk of bleeding in people with bleeding disorders. Also, the supplement must be stopped at least 2 weeks before surgery due to these bleeding risks.

Chamomile

Chamomile is an herb obtained from a daisy-like plant of the family *Asteraceae* (see Fig. 6.7). It is used as a flavoring agent and herbal medicine. Its primary indications are to treat anxiety, nausea, intestinal gas, diarrhea, and mouth ulcers caused by chemotherapy or radiation treatment. It has also been used for insomnia, gingivitis, and skin irritations. The dry powder obtained from chamomile has been used for many health conditions because of its antiinflammatory, antioxidant, and mild astringent properties. The main constituents of the flowers of the chamomile plant are polyphenol compounds, which include *apigenin*, *luteolin*, *patulin*, and *quercetin*.

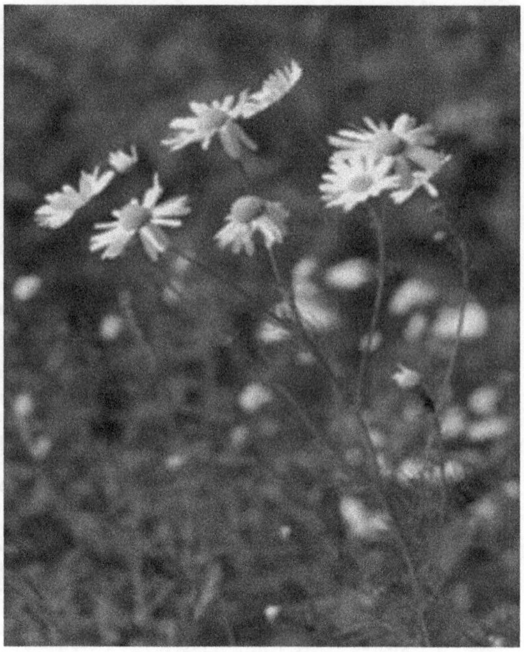

FIG. 6.7 Chamomile.

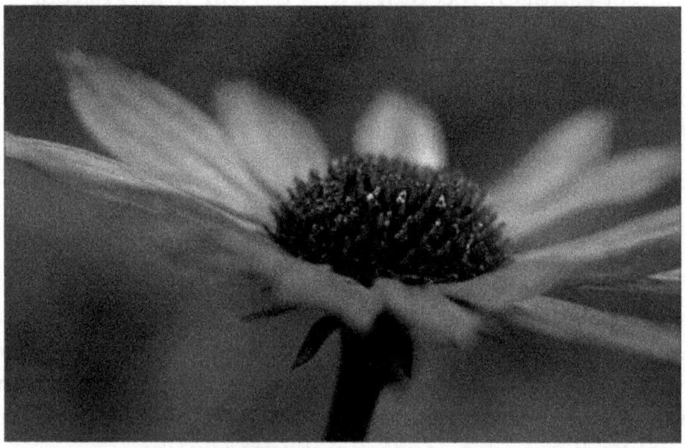

FIG. 6.8 Echinacea.

There have been adverse interactions with other herbal products and prescription drugs. Chamomile may worsen pollen allergies, and people allergic to *ragweed, in the same plant family,* may also be allergic to chamomile. The apigenin in chamomile may interact with anticoagulants and nonsteroidal antiinflammatory drugs. The other polyphenols in chamomile may interact with vitamins and sleep-enhancing **herbal supplements**. Chamomile also contains coumarin, increasing the chance for interactions with anticoagulants and antiplatelet drugs. Chamomile should not be used by people with a history of or current breast, ovarian, or uterine cancers, endometriosis, or uterine fibroids.

Echinacea

Echinacea is also called purple coneflower, one of the most popular herbs worldwide (see Fig. 6.8). Native Americans have used it for centuries to treat various ailments. Today, it is best known as an over-the-counter herbal remedy for the common cold or flu. However, it also treats pain, inflammation, migraines, and other health issues. Other uses include preventing upper respiratory infection and treating cancer, genital herpes, and otitis media in children.

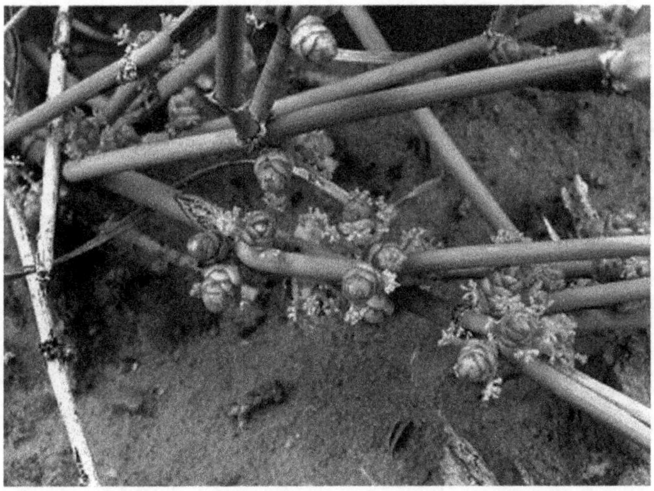

FIG. 6.9 Ma huang.

Sales of echinacea were about $110 million in 2019. The exact mechanism of action of the herb is unclear. Still, it may enhance phagocytosis, T-lymphocyte activity, and the release of inflammatory mediators such as **cytokines** and **tumor necrosis factor**. Both the root and the plant are used in various preparations.

Adverse effects of echinacea include anaphylaxis, and those with asthma appear at higher risk for this event. Other side effects include rash, urticaria, dyspepsia, nausea, and vomiting. Echinacea seems to modulate immune function, so it should not be used in patients who are undergoing treatment for cancer and HIV or who are taking other immunosuppressive drugs.

Ma huang

Ma huang (*Ephedra sinica)* is another herb used for thousands of years in Chinese medicine (see Fig. 6.9). The active ingredients are ephedrine and pseudoephedrine, primarily as sympathetic nervous system stimulants. Typical uses include appetite suppression, energy enhancement, and weight loss. In Germany, ephedra is approved to treat mild bronchospasm. Ma huang was banned by the US FDA in 2004 due to concerns that it presents a "significant and unreasonable human health risk of illness or injury." Despite this, internet vendors can obtain the herb in many preparations.

There are numerous safety concerns with ephedra's side effects related to the herb's sympathomimetic properties. Ephedra has more reported severe adverse events in the United States than any other herbal preparation. Hypertension, tachycardia, myocardial infarction, stroke, and cardiac rhythm disturbances are among the reported adverse events, and hundreds of these are reported worldwide. Other side effects include insomnia, dizziness, urinary retention, anxiety, nausea, headache, and nervousness.

You should remember

Ma huang can cause tachycardia, hypertension, palpitations, nausea, and vomiting. Over 800 dangerous reactions have been reported, including heart attacks, strokes, seizures, and sudden deaths. Approximately 1% of herbal supplement sales in the United States are products containing ma huang, but they are responsible for 62% of herbal supplement–related reports to poison control centers.

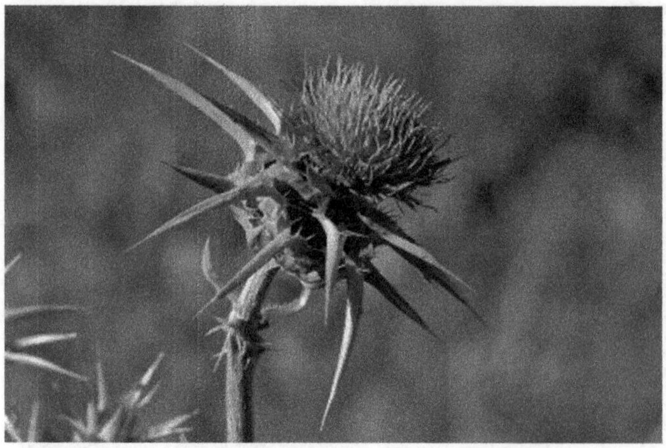

FIG. 6.10 Milk thistle.

Milk thistle

Milk thistle is an herb that is native to Kashmir but is also found in North America from Canada to Mexico (see Fig. 6.10). It is used as protection against alcoholic cirrhosis and hepatitis. Standardized extracts have shown some efficacy for preventing cirrhosis in clinical trials. It is thought that the active ingredient in milk thistle found in the seeds may have antioxidant action. Milk thistle is a reasonably safe compound with few side effects and interactions. The side effects may include nausea, abdominal pain, diarrhea, dyspepsia, and rash. There have been rare case reports of anaphylaxis and patients with allergies to other members of the milk thistle family. It should not be used during pregnancy and lactation.

Ginseng

Ginseng (*Panax ginseng*) is the primary form used in the United States and grown in Asia (see Fig. 6.11). Chinese medicine has used the root for varying purposes for thousands of years. The conditions under which the root is grown (season harvested, location where it was grown, age of the heart, and method used to dry the plant) can affect the properties of the root. Primary uses for ginseng include overall **adaptogenic** (increased energy and strength, improved memory, improved immune function, increased appetite), treatment of hyperglycemia in healthy subjects, and improved mental function. Ginseng is available in various preparations, including gum, candies, capsules, tablets, teas, and cigarettes.

Ginsenosides are 13 compounds found in the root thought to have medicinal activity, and interestingly, some of these compounds directly oppose the effects of other ginsenosides. Animal studies suggest that ginseng can affect **platelet aggregation** and enhance protein synthesis and natural killer cell activity.

The glucose-lowering effect of ginseng has been studied in small, randomized trials. Ginseng lowered fasting and postprandial glucose in healthy subjects without diabetes. However, the outcome could have been more consistent, and a dose-dependent result took time to discern. Ginseng does not appear to have the side effect of hypoglycemia, which is a promising safety benefit of the herb. Ginseng also has good evidence related to enhancing the impact of influenza vaccinations and preventing the common cold. Side effects of ginseng are few and mild but include rash, nausea, vomiting, and abdominal pain. There are reports of hypoglycemia, elevated blood pressure, low blood pressure, and breast tenderness at very high ginseng doses.

You should remember

Ginseng has a long list of adverse effects. These include diarrhea, insomnia, headaches, tachycardia, blood pressure fluctuations, vaginal bleeding, and breast tenderness. Ginseng may also produce mania and psychosis. Patients need to be hospitalized because of the development of acute mania after only 1 month of daily ginseng supplements.

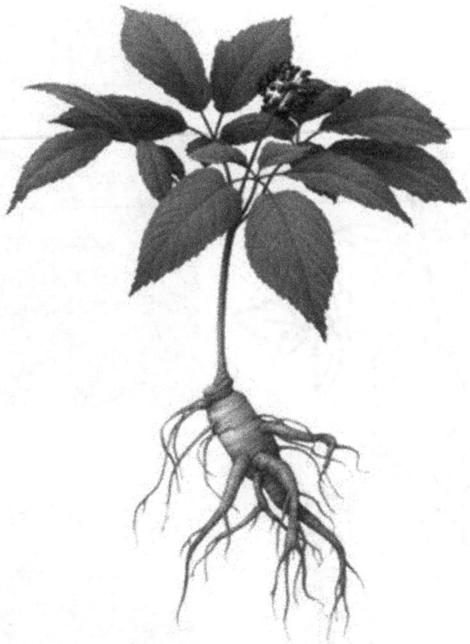

FIG. 6.11 Ginseng.

Dong quai

Dong quai is the common name for *Angelica sinensis* (female ginseng)—see Fig. 6.12. It is an herb from the family *Apiaceae*, which grows in China, Japan, and Korea. The yellow-brown root of the plant is harvested in the fall and has been used in Chinese medicine for thousands of years. It is primarily indicated for menopausal symptoms, menstrual cramps, and migraine headaches. Adverse effects of dong quai include increased skin sensitivity to sunlight, burping, flatulence, and hypertension. Taking high doses of dong quai for more than 6 months may increase the risk of developing cancer. It must be avoided during pregnancy because it can affect the uterus and increase the risk of congenital disabilities. It may also be linked to bleeding disorders, endometriosis, uterine fibroids, and cancers of the breast, uterus, and ovaries. Dong quai has a significant interaction with warfarin and can increase the risks of bruising and bleeding. Other exchanges include anticoagulant/antiplatelet drugs and estrogens.

Dong quai must be avoided if a person has chronic diarrhea or abdominal bloating or is at risk for hormone-related cancers such as breast, ovary, and uterus. In very high doses, dong quai may increase sensitivity to sunlight and cause skin inflammation or rashes. People taking dong quai are advised to stay out of the sun or use sunscreen.

Ginkgo

Ginkgo, also known as *Ginkgo biloba*, is one of the most common herbs sold in the United States, with sales topping $250 million in 2019. It is usually prepared as a leaf extract. The seeds are toxic, can induce seizures, and are not used medicinally. Ginkgo is used for the treatment of Alzheimer dementia, intermittent claudication, **premenstrual syndrome**, morning sickness, and memory improvement. The most concerning side effect of ginkgo is bleeding, with several case reports of spontaneous bleeding related to the use of ginkgo. Those on anticoagulant medications such as warfarin, aspirin, and clopidogrel may have an increased risk of bleeding. Other side effects include nausea, vomiting, diarrhea, and headache. Those who are allergic to **urushiol** may also be allergic to ginkgo. Ginkgo is a CYP3A enzyme inducer. The Ginkgo biloba tree is shown in Fig. 6.13.

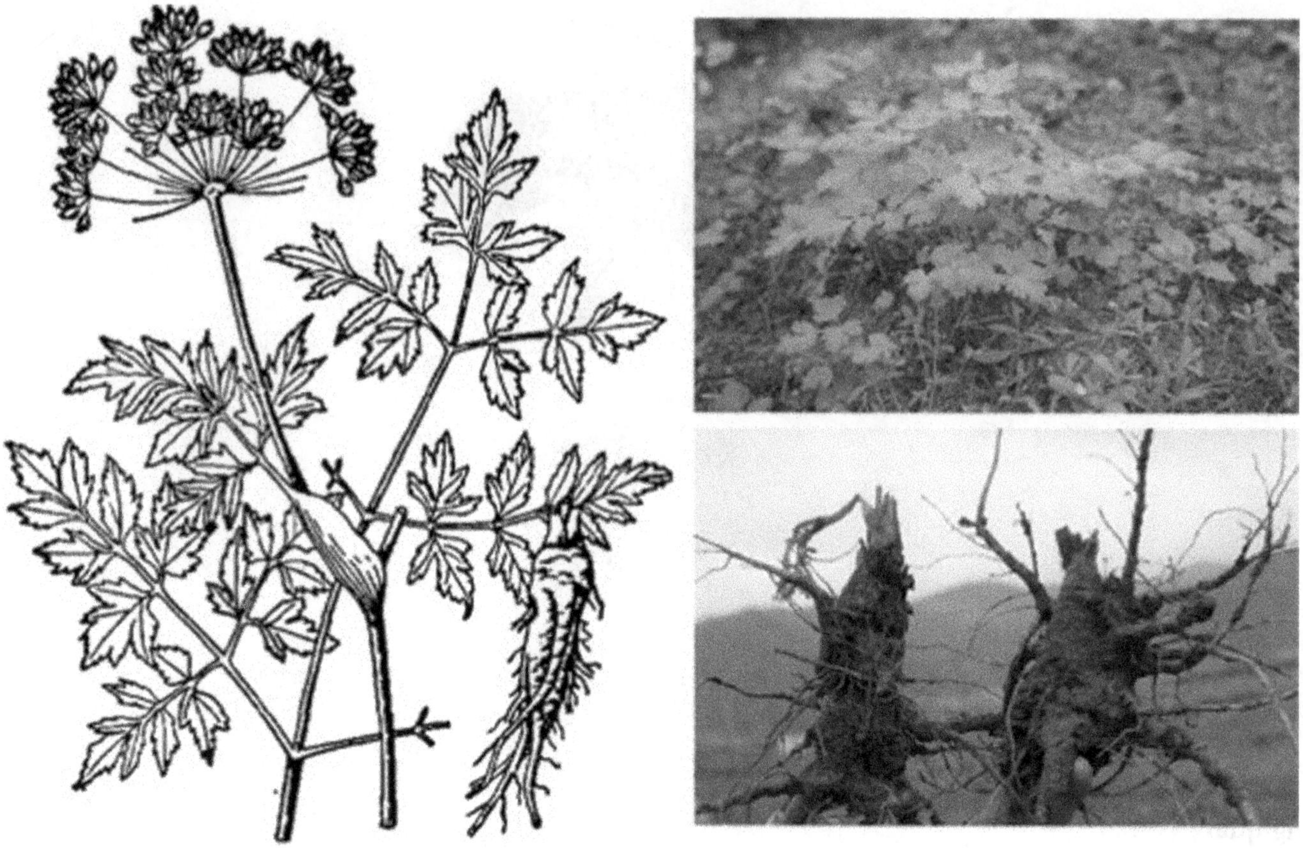

FIG. 6.12 Dong quai.

Kava kava

Kava kava is a plant found in the Pacific Islands and is most frequently used to treat anxiety. Other uses include stress reduction, insomnia, and **Parkinson disease**. Most preparations sold to consumers contain the ground root of the plant. Kava kava is sometimes mixed with alcohol or prepared as a tea in the South Pacific cultures (Australian Aboriginal cultures and Fiji) to produce relaxing effects.

Kava kava has been implicated in cases of liver toxicity and, as a result, has been removed from the market in some countries (Germany and Canada). However, it is available in the United States. Most liver toxicity cases have been related to heavy or chronic use and have involved cirrhosis, jaundice, and liver failure. Many cultures have used kava kava for hundreds of years, and it had been assumed to be safe before more recent case reports. Those who use kava tea long term in South Pacific cultures develop yellow skin, hair, and nail discoloration, which is related to the yellow pigment in the plant. Other side effects of concern also relate to chronic use and have been noted in South Pacific individuals. These include **ataxia**, azotemia, increased HDL cholesterol, hypoalbuminemia, hyperbilirubinemia, and perhaps pulmonary hypertension. Kava kava inhibits several CYP450 hepatic enzymes and thus has a high potential for adverse drug interactions. Kava kava should not be used concurrently with other hepatotoxic drugs.

You should remember

Over 100 reports of severe liver damage related to kava kava have been reported in the United States alone. Symptoms have included fatigue, nausea, jaundice, abnormal enzyme levels, rashes, and fever. Any person experiencing these symptoms must stop taking the supplement immediately. In high doses, long-term use of kava could also cause dry and scaly skin, yellowing of the skin, and abnormalities of the eyes and heart.

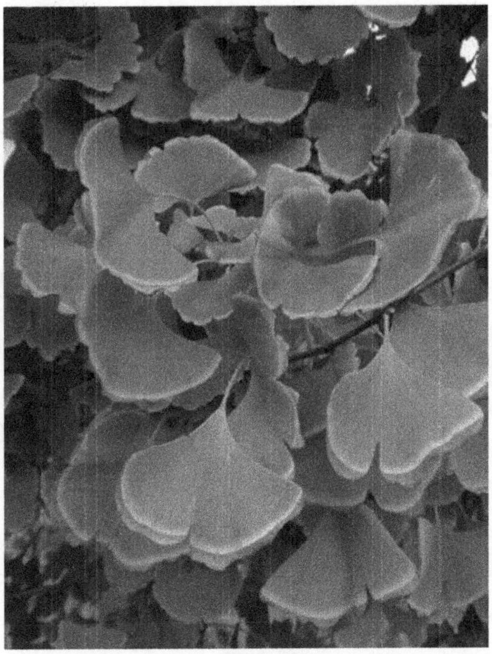

FIG. 6.13 The ginkgo biloba tree.

Valerian

Valerian is an herb found in Europe and parts of Asia, but it also grows in North America (see Fig. 6.14). It can be used to treat insomnia, anxiety, depression, and menopausal symptoms. The root and stem of the plant are used in preparations that include teas, tablets, tinctures, powders, and capsules. Valerian may also be a smooth muscle relaxant and act as a vasodilator. Daily use of valerian may be beneficial in improving sleep quality versus "as needed" help. A newer use of valerian is as a memory enhancement product for people with Alzheimer disease.

Side effects include headache, drowsiness, dry mouth, sedation, tachycardia, depression, and dyspepsia. Valerian does not appear to be metabolized by the CYP450 system; thus the potential for drug interactions is lower. Valerian may potentiate the sedative effects of other drugs that affect CNS function, including barbiturates, alcohol, and benzodiazepines.

Potential hazards of herbals

Many herbal remedies are biotransformed along the CYP450 family of metabolizing enzymes, making them an additional hazard for drug-drug and drug-herbal interactions. The most crucial advice healthcare providers can give patients is to make them aware that herbals can interact with other medications and supplements. Herbals should always be included on a medication list. Common herbal-herbal and herbal-drug interactions are listed in Table 6.1.

You should remember

It is essential to understand that the Food and Drug Administration does not regulate herbal supplements like prescription and over-the-counter drugs. This means that some accessories that can be easily purchased in drug stores are potentially dangerous, mainly when used with prescription medications. Discussing herbal supplements with a healthcare provider before taking them is always advised. The most common risks include drug interactions and damage to the liver or kidneys.

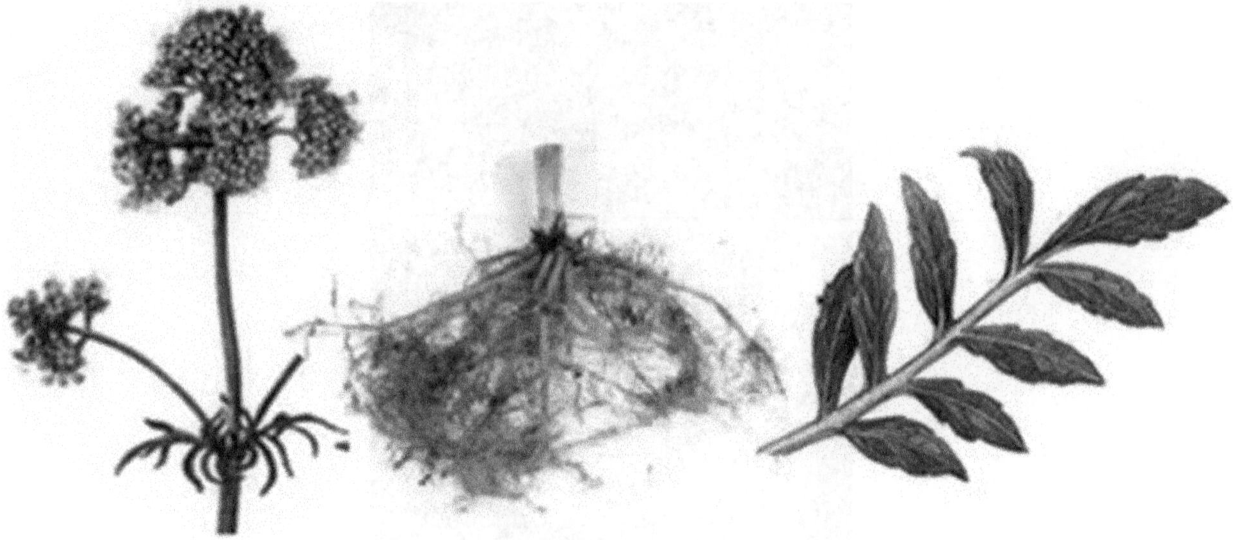

FIG. 6.14 Valerian.

TABLE 6.1 Common herbal-herbal and herbal-drug interactions.

Herbal	Interactions
Cinnamon	Antidiabetes drugs (severe hypoglycemia)
Saw palmetto	Androgens (antagonizes action of these drugs)
Goldenseal	Digoxin, cytochrome P450 2D6 substrates, cytochrome P450 3A4 substrates, P-glycoprotein substrates, dextromethorphan, losartan (altered clinical effects)
Chamomile	Sedatives, opioids, muscle relaxants, antianxiety drugs, antidepressants, anticonvulsants (increased sedation)
Garlic	Anticoagulants (increased bleeding risk) NSAIDs, platelet inhibitors such as ASA and clopidogrel, protease inhibitors (decreased drug concentrations)
Milk thistle	Ethanol (may negate the liver-protective actions of milk thistle)
Dong quai	Warfarin (increased potency and risks) Hormones (decreased or increased effects) Other herbs such as garlic, ginger, ginkgo, and ginseng (increased blood-thinning effects) St. John's wort (increased sensitivity to sunlight)
Ginkgo	Platelet inhibitors, anticoagulants, NSAIDs (increased risk for bleeding) Trazadone (excessive sedation)
Kava kava	Ethanol, other CNS sedatives (increased intoxication, sedation) Warfarin (increased INR, increased risk for bleeding) Parkinson drugs such as levodopa, apomorphine (decreased clinical effect)
St. John's wort	Linezolid, SSRIs, SNRIs (serotonin syndrome) MAO inhibitors (hypertensive crisis, convulsions, hyperthermia) Tramadol (decreased efficacy) General anesthesia (prolonged anesthesia effect, hypotension) Warfarin (decreased INR, increased risk of thrombosis) Protease inhibitors (decreased effectiveness)
Black cohosh	Oral contraceptives (may interfere with activity of estrogens) SERMs such as tamoxifen, raloxifene, toremifene (may interfere with actions)
Valerian	Ethanol, other CNS sedatives (increased intoxication, sedation)
Echinacea	Antineoplastic agents, antiretroviral protease inhibitors, antiretroviral nucleoside reverse transcriptase inhibitors, antiretroviral nonnucleoside reverse transcriptase inhibitors (monitor therapy for decreased clinical effects)

TABLE 6.1 Common herbal-herbal and herbal-drug interactions.—cont'd

Herbal	Interactions
Ginger	Platelet inhibitors, anticoagulants (increased risk of bleeding)
Ginseng	Warfarin (decreased INR, increased risk for thrombosis) Platelet inhibitors (increased risk for bleeding) Calcium channel blockers (inhibit metabolism, causing decreased effects)
Ma huang	Caffeine, appetite suppressants such as amphetamine, sibutramine, theophylline, MAO inhibitors (increased cardiovascular and CNS stimulation) Corticosteroids, antihypertensive drugs (decreased clinical effect)

ASA, Acetylsalicylic acid; *INR,* international normalized ratio; *MAO,* monoamine oxidase; *SERMS,* selective estrogen receptor modifiers; *SNRIs,* serotonin and norepinephrine reuptake inhibitors; *SSRIs,* selective serotonin reuptake inhibitors.

Key Terms

Adaptogenic
Alopecia
Ataxia
Black cohosh
Chamomile
Cytokines
Dong quai
Echinacea
Ginseng
Goldenseal
Herbal supplements
Leukotriene
Libido
Ma huang
Milk thistle
Parkinson disease
Platelet aggregation
Premenstrual syndrome
Prostaglandin
Saw palmetto
St. John's wort
Tumor necrosis factor
Urushiol
Valerian
Xerostomia

Clinical Case Studies

Clinical Case Study 1

A 67-year-old female was recently discharged from the hospital after a new onset of atrial fibrillation and the institution of anticoagulant therapy with warfarin. Her current daily medications include atenolol, enalapril, warfarin, and pravastatin. She is obese, with a weight of 210 pounds and a height of 5'6". Her physician has told her to lose weight and eat a cholesterol-free diet. She was also started on pravastatin (20 mg) during her recent hospitalization to help lower her LDL cholesterol (her current LDL cholesterol was 179 mg/dL). At an anticoagulation clinic, the patient is being monitored for warfarin therapy. During medication reconciliation, she asks whether it would be a good idea to start taking garlic tablets to help lower cholesterol.

Critical Thinking Questions

1. What should the patient be told about the advantages of garlic for lowering cholesterol and its other benefits?
2. What other therapy discussed in this chapter might help her lower LDL cholesterol?
3. What concerns related to side effects should be discussed?

Clinical Case Study 2

A 54-year-old male with a history of coronary artery disease, hypertension, and severe depression is brought to the emergency department by his family. The family reports that he has become increasingly confused and sweaty over the past 2 days, complaining of loose stools, headache, shivering, and palpitations. His vital signs are BP 190/120, pulse 138, respirations 32, and temperature 101.5°F. He is confused and oriented to name only, diaphoretic, shy, and restless in bed. The family brings in a bag with his home medications with them. The family also notes that he has a new St. John's wort bottle in his medication bag, with about eight tablets missing from the bottle according to a pill count. His current daily medications include citalopram, atenolol, atorvastatin, ramipril, amlodipine, and garlic (one tablet).

Critical Thinking Questions

1. What are the concerns related to his current drug regimen and the addition of St. John's wort?
2. What do you think could be causing some of his symptoms?
3. Why would a person with depression already on medication for depression add St. John's wort as self-treatment?

Further Reading

[1] F. Brinker, Herbal Contraindications and Drug Interactions plus Herbal Adjuncts with Medicines, fourth ed., Eclectic Medical Publications, 2010.
[2] M. Chandler Goldstein, M.A. Goldstein, Dietary Supplements: Fact Versus Fiction, Greenwood, 2020.
[3] S.J. Enna, S. Norton, Herbal Supplements and the Brain: Understanding Their Health Benefits and Hazards, F.T. Press – Science, 2012.
[4] A.R. Gaby, the Healthnotes Medical Team, A-Z Guide to drug-herb-vitamin Interactions, second ed., Harmony, 2006.
[5] S. Harrod Buhner, Herbal Antibiotics: Natural Alternatives for Treating Drug-Resistant Bacteria, second ed., Storey Publishing, 2012.
[6] B.B. Haycock, A.A. Sunderman, Dietary Supplements (Nutrition and Dietetics Practice Collection), Momentum Press – Health, 2016.
[7] M. Jafari, The truth about dietary supplements: an evidence-based guide to a safe medicine cabinet, Archangel Ink, 2021.
[8] L.E. Jesson, S.A. Tovino, Complementary and Alternative Medicine and the Law, Carolina Academic Press, 2010.
[9] D.C. Kailin, Quality in Complementary & Alternative Medicine, CMS Press, 2006.
[10] M.S. Micozzi, Fundamentals of Complementary, Alternative, and Integrative Medicine, sixth ed., Saunders, 2018.
[11] Physicians' Desk Reference, Inc., PDR for Nonprescription Drugs, Dietary Supplements, and Herbs, Thirtieth ed., Physicians' Desk Reference Inc, 2008.
[12] A. Sarubin Fragakis, C.A. Thompson, The Health Professional's Guide to Popular Dietary Supplements, third ed., 2007. American Dietetic Association.
[13] S.M. Talbott, K. Hughes, The Health Professional's Guide to Dietary Supplements, Lippincott, Williams, & Wilkins, 2006.
[14] R.B. Termini, Food and Drug Law: Federal Regulation of Drugs, Biologics, Medical Devices, Foods, Dietary Supplements, Personal Care, Veterinary and Tobacco Products, tenth ed., Forti Publications, 2019.
[15] K.M. Williams, Dr. Sebi's Book of Remedies. Sebi Books, 2021.
[16] P.A. Balch, Prescription for Nutritional Health – A Practical A-to-Z Reference to Drug-free Remedies Using Vitamins, Minerals, Herbs & Food Supplements, fifth ed., Avery, 2010.

CHAPTER

7

Adverse drug effects and drug interactions

OUTLINE

LEARNING OUTCOMES

After study of the chapter, readers should be able to:

1. Describe the adverse drug reaction.
2. Explain a narrow therapeutic index of drugs.
3. Identify the adverse drug reaction classifications.
4. Describe the signs and symptoms of idiosyncratic adverse drug reactions.
5. Discuss the drug-disease interaction.
6. Explain the drug-drug interaction classification.
7. Give two examples of pharmaceutical-drug interactions.
8. Describe the polypharmacy effect of drug interactions.
9. Explain the impact of prodrugs on the body.
10. Describe the role of computers in drug interactions.

Overview

The risk of dying from a drug-related incident now exceeds the risk of dying in a traffic accident. Every year in the United States, more than 4 billion prescriptions are dispensed, which is expected to increase substantially. The risk of adverse drug effects and drug interactions increases with the number of drugs a patient is taking. Forty percent of elderly patients take from five to nine medications, and 18% take 10 or more drugs. Adverse drug events cause

https://doi.org/10.1016/B978-0-443-29038-1.00007-5

approximately 1.3 million emergency department visits each year. About 350,000 patients each year need to be hospitalized for further treatment after emergency visits for adverse drug events. "Adverse drug event" is a broad term encompassing several drug mechanisms of action. However, the term is defined as any unexpected, unintended, undesired, or excessive response to a drug that requires discontinuing or changing the drug or modifying the dose; causes hospital admission or prolongs stay; requires supportive treatment; complicates diagnosis or negatively affects prognosis; or results in harm, disability, or death. Although this term is sometimes used interchangeably with "side effect," a side effect differs from an adverse drug reaction (ADR) in that it is an expected, well-known reaction resulting in little or no change in treatment.

Adverse drug effects

An **ADR** is a significant health problem worldwide, with high morbidity and mortality rates ranging from 0.5% to 16.8% in hospitalized children. It is an unpleasant or harmful reaction caused by an intervention related to the use of a drug product. Adverse effects usually predict hazards from future administration and warrant prevention, specific treatment, or alteration of the dosage regimen. The severity of ADRs varies by patient characteristics such as gender, age, genetics, ethnicity, coexisting disorders, or geographic factors. Drug factors include the type of drug, dose, dosage, administration route, treatment duration, and bioavailability. ADRs are more frequent in older adults and for those who engage in polypharmacy. In older adults, the use of anticoagulants in the presence of diabetes may cause more ADRs. The use of sedative and hypnotic drugs such as benzodiazepines and analgesics also contributes to drug-related harm.

Most ADRs are dose related and usually predictable, while ADRs unrelated to drug dose are generally unpredictable. ADRs are particularly concerning when drugs have a **narrow therapeutic index**, such as bleeding, as observed with oral anticoagulants. These ADRs may result from decreased drug clearance in patients with renal or liver impairment or from **drug-drug interactions** (DDIs).

Adverse drug reaction classifications

ADRs are increasingly common and are a significant cause of **morbidity** and **mortality**. They are classified into five categories: A, B, C, D, and E. Type A reactions are predictable from the known pharmacology of a drug and are associated with high morbidity and low mortality rates. Type B reactions are idiosyncratic, bizarre, or novel responses that cannot be predicted from the known pharmacology of a drug and are associated with low morbidity and high mortality. Type C persists for a relatively long time. An example is osteonecrosis of the jaw with bisphosphonates. Type D reactions, called delayed reactions, become apparent after using a medicine. The timing of these may make them more challenging to detect. Type E reactions are end-of-use events and are associated with the withdrawal of a drug. An example is insomnia, anxiety, and perceptual disturbances following the withdrawal of benzodiazepines. Age, gender, disease states, pregnancy, ethnicity, and polypharmacy influence susceptibility to ADRs.

Allergic reactions to medications refer to ADRs involving immune mechanisms, accounting for up to 15% of ADRs, and can be identified as a type I through IV immune reaction. The most common immunologic mechanism is an IgE-mediated type I reaction. Allergic ADRs are not dose related and require prior exposure. Allergies develop when a drug acts as an antigen or **allergen**. After a patient is sensitized, subsequent exposure to the drug produces one of several types of allergic reactions. Patient medical history and skin tests can help predict drug allergies.

Idiosyncratic ADRs have no clear definition. However, the term is used to designate an adverse reaction that does not occur in many patients treated with that drug, and these events do not involve the drug's therapeutic effect. The term may become obsolete as specific mechanisms of ADRs become known.

The signs and symptoms of an ADR manifest soon after the first dose or after chronic use. In older adults, subtle ADRs can cause functional deterioration, changes in mental status, depression, confusion, failure to thrive, and loss of appetite. Symptoms of allergic ADRs include itching, rash, upper or lower airway edema with difficulty breathing, and hypotension. Idiosyncratic ADRs can produce almost any symptom or sign and usually cannot be predicted.

Modifying the dose or eliminating or reducing triggering factors may be enough for dose-related ADRs to medications. For allergic and idiosyncratic ADRs, the drug usually should be discontinued and not tried again. Changing to a different drug class is often required for allergic ADRs and is sometimes needed for dose-related ADRs. For example, opioid-induced constipation may be improved with the use of an opioid receptor antagonist such as lubiprostone (Amitiza).

The prevention of ADRs requires understanding the medication and potential reactions to it. Computer-based analysis should be used to investigate possible drug interactions, and this investigation should be repeated when medications are changed or added. Medications and initial doses must be carefully selected for older adults, as various genes have been identified as being associated with ADRs. For example, multiple liver enzymes that affect liver metabolism of cytochrome P450 have been characterized.

You should remember

ADRs may be classified as mild, moderate, severe, or lethal. Severe or lethal ADRs may be mentioned explicitly in black box warnings in the physician prescribing information provided by the manufacturer.

Drug-drug interactions

DDI is the pharmacologic or clinical response to administering a combination of drugs that differs from the anticipated effects of the two drugs when given alone. It may result in ADRs, decreased therapeutic benefit, or patient harm. More than 100,000 types of potential drug interactions have been documented, but most do not lead to adverse effects. The incidence of ADRs is between 5% and 10% in patients. However, not all drug interactions are harmful. Some drug interactions are used therapeutically. For example, drugs used for numbing a specific area, such as local anesthetics, often contain a combination of lidocaine and epinephrine, thereby prolonging the effect of lidocaine in the area of the injection. Reversing agents such as naloxone (Narcan) are given after surgery to stop the effects of narcotics. Several drugs are given simultaneously for cancer treatment to provide a therapeutic effect at multiple sites of cancer cell growth. Beneficial drug interactions can improve treatment.

Drug-disease interaction

Sometimes interactions occur when a drug affects a preexisting disease or condition. Some disorders can interact with drugs to increase the risk of adverse effects. For example, aspirin increases bleeding in patients with peptic ulcer disease; people with hypertension may be at greater risk for tachycardia with oral decongestants found in over-the-counter cough, cold, and allergy products. Sometimes helpful drugs for one disease are harmful for another disorder. For example, some beta-blockers taken for heart disease or hypertension can worsen asthma or make it difficult for patients with diabetes to know when their blood sugar is too low. Aging can also increase drug interaction risks. For example, sedatives increase the risk of falls in older adults, and lower doses of narcotics are often most effective for pain relief. The anticoagulant warfarin causes more bleeding in elderly patients and usually requires a lower dose, too.

Interactions can also occur when a food changes the expected effect of a drug. For example, milk decreases the absorption of antibiotics such as tetracycline or ciprofloxacin; grapefruit juice increases the impact of some statin and antihypertensive medications. Drug-herb interactions occur when an herb or dietary supplement changes the expected effect of a drug. For example, **ginkgo biloba** may increase the impact of anticoagulants, and calcium supplements may reduce the absorption of thyroid supplements. This review will focus on DDI mechanisms and include examples of common drug interactions.

You should remember

Understanding potential drug interactions is an integral part of pharmaceutical care. The term "drug interactions" includes drug-disease interactions, drug-herb interactions, drug-food interactions, and DDIs.

You should remember

Drinking grapefruit juice can interact with certain statin drugs for lowering cholesterol, such as simvastatin (Zocor) and atorvastatin (Lipitor). Grapefruit juice inhibits statin metabolism, causing drug accumulation and toxicity, increasing the risk of liver and kidney failure and fibromyalgia.

Drug-drug interaction classification

DDIs can be classified outside or inside the body. Most pharmaceutical drug interactions, referred to as "unsuitable" reactions, occur outside the body, whereas pharmacological interactions may occur inside the body. Pharmaceutical interactions generally occur before drugs are administered to the patient.

Pharmaceutical drug interactions

Pharmaceutical drug interactions can be divided into chemical and physical reactions. An example of a chemical reaction is the unsuitable calcium chloride and potassium phosphate in parenteral nutrition preparations or hyperalimentation. The two drugs may interact to form calcium phosphate, resulting in a residue in the IV fluid bag. Status epilepticus is a life-threatening condition that requires medication to stop the seizures as soon as possible. Two commonly used anticonvulsant drugs, phenytoin and lorazepam, become ineffective if mixed in the same IV bag or syringe.

Physically altering a drug formulation, such as by crushing a **sustained-release** tablet, could result in the drug being released more quickly and in a more significant amount. Alcohol or food given with some sustained-release products may cause similar problems. Another example of a physical reaction is when the thyroid drug levothyroxine sticks to IV bags. Sometimes one drug can alter the formulation of another drug, for example, the combination of diazepam with the emulsion propofol. Diazepam destabilizes the propofol emulsion, causing a thin layer of oil and making it dangerous to administer intravenously.

Environmental conditions can adversely affect drugs. Ultraviolet light can cause some drugs to degrade and become less effective. This is why medicine bottles are usually amber or opaque. Humidity can have a similar effect on drugs. Other environmental conditions can affect drug absorption. For example, heating pads can increase the release of the narcotic fentanyl from transdermal patches.

Pharmacological drug interactions

DDIs are commonly identified from reactions within the body, which are pharmacological interactions, and these can be classified as pharmacodynamic or pharmacokinetic interactions.

Polypharmacy effect of drug interactions

In the United States, 48% of the population take at least one prescription medicine, and more than 10% take five or more prescription medications. Given the thousands of prescription and over-the-counter drugs and dietary supplements available, the number of possible combinations and potential DDIs is surprising. Fortunately, many potential DDIs do not have a noticeable clinical effect. For the interaction to be clinically significant, the interaction must cause a change in the expected response to the drug. DDIs may cause different reactions in different patients and are affected by many factors. Logically, the risk of a DDI is higher with the increased number of drugs a patient is taking. Older adults who have more chronic diseases are at particular risk for DDIs. Patients older than 74 years of age are six times more likely to be taking potentially interacting drugs.

Genetic factors are becoming increasingly recognized contributors to ADRs and metabolic DDIs. The CYP enzymes 2D6, 2C19, 2C9, 1A2, and 3A4 exhibit genetic polymorphism, which refers to genetic differences that produce functional or nonfunctional enzymes within a population. People who have genetically determined low enzyme activity are poor metabolizers. Other people make more enzymes than most of the population and are "ultrametabolizers." For CYP1A2 and -3A4, most people produce intermediate amounts of enzyme; this is the so-called normal population. Few people have very low or very high activity. Genetic variations of CYP2D6, -2C19, and -1A2 are considerable and may also explain differences in drug response among individual patients.

Prodrugs rely on the body for conversion to an active form. They improve a medication's efficacy and may be designed to avoid specific side effects or toxicities. Prodrugs are essential for developing new medications; certain medications only work because they are a prodrug. The antiplatelet drug clopidogrel is an example of a prodrug: it has no pharmacological activity until it is metabolized in the liver to its active form by CYP2C19. Proton pump inhibitors such as omeprazole (Prilosec), which are taken to reduce the secretion of acid in the stomach, also inhibit the activity of CYP2C19 and decrease the metabolism of clopidogrel to its active form. The interaction between drugs that inhibit CYP2C19 and clopidogrel might be significant in patients who do not adequately produce CYP2C19.

Other factors that can increase the risk for DDIs include patient-specific conditions such as kidney impairment or liver failure, which may reduce the body's ability to eliminate drugs. Comorbidity diseases or conditions such as malnutrition, severe heart failure, and dehydration could also increase DDI risk. Drug-specific factors, such as the dose of a drug or drugs with a high risk for toxicity (e.g., digoxin, cyclosporine, and warfarin), can increase DDI risk.

You should remember

Adverse effects from DDIs are more common in females than males. Females generally weigh less than males but are usually given the same dose of a drug; however, other factors, such as differences in the way females metabolize or eliminate medicines, may also be involved.

The role of computers in drug interactions

Computer programs are widely available to identify potential drug interactions. Although this seems helpful, computerized DDI alerts have not been shown to decrease the risk of adverse events caused by DDIs. Alerts are triggered so frequently that they are largely ignored. To prevent a single ADR of any severity, an estimated DDI alert must be reviewed. To avoid a single severe ADR, an estimated 2715 alerts must be reviewed. To prevent a single event leading to death, disability, or prolonged symptoms, the clinician must review 4292 to 44,350 alerts. Efforts to eliminate alerts with little clinical value are underway.

Many online pharmacy references, such as **Lexicomp** and **Micromedex**, include information on drug interactions. Trissel's Stability of Compounded Formulations is an online resource and book for nonoral drugs that provides specific compatibility and stability data. None of these resources covers all potential DDIs, but they provide information about interactions of particular clinical concerns.

You should remember

One of the most promising aspects of artificial intelligence in drug discovery is its ability to predict the efficacy and safety of a new drug candidate. Artificial intelligence uses predictive analytics to analyze vast amounts of data from various sources, including clinical trials, scientific literature, and social media, identifying trends, patterns, and potential risks. Such algorithms can speed up the identification of possible side effects and drug interactions.

Key Terms

Adverse drug reaction
Allergic reactions
Drug-drug interactions
Ginkgo biloba
Idiosyncratic adverse drug reactions
Lexicomp

Micromedex
Morbidity
Mortality
Narrow therapeutic index
Prodrugs
Sustained release

Clinical Case Studies

Clinical Case Study 1

A 14-year-old male was hospitalized for tuberculosis with no history of liver or kidney disease. The skin test was positive, and a chest X-ray confirmed the infection. Treatment with isoniazid (INH), rifampin, and pyrazinamide was initiated. After 10 days, liver enzymes were elevated. Because of liver toxicity, both INH and rifampin doses were reduced. Subsequently, liver enzymes and uric acid increased again. Therefore rifampin-INH therapy was discontinued. Allopurinol treatment was initiated, and there was suspected INH toxicity.

Critical Thinking Questions

1. What are the concepts of ADRs?
2. What are the risk factors for ADRs?
3. What are the five categories of ADRs?

Clinical Case Study 2

A 31-year-old male with HIV/AIDS had a history of injected drug use, idiopathic thrombocytopenic purpura, gastrointestinal bleeding, and chronic hepatitis C. The HIV infection was being treated with lamivudine and nevirapine. A recent chest X-ray revealed bilateral infiltrates, prompting a concern that the patient may have tuberculosis. He was treated with itraconazole, but it did not improve the symptoms, and he developed headaches, nausea, and vomiting. A drug-drug reaction was discovered to have occurred between itraconazole and nevirapine.

Critical Thinking Questions

1. What is the concept of a DDI?
2. How many DDIs have been documented?
3. How can DDIs be used therapeutically?

Clinical Case Study 3

A 59-year-old female has previously been diagnosed with chronic kidney disease. Due to familial hypercholesterolemia, she has been taking a statin for several years. Her recent blood tests revealed she needs a higher dose to manage her cholesterol. Soon after switching to the higher dose, she began to experience symptoms related to cardiovascular disease, which she did not have before. The physician reduces her statin to a lower dose, and the symptoms subside.

Critical Thinking Questions

1. How can drug-disease interactions occur?
2. How can drugs that are helpful for one disease be harmful to another disease?
3. How can drugs interact with the effects of aging?

Further Reading

[1] J.K. Aronson, Meyler's Side Effects of Drugs—The International Encyclopedia of Adverse Drug Reactions and Interactions, sixteenth ed., Elsevier, 2015.
[2] D. Barenholtz Levy, Maybe it's your medications—how to avoid unnecessary drug therapy and adverse drug reactions, Skyhorse (2023).
[3] I.H. Bowen, D. Corrigon, J.I. Cubbin, P.A.G.M. de Smet, R. Hansel, U. Sonnenborn, J. Westendorf, H. Winterhoff, H.J. Woerdenbag, Adverse Effects of Herbal Drugs, second ed., Springer-Verlag, 2012.
[4] F. Brinker, Herbal Contraindications and Drug Interactions—Plus Herbal Adjuncts with Medicines, fourth ed., Eclectic Medical Publications, 2010.
[5] J.K. Grover, Adverse Drug Reactions, CBS Publishers and Distributors Pvt Ltd, 2018.
[6] T.K.L. Kiang, K.J. Wilby, M.H.H. Ensome, Pharmacokinetic and pharmacodynamic drug interactions associated with antiretroviral drugs, Adis (2016).
[7] A. Lee, M. Cuthbert, Adverse Drug Reactions, third ed., Pharmaceutical Press, 2023.
[8] E. Ozkaya, K. Didem Yazganoglu, Adverse Cutaneous Drug Reactions to Cardiovascular Drugs, Springer, 2014.

[9] M.P. Pai, J.J. Kiser, P.O. Gubbins, K.A. Rodvold, Drug Interactions in Infectious Diseases—Antimicrobial Drug Interactions, fourth ed., Humana Press, 2018 (Infectious Disease Series).

[10] S.C. Piscitelli, K.A. Rodvold, M.P. Pai, Drug Interactions in Infectious Diseases, third ed., Humana Press, 2011 (Infectious Disease Series).

[11] S.H. Preskorn, Drug-Drug Interactions with an Emphasis on Psychiatric Medications, Professional Communications, Inc., 2018.

[12] C.L. Preston, Stockley's Drug Interactions—A Source Book of Interactions, Their Mechanisms, Clinical Importance and Management, twelfth ed., Pharmaceutical Press, 2019.

[13] J. Talbot, J.K. Aronson, Stephens' Detection and Evaluation of Adverse Drug Reactions—Principles and Practice, sixth ed., Wiley-Blackwell, 2011.

C H A P T E R

8

Drug approval and drug regulations

OUTLINE

LEARNING OUTCOMES

After study of the chapter, readers should be able to:

1. Explain the four phases of drug approval.
2. Describe the drug approval process.
3. Discuss the Harrison Narcotic Act of 1914.
4. Give four examples of diseases or conditions treated by orphan drugs.
5. Describe the benefits of the Medicare Prescription Drug, Improvement, and Modernization Act.
6. Explain why pharmacopeias were established.
7. Describe the three primary missions of the FDA.
8. List the seven branches of the FDA.
9. Describe the advantages of e-prescriptions.
10. Explain the Controlled Substances Act.

Overview

The process of new therapeutic drugs being discovered, developed, and approved for commercial use is long, complicated, and highly regulated. It can take up to 15 years and cost more than $2.6 billion to bring a new drug into the market. During this period, experts from many disciplines must interact with extreme coordination. Estimates show that up to 2000 different people may be involved in the process. All of the time, cost, and effort involved result in only about 10% of drugs being approved after clinical testing. This is often caused by toxicities that were not

The Science of Pharmacology
https://doi.org/10.1016/B978-0-443-29038-1.00008-7

anticipated or by a lack of a drug's effectiveness. However, the process is under continuing improvement so that time and costs can be reduced and better safety and efficacy can be achieved. During the early phases of drug development, some steps help detect toxicities sooner and better evaluate factors concerning drug metabolism and bioavailability. These steps help prevent the new drug from advancing to further action that will likely fail and cost millions more than needed. It is essential that for each step involved in drug development, the level of confidence is very high—to avoid moving the drug forward unnecessarily.

Drug approval

The Food and Drug Administration (FDA) reviews therapeutic drugs and biologics in four different phases: preclinical investigation, clinical investigation, new drug application review, and postmarketing surveillance. Table 8.1 further describes these phases.

You should remember

Clinical research studies determine the effects of independent and dependent variables. An *independent variable* is a treatment, such as with a drug, while a *dependent variable* is an outcome, such as a clinical effect. *Intervening variables* can interfere with the study's results, including age, sex, weight, disease state, diet, and social environment. Intervening variables must be controlled as much as possible.

Every year, the FDA holds meetings to review patient and healthcare provider feedback on new drugs. A drug can be ordered to be withdrawn when serious problems are found. The FDA offers the MedWatch subscription service and substantial drug safety information to the public. The drug approval process in the United States is being

TABLE 8.1 The four phases of FDA review of drugs and biologics.

Phase	Description	Comments
Preclinical investigation	Extensive research in a laboratory, using human and microbial cells. Cultured cells and animal studies are also used to determine dosages, effectiveness, and adverse effects. This phase usually takes 1 to 3 years, with an average of 18 months to complete. Animal pharmacology and toxicology data are obtained. Drug developers can determine **genotoxicity**, which involves damage to the genetic information in cells.	This phase is not conclusive because results may be insufficient or excessive compared to how human test subjects will react. In 2007, the FDA Critical Path Initiative improved bioinformatics, imaging, **genomics**, and **proteonomics**.
Phase 1: clinical investigation	This phase requires several months and is conducted in healthy	This phase does not include subjects who have the disease under

TABLE 8.1 The four phases of FDA review of drugs and biologics.—cont'd

Phase	Description	Comments
	volunteers who do not have the disease under investigation. Bodily fluid samples are taken to assess pharmacokinetics and pharmacodynamics and to establish safety.	investigation, so the safety established in this phase may not always be certain in future phases.
Phase 2: clinical investigation	This phase takes 2 to 10 years, with an average of 5 years, and is divided into three different subphases. *Clinical phase 1 trials* occur over several months, with doses and adverse effects being assessed on 20 to 100 volunteers who have the disease or condition for which the drug is intended to treat.	Most manufacturers begin developing the trade name during clinical phase I trials, with doses often being subtherapeutic but increasing, determining if the drug is safe, so it can be confirmed with respect to safety. About 70% of drugs can move on to the next phase.
	Clinical phase 2 trials require several months to 2 years, testing several dozen to 300 volunteers with the disease or condition. The drug is assumed not to be therapeutically useful until additional testing occurs.	Investigators come from a variety of medical specialties. Effectiveness, harmful effects, unsafe drug interactions, and different effects in various types of patients are assessed. About 33% of drugs tested will move on to the next phase.
	Clinical phase 3 trials require 1–4 years, with several hundred to about 3000 volunteers being tested. The drug is assumed to be therapeutically effective in this phase. Some drugs require a "fourth clinical phase" with testing in several thousand volunteers, but this is uncommon.	Responses vary widely. If there are no serious adverse effects, this phase can speed up the drug approval process. Sometimes with careful monitoring, the drug is approved for immediate use. However, precautions may be found that cause changes to be made to the new drug product. Only about 25% to 30% of drugs move on to the next phase. An NDA must be submitted. If the drug has significant therapeutic effects and is reasonably safe, an IND is submitted.
Phase 3: review of the NDA	The trade name is finalized. Clinical trials and more animal	If approved, the process continues. If rejected, the manufacturer must

Continued

TABLE 8.1 The four phases of FDA review of drugs and biologics.—cont'd

Phase	Description	Comments
	testing may continue if needed. The FDA must make its first NDA review within 6 months, but this phase may require 2 months to 7 years.	address any concerns, and the process resumes. Most new drugs require about 24 months for a full NDA review.
Phase IV: postmarketing surveillance	This starts after clinical trials are completed and the NDA has been reviewed. Adverse effects sometimes manifest once the drug is on the market that were not seen in clinical trials.	Drugs withdrawn because of this phase include aprotinin, gatifloxacin, propoxyphene, lumiracoxib, ozogamicin, pergolide, and sibutramine because of severe and possibly life-threatening adverse effects. Famously, valdecoxib, celecoxib, and rofecoxib were withdrawn because of causing strokes and heart attacks. Celecoxib remains on the market but with a black box warning (potentially fatal cardiovascular disease, severe gastrointestinal problems, and bleeding ulcers).

IND, Investigational new drug application; *NDA*, new drug application.

revised to streamline its activities and reduce the time required. The FDA may take years to complete drug reviews, with hundreds of millions spent on each newly developed drug. Discovering and developing new drugs is also summarized in Fig. 8.1.

Changes to the drug approval process

Because the drug approval process can take many years, volumes of experimental and clinical data, and huge costs, changes designed to improve the process are being implemented. Drug manufacturers are eager to get each drug to market to recoup their expenses. The public is also anxious to find new, safe, and effective medications for diseases and conditions of all types. The FDA is responsible for caring for the people, yet it still tries to get the drugs needed to be marketed as soon as possible. Clinical research must follow the Good Clinical Practice Consolidated Guideline, which comprises international ethics and scientific quality standards.

Beginning in the early 1990s, the federal government initiated steps to speed up the drug approval process. Guidelines were improved, communication was sped up, and enough people were added. When the Prescription Drug User Fee Act was passed in 1992, drug and biologic manufacturers were required to provide yearly product user fees. This new revenue allowed the FDA to restructure and handle new drug applications more efficiently. Priority drugs received faster approval, including those to treat severe or life-threatening conditions that lacked effective treatments, such as acquired immunodeficiency syndrome and cancer. Sometimes the FDA grants accelerated approval before a drug completes phase 3 trials, requiring the manufacturer to file additional reports confirming the drug's effectiveness.

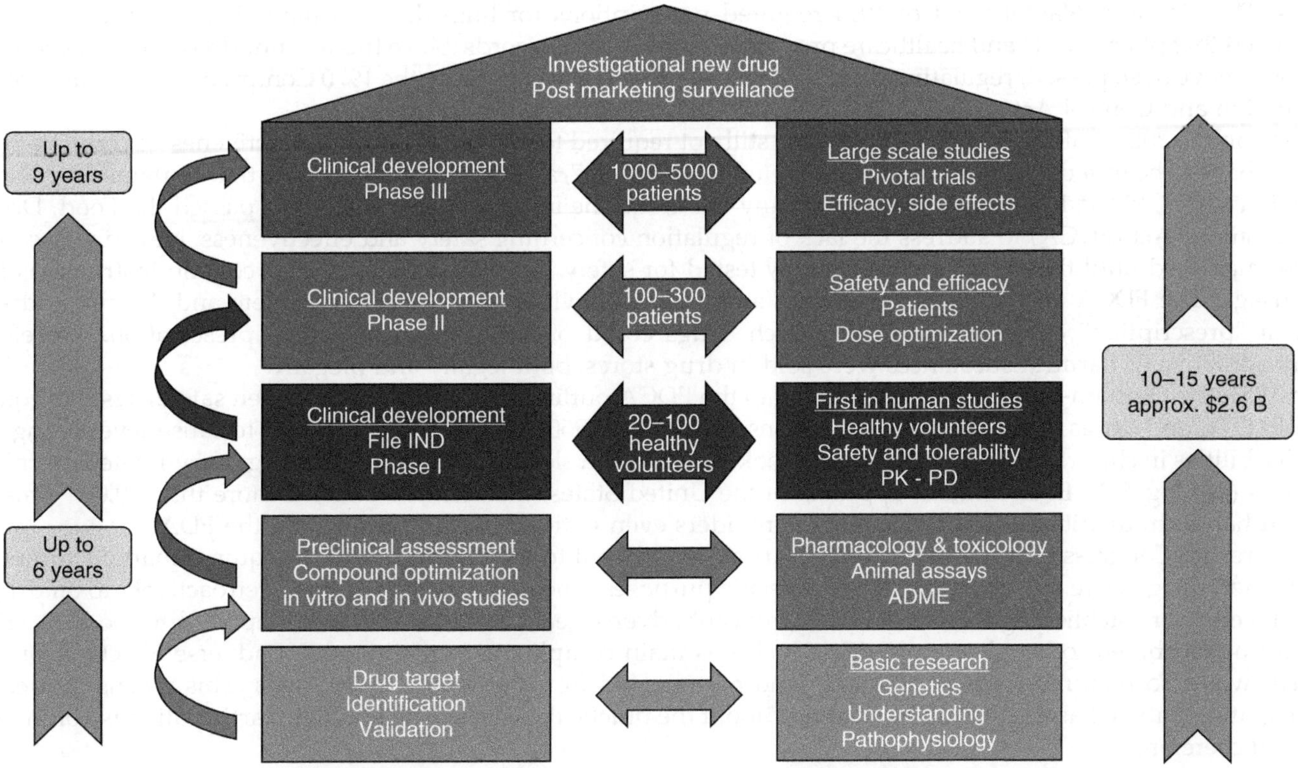

FIG. 8.1 The drug discovery and development process. *ADME*, Absorption, distribution, metabolism, excretion; *IND*, investigational new drug; *PK*, pharmacokinetics; *PD*, pharmacodynamics. *From Wecker, L., Taylor, D.A., Theobald, R.J. [2019]. Brody's human pharmacology [6th ed.]. Philadelphia: Elsevier.*

You should remember

For the first time in vaccine development, the first two vaccines for COVID-19 (by Pfizer and Moderna) were created, evaluated, and authorized for emergency use in less than 1 year. Even though their development timeline was accelerated, the vaccines went through appropriate clinical trials, and the CDC closely monitors them for safety and efficacy. The speed at which the vaccines were developed occurred because of global cooperation between scientists from many countries.

Brief history of drug legislation

Following early attempts by individual states to regulate drugs, the first federal law was the Drug Importation Act of 1848. Its goal was to stop unsafe medicines from entering the United States. Later, when 13 children died after being given diphtheria antitoxin that was contaminated with tetanus, the 1902 Biologics Control Act was passed. It focused on standardizing the quality of serums, antitoxins, and other blood-related products. The Pure Food and Drug Act (PFDA) of 1906 was passed to allow the government to regulate medication labeling. It required each drug label to reflect the actual contents accurately. Before this act, drug labels often contained no information about active ingredients or their quantities. However, the PFDA did not control any drug's marketing; therefore drugs could still be marketed for any disease the manufacturer chose.

In 1912, the PDFA was altered by the Sherley Amendment, which prohibited selling drugs with false therapeutic claims intended to defraud consumers. Many legal battles ensued, and it was evident that there was difficulty in proving that drug sellers made intentionally false claims. No attempt had yet been made to legislate any addictive drugs. The Harrison Narcotic Act of 1914 required prescriptions for high doses of narcotic medications. It also mandated that pharmacists and healthcare providers keep narcotic records. Since this act, hundreds of state and federal laws have been passed, regulating drugs with abuse potential—especially the 1970 Comprehensive Drug Abuse Prevention and Control Act.

Early in the 20th century, manufacturers were still not required to prove each drug's effectiveness. Product safety did not have to be tested before a cure was marketed. Then in 1937, an elixir of sulfanilamide that contained a poison, *diethylene glycol*, killed 107 people, including many children. The following year, Congress passed the Food, Drug, and Cosmetic Act (FDCA) to address the lack of regulation concerning safety and effectiveness. New drugs could not be marketed until they had been thoroughly tested for safety. Drug labels now had to contain instructions for safe usage. The FDCA also regulated cosmetics and medical devices. It was still incomplete and did not address what a "prescription" consisted of or list which drugs could only be acquired with a prescription. Therefore many addictive or harmful substances were sold in drug stores, both legally and illegally.

In 1951, the Durham-Humphrey Amendment to the FDCA outlined the difference between safe drugs that could be sold OTC and drugs that required prescriptions. Late in the 1950s, *thalidomide* was found to cause severe congenital disabilities in children born to females who took the drug as a sleeping pill or to treat pregnancy-related morning sickness (see Fig. 8.2). Even without approval in the United States, thalidomide affected more than 20,000 Americans. It had been distributed to US healthcare providers even without being approved by the FDA.

As a result, Congress passed the Kefauver-Harris Amendment to the FDCA in 1962. It required manufacturers to prove their drugs were effective and safe for specific purposes. The law was then applied retroactively to all drugs introduced after establishing the FDCA. All significant adverse reactions now had to be reported to the FDA. The literature distributed to healthcare providers had to contain complete information about adverse effects. *Informed consent* was also required from any patient who participated in experimental drug trials. This means that each participating patient has the right to be informed about the practical use of a drug and that participation is voluntary, with no coercion.

Informed consent includes the mutual sharing of information, showing respect for each patient, helping the patients to be involved in their care, and respecting the right to self-determination. When giving written consent, the patient must be alert and understand what is being agreed to. The duty to protect patients in research studies from harm is known as *beneficence. Autonomy* is the right to self-determination.

Every patient has the right to make healthcare decisions in their best interest. For every clinical study, all possible outcomes must be analyzed and balanced against risks and likely benefits. This is known as the **risk-benefit ratio**

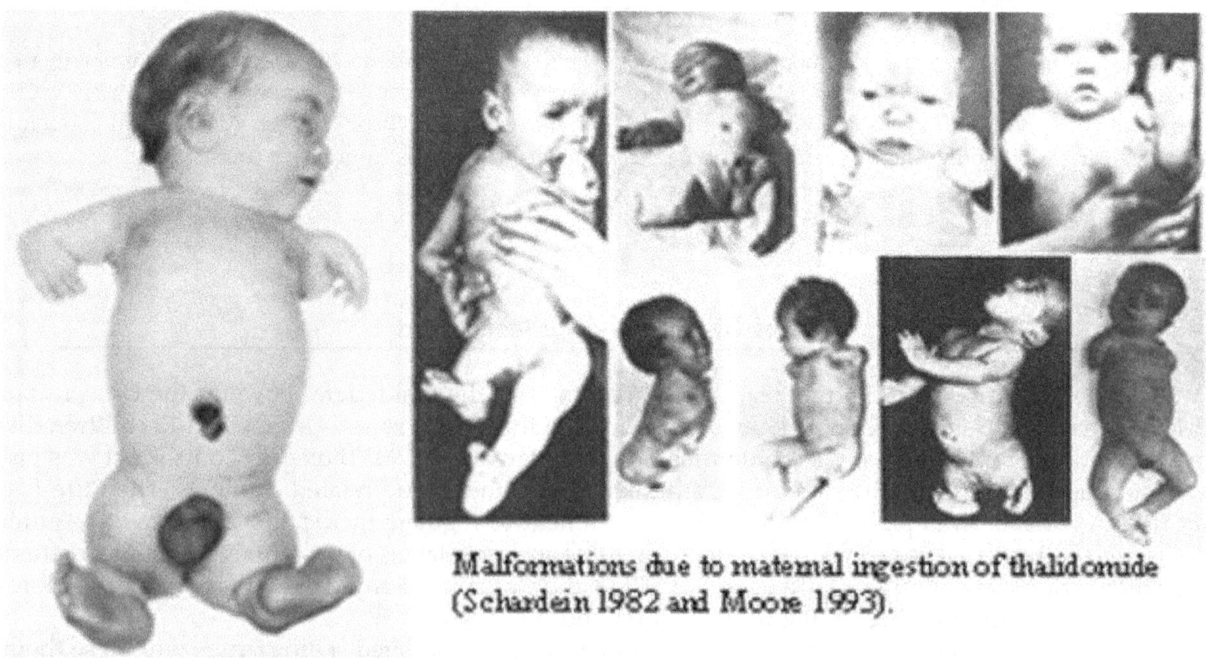

FIG. 8.2 A patient's hands affected by the thalidomide tragedy of the 1950s.

and includes physical, psychological, and social risks. Informed consent forms used in these studies include the title of the study, the principal investigator's name, an introduction of the study's purpose, background information, meaning, intended procedures, possible risks and benefits, an explanation of the right of refusal to participate and withdraw from the study, information about confidentiality, and available sources of information. So that justice is done, the selection of research subjects must be fair, with the distribution of benefits and burdens being equitable to everyone regardless of social class, race, and ethnicity.

You should remember

The experimental group in a drug trial receives the drug being tested. The control group may receive no drug, a drug, a placebo, a pharmacologically inert substance, or the actual drug being tested in a different dose, route, or frequency of administration.

The FDA joined with the National Academy of Sciences and the National Research Council in 1966, evaluating the effectiveness of 4000 drugs approved between 1938 and 1962 that had only been approved because they were considered safe. The study revealed that about 40% of these drugs were ineffective, so they were removed from the market. A 1972 review of OTC drugs examined their safety and effectiveness. In 1970, the *Comprehensive Drug Abuse Prevention and Control Act* was passed to promote drug education and research into the prevention and treatment of drug dependence, strengthen enforcement authority, establish treatment and rehabilitation facilities, and designate drug schedules for controlled substances based on their potential for abuse.

In the 1980s, the public pressured the FDA to find drugs that could treat rare or unusual disorders. Manufacturers were reluctant to develop such drugs due to the need for more profit potential. Therefore the 1983 Orphan Drug Act was passed to create drugs or biologics that treat rare diseases that affect less than 200,000 people in the United States. The government offered manufacturers grants, tax credits, and 7 years of drug exclusivity. Since then, more than 400 orphan drugs have been approved. Examples of diseases or conditions treated by orphan drugs include **acromegaly**, **amyotrophic lateral sclerosis**, cystic fibrosis, and **Tourette syndrome**.

In the 1990s, the Prescription Drug User Fee Amendments (PDUFA) assessed fees from drug manufacturers to reduce the review time for new drug applications. It was reauthorized in 1997 with the passage of the FDA Modernization Act, which accelerated the review of medical devices, regulated advertising of unapproved drug uses, and handled health claims for food products. The PDUFA has been reauthorized to improve communication between the FDA and new drug sponsors. Because of this, collected fees greatly expanded the number of people handling new drug applications at the FDA. The Dietary Supplement Health and Education Act of 1994 put into place controls against misleading claims about these products. Regulation of dietary supplements, however, remains quite relaxed because of lobbying from industry members.

In 2003, the Medicare Prescription Drug, Improvement, and Modernization Act was passed. It provided benefits that helped give better access to adequate healthcare for people who were poor, uninsured, underinsured, disabled, or elderly. Anyone qualifying for the low-income criteria may have premiums and costs subsidized by the government. In 2012, the FDA Safety and Innovation Act again reauthorized the PDUFA, requiring the FDA to implement a structured benefit-risk framework for new drug approvals. In 2013, the Drug Quality and Security Act outlined steps for an electronic, interoperable system to identify and trace prescription drugs in the United States.

You should remember

In 1862, President Abraham Lincoln appointed a chemist, Charles M. Wetherill, to the new Department of Agriculture. This was the origin of the Bureau of Chemistry, which preceded the FDA. In 1883, Dr. Harvey W. Wiley became the chief chemist and expanded the Bureau of Chemistry's food adulteration studies. He is now considered the "father" of the Pure Food and Drugs Act.

Drug standards

Originally, drugs were prepared from plants that could be found in nature. Drug strength and purity were based on the experience and integrity of the manufacturer, as well as the quality of the ingredients. Potency and safety were uncontrolled. In the 1800s, one of the first pharmaceutical standards was the **formulary**—a list of drug products and recipes. In the United States, the *United States Pharmacopeia* (USP) was established in 1820, and it contained comprehensive drug standards. A **pharmacopeia** summarizes purity, strength standards, and drug synthesis directions. From 1852 to 1975, the two major pharmaceutical publications were the USP and the National Formulary (NF), established by the American Pharmaceutical Association (APhA).

The USP covered all drug products, while the NF covered all nondrug ingredients. They were merged in 1975 into the *USP-NF*. Currently, the USP-NF contains over 300 chapters and over 4900 **drug monographs**. It is published every year, and two supplements are issued throughout each year. The USP label is found on many medications, verifying purity and precisely the correct amounts of ingredients. Drugs in the United States must conform to these standards to avoid charges of misbranding or **adulteration**. The USP also provides a voluntary program for verifying the accuracy of dietary supplement labels.

You should remember

In 2020, the CARES Act gave the FDA new tools to regulate OTC drugs after the organization complained about the previous rulemaking process that took years to update drug monographs. This limited the FDA's ability to respond to safety issues quickly. The CARES Act came about because of the COVID-19 pandemic. Its full name is the *Coronavirus Aid, Relief, and Economic Security Act*. It created a new process for updating and finalizing requirements, authority for the FDA to collect user fees supporting its activities, and an expedited process for addressing severe safety issues.

The US Food and Drug Administration

The PFDA established the FDA in 1906. The FDA was later expanded to carry out the FDCA provisions in 1938. The FDA has three primary mission statements, as follows:

- To protect public health by ensuring the safety, efficacy, and security of human and veterinary drugs, biological products, medical devices, the food supply, cosmetics, and radiation-emitting products
- To advance public health by helping to speed up innovations, making medicines and foods more effective, safer, and more affordable
- To help the public receive accurate, science-based information needed to use medicines and foods to improve health

There are seven branches of the FDA, headed by the Office of the Commissioner. These branches are summarized as follows:

- *The Center for Drug Evaluation and Research* (CDER): facilitates the availability of safe, effective drugs; keeps unsafe or ineffective drugs off the market; improves public health; provides understandable drug information for safe, effective use. All new drugs must be approved by the CDER, including prescription drugs, OTC drugs, and generic equivalents; the CDER also monitors the safety of marketed drugs and may issue warnings as additional information becomes available.
- *The Center for Biologics Evaluation and Research* (CBER): regulates the use of biologics, which are drugs derived from living sources, including serums, vaccines, and blood products. Ahe 1986 Childhood Vaccine Act authorized the FDA to acquire data on patients taking vaccines, recall biologics, and recommend civil penalties if guidelines are not followed; the CBER now also regulates **gene therapy** and treatments using human cells or tissue-based products.

- *The Center for Food Safety and Applied Nutrition* (CFSAN): oversees the administration of herbal products, dietary supplements, and cosmetics; also takes action against any herbal or dietary supplement that is found to be unsafe. Regulated cosmetics include perfumes, skin moisturizers, fingernail polishes, lipsticks, eye and facial makeup, deodorants, shampoos, and toothpaste; cosmetic manufacturers must be careful about not promoting therapeutic claims.
- *The Center for Devices and Radiological Health* (CDRH) assures patients and providers have timely, continued access to safe, effective, high-quality medical devices and safe radiation-emitting products.
- *The National Center for Toxicological Research* (NCTR): conducts research to define biological mechanisms of action underlying the toxicity of FDA-regulated products.
- *The Center for Tobacco Products* (CTP): in 2009, the CTP was created to regulate the manufacture, marketing, and distribution of tobacco products.
- *The Center for Veterinary Medicine* (CVM): regulates the manufacture and distribution of food, food additives, and drugs given to animals.

You should remember

The FDA oversees more than $2.8 trillion in food, medical products, and tobacco consumption. FDA-regulated products make up about 20 cents of every dollar consumers spend in the United States. Over 20,000 prescription drug products are approved for marketing. The FDA also oversees more than 6500 different medical device product categories. There are about 300 FDA-licensed biologic products.

The FDA approves generic drugs before they can be marketed. When a generic drug is considered *bioequivalent* to a trade-name drug, the generic drug is described as *therapeutically equivalent*. It receives an "A" rating from the FDA. A generic drug is defined as identical to a trade-name drug when there is less than a 20% variance in its absorption, distribution, metabolism, and excretion. The FDA publishes lists of approved generic drugs that are bioequivalent to trade-name drugs. The generic versions are less expensive and have the same active ingredients. All medicines have inert binders, fillers, and other **excipients** to create tablet shapes and control drug release speed. Therefore these factors may result in different drug bioavailability.

Prescription writing and regulations

Prescribers write prescriptions to instruct pharmacists to dispense a specific medication to a patient. Today, most drugs involve *e-prescribing*, meaning they originate from a computer instead of the traditional prescription pad. E-prescribing utilizes electronic creation, transmission, and filling of prescriptions. Even so, the critical required information is identical to what would appear on a paper prescription. Each prescription must communicate the medication needed and how the patient must use it.

Advantages of e-prescribing include prevention of medication errors; automation of clinical decision making; speeding up medication reconciliation; meeting meaningful use requirements; instantly notifying medical personnel about allergies, drug interactions, and duplicate therapies; tracking patient fulfillment of prescriptions; reducing numbers of lost prescriptions; simplifying the process of prescribing controlled substances; enabling better monitoring of controlled substance prescriptions; speeding up refills; reducing risks of readmissions; improving medication adherence; and making it easier to verify insurance.

The clarity of the directions on a prescription helps ensure patient compliance. It is also essential that the drug's trade name is evident because of its similarities with other medications. When the trade name is similar, the generic name should also appear on the prescription, helping to avoid confusion.

Before a prescription is prepared, the patient's medical history, any current medications being taken, and any kidney or liver dysfunction must all be evaluated. For all prescriptions, regardless of whether they are electronic or written, all of the following information must be included:

- Physician's name, address, office telephone number

- Prescription date
- Patient's full name, date of birth, address
- How the prescription is to be taken
- The age of the patient (if under 12 years or over 60 years)
- Refill information, safety cap information (if needed)
- For controlled substances, the physician's Drug Enforcement Administration (DEA) number
- Prescriber's signature

You should remember

More than 50% of all Americans use prescription drugs. About 90% of prescriptions filled today are generic drugs, not trade-name drugs. About 48% of the public has used at least one prescription drug in the past 30 days. The most frequently prescribed prescription drugs include analgesics, antihyperlipidemic, and dermatological agents.

Over-the-counter drugs

Drugs legally sold and not requiring a prescription are OTC drugs. They are safe and effective for use without the direct supervision of a healthcare provider. However, some OTC drugs have certain restrictions and must be kept behind the counter at the pharmacy. For these to be purchased, the customer's age and identity must be verified, and the pharmacist must educate the customer about the proper use of the drug. The FDA standardized the labeling of OTC drugs in 2002 to give customers better information about benefits and risks. All OTC drug labels must follow this format.

The OTC drugs may be involved in drug-drug interactions, such as nonsteroidal antiinflammatory drugs, food supplements, antacids, proton-pump inhibitors, H_2 antihistamines, laxatives, antidiarrheal drugs, and herbal drugs. The following five combinations should never be taken together:

- Acetaminophen (Tylenol) with alcohol can lead to severe liver damage.
- Ibuprofen with naproxen and aspirin because all of these are nonsteroidal antiinflammatory drugs and utilize the same pathways to be effective; taking more than one of these simultaneously increases the likelihood of adverse effects, from mild nausea to severe gastrointestinal bleeding.
- Antihistamines (such as Benadryl) with motion-sickness medications (such as Dramamine) because they can result in excessive drowsiness; when taking an antihistamine, it is essential to take a nondrowsy motion-sickness medicine instead.
- Antidiarrheal medicines (such as Imodium AD) with calcium supplements; this combination can result in constipation.
- The herbal supplement St. John's wort with cough medicine. This combination can trigger *serotonin syndrome*, which involves sweating, confusion, discomfort, movement difficulties, and, rarely, death.

You should remember

Because OTC drugs are generally safer than prescription drugs, it does not mean they cannot cause potentially serious problems. Many OTC drugs have addictive ingredients. Cough medicines, for example, often contain dextromethorphan. In higher-than-average doses, this drug can result in a "high" that can lead to intoxication and toxicity. Children and teenagers are at the highest risk of abusing these OTC preparations. Addition to OTC drugs may be challenging to identify, and these agents can also cause withdrawal symptoms if they are stopped quickly.

Controlled substances

For most drugs, prescriptions are not highly restricted—except for those with a significant potential for abuse. These **scheduled drugs** are prescribed with certain limitations based on the schedule in which they are classified. In the United States, the Comprehensive Drug Abuse Prevention and Control Act included the *Controlled Substances Act*, which established policies governing certain drugs' manufacture, importation, possession, use, and distribution. Five drug schedules were created in which potentially abused drugs were classified. These controlled drugs include compounds such as opioids, sedative-hypnotics, and stimulants in the most rigidly controlled schedules and substances such as cough medications and anticonvulsants in the least owned schedules. The five drug schedules are briefly summarized as follows:

- *Schedule I*: high abuse potential and lack of accepted safety, no currently accepted medical use
- *Schedule II*: high abuse potential that may lead to severe psychological or physical dependence, such as some opioids and stimulants. However, with accepted medical uses, drugs in this schedule cannot be refilled or prescribed by telephone.
- *Schedule III*: moderate abuse and dependence potential, including low doses of opioids and drugs such as anabolic steroids and testosterone; up to five refills are allowed, and prescriptions become invalid 6 months after being issued.
- *Schedule IV*—low to moderate abuse and dependence potential, including benzodiazepines; up to five refills are allowed, and prescriptions become invalid 6 months after being issued.
- *Schedule V*—low abuse and dependence potential, including some anticonvulsants and antidiarrheal drugs; for patients 18 years of age or older, these drugs may be dispensed in limited quantities by pharmacists.

Hospitals and pharmacies must register with the DEA and use their registration numbers to purchase scheduled drugs. Complete records of all quantities bought and sold must be kept. To obtain a Schedule II drug, a provider must use a particular order form that they fill out and sign. Refills for Schedule II drugs are not permitted. Patients must visit their healthcare provider each time a new Schedule II prescription is needed. Any provider convicted of unlawful manufacturing, distribution, or dispensing of controlled substances beyond the DEA policies and limitations will face severe penalties.

Table 8.2 summarizes the drugs that are listed in the five federal controlled substance schedules in the United States.

TABLE 8.2 The five federal controlled substance schedules.

Schedule	Examples
I	Methylenedioxymethamphetamine (ecstasy), heroin, LSD, methaqualone, peyote, marijuana (cannabis)—though individual states have different regulations today
II	Amobarbital, amphetamine, cocaine, codeine, fentanyl, glutethimide, hydrocodone, hydromorphone, meperidine, methadone, methamphetamine, methylphenidate, morphine, opium, oxycodone, pentobarbital
III	Anabolic steroids, benzenediamine, buprenorphine, ketamine, phendimetrazine, testosterone, and products that contain more than 90 mg of codeine per dosage unit (such as Tylenol with codeine)
IV	Alprazolam, benzodiazepines, carisoprodol, clonazepam, clorazepate, diazepam, lorazepam, midazolam, temazepam, triazolam
V	Cough preparations that contain less than 200 mg of codeine per 100 mL, or 100 g (such as Robitussin AC or Phenergan with codeine); ezogabine

LSD, Lysergic acid diethylamide.

You should remember

Drug dependence or addiction does not always begin with the abuse of illegal drugs. Many people who become dependent or addicted to drugs start with a legal prescription given to them by their physician. Also, leftover medications from medicine cabinets are often stolen or given to friends or family members. Prescription narcotic analgesics are also involved in many fatal overdoses.

Key Terms

Acromegaly
Adulteration
Apothecary system
Amyotrophic lateral sclerosis
Drug monographs
Excipients
Formulary
Gene therapy
Genomics
Genotoxicity
Pharmacopeia
Proteonomics
Risk-benefit ratio
Scheduled drugs
Tourette syndrome

Clinical Case Study

A female pharmacist met a male at a social gathering and, over a few weeks, started dating him. He told her about a recent car accident he had been involved in and that he was suffering from severe pain. He said his doctor had prescribed him oxycodone for his pain and asked his new acquaintance if she could fill his prescription at her pharmacy. She agreed, but because of their relationship, she did not call the physician's office to verify the accuracy of the prescription. About 90 days later, he gave her another prescription and asked for it to be filled. Eventually, the man was convicted of forging prescriptions and sentenced to a 5-year prison term. The court case revealed that the prescription pad was stolen from a physician's office, and the man had been writing them himself after learning about the wording needed to make them appear genuine.

Critical Thinking Questions

1. Which significant development in the field of pharmacy has helped to reduce illegal and forged prescriptions?
2. What is the significance of scheduled drugs in comparison to other drugs?
3. Why is oxycodone, a Schedule II drug, classified as such?

Further Reading

[1] D.G. Adams, R.M. Cooper, M.J. Hahn, J.S. Kahan, Food and Drug Law and Regulation, third ed., Food and Drug Law Institute, 2015.
[2] S. Ainsworth, Neonatal Formulary: Drug Use in Pregnancy and the First Year of Life, eighth ed., OUP Oxford, 2020.
[3] J.J. Berman, Rare Diseases and Orphan Drugs: Keys to Understanding and Treating the Common Diseases, Academic Press, 2014.
[4] C. Chang, Violations of 21 CFR Part 50—Protection of Human Subjects—Letters Issued by U.S. Food and Drug Administration, CreateSpace Independent Publishing Platform, 2015.
[5] L. Endrenyi, P. Declerck, S.C. Chow, Biosimilar Drug Product Development (Drugs and the Pharmaceutical Sciences Volume 216), CRC Press, 2017.
[6] L.T. Friedhoff, New Drugs: An Insider's Guide to the Fda's New Drug Approval Process for Scientists, Investors and Patients, PSPG Publishing, 2009.
[7] M. George, L. Joseph, K. Sujith, Drug Formulary, Jaypee Brothers Medical Publishers Ltd, 2015.

[8] N.W. Goodman, M.B. Edwards, A. Black, E. Landon-Neuner, Medical Writing: A Prescription for Clarity, fourth ed., Cambridge University Press, 2014.
[9] R.A. Guarino, New Drug Approval Process (Drugs and the Pharmaceutical Sciences Volume 190), fifth ed., CRC Press, 2016.
[10] E. Hernberg-Stahl, M. Reljanovic, Orphan Drugs: Understanding the Rare Disease Market and its Dynamics (Series in Biomedicine Book 46), Woodhead Publishing, 2013.
[11] P. Hutt, R. Merrill, L. Grossman, Food and Drug Law: Cases and Materials, fourth ed., Foundation Press, 2013.
[12] S.M. Kanovsky, W.L. Pines, A Practical Guide to Fda's Food and Drug Law and Regulation, seventh ed., Food and Drug Law Institute, 2020.
[13] T.I. King, T.R. Baker, FDA Drug Approval: Elements and Consideration (Pharmacology Research, Safety Testing and Regulation), Nova Biomedical, 2012.
[14] Law Library, The, Exclusion of Orphan Drugs for Certain Covered Entities Under 340B Program (US Department of Health and Human Services (HHS) Regulation), The Law Library, 2018.
[15] A.S. Meyers, Orphan Drugs: A Global Crusade, Meyers, 2016.
[16] R. Ng, Drug: From Discovery to Approval, third ed., Wiley-Blackwell, 2015.
[17] J.J. O'Donnell, J. Somberg, V. Idemyor, J.T. O'Donnell, Drug Discovery and Development, third ed., CRC Press, 2019.
[18] K.R. Pina, W.L. Pines, A Practical Guide to Fda's Food and Drug Law and Regulation, sixth ed., Food and Drug Law Institute, 2017.
[19] S.O.L. Potter, Potter's Compend of Materia Medica Therapeutics and Prescription Writing, University of Michigan Library, 2009.
[20] D.C. Pryde, M. Palmer, D. Fox, A. Kent, R. Boyd, Orphan Drugs and Rare Diseases: RSC Drug Discovery (Volume 38), Royal Society of Chemistry, 2014.
[21] J. Teitelman, K. Detweiler, AAHA Guide to Safeguarding Controlled Substances, AAHA Press, 2020.
[22] N. Ting, D.G. Chen, S. Ho, J.C. Cappelleri, Phase II Clinical Development of New Drugs (ICSA Book Series in Statistics), Springer, 2017.
[23] United States Department of Justice, Pharmacist's Manual: An Informational Outline of the Controlled Substances Act, Lulu.com, 2019.
[24] United States Government Accountability Office, Health Care: Food and Drug Administration's Drug Approval Process, BiblioGov, 2013.
[25] United States Pharmacopeial Convention, The Pharmacopeia of the United States of America, Forgotten Books, 2018.

UNIT II

Drug effects on the central nervous system

CHAPTER

9

Antimigraine drugs

OUTLINE

LEARNING OUTCOMES

After study of the chapter, readers should be able to:

1. Describe the classifications of migraines.
2. Explain the silent migraines and their treatment.
3. Discuss the causes of retinal migraine.
4. Describe the risk factors for chronic migraine.
5. Explain the pathophysiology of migraine.
6. List the trade names of eletriptan, sumatriptan, and ergotamine.
7. Explain the clinical indication of triptans.
8. Discuss the contraindications of ergot alkaloids and triptans.
9. Explain the toxicities of triptan drugs.
10. Describe the medications used for migraine prevention.

Overview

A migraine is a complicated condition with a severe headache, most often unilateral on one side of the head. The pain is much worse than a typical headache and is usually accompanied by various neurological symptoms.

The Science of Pharmacology
https://doi.org/10.1016/B978-0-443-29038-1.00009-9

Headaches are only considered migraines if the typical symptoms have occurred at least five times. Migraines can significantly affect everyday life. Some individuals only get them occasionally, while others may have migraines several days of every month. Some patients with migraines experience numbness in their bodies and have difficulties with speaking typically. The most common type of migraine is without aura in about 75% of cases. Migraines affect approximately 1 billion people globally and more than 37 million people of all ages annually in the United States.

Classifications of migraines

Migraines are classified into several general forms, though a few less common forms exist. The most common migraines are those that do not have the perception of an **aura**, followed by migraine with aura, migraine with brainstem aura, silent migraine, chronic migraine, and status migrainosus. The rarer forms of migraines include hemiplegic migraine and retinal migraine.

Migraine without aura

Migraine without aura is by far the most common type of migraine, affecting 75% of all migraine sufferers. It involves a pulsating headache on one side of the head, which is of moderate to severe intensity. Regular physical activity, bright lights, and loud sounds aggravate this migraine. The risk factors are anxiety, depression, obesity, and snoring. Several triptans are available with different pharmacokinetics and routes of administration. The choice of triptan should be individualized based on the patient's migraine characteristics and the route of administration, pharmacokinetics, and cost. Treatments for migraine without aura include over-the-counter painkillers or triptans. Preventive treatments include beta-blockers, tricyclic antidepressants, or antiepilepsy drugs. These medications can reduce the frequency and severity of attacks.

Migraine with aura

Migraine with aura is less common than migraine without aura. Symptoms start about 30 minutes before the actual headache begins. They are usually visual and may include the perception of flashing lights or wavy lines or losing some or all vision for a short period. An aura may involve losing the ability to speak, tingling, numbness, and weakness in the extremities. Some patients experience the aura without having the headache or other symptoms—this is most common in people aged 50 or older. This situation becomes more familiar with continued aging. Migraine with aura usually lasts for less than 1 hour. Learning relaxation techniques, regular sleeping and eating routines, and appropriate hydration may help patients without medications.

Silent migraine

Silent migraines are infrequent and lack the characteristic headache. Vision problems and altered color perception are the most common symptoms. Silent migraines are more common in adults over age 50 and have been misdiagnosed as strokes. Even though the headache is absent, the aura symptoms can be highly debilitating. There can be nausea and extreme sensitivity to light and sound. The aura evolves over several minutes, usually lasting between 5 and 60 minutes. Treatment can be complex because oral triptans and NSAIDs take longer to work than the duration of the aura. Some patients find that treatment relieves nausea and sensitivity to light and sound. Silent migraine is managed on a case-by-case basis.

Migraine with brainstem aura

This form usually affects children and adolescents. It is characterized by throbbing pain on both sides and the back of the head. There is temporary or double vision loss, **slurred speech**, dizziness or **vertigo**, poor muscle coordination, **tinnitus**, and fainting. This condition affects all age groups, without a female predominance like the other types. Symptoms originate from the brainstem or both cerebral hemispheres at the same time. Typical aura symptoms are present, lasting for up to 1 hour. Additional symptoms of *migraine with brainstem aura* include **ataxia**, decreased level of consciousness, **dysarthria**, **hyperacusis**, tinnitus, and vertigo. Anxiety and hyperventilation sometimes occur. For acute treatment, combinations of NSAIDs with antiemetics are usually adequate. Preventive medications include lamotrigine, topiramate, and verapamil. This condition often becomes more common in later middle age. Symptoms, however, are usually more frightening than harmful.

Hemiplegic migraine

Hemiplegic migraine is characterized by unilateral paralysis, vertigo, and problems seeing, speaking, or swallowing. A concurrent headache is also common. The weaknesses caused by hemiplegic migraine are related to an aura. *Familial hemiplegic migraine* occurs in families, while *sporadic hemiplegic migraine* occurs in individuals with no family history. Females are three times more likely to have this type of migraine. Any weakness developing after a headache must prompt the individual or a caregiver to seek immediate medical attention.

Hemiplegic migraine often begins in childhood, between 12 and 17 years of age. Symptoms last for hours to days but rarely over weeks. Usually, they resolve entirely. Primary symptoms include hemiplegia, headache, vision changes, numbness, tingling, and difficulty speaking. Secondary symptoms include fever, changes in consciousness (confused with profound coma), coordination problems, nausea, vomiting, and increased sensitivity to sound and light. Short-acting NSAIDs, antiemetics, or intranasal ketamine may be required. A new class of medications known as *detans* may be used. Preventive medications also used for typical migraine with aura are helpful.

Retinal migraine

Retinal migraine is distinguished by vision loss or visual disturbances in only one eye. It is also known as *ocular migraine*. Most episodes, while frightening, are harmless and transient, with full eyesight returning. Retinal migraines may occur every few months but can vary in frequency. One eye's partial or total vision loss usually lasts 10 to 20 minutes. A headache may occur before, during, or after vision loss.

In most cases, the same eye is affected every time. Rarely, vision loss lasts for more than 1 hour. It may become blurred or dimmed slowly, or there may be light flashes. Sometimes, **scotomas** appear initially, enlarging to cause total vision loss.

Retinal migraine is caused by a sudden constriction of the eye's blood vessels. This may be triggered by simply bending over, dehydration, exercise, excessive heat, high altitudes, hypertension, hypoglycemia, use of oral contraceptives, smoking, and stress. Retinal migraines are more common in females, individuals under age 40, or those with a personal or family history of migraines or headaches. Treatments include aspirin, beta-blockers, calcium channel blockers, tricyclic antidepressants, and anticonvulsants. Possible complications include damage to the retina and ocular blood vessels, though permanent vision loss is rare.

Chronic migraine

Chronic migraine affects about 1% of the US population. About 2.5% of people with episodic migraine will transition to chronic migraine. This condition is diagnosed when migraines occur 15 or more days per month over 3 months or longer. Chronic migraine is also called **transformed migraine**. Over time, increased amounts of headaches develop for different reasons, which include hormonal changes, increased stress, illness, and increased use of pain medications. The increased number of headaches decreases the threshold for new headaches, making the condition chronic and less likely to respond to medications. Risk factors for chronic migraine include anxiety, depression, acute medication overuse, asthma, excessive caffeine, head or neck injuries, other pain disorders, obesity, frequent nausea, snoring, and stress.

Treatments are similar to those of episodic migraine but with only a limited number of uses of acute medications, onabotulinumtoxin A, anticonvulsants, antidepressants, antihypertensives, biofeedback, cognitive behavioral therapy, and reducing risk factors.

Status migrainosus

Status migrainosus affects about 1% of all migraine patients. It is painful and debilitating, lasting for 72 hours or longer. When moderate to severe pain lasts longer than this, with less than a 4-hour pain-free period while being awake, it is an emergency condition. The patient must be taken to an emergency department for treatment because this condition is potentially life-threatening. Its prolonged symptoms, such as vomiting, can cause dangerous dehydration and electrolyte imbalance. Hospitalization is required to provide solid medications and intravenous (IV) fluids. A typical migraine can evolve into status migrainosus without proper treatment, with treatment occurring too late, or if excessive amounts of headache medications are taken to relieve pain.

Symptoms are similar to other types of migraine and include vision changes, difficulty concentrating, nausea, and vomiting. The headache may be on one or both sides of the head. The visual aura can also affect the other senses. **Photophobia** and **phonophobia** are common, as are changes in consciousness, weakness, and tingling. Complications of status migrainosus include stroke, **aneurysm**, permanent vision loss, severe dental problems, anxiety, depression, suicidal thoughts, coma, and death.

Because of the common nausea, medications are usually given IV or via nasal spray or suppository. Some patients require Botox injections or minimally invasive migraine surgery, which helps remove abnormal nerve signals that cause the attacks.

You should remember

In the United States, about 1.2 million emergency department visits annually are for acute migraine attacks. Most people experience attacks once or twice per month. The overall condition of migraine is most prevalent in females (18%), children (10%), and males (6%). It is most common between the ages of 18 and 44. About 90% of migraine sufferers have a family history of migraine.

Pathophysiology

Migraine is a primary brain disorder that most likely involves an ion channel in the aminergic brain stem nuclei. It is a neurovascular headache in which neural events result in dilation of blood vessels and aura by vasoconstriction, aggravating the pain, and further nerve activation. Migraine is a genetically influenced complex disorder characterized by episodes of moderate to severe headache, most often unilateral and generally associated with nausea and light and sound sensitivity.

Serotonin released may play a role in migraines. However, the exact role of its mechanisms is unknown. Serotonin levels are most likely low between attacks because they may cause a deficiency in the serotonin pain inhibition system. Pituitary adenylate cyclase–activating polypeptide may also play an essential role in mediating migraine attacks, as its concentration is elevated during the attacks.

Pharmacotherapy

For migraine, different goals are to stop an acute migraine while it is progressing and to prevent or reduce migraines and how often they occur. Table 9.1 summarizes drugs to treat acute migraine. Pharmacotherapy is most successful if it begins before the pain becomes severe. It is different for mild, moderate, and severe migraines, as follows:

- *Mild migraine* –NSAIDs are usually tried first. Acetaminophen is not effective on its own but is better when combined with an NSAID and caffeine. The oral serotonin (5-HT) agonists, including triptans or ergot alkaloids, are used when a mild migraine persists and is not relieved by NSAIDs.

TABLE 9.1 Triptans and ergot alkaloids used to treat acute migraines.

Generic name	Trade name
Triptans	
almotriptan	Axert
eletriptan	Relpax
frovatriptan	Frova
naratriptan	Amerge
rizatriptan	Maxalt
sumatriptan	Imitrex, Imitrex Statdose, Tosymra
zolmitriptan	Zomig, Lasmiditan
Ergot alkaloids	
dihydroergotamine	Migranal
Ergotamine	Ergomar

- *Moderate migraine*: the preferred agents are 5-HT agonists orally, intranasally, or subcutaneously. If these are contraindicated or do not work, then dopamine agonists can be prescribed. These include *prochlorperazine (Compazine)* and *metoclopramide (Reglan)*.
- *Severe migraine*: Serotonin agonists are usually administered (subcutaneous, intramuscular, or IV). Another choice is a parenteral dopamine agonist, which may be combined with a serotonin agonist or used alone. Narcotic analgesics can stop migraine pain that has not responded to other therapies.

The primary drug classes for acute migraines are serotonin receptor agonists (triptans and ergot alkaloids). Table 9.1 summarizes these medications.

The first triptan ever marketed was sumatriptan in 1992. In 1997, the second-generation triptans (beginning with naratriptan) were sold and offered better absorption, a quicker onset of action, and longer duration.

New medications known as calcitonin gene–related peptide inhibitors are available today. These injectable medications can be taught about so that patients can self-inject as needed. Though they may not entirely stop a migraine attack, they make it much less severe. Over time, they also reduce the frequency of migraine attacks.

Pharmacokinetics

The triptans generally have similar pharmacokinetics. Their absorption percentages differ based on the route—via oral (15%) and intranasal or subcutaneous (97%). They are widely distributed, cross the placenta, and are secreted in breast milk. These agents are less than 21% bound to plasma protein. The triptans are metabolized in the liver and primarily excreted in the urine (60%) and feces (40%). The onset of oral action is 30–60 minutes, intranasal action is 30 minutes, and subcutaneous action is 10–15 minutes. The oral duration of action is 6–8 hours, subcutaneous is 4–6 hours, and intranasal is unknown.

Mechanism of action

The triptans are selective for the 5-HT_1 receptor subtype. They are believed to act by constricting intracranial vessels and stopping migraines, whether auras are present or not. The ergot alkaloids promote vasoconstriction, stopping a migraine as it is in progress.

Clinical indications

Triptans are also indicated for migraines, **cluster headaches**, and altitude sickness. They are shown to be effective for acute migraines but are not effective for long-term prevention. The ergot alkaloids are also indicated for Parkinson disease.

Contraindications

The triptans and ergot alkaloids are contraindicated with peripheral vascular disease, coronary artery disease, and cerebrovascular disease. Triptans are contraindicated with uncontrolled hypertension, hypercholesterolemia, or a strong family history of cardiovascular disease. They are also contraindicated with severe chronic kidney disease or hepatic impairment. They must be used cautiously in patients with epilepsy. However, ergot alkaloids are also contraindicated with severe hypertension. The ergot alkaloids are pregnancy category X drugs and must be avoided during pregnancy.

Adverse effects

The triptans commonly cause **paresthesia**, dry mouth, tingling, dizziness, a warming sensation, and **vertigo**. Their adverse severe effects include coronary artery vasospasm, cardiac arrest, and myocardial infarction. The ergot alkaloids commonly cause nausea, vomiting, weakness, abnormal pulse, nasal or throat irritation, and **dysgeusia**. Their adverse severe effects include delirium, cerebrovascular events that include bleeding, seizures, congenital disabilities, intermittent claudication, inhibition of lactation or the cause of infant vomiting, physical dependence, and withdrawal that resembles migraine.

Toxicities

The triptans do not have significant toxicities when used on their own. It is only the drugs with which they interact that can result in problems when used concurrently. Ergot alkaloid toxicity is signified by constriction of the peripheral arteries to cause coldness, paleness, numbness of the extremities, and muscle pain. Overall, there have seldom been overdoses of these agents, and treatment is generally supportive.

You should remember

Though the orally administered triptans are preferred due to convenience, if a patient has nausea and vomiting during the migraine, another route of administration may be needed. Intranasal formulations and prefilled syringes may be used if the patient can self-administer them.

You should remember

The ergot alkaloids are used today after triptans have failed but must only be used 24 hours after a triptan was administered. The first purified ergot alkaloid was *ergotamine*, isolated from the *ergot fungus* in 1920, though these alkaloids have been known for thousands of years. Ergotamine is inexpensive and available in oral, sublingual, and suppository forms. The drug modified from it, *dihydroergotamine*, is available as a nasal spray and an injection. The ergot alkaloids have many actions and adverse effects because they interact with adrenergic, dopaminergic, and serotonergic receptors.

Drugs used for migraine prophylaxis

Preventive treatment helps to reduce attack frequency, improve responsiveness to acute attacks' severity and duration, and reduce disability.

Antidepressants, beta-blockers, calcium channel blockers, and anticonvulsants are used for migraine prevention. Table 9.2 summarizes medications used for migraine prevention.

Novel therapeutics are available for both the prevention and acute treatment of migraine headaches. These new medications and neuromodulatory devices appear overall to be safe and effective in the management of migraine headaches.

TABLE 9.2 Drugs used for migraine prevention.

Generic name	Trade name
Antiseizure drugs	
gabapentin	Neurontin
topiramate	Topamax
valproic acid	Depakene, Depakote
Beta-adrenergic blockers	
atenolol	Tenormin
metoprolol	Lopressor
propranolol	Inderal
timolol	Blocadren
Calcium channel blockers	
nifedipine	Procardia
nimodipine	Nimotop
verapamil	Isoptin
Tricyclic antidepressants	
amitriptyline	Elavil
imipramine	Tofranil
protriptyline	Vivactil
Miscellaneous	
Methysergide	Sansert

Key Terms

Aneurysm
Antiphospholipid syndrome
Ataxia
Aura
Cluster headaches
Diplopia
Dysarthria
Dysgeusia
Hemiplegic migraine
Hyperacusis
Lupus erythematosus
Paresthesia
Phonophobia
Photophobia
Retinal migraine
Scotoma
Silent migraine
Slurred speech
Status migrainosus
Tension headache
Tinnitus
Transformed migraine
Vertigo

Clinical Case Studies

Clinical Case Study 1

A 24-year-old female experienced her first migraine, which lasted for 5 days. It caused nausea, vomiting, and severe, continually throbbing pain. She had a positive family history of migraines and also found that oral contraceptives made the headaches much worse. The patient always experienced an aura before each migraine and stated to the examining physician that any amount of alcohol regularly triggered an attack. She was diagnosed with "migraine with aura" and started on appropriate treatment.

Critical Thinking Questions

1. What are the signifying factors of migraines?
2. How is migraine with aura described?
3. What are the pharmacotherapies used for severe migraines?

Clinical Case Study 2

A 35-year-old female had a history of endometriosis and migraine without aura. Her husband brought her to the emergency department because she had suffered from continual migraines for about 3 weeks, with neurological features. She described the pain as bilateral, squeezing, and frontal in location. She also had scotomas that lasted for 2–3 hours per day, along with tongue numbness and left facial paresthesia. A neurologist diagnosed the patient with status migrainosus with aura. A CT scan of the patient's head revealed a thickening of the bilateral optic nerves. An MRI revealed a venous anomaly. Several regimens of medications were tried, and the patient's condition was resolved with a combination of topiramate, naproxen, and ubrogepant.

Critical Thinking Questions

1. How common is the occurrence of migraines without aura?
2. What are the drugs used for preventive migraines without aura?
3. What is the treatment for acute migraines without aura?

Clinical Case Study 3

A 57-year-old female had a history of chronic migraines for several years. She had seen many physicians, changed her diet, and tried many oral medications, but nothing seemed to work. Her family history revealed that migraines affected several of her relatives. She was started on therapy with the self-injectable (subcutaneous) form of sumatriptan, which she was taught to inject initially as a single dose, with a second dose allowed after 1 hour if needed. The maximum amount allowed was two doses per day, and that was all she was prescribed to see the results. Fortunately, the patient found quick relief from the next migraine attack she experienced with just a single dose of the new medication.

Critical Thinking Questions

1. How common is chronic migraine, and how is it diagnosed?
2. How are the triptans believed to act in the treatment of migraines?
3. What are the contraindications of sumatriptan?

Further Reading

[1] S.D. Brain, P. Geppetti, Calcitonin Gene-Related Peptide (CGRP) Mechanisms (Handbook of Experimental Pharmacology, 255, Springer, 2019.
[2] S. Diamond, R.K. Cady, M.L. Diamond, M.W. Green, V. Martin, Headache and Migraine Biology and Management, Academic Press, 2015.
[3] R. Grossinger, K. Podoll, M. Dahlem, Migraine Auras: When the Visual World Fails, North Atlantic Books, 2006.
[4] R.S. Lee, Headaches: Amazing Natural Remedies to Alleviate Migraines, Cluster, Sinus, Tension, and Rebound Headaches, Maria Fernanda Moguel Cruz, 2019.
[5] A. Maassen van den Brink, E.A. MacGregor, Gender and Migraine (Headache Series), Springer / European Headache Federation, 2019.
[6] M. Neeley, D. Greenberg, Cracking the migraine code: the mystery of migraine & chronic headaches, Neeley Dental Group (2018).
[7] K. Ravishankar, Modern Day Management of Headache – Questions and Answers, Jaypee Brothers Medical Publishers Pvt. Ltd, 2018.
[8] L. Robbins, Advanced Headache Therapy: Outpatient Strategies, Springer, 2015.
[9] S. Shah, Migraine: Emerging Innovations and Treatment Options, Springer, 2021.
[10] B. Talley Daniel, The Mini Neurology Series Volume 1: Migraine, CreateSpace Independent Publishing Platform, 2014.
[11] A. Vasquez, Pain revolution for migraine and fibromyalgia: the paradigm-shifting guide for doctors and patients dealing with chronic pain (A three-part learning system of text. Images, and Video), third ed., CreateSpace Independent Publishing Platform, 2015.
[12] W.B. Young, S.D. Silberstein, Navigating Life with Migraine and Other Headaches, Oxford University Press, 2018.

CHAPTER

10

The Science of Pharmacology Antiseizure drugs

OUTLINE

LEARNING OUTCOMES

After study of this chapter, readers should be able to:

1. Describe the classifications of seizures.
2. Identify the causes of seizures.
3. List medications that are used for generalized seizures.
4. Compare characteristics of partial and absence seizures.
5. List medications used for tonic-clonic seizures.
6. Identify the pharmacokinetics of ethosuximide.
7. Explain the long-term treatment of status epilepticus.
8. Describe the characteristics of typical absence seizures.
9. Explain the contraindications of clonazepam.
10. Discuss new antiseizure medications for the treatment of epilepsy.

The Science of Pharmacology
https://doi.org/10.1016/B978-0-443-29038-1.00010-5

Overview

A seizure is an abnormal, uncontrolled electrical discharge in the brain's cortical gray matter, transiently interrupting normal function. Seizures usually cause odd sensations, altered awareness, involuntary focal movements, or generalized convulsions. Approximately 2% of all adults will have a seizure during their lifetimes, but two-thirds of these people will never have another seizure. Epilepsy is a chronic brain disorder that is also called *epileptic seizure disorder.* It mainly involves two or more recurrent, unprovoked seizures unrelated to reversible stressors. It is often idiopathic. Classifications of seizures include tonic-clonic, partial, absence, febrile, atonic febrile, atonic, and myoclonic seizures. The term "epilepsy" refers to chronic neurologic disorders with recurring seizures. A "seizure" refers to all epileptic events, but a "convulsion" is only the abnormal motor activity. Temporary stressors or disorders cause nonepileptic seizures. Fever can provoke seizures in children. They are most common in infants and older people. *Psychogenic seizures* or *pseudoseizures* are older terms for nonepileptic seizures most often seen in patients with psychiatric disorders. Still, there are no abnormal electrical discharges in their brains.

Causes of seizures

Seizure disorders may be caused by various factors such as trauma, infectious disease, fever, neoplastic disorders, metabolic disorders, vascular disorders, and miscellaneous substances. Head injuries and trauma can also be caused by toxic fumes or substances and ingesting poisons, with damaged brain tissue linked to seizures. Encephalitis and meningitis cause brain inflammation and seizures. Rapid increases in body temperature can cause febrile seizures, especially common in infants and toddlers. Brain tumors, significantly when overgrowing, stop sufficient oxygenated blood to brain tissues and increase intracranial pressure, leading to seizures.

Altered fluid and electrolyte levels can cause seizures; electrical impulse transmission in cells can be changed by hypoglycemia, hyponatremia, and water intoxication. Seizures are caused by hypoxia of brain tissue when electrical impulses are interrupted. carbon monoxide poisoning results in cerebral hypoxia; brain tissue ischemia changes impulse transmission and adds to the likelihood of seizures. Other vascular causes include hypotension, cardiac dysrhythmias, shock, and stroke. Withdrawal from alcohol and sedative/hypnotics can also cause seizures.

Classifications of seizures

Seizures have various classifications, including tonic-clonic, partial, absence, and myoclonic seizures. They are treated by multiple backup and adjunctive drugs based on the actual type of seizure present. The condition known as epilepsy is commonly associated with seizure disorders. It refers to chronic neurologic disorders with recurring seizures due to excessive excitability of brain neurons. Various types of seizures can involve a brief lack of consciousness or cause violent convulsions. Some patients also have problems with memory, mood, and learning. More than 3.4 million people in the United States have epilepsy. It is essential to understand that a *seizure* refers to all forms of epileptic events, while a *convulsion* refers only to abnormal motor activity that occurs during an attack. While all convulsions can also be called seizures, the reverse is untrue.

Generalized seizures

Generalized seizures occur when abnormal electrical activity begins in both of the brain hemispheres at the same time. They are the most common and dramatic form, formerly called grand-mal seizures. The symptoms include loss of consciousness, which can be accompanied by the patient crying out or groaning, sudden collapse, spasms, shaking, stiffening, loss of muscle tone, muscle contractions, loss of bladder or bowel control, limited breathing or stoppage of breathing, and cyanosis of the lips. Generalized seizures are diagnosed by the patient's medical history, electroencephalogram, magnetic resonance imaging, and blood tests.

Tonic-clonic seizures

A **tonic-clonic seizure** usually begins with little warning on both sides of the brain but may sometimes start on one side and then spread to the entire brain. A **prodrome** of several subjective phenomena may precede them. There may be a few hours of feelings of **apathy**, depression, and irritability. The affected individual then experiences muscle stiffening and jerking movements. The individual may cry out loudly because of whole-body muscle spasms. The lateral part of the tongue is often bitten, and air is forced out through the vocal cords. Due to respiratory muscle spasms, breathing is suspended, and cyanosis may follow.

The patient seldom remembers anything that has occurred and often falls asleep again, up to several hours, repeatedly awakening with a pulsing headache. If the contractions were severe during the episode, there may be crushing of the spinal vertebral bodies, fractures, periorbital hemorrhages, **subdural hematoma**, shoulder dislocations, or **skin abrasions**. Tonic-clonic seizures usually last for 1 to 3 minutes, and a more extended period is required for an individual to recover compared to other seizures. If a tonic-clonic seizure lasts more than 5 minutes, it is a true medical emergency. This is referred to as **status epilepticus**. Certain seizure conditions are more likely to occur as nocturnal seizures.

Partial seizures

A **partial seizure** may be simple or complex. A *simple partial seizure* affects only one area of the brain, does not cause loss of consciousness, and lasts for only 1 to 2 minutes. A *complex partial seizure* is the most common type in adults with epilepsy. The affected person may be unable to talk or control movements and may not remember having the seizure after it stops.

Absence seizures

An **absence of seizure** begins in both sides of the brain simultaneously. It causes lapses in awareness. The older term for absence seizures was petit mal seizures. Absence seizures start and end quickly, lasting only a few seconds. They can be so short that they are often mistaken for "daydreaming" and may not be detected for months. Most patients with absence seizures continue to move somewhat, with delicate clonic eyelids, facial muscles, or finger movements. There may be small, synchronized movements of both arms. All of these types of activities occur at about three per second.

Typical absence seizures are the most common form of childhood epilepsy. The seizures do not usually begin before age 4 or after puberty. Up to several hundred absence seizures can occur in 1 day, often in clusters at certain repeated times. The child may appear to be inattentive. If they occur frequently, the child's school performance becomes impaired. Less often, the attacks last for hours without a break in between.

Myoclonic seizures

A **myoclonic seizure** involves brief, shock-like jerks of a muscle or a group of muscles. It occurs in various epilepsy syndromes with different features. During a myoclonic seizure, the affected person is usually awake and able to think clearly. These seizures typically do not last longer than 1 or 2 seconds. There can be just one seizure, or many can occur quickly. Myoclonic seizures cause abnormal movements on both sides of the body simultaneously.

Antiseizure drugs

There is no formula to choose which seizure medicine to use for a particular patient. No one medicine dominates for effectiveness, and all have various side effects. Antiseizure medications (ASMs), previously called antiepileptic drugs, consider which side effects should be avoided in particular cases as well as the convenience of use, cost, and physician experience. An important start is to know which ASMs work for which seizure types. The narrow-spectrum ASMs primarily work for specific types of seizures (such as focal, absence, or myoclonic seizures). Broad-spectrum ASMs are also effective for various seizures (focal plus absence myoclonic seizures). Some types of seizures are difficult to treat with any ASM. Narrow-spectrum and broad-range ASMs are summarized in Table 10.1.

Pharmacokinetics

Generally, antiseizure drugs given orally are well absorbed. They have substantial bioavailability and cross the blood-brain barrier easily. Liver enzymes metabolize most ASMs, and sometimes active metabolites are formed.

TABLE 10.1 Narrow-spectrum and broad-spectrum antiseizure drugs.

Narrow-spectrum AEDs	Broad-spectrum AEDs
phenytoin (Dilantin)	valproic acid (Depakote)
phenobarbital (Luminal)	lamotrigine (Lamictal)
carbamazepine (Tegretol)	topiramate (Topamax)
oxcarbazepine (Trileptal)	zonisamide (Zonegran)
gabapentin (Neurontin)	levetiracetam (Keppra)
pregabalin (Lyrica)	clonazepam (Klonopin)
lacosamide (Vimpat)	rufinamide (Banzel)
vigabatrin (Sabril)	fosphenytoin (Cerebyx)
tiagabine (Gabitril)	

AED, Antiepileptic drug.

The pharmacokinetics of *carbamazepine* include nearly 100% bioavailability, 70%–80% protein binding, and metabolism in the liver. Carbamazepine may increase clearance of anticonvulsants such as clonazepam, lamotrigine, and valproic acid. The elimination half-life is 36 hours for a single dose and 16–24 hours with repeated doses. Carbamazepine is excreted 72% via the urine and 28% via the feces.

The pharmacokinetics of *lamotrigine* include 98% bioavailability, 55% protein binding, and metabolism primarily by liver enzymes. Its elimination half-life is 29 hours, excreted mainly via the urine and 2% via the feces. The pharmacokinetics of *phenytoin* include 70%–100% bioavailability for oral doses. Its oral bioavailability is variable due to individual differences in first-pass metabolism. Protein binding is 98%, and the liver metabolizes the drug. Metabolism of phenytoin is enhanced by drugs that induce liver metabolism, such as phenobarbital or rifampin, and inhibited by cimetidine and isoniazid.

Phenytoin decreases the effects of carbamazepine, clonazepam, and lamotrigine. The elimination half-life is 10 to 22 hours, and the duration of action is 24 hours. Elimination kinetics change from first order to zero order at moderate to high doses. Phenytoin is excreted mainly via the urine and to an uncertain percentage in the bile. *Fosphenytoin* is a water-soluble prodrug of phenytoin and is administered parenterally. The pharmacokinetics of *valproic acid* include rapid absorption and bioavailability, 80%–90% protein binding, and metabolism by the liver. The elimination half-life is 9–16 hours, and excretion is via the urine at 30%–50%.

Ethosuximide has a bioavailability of 93%. It is metabolized in the liver, and the elimination half-life is 53 hours. This drug is excreted via the kidneys. *Clonazepam* is lipid soluble and quickly crosses the blood-brain barrier. It also penetrates the placenta. It is metabolized extensively by the cytochrome P450 enzymes in the liver. Clonazepam has an elimination half-life of 19–60 hours. Peak blood concentrations usually reach within 1–2 hours after a single oral dose. Some patients experience peak blood concentrations within 4–8 hours. Clonazepam has plasma protein binding of 85%, and its metabolites are excreted via the kidneys.

Mechanism of action

Antiseizure drugs generally act by suppressing repetitive action potential in the brain's epileptic foci. They include sodium channel blockade, gamma-aminobutyric acid (GABA)–related targets, calcium channel blockade, glutamate synapses, and other mechanisms. Two other significant mechanisms include enhancing inhibitory GABA synapses and inhibiting excitatory glutamate activity. Sometimes several mechanisms work together. The mechanisms of action of antiepileptic drugs that affect GABA are shown in Fig. 10.1.

Ethosuximide utilizes calcium channel blockade by inhibiting low-threshold calcium ion currents, primarily in the thalamic neurons that serve as pacemakers and generate rhythmic cortical discharge. *Valproic acid* may also use this mechanism of action. *Clonazepam* binds to $GABA_A$ receptors, increasing the effect of GABA. It attaches to the benzodiazepine site of the GABA receptors, enhancing the development of GABA binding upon neurons and causing an increased influx of chloride ions into the neurons.

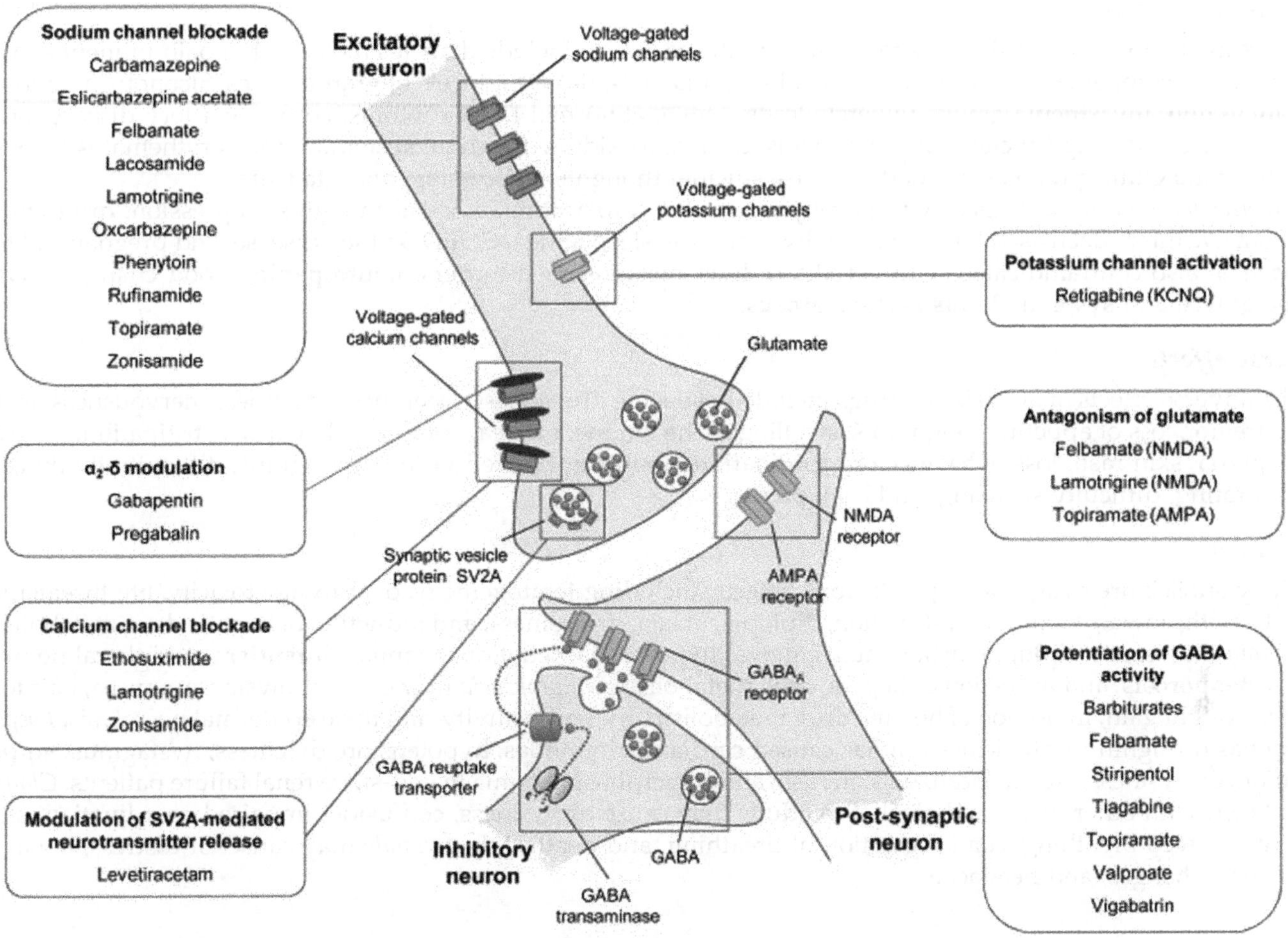

FIG. 10.1 Mechanisms of action of antiepileptic drugs that affect gamma-aminobutyric acid (GABA).

Clinical indications

To prescribe medications correctly, it is essential to accurately diagnose the specific types of seizures occurring. Choices of medications are usually based on established efficacy in the diagnosed seizures, patient responsiveness, anticipated toxicities, and possible drug interactions. Treatments may involve drug combinations with agents that are understood to be effective being added when an initial drug or drugs are not sufficient. The medicines of choice for generalized tonic-clonic and partial seizures include carbamazepine, lamotrigine, phenytoin, and valproic acid.

Ethosuximide and *valproic acid* are preferred over *clonazepam* because they only cause slight sedation. However, ethosuximide must be considered carefully due to GI adverse effects. Valproic acid is preferred if the patient has concurrent generalized tonic-clonic or myoclonic seizures. Clonazepam's effectiveness must be assessed against the likelihood of tolerance. Also effective for absence seizures are *lamotrigine*, *levetiracetam*, and *zonisamide*.

You should remember

For status epilepticus, IV *diazepam* or *lorazepam* is usually adequate. For long-term therapy, IV *phenytoin* is often preferred, though there is potential cardiotoxicity. Therefore *fosphenytoin* may be an even safer choice. For children with status epilepticus, *phenobarbital* has been successful. For extraordinarily severe and unresponsive status epilepticus, general anesthetics may be required.

Contraindications

There are many contraindications to antiseizure drugs, which include diabetes mellitus, hypoalbuminemia, osteomalacia, pancytopenia, porphyria, decreased blood platelets, deficient levels of granulocytes, alcoholism, myocardial infarction, myasthenia gravis, hypercholesterolemia, abnormal heart rhythms, coronary artery disease, heart failure, decreased lung function, liver problems, decreased kidney function, systemic lupus erythematosus, overgrowth of the gums, pregnancy, mood changes, suicidal thoughts, depression, and **glaucoma**.

Clonazepam is contraindicated with porphyria, alcohol intoxication, suicidal thoughts, depression, drug abuse, glaucoma, asthma, decreased lung function, liver disease, sleep apnea, COPD, kidney disease, and pregnancy. *Ethosuximide* is also contraindicated with hereditary liver metabolism disorders, **neutropenia**, mood changes, myasthenia gravis, and **systemic lupus erythematosus**.

Adverse effects

The adverse effects of antiseizure drugs include headache, drowsiness, sleepiness, dizziness, nervousness, instability, tremor, loss of appetite, weight loss, swelling of the tongue, nausea, vomiting, diarrhea, constipation, gingival hyperplasia, skin rash, loss of balance or coordination, double or blurred vision, nystagmus, difficulty thinking or concentrating, difficulty speaking, and back pain.

Toxicities

Many antiseizure drugs have specific toxic effects, including teratogenicity, overdosage toxicity, life-threatening toxicity, withdrawal, cognitive dysfunction, diplopia, ataxia, drowsiness, and induction of hepatic drug metabolism. *Phenytoin* may cause **diplopia**, nystagmus, gingival hyperplasia, sedation, anemias, **hirsutism**, peripheral neuropathy, **osteoporosis**, and induction of hepatic drug metabolism. *Valproic acid* may cause drowsiness, nausea, hair loss, tremor, weight gain, inhibition of hepatic drug metabolism, hypersensitivity, and toxic epidermal necrolysis. *Fosphenytoin* has no significant toxicities but has caused cardiac arrhythmias, hypotension, dizziness, nystagmus, **stupor**, sedation, drowsiness, **ataxia**, localized skin rash, and hyperphosphatemia in end-stage renal failure patients. *Clonazepam* taken with other drugs and alcohol in adults may cause drowsiness, confusion, impaired coordination, slow reflexes, slowed breathing, coma, cessation of breathing, and death. *Ethosuximide* may cause GI distress, lethargy, behavioral changes, and headache.

You should remember

Absence seizures cause patients to "blank out" or continually stare for a few seconds. They are most common in children and usually do not cause long-term problems. They are often initiated by hyperventilation. Some children have 10 to 100 absence seizures within 1 day, and these are often not noticed by others. The absence seizures can significantly affect learning and concentration, so prompt treatment is essential.

Backup and adjunctive drugs

Various backup and adjunctive drugs are used for multiple types of seizures (see Table 10.2). These drugs include *felbamate, gabapentin, lacosamide, levetiracetam, perampanel, phenobarbital, rufinamide, tiagabine, topiramate, vigabatrin,* and *zonisamide*.

Pharmacokinetics

Tiagabine, topiramate, and *vigabatrin* are metabolized in the liver and eliminated by the kidneys. *Perampanel* has a long half-life. CYP3A4 metabolizes it in the liver and then undergoes glucuronidation. *Felbamate* has over 90% bioavailability and is metabolized by the liver. Its elimination half-life is 20–23 hours. *Lacosamide* has high bioavailability and an elimination half-life of 13 hours and is secreted by the kidneys. *Phenobarbital* has over 95% bioavailability and protein binding of 20%–45%. It is metabolized in the liver mainly by CYP2C19 and has an onset of action within 5 minutes intravenously and within 30 minutes orally. Its elimination half-life is 53–118 hours, and the duration of action is between 4 hours and 2 days. *Rufinamide* has a maximum bioavailability of 85% over 4–6 hours and

TABLE 10.2 Backup and adjunctive drugs for various types of seizures.

Generic name	Trade name
cenobamate	Ontozry, Xcopri
felbamate	Felbatol
fenfluramine	Fintepla
gabapentin	Neurontin
lacosamide	Vimpat
levetiracetam	Keppra
perampanel	Fycompa
phenobarbital	Luminal
rufinamide	Banzel
tiagabine	Gabitril
topiramate	Topamax
vigabatrin	Vigadrone
zonisamide	Zonegran

34% protein binding. It is metabolized via carboxylesterase-mediated hydrolysis, with CYP not being involved. Its metabolites are inactive; the elimination half-life is 6–10 hours. Rufinamide is excreted in the urine at 85%.

Zonisamide has close to 100% bioavailability and 40% protein binding. It is metabolized in the liver via CYP3A4, and its elimination half-life is 63 hours in the plasma. Zonisamide is excreted at 62% in the urine and 3% in the feces.

Mechanism of action

Felbamate is believed to have a unique dual mechanism of action as a positive modulator of $GABA_A$ receptors and a blocker of NMDA receptors. *Gabapentin, lacosamide, levetiracetam, rufinamide,* and *vigabatrin* have uncertain mechanisms of action. The precise mechanism of action for *perampanel* has yet to be fully understood. *Phenobarbital* acts on $GABA_A$ receptors to increase synaptic inhibition. *Tiagabine* binds to recognition sites related to the GABA uptake carrier. *Topiramate* affects voltage-dependent sodium channels, GABA receptors, and glutamate receptors. *Zonisamide* targets sodium and calcium channels.

Clinical indications

Felbamate is used as monotherapy or adjunctive therapy in treating adult partial seizures, with and without generalization. It is an adjunctive therapy in treating partial and generalized seizures in children. *Gabapentin* is approved for treating focal and mixed seizures, but there is no evidence for its use in generalized epilepsy. *Lacosamide* is approved for adjunctive treatment of partial-onset seizures and neuropathic pain and conversion to monotherapy for partial-onset seizures. *Levetiracetam* is an effective monotherapy for newly diagnosed focal epilepsy in adults and is an adjunct drug for partial, myoclonic, and tonic-clonic seizures. *Perampanel* is used with other medicines for partial and generalized tonic-clonic seizures in patients older than 12.

Phenobarbital is used for all types of seizures except absence seizures. It is the first-line choice for neonatal seizures. *Rufinamide* is used for various types of seizures. *Tiagabine* is approved as an adjunctive treatment for partial seizures in patients 12 years and older. *Topiramate* is used to treat epilepsy in patients 2 years and older.

Vigabatrin is approved as monotherapy for pediatric patients 1 month to 2 years of age with infantile spasms when the benefits are likely to exceed the risk of vision loss. It is also adjunctive therapy for adults with refractory complex partial seizures who have not responded well to other treatments. *Zonisamide* is approved for adjunctive treatment of partial seizures in adults.

Contraindications

Felbamate is contraindicated with any history of hematological diseases, including leukopenia, agranulocytosis, neutropenia, bone marrow suppression, anemias, and thrombocytopenia because of increased risks for hematologic toxicity. *Gabapentin* is contraindicated with suicidal thoughts, depression, myasthenia gravis, COPD, and kidney disease.

Lacosamide is also contraindicated with coronary artery disease, low supplies of oxygen-rich blood to the heart, atrial fibrillation, and flutter. *Levetiracetam* is contraindicated with anemia, low levels of white blood cells, psychosis, and hallucinations.

Perampanel is contraindicated with behavioral changes, bipolar disorder, schizophrenia, driving or operating machinery, liver or kidney disease, substance abuse, and in older adults. *Phenobarbital* is contraindicated with high blood ammonia, porphyria, alcohol intoxication, and coma from liver failure.

Adverse effects

Felbamate commonly can cause drowsiness, dizziness, nausea, vomiting, diarrhea, constipation, insomnia, and headache. *Gabapentin* can cause uncontrollable tremors, double or blurred vision, and anxiety. *Lacosamide* uniquely causes nystagmus. *Levetiracetam* can cause tiredness, weakness, aggressiveness, irritability, loss of appetite, increased likelihood of infections, and stuffy nose. *Perampanel* has been uniquely linked to coordination problems and falling.

Toxicities

Felbamate may cause aplastic anemia or hepatic failure. *Gabapentin* may cause dizziness, sedation, ataxia, and nystagmus, but this does not affect drug metabolism, similar to *pregabalin*. *Lacosamide* may cause diarrhea, nausea, vomiting, dizziness, headache, drowsiness, blurred vision, diplopia, involuntary movements, memory problems, ataxia, panic attacks, agitation, restlessness, irritability, aggression, anxiety, depression, suicidal thoughts, insomnia, mania, altered mood, postural hypotension, and pruritus.

Levetiracetam may cause dizziness, sedation, irritability, weakness, hallucinations, and psychosis. *Perampanel* may cause dizziness, drowsiness, behavioral hostility, and headache. *Phenobarbital* may cause cognitive dysfunction, sedation, dependence, tolerance, and induction of hepatic drug metabolism. *Rufinamide* has caused low rates of transient serum enzyme elevations.

Tiagabine may cause abdominal pain, nausea, dizziness, tremor, and asthenia. *Topiramate* may cause dizziness, drowsiness, ataxia, psychomotor slowing, memory impairment, paresthesias, acute myopia, and weight loss. *Vigabatrin* can cause dizziness, sedation, weight gain, and irreversible visual field defects. *Zonisamide* may cause confusion, dizziness, agitation, diarrhea, rash, and weight loss.

You should remember

Five new ASMs were approved between 2018 and 2020 for the daily treatment of epilepsy. Three are for patients 2 years of age and older: everolimus (Afinitor), stiripentol (Diacomit), and fenfluramine (Fintepla). One is for patients 1 year of age and older: cannabidiol (Epidiolex). One is for adults only: cenobamate (Xcopri).

Clinical Case Studies

Clinical Case Study 1

A 38-year-old female had been having nocturnal seizures since the age of 29. She also experienced dizziness, confusion, depression, and severe joint pain. Her previous medication was phenobarbital, but the patient disliked its effects. She tried to wean off the medication but experienced more nocturnal seizures. There was no indication of head trauma, infections, or fever. No family history of seizure disorders was present. The patient's medication was switched slowly to carbamazepine, and the intensity and duration of his nocturnal seizures greatly improved.

Critical Thinking Questions

1. Which types of seizure conditions are more likely to occur as nocturnal seizures?
2. What is the primary indication for carbamazepine?
3. If toxic levels are reached, what can carbamazepine cause?

Clinical Case Study 2

A 21-year-old female had a history of absence seizures that started when she was 10. At that time, she was diagnosed with generalized epilepsy. Valproic acid was initiated, and she had no seizures for 11 years. When she was 19, she started taking oral contraceptives and had daily absence seizures and a few generalized tonic-clonic seizures. Lamotrigine was tried, but the seizures worsened. Eventually, seizure control was provided by a combination of valproic acid and levetiracetam. Intending to start a family, the patient went to a specialist in epilepsy and asked if this would be possible along with her condition. The specialist explained that her ability to become pregnant and deliver a healthy baby was very likely with modern medications and careful management.

Critical Thinking Questions

1. What is an absence seizure?
2. What are the drugs of choice for generalized tonic-clonic seizures?
3. What are the indications of levetiracetam?

Key Terms

Absence seizure
Action potential
Apathy
Asthenia
Ataxia
Carboxylesterase
Diplopia
Epilepsy
Generalized seizures
Glaucoma
Grand mal seizures
Hirsutism
Myoclonic seizure
Neutropenia
Nocturnal seizures
Nystagmus
Osteomalacia
Osteoporosis
Partial seizure
Porphyria
Prodrome
Skin abrasions
Status epilepticus
Stupor
Subdural hematoma
Systemic lupus erythematosus
Tonic-clonic seizure

Further Reading

[1] C.W. Bazil, Living Well with Epilepsy and Other Seizure Disorders: An Expert Explains what You Need to Know (Living Well), HarperResource, 2004.
[2] T. Betts, L. Greenhill, Managing Epilepsy with Females in Mind, CRC Press, 2005.
[3] J. Cafer, J. Link, Cafer's Mood Stabilizers and Antiepileptics: Drug Interactions and Trade/Generic Name Pairings of Medications for Bipolar and Seizure Disorders (Visualize to Memorize), CaferMed LLC, 2020.
[4] G. Coppola, Pediatric Neurology Part I: Chapter 62. Malignant Migrating Partial Seizures in Infancy (Handbook of Clinical Neurology 111), Elsevier, 2013.
[5] T. Deonna, E. Roulet-Perez, The Epilepsy Aphasia Spectrum: From Landau-Kleffner syndrome to Rolandic Epilepsy. (Clinics in Developmental Medicine), Mac Keith Press, 2016.
[6] O. Devinsky, Epilepsy: A Patient and Family Guide, third ed., Demos Health, 2007.
[7] O. Devinsky, E. Conway, C. Schnabel Glick, Epilepsy in Children: What Every Parent Needs to Know, Demos Health, 2015.
[8] M.J. Eadie, F.J.E. Vajda, Antiepileptic drugs and pregnancy: a guide for prescribers, Adis (2015).

[9] C.L. Faingold, G.H. Fromm, Drugs for the Control of Epilepsy: Actions on Neuronal Networks Involved in Seizure Disorders, CRC Press, 2019.

[10] B. Fisch, Epilepsy and Intensive Care Monitoring: Principles and Practice, Demos Medical Publishing, 2009.

[11] V.K. Harpale, V. Bairagi, Brain Seizure Detection and Classification Using EEG Signals, Academic Press, 2021.

[12] R.T. Johnson, J.W. Griffin, J.C. McArthur, Current Therapy in Neurologic Disease, seventh ed., Mosby, 2005.

[13] M.Z. Koubeissi, N.J. Azar, Epilepsy Board Review: A Comprehensive Guide, Springer, 2017.

[14] H.B. McIntyre, The Primary Care of Seizure Disorders: A Practical Guide to the Evaluation and Comprehensive Management of Seizure Disorders, Butterworth-Heinemann, 2013.

[15] P.N. Modur, P.K. Gupta, D. Sirsi, Epilepsy Board Review, Demos Medical, 2016.

[16] P.N. Patsalos, E.K. St. Louis, The Epilepsy Prescriber's Guide to Antiepileptic Drugs, third ed., Cambridge University Press, 2018.

[17] J.E. Pina-Garza, Fenichel's Clinical Pediatric Neurology, seventh ed., Saunders, 2013.

[18] A. Pitkanen, P. Buckmaster, A.S. Galanopoulou, S.L. Moshe, Models of Seizures and Epilepsy, second ed., Academic Press, 2017.

[19] S.K. Satapathy, S. Dehuri, A. Kumar Jagadev, S. Mishra, EEG Brain Signal Classification for Epileptic Seizure Disorder Detection, Academic Press, 2019.

[20] M. Sazgar, C.L. Harden, Controversies in Caring for Females with Epilepsy: Sorting Through the Evidence, Springer, 2016.

[21] B.E. Skolnick, W.M. Alves, Handbook of Neuroemergency Clinical Trials, second ed., Academic Press, 2017.

[22] E.A.P. Steegers, M.J. Cipolla, E.C. Miller, Neurology and Pregnancy: Neuro-Obstetric Disorders (Handbook of Clinical Neurology 172), Elsevier, 2020.

[23] M.B. Sterman, L.M. Thompson, Clinical Neurotherapy: Chapter 12. Neurofeedback for Seizure Disorders: Origins, Mechanisms and Best Practices, Academic Press, 2013.

[24] A.N. Wilner, Epilepsy, 199 Answers: A Doctor Responds to Patients' Questions, third ed., Demos Health, 2008.

[25] E. Wyllie, B.E. Gidal, H.P. Goodkin, L. Jehi, T. Loddenkemper, Wyllie's Treatment of Epilepsy: Principles and Practice, seventh ed., Lippincott, Williams, and Wilkins, 2020.

CHAPTER

11

General anesthetics

OUTLINE

LEARNING OUTCOMES

After study of this chapter, readers should be able to:

1. Describe the main classes of anesthetic agents.
2. Explain the various stages of anesthesia.
3. Explain the purposes of general anesthesia.
4. Describe the advantage of combining IV and inhaled anesthetics.
5. Discuss the benefits of propofol.
6. Identify the contraindications of general anesthesia.
7. Explain the potency of inhalation anesthetics.
8. Describe the indications of nitrous oxide.
9. Explain the contraindications of isoflurane.
10. Discuss the symptoms of anesthesia adjuncts.

The Science of Pharmacology
https://doi.org/10.1016/B978-0-443-29038-1.00011-7

Overview

General anesthesia brings on a sleeplike state with a combination of medicines. The medicines, known as anesthetics, are given before and during surgery or other medical procedures. General anesthesia usually uses a variety of intravenous (IV) drugs and inhaled gases. It allows surgical and other interventional procedures to be performed quickly and safely, producing analgesia, no anxiety, and adequate muscle relaxation. Medications used to block pain are called anesthetics. Different types of anesthesia have varying mechanisms of action. Some anesthetic medications numb certain body parts, while others numb the brain, inducing sleep for more invasive surgical procedures. General anesthesia is given by IV injection or inhalation. The components of general anesthesia are analgesia, amnesia, muscle relaxation, control of vital signs, and unconsciousness. The depth of anesthesia is planned to allow the surgical procedure to be performed without the patient experiencing pain, moving, or having any recall of the process. Endotracheal intubation or insertion of another artificial airway device and respiratory support are often necessary. General anesthesia may be administered only by an anesthesiologist with or without an assistant or a certified registered nurse anesthetist or by a dentist with postgraduate training and licensing.

Stages of anesthesia

Anesthesia is the production of a controlled loss of sensation as a part of surgery or diagnosis. **General anesthesia** of the entire body occurs in distinct stages. There are four stages of general anesthesia, which include the following:

- **Stage I (analgesia):** The general sensation is lost, but the patient may remain awake; this stage continues until there is a loss of consciousness.
- **Stage II (excitement):** The patient can become delirious and try to "fight back" and resist treatment; heart rate and respiratory rate may become irregular, and blood pressure may increase; administration of IV agents may help to calm the patient; the patient should progress into stage III quickly to avoid experiencing feelings of panic; and there is close monitoring for irregularities of heart rate and increased blood pressure.
- **Stage III (surgical anesthesia):** The skeletal muscles relax, and **delirium** is stabilized, as well as cardiopulmonary effects; the patient is motionless, and eye movements are limited; it is at this point that the surgery begins, and the patient remains in this stage until the procedure is completed.
- **Stage IV (medullary paralysis):** This stage is avoided because if breathing and cardiac function stop, death could occur.

The best medications used for anesthesia can quickly induce all of the stages of anesthesia, while weaker drugs can only induce stage I. As the patient recovers after surgery, they move back up through the four stages until awakening. Newer inhaled and IV general anesthetics often have a much faster onset of action and distribution throughout the body. Therefore specific stages of anesthesia may not be as readily observable as with older drugs.

Classifications of medications

There are five classifications of medications used in anesthesia: IV anesthetics, inhalational anesthetics, IV sedatives, synthetic opioids, and neuromuscular blocking drugs. Each type is based on the sedation and analgesia needed for the intended procedure. The primary goal of general anesthesia is loss of sensation, along with loss of consciousness. General anesthesia is used for major surgical procedures. **Regional anesthesia** affects an entire limb or relatively large portion of the body, with fewer adverse effects than general anesthesia. It is often the chosen method because of this factor. Examples of regional anesthesia include epidural and spinal anesthesia. **Monitored anesthesia care** utilizes analgesics, sedatives, and low doses of other drugs, which allow the patient to remain responsive and breathe without assistance as a procedure is being performed. It supplements regional or local anesthesia during diagnostic procedures and minor surgeries. There are subtypes of monitored anesthesia care that include the following:

- **Anxiolysis** (minimal sedation): The patient can respond to verbal commands and has normal airway, cardiovascular, and ventilation functions.

- **Conscious sedation** (moderate sedation): The patient can respond to verbal commands, light, and touch. There is normal airway, cardiovascular, and ventilation function.
- **Deep sedation and analgesia**: The patient can be aroused by repeated or painful stimulation, but airway and ventilation interventions may be needed. Cardiovascular functions are primarily adequate.

You should remember

Without anesthesia, surgical incisions would cause reflexes in the body and damage to the site being operated upon. There would be increases in heart rate and changes in blood pressure. All of these are automatic defense mechanisms.

Methods of anesthesia

The medicine is inhaled through a breathing mask or tube or given through an IV line. Four main categories of anesthesia are used during surgery and other procedures: general anesthesia, regional anesthesia, sedation, and local anesthesia (see Chapter 12). A variety of medications are administered to achieve general anesthesia. The five purposes of general anesthesia are analgesia, relaxation, hypnosis, **amnesia**, and loss of **reflexes**. Analgesia is the blocking of pain sensations. Relaxation is the removal of extreme anxiety that is linked to medical procedures. Hypnosis is the production of unconsciousness. Amnesia is the blocking of memories in the system. Loss of reflexes involves the blockade of autonomic and other reflexes that can be affected by the medical process. No individual drug can safely achieve all five of these purposes. Therefore the method of **balanced anesthesia** is used, in which a combination of medications work together to produce general anesthesia.

These medications include neuromuscular blockers, opioids, short-acting benzodiazepines, and general anesthetics. Their combination provides sedation, a fast induction of unconsciousness, muscle relaxation, and analgesia. The medication combination also lessens the need for many inhaled drugs, which are not as safe. Balanced anesthesia begins with administering IV medications before the general anesthetic is given. Muscle relaxation, pain reduction, and sleep occur. After losing consciousness, the patient is given an inhaled prevalent drug to remain anesthetized. Less anesthesia is required for shorter procedures; sometimes injected agents alone are adequate.

Intravenous anesthetics

IV anesthetics are crucial to balanced anesthesia; these include opioids, benzodiazepines, and miscellaneous agents. When a single IV bolus is given, it enters the brain, allowing the patient to progress quickly through stages I and II. Sometimes they are used alone for minor diagnostic or surgical procedures. The simultaneous use of IV and inhalation anesthetics allows for lower doses of the inhalation drugs. This provides a better surgical outcome and reduces risks of serious adverse effects from inhaled anesthetics. Also, combining IV and inhaled anesthetics allows more analgesia and muscle relaxation than when inhalation anesthetics are used independently. Less than 12 drugs are used as IV anesthetics; some have nonanesthetic uses. Table 11.1 summarizes the effects of IV and inhaled general anesthetics.

Opioids, also called *narcotic analgesics*, are the most effective drugs for analgesia. They must be combined with other anesthetics for deep anesthesia to be provided. This allows for lower doses and adequate analgesia to prevent pain from being perceived. Generally, opioids used as IV anesthetics include *fentanyl*, *alfentanil*, *remifentanil*, and *sufentanil*. The opioid receptor agonists cause a rapid onset of action, with a short duration of only 10–30 minutes. Their main disadvantage is respiratory depression. Also, muscle rigidity can develop, which may further restrict ventilation. **Neuroleptanalgesia** occurs when fentanyl is combined with the antipsychotic drug known as *droperidol or haloperidol*. This causes the patient to feel indifferent or unaffected by the surrounding environment. The patient does not lose consciousness yet appears to be asleep. Fentanyl is a potent opioid agonist that acts similar to morphine. Droperidol is identical to *haloperidol* and can reduce nausea and vomiting caused by opioids while

TABLE 11.1 The effects of intravenous and inhaled general anesthetics.

Effects	Organ or body system involved
Brain and spinal cord depression, blurred vision, nystagmus, progression of depression to decreased alertness, decreased level of consciousness and sensation	Central nervous system
Decreased glomerular filtration	Renal system
Depressed myocardium, hypotension and tachycardia, bradycardia as a response to vagal stimulation	Cardiovascular system
Impaired oxygenation, airway irritation, possible laryngospasm, depressed airway-protective mechanisms	Respiratory system
Increased intracranial pressure	Cerebrovascular system
Reduced liver blood flow and clearance	Gastrointestinal system
Skeletal muscle relaxation	Musculoskeletal system
Vasodilation	Integumentary system

FIG. 11.1 Context-sensitive halftime of various IV anesthetics.

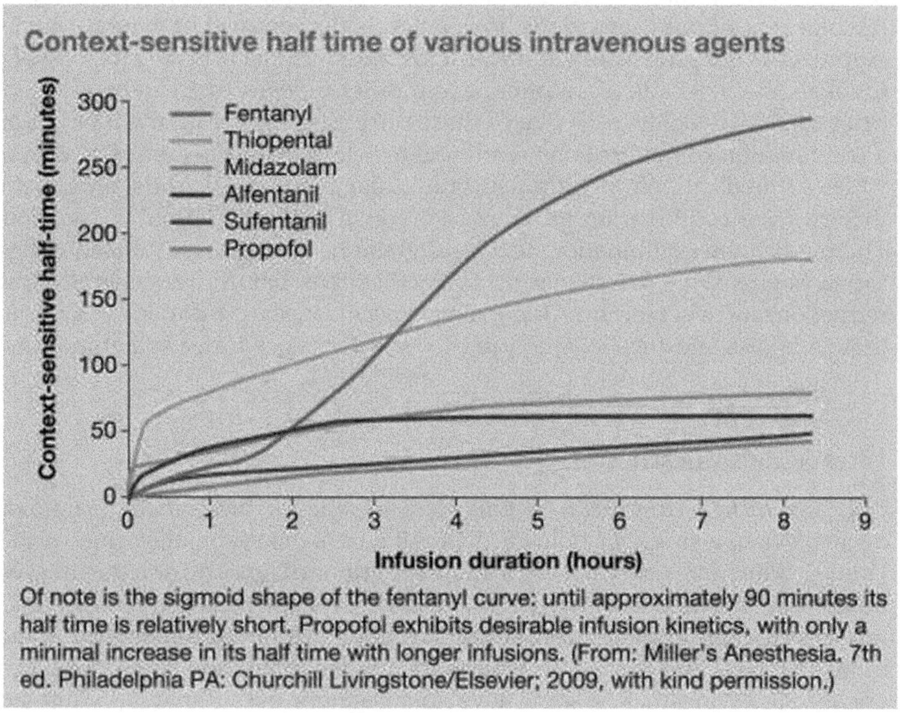

Of note is the sigmoid shape of the fentanyl curve: until approximately 90 minutes its half time is relatively short. Propofol exhibits desirable infusion kinetics, with only a minimal increase in its half time with longer infusions. (From: Miller's Anesthesia. 7th ed. Philadelphia PA: Churchill Livingstone/Elsevier; 2009, with kind permission.)

producing sedation by reducing motor activity and anxiety. Fig. 11.1 illustrates the context-sensitive half-time of various IV anesthetics. Opioid analgesics are discussed in detail in Chapter 15.

Sedative and hypnotic drugs are injected as preoperative and dental procedures. They have sedative, hypnotic, anxiolytic, anticonvulsant, and muscle relaxant properties. Benzodiazepines are commonly used for patients on a mechanical ventilator (see Chapter 9). Miscellaneous drugs used as IV anesthetics include *propofol* and *ketamine*. They both have short durations of action and quickly induce anesthesia. IV narcotics (opioids, benzodiazepines, and miscellaneous drugs) are listed in Table 11.2.

TABLE 11.2 Intravenous anesthetics.

Generic name	Trade name
Opioids	
alfentanil	Alfenta
fentanyl	Sublimaze
remifentanil	Ultiva
sufentanil	Sufenta
Benzodiazepines	
diazepam	Valium
midazolam	Versed
lorazepam (in the hospital)	
Miscellaneous	
etomidate	Amidate
ketamine	Ketalar
methohexital	Brevital
propofol	Diprivan

You should remember

In older adults, IV anesthetics must be used carefully because organ systems deteriorate with aging. For example, reduced liver function causes decreased metabolism of many drugs, and reduced kidney function results in decreased drug excretion. Both of these conditions can lead to drug toxicity and even overdose. Older adults are also more sensitive to drugs that affect the CNS. Cardiac and respiratory disease also increase risks for anesthetic-related dysrhythmias, hypotension, atelectasis, respiratory depression, and pneumonia. Polypharmacy is another factor to consider when an older adult requires IV anesthetics.

Pharmacokinetics

Injected opioids such as fentanyl may be given by IV, intramuscular (IM), epidural, transdermal, or transmucosal routes with rapid absorption. They cross the placenta and can be secreted in breast milk. Injected opioids are 80% bound to plasma protein. Primary metabolism occurs in the liver by the cytochrome P450 enzyme and is excreted by the kidneys. The onset of action for the IV form is immediate. Via IM injection, they start to work in 7–15 minutes and via epidural injection in 10–15 minutes. Via the transmucosal route, effects peak in 20–30 minutes, and via the transdermal route, they peak within 24–72 hours. The IV duration of action is 30 minutes to 1 hour, and the IM duration is 1–2 hours. The epidural duration of action is 2–3 hours. The transdermal route has a 17-hour half-life; the transmucosal course is unknown.

Benzodiazepines may be administered IV or IM. They are rapidly absorbed and widely distributed. These drugs cross the blood-brain barrier and the placenta and are secreted in breast milk. Injected benzodiazepines are 97% bound to plasma protein. They metabolize in the liver and are eliminated via the kidneys. The IV onset of action is 1.5 minutes, while the IM onset is 5–15 minutes. The miscellaneous drugs, including *propofol*, are rapidly absorbed and widely distributed, with high protein binding. Primary metabolism is via the liver, and excretion is via the kidneys. There is an immediate onset of action, lasting 10–15 minutes.

Mechanism of action

Opioid agonists act at the mu and kappa receptors, with the mechanism of action being the same as that of other opioids, including morphine. However, fentanyl has a much more rapid onset of action. *Midazolam* acts at the brain's hypothalamic, limbic, and thalamic regions, producing CNS depression and skeletal muscle relaxation. For *propofol*, the exact mechanism of action is not precise. It is believed to act via activation of the GABA receptors, resulting in a general inhibition of the CNS.

Clinical indications

Fentanyl is administered with oxygen for high-risk patients, including those having open-heart surgery or complex neurologic or orthopedic surgeries. In oral, buccal, sublingual, transmucosal, intranasal, and transdermal forms, fentanyl is prescribed for treating pain in patients who are receiving constant opioid therapy and have become tolerant. *Alfentanil* is used as a component of balanced anesthesia. It is used to assist with intubation and promote anesthesia induction and as an infusion to maintain anesthesia. It is indicated for managing severe postoperative pain when administered as an epidural injection. *Remifentanil* is given during installation and maintenance of general anesthesia to provide pain relief after surgery and can be used alone or in combination with *midazolam*. *Sufentanil* is used as part of balanced anesthesia or as a primary anesthetic, along with 100% oxygen administered concurrently. It is sometimes indicated, along with *bupivacaine*, as an epidural anesthetic during labor and delivery. Sufentanil is 5–10 times more potent than fentanyl.

Benzodiazepines are mainly indicated to treat anxiety, but high doses cause sedation and unconsciousness. They are used as part of balanced anesthesia, often given with inhalation anesthetics. They are sometimes given orally as a premedication before surgery to relax the patient. The most commonly used benzodiazepine for surgery is midazolam, though diazepam (Valium) and lorazepam are sometimes used. Midazolam is approved for the induction of amnesia, installation, maintenance of general anesthesia, and sedation.

Propofol is now the most widely used IV anesthetic because of its high effectiveness and relative safety. It is indicated for induction and maintenance of general anesthesia. In intensive care, propofol is given to intubated and mechanically ventilated adults, providing continuous sedation and control of stress responses. It is also effective for conscious sedation. *Etomidate* is indicated for induction of general anesthesia for short medical and surgical procedures, including cardioversion, endotracheal intubation, and reduction of dislocated joints. It is also used as a supplement for anesthesia and nitrous oxide. *Ketamine* produces a trancelike state. When used alone, it is used for surgeries and diagnostic procedures that do not require relaxation of the skeletal muscles. Ketamine is also given before other general anesthetics are administered. *Methohexital* is a barbiturate that is sometimes used as a supplement form of anesthesia with nitrous oxide.

Contraindications

There are no absolute contraindications to general anesthesia other than patient refusal or the lack of availability of trained personnel. However, there are some relative contraindications. IV anesthetics are contraindicated if there are known drug allergies, with narrow-angle glaucoma, acute **porphyria**, and if the patient has a known susceptibility to **malignant hyperthermia**.

Adverse effects

Propofol may cause dose-dependent hypotension or respiratory depression. It can also cause anaphylaxis, injection site pain, and infusion syndrome, including severe metabolic acidosis, rhabdomyolysis, kidney failure, and heart failure. *Etomidate* may cause injection site pain, myoclonus, averting movements, tonic movements, ocular movements, and postoperative nausea and vomiting. *Ketamine* may cause nystagmus, increased oxygen demand and pulmonary arterial pressure, disorientation, hallucinations, nightmares, vivid dreams, abnormal electroencephalogram results, increased salivation, and, with rapid injection or high doses, respiratory depression.

Methohexital may cause dose-dependent hypotension, apnea, or respiratory depression, as well as bronchospasm, laryngospasm, myoclonus, injection site pain, visual hallucinations, vivid dreams, and arrhythmias. Patients who are older, sicker, and undergoing lengthy procedures are at increased risk of serious complications, including persistent confusion, memory loss, pneumonia, thromboembolism, myocardial infarction, and cerebrovascular accidents. General anesthesia deaths are rare and estimated to be approximately 1 in 150,000.

Toxicities

Opioids do not cause specific organ toxicity and are not associated with upper GI bleeding or kidney toxicity. In medical use, any potential for toxicity is unseen because effects end long before the elimination half-life. Benzodiazepines have a potential for toxicity when combined with other CNS depressants, including alcohol and opioids, as well as with tricyclic antidepressants. There have been fatal overdoses from these combinations. There are sporadic reports of liver toxicity from benzodiazepines. There may be a slight possibility of carcinogenesis with these drugs. Symptoms of benzodiazepine toxicity include drowsiness, nystagmus, slurred speech, ataxia, hypotension, respiratory depression, cardiorespiratory arrest, and coma. While most of the miscellaneous drugs used for anesthesia have no severe toxicities, ketamine has been linked to urotoxicity and hepatotoxicity.

You should remember

Fentanyl is given IV for short-duration analgesia as a component of premedication, balanced anesthesia, induction and maintenance, and postoperative pain. Propofol starts and maintains general anesthesia and provides sedation for mechanically ventilated adults and various surgical procedures.

Inhalation anesthetics

Inhalation anesthetics, classified as volatile liquids or gases, also provide general anesthesia and are administered through a facemask, laryngeal mask airway, or tracheal tube connected to an anesthetic vaporizer and delivery system. After IV medications, inhalation anesthetics are administered, quickly producing unconsciousness and total analgesia. Table 11.3 lists the generic and trade names of inhalation anesthetics.

The potency of inhalation anesthetics is described via their minimum alveolar concentration, the amount of drug vapor in the lung's alveoli that prevents motor responses in 50% of patients exposed to a painful stimulus. If the concentration is low, it shows that only a tiny amount of the anesthetic is required to immobilize a patient. Inhalation anesthetics are very potent because they have such low minimum alveolar concentrations—except for nitrous oxide, which has low potency and a high minimum alveolar concentration value. Minimum alveolar concentrations change with age and are most lacking in newborns, highest in infants, and gradually decline over the lifespan.

Inhalation anesthetics are quickly absorbed from the alveoli into systemic blood circulation. An anesthesiologist controls anesthesia by delivering the correct concentration of the required drug. These highly lipid-soluble anesthetics rapidly cross the blood-brain barrier to produce sedation. Their oil-to-gas partition coefficient measures the potency of these anesthetics. Metabolism of the drugs is only minimal, and exhalation is responsible for most drug elimination. Today's inhalation anesthetics are designed to allow patients to regain consciousness soon after stopping the infusion. Because these anesthetics are stored in fat and released slowly, obese patients may need more time to recover from anesthesia.

Volatile liquids are used as inhalation anesthetics because they have a low vapor pressure. This allows them to vaporize into a gas at low temperatures and pressure. An anesthesia machine vaporizes the liquids, mixing the vapors with oxygen and air, and then carefully delivers them to the patient. Anesthesia machines establish a **partial-pressure** gradient, ensuring the anesthetic flows to the alveoli, blood, and brain. *Isoflurane, desflurane,* and *sevoflurane* all have a rapid onset of action. The minimum alveolar concentrations of these drugs are deficient and have high potency. Therefore they quickly produce unconsciousness at low doses. They make only a slight amount of analgesia, usually combined with nitrous oxide and opioids in balanced anesthesia. Some volatile liquids sensitize the heart to catecholamines, including dopamine, epinephrine, and norepinephrine, to cause serious dysrhythmias. They also depress pulmonary and cardiovascular function, which can result in laryngospasm or respiratory arrest.

Pharmacokinetics

With inhalation anesthetics, the depth of anesthesia is measured via the partial pressure of the inhaled drug within the brain. An adequate amount of anesthetic must reach the brain to produce concentrations needed for surgery. A rigid set of physical principles applies because these drugs are administered as gases or vapors. The lungs rapidly absorb inhalation anesthetics and cross the blood-brain barrier to become concentrated in the neurons. There

TABLE 11.3 Inhalation anesthetics.

Generic name	Trade names
desflurane	Suprane
enflurane	Ethrane
isoflurane	Forane, others
nitrous oxide	Entonox
sevoflurane	Ultane, others

is minimal metabolism, and 95% of its excretion is via the lungs (see Fig. 11.2). The onset of action is 2–5 minutes. The patient begins to return to consciousness in less than 1 hour. Action duration is a variable half-life, and their peak effect is less than 10 minutes.

Mechanism of action

Inhalation anesthetics inhibit the flow of sodium into neurons, delaying nerve impulses and considerably slowing the activity of neurons. Inhibitory gamma-aminobutyric acid (GABA) receptors in the brain are activated. *Isoflurane* interacts with many brain receptors, including the GABA and glutamate receptors. *Desflurane* also affects ligand-gated ion channels. *Nitric oxide* may activate opioid receptors in the midbrain. Its relaxation properties are believed to be due to activation of GABA receptors and inhibition of the firing of neurons.

Clinical indications

Isoflurane is a very safe and effective inhaled anesthetic that provides general anesthesia quickly, with a low amount of metabolism by the body. The lungs nearly eliminate it and provide extreme muscle relaxation. Isoflurane is indicated for induction and maintenance of general anesthesia and status asthmaticus. It does not sensitize the myocardium for dysrhythmias and produces few cardiovascular effects. *Desflurane* has the most rapid onset and offset of all volatile liquids used for general anesthesia due to its low solubility in the blood. *Sevoflurane* is one of the most commonly used flammable liquids and is often administered in a mixture of nitrous oxide and oxygen.

Nitrous oxide is an inorganic, nonirritating, odorless gas used for medical and surgical procedures. Used alone, it cannot induce deep anesthesia at therapeutic doses. Therefore nitrous oxide is used for minor surgical procedures or combined with IV anesthetics for more complicated surgeries. Most patients who need to be sedated for surgical, diagnostic, or dental procedures are given nitrous oxide. The agent has powerful analgesic properties. At only 20% concentration, it delivers as much analgesia as morphine. It does not produce loss of consciousness or any extreme skeletal muscle relaxation. Nitrous oxide is combined with 25%–30% oxygen. A patient may be given an IV anesthetic to produce sedation and then given nitrous oxide via a mask or tube. For dental procedures, the show is placed

FIG. 11.2 Pharmacokinetics of inhaled anesthetics.

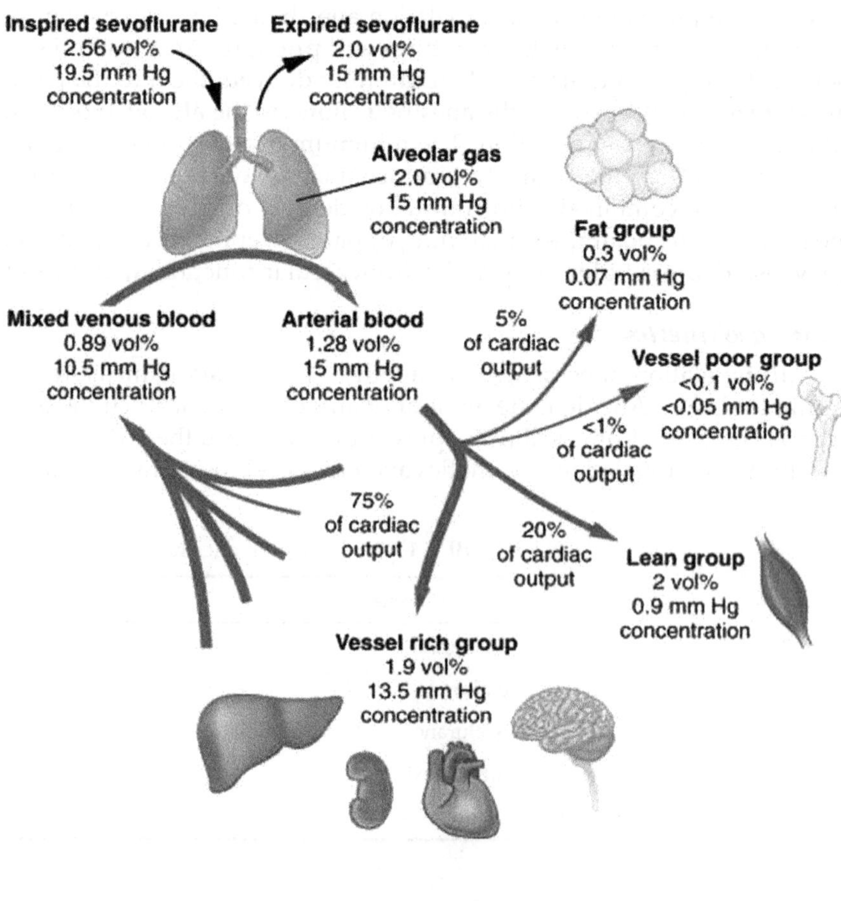

over the patient's nose. Nitrous oxide is also indicated for obstetric procedures. It lowers the minimum alveolar concentration of other anesthetics, increasing their potency. Therefore their dosages can be decreased.

Contraindications

Isoflurane is contraindicated in patients with hyperkalemia and muscle or nerve diseases, including **Duchenne muscular dystrophy**, hypotension, liver abnormalities, and malignant hyperthermia. *Desflurane* is contraindicated with malignant hyperthermia in patients who cannot tolerate general anesthesia, children with known sensitivity to this drug or similar agents, and patients with moderate to severe liver dysfunction after previous administration of anesthesia. *Sevoflurane* is contraindicated with hyperkalemia; muscle or nerve diseases, including Duchenne muscular dystrophy; prolonged QT interval; abnormal EKG with QT changes over time; hypotension; liver abnormalities; decreased kidney function; seizures; elevated urine proteins; excessive sugar in the urine; malignant hyperthermia; or high intracranial pressure. *Nitrous oxide* is contraindicated in patients with pneumothorax or pulmonary hypertension.

Adverse effects

The adverse effects of inhalation anesthetics include postoperative shivering, nausea, vomiting, and a risk of malignant hyperthermia. *Isoflurane* may cause shivering, infrequent hypotension, decreased peristalsis, delirium, nausea, vomiting, and headaches. *Desflurane* may cause increased blood pressure and heart rate. *Sevoflurane* may cause nephrotoxic breakdown products known as *compounds A to E*. *Nitrous oxide* can diffuse into gas-filled body areas, causing the present gas to expand, possibly damaging organs and tissues. It also causes mild myocardial depression and increased pulmonary vessel resistance.

Toxicities

No significant toxicities are listed for *isoflurane* or *desflurane*. *Sevoflurane* is under review for potential neurotoxicity, primarily in infants and children, and there are rare reports of hepatotoxicity. *Nitrous oxide* is relatively nontoxic but has produced neurotoxicity in test animals, not humans. However, nitrous oxide depletes the body's levels of vitamin B_{12}, which can cause severe neurotoxicity if the individual has a preexisting vitamin B_{12} deficiency.

You should remember

Inhalation anesthetics are passively absorbed via diffusion, which depends upon the drug's blood solubility and ventilation, volume, and lung perfusion. Distribution and uptake into the brain are based on cerebral perfusion and the fat solubility of the inhalation anesthetic.

Anesthesia adjuncts

Anesthesia adjuncts are agents used during the perioperative phase of surgery to enhance anesthesia or to treat possible adverse effects of anesthetics. Reduced autonomic function can seriously harm the cardiovascular and gastrointestinal systems. Anxiety is a common symptom before a surgical procedure. Therefore oral benzodiazepines may be given for several days before the surgery date. Before surgery, midazolam is often injected to sedate the patient and cause amnesia. Some patients lose protective airway reflexes during surgery, making aspiration pneumonia a possibly serious problem. Histamine receptor antagonists such as famotidine may be used to reduce the likelihood of aspiration pneumonia because they decrease gastric fluid volume and reduce acidity.

Histamine may be given the night before surgery and via IV infusion 1 hour before. Anticholinergics such as atropine may be given before surgery to reduce salivary and airway secretion. This drug also prevents bradycardia, which is caused by some anesthetics. It is administered IM about 45–60 minutes before anesthesia is given. Also, neuromuscular blockers may relax skeletal muscles during surgical procedures. For severe pain management after anesthesia, opioids are used. Nonsteroidal antiinflammatory drugs are sufficient for moderate or mild pain. Table 11.4 lists the generic and trade names of anesthesia adjuncts.

TABLE 11.4 Anesthesia adjuncts.

Generic name	Trade names
atracurium	Tracrium
atropine	Atreza
cisatracurium	Nimbex
clonidine	Catapres
rocuronium	Zemuron, Esmeron
famotidine	Pepcid
metoclopramide	Reglan, Metozolv ODT
ondansetron	Zofran
promethazine	Phenergan
succinylcholine	Anectine

Pharmacokinetics

When administered orally, famotidine has a 40%–45% bioavailability. The liver metabolizes it. The elimination half-life is 2.5–3.5 hours, and after oral dosing, it is excreted by the kidneys, with 25%–30% remaining unchanged. The bioavailability of atropine is 25%. The action is within one minute, and its elimination half-life is 2 hours. The duration of action is 30–60 minutes, and 15%–50% is excreted unchanged in the urine.

Mechanism of action

Famotidine blocks the action of histamine on the parietal cells, reducing acid secretion into the stomach. *Atropine* competitively binds to receptors with acetylcholine and other agonists. *Cisatracurium* binds competitively to cholinergic receptors, resulting in the blockade of neuromuscular transmission. *Promethazine* blocks the histamine-H_1 receptors and produces clinically beneficial antiemetic and sedative effects. *Ondansetron* is a serotonin antagonist and blocks serotonin receptors in the chemoreceptor-triggering area of the medulla oblongata, reducing or preventing nausea and vomiting.

Clinical indications

Famotidine reduces acid production in the stomach during surgery to reduce risk of aspiration pneumonitis. *Atropine* is indicated for temporary blockade of severe or life-threatening muscarinic effects. *Atracurium* is used to provide skeletal muscle relaxation during surgery. *Cisatracurium* is used as a neuromuscular-blocking drug or skeletal muscle relaxant, and it is used adjunctively in anesthesia to allow for endotracheal intubation and to provide skeletal muscle relaxation during surgery or mechanical ventilation.

Succinylcholine is also used for short-term muscle relaxation in anesthesia, often for the endotracheal intubation procedure. *Promethazine* has many medical uses, including sedation, relieving nausea and vomiting, treating allergic conditions and anaphylaxis, and relieving anxiety before surgery. *Metoclopramide* is often used to treat nausea and vomiting. *Ondansetron* is another effective antiemetic that eases nausea and vomiting in many patients.

Contraindications

Famotidine is contraindicated if there is a history of severe hypersensitivity reactions to famotidine or other histamine-2 receptor antagonists. *Atropine* has no significant contraindications, though warnings and precautions for its use include tachycardia, acute glaucoma, pyloric obstruction, complete urinary retention, and viscid plugs. *Atracurium* is contraindicated if there is a known hypersensitivity to the drug or to benzyl alcohol. *Cisatracurium* is contraindicated if there is a known hypersensitivity to the drug or its components. *Succinylcholine* is avoided with malignant hyperthermia, skeletal muscle myopathies, multiple trauma, upper motor neuron injury, extensive or severe burns, extensive denervation of skeletal muscle due to CNS disease or injury, and known hypersensitivity to the drug or its components.

Promethazine is contraindicated in children under 2 years of age, with large doses of other CNS depressants, in comatose patients, with known hypersensitivity or idiosyncrasy to this drug or other phenothiazines, or if the patient has asthma or other lower respiratory symptoms. Promethazine should not be given via subcutaneous or intra-arterial injection. Some manufacturers state promethazine is contraindicated with angle-closure glaucoma, bone marrow depression, and prostatic hypertrophy. *Metoclopramide* is contraindicated with GI bleeding, mechanical obstruction, or perforation. *Ondansetron* should be avoided with known hypersensitivity to the drug or its components and in patients receiving apomorphine.

Adverse effects

Famotidine usually has insignificant adverse effects, which include headache, dizziness, and constipation. *Atropine* may cause blurred vision, mouth dryness, photophobia, tachycardia, and heat intolerance. In elderly patients, atropine can cause constipation and difficulty with urination. Occasional skin rashes that progress to **exfoliation** may occur. *Clonidine* may cause mild adverse effects, including mouth dryness, drowsiness, dizziness, constipation, and sedation. *Atracurium* has no significant adverse effects except for skin flushing. *Cisatracurium* has no significant adverse impact except in intensive care patients, which may prolong recovery from neuromuscular blockade.

Succinylcholine may cause varying degrees of skeletal muscle weakness. *Promethazine* may cause extreme sedation, drowsiness, confusion, or disorientation. *Metoclopramide* may cause drowsiness or restlessness, fatigue, and, less often, headache, insomnia, confusion, dizziness, depression with suicidal ideation, convulsions, hallucinations, and extrapyramidal reactions that involve involuntary muscle movements. *Ondansetron* causes headaches, diarrhea, malaise, fatigue, and constipation.

Toxicities

Famotidine has no significant toxicities. *Atropine* toxicity may result in paralysis of the organs innervated by the parasympathetic nervous system, resulting in drying of the mucous membranes, dilation and unresponsiveness of the pupils, increased heart rate, fever, mania, disorientation, hallucinations, depressed respiration, circulatory system collapse, coma, and eventual death. *Clonidine* toxicity may result in dizziness, orthostatic hypotension, drowsiness, dry mouth, headache, fatigue, skin reactions, and hypotension. *Atracurium* may cause skin flushing—usually of the face and arms, hypotension and reflex tachycardia, bronchospasm, and, in rare cases, seizures. *Cisatracurium* has the same toxicities as atracurium.

Succinylcholine toxicity may result in malignant hyperthermia, muscle pain, acute rhabdomyolysis, hyperkalemia, transient ocular hypertension, constipation, and changes in cardiac rhythm, including slow heart rate and cardiac arrest. With succinylcholine, there is the possibility of apnea occurring, so its use is rigidly controlled. *Promethazine* toxicity results in tardive dyskinesia, pseudoparkinsonism, acute dystonia, confusion, drowsiness, dizziness, fatigue, vertigo, dry mouth, nausea, respiratory depression, blurred vision, dry nasal passages, dilated pupils, constipation, urinary retention, chest discomfort or pressure, and **akathisia**. *Metoclopramide* toxicity may cause akathisia, focal dystonia, hypertension or hypotension, hyperprolactinemia that leads to galactorrhea, headache, and extrapyramidal effects such as **oculogyric crisis**. It can also induce tardive dyskinesia. Rarely, metoclopramide has been linked with panic disorder, major depressive disorder, agranulocytosis, supraventricular tachycardia, **hyperaldosteronism**, and neuroleptic malignant syndrome. *Ondansetron* toxicity may cause headaches, constipation, diarrhea, dizziness, and ototoxicity.

You should remember

Anesthesia adjuncts augment specific components of anesthesia, allowing lower doses of general anesthetics to reduce adverse effects. Standard anesthesia adjuncts include hydromorphone, fentanyl, atracurium, butorphanol, and methohexital. Hydromorphone, fentanyl, and butorphanol are opioids. Atracurium is a neuromuscular blocking agent. Methohexital is a barbiturate.

Key Terms

Akathisia
Amnesia
Balanced anesthesia
Delirium
Duchenne muscular dystrophy
Exfoliation
General anesthesia
Hyperaldosteronism
Malignant hyperthermia
Monitored anesthesia care
Neuroleptanalgesia
Oculogyric crisis
Partial pressure
Porphyria
Reflexes
Regional anesthesia
Volatile liquids

Clinical Case Studies

Clinical Case Study 1

A 52-year-old male was scheduled for partial gastrectomy under general anesthesia. The anesthesiologist evaluated the patient, who had a short and thick neck, and anticipated that endotracheal intubation might be difficult. Anesthesia was induced with IV propofol and fentanyl, and a neuromuscular block was obtained with IV. A second-year resident failed when attempting to intubate the patient. The anesthesiologist took over, but the patient started to cough before intubation could be done and desaturated to 40%–50%. Additional drugs were administered to make intubation easier, but it failed again. The neuromuscular block was reversed with an agent that opposed the effects of suxamethonium, and the patient started to cough up bloody secretions. The mask gave oxygen (100%), and the patient's arterial saturation quickly increased to 100%. There was fortunately no neurological damage even though the arterial saturation had been too low for at least 10 minutes. The procedure was rescheduled for the next week and was completed successfully.

Critical Thinking Questions

1. In general anesthesia, which combined medications are used to achieve balanced anesthesia?
2. What are the respiratory system effects of IV and inhaled general anesthetics?
3. How common is propofol as an IV anesthetic?

Clinical Case Study 2

A 34-year-old obese female with type II diabetes mellitus was scheduled for knee surgery. She had two surgeries during childhood for other reasons, without complications, and had no history of drug allergies. She was premedicated with oral hydroxyzine for this surgery and then given IV sufentanil and propofol. Tracheal intubation was facilitated with IV succinylcholine. Chest auscultation revealed a total absence of bilateral breath sounds and low initial carbon dioxide concentrations. An esophageal intubation was suspected, and the tube was immediately removed, with mask ventilation applied. This was difficult due to significantly reduced lung compliance. Bronchospasm was considered. Rapid arterial oxygen desaturation and arterial hypotension occurred. These were corrected by administration of epinephrine and lactated Ringer solution. The patient recovered, but the surgery was rescheduled. The patient returned to normal in the intensive care unit with inhaled albuterol and IV hydrocortisone. It was discovered that the patient had suffered succinylcholine-induced anaphylaxis.

Critical Thinking Questions

1. What type of drug is succinylcholine classified as, and what is it indicated for?
2. What are the contraindications of succinylcholine?
3. What are the complications of succinylcholine toxicity?

Further Reading

[1] A.R. Absalom, K.P. Mason, Total Intravenous Anesthesia and Target Controlled Infusions: A Comprehensive Global Anthology, Springer, 2017.
[2] D.B. Andropoulos, G.A. Gregory, Gregory's Pediatric Anesthesia, sixth ed., Wiley-Blackwell, 2020.
[3] ASA Publications – Anesthesiology Volume 114, Issue 5, Case Scenario: Bronchospasm During Anesthetic Induction, American Society of Anesthesiologists – Wolters Kluwer Health – Lippincott, Williams, & Wilkins – Silverchair, 2011. https://pubs.asahq.org/anesthesiology/article/114/5/1200/14189/Case-Scenario-Bronchospasm-during-Anesthetic.
[4] P.G. Barash, B.F. Cullen, R.K. Stoelting, M.K. Cahalan, M.C. Stock, R. Ortega, S.R. Sharar, N.F. Holt, Clinical Anesthesia, eighth ed., Lippincott, Williams, and Wilkins, 2017.
[5] A.P. Boezaart, P.E. Bigeleisen, D.S. Bohannon, S.V. Chembrovich, D.A. Edwards, B.V. Inhatsenka, L. Le-Wendling, J.P. Reyneke, Y. Zasimovich, M.K. Bryson, Must Know Anatomy for Regional Anesthesia and Acute Pain Medicine: Macroanatomy – Microanatomy – Sonoanatomy – Functional Anatomy, RAEducation.com LLC Publications, 2018.
[6] V. Chan, B.T. Finucane, T. Grau, A. Walji, B.C.H. Tsui, C.T.S. Chan, R. Bhargava, D. Dillane, S. Ganapathy, L. Lou, M. Noga, Atlas of Ultrasound- and Nerve Stimulation-Guided Regional Anesthesia, Springer, 2008.
[7] D.H. Chestnut, C.A. Wong, L.C. Tsen, W.D. Ngan Kee, Y. Beilin, J.M. Mhyre, B.T. Bateman, Chestnut's Obstetric Anesthesia: Principles and Practice, sixth ed., Elsevier, 2019.
[8] P.J. Davis, F.P. Cladis, Smith's Anesthesia for Infants and Children, ninth ed., Elsevier, 2016.
[9] J. Ehrenwerth, J.B. Eisenkraft, J.M. Berry, Anesthesia Equipment: Principles and Applications, third ed., Saunders, 2020.
[10] J.L. Fellahi, M. Leone, Anesthesia in High-Risk Patients, Springer, 2018.
[11] S.A. Grant, D.B. Auyong, Ultrasound Guided Regional Anesthesia, second ed., Oxford University Press, 2016.
[12] G.P. Gravlee, A.D. Shaw, K. Bartels, Hensley's Practical Approach to Cardiothoracic Anesthesia, sixth ed., Lippincott, Williams, and Wilkins, 2018.
[13] M.A. Gropper, L.I. Eriksson, L.A. Fleisher, J.P. Wiener-Kronish, N.H. Cohen, K. Leslie, Miller's Anesthesia, 2-Volume Set, ninth ed., Elsevier, 2019.
[14] A. Hadzic, Hadzic's Textbook of Regional Anesthesia and Acute Pain Management, second ed., McGraw-Hill Education/Medical, 2017.
[15] R.A. Jaffe, C.A. Schmiesing, B. Golianu, Anesthesiologist's Manual of Surgical Procedures, sixth ed., Lippincott, Williams, and Wilkins, 2019.
[16] J.A. Kaplan, Kaplan's cardiac anesthesia, in: Cardiac and Noncardiac Surgery, seventh ed., Elsevier, 2016.
[17] B.M. Keech, R.D. Laterza, Anesthesia Secrets, sixth ed., Elsevier, 2020.
[18] K. Marschall, R.L. Hines, Stoelting's Anesthesia and Co-Existing Disease, seventh ed., Elsevier, 2017.
[19] Mayo Foundation for Medical Education, B.A. Hall, R.C. Chantigian, Anesthesia: A Comprehensive Review, sixth ed., Elsevier, 2019.
[20] Mayo Foundation for Medical Education, Faust's Anesthesiology Review, fifth ed., Elsevier, 2019.
[21] W. Owens, The Advanced Ventilator Book, First Draught Press, 2017.
[22] Peertechz – Open Journal of Pain Medicine, Case Study: Local Anesthetic Toxicity After Bier Block. was Intralipid Therapy the Correct Remedy? Peertechz Publications Inc, 2017. https://www.peertechzpublications.com/articles/OJPM-1-102.php.
[23] J. Schuttler, H. Schwilden, Modern Anesthetics (Handbook of Experimental Pharmacology 182), Springer, 2010.
[24] P. Slinger, Principles and Practice of Anesthesia for Thoracic Surgery, second ed., Springer, 2019.
[25] C.E. Smith, Trauma Anesthesia, second ed., Cambridge University Press, 2015.
[26] S.D. Waldman, Atlas of Interventional Pain Management, fifth ed., Elsevier, 2020.
[27] F.S.F. Yao, Jr.,H.C. Hemmings, V. Malhotra, J. Fong, Yao & Artusio's Anesthesiology: Problem-Oriented Patient Management, ninth ed., Lippincott, Williams, and Wilkins, 2020.

CHAPTER

12

Local anesthetics

OUTLINE

LEARNING OUTCOMES

After study of this chapter, readers should be able to:

1. Describe the indications of local anesthesia.
2. Identify various types of regional anesthesia administration.
3. List three names for the ester and amide drugs used as local anesthesia.
4. Compare nerve block anesthesia with topical anesthesia.
5. Describe infiltration anesthesia and epidural anesthesia.
6. Discuss the indications of spinal anesthesia.
7. List the trade names of bupivacaine, lidocaine, and tetracaine.
8. Describe the toxicities of local anesthetics.

Overview

Local anesthesia provides reversible nerve blockade, leading to pain sensation loss. Local anesthetics are classified as esters or amides. Topical application and direct infiltration anesthetizes the immediate area. Regional blocks anesthetize larger sizes via a nerve or field block. Local anesthesia is used for many reasons, including the elimination of pain so that the following can be carried out: repair of lacerations, skin surgery, treatment of painful oral or

https://doi.org/10.1016/B978-0-443-29038-1.00012-9

genital lesions, and the removal of superficial lesions by chemical or physical means. Nearly painless anesthesia may be achieved when the location, surface area involved, and estimated length of time for the procedure are considered. The patient's emotional response is critical in ensuring nearly painless anesthesia, as most patients fear the injection will be painful. The spinal anesthetics must be used carefully if the patient has cardiac disease, abnormal coagulation studies, or preexisting neurological disorders such as multiple sclerosis.

Local anesthetics

Local anesthetics stop the nerves in a part of the body from sending signals to the brain. The patient will not be able to feel any pain after having a local anesthetic, although they may still feel some pressure or movement. It usually only takes a few minutes to lose feeling in the area where a local anesthetic is given. They can also prevent motor and autonomic function in this area. The effect is transient (time limited). Drugs available for local anesthesia are classified as members of the ester or amide families (see Table 12.1). **Amide** local anesthetics are generally more therapeutic than **ester** local anesthetics but can produce more toxic reactions than ester derivatives. Specific preparations are available for topical administration, infiltration, and various regional administrations, including field block, regional block, epidural block, and spinal block—see Table 12.2. People sensitive to one group of local anesthetics often can tolerate those of the other group. The vascularity of the injection site, the speed with which the drug is given, the rapidity of action of the drug, and the presence of epinephrine may affect any adverse response. Table 12.3 lists the generic and trade names for local anesthetics.

TABLE 12.1 Classifications of ester and amide drugs.

Ester group	Amide group
benzocaine	bupivacaine
chloroprocaine	dibucaine
cocaine	etidocaine
procaine	lidocaine
proparacaine	mepivacaine
tetracaine	prilocaine
	ropivacaine

TABLE 12.2 Specific methods for delivering local and regional anesthesia.

Methods or technique	Description
Topical (surface) anesthesia	A drug is applied to or sprayed directly onto the surface of skin or mucous membranes and does not penetrate deeper layers. This provides relief for minor skin irritation or before a needlestick.
Nerve block	A drug is injected around a peripheral nerve; all regions that are innervated by the nerve lose sensation, as in dental procedures or regional anesthesia.
Infiltration anesthesia	A drug is injected into deeper skin layers and moves to surrounding areas, providing pain relief during minor skin surgeries or dental procedures or before a deep needlestick.
Spinal anesthesia	A drug is injected into the cerebrospinal fluid, most often via the lumbar region; this blocks sensation to larger areas of the lower abdomen or pelvis.
Epidural anesthesia	A drug is injected into the epidural space that surrounds the spinal cord, blocking sensation to many nerve roots that supply limited portions of the chest, limbs, abdomen, or pelvis; this is often used for urologic and obstetric procedures.

TABLE 12.3 Generic and trade names of local anesthetics.

Generic name	Trade names
articaine	Septocaine
benzocaine	Dendracin
bupivacaine	Marcaine
chloroprocaine	Nesacaine
cocaine	Goprelto
dibucaine	Nupercainal
etidocaine	Duranest
lidocaine	Xylocaine
mepivacaine	Carbocaine
prilocaine	Citanest
procaine	Novocain
proparacaine	Alcaine
ropivacaine	Naropin
tetracaine	Niphanoid

You should remember

A new method of administering local anesthesia involves a peripheral nerve catheter attached to a pump containing the anesthetics. The pumps infuse the drugs around the nerves several days after surgery, innervating the surgical site. The catheter is implanted during surgery and usually taken out by the patient at home once the anesthetics have been infused.

Pharmacokinetics

Many local anesthetics can be easily absorbed into the bloodstream after being injected. The duration of local action is limited unless blood flow to the area is reduced. They metabolize in the liver. The metabolism is speedy for *procaine*, with a half-life of 1–2 minutes, and slower for *cocaine* and *tetracaine (10 mins for cocaine, not established for tetracaine)*. The amide local anesthetics are metabolized in the liver, partly by the cytochrome P450 isozymes. *Lidocaine* and *prilocaine* have half-lives that are about 1.5 hours in length. The most prolonged half-lives are for *bupivacaine* (3.5 hours) and *ropivacaine* (4.2 hours). If the liver is not functioning normally, this may increase the elimination of half-lives of the amide local anesthetics, resulting in higher toxicity risks. If the urine is acidified, this promotes ionization of the local anesthetics. The altered drug forms are excreted more quickly than their nonionized forms.

Mechanism of action

The local anesthetics block voltage-dependent sodium channels, reducing the **influx** of sodium ions and preventing **depolarization** of the membrane while blocking the conduction of action potentials. These anesthetics access their receptors via the cell membrane or cytoplasm. Because drug molecules must cross lipid membranes to reach the cytoplasm, more lipid-soluble forms run effective intracellular concentrations more quickly than ionized forms. However, when the ionized drugs are inside axons, they can better block the channels. Therefore ionized drug forms are essential. The affinity of a receptor site in a sodium channel for a local anesthetic occurs because the track is open, resting, or inactivated. High extracellular potassium ions can enhance local anesthetic activities, while elevated extracellular calcium ions may have antagonistic effects. Esters such as *procaine* act mainly by inhibiting sodium influx but also bind or antagonize the function of *N*-methyl-*D*-aspartate receptors, plus nicotinic acetylcholine receptors and the serotonin receptor-ion channel complex.

Clinical indications

Local anesthetics are indicated to reduce the stress associated with surgery and provide relief after surgery for pain caused by hemorrhoids; fissures; insect bites; minor burns; vaginal, rectal, and ontological examinations; **cystoscopy**; and catheterization. Local anesthetics are also used for dental procedures. Dentists commonly use two types of injections: infiltration and nerve block (see Fig. 12.1). The effects of the injections can last up to several hours. The most common anesthetic agent used by dentists is *lidocaine 2%*.

Contraindications

Local anesthetics are contraindicated with a history of hypersensitivity to local painkillers, sunscreens, sulfa drugs, or hair dyes.

Adverse effects

The adverse effects of local anesthetics are usually insignificant. However, too much of a local anesthetic can be absorbed. In that case, there can be vision abnormalities, confusion, convulsions, dizziness, lightheadedness, drowsiness, headache, abnormal body temperature, numbness, sweating, tinnitus, shivering, irregular heartbeat, difficulty breathing, anxiety, excitement, nervousness, restlessness, paleness, tiredness, weakness, and swollen areas of the skin, mouth, or throat. *Procaine* may also cause hives, chest pain, nausea, vomiting, trembling, and shaking. Allergic reactions to procaine are usually not in response to the actual drug but to its metabolite, which is known as *para-aminobenzoic acid.*

Toxicities

Most local anesthetics have significant CNS toxicities. All of them can produce central effects that include lightheadedness, restlessness, sedation, nystagmus, tonic-clonic convulsions, and coma. Other toxicities with local anesthetics include respiratory and cardiovascular depression. Except for *cocaine,* all local drugs are vasodilators, resulting in hypotension. A person with preexisting cardiovascular disease may develop a heart block. Local anesthetics may also cause arrhythmias, myocardial infarction, and cerebral hemorrhage. The ester local anesthetics are metabolized into products that may cause the formation of antibodies. Allergic responses to local anesthetics, however, are rare. At high levels, local anesthetics can cause a local neurotoxic action—dangerous in the spinal cord—including cell and tissue damage and permanently impaired functions.

When toxicity is severe, it is treated symptomatically because there are no antidotes available. Convulsions are managed with IV diazepam or short-acting barbiturates. Hyperventilation can be treated with oxygen. Sometimes, a neuromuscular blocker is used to control violent convulsions. Cardiovascular toxicity from *bupivacaine* overdose is hard to treat and fatal in younger adults.

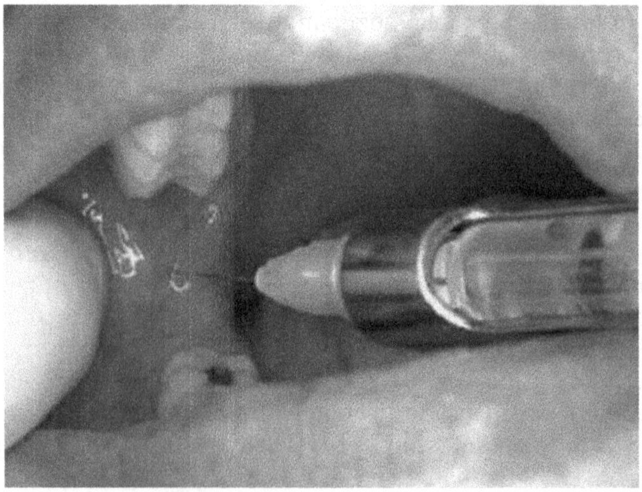

FIG. 12.1 Block injection during a dental procedure.

You should remember

Nerve blocks are used to diagnose and treat many painful conditions. They reduce acute pain from surgery, nerve trauma, and injuries. They also help to alleviate chronic pain. Nerve blocks work directly at the source of pain by stopping pain signals from reaching the spinal cord and brain. The benefits of nerve blocks include pinpointing the source of pain, predicting future treatment outcomes, and preventing chronic pain after a surgical procedure. A single nerve block is injected around one nerve, while a ganglion (plexus) block is injected around interconnected nerves. A sympathetic nerve block is injected along a chain of nerves controlling general body functions.

Spinal anesthesia

Spinal anesthesia involves the injection of a local anesthetic into the subarachnoid space between the L3 and L4 segments to avoid spinal cord injury. For a nerve block, various sites of the spinal column can be used (see Fig. 12.2). Spinal **block anesthesia** occurs when the local anesthetic penetrates the subarachnoid space between the pia mater and arachnoid membranes. In an **epidural block anesthesia**, the local anesthetic is placed into the epidural space, just posterior to the spinal cord or dura mater. The epidural space lies between the posterior longitudinal ligament on the anterior side and the **ligamentum flavum** posteriorly. A **caudal block anesthesia** is an epidural block in which a local anesthetic is administered through the **sacral hiatus**. A **saddle block anesthesia** is done at the lower end of the spinal column to block the perineal area. Blood pressure must be monitored for all types of spinal anesthesia.

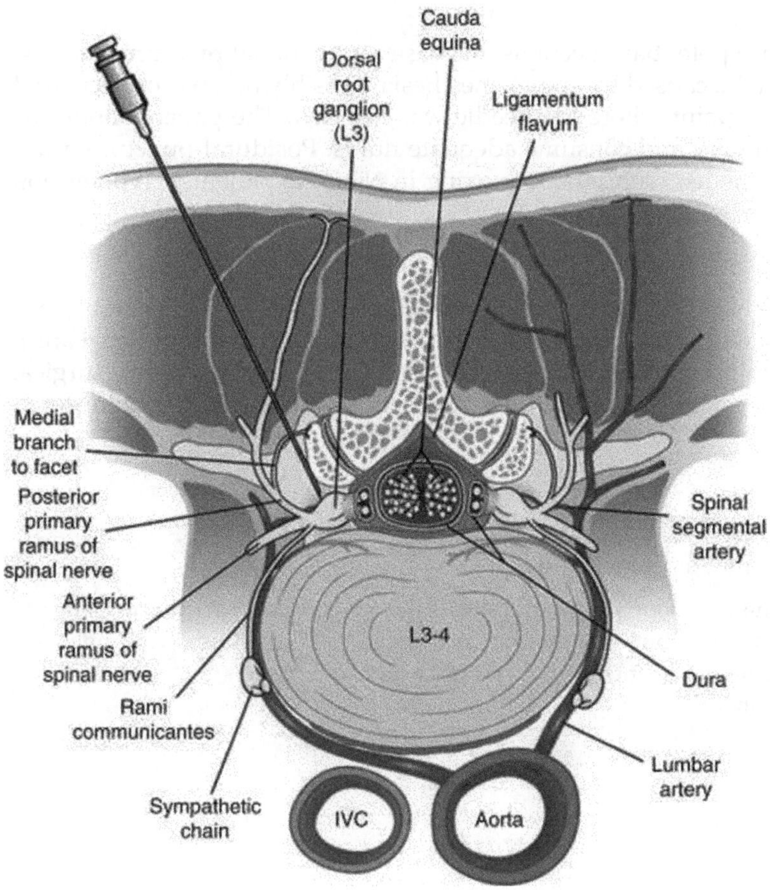

FIG. 12.2 Spinal nerve block sites.

Pharmacokinetics

The pharmacokinetics of local anesthetic agents are different than for most other drugs, as these agents are applied directly to their site of action rather than being transported in the bloodstream to this site. Toxic reactions to local anesthetics are usually associated with accidental intravenous injection, but harmful effects can occur with regular usage. The systemic absorption of *lidocaine*, *bupivacaine*, and *etidocaine* after lumbar epidural administration is biphasic, with a rapid initial absorption phase followed by a much slower absorption phase. Initial absorption rates of lidocaine and bupivacaine after subarachnoid injection are much slower, but the late absorption rates are similar to those after epidural administration. These drugs are metabolized in the liver and eliminated via the kidneys.

Mechanism of action

Spinal anesthetics work by initially blocking tiny, unmyelinated sympathetic fibers. After this occurs, the myelinated sensory and motor fibers are blocked. The sympathetic block can exceed the motor/sensory block by a **dermatome**. There is little effect upon ventilation, though high levels of anesthesia can affect the abdominal and intercostal muscles and the ability to cough. The patient may be unable to feel the sensations of breathing, resulting in dyspnea. Any procedure above T5 inhibits the sympathetic nervous system's effects on the GI tract.

Clinical indications

Spinal anesthesia is used to control pain during surgical procedures and childbirth. Nerve block anesthesia is used for diagnostic and surgical procedures and chronic pain management. Clinical indications include lower abdominal, perineal, and lower extremity surgery.

Contraindications

Contraindications for local anesthetics used in spinal anesthesia include known drug allergies and patient refusal. Relative contraindications include cardiac disease and abnormal coagulation studies. There is controversy about using spinal anesthesia in patients with preexisting neurological disorders such as multiple sclerosis.

Adverse effects

The adverse effects of spinal anesthesia may cause potential infections, increased intracranial pressure, and respiratory failure. A postdural-puncture headache can be caused by spinal anesthesia, possibly because of decreased cerebrospinal fluid pressure from a fluid leak at the point where the needle was inserted. The patient should be encouraged to remain flat after spinal anesthesia surgery and consume adequate fluids. Postdural-puncture headaches are most common in females and younger patients, with most occurring in obstetric patients. Hypotension may also occur after spinal anesthesia.

Toxicities

In most circumstances, local anesthetics are unlikely to cause toxicities. Systemic reactions can occur if large quantities are absorbed into the blood circulation. This is why *epinephrine* is often given concurrently with the local anesthetic to maintain localized drug activity. Epinephrine also reduces local blood loss during minor surgical procedures. Cardiovascular and respiratory function can be compromised if large amounts of a locally administered anesthetic are absorbed systemically.

You should remember

Spinal anesthesia is indicated for lower abdominal, perineal, and lower extremity surgery. Indications for epidural anesthesia include abdominal or lower extremity, but because of its segmental nature, it may be less than optimal for procedures that involve the lower sacral distribution. Epidural anesthesia is also often used to supplement general anesthesia and labor pain.

Key Terms

Caudal block anesthesia
Cystoscopy
Depolarization
Dermatome
Epidural block anesthesia
Infiltration injections
Influx
Ligamentum flavum
Nerve block anesthesia
Sacral hiatus
Saddle block anesthesia
Spinal block anesthesia

Clinical Case Studies

Clinical Case Study 1

A 35-year-old female required an emergency cesarean section under spinal anesthesia to deliver her baby safely. Spinal anesthesia was given at L3/L4 with a sensory block of T4, and the delivery was uneventful. However, the woman developed difficulty breathing, hypotension, bradycardia, hypoxia, and loss of consciousness. Resuscitation was successful with vasopressors, endotracheal intubation, and mechanical ventilation. Over 1 week, she slowly regained motor and sensory functions. She was discharged without any neurological or clinical sequelae.

Critical Thinking Questions

1. What are the differences between spinal and epidural blocks?
2. How do spinal anesthetics work?
3. How can a local anesthetic spread in the spinal column to affect respiration and cause hypotension?

Clinical Case Study 2

A 9-year-old male had been given the procaine local anesthetic to extract a tooth from the upper right portion of his mouth. There was an immediate hematoma of the right cheek, hypotension, bradycardia, and hypoxia, so the boy was transferred to the local hospital with a suspected allergic reaction. A systemic corticosteroid was administered. In 4 days, an acute bacterial infection had developed. A local dentist performed an intraoral incision and drainage. He prescribed an antibiotic as well. The swelling started to regress slowly, and the hematoma diminished. After 8 days, the boy still had a discrete swelling, but the hematoma was regressing. It was resolved within 2 weeks.

Critical Thinking Questions

1. What is the popularly known trade name for procaine?
2. What are the comparisons between esters and amides as local anesthetics?
3. How do allergic reactions to procaine occur?

Clinical Case Study 3

A 48-year-old male had been diagnosed with carpal tunnel syndrome in both hands, which would become numb in the morning after awakening. He initially tried chiropractic therapy, which provided some relief, but his job as a computer programmer required long and repetitive use of his hands and wrists. The condition only worsened over time. Eventually, the patient was evaluated for surgery under local anesthesia and found to be a good candidate for a successful outcome. Unlike under general anesthesia, the procedure does not require patients to fast or undergo complicated blood studies. The patient underwent surgery after the local anesthetic *lidocaine* was administered. Each wrist took only about 20 minutes. His postoperation recovery only required a small dressing on each wrist and acetaminophen for pain, which was minimal.

Critical Thinking Questions

1. What are the classifications of the different types of local anesthetics?
2. What is the half-life of lidocaine, and what is its length of action?
3. What are the potential CNS toxicities of local anesthetics?

Further Reading

[1] A. Alban, Y. Gutfreund, H. Grotbo, N. Fuster, Peripheral Nerve Blocks: In Emergency Medicine and Urgent Care, Harper Duz Press, LLC, 2021.
[2] H. Barop, Textbook and Atlas of Neural Therapy: Diagnosis and Therapy with Local Anesthetics, Thieme, 2017.
[3] G. Capogna, Epidural Technique in Obstetric Anesthesia, Springer, 2020.
[4] D. Chiumello, Topical Issues in Anesthesia and Intensive Care, Springer, 2016.
[5] M. Dosch, Atlas of Neural Therapy: With Local Anesthetics, third ed., Thieme, 2012.
[6] S. Elisha, J.J. Nagelhout, J.S. Heiner, Current Anesthesia Practice – Evaluation & Certification Review, Elsevier, 2020.
[7] R. Fernando, P. Sultan, S. Phillips, Quick Hits in Obstetric Anesthesia, Springer, 2021.
[8] A. Hadzic, Hadzic's Peripheral Nerve Blocks and Anatomy for Ultraasound-Guided Regional Anesthesia, second ed., McGraw-Hill Education / Medical, 2011.
[9] C.W. Hanke, B. Sommer, G. Sattler, Tumescent Local Anesthesia, Springer, 2012.
[10] M. Huntoon, H. Benzon, S. Nauroze, T.R. Deer, Spinal Injections and Peripheral Nerve Blocks, vol. 4, Elsevier, 2011.
[11] S.F. Malamed, Handbook of Local Anesthesia, seventh ed., Elsevier, 2019.
[12] Open Anesthesia, Spinal vs. Epidural, OpenAnesthesia / Improving Health through Discovery and Education, 2021. https://www.openanesthesia.org/spinal_anesthesia/.
[13] R.T. Parmley, J. Adriani, Saddle Block Anesthesia: American Lecture Series, Number 258. Literary Licensing, LLC, 2013.
[14] K. Sairyo, Transforaminal Full-Endoscopic Lumbar Surgery Under the Local Anesthesia – State of the Art, Springer, 2021.
[15] E. Silvestri, F. Martino, F. Puntillo, Ultrasound-Guided Peripheral Nerve Blocks, Springer, 2018.

CHAPTER

13

Skeletal muscle relaxants

OUTLINE

LEARNING OUTCOMES

After study of this chapter, readers should be able to:

1. Describe the components of the musculoskeletal system.
2. Explain muscle cramps.
3. List examples of medications that can cause muscle spasms.
4. Discuss diseases that cause muscle spasticity.
5. Explain the various types of muscle relaxants.
6. Identify the clinical indications of skeletal muscle relaxants.
7. Discuss the pharmacokinetics of direct-acting muscle relaxants.
8. Identify the clinical indications of botulinum toxins.
9. List the common adverse effects of dantrolene.
10. Describe the contraindications of baclofen.

The Science of Pharmacology
https://doi.org/10.1016/B978-0-443-29038-1.00013-0

Overview

The skeletal muscles are essential structures that produce the force needed to move and function. The central nervous system (CNS) voluntarily controls the skeletal muscles to create movement, maintain posture and body position, stabilize joints, and generate heat. The skeletal system comprises bones, cartilage, ligaments, and other connective tissues. Primary muscle diseases result from actual muscle abnormalities. Secondary muscle diseases are caused by other conditions that trigger muscle disease. Both types of diseases sometimes also affect the nerves that supply the muscles. They may eventually result in muscle wasting or loss of muscle mass. This can involve loss of strength and function in one or more muscles.

In some cases, paralysis occurs. A muscle spasm is a sudden, involuntary movement in one or more muscles and is sometimes referred to as a Charley horse or a muscle cramp or twitch. These movements can happen in any muscle and are common in all ages. Muscle spasms often occur from stress, exercise, or dehydration. Spasticity is abnormal muscle tightness due to prolonged muscle contraction. It is associated with brain, spinal cord, and motor nerve damage. Spasticity is seen with neurological conditions such as cerebral palsy (CP), multiple sclerosis (MS), stroke, and amyotrophic lateral sclerosis (ALS).

Musculoskeletal system

The muscular system includes skeletal, cardiac, and smooth muscles. The skeletal muscles are voluntary under the CNS control. The skeletal muscles produce movement, maintain posture and body position, stabilize joints, and generate heat. The skeletal system includes the bones, cartilage, ligaments, and other connective tissues that stabilize or connect the bones. Skeletal muscles perform essential functions for the body. Transmission of impulses from motor nerves to muscle cells occurs across **neuromuscular junctions** (see Fig. 13.1). These spaces are sensitive to localized chemical changes. Therefore bodily motor nerve impulses cannot be generated. This may also decrease the availability of calcium ions to the myofibrillar contractile system.

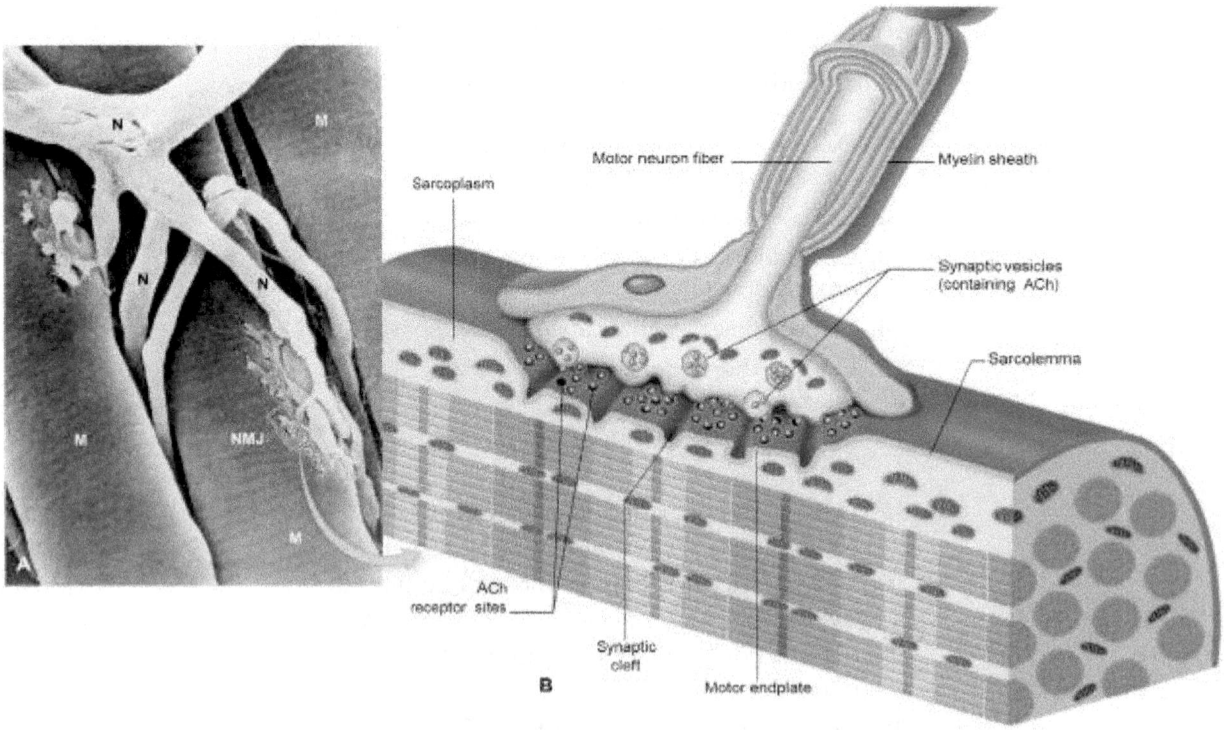

FIG. 13.1 Neuromuscular junction.

Muscle spasms and spasticity

Muscle spasms (muscle cramps) involve painful contractions and tightening. They are common, involuntary, and unpredictable. Although steps can be taken to prevent or treat a muscle spasm, the results are unreliable. Muscle relaxants, stretching, and massage are often helpful. Muscle spasms range from mild, uncomfortable twitches to intense, severe pain. Cramps typically last from a few seconds to 15 minutes or longer and may recur multiple times before going away. Some muscle spasms are idiopathic. Causes of muscle spasms include muscle fatigue, dehydration, depletion of electrolytes, exercising in the heat, restriction in the blood supply, and stress.

There are two types of muscle spasms: *tonic* and *clonic*. A single, prolonged contraction is called a **tonic spasm**, while multiple rapidly repeated contractions are known as **clonic spasms**. Most muscle spasms and strains respond to rest, physical therapy, and the short-term use of aspirin and other analgesics. Medications may also cause muscle spasms, which usually develop slowly after several months of taking medicine. Examples of drugs that can cause muscle spasms include the following:

- Antihyperlipidemics: statins, such as rosuvastatin (Crestor), atorvastatin (Lipitor), and simvastatin (Zocor); excessive niacin (vitamin B_3)
- Antifungals: fluconazole (Diflucan), ketoconazole (Nizoral)
- Antineoplastics: cisplatin (Platinol), imatinib (Gleevec), vincristine (Oncovin)
- Adrenergic agonists: albuterol (Proventil), terbutaline (Brethine)
- Calcium channel blockers: nifedipine (Procardia)
- Cholinesterase inhibitors: donepezil (Aricept)
- Diuretics: furosemide (Lasix), hydrochlorothiazide (Microzide)
- Immunosuppressants: leflunomide (Arava), corticosteroids such as prednisone (Deltasone)
- Proton pump inhibitors: esomeprazole (Nexium), omeprazole (Prilosec)

Statins are the most critical drugs that cause muscle spasms and are used widely to lower cholesterol in the bloodstream. They can cause **rhabdomyolysis**, which can result in extreme morbidity and disability. Fortunately, most drug-induced myopathies can be reversed early in their course. Doses can be lowered, or the drug can be discontinued entirely.

You should remember

Various conditions, including nervous system diseases, diabetes mellitus, anemia, kidney disease, thyroid abnormalities, hormone imbalances, and certain medications, may cause muscle spasms. Rapid muscle spasms are usually caused by dehydration, overexercising, and stress. Cramps can affect any muscle, but the calf and foot muscles are most often involved.

Muscle spasticity may be seen in individuals who have experienced severe trauma to the head or spinal cord, MS, CP, stroke, and ALS. Muscle spasticity due to a spinal cord injury occurs from an imbalance of excitatory and inhibitory signals. The area distal to the injury, or lesion becomes disassociated from the inhibitory portion of the brain. Excitatory impulses dominate the affected muscles. Spastic paralysis may occur with flexor muscles tightening. Extension of the muscles may then be challenging. If they are extended, they often flex back immediately. Even though symptoms appear to be related to the involved muscles, a neurologic injury caused them. With MS, spasticity occurs in the advanced stages of the disease as myelin sheaths are destroyed. The main motor pathways from the spinal cord to the muscles become interrupted. The affected person's gait is stiff and unbalanced, and they usually eventually use a wheelchair.

CP is a neurologic disorder that causes severe muscular spasticity. The facial muscles may be affected, and the individual's gait becomes unsteady and scissoring (see Fig. 13.2). There are painful deformities and joint contractures. Congenital brain or spinal cord trauma is the leading cause of spasticity. With stroke, about 35% of patients have muscle spasticity. Often, the spasticity is permanent, signified by clenching of the fist, permanent flexing of the elbow, or pointed toes.

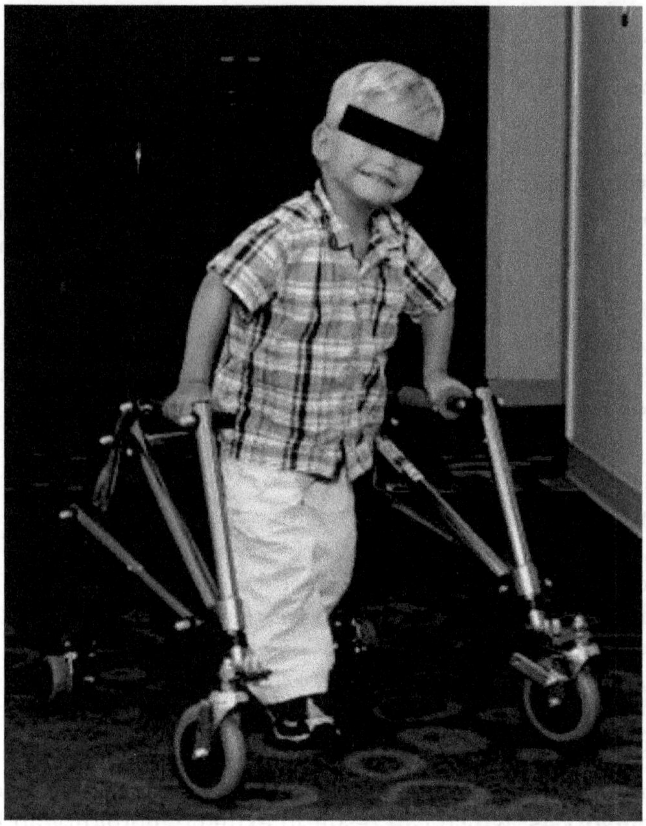

FIG. 13.2 A child with cerebral palsy.

The disease known as ALS, or **Lou Gehrig disease**, causes muscle spasticity, spasms, and twitching because of degeneration and loss of upper and lower CNS motor neurons. The disorder progresses until the death of the patient occurs. During periods of extreme muscle spasticity, muscle relaxants may relieve some of the pain. **Dystonia** is a chronic neurologic disorder. Involuntary muscle contractions cause body parts to assume abnormal and painful postures or movements. All of the body is affected by *generalized dystonia*. This is treated with high doses of anticholinergic drugs, including baclofen, benzodiazepines, and benztropine. The disorder affects one body region in focal dystonia, including the eyelids, face, vocal cords, neck, trunk, arms, or legs. MS, CP, or stroke may cause dystonia. The patient becomes unable to perform activities of daily living. Focal dystonia can be partially relieved by administering botulinum toxin type A.

You should remember

A muscle spasm is a sudden, involuntary tightening or contraction of a muscle, usually of the legs, arms, trunk, or back. Spasticity is described as muscle stiffness, heaviness, and difficulty in moving the muscles. It can be challenging to bend a limb to any degree, if severe. Spasticity and spasms range from mild to severe, varying over time. Symptoms can be annoying, uncomfortable, and unpredictable. Sometimes they affect walking and can even cause falling.

Skeletal muscle relaxants

Treating muscle spasms may be nonpharmacologic or pharmacologic (muscle relaxants). Nonpharmacologic treatments include immobilizing the affected muscle, applying heat or cold, hydrotherapy, and massage. Local anesthesia may also affect the relaxation of limited muscle groups. The local anesthetic block of efferent somatic motor outflow is sometimes used to relieve localized skeletal muscle spasms. Spasticity results from increased muscle tone because of hyperexcitable neurons or a lack of inhibition in the spinal cord (or at the skeletal muscles). Many neurologic disorders that cause spasticity require long-term use of muscle relaxants. Skeletal muscle relaxants block somatic motor nerve impulses through the depression of specific neurons within the CNS. These relaxants are subdivided into the *centrally acting* and *direct-acting* skeletal muscle relaxants. Also, *nonsteroidal antiinflammatory drugs (NSAIDs)* may be used for some relief.

Centrally acting muscle relaxants

The centrally acting muscle relaxants relieve symptoms of muscular stiffness and rigidity. They have CNS actions that reduce muscle spasms but do not affect neuromuscular junctions or the actual muscles. They may help restore excitatory and inhibitory impulse balancing from CNS motor neurons and have sedating effects. These agents improve the mobility of the body's affected part. They can be combined with analgesics and antiinflammatory medications. The centrally acting muscle relaxants are listed in Table 13.1.

Pharmacokinetics

Baclofen is very well absorbed and has a protein binding of 30%. It is 85% excreted in the urine and feces unchanged, and 15% is metabolized via deamination. The elimination half-life is 1.5 to 6 hours. *Carisoprodol* has protein binding of 60%, and it is metabolized in the liver by CYP2C19. There is a rapid onset of action within 30 minutes. The elimination half-life is about 2.5 hours, and it is excreted in the urine. *Chlorzoxazone* is very well absorbed and has 13% to 18% protein binding. It is metabolized in the liver and has an elimination half-life of 1.1 hours and a duration of action of 3–4 hours. It is excreted very little via the urine (less than 1%). *Cyclobenzaprine* is well absorbed in the GI tract and is 93% protein bound. It has extensive liver metabolism via the CYP450 enzymes to inactive metabolites and is mainly excreted in the urine. The onset of action is 1 hour and lasts 12–24 hours.

Deutetrabenazine is absorbed by 80% or more after oral administration and quickly metabolizes in the liver. The bioavailability of *metaxalone* is unknown. It is metabolized in the liver and has an elimination half-life of 9.2 hours, with a variance of ±4.8 hours. It is excreted in the urine. *Methocarbamol* is metabolized in the liver and has an elimination half-life of 1.14–1.24 hours. *Orphenadrine* has 90% bioavailability and 95% protein binding. It undergoes hepatic demethylation and has an elimination half-life of 13–20 hours. It is excreted via the urine and biliary tract. *Tetrabenazine* has low bioavailability and an extensive first-pass effect. It has 82%–85% protein binding and is metabolized in the liver via CYP2D6. Its elimination half-life is 10 hours for the parent drug and 2–8 hours for its active

TABLE 13.1 Centrally acting muscle relaxants.

Generic drugs	Trade name	Average dosage range (mg/day)	Dosage form (mg)
baclofen	Lioresal	5–80	Oral: 5, 10, 20; intrathecal injection: 0.05 mg/mL, 0.5 mg/mL, 1 mg/mL, 2 mg/mL, 5 mg/mL, 5 mg/5 mL
carisoprodol	Soma	250–1400	Oral: 250, 350
chlorzoxazone	Lorzone	750–3000	Oral: 250, 375, 500, 750
cyclobenzaprine	Amrix	5–30	Oral, immediate release: 5, 10; Oral, extended release: 15, 30
deutetrabenazine	Austedo	6–48	Oral: 6
metaxalone	Skelaxin	800–3,200	Oral: 400, 800
methocarbamol	Robaxin	500–6000	Oral: 500, 750
orphenadrine	Norflex	Oral: 100–200 Parenteral: 60–120	Oral: 100; parenteral: 30 mg/mL
tetrabenazine	Xenazine	12.5–50	Oral: 12.5, 25
tizanidine	Zanaflex	2–36	Oral: 2, 4, 6

metabolites. The drug is mainly excreted in the urine and also in the feces. *Tizanidine* has a bioavailability of about 40% and protein binding of about 30%. It is 95% metabolized in the liver via CYP1A2. Its elimination half-life is 2.54 hours for the parent drug. Its inactive metabolites have an elimination half-life of 20–40 hours. The drug is 60% excreted in the urine and 20% in the feces.

Mechanism of action

The exact mechanism of action of the centrally acting muscle relaxants is unknown, but they may affect the brain or spinal cord to inhibit upper motor neuron activity. *Baclofen* inhibits neuronal activity within the brain and spinal cord in ways that mimic the inhibitory neurotransmitter gamma-aminobutyric acid. *Carisoprodol* produces significant sedation, which is likely responsible for its relief of pain from muscle spasms. *Chlorzoxazone* acts on the spinal cord by depressing reflexes, though its actual mechanism of action is uncertain. *Cyclobenzaprine* increases norepinephrine activity by blocking its synaptic reuptake, resulting in anticholinergic effects. *Orphenadrine* binds and inhibits histamine H1 receptors. *Tetrabenazine* promotes serotonin, norepinephrine, and dopamine depletion while decreasing uptake into the synaptic vesicles. *Tizanidine* causes presynaptic inhibition of motor neurons via agonist actions at alpha-2 adrenergic receptor sites.

Clinical indications

Skeletal muscle relaxants treat local spasms to reduce pain and increase range of motion. *Baclofen* is often the drug of first choice because of its comprehensive safety margin. It is mainly used for spastic movement disorders, primarily caused by spinal cord injury, MS, or CP. *Carisoprodol* and *metaxalone* are used for muscle strains, sprains, and injuries. *Chlorzoxazone* is used for muscle spasms and their related pain or discomfort. *Cyclobenzaprine* is indicated for short-term therapy of acute musculoskeletal conditions unrelated to CNS diseases. *Deutetrabenazine* and *tetrabenazine* are used for chorea associated with **Huntington disease** and **tardive dyskinesia**. *Methocarbamol* is used to treat short-term musculoskeletal pain. *Orphenadrine* is primarily used for acute back or neck pain. *Tizanidine* is used for muscle spasticity due to spinal cord injury or MS.

Contraindications

Baclofen is contraindicated in patients with bacteremia and clotting disorders. *Carisoprodol* is contraindicated with alcohol and other CNS depressants. *Chlorzoxazone* is contraindicated with liver disease and CNS depressants. *Cyclobenzaprine* should be avoided in patients with acute intermittent porphyria and children younger than age 5 years. It is used cautiously in patients over 65 because they are more likely to experience adverse effects. None of the centrally acting muscle relaxants should be used during pregnancy and lactation. *Deutetrabenazine* is contraindicated with liver impairment and in Huntington disease patients with depression or suicidal thoughts. *Metaxalone* is contraindicated with hemolytic anemia, acute or severe liver disease, and chronic kidney disease. *Methocarbamol* is also contraindicated with liver or kidney abnormalities. *Orphenadrine* is contraindicated with arrhythmias, **necrotizing enterocolitis**, severe liver disease, seizures, and chronic kidney disease. *Tetrabenazine* is contraindicated with suicidal thoughts, parkinsonism, **neuroleptic malignant syndrome**, arrhythmias, and liver disease. *Tizanidine* is contraindicated with psychosis, bradycardia, hypotension, severe liver disease, and decreased kidney function.

Adverse effects

All of the centrally acting agents can cause sedation. Common adverse effects include drowsiness, dizziness, weakness, and fatigue. *Baclofen* also causes headaches, insomnia, dysrhythmias, nausea, vomiting, constipation, and urinary retention. The most severe adverse effects of *carisoprodol* include anaphylactic shock, profound sedation, and physical dependence. *Chlorzoxazone* has serious adverse effects, including anemia, hepatotoxicity, jaundice, and neutropenia. *Cyclobenzaprine* has serious adverse effects, including hallucinations, **serotonin syndrome**, and tongue edema. *Deutetrabenazine* and *tetrabenazine* may cause a profound negative impact on neurologic malignant syndrome. *Metaxalone* causes severe adverse effects such as anaphylaxis, hemolytic anemia, hepatotoxicity, and jaundice. *Methocarbamol* may cause anaphylactic shock and sloughing of the skin with extravasation. *Orphenadrine* may cause anaphylactic shock and hallucinations. *Tizanidine* may cause hallucinations, bradycardia, hepatotoxicity, and hypotension.

Toxicities

Baclofen toxicity may cause vomiting, general weakness, sedation, respiratory insufficiency, seizures, abnormal pupil size, dizziness, headaches, itching, hypothermia, bradycardia, hypertension, hyporeflexia, and even coma or death. *Carisoprodol* toxicity may cause **lethargy**, double vision, nystagmus, and tachycardia. *Chlorzoxazone* toxicity may cause nausea, vomiting, diarrhea, significant loss of muscle tone, and respiratory depression. *Cyclobenzaprine* toxicity is signified by CNS depression and tachycardia. *Deutetrabenazine* toxicity may cause nausea, vomiting, diarrhea, hallucinations, and suicidal thoughts. *Metaxalone* toxicity can cause serotonin syndrome. *Methocarbamol* toxicity causes nausea, sedation, and seizures and can lead to coma and death, but this is rare. *Orphenadrine* toxicity may cause palpitations, nausea, vomiting, constipation, hypersensitivity reactions, hallucinations, and, rarely, aplastic anemia. *Tetrabenazine* at toxic levels can cause QT prolongation and cardiac arrhythmias. *Tizanidine* toxicity is signified by shallow breathing, syncope, chest pain, cyanosis, and severe sedation.

You should remember

Centrally acting muscle relaxants work in the CNS to reduce tension and spasms in the skeletal muscles. They are structurally heterogeneous and work upon many CNS receptors. These agents may act at the level of the spinal cord or peripherally. They are also called antispasmodics and are safe for up to 2–3 weeks.

Direct-acting muscle relaxants

The direct-acting muscle relaxants relieve muscle spasticity. *Dantrolene (Dantrium)* and the various botulinum toxins act directly on skeletal muscle for this purpose. The prototype drug for these agents is dantrolene. It acts as a calcium release blocker within skeletal muscle cells. Botulinum toxins are neurotoxins that affect nerves and cause muscle paralysis. They are used as skeletal muscle relaxants and include *abobotulinumtoxinA (Dysport)*, *incobotulinumtoxinA (Xeomin)*, *onabotulinumtoxinA (Botox Cosmetic)*, and *rimabotulinumtoxinB (Myobloc)*. They are the most poisonous substances known, requiring extreme caution.

Pharmacokinetics

Dantrolene has 70% bioavailability and is metabolized in the liver. It is absorbed from the GI tract slowly and bound to plasma protein. *Dantrolene* is excreted in the urine and feces. Peak concentration is at 5 hours after administration. Its half-life is 8.7 hours if given orally and 4–8 hours intravenously. For the botulinum toxins, the onset and duration of action are based on each drug's clinical use. The recommended quantities of each neurotoxin administered per treatment are not large enough to cause systemic or apparent effects such as muscle weakness, as long as the patient has no other neuromuscular dysfunction.

Mechanism of action

Dantrolene directly relaxes spastic muscles via interference with calcium ion release from the sarcoplasmic reticulum of skeletal muscles. *Botulinum toxins* bind with high affinity to peripheral cholinergic nerve endings, such as those at the neuromuscular junction and in the autonomic nervous system, preventing the release of neuromuscular transmission of acetylcholine.

Clinical indications

Dantrolene is indicated for spasticity, especially in the head and neck, after spinal cord injury, stroke, MS, or CP. It is also used off label for malignant neuroleptic syndrome or to treat pain after heavy exercise. In 1989, the FDA approved botulinum toxins to treat strabismus, blepharospasm, and hemifacial spasm. Later, they were approved for treating cervical dystonia, glabellar facial lines, axillary hyperhidrosis, chronic migraine, and cosmetic uses.

Contraindications

Dantrolene is contraindicated with active liver diseases such as hepatitis or cirrhosis. The medication cannot be used when spasticity is needed to maintain an upright posture and balance while walking or if it is required to obtain or sustain increased function. *Botulinum toxins* are contraindicated in preexisting motor neuron disease, myasthenia gravis, Eaton-Lambert syndrome, neuropathies, psychological conditions, history of reactions to toxins or albumin, and during pregnancy or lactation.

Adverse effects

The most common adverse effects of *dantrolene* include transient dizziness, drowsiness, general malaise, weakness, diarrhea, and fatigue. However, diarrhea can be severe, and the drug may need to be stopped. Common adverse effects of the *botulinum toxins* include dysphagia, headaches, myasthenia, nasopharyngitis, voice changes, and xerostomia.

Toxicities

Dantrolene toxicity may cause muscular weakness, lethargy, vomiting, diarrhea, crystalluria, and coma. *Botulinum toxins* in excessive doses can cause severe muscle weakness, hoarseness, drooping eyelids, vision changes, difficulty swallowing or talking, loss of bladder control, and weak or shallow breathing.

You should remember

Direct-acting muscle relaxants inhibit muscle contraction by decreasing calcium release from the sarcoplasmic reticulum of muscle cells. A gradually increasing dosing regimen is required when one of these drugs is used for muscle spasms and spasticity. These agents are less helpful for immediate treatments but are of better value for longer-term management. Some affect liver function, requiring periodic blood samples to check for abnormalities.

Nonsteroidal antiinflammatory drugs

NSAIDs include aspirin, ibuprofen, and naproxen. They are usually the first-line drugs for minor to moderate pain caused by muscle overexertion. They can relieve muscle pain and reduce inflammation, relieving nerve pressure and enhancing mobility. For a more significant discussion of NSAIDs, see Chapter 55.

Key Terms

Clonic spasms
Dystonia
Hemifacial spasm
Huntington disease
Lethargy
Lou Gehrig disease
Necrotizing enterocolitis
Neuroleptic malignant syndrome
Neuromuscular junctions
Rhabdomyolysis
Serotonin syndrome
Strabismus
Tardive dyskinesia
Tonic spasm

Clinical Case Studies

Clinical Case Study 1

A 44-year-old male began having muscle spasms in his legs and trunk every 10 minutes to every 2 hours, always during the night. The cramps caused him to become sleep deprived and were mainly triggered by cold exposure, coughing, and sneezing. The patient was treated with oral baclofen, taken before going to bed, and botulinum toxin injections, but he had no relief. A decision was made to administer baclofen directly into his spinal canal, and after a few treatments, his muscle spasms began to decrease in severity and frequency.

Critical Thinking Questions

1. What type of muscle spasms occur multiple times?
2. Why is baclofen often the skeletal muscle relaxant of first choice?
3. What are the potential adverse effects of baclofen?

Clinical Case Study 2

A 35-year-old female with MS had developed muscle spasticity and fatigue for several years with no family history. Her condition had progressed so much that the patient began falling at home and had increased difficulty walking. The spasticity pain had also increased, and the patient reported losing sensation. Specific exercises made her symptoms worse. The patient was started on a course of gait training, using a walker and home-based physiotherapy and administering tizanidine.

Critical Thinking Questions

1. With MS, how does spasticity occur?
2. What other drug besides tizanidine is indicated for muscle spasticity?
3. What are the contraindications of tizanidine?

Further Reading

[1] M. Bakheit, Botulinum Toxin Treatment of Muscle Spasticity, AuthorHouse, 2007.

[2] M.P. Barnes, G.R. Johnson, Upper Motor Neurone Syndrome and Spasticity: Clinical Management and Neurophysiology, second ed., Cambridge University Press, 2008.

[3] G. Bavikatte, D. Mackarel, C. Shippen, R. Roberts, S. Mahendran, S. Mackarel, et al. Spasticity Early & Ongoing Management: Common Patterns, Botulinum Toxin Treatment, Ultrasound Localization, Post-Treatment Exercises, The Walton Centre NHS Foundation, 2018.

[4] J. Bedi, K. Kumar Malhotra, N. Mehta, Effect of an Adjuvant on the Properties of Muscle Relaxant, Lap Lambert Academic Publishing, 2017.

[5] A. Brashear, Spasticity: Diagnosis and Management, second ed., DemosMedical, 2015.

[6] A. Buvanendran, S. Diwan, T. Deer, Intrathecal Drug Delivery for Pain and Spasticity: Interventional and Neuromodulatory Techniques for Pain Management, Elsevier, 2011.

[7] F.F. Foldes, J. Adriani, Muscle Relaxants in Anesthesiology: American Lecture Series, Number 294, Literary Licensing, LLC, 2013.

[8] A. Ghai, R. Aggarwal, Ultrasound Guidance in Obturator Nerve Block in Lower Limb Spasticity, Lap Lambert Academic Publishing, 2016.

[9] M.W. Jann, S.R. Penzak, L.J. Cohen, Applied Clinical Pharmacokinetics and Pharmacodynamics of Psychopharmacological Agents, Adis, 2016.

[10] R.A. Jil, Sciatica Treatments: Chiropractic Care, Antibiotics, Corticosteroids, Analgesics, Epidural Steroid Injections, Muscle Relaxants, Physical Therapy, Surgery, Massage, Other Therapies and Options, CreateSpace Independent Publishing Platform, 2020.

[11] A.D. Pandyan, H.J. Hermens, B.A. Conway, Neurological Rehabilitation: Spatisticity and Contractures in Clinical Practice and Research (Rehabilitation Science in Practice Series), CRC Press, 2018.

[12] F.M. Pottenger, Muscle Spasm and Degeneration in Intrathoracic Inflammations: Their Importance as Diagnostic Aids and Their Influence in Producing and Altering the Well Established Physical Signs, Also a Consideration of Their Part in the Causation of Changes in the Body, Ulan Press, 2012.

[13] R.L. Rosales, D. Dressler, Botulinum Toxin Therapy Manual for Dystonia and Spasticity, InTechOpen, 2016.

[14] M. Sindou, G. Georgoulis, P. Mertens, Neurosurgery for Spasticity: A Practical Guide for Treating Children and Adults, Springer, 2014.

[15] V.L. Stevenson, L. Jarrett, Spasticity Management: A Practical Multidisciplinary Guide, second ed., CRC Press, 2018.

[16] H. Winchell Magoun, R. Rhines, R.F. Pitts, Spasticity: The Stretch Reflex and Extrapyramidal Systems, Literary Licensing, LLC, 2013.

CHAPTER

14

Drugs used in Parkinson and Alzheimer diseases

OUTLINE

LEARNING OUTCOMES

After study of the chapter, readers should be able to:

1. Describe the four primary signs of Parkinson disease.

The Science of Pharmacology
https://doi.org/10.1016/B978-0-443-29038-1.00014-2

2. Explain the two parts of the basal nuclei involved in developing Parkinson disease.
3. Identify the causes of Parkinson disease.
4. Compare dopaminergic and anticholinergic drugs.
5. Describe the dopaminergic first-line medicines for the treatment of Parkinson disease.
6. Explain the adverse effects of the anticholinergic drugs.
7. Describe the causes of Alzheimer disease and the risk factors.
8. Explain the pathophysiology of Alzheimer disease.
9. List three generic and trade names of the catechol-*O*-methyltransferase inhibitors.
10. Describe the adverse effects of memantine.

Overview

Parkinson disease (PD) is a common progressive neurodegenerative condition associated with significant disability and negatively impacting quality of life. Although the cause of PD is unknown, the pathologic manifestation involves the loss or dysfunction of dopaminergic neurons in the substantia nigra pars compacta. It is most commonly seen in persons 60 and older. However, up to 10% of patients are diagnosed before age 50, with males generally affected more than females. It may occur idiopathically and is most common in Caucasians out of all racial or ethnic groups. Many cases of PD have developed after repeated head trauma, especially in athletes. Characteristic clinical manifestations include difficulty with coordinated movements, such as asymmetric resting tremor, rigidity, and bradykinesia. Alzheimer disease (AD) causes a decline in memory, thinking, learning, and organizing skills. It's the most common cause of dementia and usually affects people over 65. AD affects approximately 24 million people across the world. One in 10 people older than 65 and nearly a third of people older than 85 have the condition. There is no cure for PD or AD, but certain medications and therapies can help manage symptoms temporarily.

Parkinson disease

PD was first identified in 1817 by British physician James Parkinson. The condition is the second most common degenerative disease in the nervous system. In older adults, it is the third most common neurologic disorder, peaking between the ages of 58 and 62, and it is 1.5 times more common in males than females. The most common subtype is *idiopathic PD*, which is of unknown cause and causes progressive neuronal destruction in specific brain areas. There is sometimes a family history indicating a genetic link. *Secondary PD* may be caused by brain infections or tumors, head trauma, and neurotoxin exposure. However, the most frequent cause is the use of antipsychotic and anesthetic drugs. If a patient taking these drugs develops signs of Parkinsonism, the drugs are discontinued. The symptoms usually resolve, though they can be permanent if the use of the drugs is long term.

Characteristic neuropathologic findings and clinical presentation signify PD. These include motor deficits and sometimes mental deterioration. The condition is relatively asymptomatic until 70%–80% of neurons of the substantia nigra are depleted. Reduced activation of dopamine receptors causes increased inhibition of the thalamus. Though its cause is not entirely understood, genetic and environmental factors are believed to be involved in an imbalance of neurotransmitters in the brain.

PD develops insidiously and slowly progresses from several months to several years. Approximately 1 million people in the United States have PD. This number is predicted to reach 1.2 million by 2030. About 60,000 new cases of PD are diagnosed in the United States each year. The disease affects one in 100 people over age 60. There is no definitive PD testing method; diagnosis is clinical once other neurologic disorders have been ruled out. The four primary signs of PD are muscle rigidity, **bradykinesia**, tremor, and postural instability, which are further explained as follows:

- *Muscle rigidity*: Resistance to passive movements of the extremities that may resemble the stiffness of arthritis. The individual may have problems moving the limbs and bending over. The rigidity of facial muscles causes a lack of expression or changes in expression. When the pharyngeal muscles are involved, chewing and swallowing problems can develop, and uncontrolled drooling may occur. A prominent symptom is a lack of arm swinging when the individual walks. The arms are instead held close to the sides of the body. Muscle rigidity occurs early in the disease but becomes more evident over the years.
- *Bradykinesia* is an uncontrolled slowness of voluntary movement and speech that is highly noticeable and results in difficulty speaking, chewing, and swallowing. There are problems initiating activities and controlling fine muscle movements. The individual shuffles their feet while walking and no longer takes normal strides. This makes walking much more difficult.
- *Tremor*: The head and hands develop continuous shaking or motions while at rest. The tremors may become so severe that holding objects becomes difficult, and bringing eating utensils to the mouth is hard. As the disease progresses, there are **pill-rolling motions**, with the thumbs and forefingers rubbed together in circular motions.
- *Postural instability*: There is often a "stooped-over" body position, and balance can easily be lost. If the patient stumbles, falling is likely, resulting in injuries.

The prominent features of PD are illustrated in Fig. 14.1.

Additional health problems may include anxiety, sleep disturbances, and autonomic abnormalities resulting in constipation, sexual dysfunction, and problems urinating. Over 50% of patients become clinically depressed, and many have disorders of sensations and thoughts. Dementia may develop, especially if the individual is over age 70. Medications are often required, which increases the likelihood of drug interactions and adverse effects.

The **basal nuclei** control involuntary muscle movements and are the interconnected neuronal clusters in the brain. They regulate information from the cerebral cortex to the spinal cord's motor neurons and help stop and start activity while walking. The two parts of the basal nuclei involved in the development of PD are the substantia nigra and the striatum. The substantia nigra is the main production area of dopamine and appears as a dark band of gray matter in the midbrain. Dopamine moves through the axons of the **nigrostriatal pathway** to the **striatum**, also called

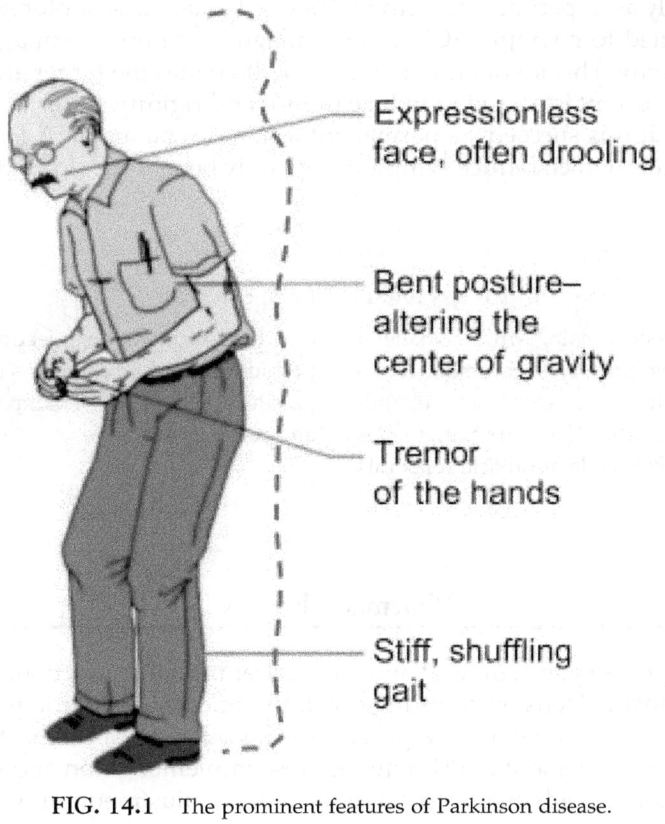

FIG. 14.1 The prominent features of Parkinson disease.

the **corpus striatum**. It is here where dopamine is released. In the striatum, dopamine contacts its receptors to produce various actions. Concerning PD, the planning and regulation of motor pathways involved in unconscious muscle movements are affected, with dopamine inhibition slowing impulses that move down the spinal neurons.

Average amounts of dopamine regulate the flow of motor impulses from the striatum, producing unconscious, coordinated muscle movements. When levels of dopamine decrease, the symptoms appear. The body can function normally when up to 50% of these neurons stop producing dopamine, but PD symptoms are seen once 60%–80% lose function. Acetylcholine (ACh) is another neurotransmitter that modulates the effects of the neuronal outflow from the striatum with excitatory functions. The effects of dopamine and ACh typically balance each other out, resulting in smooth and coordinated muscle movements. However, with a decline in dopamine, ACh has a more extreme stimulatory effect, and the abnormal muscle movements of PD are then seen.

Therefore antiparkinson medications are required to balance out dopamine and acetylcholine levels in various brain regions. The two primary types of drugs for PD are dopaminergics and anticholinergics. They help patients perform routine daily activities, including walking, eating, bathing, and dressing. They also help to decrease the likelihood of falling. The medications improve PD symptoms, self-worth, quality of life, and the ability for self-care. However, long-term medications occasionally lose their effects gradually near the end of dosing intervals. Symptoms temporarily worsen as drug concentrations decrease below the therapeutic level. Adjusting dosing intervals for more frequent doses can reduce this wearing-off effect. There is no cure for PD. However, medications and other treatments can help relieve some of the symptoms. Exercise can help Parkinson symptoms significantly, along with physical and occupational therapy.

The **on-off phenomenon** is a syndrome of alternating periods of being symptom free (the "on" period) and an abrupt reappearance of symptoms (the "off" period). These on-off periods can range from a few minutes to several hours. The off periods can occur sometimes even if the serum drug level is high, and the overall phenomenon is difficult to control. For patients taking carbidopa-levodopa, doses can be scheduled closer together, or another adjunct medication can be taken during the off period to handle the phenomenon better. When drugs become ineffective, four nonpharmacologic methods may be helpful. These include deep brain stimulation, *fetal tissue transplantation*, **pallidotomy**, and thalamotomy.

Deep brain stimulation involves an electrode implanted in the thalamus or subthalamus, delivering electric currents that interfere with tremor-creating cells, and an implanted generator inserted under the patient's skin that can be adjusted using a magnet placed over it. Fetal tissue from humans or pigs can be transplanted into the brain's caudate nucleus, but this is only an experimental method designed to decrease motor symptoms of PD. After a target area is identified via a computed tomography (CT) scan or magnetic resonance imaging (MRI), the patient can be sedated to perform a pallidotomy. This involves making a burr hole into the target area and inserting an electrode, through which a mild electric current is passed to reduce tremor and rigidity. If this does not occur, the probe can be moved until the effects occur. If this succeeds, a permanent lesion can be made. A *thalamotomy* involves surgically produced lesions in the thalamus, which reduce symptoms but only benefit the side of the body that is most affected.

You should remember

Most patients with PD report pain. Musculoskeletal pain from mobility limitations is the most common. Treatments include acetaminophen, NSAIDs, physical rehabilitation, and low doses of opioids. When the patient has dystonia as a component of PD, skeletal muscle relaxants and botulinum toxin injections may be needed. Neuropathic pain is less joint and is treated with gabapentin, pregabalin, duloxetine, venlafaxine, spinal cord stimulation, and nerve blocks.

Pharmacotherapy

Medications for PD can improve symptoms and allow for better mobility, functionality, and performance of daily living tasks. The current treatments focus on restoring dopaminergic activity through different mechanisms. However, treatment benefits are reduced as the disease progresses, and the use of medications then becomes very challenging. The pharmacological management of PD requires close implementation and monitoring to balance clinical effectiveness and the minimization of adverse events. Frequent dose adjustments and combination therapies achieve the best control of motor and nonmotor symptoms. The dopaminergic agents benefit motor symptoms, known as improvement in "on time" or reduced "off time."

Dopaminergic drugs

Dopaminergic agents directly or indirectly cause the activation of dopamine receptors. These agents are more widely used than the anticholinergic agents. Mild symptoms are usually treated, beginning with selegiline or rasagiline. More severe symptoms are treated with either carbidopa-levodopa or a dopamine agonist. While levodopa is more effective, long-term use carries a greater risk of disabling **dyskinesias**. Unfortunately, the beneficial effects of levodopa diminish over time, hence the combination of levodopa with carbidopa because carbidopa increases the plasma levels and half-life of levodopa. The first-line dopaminergics for PD are carbidopa-levodopa, pramipexole, and ropinirole. Combining *carbidopa* and *levodopa* is the most effective therapy for PD. It is much more effective than when levodopa is used alone. Levodopa without carbidopa is no longer available.

Pharmacokinetics

Of the dopamine agonists, *apomorphine* has lower bioavailability when taken orally because it is not absorbed well in the GI tract and undergoes heavy first-pass metabolism. It has a bioavailability of 100% when given subcutaneously, reaching peak plasma concentration in 10–60 minutes. Its lipophilic structures help it to cross the blood-brain barrier, and the medication has an affinity for dopamine, serotonin, norepinephrine, and epinephrine receptors. Apomorphine is metabolized in the liver and eliminated via urine and feces. *Bromocriptine* has extensive hepatic first-pass extraction and metabolism. Only 5%–10% of the ingested dose reaches the systemic circulation, and only about 28% of oral doses are absorbed. The elimination half-life is 12–14 hours, with 85% excreted in the bile in the feces and 2.5%–5.5% excreted in the urine.

Pramipexole has linear pharmacokinetics over the clinical dosage range, with a terminal half-life of about 8 hours in younger and 12 hours in elderly patients. It has about 90% bioavailability and 15% protein binding. Excretion is 90% via the urine and 2% via the feces. *Ropinirole* is rapidly absorbed after oral administration and reaches peak concentration in about 1–2 hours. It also has a first-pass effect, with absolute bioavailability of 50%. Elimination half-life is 5–6 hours. Metabolism is via the liver enzyme cytochrome P450 (CYP) 1A2. *Rotigotine* is another option, administered via a transdermal patch that is replaced daily. It has 37% bioavailability, 92% protein binding, and CYP-mediated liver metabolism. The elimination half-life is 5–7 hours, and excretion is 71% in the urine and 23% in the feces. The dopaminergics used for PD are summarized in Table 14.1.

Mechanism of action

The dopamine agonists work by imitating the actions of dopamine when levels are low. They activate postsynaptic dopamine receptors in the corpus striatum and may allow for reduced maintenance doses of levodopa, even in combination products such as carbidopa-levodopa. The exact mechanisms of action of *pramipexole* and *ropinirole* for PD are unknown.

You should remember

Though dopaminergic medications are the most effective drugs for patients with PD, their long-term use is related to debilitating motor fluctuations. Strategies are required to identify and alleviate motor dysfunction because patients may not spontaneously seek assistance when they experience changes. Motor fluctuations include "wearing off," unpredictable "off" periods, freezing of gait, failure of the "on" response, and acute akinesia.

Clinical indications

Carbidopa-levodopa is indicated for treating PD, postencephalitis parkinsonism, and symptomatic parkinsonism following carbon monoxide or manganese intoxication. *Carbidopa-levodopa-entacapone* is only meant for treating PD to relieve nausea and vomiting. *Apomorphine* is indicated for PD and alcoholism as an emetic and is also used for erectile dysfunction. *Bromocriptine* is indicated for PD, pituitary tumors, hyperprolactinemia, neuroleptic

TABLE 14.1 Dopaminergics used for Parkinson disease.

Generic name	Trade name	Average dosage range (mg/day)	Dosage forms (mg)
Carbidopa-levodopa products			
carbidopa-levodopa	Sinemet	300–1000	10/100, 25/100, 25/250
carbidopa-levodopa	Parcopa	300–1000	10/100, 25/100, 25/250
carbidopa-levodopa	Sinemet CR	400–1000	25/100, 50/200
carbidopa-levodopa	Rytary ER	400–855	23.75 mg, 36.25 mg
carbidopa-levodopa/ entacapone	Stalevo	600–1600	12.5/50/200, 18.75/75/ 200, 25/100/200, 31.25/ 125/200
carbidopa	Lodosyn	25–75	25
Dopamine agonists			
apomorphine	Apokyn	3–12	30/3 mL
bromocriptine	Parlodel	15–40	2.5, 5
pramipexole	Mirapex	1.5–4.5	0.125, 0.25, 0.5, 1, 1.5
pramipexole	Mirapex ER	1.5–4.5	0.375, 0.75, 1.5, 3, 4.5
ropinirole	Requip	9–24	0.25, 0.5, 1, 2, 3, 4, 5
ropinirole	Requip XL	8–24	2, 4, 6, 18, 12
rotigotine	Neupro	2–8	2, 4, 6, 8

malignant syndrome, and adjunctively for type 2 diabetes. *Pramipexole* and *ropinirole* are indicated for PD and restless legs syndrome. *Rotigotine* is meant for early- and late-stage PD and restless legs syndrome. It reduces the on-off periods of PD.

Contraindications

The contraindications of dopamine agonists include known hypersensitivity, **narrow-angle glaucoma**, suspicious undiagnosed skin lesions, and a history of **melanoma**. *Apomorphine* is contraindicated with adrenergic receptor antagonists, alcohol, and dopamine antagonists. Contraindications of *bromocriptine* include uncontrolled hypertension, use of other medications that lower blood pressure, and a history of psychosis or cardiovascular disease. *Pramipexole* is contraindicated with recurrent daytime sleep episodes, orthostatic hypotension, rhabdomyolysis, drowsiness, hallucinations, sleep apnea, dyskinesia, breastfeeding, uncontrolled impulsive behaviors, and kidney disease. *Ropinirole* is contraindicated with psychosis, bradycardia, orthostatic hypotension, drowsiness, hallucinations, dyskinesia, unruly impulsive behaviors, and kidney failure.

Adverse effects

The adverse effects of *carbidopa-levodopa* and *carbidopa* on its own include dyskinesias, nausea, vomiting, constipation, headaches, and asthenia. The adverse effects of the *dopamine agonists* include abnormal involuntary movements, vertigo, peripheral edema, GI ulcers, pulmonary fibrosis, psychosis, hallucinations, hypotension, myocardial infarction, congestive heart failure, cardiac fibrosis, tachycardia, and pericardial effusion. Other adverse effects of the *dopamine agonists* are insomnia, impulse control disorder, confusion, the on-off phenomenon, dizziness, drowsiness, asthenia, fainting, visual disturbances, ataxia, and shortness of breath. With *rotigotine*, there can be unexpected sleep attacks that can result in injury to the patient.

Toxicities

In addition to the long-term adverse effects described, carbidopa, levodopa, entacapone, apomorphine, bromocriptine, pramipexole, and ropinirole have no significant toxicities.

You should remember

Research about PD is developing rapidly, partly because of the Michael J. Fox Foundation, which was started in 2000. It is the largest nonprofit organization funding PD research and development globally. Aside from Fox, other famous people diagnosed with PD include actor Alan Alda, singer Neil Diamond, singer Ozzy Osbourne, singer Linda Ronstadt, and boxer Muhammed Ali.

Anticholinergic drugs

Anticholinergic agents are antiparkinsonian drugs that block receptors for acetylcholine. These agents are rarely effective for bradykinesia and other disabilities and can be used either as monotherapy or with other antiparkinsonian drugs. Anticholinergics used for PD include benztropine and trihexyphenidyl (see Table 14.2).

Pharmacokinetics

Benztropine is absorbed from the GI tract and metabolized in the liver, and a small part of the dose passes through the GI tract unchanged into the feces. It crosses the blood-brain barrier. Elimination half-life is 12 to 24 hours, and most of the drug is excreted as the drug and its metabolites. *Trihexyphenidyl* is quickly absorbed from the GI tract, with an onset of action within 1 hour and a duration of 6–12 hours. Elimination half-life is 3.3–4.1 hours. It is principally excreted in the urine, mainly as an unchanged drug.

Mechanism of action

All anticholinergic agents share the exact mechanism of action: they block muscarinic receptors in the striatum. *Benztropine (Cogentin)* has antimuscarinic, antihistaminic, and local anesthetic effects, competing with acetylcholine and other cholinergic mediators at muscarinic receptors in the CNS. By blocking muscarinic cholinergic receptors, benztropine reduces excessive cholinergic activity in parkinsonism and related states. The medication can also block dopamine reuptake and storage, prolonging dopamine's effects. *Trihexyphenidyl (Artane)* has atropine-like action, exerting antispasmodic effects upon parasympathetic-innervated peripheral structures. Its exact mechanism of action in PD is not fully understood.

Clinical indications

Benztropine and trihexyphenidyl are used for PD and dyskinesias caused by certain medications. Benztropine is approved as adjunctive therapy for all forms of parkinsonism and is also used for drug-induced **extrapyramidal symptoms**, prevention of dystonic reactions, and treatment of acute dystonic reactions. Trihexyphenidyl treats tremors, spasms, stiffness, and weak muscle control.

Contraindications

Benztropine is contraindicated with intestinal infections caused by *Shigella* bacteria or *Clostridium difficile*, thyrotoxicosis, tardive dyskinesia, autonomic neuropathy, myasthenia gravis, wide-angle or closed-angle glaucoma, hypertension or hypotension, coronary artery disease, dysrhythmia, chronic heart failure, **achalasia** of the esophagus, gastroesophageal reflux disease, hiatal hernia, stomach ulcers, ulcerative colitis, **toxic megacolon**, intestinal paralysis, liver disease, decreased kidney function, enlarged prostate, dysuria, and chronic obstructive pulmonary disease. *Trihexyphenidyl* is contraindicated with known hypersensitivity, glaucoma, tardive dyskinesia, cardiac disease, hypertension, prostatic hypertrophy, and liver or kidney impairment.

TABLE 14.2 Anticholinergics used for Parkinson disease.

Generic name	Trade name	Average dosage range (mg/day)	Dosage forms (mg)
Benztropine	Cogentin	0.5–4	0.5, 1, 2
Trihexyphenidyl	Artane	1–6	2, 5, 2/5 mL

Adverse effects

Adverse effects of the anticholinergics include blurred vision, dry mouth, nausea, nervousness, constipation, and urinary retention. Patients with preexisting cognitive deficits and older adults have a higher risk for central anticholinergic adverse effects.

Toxicities

Benztropine is toxic only in younger children, so it should not be used in children younger than 3. *Trihexyphenidyl* has caused toxic symptoms such as **xerostomia**, mydriasis, **anhidrosis**, nausea, vomiting, tachycardia, decreased bowel movements, rash, and hyperthermia. It must also be used with caution in younger children.

You should remember

Anticholinergics treat many medical conditions affecting muscle contraction and relaxation, including Parkinson. The Parkinson's Foundation has found that cognitive slowing is a side effect of these drugs. They should be avoided in people older than age 70 because these individuals are especially susceptible to confusion and hallucinations.

Monoamine oxidase type B inhibitors

Monoamine oxidase type B (MAO-B) is an enzyme in the body that breaks down several chemicals in the brain, including dopamine. Therefore, by using a medication that blocks the effect of MAO-B inhibitor, more dopamine is available to be used by the brain, which can slightly improve many of the motor symptoms of PD. The MAO-B inhibitors are also helpful as early monotherapy or can be used with medications such as carbidopa-levodopa to reduce the "off" time and extend the "on" time of the effects. The primary MAO-B inhibitors are *rasagiline, safinamide,* and *selegiline* (see Table 14.3).

Pharmacokinetics

Rasagiline has 36% bioavailability and protein binding of 88%–94%. It metabolizes in the liver, and the elimination half-life is 3 hours. Excretion is via the urine and feces. *Safinamide* has the pharmacokinetic properties of these drugs but also has an antiglutamatergic effect. It has 95% bioavailability and 88%–90% protein binding. The amidases metabolize via glucuronidation in the liver and have an elimination half-life of 20–30 hours. Excretion is mainly via the urine and less in the feces. *Selegiline* has 10% oral bioavailability, 73% transdermal patch bioavailability, and 94% protein binding. It is metabolized in the liver. The elimination half-life of the oral form is 1.5–3.5 hours and 18–25 hours of the transdermal form, and it is excreted in the urine.

Mechanism of action

The MAO-B inhibitors have a complex mechanism of action. When used as monotherapy, they provide a slight yet significant improvement of motor function and delay the need for levodopa. They significantly reduce off time and achieve improvements in some nonmotor symptoms as well. Rasagiline prevents the breakdown of dopamine by irreversibly binding to MAO-B. Safinamide has similar actions but is reversible, unlike rasagiline and selegiline.

TABLE 14.3 MAO-B inhibitors used for Parkinson disease.

Generic name	Trade name	Average dosage range (mg/day)	Dosage forms (mg)
rasagiline	Azilect	0.5–1	0.5, 1
safinamide	Xadago	50–100	50, 100
selegiline	Eldepryl	5–10	5
selegiline	Zelapar	1.25–2.5	1.25, 2.5

It also binds to *sigma receptors* and blocks sodium and calcium channels. Selegiline inhibits MAO-B and other MAOs at higher doses.

Clinical indications

Rasagiline is used as monotherapy to treat symptoms of early PD or as an adjunct therapy for more advanced cases. Safinamide is used for idiopathic PD as an add-on medication with carbidopa-levodopa to assist with the "off" episodes when the other drugs stop working. Selegiline is used for PD, usually as an adjunct to different medications, but can be used as a monotherapy. It is also indicated for off-label use as a palliative treatment for dementia in AD.

Contraindications

Rasagiline is contraindicated with malignant melanoma, bipolar disorder, psychosis, hypertension, orthostatic hypotension, liver abnormalities, and dyskinesia. Safinamide is contraindicated with hypersensitivity and Child-Pugh liver impairment. Selegiline is contraindicated with melanoma, severe mental disorders involving loss of personality and reality, orthostatic hypotension, liver abnormalities, and **Child-Pugh liver impairment**.

Adverse effects

The adverse effects of rasagiline include dizziness or fainting; hallucinations; sore throat; lip or mouth abnormalities; tachycardia; stomach pain; muscle pain; chest pain; coughing, chills, or fever; difficulty swallowing; loss of appetite; nausea; cloudy urine; dysuria; sweating; liver abnormalities; and unusual bleeding, bruising, tiredness, or weakness. The common adverse effects of safinamide include nausea, dizziness, orthostatic hypotension, fatigue, sleepiness, and headache. The most common adverse effects of selegiline are various dyskinesias of the tongue, lips, face, arms, or legs.

Toxicities

The signs of MAO-B inhibitor toxicity are nonspecific. They may include agitation, **diaphoresis**, tachycardia, mild temperature elevation or hyperthermia, altered mental status, tachypnea, vomiting, dysrhythmias, and hypertension.

You should remember

It is essential to understand that in large doses, some MAO-B inhibitors interact with foods high in tyramine and can increase blood pressure to dangerous levels. These foods include cheeses, dried or cured meats, fava beans, beer, sauerkraut, and soybeans.

Catechol-O-methyltransferase inhibitors

The *catechol-O-methyltransferase (COMT) inhibitors* have no direct effect on PD symptoms but prolong the effect of levodopa by blocking its metabolism. They are mainly used to help with the "wearing-off" phenomenon in which the effects of levodopa become short lived. The primary COMT inhibitors are summarized in Table 14.4.

TABLE 14.4 Catechol-O-methyltransferase inhibitors.

Generic name	Trade name	Average dosage range (mg/day)	Dosage forms (mg)
Entacapone	Comtan	200–1600	200
Tolcapone	Tasmar	300–600	100, 200
Opicapone	Ongentys	25–50	25, 50 (though mostly given as 50 mg once daily at bedtime)

Pharmacokinetics

The pharmacokinetics of *entacapone* are linear over the dosage range and independent of levodopa and carbidopa concurrent administration. Bioavailability is 35%, protein binding is 98%, and it is metabolized in the liver. The elimination half-life is 0.4–0.7 hours based on the beta phase and 2.4 hours based on the gamma phase. The drug is 90% excreted in the feces and 10% in the urine. *Tolcapone* has absolute bioavailability after oral administration of about 65%, protein binding of 99.9%, and metabolism in the liver, mainly via glucuronidation. Peak plasma concentrations are usually attained within 2 hours. The COMT inhibitory activity persists for 16–24 hours. Elimination half-life is 2–3 hours, excretion is 60% in the urine and 40% in the feces, and only 0.5% is in its unmetabolized form. *Opicapone* attains its peak plasma concentrations in about 2 hours after oral administration. It has about 20% bioavailability and 99.9% protein binding, and metabolism is mainly via sulfation, followed by reduction, glucuronidation, and methylation. Elimination half-life is 0.7–3.2 hours, with a duration of action of about 24 hours. Excretion is mainly via the feces and some from urine.

Mechanism of action

The mechanism of action of *entacapone* is believed to be through its ability to inhibit COMT and alter the plasma pharmacokinetics of levodopa. The precise mechanism of action of *tolcapone* is unknown. Still, it is believed to be related to its ability to inhibit COMT and alter the plasma pharmacokinetics of levodopa, increasing plasma levodopa concentrations. *Opicapone* blocks COMT effectively, selectively, reversibly, and only outside the CNS. It dissociates slowly from COMT, with a duration of action longer than 24 hours, even though it has a short blood plasma half-life.

Clinical indications

Entacapone is indicated as a combination therapy with levodopa for motor fluctuations. It is not used without levodopa. Tolcapone has the same indications but should only be used after all Parkinson medications have been tried. If it shows no benefit, it should be discontinued in 3 weeks. Opicapone is indicated as adjunctive therapy for PD and end-of-dose motor fluctuations or "off" episodes whose symptoms cannot be stabilized on the combination therapy of levodopa and DOPA decarboxylase inhibitor (such as carbidopa).

Contraindications

Entacapone is contraindicated in patients with known hypersensitivity to the drug or its ingredients. Tolcapone is contraindicated in patients with liver disease, related hepatocellular injury, a history of nontraumatic rhabdomyolysis, drug-related confusion and hyperpyrexia, and known hypersensitivity to the drug or its ingredients. Opicapone is contraindicated in patients with catecholamine-secreting cancers such as pheochromocytoma or paraganglioma and a history of neuroleptic malignant syndrome or nontraumatic rhabdomyolysis.

Adverse effects

Entacapone may cause diarrhea, discolored urine, and enhanced adverse effects of levodopa, such as confusion and dyskinesia. Negative impacts of tolcapone include the same ones as for entacapone plus risks of liver damage, so regular blood tests to check liver function are required. Common adverse effects of the combination agent carbidopa-levodopa/entacapone include hypotension, confusion, nausea, diarrhea, discolored urine, and dyskinesia. Negative impacts of opicapone include constipation, dyskinesia, hypotension with dizziness, and weight loss.

Toxicities

Entacapone can cause renal toxicity in substantial doses. Patients with hepatic impairment should be closely monitored with its use. Hepatotoxicity is a severe concern with tolcapone. There is a risk of potentially fatal acute fulminant liver failure. Signs of hepatic toxicity must be closely monitored. Other toxicities include worsening of levodopa-associated adverse effects, orthostatic hypotension, hallucinations, excessive sedation, compulsive behaviors, extreme nausea, and possible adverse effects upon pregnancy. With *opicapone*, no significant liver toxicity has been found.

You should remember

The COMT inhibitors are helpful because they extend the effectiveness of carbidopa-levodopa therapy. They also allow for lower doses of carbidopa-levodopa and can reduce motor fluctuations seen in PD.

Amantadine

Amantadine is an antidyskinetic agent. It is used to treat early and advanced PD because it helps reduce tremors. More recently, amantadine (Symmetrel) has also been found to help lower dyskinesias caused by dopamine-based medications. It is available in 100-mg capsules or tablets and 50-mg/5-mL syrup. The typical treatment regimen is 100 mg twice to three times per day. In 2017, an extended-release capsule form known as the FDA-approved Gocovri to treat Parkinson's dyskinesias. There are also extended-release tablets available under the trade name Osmolex ER.

Pharmacokinetics

Amantadine is well absorbed orally and has a half-life of 9.7–31 hours for elimination. Bioavailability is 86%–90%, protein binding is 67%, and metabolism is minimal, primarily to acetyl metabolites. Excretion is via the urine. It should be noted that in compromised patients, amantadine is eliminated over a more extended period of 18.5 hours to 33.8 days.

Mechanism of action

The mechanism of action of amantadine in PD is poorly understood. It acts as an anticholinergic, binding to and acting as an agonist of the sigma-1 receptor. It increases dopamine release and blocks dopamine reuptake.

Clinical indications

Amantadine was first used to treat influenza A. However, it is no longer recommended for this purpose. In 1973 the FDA approved amantadine for treating PD. The immediate-release form of amantadine is indicated as monotherapy for slowness, stiffness, and tremor. It is also used in combination therapy with levodopa for dyskinesias. The extended-release capsules and tablets are used for dyskinesias as part of the "off" episodes of the disease.

Contraindications

Amantadine is contraindicated with end-stage kidney disease and must be used cautiously in people with an enlarged prostate or glaucoma. Also, live attenuated vaccines are contraindicated while taking amantadine.

Adverse effects

Adverse effects of amantadine include arrhythmia-related symptoms, confusion, constipation, dizziness, dry mouth, hallucinations, insomnia, leg discoloration, nausea, orthostatic hypotension, paranoia, and urinary retention.

Toxicities

In excessive quantities, amantadine can cause irregular heart rhythms, tachycardia, difficulty breathing, decreased urination, swelling of the extremities, stiffness of the arms or legs, dyskinesias, tremors, coordination problems, confusion, a feeling of being "outside" the self, fear, irritability, aggression, hallucinations, and fatigue.

You should remember

In the treatment of PD, amantadine acts on dopamine neurons. It may be given alone or in combination with other medications. By improving muscle control and reducing stiffness, amantadine allows for more normal body movements as the disease's symptoms are relieved. Improvements in symptoms usually occur in a few days, though some patients must take amantadine for up to 2 weeks before complete benefits will be seen.

Alzheimer disease

AD is a brain disorder that slowly destroys memory, thinking skills, and the ability to carry out the simplest tasks. Senile plaques, beta-amyloid deposits, and tangles of neurofibrils in the cerebral cortex and the subcortical gray matter signify it. These tangles can only be identified via biopsy or autopsy because they cannot be seen in CT or MRI scans. More than 80% of elderly dementia patients have AD, and more than 6.2 million Americans have the condition.

AD is the most expensive in the United States, surpassing cancer and heart disease. It is estimated that the cost of caring for people with dementia in the United States totaled $305 billion in 2020. Medicare and Medicaid are responsible for approximately 67% of these costs each year and will spend an estimated $65 billion in 2023 to care for those with dementia. On a per-person basis, the average individual spending for seniors with dementia is more than three times higher than for seniors without dementia.

It is more common in advanced age (usually beginning after age 60), with up to 50% of patients over age 85 affected. It is the fifth leading cause of death for people over 65 and the sixth overall cause of death in the United States. However, though a terminal condition, most deaths of Alzheimer patients occur from aspiration, sepsis, other concurrent chronic illnesses, or pneumonia. Though the disease can range from 3 to 20 years before causing death, most patients live for 4–6 years after being diagnosed. Other common types of dementia include vascular dementia, **Lewy body dementia**, **Pick disease**, and dementia related to PD.

Etiology and risk factors

The exact cause of dementia is largely unknown, but multiple factors are thought to cause the development of dementia. AD is believed to be caused by genetic and environmental factors, including gene changes and a family history of dementia. The changes in chromosomes lead to two specific changes in the brain of patients with AD: the formation of plaques and tangles. Proteins in the brain group together and form plaques outside and around the brain's neurons, and twisted strands of protein (tangles) collect inside the brain's nerve cells. These changes to neurons in the brain lead to damage to the brain tissue and death of the neurons, which cause the symptoms of dementia in these patients. AD is a slowly progressive disease, so these changes occur years before symptoms appear.

Pathophysiology

The classic characteristic findings in the brain of people with AD include senile plaques and neurofibrillary tangles in the cerebral cortex (the outermost tissue of the brain). These findings do not appear in imaging studies such as CT or MRI scans and can only be identified from biopsy or autopsy. The development of senile plaques is thought to be closely related to the production of a protein called β-amyloid (beta-amyloid). β-amyloid is produced from another protein called amyloid precursor protein. How β-amyloid causes brain nerve cell problems is not completely clear. However, numerous agents that decrease production or reduce the deposits of β-amyloid in the brain are being investigated to prevent or treat AD. Overproduction of β-amyloid is associated with earlier-onset AD (before age 65) and is thought to have a genetic component, with alterations linked to chromosomes 1, 14, and 21.

Late-onset AD (after age 65), which is much more common, is also linked to genetic variations. A protein called apolipoprotein E is associated with the neurofibrillary tangles found in people with known AD brains. The gene responsible for producing apolipoprotein E is located on chromosome 19.

Diagnosis

To make an appropriate diagnosis, providers must complete a thorough medical assessment and patient interview and rule out other potential causes of memory impairment. This can include obtaining bloodwork (vitamins, thyroid levels) and assessing changes in alcohol intake, water intake, and medications.

There may be increased brain and cerebrospinal fluid concentrations of the **tau protein** and reduced levels of choline acetyltransferase and neurotransmitters such as somatostatin. The disease primarily affects memory. Damage occurs initially in the hippocampus and entorhinal cortex, parts of the brain that are essential in forming memories. Regular brain changes related to aging are accelerated. These include decreased brain size, ventricle enlargement, cerebral sulci enlargement, fissure enlargement, and abnormalities of the hippocampus, superior temporal gyrus, precentral frontal lobe gyrus, and substantia nigra.

You should remember

The Alzheimer's Association predicts that by 2050, the number of people in the United States who will have AD will surpass 13 million, with a projected 1 million new cases yearly. Without changes in the treatment or prevention of AD by 2050, someone in the United States will develop the disease every 33 seconds.

Pharmacotherapy

AD is a complicated disease that is unlikely to be successfully treated by a single medicine or other intervention. Current pharmacotherapeutic techniques are centered on assisting patients in preserving mental capacities, managing behavioral manifestations, and delaying the progression, thereby slowing the emergence of illness symptoms. Currently, two classes of FDA-approved medications help delay the progression of dementia: cholinesterase inhibitors and *N*-methyl-*D*-aspartate (NMDA) antagonists. There are also newer drugs called monoclonal antibodies (Aduhelm and Leqembi) that remove specific forms of beta-amyloid.

Acetylcholinesterase inhibitors

Acetylcholinesterase inhibitors, starting with tacrine, were the first medications approved for treating the cognitive symptoms of AD. Approved in the 1990s, these agents target reductions in acetylcholine that cause reduced communication between nerve cells and increased cognitive symptoms. These agents include tacrine (Cognex), donepezil (Aricept), rivastigmine (Exelon), and galantamine (Razadyne). However, tacrine is seldom used today because of its excessive toxicity. Overall, the acetylcholinesterase inhibitors only have a modest effect on AD, do not cure the disease, and may result in slight cognitive improvement. The expected benefits are not highly significant.

Pharmacokinetics

Acetylcholinesterase inhibitors are rapidly absorbed through the GI tract, with the peak concentration usually being less than 2 hours. They are highly protein bound, but the protein binding of *rivastigmine* and *galantamine* is less than 40%. These inhibitors are metabolized by hepatic CYP. Clinical improvement occurs with 40% and 70% of these agents' cholinesterase inhibition.

Mechanism of action

Acetylcholinesterase inhibitors prevent the enzyme acetylcholinesterase from breaking the neurotransmitter acetylcholine into choline and acetate. This increases the level and duration of action of acetylcholine in the CNS, autonomic ganglia, and neuromuscular junctions, which have many acetylcholine receptors.

Clinical indications

Tacrine, donepezil, and *galantamine* are indicated for treating mild to moderate dementia of the Alzheimer's type. *Rivastigmine* is also indicated for this and for mild to moderate dementia associated with Parkinson's disease. Tacrine is rarely used in the United States.

Contraindications

Tacrine is contraindicated for parkinsonism, sick sinus syndrome, bradycardia, hypotension, asthma, stomach ulcers, intestinal or stomach blockage, liver disease, seizures, hyperbilirubinemia, diarrhea, abnormal liver function tests, and jaundice. *Donepezil* is contraindicated with epilepsy, hypersensitivity, atrioventricular heart block, sick sinus syndrome, asthma, sinus bradycardia, bronchi muscle spasm resulting from chronic obstructive pulmonary disease, stomach or intestinal bleeding or ulceration, blockage of the urinary bladder, and lightheadedness. Rivastigmine is contraindicated with hypersensitivity. Galantamine is contraindicated with hypersensitivity, concurrent use of succinylcholine-type and similar neuromuscular blocking agents during anesthesia, supraventricular cardiac conduction disorders, use of drugs that slow the heart rate, high risk of gastrointestinal ulcers, concurrent use of nonsteroidal antiinflammatory drugs, and history of severe asthma or obstructive pulmonary disease.

Adverse effects

Tacrine causes extreme nausea, vomiting, and diarrhea, making it unlikely to be chosen over the newer, safer options. Donepezil is best taken with food to minimize GI adverse effects. During the first few weeks of administration, donepezil may cause agitation. Other adverse effects include generalized pain, dizziness, headache, fatigue, nausea, vomiting, diarrhea, loss of appetite, muscle cramps, insomnia, weight loss, joint pain, and increased urination. Rivastigmine is best administered with food to minimize GI adverse effects. Adverse effects include nausea, vomiting, anorexia, dizziness, asthenia, dyspepsia, diarrhea, weight loss, abdominal pain, fatigue, insomnia, and tremors. Adverse effects of galantamine include nausea, vomiting, anorexia, diarrhea, weight decrease, fatigue, dizziness, headache, abdominal pain, depression, insomnia, and urinary tract infections.

Toxicities

Tacrine is highly toxic to the liver; periodic liver function testing is required. It has caused fatty liver degeneration, impaired liver function tests, changes in blood cell counts, and hepatocellular necrosis. Donepezil has induced minor hepatotoxicity in a small number of patients. The transdermal form of rivastigmine caused mild hepatoxicity in one or more patients, resulting in mild jaundice. Galantamine has caused isolated cases of elevated liver enzymes and hepatitis.

You should remember

Acetylcholinesterase inhibitors boost the acetylcholine available to nerve cells by preventing it from breaking down in the brain. These medications cannot reverse AD or stop the destruction of nerve cells. Over time, they lose effectiveness because less viable brain cells are present, and the production of acetylcholine continually drops as the disease progresses.

N-methyl-*D*-aspartate receptor modulators

Other drugs used for AD include the NMDA receptor modulator called memantine (Namenda), vitamin E, antidepressants, anxiolytics, and antipsychotic agents. Memantine is a receptor modulator that appears to slow the disease's progression. Other substances being studied for AD include NSAIDs, Ginkgo biloba extracts, and statins. Memantine is the only FDA-approved NMDA antagonist (see Table 14.5).

Pharmacokinetics

Memantine interferes with the metabolism of the neurotransmitters dopamine, norepinephrine, and serotonin while modulating synaptic transmission. It reduces membrane resistance and membrane conductance of sodium, potassium, and chloride ions, so this medication may be directly involved in generating action potentials.

TABLE 14.5 Drug therapy for dementia.

Generic name	Trade name
Cholinesterase inhibitors	
donepezil	Aricept
galantamine	Razadyne, Razadyne ER
rivastigmine	Exelon
NMDA antagonist	
memantine	Namenda, Namenda XR

NMDA, *N*-methyl-*D*-aspartate.

Mechanism of action

Memantine blocks the excitatory neurotransmitter glutamate's effects in the brain, which is implicated in everyday learning and memory. As glutamine binds to NMDA receptors, calcium moves into nerve cells, allowing them to communicate and process information. With AD, glutamate is likely available in excessive amounts, and enormous levels of calcium move into the nerve cells, resulting in cell death from toxicity. Memantine safely reduces the effects of glutamate without completely blocking glutamate binding. It is available as 5-mg and 10-mg oral tablets in 2 mg per mL oral solution. Initial dosing is 5 mg once per day, titrated in 1-week intervals to 5 mg twice daily, then 10 mg in the morning and 5 mg in the evening, to the target dose of 10 mg twice daily. A dose of 5 mg twice daily is recommended if there is renal impairment and a creatinine clearance of less than 30 mL per minute. Memantine can be used along with acetylcholinesterase inhibitors (with careful monitoring) because of its different mechanism of action. Memantine also does not cure AD but helps to manage some symptoms.

Clinical indications

Memantine is indicated for treating moderate to severe dementia of the Alzheimer type. It is used to slow the neurotoxicity believed to be involved in AD and other neurodegenerative diseases. It is classified as an NMDA receptor antagonist.

Contraindications

Memantine is contraindicated in patients with known hypersensitivity to the drug or any excipients used in the formulation. The patient must alert the physician if there has ever been an allergic reaction to the drug or other medicines, epilepsy, heart attack, heart failure, hypertension, and kidney or liver problems.

Adverse effects

Adverse effects of memantine include dizziness, nausea, vomiting, diarrhea, headache, weight loss, sleep changes, bradycardia, confusion, excitement, talkativeness, and hyperactivity. Less common adverse effects include coughing, fatigue, and dyspnea. Memantine appears to have no significant toxicities.

You should remember

Most patients start seeing some improvement in the first few weeks after beginning memantine, though it may take a few months for complete effects to occur. The less severe the symptoms, the sooner that improvement occurs. The medication has been shown to improve memory temporarily.

Aducanumab

Aducanumab (Aduhelm) is an amyloid beta-directed antibody. It is indicated to treat AD and is approved under the accelerated approval pathway. This gives patients earlier access to the drug when there are expected clinical benefits but not proven clinical benefits. Accelerated approval is based on how the medication affects a surrogate endpoint, which reflects the drug's effect on an essential aspect of the disease. The drug's development is not yet established to predict a particular clinical benefit. With aducanumab, the surrogate endpoint is the reduction of amyloid beta plaque. Clinical benefits must still be verified in a postapproval trial. If the manufacturer (Biogen) cannot prove this, the FDA could withdraw the drug's accelerated approval.

Aducanumab is the first therapy that targets the underlying disease process of AD and not only the symptoms. The drug showed significant dose- and time-dependent reduction of amyloid beta plaque in the clinical trials. Levels of plaque were determined by using positron emission tomography imaging in brain regions expected to be widely affected by AD pathology. Prescribing information for the medication includes a warning for amyloid-related imaging abnormalities, which usually involve temporary swelling in some areas of the brain that generally resolves over time. There are usually no symptoms, but some people have developed headaches, confusion, dizziness, vision changes, and nausea. Another warning is for a risk of hypersensitivity reactions, including angioedema and urticaria. The most common adverse effects included falling, diarrhea, delirium, altered mental status, and disorientation.

You should remember

Recent studies have shown that some antihypertensive medications, especially diuretics, are linked to reduced neuropathology and other degenerative processes of AD. These drugs reduce the TAR DNA-binding protein 43 by 40%, Lewy bodies by 22%, and the neuropathology of AD by 18%. These findings were presented at the 2021 Annual Meeting of the American Neurological Association.

You should remember

In January 2023, the FDA approved a second amyloid beta-directed antibody for treating Alzheimer. *Lecanemab-irmb (Leqembi),* like Aducanumab, was also supported through the Accelerated Approval pathway. Phase 3 test results showed that the drug is highly clinically beneficial. Patients receiving it have significant dose- and time-dependent reduction of amyloid beta plaques. The drug is given every 2 weeks.

Key Terms

Achalasia
Anhidrosis
Asthenia
Child-Pugh liver impairment
Diaphoresis
Dyskinesias
Melanoma
Narrow-angle glaucoma
On-off phenomenon
Pallidotomy
Parkinson disease
Pill-rolling motions
Toxic megacolon
Xerostomia

Clinical Case Studies

Clinical Case Study 1

A 79-year-old female was diagnosed with PD 9 years ago. Recently, her balance, gait, and strength have decreased dramatically. She was hospitalized for monitoring, and her medications were adjusted as needed. The patient was then transferred to a rehabilitation facility, where she stayed for several weeks, followed by 4 weeks of physical therapy. Today, she starts her outpatient physical therapy. The patient has also battled with depression because of her PD. She lives with her 86-year-old husband in a house with no staircases and regularly uses a cane, walker, and protective devices in her bathroom to keep from falling. She has begun having difficulty standing up from a sitting position, controlling utensils while eating, and getting dressed or undressed.

Critical Thinking Questions

1. What are the four primary signs of PD?
2. What are the two primary types of medications for PD?
3. Which type of drugs for PD should be avoided in people older than age 70?

Clinical Case Study 2

A 62-year-old male was diagnosed with middle-stage PD. He has extreme gait difficulties, increased stiffness, reduced range of motion, resting tremors, cogwheel rigidity, and coordination difficulties. Even with all these problems, the patient sometimes goes out dancing with his wife, something they have always enjoyed and don't want to lose. The patient is having a supervised training problem and performs daily home exercises. These efforts have improved his balance and gait. His current medications include carbidopa-levodopa and trihexyphenidyl.

Critical Thinking Questions

1. What are the drug classifications of carbidopa-levodopa and trihexyphenidyl?
2. What is the on-off phenomenon of PD?
3. Are there any contraindications with trihexyphenidyl?

Further Reading

[1] J.E. Ahlskog, The New Parkinson's Disease Treatment Book: Partnering to Get the Most from Your Medications, second ed., Oxford University Press, 2015.
[2] J.E. Ahlskog, Parkinson's Disease Treatment Guide for Physicians, Oxford University Press, 2009.
[3] B. Alexander, Understanding and Treating Parkinson's Disease: The Beginners Guide on Parkinson's Disease Treatment Management and Strategies for Surviving with Parkinson's Disease and Other Disease, Alexander, 2021.
[4] K. Bhatia, K.R. Chaudhuri, M. Stamelou, International Review of Neurobiology – Parkinson's Disease, vol. 132, Academic Press, 2017.
[5] M.J. Edwards, M. Stamelou, N. Quinn, K.P. Bhatia, Parkinson's Disease and Other Movement Disorders (Handbooks in Neurology), second ed., Oxford University Press, 2016.
[6] J.P.M. Finberg, M.B.H. Youdim, P. Riederer, K.F. Tipton, MAO – The Mother of All Amine Oxidases (Journal of Neural Transmission – Supplement), Springer, 2003.
[7] R. Griffiths, Parkinson's Disease: An In-depth Metabolic Guide, Griffiths, 2019.
[8] M.O.F. Khan, A.E. Philip, Medicinal Chemistry of Drugs Affecting the Nervous System (For Pharmacy Students), Book 2, Bentham Books, 2020.
[9] G. Leader, L. Leader, L. Findley, Parkinson's Disease: Reducing Symptoms with Nutrition and Drugs, third ed., Denor Press, 2017.
[10] F. Lindop, R. Skelly, Parkinson's Disease: A Multidisciplinary Guide to Management, Elsevier, 2022.
[11] C.R. Martin, V.R. Preedy, Genetics, Neurology, Behavior, and Diet in Parkinson's Disease – the Neuroscience of Parkinson's Disease, vol. 2, Academic Press, 2020.
[12] J.A. Obeso, R. Horowski, C.D. Marsden, Continuous Dopaminergic Stimulation in Parkinson's Disease – Journal of Neural Transmission – Supplementum 27, Springer, 2013.
[13] M.S. Okun, 10 Breakthrough Therapies for Parkinson's Disease, Books4Patients, 2015.
[14] D. Playford, Neurological Rehabilitation of Parkinson's Disease (Queen Square Neurological Rehabilitation Series), CRC Press, 2019.
[15] S.G. Reich, S.A. Factor, Therapy of Movement Disorders – A Case-based Approach – Current Clinical Neurology, Humana Press, 2019.
[16] M. Tiberi, Dopamine Receptor Technologies (Neuromethods, 96), Humana Press, 2015.
[17] J.M. Vine, A Parkinson's Primer: An Indispensable Guide to Parkinson's Disease for Patients and Their Families, Paul Dry Books, 2017.
[18] W.J. Weiner, L.M. Shulman, A.E. Lang, Parkinson's Disease: A Complete Guide for Patients and Families (Press Health Book), third ed., Johns Hopkins University Press, 2013.
[19] D. Zid, J. Russell, OhioHealth, Exercise and Parkinson's Disease ' Delay the Disease – the #1 Parkinson's Exercise Program, OhioHealth, 2017.

CHAPTER

15

Opioid analgesics and antagonists

OUTLINE

LEARNING OUTCOMES

After study of the chapter, readers should be able to:

1. Describe the classifications of pain.
2. Discuss the development of pain.
3. Explain different modal treatments for chronic pain.
4. Describe chronic pain and nociceptive somatic pain.
5. Identify pain processing and substance P.
6. Describe opioid analgesics and their indications.
7. Identify the common adverse effects of opioids.
8. Explain narcotic antagonists and common reactions of naltrexone.
9. Describe the effects of buprenorphine.
10. Explain the potential risks of methadone.

The Science of Pharmacology
https://doi.org/10.1016/B978-0-443-29038-1.00015-4

Overview

Pain is an uncomfortable feeling that indicates something may be wrong in the body. It can be described as steady, throbbing, stabbing, aching, pinching, or by other terms. Sometimes, pain is not intense, like a mild headache, but it can be so severe that it becomes debilitating. Pain is the most common symptom that people see physicians for. Generally, it is classified as acute pain, chronic pain, and the pain of malignancy. It is a vital nervous system function, warning of potential bodily injury. Pain is a sensory and emotional experience affected by psychological factors, including past experiences, beliefs about pain, fear, and anxiety. Opioids are used for many different types of pain. Opioid analgesics are now among the most commonly prescribed medications for patients in the United States. Healthcare professionals must understand appropriate and effective pain management strategies and be able to differentiate between medication management used for pain as opposed to opioid-use disorder.

Classifications of pain

Pain is an "unpleasant sensory and emotional experience associated with or described in terms of actual or potential tissue damage." Pain is a subjective experience. Its signals are transmitted from the peripheral nervous system to the central nervous system, where they are perceived. Often, this experience is affected and modified by environmental, emotional, cultural, spiritual, and cognitive factors.

Acute pain is considered temporary or short-term pain. It is a complex, unpleasant experience with emotional, cognitive, and sensory features that occur in response to tissue trauma. Acute pain occurs immediately after the injury and typically resolves with the healing of the underlying problem.

Chronic pain is a prolonged, painful experience that may or may not be associated with a disease process and is characterized by pain lasting 3 months or longer or beyond the time of healing. Chronic pain can be prolonged by trauma, surgery, cancer, or painful disease processes such as arthritis, **fibromyalgia**, and nerve damage.

Pain can be characterized as nociceptive or neuropathic. **Nociceptive pain** is caused by actual or potential tissue damage to the somatic or visceral anatomy. It is often described as dull, sharp, throbbing, achy, or squeezing. Somatic pain results from injury to skin, joints, bones, muscles, or tendons and is typically well localized. Visceral pain results from distention, stretching, or ischemia of internal organs and is generally not well localized.

Neuropathic pain is caused by dysfunction or nervous system damage. It may be described as squeezing, numbing, tingling, burning, or pricking. Neuropathic pain can be *central* or *peripheral.* Central neuropathic pain results from brain damage, such as a stroke. Peripheral neuropathic pain results from damage to the spinal cord. This type of pain can often be limited to damage to the extremities, such as hands or feet.

Development of pain

Pain is an essential adaptive and protective mechanism of the body. There are several theories about the development of pain, which include the following:

- *Specificity theory*: an injury activates pain receptors and fibers that project to the brain. The intensity of pain is directly related to the amount of tissue injury. This theory is helpful if applied to specific injuries and related acute pain. It is not associated with chronic pain or emotional and cognitive elements contributing to more complex types of pain.
- *Pattern theory* describes the role of impulse intensity and repatterning of the CNS. It does not account for all the different types of pain.
- *Gate control theory* combines features of other pain theories to explain pain perception and modulation. The transmission of pain is regulated by balanced impulses that travel to the spinal cord, where cells of the **substantia gelatinosa** act as a "gate." This spinal gate modulates pain transmission to higher parts of the CNS. Large, myelinated, and small, unmyelinated fibers respond to mechanical, thermal, and chemical stimuli. Nociceptive transmission on fibers opens the spinal gate, increasing pain **perception**. Closure or partial closure of spinal gates may be due to nonnociceptive stimulation, such as the skin's touch sensors. Signals are carried on nonnociceptive larger fibers to decrease pain perception.

- *Neuromatrix theory*: The brain creates patterned nerve impulses from genetic, psychological, and cognitive experiences. Pain can be felt due to insufficient inputs, such as **phantom limb pain**. Stimuli can trigger patterns but not produce them.

Pain processing

The first step in pain processing is **transduction**. A painful stimulus is received by pain receptors near where the cause of the pain occurs. There is a release of chemicals that cause an action potential to be conducted from nerve fibers to the spinal cord. The second step is *transmission,* when the nerve signal reaches the spinal cord. There is a release of excitatory chemicals, including glutamate and substance P, which are involved in slower neurotransmission by the C fibers. Destruction of substance P fibers results in analgesia. The pain signal is then transported to the brain via the ascending spinal cord pathways. Once reaching the brain, it is perceived by the patient in the third step, called perception, which is the conscious awareness of pain impulses.

Various people perceive pain differently, and it can be modified via cognitive and behavioral functions, including relaxation and meditation. The last step is modulation, in which the brain and spinal cord interact to influence the pain intensity. Excitatory chemicals can be released, increasing the amount of perceived pain. Other chemicals, including endogenous opioids (endorphins and enkephalins), norepinephrine, gamma-aminobutyric acid, and serotonin, take effect via the descending nerve pathways to decrease pain intensity. Some medications used for pain management work by reducing excitatory chemicals or increasing inhibitory chemicals in the nervous system.

Chronic pain

More than 100 million Americans suffer from chronic pain, closely representing a third of the US population. The financial impact of chronic pain in the United States is staggering and goes beyond the cost of healthcare utilization. Chronic pain can lead to decreased work productivity, increased "sick days" utilized, and, in some cases, may result in permanent disability. These consequences can cost society 300 billion dollars annually, emphasizing the need for effective treatment of chronic pain and a focus on improving function in these patients.

A significant problem in treating chronic pain is that not all pain is the same. It can be described as nociceptive or neuropathic, somatic or visceral, and central or peripheral. *Nociceptive somatic* chronic pain conditions include degenerative disc disease, muscle pain, nonspecific lower back or neck pain, and **osteoarthritis**. *Nociceptive visceral* chronic pain conditions include angina, **Crohn disease**, pelvic pain, and **irritable bowel syndrome**.

Neuropathic central chronic pain conditions include fibromyalgia, poststroke pain, **multiple sclerosis**, and spinal cord injury. *Neuropathic peripheral* chronic pain conditions include chemotherapy-induced neuropathy, diabetic neuropathy, postherpetic neuralgia (**shingles**), and **radiculopathy**. About three out of every four chronic pain patients also report depression, and 86% have difficulty sleeping. Chronic pain is most prevalent in adults who live in poverty, those who did not finish high school, and people insured through public health programs. Age-adjusted prevalence is much higher in females, the unemployed, and rurally located residents. Non-Hispanic Caucasian adults have a much higher age-adjusted prevalence of chronic pain.

The most common chronic pain condition is persistent low back pain, followed by **myofascial pain syndromes**. In most cases of chronic pain, physical processes help sustain it and may be the primary factor, such as in cancer patients. Chronic pain can cause or worsen psychological problems, including anxiety and depression. It often leads to vegetative signs such as **lassitude**, loss of taste, decreased appetite, weight loss, and reduced **libido**.

Various modal treatments for chronic pain

Different treatments are often needed for chronic pain, including physical medicine/rehabilitation, interventional analgesia, behavioral medicine, and medication management. Early, aggressive treatments can reduce or prevent sensitization and remodeling, stopping acute pain from becoming chronic. A multidisciplinary team is often required. Analgesics include nonsteroidal antiinflammatory drugs and opioid analgesics. Opioids used for chronic pain must be prescribed very carefully, primarily for continuing moderate-to-severe pain that impairs function. The factors that must be considered include the appropriate, conventional treatments, other reasonable treatments, any high risk of opioid-related adverse effects, and whether the patient is at risk of misuse, diversion, or abuse.

Physical medicine/rehabilitation

Physical medicine/rehabilitation includes physical therapy, occupational therapy, chiropractic manipulation, **acupuncture**, heat and cold application, and transcutaneous electrical nerve stimulation (see Fig. 15.1). Physical and occupational therapies involve patient-individualized exercise regimens to improve and restore a normal range of motion, often with passive and active stretching.

Interventional analgesia

Interventional analgesia may refer to spinal injections such as **epidural**, **facet joint**, or **sacroiliac joint** injections, nerve blocks such as medial branch and peripheral nerve blocks, and neural ablation techniques such as radiofrequency ablation (see Fig. 15.1).

Behavioral medicine

Self-management of chronic pain is a crucial skill for all chronic pain patients. Self-care education books can teach this skill but may not be appropriate or effective for all patients. For those unable to gain this skill independently, more intensive behavioral treatment with a psychologist or counselor may be necessary to promote appropriate coping skills. Patients with chronic pain often have multiple behavioral health abnormalities, including sleep disorders, depression, anxiety, and learned maladaptive behaviors such as **kinesophobia**. Therefore psychological interventions such as cognitive behavioral therapy can help improve function, quality of life, and pain score outcomes. Similarly, education by healthcare providers regarding pain processes and treatment methods may help decrease pain.

You should remember

When acute pain transforms into chronic pain, the biological benefit of pain is less appreciated or even worthy of acknowledgment. For example, the case of a traumatic motor vehicle accident is a significant contributor to chronic pain. These accidents can often lead to substantial bone fractures and mechanical rearrangement of muscles, bones, and nerves.

You should remember

Females are more likely to experience chronic pain than males. They are more likely to suffer from chronic pain conditions such as migraine headaches, osteoarthritis, fibromyalgia, chronic fatigue syndrome, and rheumatoid arthritis. Females also suffer from gender-specific chronic pain conditions such as endometriosis.

Classification of opioids

Opioids are classified into three basic types of formulations: *natural*, *semisynthetic/manmade*, and *fully synthetic/manmade*. These are further explained as follows:

- *Natural* (opiates): occurring in plants such as the *opium poppy*, containing base chemical compounds that include nitrogen as a component; examples include codeine, morphine, and thebaine.

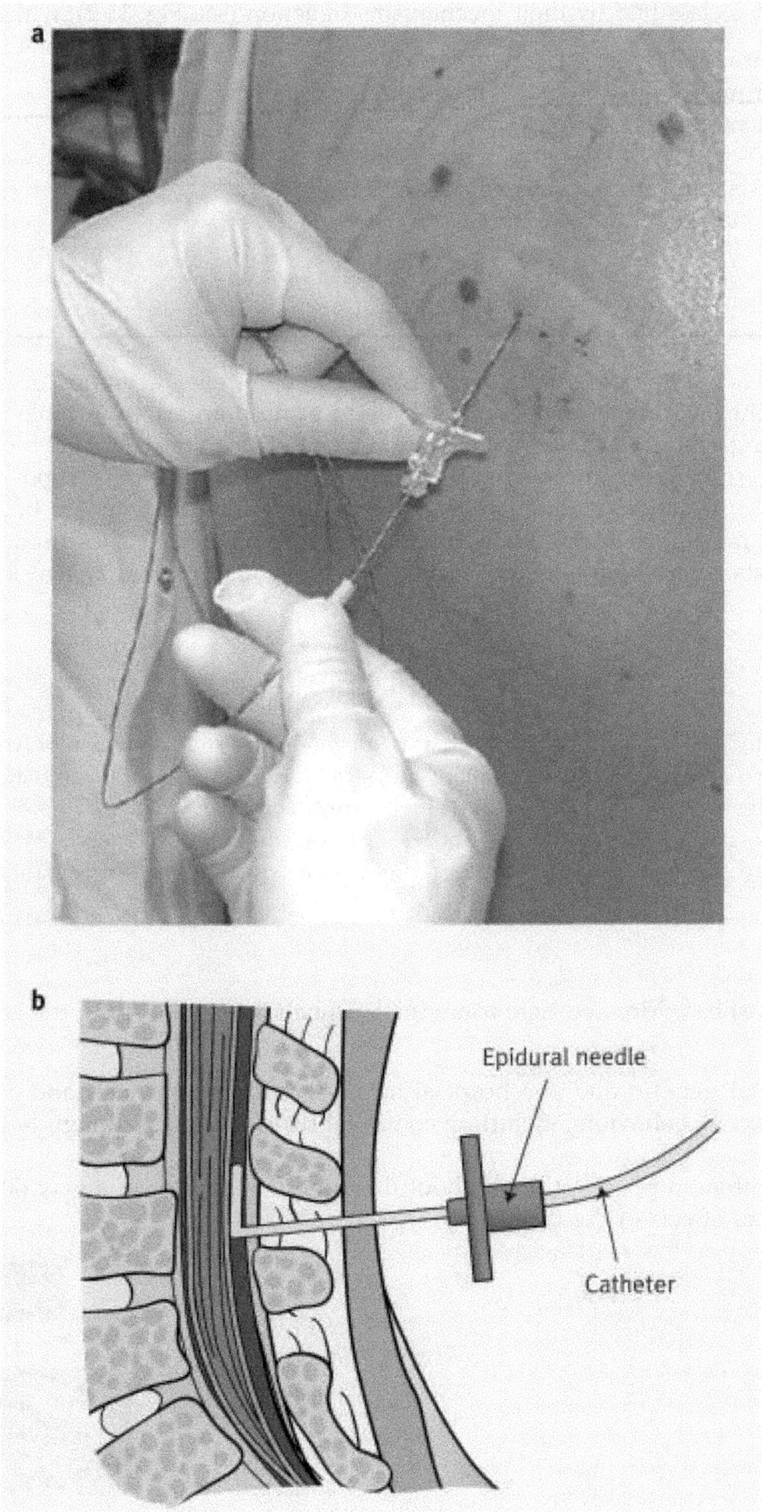

FIG. 15.1 Epidural injection.

- *Semi-synthetic/manmade*: created in laboratories from natural opiates; examples include heroin (made from morphine), hydrocodone, hydromorphone, and oxycodone.
- *Fully synthetic/manmade*: synthesized drugs; examples include dextropropoxyphene, fentanyl, levorphanol, methadone, pethidine, and tramadol.

However, opioids are also classified by their mechanisms of action (see Fig. 15.2), which include the following:

- Agonists, which have three subtypes:
  - Potent: fentanyl, hydromorphone, meperidine, methadone, morphine, sufentanil
  - Moderate: codeine, oxycodone
  - Weak: propoxyphene
- Mixed agonist-antagonists: buprenorphine, nalbuphine
- Antagonists: nalmefene, naloxone, naltrexone

Opioid analgesics

Opioid analgesics directly act upon opioid receptors, resulting in pain relief. Common examples include morphine, hydrocodone, and oxycodone. Various dosing of opioid analgesics are summarized in Table 15.1. Opioids are typically not the first step in managing acute and cancer-related chronic pain. Due to the potential for addiction and abuse and the current opioid crisis, prescribing recommendations for opioids have become more rigid. Opioid analgesics bind to opioid receptors and mimic the actions of endogenous opioids (naturally made by the body). Opioid receptors are divided into three classes: mu (μ), delta (δ), and kappa (κ). Most opioid analgesics used in treatment bind to the μ-opioid receptor as agonists, which results in a reduction of pain signals. Opioid analgesics have many risks.

You should remember

Opioid analgesics include strong medications such as morphine, codeine, oxycodone, hydrocodone, fentanyl, methadone, and many others. The legitimate use of these drugs reduces pain successfully, but they can also cause extreme euphoria or an intense "high," leading to dependence and addiction. Overdose effects include severe respiratory depression that can lead to respiratory arrest, coma, and death. Opioid dependence and withdrawal are signified by nausea, confusion, drowsiness, extreme sweating, and constipation.

Some medical terms must be addressed here to understand better the concept of the adverse effects of opioids. They include:

- **Addiction:** environmental, genetic, and psychosocial factors influence a primary and chronic disease. It is often concurrent with maladaptive behaviors, including continual drug use, even though harm and severe consequences occur.
- **Abuse:** use of a drug without a prescription, without therapeutic intent, or in a way other than prescribed to achieve certain feelings or effects of the drug.

FIG. 15.2 Classification of opioids.

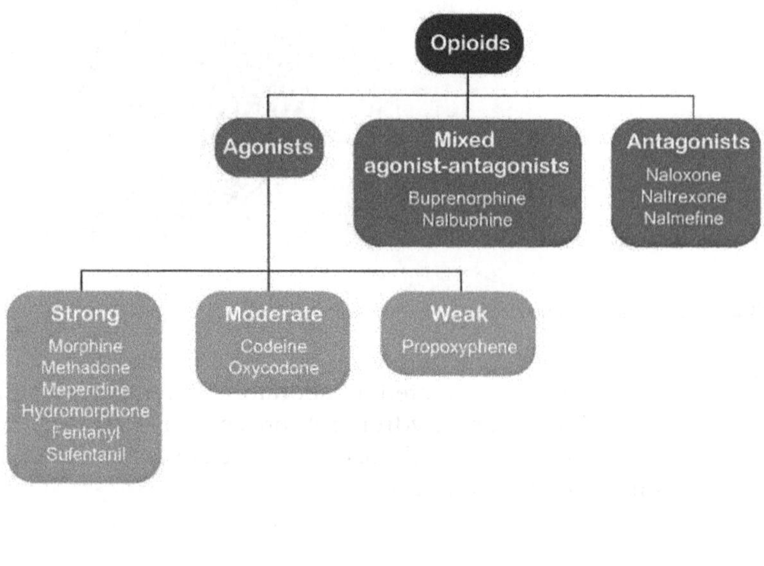

TABLE 15.1 Opioid analgesic dosing

Generic name	Trade name	Average dosage range (mg/day, except as noted)	Dosage form (mg, except as noted)
codeine	(generic only, also in many combination drugs)	15–120	15, 30, 60
fentanyl	Actiq	Micrograms: 200–1600	Micrograms: 200, 400, 600, 800, 1,200, 1600
hydrocodone	Zohydro	10–30	10, 15, 20, 30
meperidine	Demerol	50–1200	50, 100
methadone	Methadose	10–40	5, 10, 40
morphine	Avinza, MS-Contin	30–1600	30, 45, 60, 75, 90, 120
oxycodone	Oxycontin, Oxecta	5–90	5, 7.5
oxymorphone	Opana	5–20	5, 10, 15, 20
tapentadol	Nucynta	50–500	50, 75, 100, 150, 200, 250
tramadol	Ultram	50–400	50, 75, 100, 150, 200, 300, 400

- **Misuse:** involves any drug use outside of prescription goals or self-medication for reasons outside of the intent of the prescription.
- **Diversion:** transfer of a controlled substance, such as an opioid analgesic, from a lawful to an unlawful distribution method.
- **Dependence:** occurs due to chronic drug use, and use must continue to avoid withdrawal symptoms.
- **Opioid withdrawal**: causes diarrhea, restlessness, eye tearing, muscle pain, sweating, tachycardia, and insomnia. It occurs after abrupt cessation of a drug after the body has become physically dependent upon it.
- **Tolerance**: either a need for highly increased amounts of a drug to achieve a desired effect or intoxication or a significantly reduced effect with continual use of the same amount of the drug; tolerance is additionally described as the length of time or pain intensity that can be tolerated before extreme pain responses are initiated. It is influenced by cultural perceptions, expectations, fatigue, gender, physical and mental health, anger, apprehension, role behaviors, boredom, and sleep deprivation; tolerance can be increased by a variety of factors, which include consuming alcohol, regular use of pain medications, hypnosis, distracting activities, solid beliefs or religious faith, and warmth.

Pharmacokinetics

The wide bioavailability range amongst different opioids is partially attributable to differences in first-pass metabolism when the drug is metabolized directly by the liver from the GI tract before it reaches the systemic circulation. Clinicians should be aware of the bioavailability of the opioid being prescribed because it indirectly affects oral-intravenous conversion ratios. Opioids are more likely to distribute faster and more intensely in and out of the blood-brain barrier. They also tend to have a quicker onset and shorter duration of analgesic action. The most critical area of opioid pharmacokinetics is metabolism. The metabolism process may involve the cytochrome (CYP) P450 enzymes, particularly CYP 2D6 and 3A4.

Mechanism of action

Opioids mimic the actions of endogenous opioid peptides by interacting with mu, delta, or kappa opioid receptors. The opioid receptors are coupled to G1 proteins, and the activities of the opioids are mainly inhibitory. Most clinically relevant opioid analgesics bind to mu-opioid receptors in the central and peripheral nervous systems in an agonist manner to elicit analgesia.

Clinical indications

Opioids are used for acute, chronic, cancer-related, postsurgical, and vascular pain. The FDA has also approved the use of opioids as antitussive and antidiarrheal medications. Loperamide, or the over-the-counter medication Imodium, is an opioid used to treat diarrhea and irritable bowel syndrome. It exerts this effect by decreasing intestinal motility and increasing absorption time. Opioids such as codeine and dextromethorphan are useful as cough suppressants. Codeine is considered the standard cough suppressant against which new drugs get tested. Codeine is also a valuable antitussive, as it provides additional benefits of analgesia and sedation. The use of opioids for analgesia is controversial due to the risk of addiction and tolerance.

Contraindications

Opioids are contraindicated in true allergies, severe respiratory depression, acute or chronic bronchial asthma, increased intracranial pressure, acute psychiatric fluctuation, uncontrolled suicide risk, or increased risk of prescription misuse.

Adverse effects

Adverse effects of opioid use include drowsiness, constipation, euphoria, nausea, vomiting, dizziness, and slowed breathing. A person using opioids over time can develop tolerance, physical dependence, and opioid use disorder, with the risk of overdose and death.

Toxicities

Opioid overdose typically causes pinpoint pupils, respiratory depression, and decreased levels of consciousness.

You should remember

Opioids come in several forms and can be administered orally, rectally, topically (transdermal patches), intravenously, in the epidural space, or into the dura. The mode of administration and duration of action depend on the opioid's lipophilicity and hydrophilicity. For example, codeine can be administered via oral, intramuscular, and rectal routes. In most adults, oral codeine absorbs rapidly and reaches a peak concentration within 1 hour.

You should remember

Multiple label warnings are required, most notably a risk of serious, life-threatening, or fatal respiratory depression. There is a warning to avoid combined use of opioids with benzodiazepines or other CNS depressants such as alcohol because these combinations can lead to further sedation, respiratory depression, coma, and death. The warnings also discuss the potential risk of addiction, abuse, and misuse.

You should remember

Babies exposed to opiates during pregnancy are at risk for low birth weight, behavioral problems, developmental delays, learning disabilities, congenital disabilities, and stillbirth.

Narcotic antagonists

Opioid receptor antagonists block one or more opioid receptors in the central or peripheral nervous system. Opioid receptors are specific transmembrane neurotransmitter receptors that couple **G-proteins**, which, upon stimulation by endogenous or exogenous opioids, lead to the intracellular signal transduction process. The two most commonly used centrally acting opioid receptor antagonists are naloxone and naltrexone. The opioid receptor antagonists include methylnaltrexone, nalbuphine, nalmefene, nalorphine, naloxone, naltrexone, and nalorphine. Narcotic antagonists such as naloxone (Narcan), naltrexone, and nalmefene are commonly prescribed. They are designed to reverse opioid overdose rapidly.

Pharmacokinetics

Opioid receptor antagonists block one or more opioid receptors in the central or peripheral nervous system, stimulating central mu receptors that cause respiratory depression, analgesia, and euphoria.

Mechanism of action

The opioid antagonist binds to opioid receptors and can change and block the effects of other opioids such as heroin, morphine, and oxycodone.

Clinical indications

Narcotic antagonists have clinical applications in diagnosing addiction, prophylactic treatment of narcotic abuse, and emergency treatment of narcotic overdosage. They are used to help reduce cravings for the opioid analgesic that is being abused. Narcotic antagonists also decrease the risks of continuing opioid abuse and opioid overdose.

Contraindications

Opioid antagonists are contraindicated in patients with liver disease. Possible side effects of opioid antagonists include increased anxiety and gastrointestinal problems such as abdominal cramps, nausea, vomiting, and constipation.

Adverse effects

Adverse drug reactions of opioid analgesics include respiratory depression, itching, increased sphincter tone (biliary spasm, urinary retention), inability to concentrate, sedation, mood changes (dysphoria or euphoria), constipation, nausea, vomiting, tolerance, addiction, and dependence.

Toxicities

Opioid toxicity should be suspected when the clinical triad of CNS depression, respiratory depression, and pupillary miosis is present; respiratory depression is the most specific sign of opioid toxicity.

Opioid-use disorder pharmacotherapy

Opioid-use disorder pharmacotherapy is often referred to as medication-assisted treatment. The medications used in medication-assisted treatment can help reduce cravings for opioid abuse, decrease the risk of continued opioid abuse, and decrease the risk of opioid overdose. The 2016 American Society of Addiction Medicine Guideline recommends a choice between methadone and buprenorphine/naloxone as a patient and provider-specific choice as the first-line treatment and to use naltrexone cautiously after stopping opioid use.

Buprenorphine products

Buprenorphine (Buprenex) is used for opioid detoxification, opioid maintenance, and pain management. It is also used for acute, chronic, and opioid dependence. It is an agonist substitution treatment agent that treats addiction by using a substance (such as buprenorphine or methadone) to substitute for a more potent full-agonist opioid (such as heroin). Buprenorphine is a partial opioid receptor agonist that detoxifies and maintains opioid tolerance. It is combined with *naloxone* in products such as *Suboxone*. The naloxone is orally inactive, but if snorted or injected, it acts as an opioid antagonist and reverses the effects of buprenorphine, limiting euphoria and risks of an overdose. There are also transdermal implant and intramuscular injection forms of buprenorphine. The most common adverse drug reactions of buprenorphine products are related to opioid agonist activity, including CNS depression, orthostatic hypotension, and respiratory depression. Buprenorphine can also cause liver impairment.

Methadone

Methadone is a long-acting opioid receptor agonist that may be used to detoxify or maintain opioid tolerance. It is illegal to dispense from community pharmacies to treat opioid-use disorders. It can be prescribed from these pharmacies for pain management, limiting potential diversion. Potential risks of methadone include serious arrhythmias, but this mainly occurs with large, multiple daily doses. The drug can also cause respiratory depression, so proper dosing and titration are required. The medication should only be prescribed by providers experienced in methadone for detoxification and maintenance treatment of opioid addiction.

Most cases involve patients being treated for pain with large, multiple daily doses of methadone. However, cases have been reported in patients receiving doses commonly used for maintenance treatment of opioid addiction. Additionally, like other opioid agonists, methadone can cause respiratory depression, which is more likely during the initiation and conversion of patients to methadone and even when the drug has been used as recommended and not misused or abused.[61] Proper dosing and titration are essential, and methadone should only be prescribed by healthcare professionals knowledgeable in the use of methadone for detoxification and maintenance treatment of opioid addiction.

Naltrexone

Naltrexone is a competitive opioid antagonist. It blocks the ability of opioids to take effect. It does not maintain opioid tolerance, so patients are at a higher risk of overdose and death if they stop naltrexone and start retaking opioids. Common reactions include anxiety, nausea, dizziness, headaches, and sleep disturbances. There is a risk of liver damage and increased liver function test results. The drug causes opioid withdrawal if the patient is still taking opioids. The patient must be clear of opioids before starting naltrexone. The preferred dosage form is an intramuscular injection given once per month by a healthcare provider.

You should remember

Naloxone and naltrexone are both opioid blockers. But naloxone is a fast-acting medication that reverses the effects of an opioid overdose and is available over the counter. Naltrexone does not work in overdose situations. It is a once-daily or once-monthly medication that can treat alcohol use disorder or opioid use disorder.

Key Terms

Acupuncture
Acute pain
Chronic pain
Crohn disease
Epidural
Facet joint
Fibromyalgia
G-proteins
Irritable bowel syndrome
kinesiophobia
Lassitude
Libido
Modulation
Multiple sclerosis
Myofascial pain syndromes
Nociceptive pain
Opioid crisis
Osteoarthritis
Perception
Phantom limb pain
Radiculopathy
Sacroiliac joint
Shingles
Somatic pain
Substantia gelatinosa
Transduction
Visceral pain

Clinical Case Studies

Clinical Case Study 1

An 81-year-old female who lived in an assisted living community had recently experienced a fall but was not severely injured. She admitted to drinking wine in the evening nearly every day, often staying up most of the night watching television as she did this. The female usually slept through much of the daytime. The community's medication technician did not know about her wine consumption but reported to the community's medical facility that the patient was taking 15 different prescription medications concurrently. These included drugs for hypertension, edema, thyroid replacement therapy, asthma, gastroesophageal reflux disease, urinary incontinence, depression, insomnia, and chronic pain caused by osteoarthritis. The patient was evaluated because four of her medications (bupropion, quetiapine, trazodone, and tramadol) can interact with alcohol, increasing CNS depression and the likelihood of falling. The patient was educated about the risks of mixing alcohol with her medications. She voluntarily agreed to enter an alcohol-use disorder treatment program.

Critical Thinking Questions

1. What is the chronic pain of osteoarthritis classified as, regarding the type of chronic pain condition?
2. Is there a link between chronic pain and depression?
3. What are the dangers of using opioid analgesics with alcohol?

Clinical Case Study 2

A 48-year-old male had been involved in a motorcycle accident with multiple organ damage and bone fractures. Before the accident, he had been diagnosed with hypertension, chronic lower back pain due to spinal stenosis, anxiety, and depression. He had also undergone a laminectomy procedure of his L4 and L5 spinal regions. The patient has a history of prescription drug abuse, using oxycodone after his back surgery. He has been on buprenorphine/naloxone for the past 6 months. As he recovered from the acute trauma, the medication was stopped. Fentanyl was administered as a continuous infusion instead, with dose escalation to treat the patient's acute pain and need for sedation. The patient was eventually slowly weaned off the opioids. Finally, the suboxone was restarted. Nonopioid adjuvants were considered required, and after discharge, the patient started an addiction treatment program.

Critical Thinking Questions

1. What is the most common chronic pain condition?
2. When an opioid analgesic such as oxycodone is prescribed, what factors must be considered?
3. What are the indications for buprenorphine/naloxone?

Further Reading

[1] P. Almela Rojo, Opioids: From Analgesic Use to Addiction, Intechopen, 2020.
[2] J.K. Aronson, Meyler's Side Effects of Analgesics and Anti-inflammatory Drugs, Elsevier Science, 2009.
[3] J.C. Ballantyne, D.J. Tauben, Expert Decision Making on Opioid Treatment, Oxford University Press, 2013.
[4] R.A. Cruiciani, H. Knotkova, Handbook of Methadone Prescribing and Buprenorphine Therapy, Springer, 2013.
[5] T.R. Deer, M.S. Leong, A. Buvanendran, V. Gordin, P.S. Kim, S.J. Panchal, et al., Comprehensive Treatment of Chronic Pain by Medical, Interventional, and Integrative Approaches, Springer, 2013.
[6] E. Freye, J.V. Levy, Opioids in Medicine – A Comprehensive Review on the Mode of Action and the Use of Analgesics in Different Pain States, Springer, 2008.
[7] A. Javaherian, P. Latifpour, Acetaminophen: Properties, Clinical Uses and Adverse Effects, Nova Biomedical, 2012.
[8] S. Kaplan, A Comprehensive Guide to Non-steroidal Anti-inflammatory Drugs, Nova Biomedical, 2015.
[9] D. Lussier, P. Beaulieu, Adjuvant Analgesics (American Pain Library), Oxford University Press, 2015.
[10] P.E. Macintyre, S.A. Schug, Acute Pain Management – A Practical Guide, fifth ed., CRC Press, 2021.
[11] J.L. Murphy, S. Rafie, Chronic Pain and Opioid Management: Strategies for Integrated Treatment, American Psychological Association, 2019.
[12] M.J. Parnham, Non-Opioid Analgesics in the Treatment of Acute Pain, Springer/Birkhauser, 2012.
[13] R.S. Sinatra, J.S. Jahr, J.M. Watkins-Pitchford, The Essence of Analgesia and Analgesics, Cambridge University Press, 2010.
[14] V.B. Stolberg, Painkillers: History, Science, and Issues (The Story of a Drug), Greenwood, 2016.
[15] U.S. Department of Health and Services, Substance Abuse and MENT Administration, Medications for Opioid Use Disorder – for Healthcare and Addiction Professionals, Policymakers, Patients, and Families, 2020. Lulu.com.
[16] S.E. Wakeman, J.D. Rich, Treating Opioid Use Disorder in General Medical Settings, Springer, 2021.

CHAPTER

16

Substance use disorders

OUTLINE

LEARNING OUTCOMES

After study of this chapter, readers should be able to:

1. Define addiction.
2. Identify commonly abused drugs in the United States.
3. List five substances that cause relaxation or sedation.
4. Identify the medication used to lessen opioid withdrawal.
5. Discuss the most psychoactive agent found in cannabinoids.
6. Identify the prototype hallucinogen and how it is used.
7. Explain the signs that a substance abuse problem is present.
8. Describe what withdrawal from nicotine causes.
9. Explain the physical effects of alcoholism.
10. Discuss signs and symptoms of withdrawal from alcohol.

The Science of Pharmacology
https://doi.org/10.1016/B978-0-443-29038-1.00016-6

Overview

Substance abuse is a pervasive human problem, magnified by negative perceptions that affect individuals with antidepressants or atypical antipsychotics and show them aas "weak" or lacking moral character. However, data show that addiction is a brain disease that controls behaviors. Addiction is a severe medical condition, perhaps the most serious health problem facing humans worldwide. Approximately $532 billion is spent annually on addiction-related costs in the United States alone. In 2019, there were 21.6 drug-related deaths per 100,000 population and 28.5 alcohol-related deaths per 100,000 in the United States. Substance abuse affects people of all ages to varying degrees. For instance, babies born to drug- or alcohol-addicted mothers are often born prematurely, are underweight, or both. Affected adolescents do poorly in school, have more unplanned pregnancies, and have a greater incidence of disease and violence. Addicted adults often have poor home environments; suffer job loss, financial problems, and preventable accidents; and have low self-esteem. Substance abuse therefore is a serious concern that requires better monitoring and more novel treatments.

Substance abuse

Substance abuse affects every aspect of a person's life and becomes a problem when an individual experiences significant distress in life and when any of the following things occur:

1. Failure to fulfill parenting, school, or work obligations
2. Hazardous behaviors, such as driving under the influence
3. Recurrent legal problems related to dangerous behaviors
4. Continued use of substances despite continuing social or interpersonal problems

People are considered *substance dependent* when they exhibit tolerance, fewer social activities, a desire to quit, and **withdrawal**. A substance abuse disorder includes substance abuse and dependence, which are pharmacokinetic properties and withdrawal. Addiction, in contrast, is the progressive, chronic abuse of a substance despite severe health and social consequences, so poor and dangerous choices may occur. It depends on various factors, based on the drug or drugs used. These factors include availability, cost, dose, and method of administration. Other factors that influence addiction include drug experience, risk-taking behaviors, diseases requiring the use of scheduled drugs, educational opportunities, and peer influences. Sedatives and hypnotics promote relaxation in small doses but can induce sleep and confusion when used in higher doses. Very high amounts can result in coma and even death. Any combination of these agents can be lethal due to their **additive effect**.

You should remember

Withdrawal syndrome is the unpleasant symptoms experienced when a person with physical dependence discontinues using an abused drug. It is also known as "discontinuation syndrome." It is not proof of addiction but suggests drug misuse or excessive use.

Substance misuse

Substance misuse is often challenging to identify. Patients should be screened for the hazardous use of substances, actual substance abuse, and substance dependence. Substance use disorders usually are involved in cases of mental illness and domestic violence. Prescription opioids are commonly misused and may include taking these drugs in larger doses than prescribed, taking another person's prescription drugs, or simply taking drugs to experience euphoria or pleasant effects, and not for therapeutic reasons.

Addictive drugs

Some drugs that are abused may be addictive. These drugs cause intense cravings, making them difficult to use. According to the Drug Enforcement Administration (DEA), the most commonly abused substances include alcohol, tobacco, marijuana, cocaine, psychoactive "club drugs," hallucinogens, heroin, methamphetamine, opioids, sedatives, synthetic **cannabinoids**, and anabolic steroids. Addictive drugs include cannabinoids, depressant medications, dissociative anesthetics, hallucinogen substances, opioids and morphine derivatives, stimulant drugs, and anabolic steroids. Misuse of prescription drugs occurs more often than the combined use of all street drugs except marijuana. About 11.7% of Americans age 12 or older depend on drugs or alcohol. The use of two or more different abused substances is called polysubstance abuse.

Central nervous system depressants

Central nervous system (CNS) depressants cause relaxation or sedation and include barbiturates, benzodiazepines, nonbarbiturate hypnotics, opioids, and gamma-hydroxybutyrate (GHB). The CNS depressants approved for medical use are controlled drugs because of their abuse potential.

Barbiturates and nonbarbiturate sedative-hypnotics

There are two major types of sedative drugs, which include barbiturates and nonbarbiturate sedative-hypnotics. They are used for sleep disorders and some types of epilepsy. Those addicted often switch between these drugs and amphetamines to control their wakefulness and sleep patterns. Some sedatives last an entire day, with higher doses causing similar effects to alcohol intoxication. Overdoses are dangerous, potentially causing respiratory arrest, coma, and death. Barbiturates were responsible for the deaths of entertainers such as Marilyn Monroe, Judy Garland, and Jimi Hendrix. Sedative-hypnotic drugs are discussed in more detail in Chapter 9.

Benzodiazepines

Benzodiazepines are CNS depressants that are widely prescribed and have replaced mainly barbiturates for various conditions due to their higher safety margin. They are usually used for anxiety but also for muscle relaxation and to prevent seizures. Their potential for abuse is high. Benzodiazepines may cause individuals to appear remote from others, lightheaded, disoriented, or sleepy. Withdrawal is not as severe compared with withdrawal from barbiturates or alcohol. However, benzodiazepines remain in circulation for several weeks because, as a class, they have a mean half-life of about 12–40 hours, making abuse extremely dangerous. Benzodiazepines are also discussed in more detail in Chapter 9.

Opioids

Opioids and opiates are taken for severe pain, diarrhea, and persistent cough and are commonly referred to as *narcotics*. Opiates include codeine, morphine, and opium. Synthetic forms, or opioids, include fentanyl, meperidine, methadone, oxycodone, and illegal drugs such as heroin. Injected heroin causes a euphoric rush, intense sedation, and abnormally slow body functions. Overdose is hazardous and potentially fatal. Famous deaths from heroin have included singer Janis Joplin (who also had been drinking alcohol excessively) and actor Philip Seymour Hoffman, who died from a toxic mixture of heroin, cocaine, amphetamines, and benzodiazepines. Approximately 50,000 people die every year in the United States from opioid overdoses. Opioid addiction can develop rapidly, and withdrawal is very unpleasant. Methadone and buprenorphine are often used to treat patients with addiction to opioids because both stop withdrawal while avoiding the same degree of euphoria. They are also longer lasting than abusable opioids. Opioids are discussed in more detail in Chapter 15.

You should remember

Fentanyl is an opioid 100 times more potent than morphine. In the fiscal year 2021, US Customs and Border Protection seized 10,586 lbs of the drug at the Mexican border. This figure was much higher than the total held in 2020 (4558 lbs) or 2019 (2633 lbs). There are enough doses of fentanyl in the United States to kill more than 222 million people.

Gamma-hydroxybutyrate

GHB is a CNS depressant. It is famous as a club or party drug of abuse. It has often been put into someone's alcoholic beverage without their knowledge, resulting in euphoria, increased sex drive, or tranquility. Adverse effects include sweating, loss of consciousness, nausea, hallucinations, **amnesia**, and coma. GHB is available in odorless, colorless, and tasteless liquid or powder forms. It has anabolic effects, aiding in fat reduction and muscle building. Therefore those in the physique community use this drug to induce surges in growth hormones when they are asleep under the influence of GHB. The prescription formulation of GHB, Xyrem, was approved by the FDA in 2002 to treat narcolepsy and is a Schedule III controlled substance. The legitimate use of this drug requires patient enrollment in a restricted-access program to receive the drug.

Inhalants

Inhalants are volatile substances that quickly reach the brain without losing their potency. They include aerosol propellants found in spray paint cans, hairspray, and computer keyboard cleaners; gases such as nitrous oxide; nitrates such as amyl nitrate "poppers"; and volatile solvents such as gasoline or paint thinner. Most solvent abuse occurs in adolescents. When an inhalant is insufflated from a container or bagged (sprayed into and huffed from a plastic bag), the effects resemble those of alcohol, including staggering and slurred speech. If used heavily, inhalants can cause physical dependence. Withdrawal from inhalants can be life-threatening. Long-term use can cause brain, liver, and kidney damage; vision and hearing loss; and heart failure. Finally, *sudden sniffing death* has killed first-time users, mostly when they inhale aerosol propellants, methane, or propane. This is characterized by cardiac arrest upon an initial inhalation, and it cannot be predicted.

Cannabinoids

Cannabinoids are obtained from the hemp plant (*Cannabis sativa*) and are usually smoked to get their effects. Examples of cannabinoids include marijuana, hashish, and hash oil. The most psychoactive agent contained in these drugs is delta-9-tetrahydrocannabinol (THC). There are also synthetic cannabinoids and **designer drugs** that have been chemically altered to avoid federal regulatory laws. Synthetic cannabis is sold as *Spice* and *K2*. It binds to the same receptors in the brain that actual cannabinoids bind to, with potentially more dangerous outcomes that include psychosis, paranoia, and hallucinations.

Marijuana

Marijuana is a natural substance and the most commonly used illicit drug in the United States. It is regularly referred to as "weed," "pot," "grass," "dope," or "reefer." The effects of marijuana include decreased coordination and motor activity, confusion, euphoria, paranoia, increased thirst and hunger, and bloodshot eyes. Results occur in a few minutes and last for up to 24 hours. Marijuana smoke is usually inhaled more deeply than cigarette smoke, introducing four times the amount of tar particulates into the lungs. Daily use increases the risk of lung cancer and respiratory conditions, resulting in a lack of motivation. Marijuana produces little physical dependence or tolerance, with nearly nonexistent withdrawal symptoms. The metabolites of THC remain in the body for many months (or years, depending on usage), so tests can easily show that a person has been using marijuana or has quit before the tests. Also, THC is detectable in the urine for several days after using marijuana.

Medical marijuana treats many diseases as long as each patient meets specific requirements. Conditions treated with medical marijuana include Alzheimer disease, **amyotrophic lateral sclerosis**, cancer, **Crohn disease**, epilepsy, glaucoma, human immunodeficiency virus (HIV)/AIDS, **multiple sclerosis**, muscle spasms, seizures, severe and chronic pain, and severe nausea. As of November 2021, the United States has changed dramatically in its state-by-state attitudes about the use of marijuana. Fig. 16.1 shows the states that have fully legalized the use of marijuana or approved its medical use and decriminalized its possession. Even so, marijuana is still federally classified as a Schedule I drug.

You should remember

Marijuana is currently allowed for medical use in 39 states and the District of Columbia, Puerto Rico, and Guam. State penalties for the service, possession, and cultivation of marijuana have been decriminalized for patients with written documentation from a physician that their health may benefit from its medical use. The amount of THC contained varies widely based on the type of marijuana harvested and the methods used. Marijuana is generally more potent today than in earlier decades.

You should remember

Marijuana appears to increase the risk of cardiovascular disease. Adults who are addicted to marijuana are at a 60% higher risk of having their first heart attack, stroke, or another major cardiovascular event compared with people without cannabis use disorder. Chronic addiction to marijuana may cause a 20% increased occurrence of psychosis.

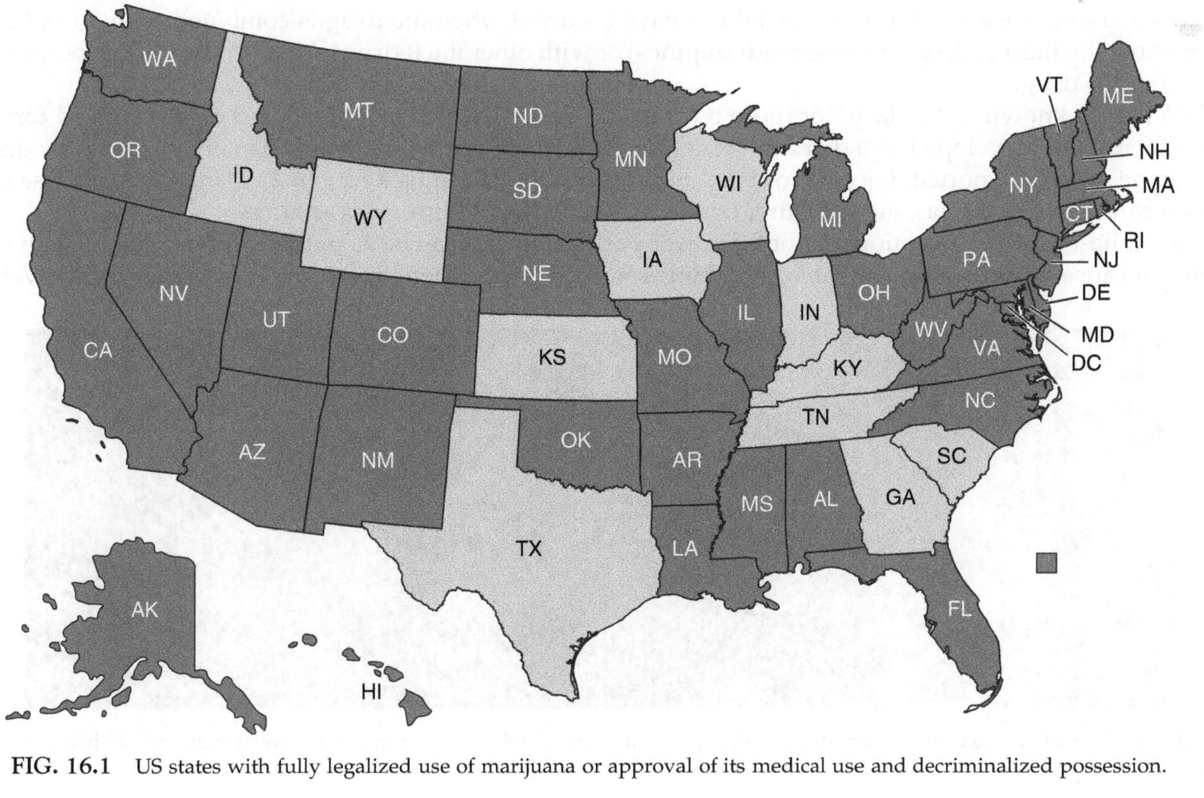

FIG. 16.1 US states with fully legalized use of marijuana or approval of its medical use and decriminalized possession.

Hallucinogens

Hallucinogens are incredibly diverse but produce similar effects, including altered consciousness, which may appear "dreamlike." All hallucinogens are Schedule I drugs with no approved medical use. The prototype hallucinogen is lysergic acid diethylamide (LSD).

LSD

LSD has widely variable effects based on the user's mood, expectations, and environment. Repeated use may cause entirely different results. Generally, common effects include laughter, hallucinations or "visions," deep personal insight, afterimages (trailing images of objects or people as they move), or religious "revelations." Colors, lights, sounds, and other sensations are often greatly intensified. Hallucinogens also have the potential to bring about terrifying experiences, including anxiety, confusion, panic attacks, paranoia, and severe depression. Commonly referred to as "acid," LSD was derived from a fungus growing on the grain known as *rye*. It can also be obtained from fungal growths on other grains. The drug is usually used orally as a liquid, capsule, or tablet. It is often placed in droplet form onto paper containing cartoon images related to the drug culture. After drying, the user ingests a piece of drug-treated paper to experience the drug's effects. There is immediate distribution throughout the body, with results usually beginning within 1 hour. The products may last up to 12 hours, increasing blood pressure and heart rate, raising body temperature, and dilating the pupils. Repeated use may lead to impaired memory, reasoning ability, and psychoses. Flashbacks sometimes occur when the drug's effects reoccur without further administration. Tolerance may occur, but little or no dependence has been seen.

Other hallucinogens

Other hallucinogens with similar effects to LSD include ketamine, methylenedioxymethamphetamine (MDMA), flakka, mephedrone, methylenedioxyamphetamine (MDA), mescaline, psilocybin, and phencyclidine (PCP). These are summarized as follows:

- Ketamine (also known as "special K," or "cat valium") is legally used as a dissociative anesthetic, but it also produces unconsciousness and amnesia. This drug is primarily lawfully used by veterinarians; the incidence of abuse is increasing in clubs or at parties; people with addiction only consume about 10%–25% of the therapeutic dose needed to induce anesthesia, but fatalities have occurred when the drug is combined with other CNS depressants (including alcohol and benzodiazepines) or with other illicit drugs. Unlike other hallucinogens, this is a Schedule III drug.
- MDMA is also known as "ecstasy," or more recently as "molly," which is a powdered or crystallized form. The drug was initially developed as a diet aid. It is often swallowed as a tablet (which usually glows in the dark) but can also be crushed, snorted, injected, or used in a suppository form (see Fig. 16.2). Dangerous adverse effects include cardiac arrhythmias, heart failure, hypertension, kidney failure, and seizures.
- Flakka (alpha-Pyrrolidinopentiophenone): a newer party drug that can be as potent as crystal meth, bath salts, or cocaine; it causes erratic, uncontrollable, and dangerous behaviors when injected, snorted, smoked, or swallowed;

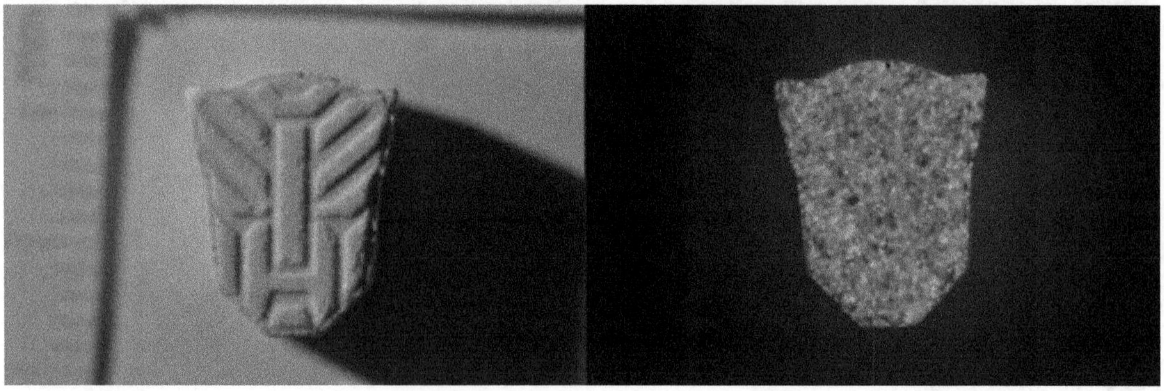

FIG. 16.2 A tablet of "ecstasy" (methylenedioxymethamphetamine, or MDMA), shown in normal room light and with luminescence in the dark.

body temperature may reach 105°F; the individual becomes psychotic and violent, often removing all clothing, with intensified strength; it is a synthetic version of the stimulant cathinone, which is grouped with bath salts.

- Mephedrone (4-methyl methcathinone) is also known as "drone" and "M-CAT." Mephedrone is a white, powdery drug that is swallowed, snorted, or injected. It causes intense cravings, hallucinations, paranoia, and rapid heart rate; it may also cause seizures, suicidal thoughts, coma, and death, especially if taken with alcohol.
- MDA is also known as "sally," "sass," and "sassafras."
- Mescaline is found in the peyote cactus of Mexico and Central America; it is used by Native Americans as part of traditional religious ceremonies. As a party drug, it is used to produce hallucinations and altered consciousness for 4–6 hours; it may also cause anxiety, tachycardia, dizziness, diarrhea, vomiting, and headache; it is not physically addictive.
- Psilocybin is the active ingredient in Mexican and southwestern US mushrooms referred to as "shrooms" by users; hallucinogenic properties are very similar to LSD.
- PCP, also known as "angel dust" and "ozone," produces a prolonged, **trancelike state** that can cause severe brain damage; it has a distinctive bitter taste and is available as tablets, capsules, and colored powders, which are taken orally or snorted. A liquid form is also available, which is highly flammable; deaths linked to this have involved accidental drownings, leaping from tall buildings, vehicular accidents, self-mutilation, suicides, and homicides. Unlike the other hallucinogens, this Schedule II drug was initially marketed as an anesthetic.

Central nervous system stimulants

CNS stimulants increase CNS activity and are legally available by prescription to treat narcolepsy, attention-deficit/hyperactivity disorder (ADHD), and obesity. These drugs improve mental and physical performance and provide a sense of exhilaration and prolonged wakefulness. However, they are often used illegally to "get high." Stimulants increase the effects of norepinephrine, dopamine, and serotonin in the central and peripheral nervous systems. Overdoses of some CNS stimulants may cause seizures and cardiac arrest. Examples include amphetamines, methylphenidate, cocaine, and caffeine. Long-term abuse can cause irreversible heart damage and extreme brain damage.

Amphetamines

In high doses and short-term use, amphetamines cause euphoria, self-confidence, alertness, and empowerment. Long-term use usually results in anxiety, restlessness, and rage (especially when "coming down" from the effects). After patients are prescribed amphetamines and dextroamphetamine for years, the drugs' risks began to outweigh their medical uses. Newer agents are much safer and have replaced these agents except for specific conditions. Illegally produced amphetamines continue to be popular drugs in substance abuse. Dextroamphetamine (Dexedrine) is used for short-term weight loss after other methods have failed and for narcolepsy. Methamphetamine (commonly known as "ice" when it is in the form of *crystal meth*) is a common recreational drug taken in a powdered or crystallized form that gives users a "rush." While its effects are similar to those of cocaine, they last much longer. It may be smoked, snorted, injected, or orally ingested—disastrously affecting health and appearance (see Fig. 16.3). Unlike other hallucinogens, it is a Schedule II drug (marketed as Desoxyn). Methamphetamine is often obtained from illegal "meth" laboratories. Another variant, methcathinone (known as "cat"), is a Schedule I agent. It is illegally made for injection, inhalation, or oral administration.

Methylphenidate

Methylphenidate (Ritalin) is a CNS stimulant used for children with ADHD. For those who are hyperactive or inattentive, Ritalin has a calming and focusing effect, helping individuals concentrate on specific tasks for longer periods than they normally can. When taken by adults, Ritalin usually causes the opposite effects, especially if they have no diagnosis of ADHD. Methylphenidate is a Schedule II drug with similar results to amphetamines and cocaine. Illegally, the drug is administered by inhalation or injection.

Cocaine

Cocaine is obtained from the leaves of the South American coca plant. It has been used since 2500 BCE. Users who chew coca leaves or make teas from them receive slow absorption of the drug because only tiny amounts of cocaine

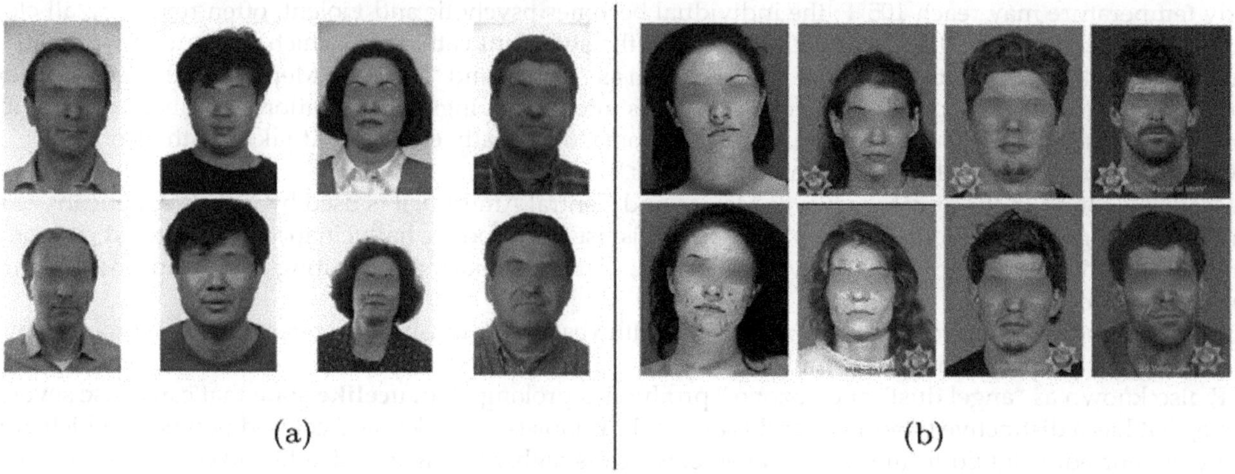

FIG. 16.3 The long-term effects of methamphetamine abuse, with each person's "before" picture above their "after" picture.

are present in the leaves. In the United States, cocaine is a Schedule II drug used entirely differently. Most users inhale the drug by "snorting" it, taking it orally, or injecting it. The rock form of cocaine is often called *crack* or *crack cocaine* and is smoked. Regardless of the state, cocaine produces rapid, intense effects similar to but more significant than amphetamines. Cocaine produces intense euphoria, analgesia, decreased hunger, increased sensory perception, and illusions of physical strength. Large doses increase these effects and cause rapid heartbeat, pupil dilation, elevated body temperature, and sweating.

When the euphoric feelings diminish, there is insomnia, irritability, depression, and extreme distrust of others. A "crawling" skin sensation may occur, and chronic inhalation results in many nasal problems. These include continual rhinorrhea, a reddened "crusting" around the nostrils, and nasal cartilage deterioration. Overdose may cause convulsions, dysrhythmias, severe heart abnormalities, stroke, and respiratory arrest deaths (see Fig. 16.4). Withdrawal from amphetamines and cocaine, however, is usually less intense than from barbiturates or alcohol. Celebrity deaths linked to cocaine use have included musician John Entwistle and singer Whitney Houston.

Caffeine

Caffeine is naturally present in the seeds, fruits, or leaves of more than 63 different plants. Coffee, chocolate, ice cream, soft drinks, and tea contain significant amounts. It increases the effectiveness of OTC pain relievers and is often added to their formulations. Two or three cups of coffee daily are suitable for the heart, while excessive amounts are not. The body metabolizes caffeine after several hours. The drug causes **diuresis**. It increases mental alertness, restlessness, irritability, nervousness, and insomnia. Physical effects include bronchodilation, increased blood pressure, increased production of stomach acid, and increased blood glucose levels. Repeated use results in physical dependence and tolerance. Withdrawal produces fatigue, headaches, depression, and impaired physical and mental performance.

Effects of substance abuse

Substance abuse often develops because of mental states such as anxiety and depression. Abuse usually prevents users from seeking treatment for the reason they chose to abuse drugs in the first place. Anxiety, panic disorder, and insomnia are all increased by using stimulants. While depression is numbed by alcohol, opioids, and sedatives initially, these agents *cause* depression over more extended periods. Hallucinogens and stimulants can bring on psychoses and related strange behaviors. Drug abuse may result in cognitive dysfunction, imprisonment, unemployment, family problems, financial loss, poor decisions, and sexual relationships that otherwise would not have occurred.

The physical effects of substance abuse include sexually transmitted infections such as hepatitis B and C and HIV. Drug use is more prevalent in victims of sexual assault. Intravenous drug abuse may be associated with hepatitis, HIV, and *Staphylococcal endocarditis*. Smoking and alcohol use have been linked to more severe drug abuse. Heart attacks and strokes are often related to the use of cocaine. Drug overdoses can cause respiratory depression, confusion, pneumonia, seizures, coma, and death. Drugs can also result in motor vehicle accidents, fetal impairment, suicide, and violence.

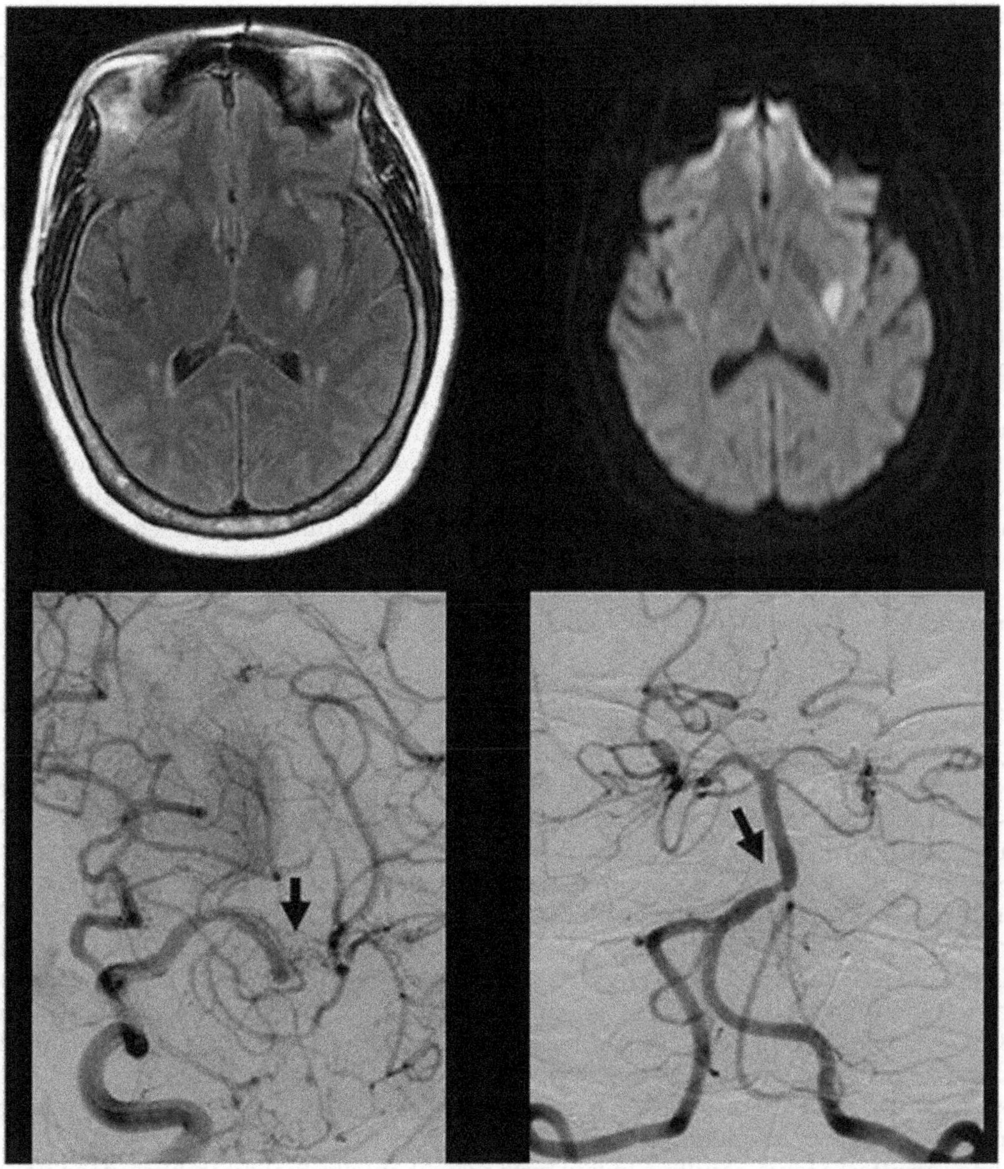

FIG. 16.4 Neurovascular complications of cocaine use, which resulted in a stroke.

You should remember

The COVID-19 pandemic presented unique challenges for individuals with substance use disorders who are at increased risk for poor COVID-19 outcomes. Also, researchers have observed increases in substance abuse and drug overdoses since the pandemic was declared a national emergency. Loneliness, confusion, and unemployment started more people to use or increase their use of substances, all when treatment centers and support groups were temporarily shut down.

Prevention and treatment for substance abuse

The risk of drug use increases significantly during times of transition. For an adult, a divorce or loss of a job may increase the risk of drug use. For a teenager, risky times include moving, family divorce, or changing schools.

Children who advance from elementary through middle school face new and challenging social, family, and academic situations. Often during this period, children are exposed to substances such as cigarettes and alcohol for the first time. When they enter high school, teens may encounter greater availability of drugs, drug use by older teens, and social activities where drugs are used. When individuals leave high school and live more independently, either in college or as an employed adult, they may find themselves exposed to drug use while separated from the protective structure provided by family and school.

Prevention is the key to substance abuse. Activities work to educate and support individuals and communities to prevent the use and misuse of drugs and the development of substance use disorders. Substance use and mental illnesses can make daily activities difficult and impair a person's ability to work, interact with family, and fulfill other primary life functions. Mental and substance use disorders are among the top conditions that cause disability in the United States.

Drug removal and detoxification is the first step when treating addiction patients. Withdrawal may cause physical and psychological symptoms and can require hospitalization. Detoxification is overcoming physical withdrawal when a person with an addiction stops taking a drug, and medical management may be necessary to prevent serious health problems. Methadone is often used for the ongoing management of withdrawal. However, the majority of treatment is psychological. Pharmacologic treatment involves substances similar to addictive drugs but have no addiction potential and may reduce or stop withdrawal. This type of treatment is not used for hallucinogens or stimulants. For opioid addiction, methadone eliminates the physical craving for heroin. Buprenorphine is similar but induces nausea if the user tries to use or abuse an addictive opioid. Frequent urine toxicology screens are used to find if the person with an addiction occasionally uses addictive substances.

Cigarette smoking

The most significant cause of preventable death and illness in the United States is the smoking of tobacco products. Nicotine addiction is the most common of all likely because nicotine is highly positively reinforcing. Continued tobacco use despite significant physical, economic, or social side effects is *tobacco dependence.* The physical adverse effects of smoking are usually severe later in life and include cancer, **emphysema**, and heart attacks. About 14% of Americans smoke, and because it is still legal, smoking is not perceived as an addiction by many.

Smoking increases alertness, focus, and relaxation but produces lightheadedness. Directly stimulating the CNS, nicotine accelerates the heart rate and hypertension. Nicotine also increases the **basal metabolic rate**, leading to weight loss and appetite reduction over time. Physical and psychological dependence occur relatively quickly. Withdrawal causes anxiety, cravings, poor attention, insomnia, cravings, GI disturbances, irritability, and headaches.

More than 480,000 people die annually in the United States from various effects of smoking. Half of the Americans who continue to smoke will die from a smoking-related disease. Smoking affects all body systems, primarily the respiratory, cardiovascular, and nervous systems. It is the primary cause of lung cancer deaths. Other cancers are also much more significant in occurrence due to smoking.

Passive smoking can affect a fetus, resulting in low birth weight, intellectual disabilities, neonatal death, and **stillbirth**. Children of smokers have a higher incidence of **asthma**, pneumonia, **bronchitis**, growth retardation, and **sudden infant death syndrome**.

Alcoholism

Ethyl alcohol is a commonly abused drug that is legal and readily available. Abuse of alcohol has enormous economic, health, and social consequences. In small quantities, red wine has been proven to reduce the risk of heart attack and stroke, but long-term abuse of alcohol can have devastating effects.

Alcohol is a CNS depressant that readily crosses the blood-brain barrier, with effects starting within 5 and 30 minutes. The results are based on the amount consumed, including relaxation, impaired memory, sedation, loss of coordination, decreased inhibition, and reduced judgment. Alcohol mimics the effects of antidepressants, antianxiety agents, and sedatives. Therefore healthcare personnel should verify which drugs a patient has consumed before treatment.

Acute overdoses of alcohol cause vomiting, severe hypotension, respiratory failure, and coma. More than 95,000 Americans die yearly due to alcohol use and related behaviors. Excessive alcohol consumption produces severe depressant effects on the brain. Therefore alcohol should never be combined with other CNS depressants because the results are cumulative, potentially leading to profound sedation and coma. Withdrawal from alcohol can be severe and possibly life-threatening, causing anxiety, insomnia, or seizures. Long-term alcoholics often experience **delirium tremens**. Symptoms include agitation, confusion, disorientation, hallucinations, anxiety, panic, a "crawling" sensation of the skin, and **paranoia**.

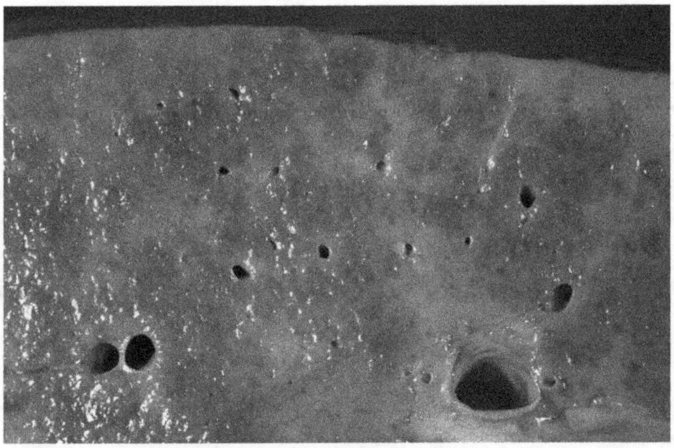

FIG. 16.5 Cirrhosis of the liver.

Chronic alcohol abuse primarily affects the liver through repeated insult and resultant scarring or cirrhosis. **Cirrhosis** is the liver's debilitating and potentially fatal failure to function normally. When the organ becomes impaired, blood clotting and nutritional states are affected (see Fig. 16.5). Impairment makes the liver more sensitive to all substances it metabolizes. Patients should be honest with their physicians about their use of alcohol because drug dosing must be determined based on this information.

You should remember

Alcohol is the most commonly used addictive substance, with about 1 in every 12 adults suffering from alcohol abuse or dependence. Psychiatric disorders are common in people who also have alcohol use disorders. Up to 25% suffer severe psychiatric disturbances. The most prevalent of these symptoms include anxiety and depression disorders. People hospitalized with an alcohol use disorder die 24–28 years earlier than the general population.

Key Terms

Additive effect
Amnesia
Amyotrophic lateral sclerosis
Asthma
Basal metabolic rate
Bronchitis
Cannabinoids
Cirrhosis
Crohn's disease
Delirium tremens
Designer drugs
Diuresis
Euphoria
Emphysema
Multiple sclerosis
Paranoia
Substance abuse
Substance misuse
Sudden infant death syndrome
Stillbirth
Trancelike state
Withdrawal

Clinical Case Studies

Clinical Case Study 1

An 18-year-old female has signs of irritability and depression. She spends more time alone in her room. She comes home later than she was supposed to. After several weeks, her mother received a phone call from the school after the girl was found having seizures on the classroom floor. The principal stated she was transported by ambulance to the emergency department. After examining, testing, and verifying that the girl had no history of epilepsy, the physician informed the mother that there was cocaine in her daughter's system.

Critical Thinking Questions

1. How do users usually take cocaine?
2. What are the effects of cocaine?
3. Aside from convulsions, what are the signs of a cocaine overdose?

Clinical Case Study 2

A 21-year-old medical assistant applied for a job. When she was hired, the office manager told her that the facility conducted random drug screenings for all employers, and she signed an agreement indicating her compliance. After a few months, the office manager noticed that she occasionally behaved strangely while at work. She was sometimes late or did not show up and did not call to inform the office of her impending absence. One day, the physician ordered a urine test for her. After the results came back, it indicated the presence of nicotine and MDMA in her system.

Critical Thinking Questions

1. Can hallucinogens such as MDMA result in behavior changes?
2. What are the two common street names for MDMA?
3. What are the dangerous adverse effects of MDMA?

Further Reading

[1] F. Brooks, B. McHenry, A Contemporary Approach to Substance Use Disorders and Addiction Counseling, second ed., American Counseling Association, 2015.
[2] G.J. Connors, C.C. DiClemente, M. Marden Velasquez, D.M. Donovan, Substance Abuse Treatment and the Stages of Change – Selecting and Planning Interventions, second ed., Guilford Press, 2015.
[3] G. Coughlin, S.S. Kimbrough, L.L. Kimbrough, Patient Records and Addiction Treatment, fourth ed., Southworth Press, 2008.
[4] R. Eskapa, C. Christian, D. Sinclair, The Cure for Alcoholism: The Medically Proven Way to Eliminate Alcohol Addiction, BenBella Books, 2012.
[5] G. Fisher, T. Harrison, Substance Abuse: Information for School Counselors, Social Workers, Therapists, and Counselors, sixth ed., Pearson, 2017.
[6] G.F. Koob, M.A. Arends, M. Le Moal, Drugs, Addiction, and the Brain, Academic Press, 2014.
[7] C. Kouimtsidis, M. Reynolds, C. Drummond, P. Davis, N. Tarrier, Cognitive-Behavioral Therapy in the Treatment of Addiction – A Treatment Planner for Clinicians, Wiley, 2007.
[8] T. MacMillan, A. Sisselman-Borgia, New Directions in Treatment, Education, and Outreach for Mental Health and Addiction (Advances in Mental Health and Addiction), Springer, 2018.
[9] M. Marden Velasquez, C. Crough, N. Stokes Stephens, C.C. DiClemente, Group Treatment for Substance Abuse: A Stages-of-Change Therapy Manual, second ed., Guilford Press, 2015.
[10] R.R. Perkinson, The Alcoholism and Drug Abuse Client Workbook, Sage Publications, Inc, 2016.
[11] T. Pichot, S.A. Smock, T.S. Nelson, Solution-Focused Substance Abuse Treatment, Routledge, 2011.
[12] D.J. Powell, A. Brodsky, Clinical Supervision in Alcohol and Drug Abuse Counseling: Principles, Models, Methods, Jossey-Bass, 2004.
[13] M.D. Reiter, Substance Abuse and the Family: Assessment and Treatment, second ed., Routledge, 2019.
[14] P. Ruiz, E. Strain, Lowinson and Ruiz's Substance Abuse: A Comprehensive Textbook, fifth ed., Wolters Kluwer Health / Lippincott, Williams, & Wilkins, 2011.
[15] R.L. Smith, Treatment Strategies for Substance and Process Addictions, American Counseling Association, 2015.
[16] D. Yalisove, Developing Clinical Skills for Substance Abuse Counseling, American Counseling Association, 2010.

UNIT III

Autonomic drugs

CHAPTER

17

Neurotransmitters

OUTLINE

LEARNING OUTCOMES

After study of the chapter, readers should be able to:

1. Explain the classifications of neurotransmitters.
2. Identify the three types of dopamine receptors.
3. Explain the two types of GABA receptors.
4. Describe the variety of epinephrine.
5. Identify the functions of serotonin.
6. Discuss the synthesis of neurotransmitters.
7. List five substances that inhibit serotonin reuptake.
8. Identify the primary parts of histamine.

Overview

Neurotransmitters are the essential chemical messengers that the body needs to function. They carry chemical signals from neurons to target cells, which can be another neuron, a muscle cell, or a gland. Their messages help us move, feel sensations, keep the heart beating, and respond to all information from the body's internal parts and the external environment. Synaptic transmission is the process at synapses by which a chemical signal is released from a neuron and diffuses to other neurons or target cells. Their signals are generated that excite, inhibit, or moderate cellular activity. Neurotransmitters allow brain cells to communicate. Some of them are *excitatory*, making cells more active. Others are *inhibitory* and block or dampen cell activities. Neurotransmitters are located in the axon terminals of neurons; they are stored in the thin-walled synaptic vesicles, each containing thousands of neurotransmitter molecules. Once released into synaptic junctions, neurotransmitters carry messages and eventually bind

The Science of Pharmacology
https://doi.org/10.1016/B978-0-443-29038-1.00017-8

to specific receptors on target cells, triggering changes or actions in the cells. More than 50 of these substances have been identified.

Classifications of neurotransmitters

Neurotransmitters are the body's chemical messengers. They are molecules used in the nervous system to transmit messages between **neurons** or from neurons to muscles. They affect thoughts, emotions, memories, movements, and sleep patterns. Synaptic transmission is mainly influenced by enhancing or inhibiting neurotransmitter release, destruction, and reabsorption and by blocking neurotransmitter binding to receptors. Neurotransmitters include amino acids, small peptides, or derivative chemicals, such as acetylcholine (ACh), dopamine, gamma-aminobutyric acid (GABA), glutamine, norepinephrine (NE), and serotonin. More than 50 neurotransmitters, or potential neurotransmitters, have been identified.

Neurotransmitters can be classified by their function or by their chemical components. They are excitatory inhibitory or sometimes both. **Excitatory neurotransmitters** trigger depolarization, which increases the likelihood of a response. **Inhibitory neurotransmitters** trigger hyperpolarization, which decreases the possibility of a reply. Neurotransmitters include ACh, dopamine, glutamine, GABA, biogenic amines, NE, epinephrine, histamine, and serotonin.

Acetylcholine

ACh is a neurotransmitter utilized by somatic efferent neurons, preganglionic sympathetic neurons, and the parasympathetic nervous system. It was the first neurotransmitter ever identified and is released at neuromuscular junctions, which are more accessible locations to study than the deeply buried CNS synapses. ACh is synthesized within nerve terminals by choline acetyltransferase. This enzyme catalyzes reactions between **acetyl coenzyme A** and **choline**. The next step is the transport of ACh into the synaptic vesicles. After being released by the presynaptic terminal, ACh is briefly bound to postsynaptic receptors. Next, it is released and degraded by **acetylcholinesterase**, becoming acetic acid and choline. The AChE enzyme is located in the synaptic cleft and upon postsynaptic membranes. The presynaptic terminals recapture the released choline and reuse it to synthesize more ACh. All neurons that stimulate skeletal muscles and many autonomic nervous system neurons release ACh. Also, ACh-releasing neurons are within the CNS. The effects of ACh are lengthened when acetylcholinesterase is blocked by nerve gas or organophosphate insecticides such as **malathion**. This results in tetanic muscle spasms. The use of botulinum toxin can inhibit the release of ACh. Levels of ACh are decreased in some brain areas in patients with Alzheimer disease.

Cholinergic receptors are those that bind with ACh. They are divided into muscarinic and nicotinic receptors. The **muscarinic receptors** activate end-organ effector cells in bronchial smooth muscle, the salivary glands, and the sinoatrial node. The binding of ACh to the muscarinic receptors is inhibited by atropine. The **nicotinic receptors** are located in the **somatic system**, on the motor end plates of skeletal muscle cells, the **adrenal medulla**, and all **postganglionic neurons**—the binding of ACh to the nicotinic receptor results in an excitatory effect. The nicotinic receptors are destroyed in the condition known as **myasthenia gravis**.

You should remember

ACh is essential for brain and muscle function. Imbalances are linked to chronic conditions such as Alzheimer disease and Parkinson disease. ACh is the chief neurotransmitter of the parasympathetic nervous system, the part of the autonomic nervous system that contracts smooth muscles, dilates blood vessels, increases secretions, and slows the heart rate.

You should remember

Myasthenia gravis is a chronic autoimmune neuromuscular disease that causes weakness in the skeletal muscles. The hallmark of myasthenia gravis is muscle weakness that worsens after periods of activity and improves after periods of rest. Specific muscles, such as those that control eye and eyelid movement, facial expressions, chewing, talking, and swallowing, are often involved in the disorder.

Dopamine

Dopamine is a monoamine synthesized from the amino acid tyrosine. Many enzymatic reactions are needed that produce levodopa, dopamine, NE, and epinephrine. Dopamine can be excitatory or inhibitory, based upon which receptor subtype is activated. Dopamine in the brain plays a part in behavior, cognition, learning, mood, sleep, and voluntary movements. Its actions are primarily in the hypothalamus, substantia nigra, arcuate nucleus, and the midbrain's ventral tegmental portion. Dopamine is an essential component of the reward system of the body. It is inactivated via reuptake, which uses the dopamine transporter. This is followed by enzymatic breakdown. Enzymes in this process include *catechol-O-methyltransferase* and monoamine oxidase. Typically, dopamine is used for smooth and coordinated muscle movements. Amphetamines and levodopa enhance dopamine release, and its reuptake is blocked by cocaine.

The $D_{1\text{-}5}$ dopamine receptors are essential for the increase in actions of the direct basal ganglia pathway. The receptors are summarized as follows:

- *D_1 receptors*: help regulate the growth and development of neurons, behavioral responses, and D_2-receptor signaling. They activate a G_s protein, activating adenyl cyclase and cAMP signaling.
- *D_2 receptors*: may be involved in muscle tone regulation and are associated with schizophrenia. They activate a G_i protein, inhibiting cyclic adenosine monophosphate (cAMP) production.
- *D_3 receptors*: may be involved in emotions, depression, cognition, drug addiction, and schizophrenia. They also activate a G_i protein, inhibiting cAMP production.
- *D_4 receptors*: may be involved in thrill-seeking behaviors and schizophrenia. They also activate a G_i protein, inhibiting cAMP production.
- *D_5 receptors*: may be involved in blood pressure regulation, decision making, and cognition. They also activate a G_s protein, followed by activation of adenyl cyclase and cAMP signaling.

When there is a lack of dopamine biosynthesis in the dopaminergic neurons, **Parkinson disease** may develop. In the brain's frontal lobes, dopamine controls information from other areas. Dopamine disorders may result in reduced neurocognitive functions. These include memory, attention, and the ability to solve problems. A dopamine imbalance is linked to mental illness, such as the overactive dopamine signaling in schizophrenia. Some psychoactive drugs, such as mescaline and LSD, can bind to biogenic amine receptors, resulting in hallucinations. Addictions to food, love, gambling, and drugs are all associated with dopamine. The amino acids in vegetables stimulate dopamine production. While very few neurons manufacture dopamine, many of them transmit it. Regulation and stimulation of dopamine levels can be modulated by tyrosine, found in many types of meat and fruit.

You should remember

Addictions to food, love, gambling, and drugs are all associated with dopamine. The amino acids contained in vegetables stimulate dopamine production. Though very few neurons manufacture dopamine, many of them transmit it. Tyrosine, found in many types of meat and fruit, can modulate the regulation and stimulation of dopamine levels.

Glutamine

Glutamine is the brain's principal excitatory neurotransmitter, with an estimated 50% or more of synapses utilizing the neurotransmitter. Glutamine is essential in learning and memory, among other functions. Excessive release of glutamine causes **excitotoxicity**, with neurons being stimulated continuously. Via **glutaminergic receptor** opening of nonselective ion channels, glutamine is generally excitatory. Its stimulation is terminated by a membrane transport system, which is utilized in the reabsorption of glutamine over the presynaptic membrane. An imbalance in synaptic excitation and inhibition is thought to contribute to the pathophysiology of **autism**. It is also called autism spectrum disorder.

Gamma-aminobutyric acid

GABA is an amino acid neurotransmitter synthesized from glutamic acid. It is the most prevalent inhibitory brain neurotransmitter, important in presynaptic inhibition at the **axoaxonal synapses**. GABA is predominantly concentrated within the substantia nigra, hypothalamus, and hippocampus. It reduces the excitability of neurons via hyperpolarization. There are two types of GABA receptors, as follows:

- *$GABA_A$*: activation opens chloride channels
- *$GABA_B$*: acts through a second messenger, either opening potassium channels or closing calcium channels

GABA is inactivated via active transport into the astrocyte glial cells close to the synapses. Alcohol, benzodiazepines, and barbiturates affect its inhibitory effects. Any substance that blocks GABA synthesis, release, or action results in convulsions. Many abused drugs affect **glutamate**, GABA, or both, stimulating or tranquilizing the brain.

Glycine is a widely distributed neurotransmitter in the brainstem, spinal cord, and retinas. It is the primary *inhibitory neurotransmitter* in the spinal cord. Its receptor is a gated channel comprising five protein subunits, allowing for an influx of chloride ions. The influx inhibits postsynaptic potential, reducing future postsynaptic or motor neuron action potentials. Competitive inhibitors of glycine receptors include caffeine and the poison strychnine. Glycine is an essential coagonist for the glutamate receptor.

You should remember

GABA and glycine are arguably the most important inhibitory neurotransmitters in the brain and the brainstem/spinal cord—many therapeutically useful drugs work by selectively affecting these two neurotransmitter systems. Many psychoactive drugs that increase or decrease CNS excitability do so by affecting GABAergic or glycinergic neurotransmission.

Biogenic amines

Biogenic amine neurotransmitters are found throughout the brain, with roles in emotions and regulating the body's biological clock. The biogenic amines include the catecholamines and indolamines. Dopamine, epinephrine, and NE are examples of catecholamines. NE and dopamine play a role in feeling good and euphoric. Via a common pathway, dopamine and NE are synthesized from the tyrosine. The adrenal medulla and the brain's epinephrine-releasing cells use the same path. Histamine and serotonin are examples of indolamines. Histamine is synthesized from the amino acid called *histidine*. Serotonin is synthesized from *tryptophan*, another amino acid. Postganglion of sympathetic nerves and adrenal medulla release NE.

Norepinephrine and epinephrine

NE, *noradrenaline*, is synthesized from tyrosine in the cytoplasm. It is contained by postganglionic fiber vesicles and released through exocytosis. NE reuptake terminates via postganglionic nerve endings, receptor site diffusion, or enzyme metabolism. The sympathetic postganglionic neurons utilize NE. Amphetamines enhance the release of

NE. Removal of NE from the synapse is stopped by cocaine and tricyclic antidepressants. The antihypertensive drug reserpine decreases brain levels of NE, which results in depression.

Epinephrine, also called *adrenaline*, is the final product of the tyrosine pathway in the **chromaffin cells** of the adrenal medulla. These cells produce dopaminc and NE as well as epinephrine. The neurotransmitter has many effects on various organ systems and metabolic functions. The degradation pathways of NE and epinephrine are very similar. They act as hormones, neurotransmitters, and adrenergic receptors, classified as alpha (α) and beta (β). Epinephrine and NE bind to all types of adrenergic receptors but with various levels of affinity. The receptors associated with NE and epinephrine vitamin A toxicity can be caused by ingesting high doses of vitamin A—acutely (usually accidentally by children) or chronically (e.g., as megavitamin therapy or treatment for skin disorders). The receptors include:

- *α_1-receptors*: postsynaptic adrenoreceptors located in the eyes, smooth muscles, blood vessels, lungs, gut, and genitourinary system. Stimulation activates a G_q protein, increasing phospholipase activity, which releases *diacylglycerol*. It also releases *inositol trisphosphate*, promoting increased calcium release. The signals are excitatory, indicated by bronchodilation, pupil dilation, blood vessel constriction, increased heart contraction strength (positive **inotropy**), and decreased heart rate (negative **chronotropy**). NE binds better than epinephrine to these receptors.
- *α_2-receptors*: mainly located on presynaptic nerve terminals. Activation of G_i proteins inhibits **adenyl cyclase** activity and cAMP production. This decreases the entry of free calcium into the neuronal terminal, reducing the amount of NE released. It also causes vasoconstriction and reduced sympathetic outflow in the CNS. Epinephrine binds better than NE to these receptors.
- *β_1-receptors*: stimulation activates a G_s protein. This increases activities of adenyl cyclase, adenosine triphosphate conversion into cAMP, and protein kinase phosphorylation of many proteins. It causes positive chronotropy, inotropy, and **dromotropy**. It is not fully understood if epinephrine and NE bind equally to this receptor or if there is a preference for epinephrine binding.
- *β_2-receptors*: primarily, these are postsynaptic adrenoceptors in glands and smooth muscles. They activate adenyl cyclase using a G_s protein and inhibit the same enzyme via a G_i protein. These opposing effects may allow for different cell and tissue functions. Smooth muscle is relaxed by B_2 stimulation, causing bronchodilation, insulin release, vasodilation, and induction of **gluconeogenesis**. Epinephrine binds to these receptors with a much higher affinity than NE.
- *β_3-receptors*: primarily found in fat and adipose tissue. These receptors also activate adenyl cyclase via the use of a G_s protein. They induce the breakdown of fats and lipids via lipolysis and help regulate thermogenesis, primarily in skeletal muscle. NE binds better than epinephrine to these receptors.

Histamine

Histamine is a vasoactive, biogenic amine involved in local immune responses, appetite control, learning, memory, and wakefulness. It is synthesized from the amino acid *histidine*. Histamine is involved in the inflammatory response and plays a central role in the mediation of itching. It causes temporary and rapid constriction of large blood vessel walls and dilation of postcapillary venules. These actions result in increased blood flow into the body's microcirculation. Vascular permeability is raised from the retraction of endothelial cells that line the capillaries. The pharmacologic effects of histamine are partly based on histamine receptors located on target cells. The two primary receptors are *H1* and *H2*, but there are also *H3* and *H4* receptors. When histamine binds to the H1 receptor, the effect is primarily proinflammatory. When it binds to the H2 receptor, an antiinflammatory effect occurs due to suppression of leukocyte functions. The H1 receptor is located on smooth muscle cells—primarily in the bronchi—causing bronchoconstriction. Both receptor types are found in many different cells, often upon the same cells, and can act antagonistically. Neutrophils usually have H1 and H2 receptors, with H1 stimulation causing chemotaxis and H2 stimulation causing inhibition. The H2 receptors are significant in stomach mucosa parietal cells, inducing gastric acid secretion.

Serotonin

Serotonin is also called *5-hydroxytryptamine*, or *5-HT*. It is a monoamine neurotransmitter involved in eating, sleeping, arousal, dreaming, mood regulation, temperature regulation, and pain transmission. Serotonin is synthesized from the amino acid known as **tryptophan** via a short metabolic pathway. This comprises the enzymes known as tryptophan hydroxylase and amino acid decarboxylase. Serotonin is terminated via uptake at the synapse of the presynaptic neuron. LSD blocks the activity of serotonin. Many different substances inhibit serotonin reuptake to relieve anxiety and depression. These include the following:

- Amphetamine
- Cocaine
- Dextromethorphan
- Ecstasy (MDMA)
- Selective serotonin reuptake inhibitors
- Tricyclic antidepressants

You should remember

Neuromodulators are neurotransmitters that diffuse through neural tissue. They affect the slow-acting receptors of many different neurons. The major CNS neuromodulators include dopamine, ACh, serotonin, histamine, and NE. Neuromodulators have modulatory effects on target areas.

Functional considerations

The function of a neurotransmitter is determined by the receptor that it binds with. If a neurotransmitter is *excitatory,* it causes **depolarization**. If it is *inhibitory,* it causes **hyperpolarization**. Some neurotransmitters have both effects based on specific receptors interacting with them. Glutamate, for example, is a neurotransmitter with mostly excitatory effects. The amino acids GABA and glycine have primarily inhibitory effects. ACh and NE bind to two or more receptor types, resulting in opposing impacts. For example, ACh has excitatory effects at neuromuscular junctions in skeletal muscles but inhibitory effects in cardiac muscle.

Neurotransmitters may be classified as having direct or indirect actions. Neurotransmitters that act directly bind to ion channels and also open them. They cause fast responses in postsynaptic cells through alteration of membrane potential. ACh and the amino acid neurotransmitters usually have direct actions. The indirect-acting neurotransmitters cause broader, longer-lasting effects. They act via intracellular second-messenger molecules, usually through G-protein pathways. Therefore the actions of these neurotransmitters resemble those of hormones. Indirect neurotransmitters include biogenic amines and dissolved gases.

You should remember

Epinephrine and NE are chemically similar and affect alpha and beta receptors. However, NE has a more significant effect on beta receptors than epinephrine. Beta receptors are found in the heart, lungs, and arteries of skeletal muscles. Serotonin is found mainly in the CNS, digestive system, and platelets. Epinephrine and NE deficiency can lead to mood disorders such as anxiety or depression.

Synthesis of neurotransmitters

Most neurotransmitters are small molecules, including amines or amino acids, while others are larger neuropeptides or modified lipids. The amines and amino acids are synthesized in the presynaptic cytoplasm. This usually means local substrates such as acetate or choline are required, and soluble enzymes are carried via slow axonal transport. The synthesis of peptide transmitters is different. It needs protein synthesis in a neuronal cell body. Neuropeptides start in the neuronal cell body as larger precursor proteins.

You should remember

Various conditions may be linked to neurotransmitters. ACh is related to myasthenia gravis. Dopamine production is associated with Parkinson disease and may be related to schizophrenia and ADHD. Problems with the display or use of glutamate are also linked to schizophrenia, autism, obsessive-compulsive disorder, and depression. Depressive disorders are related to imbalances of dopamine, NE, and serotonin. Other neurotransmitter-related conditions include bipolar disorder and cyclothymic disorder.

Key Terms

Acetylcholine
Acetylcholinesterase
Acetyl coenzyme A
Active zone
Adenyl cyclase
Adrenal medulla
Amino acid decarboxylase
Autism
Autoreceptors
Choline
Choline acetyltransferase
Cholinergic receptors
Chromaffin cells
Chronotropy
Dopamine
Dromotropy
Endocytosis
Epinephrine
Excitatory
Excitatory postsynaptic potential
Excitotoxicity
Exocytosis
Gamma-aminobutyric acid
Gluconeogenesis
Glutamate
Glutamine
Glutaminergic receptor
Glycine
Hallucinations
Inhibitory postsynaptic potential
Inhibitory
Inotropy
Lipolysis
Malathion
Molar
Muscarinic
Myasthenia gravis
Neuromodulators
Neurotransmitters
Nicotinic
Norepinephrine
Paracrine hormones
Parkinson disease
Postganglionic neurons
Serotonin
Somatic system
Strychnine
Thermogenesis
Tryptophan

Clinical Case Studies

Clinical Case Study 1

A 36-year-old female began to notice that her eyelids had started drooping. She then developed double vision and arm weakness, which progressively worsened. Her primary care physician referred her to a neurologist, who ran a blood test and found high levels of ACh receptor antibodies. The patient was diagnosed with myasthenia gravis. A cholinesterase inhibitor medication was prescribed, and the patient was instructed to rest and relax as much as possible. Her condition slowly improved, but upon returning to work, she developed right shoulder pain and daily exhaustion. She was enrolled in physiotherapy to address these symptoms.

Critical Thinking Questions

1. Where are the nicotinic receptors located?
2. How are the nicotinic receptors involved in the development of myasthenia gravis?
3. What is myasthenia gravis?

Clinical Case Study 2

A 6-year-old male was referred to an autism clinic because of behavioral problems that included physical harm to his teacher and classmates. The child could not complete his schoolwork because he could not remain seated for more than 2 minutes at a time. In the school hallways, the boy would run, crashing into other students. He would refuse to stand in line for the cafeteria, pushing or hitting anyone who tried to get him to behave. The boy engaged in the same behaviors at home, lashing out at his parents and sister.

Critical Thinking Questions

1. Which neurotransmitter is implicated in autism?
2. What other conditions are related to problems with this same neurotransmitter?
3. What is the definition of autism?

Further Reading

[1] A. Akaike, S. Shimohama, Y. Misu, Nicotinic Acetylcholine Receptor Signaling in Neuroprotection, Springer, 2018.
[2] M. Bancroft, Dopamine Vs. Serotonin: A Neurologist Breaks down the Two Happy Hormones, Bancroft, 2022.
[3] BioNinja, Types of Neurotransmitters, BioNinja, 2021.
[4] A. Eros Gupta, Acetylcholine Receptors in Health and Disease, Nova Science Publishers, Inc, 2019.
[5] N. Graziane, Y. Dong, Electrophysiological Analysis of Synaptic Transmission (Neuromethods 112), Humana Press, 2016.
[6] L. Iversen, S. Iversen, S. Dunnett, A. Bjorklund, Dopamine Handbook, Oxford University Press, 2009.
[7] P. Kumar, P. Kishore Deb, Frontiers in Pharmacology of Neurotransmitters, Springer, 2020.
[8] J. Lee, Better Living Through Neurochemistry – A Guide to the Optimization of Serotonin, Dopamine, and the Neurotransmitters that Color Your World, Lee, 2014.
[9] M. Macaluso, S.H. Preskorn, Antidepressants: From Biogenic Amines to New Mechanisms of Action (Handbook of Experimental Pharmacology 250), Springer, 2019.
[10] S.D. Meriney, E. Fanselow, Synaptic Transmission, Academic Press, 2019.
[11] M.J. Michelson, E.V. Zeimal, P. Alexander, Z.M. Bacq, Acetylcholine: An Approach to the Molecular Mechanism of Action (International Series of Monographs in Pure and Applied Biology; Division: Modern Trends in Physiological Sciences), Pergamon, 2014.
[12] S. Mochida, Presynaptic Terminals, Springer, 2015.
[13] E.J. Nestler, S.E. Hyman, R.C. Malenka, Molecular Neuropharmacology: A Foundations for Clinical Neuroscience, third ed., McGraw-Hill Education/Medical, 2015.
[14] A. Schousboe, U. Sonnewald, The Glutamate/GABA-Glutamine Cycle: Amino Acid Homeostasis (Advances in Neurobiology Book 13), Springer, 2016.
[15] V.I. Skok, A.A. Selyanko, V.A. Derkach, Neuronal Acetylcholine Receptors, Springer, 2014.
[16] J.D. Stalling, Synaptic Transmissions (Recast Impulsion Book 2), Stalling, 2020.
[17] N. Tam, Neurotransmitter Pathways: A Tutorial Study Guide, True Color Productions, 2014.
[18] S. Udenfriend, J. Meienhofer, Opioid Peptides: Biology, Chemistry, and Genetics: Analysis, Synthesis, Biology, vol. 6, Academic Press, 2014.
[19] G. Wu, Amino Acids: Biochemistry and Nutrition, CRC Press, 2013.
[20] H. Zimmermann, Cellular and Molecular Basis of Synaptic Transmission, Springer, 2011.

CHAPTER

18

Adrenergic agonists

OUTLINE

LEARNING OUTCOMES

After study of the chapter, readers should be able to:

1. Describe the classifications of catecholamines.
2. Identify the clinical indications of alpha$_1$-adrenergic agonists.
3. Explain the clinical signs of alpha$_2$-adrenergic agonists.
4. Discuss the mechanism of action of alpha$_2$-adrenergic agonists.
5. Explain the mechanism of action of beta$_1$-adrenergic agonists.
6. Describe the adverse effects of beta$_2$-adrenergic agonists in older people.

The Science of Pharmacology
https://doi.org/10.1016/B978-0-443-29038-1.00018-X

7. Discuss the mechanism of action of mirabegron (a beta$_3$-adrenergic agonist).
8. Explain the clinical indications of beta$_3$-adrenergic agonists.

Overview

Adrenergic agonists are medications that stimulate the adrenergic receptors. Their actions simulate activating certain aspects of the sympathetic nervous system, also called sympathomimetics. Adrenergic agonists are categorized as catecholamines (norepinephrine [NE], epinephrine, and dopamine) and noncatecholamines (ephedrine, phenylephrine, and terbutaline), which are more selective of receptor sites, slower acting, and have a longer duration. Many different medications in this class utilize distinct mechanisms of action. They are generally divided into groups based on whether they directly or indirectly activate adrenergic receptors. The direct-acting agonists physically bind the adrenergic receptor, simulating the binding of an endogenous ligand. The indirect agonists lead to receptor activation through various mechanisms, including promoting the release of stored NE from presynaptic terminals and inhibiting NE reuptake and degradation from synapses.

Adrenergic agonists

The adrenergic agonists are categorized as catecholamines and noncatecholamines. The catecholamines include NE, epinephrine, and dopamine. NE is the primary neurotransmitter of the sympathetic nervous system, whereas epinephrine is the primary hormone of the adrenal medulla. Dopamine is the biochemical precursor to NE in some areas of the CNS. Some synthesized drugs produce the same effects as the naturally secreted neurotransmitters. The noncatecholamines have somewhat similar actions to the catecholamines but are more selective of receptor sites, are not quite as fast acting, and have a longer duration. The medications of the adrenergic agonist class mimic the sympathetic nervous system and are also called *sympathomimetics*.

Classifications of adrenergic agonists

Adrenergic agonists were first identified when *epinephrine* was isolated from adrenal medulla extracts in 1895. It has a chemical structure comprising an aromatic ring of six carbons. Two oxygen-hydrogen groups are similar to those of the organic chemical known as *catechol*. Because the molecule also has a nitrogen-hydrogen or amino group, the name *catecholamine* was given to epinephrine by physiologists. Other adrenergic agonists with this same core chemical include NE, dobutamine, dopamine, and isoproterenol. Therefore adrenergic agonists are classified more simply as *catecholamines* or *noncatecholamines.* The *noncatecholamines* include ephedrine, phenylephrine, and terbutaline. There are two principal types of adrenoreceptors: alpha (α) and beta (β). These receptors have been further subdivided into the main subtypes of α_1, α_2, β_1, β_2, and $\beta 3$ (see Fig. 18.1).

The activation of alpha and beta receptors through the administration of adrenergic agonists produces effects consistent with sympathetic (fight-or-flight) stimulation. The *nonselective adrenergic agonists* activate alpha and beta receptors. The agonists have generally predictable actions, though stimulated receptor subtypes result in varying effects. The term *nonselective* means that two or more adrenergic receptor subtypes are stimulated. Epinephrine and NE stimulate all four types of alpha receptors. The adrenergic agonists are classified **in Table 18.1.**

The catecholamines and noncatecholamines have significant differences on a pharmacokinetic level. Catecholamines have a short duration of action because they are quickly destroyed by the enzymes *catechol-O-methyltransferase* and *monoamine oxidase (MAO)*. These destructive enzymes are active in the intestinal tract's mucosa, so catecholamines cannot be given orally. Instead, they are given parenterally or by inhalation. The oxygen-hydrogen groups on the catechol part of the molecule make the drugs **polar**, stopping them from crossing the blood-brain barrier. The noncatecholamines can be taken orally because they are not as easily destroyed by catechol-*O*-methyltransferase or MAO. Therefore this can extend their duration of action. Noncatecholamines are less polar than catecholamines, so they can enter the brain more efficiently and affect the CNS.

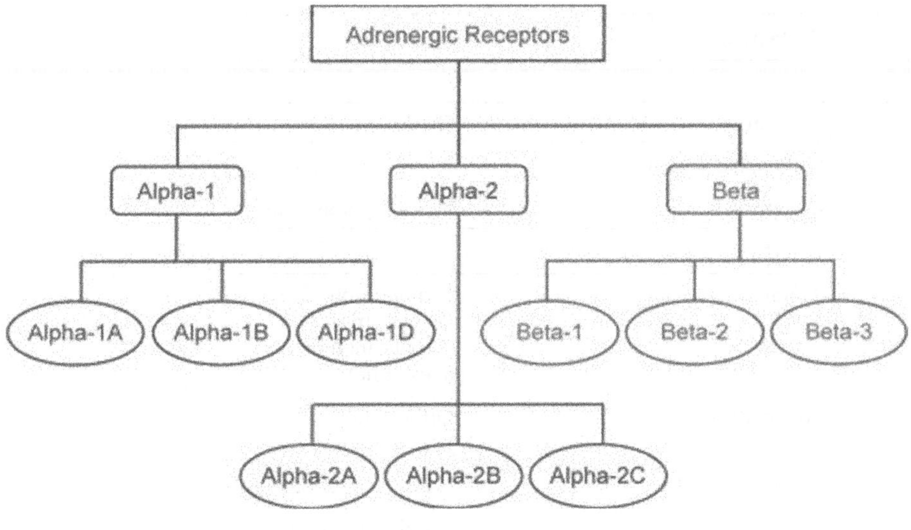

FIG. 18.1 A visual depiction of the types of adrenergic receptors.

You should remember

Adrenergic agonists work by mimicking the functions of the sympathetic nervous system. They may be direct acting, indirect acting, or dual acting. Adrenergic agonists cause a wide variety of effects. The most common are changes in heart rate and blood pressure. They are also used in ophthalmic solutions to constrict the eyes' blood vessels.

Alpha$_1$-adrenergic agonists

Alpha$_1$ receptors are located on blood vessels, influencing blood pressure and blood flow into the tissues. They are also found on the muscles of the **iris**, smooth muscle of the GI tract, male and female reproductive tracts, and sphincters of the urinary bladder. The stimulation of the alpha$_1$ receptors causes vasoconstriction of blood vessels, **mydriasis**, decreased GI motility, contraction of the external sphincter of the bladder, decreased bile secretion, and stimulation of sweat glands. Examples of alpha$_1$-adrenergic agonists include *midodrine, metaraminol,* and *phenylephrine.*

Pharmacokinetics

After oral administration, *midodrine* is quickly absorbed, with plasma levels of the prodrug peaking after about 30 minutes, declining with a half-life of about 25 minutes. The metabolite reaches peak blood concentrations approximately 1–2 hours after each dose, with a half-life of 3–4 hours. Absolute bioavailability is measured as *desglymidodrine* and is about 93%. The bioavailability of *metaraminol* is unknown, with approximately 45% protein binding and metabolism via the liver. *Phenylephrine* has 38% bioavailability through the GI tract and protein binding of 95% and is metabolized in the liver via oxidative deamination. The onset of action when given IV is rapid and within 20 minutes when given orally. Elimination half-life is 2.1–3.4 hours, and duration of action is up to 20 minutes (IV) and up to 4 hours (orally). However, in newer studies, oral phenylephrine is ineffective as a nasal decongestant, and the FDA is considering the drug's removal from OTC cough and cold products, which could significantly disrupt the market for the makers of cold medicines and affect patients. Oral phenylephrine is not dangerous in OTC doses, and patients with common cold symptoms may find some relief from the other ingredients in multiproduct formulations.

Mechanism of action

The mechanism of action of *midodrine* is via its formation of the active metabolite *desglymidodrine,* which exerts its effects by activating the alpha-adrenergic receptors of the arteriolar and venous vasculature. This increases vascular tone and elevates blood pressure. *Metaraminol* acts through peripheral vasoconstriction, increasing systolic and

TABLE 18.1 Classifications of the adrenergic agonists.

Generic name	Trade name	Primary use
Catecholamines		
dopamine	Intropin	Shock
Epinephrine	EpiPen, Adrenalin	Allergic reactions
Norepinephrine	Levophed	Shock, hypotension
Alpha$_1$-adrenergic agonists		
metaraminol	Aramine	Hypotension (especially as a complication of anesthesia)
midodrine	ProAmatine	Orthostatic hypotension
oxymetazoline	Afrin	Nasal congestion
phenylephrine	Nasop	Nasal congestion
Alpha$_2$-adrenergic agonists		
apraclonidine	Iopidine Eye	Operative eye pressure, glaucoma
clonidine	Catapres	Hypertension
dexmedetomidine	Precedex	For sedation in intensive care
guanfacine	Tenex; common causes of secondary hypertension include primary aldosteronism, **parenchymal** diseases of the kidneys, renovascular disease, and sleep apnea, Intuniv	Hypertension, ADHD
lofexidine	Lucemyra	Opioid withdrawal, postmenopausal hot flashes
methyldopa	generic only	Hypertension
tizanidine	Zanaflex	Muscle spasticity
Beta$_1$-adrenergic agonists		
dobutamine	Dobutrex	Cardiac decompensation
isoproterenol	Isuprel	Dysrhythmias, heart failure
Beta$_2$-adrenergic agonists		
albuterol	Ventolin HFA, ProAir HFA	Asthma
arformoterol	Brovana	COPD
indacaterol	Arcapta Neohaler	COPD
levalbuterol	Xopenex	Asthma, COPD
metaproterenol	Alupent	Asthma

TABLE 18.1 Classifications of the adrenergic agonists.—cont'd

Generic name	Trade name	Primary use
olodaterol	Striverdi Respimat	COPD
salmeterol	Serevent Diskus	Asthma, exercise-induced bronchospasm, COPD
terbutaline	generic only	Asthma
Beta$_3$-adrenergic agonists		
mirabegron	Myrbetriq	Overactive bladder
solabegron	(still under development)	Overactive bladder, irritable bowel syndrome
Miscellaneous adrenergic agonists		
amphetamine	Evekeo	Narcolepsy, ADHD, obesity
ephedrine	generic only	Allergies, asthma, narcolepsy
methylphenidate	Ritalin	ADHD, obesity
pseudoephedrine	Sudafed	Rhinitis, coryza, sinusitis

ADHD, Attention-deficit/hyperactivity disorder.

diastolic blood pressure. It may work by inhibiting *adenyl cyclase,* leading to an inhibition in *cyclic adenosine monophosphate (cAMP)* production. The drug also releases NE from its storage sites indirectly. *Phenylephrine* mediates vasoconstriction and mydriasis based on its route and administration location. Systemic exposure increases systolic and diastolic blood pressure and peripheral vascular resistance. Increased BP stimulates the vagus nerve, resulting in reflex bradycardia.

Clinical indications

Alpha$_1$-adrenergic agonists treat hypotension, nasal congestion, and subconjunctival hemorrhage (red eye). *Midodrine* is especially indicated for symptomatic **orthostatic hypotension**. *Metaraminol* is commonly used to treat and prevent hypotension caused by bleeding, shock due to brain damage, and spinal anesthesia. *Phenylephrine* injections are indicated for hypotension caused by shock or anesthesia. An ophthalmic formulation is shown to dilate the pupils and cause vasoconstriction, an intranasal formulation for congestion, and a topical formulation for hemorrhoids. The drug also has an off-label use in the treatment of **priapism**.

Contraindications

Alpha$_1$-adrenergic agonists are contraindicated for severe coronary or cardiovascular disease, glaucoma, hypovolemia (within 2 weeks of taking MAO inhibitors), urine retention, **pheochromocytoma**, Graves disease, sensitivity to adrenergic substances, ventricular tachycardia, and in pregnant or lactating females or children.

Adverse effects

The common adverse effects of alpha$_1$-adrenergic agonists are hypertension, blurred vision, constipation, urine retention, goosebumps, and sweating. *Midodrine* may also cause numbness, tingling, scalp itching, chills, and a skin rash. *Metaraminol* may cause headaches, nausea, vomiting, anxiety, dizziness, or nervousness. *Phenylephrine* may also cause mild nausea, insomnia, lightheadedness, tremor, and tachycardia.

Toxicity

Hypertension, piloerection, chills, and urinary retention may signify midodrine toxicity. *Metaraminol* has no significant toxicities in humans. *Phenylephrine* toxicity may be indicated by headache, hypertension, reflex bradycardia, tingling of the limbs, cardiac arrhythmias, and a feeling of fullness in the head.

You should remember

The alpha$_1$-adrenoceptors are the predominant alpha receptors located on vascular smooth muscle. Alpha$_1$-adrenergic agonists constrict arteries and veins, but their effects are more pronounced in the arterial resistance vessels. The alpha$_1$-adrenergic agonists are also referred to as systemic vasoconstrictors.

Alpha$_2$-adrenergic agonists

Alpha$_2$ receptors are located on the presynaptic neurons and seem to function as controllers of neurotransmitter release by the presynaptic neurons. The alpha$_2$-adrenergic agonists are often used in reducing blood pressure. The centrally acting agonists of this group stimulate receptors in the CNS to decrease sympathetic nervous system activity and lower BP and heart rate. Examples of these agonists include *clonidine, dexmedetomidine, lofexidine,* and *tizanidine*.

Pharmacokinetics

Clonidine has an oral bioavailability of 70%–80%. Its protein binding is 20%–40%, and it is metabolized in the liver to inactive metabolites. The most common form is the immediate release, which has an onset of action within 30–60 minutes after an oral dose. The elimination half-life is 12–16 hours in patients via the kidney. Excretion is 72% in the urine. *Dexmedetomidine* has a protein binding of 94% and is near total liver metabolism to active metabolites. Its elimination half-life is 2–4 hours and excreted in the urine. *Lofexidine* has an oral bioavailability of about 90% with extensive absorption. Peak plasma concentrations occur within 3 hours of a single administration, and the half-life is 11 hours. The drug is extensively metabolized in the liver and cleared mainly by the kidneys. It is 80%–90% plasma protein bound. *Tizanidine* has a bioavailability of about 40% and protein binding of 30% and is 95% metabolized in the liver. The elimination of the drug is 3 hours, but its inactive metabolites take 20–40 hours for this to occur. It is 80% excreted in the urine and 20% in the feces.

Mechanism of action

Alpha$_2$-adrenergic agonists stimulate alpha$_2$-adrenergic receptors in the CNS to inhibit sympathetic vasomotor centers. They reduce plasma concentrations of NE, decrease systolic blood pressure and heart rate, and inhibit **renin** release from the kidneys. *Clonidine* works by crossing the blood-brain barrier, stimulating alpha$_2$ receptors in the **brainstem** to decrease peripheral vascular resistance and lower blood pressure. It has specificity towards presynaptic alpha 2 receptors in the vasomotor center. *Dexmedetomidine* acts in the same way as clonidine. *Lofexidine* binds to the same receptors to reduce NE release and decrease **sympathetic tone**. *Tizanidine* has an unclear mechanism of action.

Clinical indications

Alpha$_2$-adrenergic agonists are used to treat hypertension alone or with diuretic agents. They are also used epidurally as an adjunct therapy for severe pain. *Clonidine* is also used to treat ADHD, alcohol, opioids, nicotine withdrawal, menopausal flushing, diarrhea, spasticity, and some pain conditions. *Dexmedetomidine* is often used in intensive care settings to achieve light to moderate sedation and has analgesic properties. Because it is opioid sparing, it does not cause significant respiratory depression. It can be used in mechanically ventilated adults, reducing the time to remove the breathing tube and the need to remain in the ICU. This drug is also used for procedural sedation, such as during **colonoscopy**, as an adjunct to other sedatives to decrease their dosages, as an adjunct to subarachnoid or epidural space to produce anesthesia for leg surgeries, and also to treat adverse cardiovascular effects of acute amphetamine or cocaine intoxication and overdose. *Lofexidine* treats opioid withdrawal over 14 days and for females suffering from postmenopausal hot flashes. *Tizanidine* is indicated for muscle spasticity due to spinal cord injury or multiple sclerosis.

Contraindications/warnings

Alpha$_2$-adrenergic agonists are contraindicated in pediatric, pregnant, and lactating patients; hypertension that is associated with **preeclampsia**; hepatitis; cirrhosis; **polyarteritis nodosa**; pheochromocytoma; **scleroderma**; and

blood dyscrasia. *Clonidine* is also contraindicated with depression, dry eye, myocardial infarction, atrioventricular block, sinus bradycardia, and stroke. *Dexmedetomidine* has no absolute contraindications but must be used carefully in higher doses if bradycardia is present. *Lofexidine* is not recommended in patients taking beta blockers or angiotensin-converting enzyme inhibitors due to decreased blood pressure or heart rate risks. *Tizanidine* is contraindicated in patients with known hypersensitivity. It must be used with caution if the patient has hypotension, renal impairment or failure, hepatic disease when driving or operating machinery, psychosis, during pregnancy and breastfeeding, and in geriatric patients. All of these drugs should never be discontinued abruptly.

Adverse effects

Adverse effects of alpha$_2$-adrenergic agonists include hypotension, peripheral edema, dry mouth or eyes, constipation, drowsiness, dizziness, rash, pruritus, impotence, nausea, vomiting, hepatitis, hallucinations, depression, and recurrent herpes simplex. *Clonidine* may also cause fatigue, generalized weakness, and irritability. *Dexmedetomidine* has induced hypertension when given via rapid IV or bolus. *Lofexidine* may also cause bradycardia and sleepiness. *Tizanidine* has caused severe effects such as bradycardia, **exfoliative dermatitis**, hepatic failure, angioedema, and anaphylactoid reactions. Moderate adverse effects include cystitis, hypotension, constipation, elevated hepatic enzymes, **dyskinesia**, excitability, blurred vision, hallucinations, hepatitis, hyperlipidemia, **leukopenia**, anemia, **thrombocytopenia**, depression, and jaundice.

Toxicity

Clonidine toxicity can cause severe cardiopulmonary instability and CNS depression. *Dexmedetomidine* toxicity from bolus injection can cause life-threatening bradycardia, hypotension, **miosis**, and hypoglycemia. *Lofexidine* during gestation can reduce birth weight, lower survival rates, and increase abortion rates. *Tizanidine* toxicity may result in signs of depressed cardiac function, including bradycardia and hypotension.

You should remember

The alpha$_2$-adrenergic agonists are centrally acting vasodilators. They block sympathetic activity, reducing sympathetic outflow to the heart and decreasing cardiac output because heart rate and contractility also decrease. The centrally acting agents are used in treating hypertension but are not considered first-line therapy, mainly because of adverse effects related to their actions in the brain. They are usually given with a diuretic to prevent fluid accumulation.

Beta$_1$-adrenergic agonists

Beta$_1$ receptors are located on the myocardium, fat cells, sphincters, smooth muscle of the GI tract, and renal arterioles. Two critical drugs represent this group: *dobutamine*, a selective beta$_1$-adrenergic agonist, and *isoproterenol*, a nonselective beta$_1$-adrenergic agonist. These agonists affect the three different beta-adrenoceptors in other cell types of many organs. The beta$_1$ subtype is mainly in the heart, kidneys, and adipocytes. Elevated heart rate and cardiac contractility occur because of beta$_1$ subtype stimulation. Beta$_2$-adrenoceptors are present in the lungs, bronchi, vascular smooth muscle, heart, uterus, bladder, adipocytes, eyes, liver, and skeletal muscle. This subtype, when activated, regulates the presynaptic release of NE, vasodilation, and bronchodilation. The beta$_3$-adrenoceptors are present in the heart, uterus, bladder, and adipocytes. They regulate cardiac contractility inhibition, bladder relaxation, uterine function, GI smooth muscle function, and lipolysis.

Pharmacokinetics

Dobutamine has an onset of action within 2 minutes, with an elimination half-life of 2 minutes. It is used for short term and up to 72 hours. It is a direct-acting agent that stimulates the beta-adrenoceptors of the heart. Dobutamine is readily metabolized in the liver. *Isoproterenol* is quickly absorbed after parenteral administration, with effects continuing for several minutes. It is metabolized in the liver and excreted in the urine. Its elimination half-life is approximately 2 minutes.

Mechanism of action

$Beta_1$-adrenergic agonists increase the rate and force of contraction of the heart, boost lipolysis in adipose tissue, decrease digestion and GI motility, and increase glomerular filtration. *Dobutamine* is a synthetic catecholamine that acts on $beta_1$ receptors to increase myocardial contractility and stroke volume, increasing cardiac output. It also has actions upon the $beta_2$ and $alpha_1$ receptors. *Isoproterenol* is a $beta_1$-adrenergic agonist that also has $beta_2$ action.

Clinical indications

$Beta_1$-adrenergic agonists treat circulatory shock, hypotension, and cardiac arrest. *Dobutamine* is used when parenteral therapy is required as **inotropic** support for short-term treatment of **cardiac decompensation** from depressed contractility, which can be due to organic heart disease or cardiac surgeries. *Isoproterenol* is used to treat heart block and episodes of Adams-Stokes syndrome that are not caused by ventricular tachycardia or fibrillation. It is also used in emergencies for cardiac arrest until electric shock can be started; for bronchospasm during anesthesia and as an adjunct to treat hypovolemic, septic, or cardiogenic shock; low cardiac output; and congestive heart failure. The drug can also improve the condition of intestinal stem cells mediated by $beta_2$-adrenoreceptors following chemotherapy.

Contraindications

Dobutamine is contraindicated in patients with idiopathic hypertrophic subaortic stenosis and those who have previously shown signs of hypersensitivity to the drug. *Isoproterenol* is contraindicated in patients with tachyarrhythmias, heart block caused by an overdose of digoxin, ventricular arrhythmias requiring inotropic therapy, or in patients with angina.

Adverse effects

The common adverse effects of $beta_1$-adrenergic agonists include hypertension, tachycardia, and constipation. *Dobutamine* may also cause **ectopic heartbeat** and phlebitis. *Isoproterenol* can also cause nervousness, headaches, dizziness, nausea, palpitations, angina, pulmonary edema, ventricular arrhythmias, tachyarrhythmias, difficulty breathing, sweating, mild tremors, weakness, flushing, and pallor. Often, isoproterenol has caused insulin resistance, leading to diabetic **ketoacidosis**.

Toxicities

Dobutamine toxicity is rare because of its short half-life. However, if symptoms of toxicity occur, they are usually due to sympathetic overstimulation and may include chest pain, headaches, palpitations, shortness of breath, tremors, nausea, and vomiting. If tachycardia occurs, it can be reversed by using IV metoprolol. *Isoproterenol* toxicity is not common either but is signified by arrhythmias, palpitations, tachycardia, headaches, flushing, and angina.

You should remember

$Beta_1$-adrenergic agonists have very selective actions upon the heart. Beta-adrenoceptors usually bind to NE released by sympathetic adrenergic nerves and to circulating epinephrine. The result is cardiac stimulation, including increased heart rate, contractility, conduction velocity, and relaxation.

$Beta_2$-adrenergic agonists

The $beta_2$-adrenoreceptors are distributed on the smooth muscle of the bronchioles; in blood vessels supplying the brain, heart, and kidneys; and in the uterus. There are four types of $beta_2$-adrenergic agonists based on their actions. One example of each class is described here: short acting (albuterol), long acting (salmeterol), ultra long acting (indacaterol), and with unknown duration of action (isoxsuprine, but this was withdrawn from the US market because of a lack of substantial evidence of its effectiveness).

Pharmacokinetics

Albuterol is a short-acting agonist, becoming effective in less than 15 minutes when inhaled and in less than 30 minutes as an oral pill. It is metabolized in the liver and has an elimination half-life of 3.8–6 hours and a duration of action of 2–6 hours. Albuterol is excreted via the urine. *Salmeterol* is a long-acting agonist with a protein binding of 96%. It is metabolized in the liver, and its elimination half-life is 5.5 hours. *Indacaterol* takes effect in about 5 minutes, reaching peak effects at 2–4 hours but lasting for 24 hours. The drug is mainly excreted in the urine and less in the feces.

Mechanism of action

Stimulation of beta$_2$ receptors results in bronchodilation; vasodilation of blood vessels to the brain, heart, kidneys, and skeletal muscle; and relaxation of the uterus in pregnancy. *Albuterol* activates the receptors, leading to the activation of adenyl cyclase and increased intracellular concentrations of cAMP. *Salmeterol* stimulates the beta$_2$ receptors in the bronchial musculature, causing them to relax. Smooth muscle tone is decreased. Salmeterol is 10,000 times more lipid soluble than albuterol. Also, salmeterol dissolves in the lipid bilayer of the cell membrane. *Indacaterol* activates its receptors to relax the bronchial tubes of the airways.

Clinical indications

Beta$_2$-adrenergic agonists are used in patients with COPD, circulatory shock, premature labor, and peripheral vascular disease. *Albuterol* is indicated explicitly for relief and prevention of bronchospasm and acute prophylaxis against anything that induces bronchospasm. *Salmeterol* is indicated for moderate-to-severe persistent asthma after previous treatment with a short-acting beta$_2$ agonist in combination with inhaled corticosteroids. The drug is also used for COPD with or without corticosteroids and can be used as monotherapy for exercise-induced bronchospasm. *Indacaterol* is indicated for the treatment of COPD.

Contraindications

Beta$_2$-adrenergic agonists are contraindicated in pediatric, pregnant, or lactating patients, in those who are sensitive to other sympathomimetic agents, and in patients with cardiac arrhythmias associated with tachycardia or digoxin intoxication, hyperthyroidism, preeclampsia, **eclampsia**, intrauterine infection, hypertension, diabetes mellitus, hypovolemia, **thyrotoxicosis**, hypersensitivity, coronary artery disease, and angle-closure glaucoma. *Albuterol* is contraindicated in patients who have arrhythmias. *Salmeterol* is contraindicated as a *monotherapy* for asthma; as a primary treatment of status asthmaticus, acute episodes of asthma, or COPD that requires intensive measures; and if the patient has severe hypersensitivity to milk proteins or with known hypersensitivity to the drug. *Indacaterol* is contraindicated with known hypersensitivity.

Adverse effects

The common adverse effects of beta$_2$-adrenergic agonists include muscle tremors, increased muscle tension, and feelings of warmth. These agents also cause hyperglycemia. *Albuterol* may cause anxiety, headaches, dry mouth, palpitations, tachycardia, flushing, alterations of sleep and behaviors, and, rarely, myocardial ischemia. *Salmeterol* may also cause dizziness, sinus infections, migraine headaches, and hypokalemia. *Indacaterol* may also cause inflammation in the extremities, tachycardia, palpitations, upper respiratory tract infections, headache, dizziness, nausea, itching, rash, and joint pain.

Toxicities

Albuterol toxicity may cause angina, seizures, hypertension or hypotension, tachycardia, arrhythmias, nervousness, headache, tremors, muscle cramps, dry mouth, palpitations, nausea, dizziness, fatigue, malaise, insomnia, hyperglycemia, hypokalemia, and metabolic acidosis. *Salmeterol* toxicity may cause tachycardia, skeletal muscle hypertrophy, and hematological and blood biochemical changes. *Indacaterol* toxicity is linked to diabetes-type changes, heart abnormalities, hypertension, hypokalemia, seizures, thyroid abnormalities, tachycardia, arrhythmias, extreme excitability, insomnia, and allergic reactions. It should not be used during pregnancy and breastfeeding or be administered to children.

You should remember

Older adults may be more sensitive to the adverse effects of $beta_2$-adrenergic agonists, including tremors, hypertension, tachycardia, and arrhythmias. Also, elderly patients with heart or blood vessel abnormalities may require particular caution when using salmeterol.

$Beta_3$-adrenergic agonists

The $beta_3$-adrenergic agonists bind selectively to the β_3-adrenergic receptors. Since the 1990s, various agonists in this class have been in development for treating obesity and type 2 diabetes, but no successful drug has made it into the market. In 2012 *mirabegron (Myrbetriq)* was approved for the treatment of overactive bladder. In 2020 *vibegron (Gemtesa)* was approved for overactive bladder. Another drug called *solabegron* is still in developmental studies, and no trade name has yet been announced.

Pharmacokinetics

Mirabegron's bioavailability is dose dependent, ranging from 29%–35% bioavailability, and peak plasma concentrations are achieved within about 3.5 hours. About 71% of the drug binds to plasma proteins. It is metabolized in the liver via dealkylation, oxidation, direct glucuronidation, and amide hydrolysis. It is eliminated in the urine and has a half-life of about 50 hours. *Vibegron* has plasma protein binding of 51% and is metabolized mainly by oxidation and glucuronidation. Its elimination half-life is 60–70 hours. Excretion is primarily in the feces but also the urine. The pharmacokinetics of *solabegron* are still being studied.

Mechanism of action

Mirabegron affects the **detrusor muscles** of the urinary bladder, decreasing their contraction so that the bladder can store more urine at a given time. The drug also influences the nonvoiding contraction by reducing its frequency. *Vibegron* causes a conformational change in its target receptors, inducing activation of adenylate cyclase via G proteins, which promotes cAMP formation. *Solabegron* works in similar ways as mirabegron and vibegron.

Clinical indications

Mirabegron is indicated for treating overactive bladder. *Vibegron* is indicated for treating overactive bladder with symptoms of urge urinary incontinence, urgency, and urinary frequency in adults. *Solabegron* has not yet been approved but is being studied for overactive bladder and irritable bowel syndrome.

Contraindications

Mirabegron and *vibegron* are contraindicated with known hypersensitivity. In Canadian labeling, mirabegron is also contraindicated in people with severe uncontrolled hypertension and pregnancy. Use is not recommended in patients with liver abnormalities, severe liver disease, urinary bladder blockage, incomplete bladder emptying, and chronic kidney disease. The contraindications of *solabegron* are still being studied.

Adverse effects

Mirabegron commonly causes bladder pain, bloody or cloudy urine, problems with urination, dizziness, urgency, blurred vision, headaches, back pain, nervousness, and heart irregularities. *Vibegron* may cause dry mouth, headaches, urinary tract infections, symptoms resembling the common cold, bronchitis, constipation, diarrhea, nausea, and upper respiratory tract infections. The adverse effects of *solabegron* are still being studied.

Toxicities

Mirabegron has no clear human toxicities, Vibegron appears to have no significant ones, and Solabegron does not yet seem to have any significant ones.

You should remember

Mirabegron should never be used in patients with uncontrolled hypertension or if there has been previous hypertension, bladder obstruction, difficulty emptying the bladder, or kidney or liver disease. Also, the drug is never used in children younger than 3.

Key Terms

Adrenergic agonists
Blood dyscrasia
Brainstem
Cardiac decompensation
Colonoscopy
Detrusor muscles
Dyskinesia
Eclampsia
Ectopic heartbeat
Exfoliative dermatitis
Inotropic
Iris
Ketoacidosis
Leukopenia
Miosis
Mydriasis

Clinical Case Studies

Clinical Case Study 1

An 82-year-old obese male with type 2 diabetes is evaluated for his general health. Though warned against it, he has smoked two packs of cigarettes daily for 40 years. He tells the physician that his brother had recently died of a heart attack. He admits that his diet is poor and that he eats many snack foods and drinks two to three cans of beer daily. The patient also describes that his feet are swollen in the morning and that he often has a snack, such as pizza, before bed. His blood pressure was 167/84 mm Hg during the visit. He is currently taking clonidine for his hypertension and describes often having a headache, shortness of breath, facial flushing, and clammy skin.

Critical Thinking Questions

1. What are the indications of alpha$_2$-adrenergic agonists?
2. How does clonidine work?
3. What are the other indications for clonidine?

Clinical Case Study 2

A 41-year-old male has a significant history of asthma. He has used a rescue inhaler that contains albuterol about three times per week over the previous year. He complains of waking up with asthma symptoms about twice a month, indicating his condition is not well controlled. The patient is prescribed low-dose fluticasone to be taken in two puffs twice daily. Over time, this does not stop all of his symptoms, so the physician switches him to a combination of fluticasone/salmeterol, which will be taken as one puff twice daily. The asthma is controlled via moderate doses of fluticasone/salmeterol.

Critical Thinking Questions

1. What types of adrenergic agonists are commonly used for asthma?
2. Where are the beta$_2$-adrenoreceptors distributed?
3. What are the indications for salmeterol?

Further Reading

[1] H. Bonisch, J.P.M. Finberg, W.W. Fleming, K.H. Graefe, S.Z. Langer, et al., Handbook of Experimental Pharmacology, Springer, 2012.
[2] W. Delius, E. Gerlach, H. Grobecker, W. Kubler, Catecholamines and the Heart: Recent Advances in Experimental and Clinical Research, Springer-Verlag, 2011.
[3] M. Dorobantu, G. Mancia, G. Grassi, V. Voicu, Hypertension and Heart Failure: Epidemiology, Mechanisms and Treatment (Updates in Hypertension and Cardiovascular Protection), Springer, 2019.
[4] L.E. Eiden, Catecholamine Research in the 21st Century: Abstracts and Graphical Abstracts, 10th International Catecholamine Symposium, 2012, Academic Press, 2013.
[5] C.M. Hai, Vascular Smooth Muscle: Structure and Function in Health and Disease, World Scientific (WSPC), 2016.
[6] F. Kummer, Treatment of Asthma: The long-acting beta-2-agonists, Springer, 2012.
[7] L. Landsberg, Catecholamines: Physiology, Pharmacology, and Pathology for Students and Clinicians, Wolters Kluwer, 2017.
[8] A.G. Lawson, R.I. Gorman, Research Progress on Epinephrine, Nova Biomedical Books, 2013.
[9] B. Madden, Treatment of Pulmonary Hypertension (Current Cardiovascular Therapy), Springer, 2015.
[10] C. Mena, S. Jayasuriya, Peripheral Vascular Disease: A Clinical Approach, Lippincott, Williams, and Wilkins, 2019.
[11] I. Mitchell, G. Govias, Asthma Education: Principles and Practice for the Asthma Educator, second ed., Springer, 2021.
[12] T. Nagatsu, T. Nabeshima, R. McCarty, D.S. Goldstein, Catecholamine Research: From Molecular Insights to Clinical Medicine (Advances in Behavioral Biology – Volume 53), Springer, 2002.
[13] D. Sidebotham, A. McKee, M. Gillham, J.H. Levy, Cardiothoracic Critical Care, Butterworth-Heinemann, 2007.
[14] R.J. Solaro, J.C. Tardiff, Biophysics of the Failing Heart: Physics and Biology of Heart Muscle (Biological and Medical Physics, Biomedical Engineering), Springer, 2013.
[15] A. Turan Isik, P. Soysal, Orthostatic Hypotension in Older Adults, Springer, 2021.
[16] A.J. Wein, C. Chapple, Overactive Bladder in Clinical Practice, Springer, 2012.

CHAPTER

19

Adrenergic antagonists

OUTLINE

LEARNING OUTCOMES

After study of this chapter, readers should be able to:

1. Explain the classifications of adrenergic antagonists.
2. Describe the mechanisms of action of the alpha-adrenergic antagonists.
3. Explain indications for pharmacotherapy with the nonselective beta-adrenergic antagonists.
4. Compare the advantages of selective beta-antagonists with nonselective beta-antagonists.
5. Discuss contraindications for the use of alpha-receptor antagonists.
6. Identify common adverse effects of beta-receptor antagonists.

https://doi.org/10.1016/B978-0-443-29038-1.00019-1

7. Discuss clinical indications of the selective adrenergic antagonists.
8. Explain the toxicities of beta-blockers.

Overview

Adrenergic compounds inhibit the action of epinephrine, norepinephrine (NE), and other catecholamines that control autonomic outflow and some functions of the CNS at the adrenergic receptors or inhibit their release. Adrenergic antagonists can act either directly or indirectly. They are also called sympatholytics. There are five adrenergic receptors, which are divided into two groups. The first group of receptors are the beta (β)-adrenergic receptors. There are β_1, β_2, and β_3 receptors. The second group contains the alpha (α)-adrenoreceptors. There are only α_1 and α_2 receptors. Adrenergic receptors are near the heart, kidneys, lungs, and GI tract. There are also α-adrenoreceptors that are located on vascular smooth muscle. Adrenergic antagonists can show specificity for one receptor or subtype. Indirect-acting agents block adrenergic nerve transmission by inhibiting neurotransmitters' release or depleting neurotransmitters' stores. Adrenergic antagonists compete with NE for adrenergic receptors. They block NE from reaching its receptors, preventing symptoms of the fight-or-flight response. As sympathetic activation is reduced, nerve impulses from the parasympathetic nervous system dominate. Most symptoms produced by adrenergic antagonists involve parasympathetic activation.

Common adrenergic antagonists

Adrenergic antagonists (adrenoblockers) are compounds that inhibit the action of adrenaline (epinephrine), noradrenaline (NE), and other catecholamines that control autonomic outflow and some functions of the CNS at the adrenergic receptors or inhibit their release. Adrenergic antagonists include alpha-adrenergic antagonists and nonselective and selective beta-adrenergic antagonists. Table 19.1 lists the common adrenergic antagonists.

Alpha-adrenergic antagonists

Alpha-adrenergic antagonists can work reversibly or irreversibly. Some are nonselective and antagonize $alpha_1$ and $alpha_2$ receptors, while others are highly selective for $alpha_1$ receptors. All antagonize the effects of endogenous catecholamines. Because their target receptors are located on arterial smooth muscle, they primarily affect the cardiovascular system.

Pharmacokinetics

The bioavailability of *doxazosin* is 65%, while protein binding is 98%. It is metabolized in the liver and has an elimination half-life of 22 hours. *Prazosin* has about 60% bioavailability, protein binding of 97%, and an onset of action of 30–90 minutes. The half-life of the elimination is 2–3 hours, and the duration of the action is 10–24 hours. *Terazosin* has protein binding of 90%–94% and an elimination half-life of 12 hours. *Phentolamine* is metabolized in the liver and has an elimination half-life of only 19 minutes. *Phenoxybenzamine* has an elimination half-life of 24 hours.

Mechanism of action

These antagonists selectively inhibit the actions of alpha-adrenoreceptors, producing vasodilation in arterioles and reducing blood pressure. The selective $alpha_1$-antagonists are much safer and are primarily indicated for hypertension. They directly lower blood pressure by blocking $alpha_1$ receptors on arterial smooth muscle. Dilating veins indirectly lowers blood pressure by decreasing venous return to the heart. Cardiac output and systemic blood pressure are reduced. For hypertension, alpha blockers are usually administered simultaneously as diuretics or other antihypertensives.

Clinical indications

Applications for alpha-receptor antagonists include control of hypertension and treatment of patients with peripheral vascular disease, **pheochromocytoma**, and urinary retention. *Doxazosin* is used to treat hypertension, **benign prostatic hyperplasia**, and perioperative management of pheochromocytoma. *Terazosin* is a less preferred

TABLE 19.1 Adrenergic antagonists.

Generic name	Trade name	Primary uses
Alpha-adrenergic antagonists		
doxazosin	Cardura	Hypertension
phenoxybenzamine	Dibenzyline	Pheochromocytoma
phentolamine	OraVerse, Regitine	Hypertension during surgery or due to pheochromocytoma
prazosin	Minipress	Hypertension
terazosin	Hytrin	Hypertension
Nonselective beta-adrenergic antagonists		
labetalol	Trandate	Hypertension
nadolol	Corgard	Hypertension and angina
pindolol	Visken	Hypertension
propranolol	Inderal	Hypertension, angina, acute MI, dysrhythmias, and tremors
timolol	Blocadren	Hypertension
Selective beta-adrenergic antagonists		
acebutolol	Sectral	Hypertension, dysrhythmias
atenolol	Tenormin	Hypertension, angina
esmolol	Brevibloc	Dysrhythmias, atrial fibrillation, atrial flutter
metoprolol	Lopressor	Angina, hypertension

MI, Myocardial infarction.

option to treat hypertension but is often used to treat symptoms of an enlarged prostate. *Phentolamine* is used primarily to treat hypertensive emergencies caused by **pheochromocytoma** and for cocaine-induced cardiovascular complications if the patient does not fully respond to benzodiazepines, nitroglycerin, and calcium channel blockers. *Phenoxybenzamine* is also used for hypertension caused by pheochromocytoma and benign prostatic hyperplasia.

Contraindications

A contraindication for alpha-receptor antagonists is known hypersensitivity to any of these drugs. *Doxazosin* is contraindicated with orthostatic hypotension, liver dysfunctions, cataract surgery, and chronic idiopathic constipation. *Prazosin* is also contraindicated with the hypotensive. *Terazosin* is also contraindicated with priapism. *Phentolamine* is contraindicated with myocardial infarction, coronary insufficiency, and angina. *Phenoxybenzamine* is also contraindicated with coronary artery disease, hypotension, pneumonia, and decreased kidney function.

Adverse effects

The common adverse effects of alpha-receptor antagonists include nasal congestion and stuffiness, postural hypotension, inhibition of ejaculation, and lack of energy. Because these drugs may cause dizziness, advise patients to change positions slowly. To determine side effects, patients should avoid driving for at least 12 hours after taking the first dose. Patients should not breastfeed while taking these drugs or take OTC drugs for coughs, colds, or allergies without discussing it with their healthcare providers. *Doxazosin* may cause inflammation, nausea, shortness of breath, and abdominal pain. Severe adverse effects include arrhythmias and priapism. *Prazosin* and *terazosin* can cause headaches and palpitations. *Phentolamine* and *phenoxybenzamine* cause orthostatic hypotension, and phenoxybenzamine may also cause tachycardia and pinpoint pupils.

Toxicity

There are only limited reports of toxicity with alpha-adrenergic antagonists. In 2005, there was an acute *doxazosin* overdose, with the patient presenting with drowsiness, hypotension, and tachycardia. Toxicity for these agents appears to be low.

You should remember

Alpha$_1$-adrenergic antagonists are also called alpha blockers. They inhibit type 1 alpha-adrenergic receptors and therefore inhibit smooth muscle contraction. Their primary uses are hypertension and symptomatic benign prostatic hypertrophy. They lower blood pressure by preventing NE from tightening the muscles in the walls of smaller arteries and veins.

Beta-adrenergic antagonists

Beta-blocking drugs reduce receptor occupancy by beta-agonists. Most of these agents are pure antagonists and occupy beta receptors, causing no activation of the receptors. **Beta-adrenergic antagonists** work against the effects of catecholamines at beta-adrenoreceptors. Beta-blockade by these antagonists results in vasodilation, decreased peripheral resistance, and orthostatic hypotension. A primary use of these *beta-blockers* is to manage hypertension. Fig. 19.1 illustrates the impact of beta-blockers on atrial fibrillation (AF) precipitation because of anger or stress. The graph shows that anger or anxiety increased the odds of AF by 20 times in people not taking beta-blockers but only by four times in people taking these medications.

Pharmacokinetics

Based on the area under the concentration curve, the medications with the highest pharmacokinetic variability are metoprolol, propranolol, carvedilol, and nebivolol. The medicines with low to moderate variability include bisoprolol (the lowest), followed by atenolol, sotalol, labetalol, nadolol, and pindolol. Beta-adrenergic antagonists have 40%–90% bioavailability. They are metabolized in the liver via the CYP2D6 and CYP3A4 enzymes. Their elimination half-life is 3–7 hours, and they are excreted in the urine.

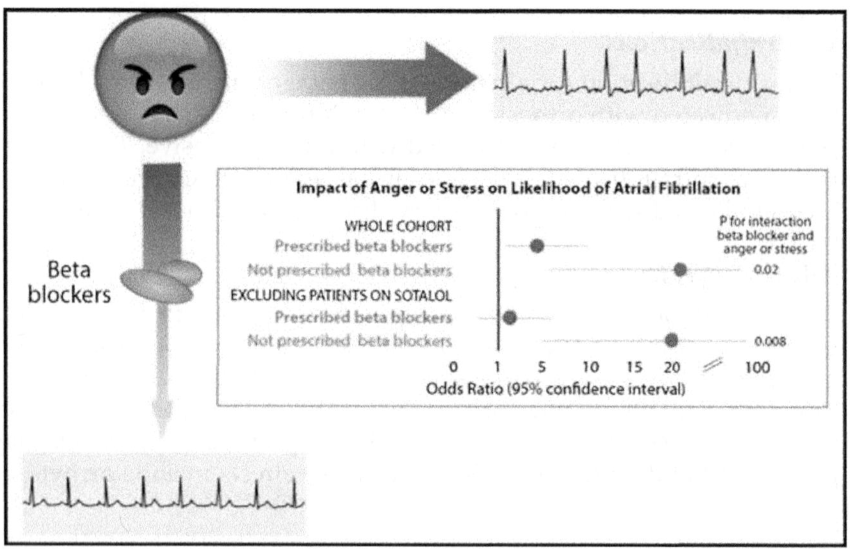

FIG. 19.1 The impact of beta-blockers on atrial fibrillation.

Mechanism of action

Metoprolol blocks beta$_1$-adrenergic receptors in heart muscle cells to decrease the slope of phase 4 in the nodal action potential. This reduces sodium ion uptake and prolongs the repolarization of phase 3, slowing the release of potassium ions. It additionally suppresses NE-induced increase in the sarcoplasmic reticulum calcium ion leak and the spontaneous sarcoplasmic reticulum calcium ion release, which are primary triggers for AF. *Propranolol* causes its effects by competitively blocking beta-adrenergic stimulation in the heart, usually induced by epinephrine and NE.

Carvedilol is a nonselective adrenergic blocker with alpha$_1$-adrenergic receptor antagonist properties. It is a nonselective cardiac beta-blocker with peripheral vasodilating effects and maintains cardiac output by decreasing afterload and a cardiac beta-blockade. It has a lesser impact on heart rate than pure selective beta-blockers. *Nebivolol* is a highly selective beta$_1$-adrenergic receptor antagonist with weak beta$_2$-adrenergic receptor antagonist activity. Its effects lead to decreased resting heart rate, exercise heart rate, myocardial contractility, systolic BP, and diastolic BP.

Bisoprolol is believed to be effective through antagonism of beta$_1$-adrenoceptors, resulting in lower cardiac output. It is a competitive, cardioselective antagonist that reduces cardiac workload by decreasing contractility and the need for oxygen through a competitive inhibitor of the beta$_1$-adrenergic receptors. *Atenolol* is a cardioselective beta-blocker, selectively binding to the beta$_1$-adrenergic receptors as an antagonist up to 26 times more than the beta$_2$ receptors. This produces cardioselectivity due to the higher population of the beta$_1$ receptor in cardiac tissue. *Sotalol* inhibits beta$_1$-adrenoreceptors in the myocardium and rapid potassium channels to slow repolarization, lengthen the QT interval, and slow as well as shorten the conduction of action potentials through the atria.

Labetalol nonselectively antagonizes beta-adrenergic receptors but selectively antagonizes alpha$_1$-adrenergic receptors. After oral administration, the beta-blocking ability is three times that of the alpha-blocking ability. This increases to 6.9 times after IV administration. Antagonism of alpha$_1$-adrenergic receptors results in vasodilation and decreased vascular resistance. *Nadolol* is described as being nonselective but does not interact with beta$_3$-adrenoreceptors. Its antagonism of beta$_1$- and beta$_2$-adrenoreceptors in the heart inhibits cyclic adenosine monophosphate, its signaling pathway to decrease the strength and speed of contractions and the rate of relaxation and conduction. Antagonism of beta$_2$-adrenoreceptors in smooth muscle cells of the vasculature inhibits their relaxation, reducing risks for severe hypotension. *Pindolol* is a nonselective beta-blocker. When it blocks beta$_1$-adrenergic receptors in the heart, BP and heart rate decrease. Blocking of beta$_1$ receptors in the juxtaglomerular apparatus inhibits the release of renin, which inhibits angiotensin II and aldosterone release. Reduced angiotensin II inhibits vasoconstriction, and reduced aldosterone inhibits water retention.

Clinical indications

These agents work primarily on cardiac muscle, competitively blocking beta-adrenergic receptors within the heart. They are used to manage hypertension—sometimes with a thiazide diuretic—for patients who have failed to respond to diet, exercise, and weight reduction. They also treat myocardial infarction (MI), tachyarrhythmias, hypertrophic subaortic stenosis, and angina pectoris.

Contraindications

Beta-blockers are contraindicated in patients with known hypersensitivity, heart block, severe heart failure, cardiogenic shock, and other severe circulatory disorders. These agents should be avoided in patients with a history of asthma or chronic obstructive airway disease unless there is no alternative. Breastfeeding must be avoided while taking these medications.

Adverse effects

Common adverse effects of beta-receptor antagonists are dizziness, lethargy, insomnia, and diarrhea. Patients must be taught to take their heart rate and BP and to report a decrease in either. Because these drugs may cause dizziness, patients are advised to change positions slowly. To determine side effects, patients should avoid driving for at least 12 hours after taking the first dose.

Toxicity

The general toxicities of the beta-adrenergic antagonists include excessive bradycardia, cardiac failure, hypotension, and bronchospasm. *Metoprolol* has also been linked to increased macrophages in the pulmonary alveoli, slight biliary hyperplasia, and small benign lung tumors. *Propranolol* can also cause hypoglycemic seizures, restlessness, euphoria, and insomnia. Patients with asthma may develop bronchospasm. *Carvedilol* may also cause cardiac insufficiency, cardiogenic shock, and cardiac arrest. *Nebivolol* can cause dizziness, hypoglycemia, fatigue, vomiting, and heart block. *Bisoprolol* can also cause hypoglycemia. *Atenolol* can cross the placenta, and fetuses exposed to this drug have been smaller than expected for gestational age. It also is carried in the breast milk and can cause bradycardia, hypothermia, and lethargy in the nursing infant. *Sotalol* toxicity may also result in congestive heart failure, hypoglycemia, cardiac asystole, prolonged QT interval, torsade de pointes, ventricular tachycardia, and premature ventricular complexes.

You should remember

Beta-adrenergic antagonists work by blocking the effects of epinephrine (adrenaline). They cause the heart to beat more slowly and with less force, lowering blood pressure. These medications also help widen veins and arteries to improve blood flow. They may take up to 2 hours to reach their full effect. They are also helpful in managing angina, hypertension, migraine, and tremor and preventing recurring heart attacks.

Nonselective beta-adrenergic antagonists

The nonselective beta-adrenergic antagonists include *labetalol, nadolol, pindolol, propranolol,* and *timolol*. Their characteristics are summarized separately as follows.

Pharmacokinetics

Labetalol has 25% bioavailability and 50% protein binding, and its metabolism in the liver is primarily through **conjugation** to glucuronide metabolites. Via oral administration, the elimination half-life is 6–8 hours. Via IV, the elimination half-life is 5.5 hours. The drug is excreted in the urine and not removed by hemodialysis. *Nadolol* has 30% protein binding and is partially metabolized in the liver. Its elimination half-life is 14–24 hours, and excretion is primarily unchanged in the urine and feces. *Pindolol* has 50%–95% bioavailability and is metabolized in the liver. Its elimination half-life is 3–4 hours and excreted in the urine. *Propranolol* has 26% bioavailability and 90% protein binding, is completely absorbed after oral administration, and is widely distributed throughout tissues. The drug is completely metabolized in the liver. Elimination occurs almost wholly by metabolic transformation in the liver and excretion of the resultant products in the urine. *Timolol* has 60% bioavailability, is 80% metabolized in the liver, and has an onset of action of 15–30 minutes. Its elimination half-life is 2.5–5 hours, the duration of action is 24 hours, and it is excreted in the urine.

Mechanism of action

Labetalol has dual alpha and beta-adrenergic antagonism, with different physiological effects over short- and long-term situations. Short-term effects include a decrease in blood pressure by decreasing systemic vascular resistance, with only a minor impact on cardiac output, heart rate, and **stroke volume**. Long-term effects include reduced heart rate during exercise while maintaining cardiac output via increased stroke volume. Labetalol competes with other catecholamines for binding to alpha and beta receptors and has potent yet reversible actions. *Nadolol* nonselectively blocks $beta_1$ and $beta_2$ receptors, though it prefers $beta_1$ receptors. It also impairs atrioventricular node conduction and decreases the sinus rate. *Pindolol* blocks $beta_1$ receptors in the **juxtaglomerular apparatus** to inhibit renin release. This inhibits the release of angiotensin II and **aldosterone**. *Propranolol* inhibits the activation of adenylate cyclase and cyclic adenosine monophosphate synthesis. *Timolol* reduces the formation of aqueous humor in the eye's **ciliary body** and works similarly to the other drugs in this classification within the heart.

Clinical indications

Labetalol is effective for hypertensive emergencies, pheochromocytoma-related hypertension, postoperative hypertension, and rebound hypertension from beta-blocker withdrawal. It is beneficial for pregnancy-induced hypertension associated with preeclampsia. Labetalol is also an alternative treatment for severe hypertension. *Nadolol* is used for hypertension, long-term treatment of angina pectoris, and as an off-label drug for AF, migraine headaches, bleeding veins with **portal hypertension** due to cirrhosis, and high thyroid hormone levels. *Pindolol* is used for hypertension, angina pectoris, arrhythmias, and prevention of acute stress reactions. *Propranolol* is indicated for hypertension, angina pectoris (except variant angina), MI, tachycardia, muscle tremor, portal hypertension, prevention of esophageal variceal bleeding and ascites, anxiety, hypertrophic cardiomyopathy, migraine and cluster headaches, excessive sweating, glaucoma, and thyrotoxicosis. *Timolol* is indicated for hypertension, prevention of MI, prevention of migraine headaches, and open angle glaucoma.

Contraindications

Labetalol is contraindicated with overt cardiac failure, higher than first-degree heart block, cardiogenic shock, severe bradycardia, history of asthma, COPD, severe hypotension, and hypersensitivity to the drug. *Nadolol* has similar contraindications, including for any severe heart disease. *Pindolol* is contraindicated with hyperthyroidism and can only be used cautiously for angina pectoris due to its intrinsic sympathomimetic activity. *Propranolol* is contraindicated with asthma, COPD, bradycardia, second or third-degree atrioventricular block, shock, severe hypotension, and cocaine toxicity. *Timolol* is contraindicated with known hypersensitivity, asthma, COPD, bradycardia, heart block, and heart failure.

Adverse effects

Common adverse effects of *labetalol* include dizziness, headaches, nausea, dyspepsia, nasal congestion, inability to ejaculate, dyspnea, fatigue, vertigo, and orthostatic hypotension. Hypotension is more severe and common when intravenous labetalol is given intravenously, which is also often why large oral doses cannot be used. *Nadolol* most commonly causes dizziness and fatigue. *Pindolol* may also cause lightheadedness, insomnia, unusual dreams, heartburn, coldness of the hands or feet, and muscle or joint pain. *Propranolol* mainly causes mild and transient dizziness, tiredness, insomnia, and nightmares. *Timolol* has serious adverse effects of cardiac arrhythmias and severe bronchospasm. It can also cause syncope, congestive heart failure, depression, confusion, impotence, and worsening of **Raynaud syndrome**. Timolol can cause burning, redness, corneal numbness, and superficial **punctate keratopathy** in the eyes (see Fig. 19.2).

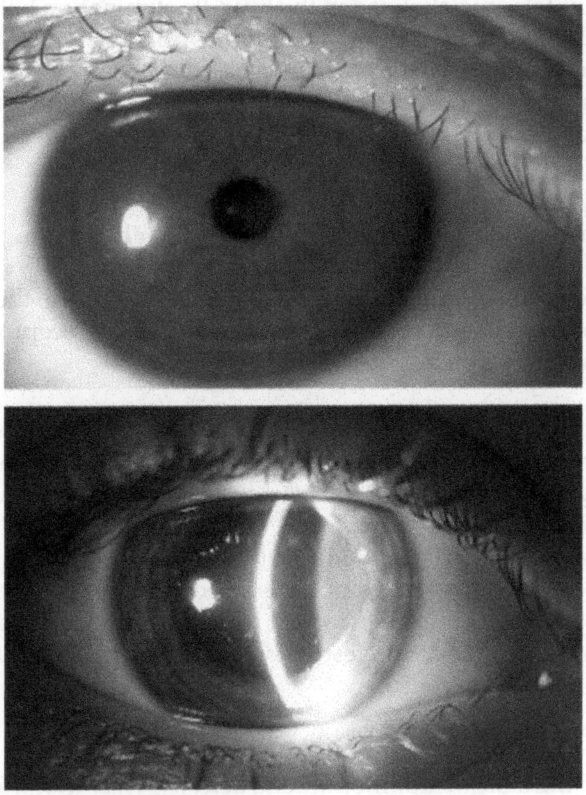

FIG. 19.2 Punctate keratopathy.

Toxicity

Labetalol toxicity may cause bradycardia, wheezing, chest tightness, difficulty breathing, extreme dizziness, seizures, and syncope. *Nadolol* toxicity is signified by severe hypotension, bradycardia, bronchospasm, heart failure, hypoglycemia, seizures, and coma. *Pindolol* toxicity may cause extreme bradycardia, cardiac failure, hypotension, and bronchospasm. *Propranolol* toxicity can cause severe hypotension, bradycardia, asystole, or profound myocardial depression. *Timolol* toxicity may cause dizziness, headaches, shortness of breath, bradycardia, bronchospasm, and, less often, cardiac arrest.

You should remember

The nonselective beta-blockers inhibit all of the body's beta receptors, resulting in decreased heart rate, heart contractions, oxygen demand by the heart, and blood pressure. They treat hypertension, angina, migraine, pheochromocytoma, supraventricular arrhythmia, and portal hypertension.

Selective $beta_1$-adrenergic antagonists

The selective adrenergic antagonists for the $beta_1$ receptor in the myocardium are used for hypertension and other cardiovascular conditions. They have fewer noncardiac adverse effects than nonselective drugs such as propranolol. The selective adrenergic antagonists include *acebutolol, atenolol, esmolol,* and *metoprolol.* Their characteristics are summarized separately below.

Pharmacokinetics

Acebutolol is well absorbed from the GI tract but undergoes substantial first-pass metabolization. The bioavailability is 40%, and peak plasma levels are reached within 2–2.5 hours after oral dosing. The elimination half-life of 3–4 hours. The drug is 60% excreted via the biliary tract and 30% in the urine. *Atenolol* has 40%–50% bioavailability and 6%–16% protein binding. Only 5% of the atenolol is metabolized in the liver. Its elimination half-life is 6–7 hours and excreted in the urine. *Esmolol* has a rapid distribution half-life of about 2 minutes and an elimination half-life of about 9 minutes. It is excreted in the urine. *Metoprolol* is absorbed via the small intestine, and over 95% of an oral therapeutic dose is generally eliminated in the urine as unchanged drug and metabolites. The bioavailability of a single dose is 50%, but in multiple quantities, it is 70%. It is metabolized in the liver, and its elimination half-life is 3–7 hours in the urine.

Mechanism of action

The selective adrenergic antagonists block the $beta_1$ receptors to lower heart rate and blood pressure, opposing the effects of epinephrine. They *block* the adrenergic activity of epinephrine and NE, decreasing inotropic contractility and conduction. They also increase atrioventricular refractory time and decrease the oxygen demand of the myocardium. The selective adrenergic antagonists also block the $beta_1$-adrenergic receptors to reduce sodium ion uptake and slow the release of potassium ions, reducing the likelihood of AF.

Clinical indications

Acebutolol is indicated for hypertension, ventricular and atrial cardiac arrhythmias, acute myocardial infarction in high-risk patients, and **Smith-Magenis syndrome**. *Atenolol* is indicated for hyperthyroidism, hypertension, angina, acute MI, supraventricular and ventricular tachycardia, and for the symptoms of alcohol withdrawal. *Esmolol* stops supraventricular tachycardia, episodic AF or flutter, and arrhythmias during anesthesia. It reduces heart rate and blood pressure during and after cardiac surgery. Esmolol is used in the early treatment of MI and to minimize the **hemodynamic response** to laryngoscopy and intubation. *Metoprolol* is indicated for hypertension, angina, acute MI, supraventricular or ventricular tachycardia, congestive heart failure, prevention of migraine headaches, and as an adjunct for hyperthyroidism.

Contraindications

Because of its partial agonist or intrinsic sympathomimetic activity, Acebutolol is contraindicated with stable or unstable angina. *Atenolol* is contraindicated with depression, myasthenia gravis, complete heart block, second-degree atrioventricular heart block, sinus bradycardia, Raynaud phenomenon, and asthma. *Esmolol* is contraindicated with sinus bradycardia, atrioventricular heart block, cardiogenic shock, pulmonary hypertension, heart failure, and known hypersensitivity. *Metoprolol* should be avoided in patients with pheochromocytoma, diabetes mellitus, hypoglycemia, depression, alcoholism, myasthenia gravis, complete heart block, and second-degree atrioventricular heart block.

Adverse effects

The adverse effects of *acebutolol include* the development of **antinuclear antibodies**, arthralgic pain, myalgias, and **systemic lupus erythematosus**. Females are more likely to develop these adverse effects. There have also been a few cases of hepatoxicity with increased liver enzymes. *Atenolol* may cause new-onset type 2 diabetes mellitus, blurred vision, coldness of the hands or feet, difficult or labored breathing, orthostatic hypotension, shortness of breath, tightness in the chest, and wheezing. *Esmolol* may cause anxiety, drowsiness, nausea, vomiting, headaches, nervousness, and reddening of the face and neck. The adverse effects of *metoprolol* also include dizziness, fatigue, diarrhea, unusual dreams, insomnia, depression, and reduced salivation. Serious adverse effects that must be reported immediately include bradycardia, persistent dizziness, fainting, unusual fatigue, cyanosis, hand and feet numbness, tingling or swelling, sexual dysfunction, hair loss, mental or mood changes, breathing difficulty, coughing, dyslipidemia, and increased thirst.

Toxicity

Acebutolol is one of the most toxic beta-blockers if an overdose occurs. It has caused deaths due to significant QT interval prolongation. *Atenolol* toxicity may cause bradycardia, hypotension, low cardiac output, cardiac failure, cardiogenic shock, bronchospasm, and respiratory depression. *Esmolol* toxicity may cause bradycardia, atrioventricular block, complete atrioventricular dissociation, decreased contractility, cardiogenic shock, asystole, and pulseless electrical activity.

You should remember

Drinking alcohol while taking any beta-blocker, such as metoprolol, is not recommended. These drugs reduce blood pressure and slow the heart rate, reducing the force of each heartbeat. Alcohol can also reduce BP, so combining it with beta-blockers creates an additive effect, and the BP can drop to a dangerously low level.

Key Terms

Aldosterone
Alpha-adrenergic antagonists
Antinuclear antibodies
Benign prostatic hyperplasia
Beta-adrenergic antagonists
Ciliary body
Conjugation
Crash cart
Hemodynamic response
Juxtaglomerular apparatus
Pheochromocytoma
Portal hypertension
Punctate keratopathy
Raynaud syndrome
Smith-Magenis syndrome
Stroke volume
Systemic lupus erythematosus

Clinical Case Studies

Clinical Case Study 1

A 61-year-old male visited his physician because of flulike symptoms, abdominal pain, and hypertension. The only abnormality that was found was increased serum alkaline phosphatase. An abdominal ultrasound revealed a cystic mass near the left kidney. A CT scan suggested that the group arose from the left adrenal gland. Past medical history included hypertension, which was controlled with medication. The patient underwent an alpha-blockage with phenoxybenzamine, an alpha-adrenergic antagonist, three times per day, followed by surgical resection of the adrenal mass. It was a pheochromocytoma with intratumoral hemorrhage and degeneration. After the resection, all levels returned to normal. The patient recovered well and required no antihypertensives.

Critical Thinking Questions

1. How does phenoxybenzamine work?
2. What is the indication of phenoxybenzamine?
3. What are the contraindications for phenoxybenzamine?

Clinical Case Study 2

A 30-year-old female went to an urgent care clinic 1 week after giving birth. She reported dyspnea and fatigue over the previous 2 days but believed them to be typical symptoms after childbirth. Her worried husband insisted she let him bring her to the urgent care clinic. She was found to be extraordinarily dyspneic and hypoxic and was referred to the local emergency department. Their medical history included obesity, but her overall health was good until the last month of her pregnancy when she developed gestational hypertension, dependent peripheral edema, and signs of an upper respiratory infection. She was given labetalol to manage her BP. Examination in the emergency department revealed a BP of 156/88 mm Hg, and chest radiographs showed cardiomegaly with increased bilateral vascular congestion. A CT scan of the patient's chest showed pleural effusion and cardiomegaly. The patient was hospitalized and given a diuretic. Her fatigue and dyspnea significantly decreased. After being released, she was prescribed labetalol and lisinopril. After 6 months, her condition was normal.

Critical Thinking Questions

1. How does labetalol work?
2. Aside from dyspnea and fatigue, what are the other adverse effects of labetalol?
3. Which drugs interact with labetalol?

Further Reading

[1] J.M. Cruickshank, The Modern Role of Beta-Blockers in Cardiovascular Medicine, PMPH-USA, Ltd, 2012.
[2] J.M. Cruickshank, The Beta-Blocker Story: Getting It Right, PMPH (People's Medical Publishing House), 2017.
[3] A.L. Gerbes, Ascites, Hyponatremia and Hepatorenal Syndrome: Progress in Treatment (Frontiers of Gastrointestinal Research, Volume 28), S, Karger, 2010.
[4] E. Juris, E. Carden, C. Toussaint, Positive Options for Complex Regional Pain Syndrome (CRPS): Self-Help and Treatment (Positive Options for Health), Hunter House, 2014.
[5] M.V. Kiselevsky, Malignant Effusions: Pleuritis, Ascites, Pericarditis, Springer, 2012.
[6] A. Lakhkar, Adrenergic Receptor Agonists and Antagonists in the Treatment of Post-Traumatic Stress Disorder, Grin Verlag, 2018.
[7] L. Loriaux, C. Vanek, Endocrine Emergencies: Recognition and Treatment (Contemporary Endocrinology), second ed., Springer, 2021.
[8] Medifocus.com Inc, Medifocus Guidebook on Reflex Sympathetic Dystrophy, CreateSpace Independent Publishing Platform, 2018.
[9] J.C. Schisler, C.H. Lang, M.S. Willis, Endocrinology of the Heart in Health and Disease: Integrated, Cellular, and Molecular Endocrinology of the Heart, Academic Press, 2016.
[10] H.M. Tabery, Keratoconjunctivitis Sicca and Filamentary Keratopathy: In Vivo Morphology in the Human Cornea and Conjunctiva, Springer, 2013.
[11] O. Tirosh, Liver Metabolism and Fatty Liver Disease (Oxidative Stress and Disease Volume 35), CRC Press, 2014.
[12] W. Wahli, H. Guillou, Metabolism and Metabolomics of Liver in Health and Disease, Mdpi AG, 2021.
[13] Q. Wang, Advances in Adrenergic Receptor Biology (Current Topics in Membranes, Volume 67), Academic Press, 2011.

CHAPTER

20

Cholinergic agonists

OUTLINE

LEARNING OUTCOMES

After study of the chapter, readers should be able to:

1. Explain the various types of cholinergic agonists.
2. Identify the mechanisms of action of the muscarinic agonists.
3. Explain the indications of the muscarinic agonists.
4. Describe the clinical indications of pilocarpine.
5. Explain the pharmacotherapy of myasthenia gravis.
6. Describe the acetylcholinesterase inhibitors and their clinical indications.
7. Explain the mechanisms of action and clinical indications of nicotine.
8. Identify what occurs from the acute toxicity of nicotine.

The Science of Pharmacology
https://doi.org/10.1016/B978-0-443-29038-1.00020-8

Overview

Cholinergic agonists are a group of medicines that mimic the actions of acetylcholine (ACh). ACh is one of the most common neurotransmitters in the human body, and it has activities in both the central and peripheral nervous systems. Cholinergic agonists have a direct action on the receptor for ACh. Some drugs are specific for the muscarinic receptors, and others are typical for the nicotinic receptors. Out of all types of autonomic nervous system medications, the cholinergic agonists make up the smallest group. They are also the least prescribed. These medications are also known as parasympathomimetics. Cholinergic synapses are very widely spread through the central and peripheral nervous systems. This means that medications that affect them have extremely diverse effects. Some cholinergic agonists are used to treat Alzheimer disease in its early stages, as well as glaucoma and myasthenia gravis.

Cholinergic agonists

Cholinergic agonists are also called **parasympathomimetics** or *cholinomimetics*. They stimulate the parasympathetic nervous system because they **mimic** the actions of ACh. The ACh is located at the ganglions and the parasympathetic terminal nerve endings. It enables the receptors in tissues, organs, and glands. The cholinergic agonists may activate cholinergic receptors directly or indirectly. Direct-acting cholinergic agonists include bethanechol, carbachol, cevimeline, and pilocarpine. Indirect-acting cholinergic agonists include donepezil, galantamine, neostigmine, physostigmine, pyridostigmine, and rivastigmine.

Classifications of cholinergic agonists

There are two types of cholinergic receptors: **muscarinic receptors** (which innervate smooth muscle and slow the heart rate) and **nicotinic receptors** (which affect the skeletal muscles). Many cholinergic drugs are nonselective and can affect the muscarinic and the nicotinic receptors. However, cholinergic selective medicines for the muscarinic receptors do not affect the nicotinic receptors. The classifications of the cholinergic agonists are summarized in **Table 20.1**.

Muscarinic agonists

The muscarinic agonists directly activate cholinergic receptors at neuroeffector junctions of the parasympathetic nervous system. ACh has little medicinal value because acetylcholinesterase (AChE) quickly destroys it in the synapses. It also has many adverse effects. The muscarinic agonists are used as medications not easily destroyed by AChE. They have a longer duration of action than ACh. These agonists have poor absorption across the GI tract and mostly do not cross the blood-brain barrier. They also have only slight effects on ACh nicotinic receptors in the ganglia. Few muscarinic agonists are widely used in pharmacotherapy because of their potentially serious adverse effects.

Nearly all of the widespread effects of these agonists are caused by parasympathetic activation. These drugs can increase the amount of smooth muscle tone and GI tract contractions. If given before meals, the increased peristalsis they cause empties the stomach more quickly. These agonists are never given to anyone with suspected GI tract obstructions because the increased peristalsis could injure or rupture the mucosa. These agents also stimulate urinary tract smooth muscles to increase ureteral peristalsis and speed up bladder emptying. Therefore they are excellent in the treatment of urinary retention. They are not given if obstructive uropathy exists because increased smooth muscle ureter and bladder contractions could improve pain and bleeding.

These agonists stimulate most exocrine glands. This increases digestive, lacrimal, salivary, and sweat secretions. Therefore they are used for xerostomia, such as in **Sjögren syndrome.** In the eyes, muscarinic agonists cause the iris muscles to contract, resulting in **miosis**. However, this is not a therapeutic goal and is therefore considered an adverse effect. Even so, these agonists contract the ciliary muscle, blurring the vision but allowing fluid to drain from the eye's anterior chamber, reducing intraocular pressure. Therefore topical agonists effectively treat **glaucoma**, though safer alternatives are available. Muscarinic agonists contract bronchial smooth muscle, so they are not used in patients with a history of asthma.

TABLE 20.1 Classifications of the cholinergic agonists.

Generic name	Trade name	Primary use
Direct acting (muscarinic agonist)		
bethanechol	Urecholine	Urinary retention
carbachol	Miostat	Reduction of pressure in the eye after surgery
cevimeline	Evoxac	Dry mouth due to Sjögren syndrome
pilocarpine	Salagen, Isopto-Carpine	Glaucoma
Indirect acting (acetylcholinesterase inhibitors)		
donepezil	Aricept	Alzheimer disease
galantamine	Razadyne	Alzheimer disease
neostigmine	Bloxiverz	To reverse effects of surgical anesthesia
physostigmine	Antilirium	To reverse effects of drugs that interfere with nerve-to-muscle communication
pyridostigmine	Mestinon	Myasthenia gravis and for exposures to nerve gas
rivastigmine	Exelon	Dementia caused by Alzheimer or Parkinson disease

When muscarinic receptors are activated in the cardiovascular system, the heart rate slows, and the blood pressure decreases. **Baroreceptors** in the carotid arteries and aortic arch signal the vasomotor center of the medulla to increase the heart rate, and **reflex tachycardia** occurs. This can also happen with any other drug that causes BP to decrease. To prevent bradycardia, oral or parenteral administration of cholinergic agonists must be closely monitored. The BP is monitored to avoid hypotension, especially with preexisting cardiovascular disease. If the patient has hyperthyroidism, atrial fibrillation is a possible outcome. The cholinergic agonists are not used if severe heart disease is present. The central muscarinic agonists used in medicine include *bethanechol, carbachol, cevimeline,* and *pilocarpine.*

Pharmacokinetics

Bethanechol is poorly absorbed but widely distributed. It does not cross the blood-brain barrier. Its primary method of metabolism is unknown, mainly excreted via the urine. The onset of action is 30–60 minutes, but the duration of action is 1–6 hours. *Carbachol* has low bioavailability. It is not well absorbed in the GI tract and does not cross the blood-brain barrier. It is not quickly metabolized by AChE and has a 2- to 5-minute onset of action. Its duration of action is 4–8 hours via topical administration and 24 hours with intraocular administration. It is poorly absorbed through topical administration, so *benzalkonium chloride* is added to promote absorption. *Cevimeline* has approximately 20% protein binding. Its mean time to peak concentration is 1.5–2 hours. It is metabolized in the liver. The mean elimination half-life is 5 hours, plus or minus 1 hour. About 97% is excreted via the urine. *Pilocarpine* has an elimination half-life of 1.35 hours for the 10-mg dose and 0.76 hours for the 5-mg dose. It is excreted via the urine.

Mechanism of action

The muscarinic agonists are direct acting. They enter the synaptic cleft, bind to ACh receptors, and produce the common rest-and-digest responses. Some of these medications cause more ACh to be released into the synaptic cleft,

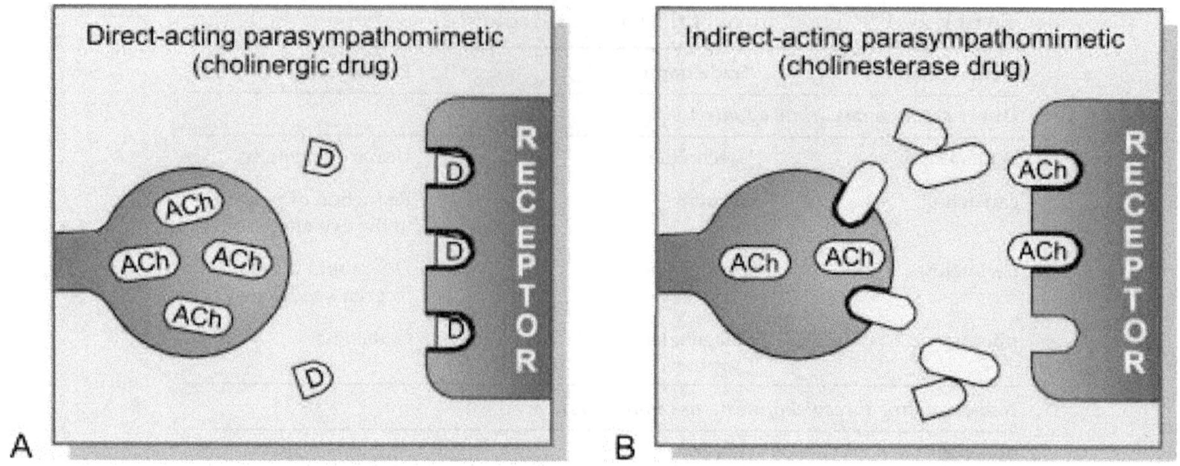

FIG. 20.1 Mechanisms of action of the (A) muscarinic (direct-acting) agonists and (B) the acetylcholinesterase (indirect-acting) inhibitors

which enhances the physiologic responses to ACh. These agonists work by using the ACh mechanism of action identically. The activities of the direct-acting agonists and those of the indirect-acting agonists are shown in **Fig. 20.1**.

Clinical indications

Bethanechol was approved in 1948 as an oral tablet to stimulate smooth muscle contraction in the digestive and urinary tracts. It is indicated for nonobstructive urinary retention with atony of the bladder. Off-label uses include treatment of adynamic ileus and gastric atony. *Carbachol* is injected into the eye's anterior chamber, promoting miosis during surgery—pupillary constriction results, which can temporarily cloud the vision. *Cevimeline* is only used for xerostomia due to Sjogren syndrome. Taken orally, it increases saliva flow to relieve dry mouth. *Pilocarpine* is given orally for xerostomia or as an ophthalmic solution for certain types of glaucoma and to counteract mydriatics and cycloplegics after eye examinations.

Contraindications

Bethanechol is used cautiously when any disorder that increases GI tract contractions, including recent GI surgery, suspected bowel obstruction, an active ulcer, and inflammatory bowel disease, could worsen. It is also avoided if suspected urinary obstruction or recent bladder surgery occurs. The drug is also contraindicated with asthma or COPD. It is additionally contraindicated with recent myocardial infarction, hypotension or hypertension, **bradycardia**, hyperthyroidism, epilepsy, Parkinson disease, and peritonitis. It should be used with caution in people with **cystitis** because the drug can cause bladder contractions to force urine up to the kidneys should the sphincter not open. *Carbachol* should be used with caution in people with asthma, coronary insufficiency, gastroduodenal ulcers, and incontinence. *Cevimeline* and pilocarpine are contraindicated with uncontrolled asthma, known hypersensitivity, acute **iritis**, and **angle-closure glaucoma**.

Adverse effects

The common adverse effects of muscarinic agonists include skin flushing, sweating, blurred vision, miosis, **sialorrhea**, abdominal cramping, nausea, and vomiting. The serious adverse effects include bradycardia, orthostatic hypotension with possible **syncope**, complete heart block, reflex tachycardia, and acute bronchospasm.

Toxicity

Bethanechol toxicity causes hypotension, salivation, nausea, vomiting, diarrhea, and abdominal cramping. Atropine is usually given subcutaneously to reverse these symptoms. Systemic toxicity is rare after topical administration or intraocular injection of *carbachol*, usually only with frequent administration. They include syncope, cardiac arrhythmia, hypotension, headaches, asthma, vomiting, diarrhea, urinary urgency, and increased sweating. *Cevimeline* toxicity may cause similar symptoms, vision problems, confusion, tremors, and shortness of breath. *Pilocarpine* toxicity may cause sweating, nausea, tremors, and bradycardia.

You should remember

Muscarinic agonists are parasympathomimetic drugs used to treat ileus, urinary retention, glaucoma, Alzheimer disease, and other conditions. They mimic the actions of ACh upon muscarinic receptors to cause cardiac slowing, contraction of smooth muscles, and increased secretions from exocrine glandular tissues.

Acetylcholinesterase inhibitors

AChE inhibitors are indirect-acting medications that inhibit AChE, the enzyme that destroys ACh. By blocking this destruction, ACh can remain and accumulate in the synaptic cleft for longer, producing increased rest-and-digest responses. Some indirect drugs bind only to AChE and have very short durations of action. These are the *reversible AChE inhibitors*. Some chemicals have *irreversible* binding to AChE and are very dangerous. Therefore the irreversible AChE inhibitors do not have significant medical uses. Examples of these chemicals include nerve gas agents and some insecticides. The AChE inhibitors differ from the muscarinic agonists in that they are nonselective. They affect ACh synapses at the autonomic ganglia, muscarinic receptors, neuromuscular junctions, and CNS synapses. Their muscarinic actions are identical to those of the direct-acting drugs. They often increase peristalsis in the urinary and GI tracts. Some of them decrease intraocular pressure.

Because of their actions in the CNS and on skeletal muscle motor nerve endings, the AChE inhibitors have other nonautonomic indications. They are used for mild to moderate Alzheimer disease by improving memory and cognitive function via increasing ACh in the brain's cholinergic synapses. However, they do not cure Alzheimer disease or slow its progression. The improvements are only limited and short lasting. Some AChE inhibitors are used to treat myasthenia gravis.

Pharmacokinetics

Donepezil has 100% bioavailability and 96% protein binding. It is metabolized in the liver by glucuronidation. The onset of action is 3–4 hours, and the elimination half-life is 70 hours. Daily doses achieve a steady-state concentration in 15–21 days. *Donepezil* is mainly excreted in the urine, with 17% remaining unchanged. About 15% to 20% is excreted in the feces. *Galantamine* has 90% bioavailability but only 18% protein binding. It is partially metabolized in the liver. Elimination half-life is 7 hours. Excretion is 95% in the urine, of which 32% is unchanged, and 5% in the feces.

Neostigmine has unclear bioavailability, which is probably below 5%. The metabolism is via slow **hydrolysis** by AChE and by plasma esterases. Via injection, the onset of action is within 30 minutes and 4 hours orally. The elimination half-life is 50–90 minutes, and the duration of action is up to 4 hours. The drug is up to 70% excreted unchanged in the urine. *Physostigmine* is absorbed from the GI tract, mucous membranes, and subcutaneous tissues. The onset of action is 3–8 minutes and lasts 30 minutes to 5 hours. The drug is widely distributed and quickly penetrates the blood-brain barrier. It is metabolized via hydrolysis by the cholinesterases. Its route of elimination has yet to be fully understood, and only tiny amounts are excreted in the urine. The half-life is 15–60 minutes.

Pyridostigmine has only 1%–2% absorption when given orally, and the oral dose is much higher than the parenteral dose. It is distributed to most body tissues and does not cross the blood-brain barrier or the placenta. Primary metabolism is in the liver via the actions of the cholinesterases. Direct excretion is via the urine. It has a 15- to 30-minute oral onset of effort and a 2- to 5-minute IV onset. Duration of action is 3–6 hours for the regular form and 6–12 hours for the extended-release form. *Rivastigmine* has an elimination half-life of about 1.5 hours, and excretion is mostly via metabolites in the urine. It is wholly and rapidly absorbed, reaching peak plasma concentrations in about 1 hour. The drug is bound at about 40% to plasma proteins and easily crosses the blood-brain barrier.

Mechanism of action

Donepezil binds and reversibly inactivates the cholinesterases to inhibit the hydrolysis of ACh, increasing ACh concentrations at cholinergic synapses. Its precise mechanism of action in Alzheimer disease is not fully understood. The drug also acts as a potent agonist of the alpha$_1$ receptor. *Galantamine, neostigmine, physostigmine, pyridostigmine,* and *rivastigmine* have similar actions. For myasthenia gravis, it is helpful because of its effects on nicotinic ACh receptors in the skeletal muscles.

Clinical indications

Donepezil treats Alzheimer disease, Lewy body dementia, traumatic brain injury, vascular dementia, and dementia associated with Parkinson disease. *Galantamine* is used for Alzheimer disease, Lewy body dementia, dementia associated with Parkinson disease, and vascular dementia. *Neostigmine* and *physostigmine* are used for myasthenia gravis to reduce the effects of nondepolarizing muscle relaxants after an operation. It is sometimes used IV to delay the impact of venom after a snakebite. *Pyridostigmine* is available in oral and parenteral forms. It is used for myasthenia gravis and indicated for possible future exposure to certain nerve gases but must be given within a few hours. When exposure has already occurred, the **antidotes** are provided instead. The IV form reverses neuromuscular blocking actions of nondepolarizing muscle relaxants. Care is taken to avoid overdosage via the IV route. *Rivastigmine* is used for mild to moderate dementia of the Alzheimer type and dementia associated with Parkinson disease.

You should remember

Gravis develops as antibodies attack nicotinic synapses on skeletal muscles. Symptoms include double vision, extreme fatigue, difficulty chewing or swallowing, impaired speech, and eyelids drooping. Muscle fatigue is worse after exercise or later in the day. The disease is progressive, with fluctuating symptoms. Treatment additionally utilizes careful use of immunosuppressants such as corticosteroids. When a *myasthenic crisis* develops, it is treated with atropine.

Contraindications

AChE inhibitors are contraindicated with known hypersensitivity and must be used cautiously during anesthesia, cardiovascular conditions, peptic ulcer disease, and GI bleeding. They must be avoided with seizure disorders, asthma or COPD, and urinary tract obstruction. *Physostigmine* is contraindicated with asthma, diabetes mellitus, **gangrene**, cardiovascular disease, mechanical obstruction of the intestines or urogenital tract, and any **vagotonic** state.

Adverse effects

The common adverse effects of AChE inhibitors include involuntary contraction or twitching of muscles, nausea, vomiting, increased salivation, and miosis. The serious adverse effects of AChE inhibitors include cardiac abnormalities such as bradycardia, atrioventricular block, torsades de pointes, and hypotension; **dyspnea**; seizures; cholinergic crisis; bronchospasm; and respiratory muscle paralysis. They may also cause diarrhea, loss of appetite, insomnia, and unusual tiredness or weakness.

Toxicity

The **cholinergic crisis** may develop from overdoses of AChE inhibitors or exposure to nerve gases such as **sarin** or organophosphate insecticides such as **malathion**. Signs of muscle paralysis signify the problem: respiratory failure, increased respiratory secretions, seizures, coma, and death. A large overdose may require mechanical ventilation to prevent death. The poisoning effects of organophosphates are classified as muscle **fasciculations**, unresponsive with pinpoint pupils, headaches, **diaphoresis**, emesis, diarrhea, salivation, anxiety, convulsions, delirium, and coma. The toxicity of AChE inhibitors is usually less severe than toxicity from organophosphates. Atropine is the drug generally used to counteract a cholinergic crisis.

You should remember

As dementia in Alzheimer disease continues to become more prevalent, AChE inhibitors provide some symptomatic benefits for cognitive decline. However, they cause various adverse effects, so they must continually be assessed carefully before being prescribed. Differences in drug formulations must be considered when determining the best route of administration for each patient.

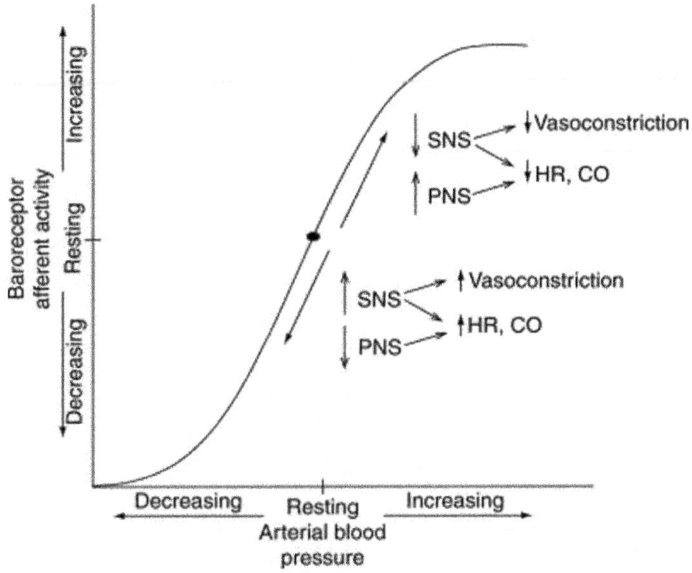

FIG. 20.2 The baroreceptor reflexes

Nicotinic agonists

Few drugs are used because of their effects on ACh nicotinic receptors in the autonomic ganglia. They can produce widespread, nonselective results on the autonomic nervous system. Therefore the only widely used drug that activates ganglionic receptors is *nicotine*. The GI tract, respiratory mucosa, and skin absorb it. Parasympathetic and sympathetic responses are stimulated because nicotine acts at the ganglia. As nicotine is absorbed, the CNS becomes more alert, and heart rate and BP increase. They may decrease soon because of the baroreceptor reflex (see **Fig. 20.2**). Nausea occurs as the emetic center of the CNS is triggered. As blood levels of nicotine decrease, the same organ systems become depressed. Nicotine is a pregnancy category D drug and is overall very dangerous. Acute toxicity may cause death because of paralysis of the respiratory muscles.

In medicine, nicotine is used as *nicotine replacement therapy (NRT)* to achieve cessation from tobacco products. It is available in forms such as transdermal patches (Habitrol), chewing gum (Nicorette), and nasal spray (Nicotrol). These products reduce uncomfortable withdrawal symptoms, including insomnia, depression, lack of concentration, headaches, and food cravings. The products are slowly withdrawn as tobacco use drops over about 8–12 weeks. The goal is to reduce physical dependence upon nicotine. Because psychological support also occurs, the best smoking cessation programs include behavior modification therapy and self-help groups. Regular use of NRT can nearly double a patient's likelihood of quitting tobacco products, but a lot of motivation and persistent follow-up are needed.

You should remember

NRT replaces some of the nicotine formerly obtained from smoking. This helps the individual feel less uncomfortable after quitting the habit. The US Food and Drug Administration approved five NRTs, and nicotine is the active ingredient in all of them. The most common forms are nicotine patches, gum, and lozenges. They can be purchased over the counter. The NRTs supply nicotine without the hundreds of harmful chemicals in cigarette smoke.

Key Terms

Angle-closure glaucoma
Antidote
Baroreceptors
Bradycardia
Cholinergic crisis
Cystitis
Diaphoresis
Dyspnea
Fasciculations
Gangrene
Glaucoma
Hydrolysis
Iritis
Malathion
Mimic
Miosis
Muscarinic receptors
Nicotinic receptors
Parasympathomimetics
Reflex tachycardia
Sarin
Sialorrhea
Sjögren syndrome
Syncope
Vagotonic

Clinical Case Studies

Clinical Case Study 1

A 44-year-old male suffers from urinary retention and a hypoactive bladder. He is questioned about any recent GI surgery, suspected bowel obstruction, an active ulcer, and inflammatory disease, and he replies that he has not had any of these. He is also not taking AChE inhibitors. The patient is prescribed bethanechol, a cholinergic agonist, and is questioned about taking any drugs it interacts with. He is not taking any of them. Over about 90 minutes after taking the first dose, the patient begins to improve.

Critical Thinking Questions

1. How do muscarinic agonists such as bethanechol work in treating urinary retention?
2. What are the indications for bethanechol?
3. What are the contraindications of bethanechol?

Clinical Case Study 2

An 83-year-old married female was assessed as to the progression of Alzheimer disease. Her husband has been her primary caretaker since her diagnosis 10 years previously. He sometimes brings her to a daycare center to interact with other people in her age group, but she shows no interest and does not want to interact. Before her diagnosis, the patient had gotten lost in her hometown and was returned home by the police. By the time of the current assessment, she had lost the ability to know what time of day it was and sometimes forgot her sons' names. She has had significant mental and physical deterioration, started wandering around the house at night, and has become verbally aggressive toward others. The patient is prescribed donepezil, which will be taken once each night at bedtime.

Critical Thinking Questions

1. How does the AChE inhibitor called donepezil improve cognitive function in Alzheimer disease?
2. For what conditions is donepezil indicated?
3. What are the signs of a cholinergic crisis caused by overdoses of AChE inhibitors?

Further Reading

[1] A. Adejare, Drug Discovery Approaches for the Treatment of Neurodegenerative Disorders: Alzheimer's Disease, Academic Press, 2016.
[2] A. Augustine, K.S. Sumana, P.J. Vazhacharickal, New Inhibitor Development for Acetylcholinesterase to Control Parkinson's Disease by CADD Method, Mar Augusthinose College Press, 2020.
[3] J. Barnard, Myasthenia Gravis: Clinical Concepts and Treatments, Foster Academics, 2015.
[4] J. Beller, J. Briggs, Dementia Overview – 2021 Update – Dementia Types, Symptoms, & Risk Factors. Dementia & Alzheimer's Handbook for Seniors, Caregivers, & Medical Professionals, Jerry Beller Health Research, 2020.
[5] T. Chen Chang, P. Ramulu, E. Hodapp, Clinical Decisions in Glaucoma, second ed., Ta Chen Chang, 2016.
[6] W.J. Collins, The Effects of Certain Parasympathomimetic Substances on the Emotions of Normal and Psychotic Individuals. Literary Licensing, LLC, 2013.
[7] D. Cozart, Alzheimer's Treatment: Acetylcholinesterase Inhibitors, Cozart, 2017.
[8] G.A.A. Dos Santos, Pharmacological Treatment of Alzheimer's Disease: Scientific and Clinical Aspects, Springer, 2021.
[9] S. Gauthier, Clive Ballard, Management of Dementia, second ed., Informa Healthcare, 2009.
[10] A. Gupta, P. Vaid, A.G. Shabana, Nicotine Replacement Therapy: A Medically Proven Way to Quit Tobacco, Lap Lambert Academic Publishing, 2019.
[11] M.A. McCrea, Mild Traumatic Brain Injury and Post-concussion Syndrome – The New Evidence Base for Diagnosis and Treatment (AACN Workshop Series), American Academy of Clinical Neuropsychology / Oxford University Press, 2007.
[12] G.E. Smith, M.W. Bondi, Mild Cognitive Impairment and Dementia – Definitions, Diagnosis, and Treatment (AACN Workshop Series), American Academy of Clinical Neuropsychology / Oxford University Press, 2013.
[13] R. Vardanyan, V. Hruby, Synthesis of Best-Seller Drugs, Academic Press, 2016.

CHAPTER

21

Cholinergic antagonists

OUTLINE

LEARNING OUTCOMES

After study of the chapter, readers should be able to:

1. Explain the classifications of cholinergic antagonists.
2. Identify a primary source of the muscarinic antagonists.
3. Explain the indications of muscarinic antagonists.
4. Describe the contraindications of atropine.
5. Identify the expression of ganglionic blocker.
6. Discussed the mechanism of action for succinylcholine.
7. List two short-acting, nondepolarizing neuromuscular blockers.
8. Identify the primary indication of succinylcholine.

Overview

The cholinergic antagonists are also known as *anticholinergics*. They inhibit acetylcholine (ACh)'s actions at the cholinergic synapses. Because there are muscarinic and nicotinic receptors, these antagonists' actions and therapeutic uses are based on their specific sites of action. The muscarinic antagonists have many more clinical indications

https://doi.org/10.1016/B978-0-443-29038-1.00021-X

than the nicotinic antagonists. These antagonists may also be subclassified as ganglionic blockers or neuromuscular blockers. The use of muscarinic antagonists has declined due to newer and safer medications being developed. There are still several pharmacologically important cholinergic antagonists. The cholinergic antagonists are used for peptic ulcer disease, irritable bowel syndrome, dilation of the pupils, bradycardia, to decrease salivary and respiratory secretions during anesthesia, for bronchodilation, to reverse poisoning with muscarinic mushrooms or organophosphate insecticides, for incontinence, and for parkinsonian symptoms.

Cholinergic antagonists

The **cholinergic antagonists** act by blocking the effects of ACh at the muscarinic or nicotinic receptors. The cholinergic antagonists are subdivided into the *muscarinic antagonists* and the *nicotinic antagonists.* The muscarinic antagonists have many more clinical indications than the nicotinic antagonists. They are also summarized in **Table 21.1**.

TABLE 21.1 Classifications of the muscarinic antagonists.

Generic name	Trade name	Primary use
aclidinium	Tudorza Pressair	COPD
atropine	AtroPen	Poisonings, to reduce salivation during surgery, for muscle spasms, and to revive the heart from bradycardia
benztropine	Cogentin	Parkinson disease
cyclopentolate	Cyclogyl	Pupil dilation
darifenacin	Enablex	Overactive bladder
dicyclomine	Bentyl	Functional bowel or irritable bowel syndrome
fesoterodine	Toviaz	Overactive bladder
glycopyrrolate	Cuvposa	To reduce salivation
hyoscyamine	Anaspaz	Peptic ulcer, irritable bowel syndrome, acute enterocolitis
ipratropium	Atrovent	COPD
Cantil	Gastrointestinal ulcers	
methscopolamine	Pamine	Peptic ulcer
oxybutynin	Ditropan	Overactive bladder
scopolamine	Transderm-Scop	Motion sickness
solifenacin	VESIcare	Overactive bladder, incontinence
tiotropium	Spiriva	COPD
tolterodine	Detrol	Overactive bladder
trihexyphenidyl	(generic only)	Parkinson disease
tropicamide	Mydriacyl	Pupil dilation
trospium	Sanctura	Overactive bladder and urinary incontinence, frequency, or urgency

COPD, Chronic obstructive pulmonary disease.

Classifications of cholinergic antagonists

There are two types of cholinergic antagonists: muscarinic antagonists and nicotinic antagonists. They are subdivided into *ganglionic blockers* and *neuromuscular blockers*. The muscarinic antagonists have more therapeutic uses than the nicotinic antagonists. The muscarinic antagonists are selective for the ACh muscarinic receptors at therapeutic doses. They do not have a significant effect on the nicotinic receptors. Cholinergic antagonists are also known as *anticholinergics*. They block cholinergic receptors from ACh. Generally the short- and long-acting antagonists are relatively safe.

Muscarinic antagonists

Muscarinic antagonists have been used in many conditions for centuries. A primary source was the *Atropa belladonna* plant, initially used to dilate the eyes or redden the cheeks, as an early form of female "beauty" techniques. The plant is shown in **Fig. 21.1.** However, it is highly toxic and has been used in suicides. With newer, safer medications being developed, the use of muscarinic antagonists has declined. They are now mainly prescribed when a safer and preferred drug is contraindicated or not well tolerated by the patient.

Pharmacokinetics

The pharmacokinetics of the muscarinic antagonists are widely similar to *atropine*, with good absorption by almost all routes of administration. Atropine is distributed and crosses the blood-brain barrier and placenta, and small amounts are secreted in the breast milk. It is primarily metabolized in the liver and mostly excreted in the urine. The onset of action is 15 minutes with subcutaneous or IM administration, 30 minutes with oral administration, and 2–4 minutes with IV administration. The half-life is 4 hours. For *ipratropium*, protein binding is 0%–9% in vitro. The drug is metabolized in the liver, and its elimination half-life is 2 hours.

Mechanism of action

The muscarinic antagonists work by suppressing the effects of ACh, allowing symptoms of sympathetic nervous system activation to dominate (the fight-or-flight response). The mechanisms of action are exemplified by the prototype drug *atropine*, based on the ability to block muscarinic receptors. Atropine increases the heart rate, which helps to treat bradycardia. In high doses, the muscarinic antagonists can block nicotinic receptors in skeletal muscle and the ganglia. Some of these drugs, such as *ipratropium*, block the receptors to decrease the production of **cyclic**

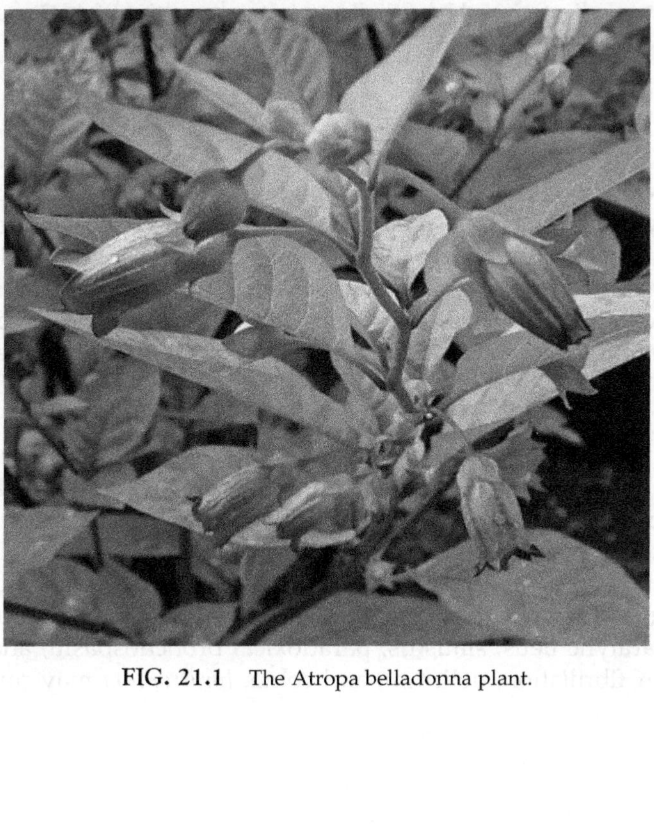

FIG. 21.1 The Atropa belladonna plant.

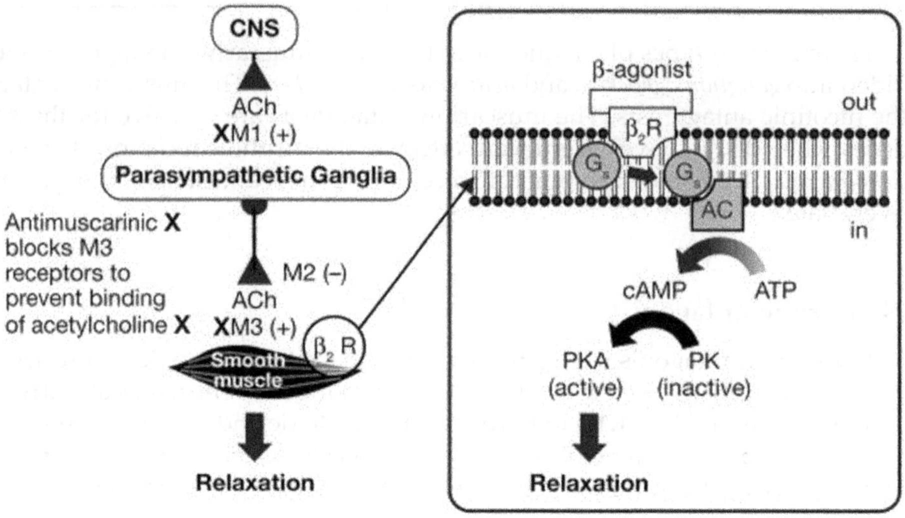

FIG. 21.2 Mechanism of action of the muscarinic agonists.

CMP, leading to reduced contraction of smooth muscles in the lung airways. Antimuscarinic antagonists block *muscarinic 3 receptors* to prevent ACh binding, resulting in relaxation (see **Fig. 21.2**).

Clinical indications

Muscarinic antagonists are used for peptic ulcers, irritable bowel syndrome, dilation of the pupils during ophthalmic examinations, bradycardia, to decrease salivary and respiratory secretions during anesthesia, for bronchodilation, to reverse poisoning with muscarinic mushrooms or organophosphate insecticides, for incontinence, and parkinsonian symptoms. The antagonists, such as *ipratropium,* are indicated primarily for treating COPD and asthma exacerbation.

You should remember

Atropine, the prototype drug, is derived from the plant belladonna. It is used to depress salivation and bronchial secretions and to dilate the bronchi, but it can thicken respiratory secretions (obstructing airways).

Contraindications

Muscarinic antagonists are contraindicated with acute angle-closure **glaucoma** because they can cause **cycloplegia**. Atropine must be carefully used in cardiovascular conditions because it accelerates heart rate. It should be used with caution in hyperthyroidism due to the risk of dysrhythmias and severe GI conditions, including ulcerative colitis and paralytic ileus, because it can worsen them. Atropine also worsens **gastroesophageal reflux disease** and hiatal hernia, making esophageal injury and aspiration more likely. Muscarinic antagonists must be used cautiously in Down syndrome patients. *Ipratropium* may also cause obstructions in the gastrointestinal tract or urinary system.

Adverse effects

Muscarinic antagonists are usually not drugs of choice for various conditions because of many adverse effects. Most of these are predictable because they are related to inhibiting the parasympathetic nervous system. Serious adverse effects include tachycardia, CNS stimulation, urinary retention, xerostomia, dry eyes, hyperthermia due to inhibition of sweating, **photophobia**, and increased intraocular pressure. Additional adverse effects may include coughing, headaches, blurred vision, mydriasis, constipation, insomnia, nasal burning, nasopharyngitis, and **allergic conjunctivitis (see Fig. 21.3)**. Other serious adverse effects may include worsening of glaucoma, paradoxical bradycardia, dysrhythmias, paralytic ileus, sinusitis, paradoxical bronchospasm, and oropharyngeal **candidiasis**. *Atropine* can lead to ventricular fibrillation, delirium, and coma. *Ipratropium* may cause dry mouth, sedation, skin

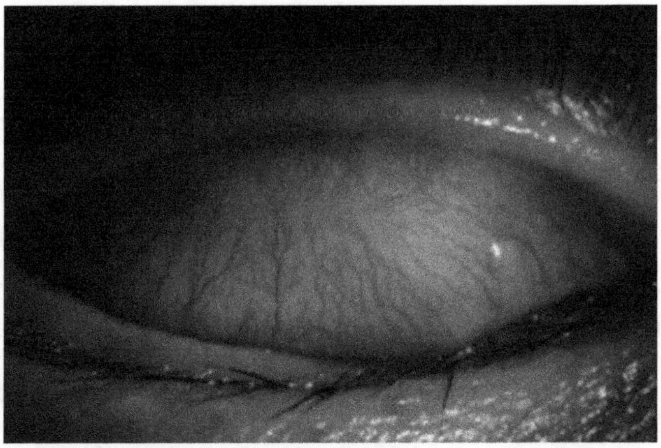

FIG. 21.3 A patient with allergic conjunctivitis.

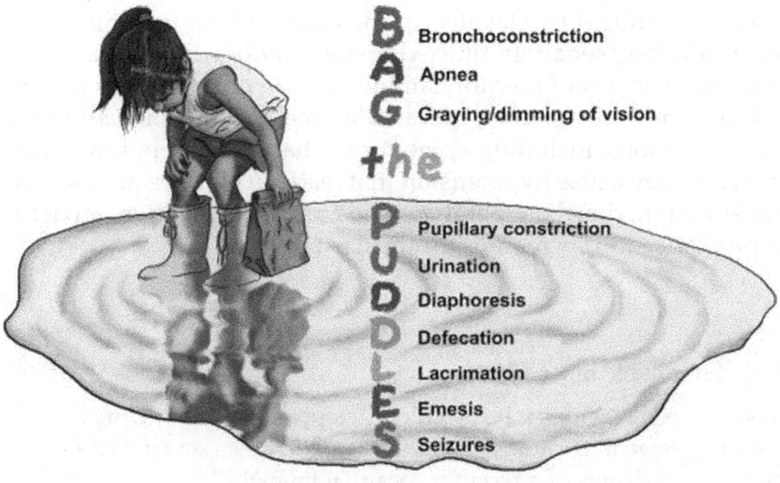

FIG. 21.4 The significant factors involved in the cholinergic crisis are remembered by using an acronym.

flushing, tachycardia, acute angle-closure glaucoma, nausea, palpitations, headache, throat irritation, and urinary retention.

Toxicity

Overdose of muscarinic antagonists leads to toxic symptoms called anticholinergic syndrome. These include blurred vision, dry mouth, photophobia, difficulty swallowing, visual changes, agitation, hallucinations, and urinary retention. Though rare, death has occurred because of high doses of these antagonists. The specific antidote for toxicity is physostigmine, which is a reversible cholinesterase inhibitor. However, it can induce a **cholinergic crisis** in high doses, so it is usually only administered when there are severe symptoms of anticholinergic syndrome such as psychoses or seizures. **Fig. 21.4** illustrates an exciting way of remembering the significant factors involved in the cholinergic crisis, known as "BAG the PUDDLES."

You should remember

Even though atropine, a muscarinic antagonist, has some medical uses, it is a poisonous crystalline substance in the *alkaloid* class of compounds. They have diverse physiological effects, including antibacterial, antimitotic, antiinflammatory, analgesic, local anesthetic, hypnotic, psychotropic, and antitumor activities.

Nicotinic antagonists: ganglionic blockers

The nicotinic antagonists known as **ganglionic blockers** act at the autonomic ganglia. They lower blood pressure and are used in emergencies. These blockers interrupt the transmission of nerve impulses at nicotinic receptors of the autonomic ganglia. Because both the sympathetic and parasympathetic nervous systems have ganglia, these blockers are nonselective. They inhibit all of the autonomic nervous system. The parasympathetic system is more highly affected because most organs' dominant baseline autonomic tone is parasympathetic. After slowing down parasympathetic nerve impulses, symptoms include constipation, urinary retention, blurred vision, dry mouth, and increased heart rate. The only therapeutic action is vasodilation, and these blockers can cause extreme hypotension, requiring emergency kits to be available that contain agents such as epinephrine to reverse extremely low BP. Because of these agents' potential toxicities, only one ganglionic blocker is currently available for medical use. It is *mecamylamine (Vecamyl)*. It is a long-acting nicotinic receptor antagonist initially used for BP reduction in cases of severe hypertension. Safer antihypertensive drugs have replaced this drug for clinical use.

Mecamylamine has more recently been approved for nicotine dependence because it reduces the brain's psychologically rewarding effects of nicotine. It is also used for Tourette syndrome when that condition is unresponsive to other medications. Mecamylamine is contraindicated in mild, moderate, or labile hypertension; coronary insufficiency; **uremia**; glaucoma; organic pyloric stenosis; known hypersensitivity; and recent myocardial infarction. The drug is only used cautiously if kidney insufficiency is signified by elevated or increasing blood urea nitrogen. Common adverse effects include fatigue, weakness, headaches, sedation, blurred vision, mydriasis, decreased libido, impotence, and urinary retention. The serious adverse effects of mecamylamine include orthostatic hypotension, precipitation of angina, **adynamic ileus**, and **choreiform movements**. Mecamylamine has a significant drug interaction with tizanidine and many moderate drug interactions, including epinephrine, haloperidol, norepinephrine, risperidone, and vasopressin. Mecamylamine toxicity may cause hypotension that leads to peripheral vascular collapse, nausea, vomiting, postural hypotension, constipation, diarrhea, paralytic ileus, urinary retention, anxiety, dizziness, dry mouth, mydriasis, blurred vision, palpitations, and increased intraocular pressure.

You should remember

Mecamylamine is a nicotine antagonist/ganglionic blocker that is highly potent and is used for severe or life-threatening blood pressure. It starts working in 1–2 hours and is only approved for use in adults. The drug is dangerous if it is suddenly stopped, has many drug interactions, and is unsafe if the patient has severe kidney problems or a recent myocardial infarction.

Nicotinic antagonists: neuromuscular blockers

The nicotinic antagonists classified as **neuromuscular blockers** are significant for many hospitalized patients, but their use is somewhat controversial. They are commonly used in surgical situations and rapid sequence intubation. Indications such as acute respiratory distress syndrome, elevated intracranial pressure, and therapeutic hypothermia are under debate. There are two classifications of these blockers: depolarizing and nondepolarizing. The medications are divided into groups by duration of action, including ultrashort-, short-, intermediate-, and long-acting forms.

There is only one drug in the class of *depolarizing neuromuscular blockers*. It is called *succinylcholine (Anectine)*. It competes with ACh for nicotinic receptors on motor end plates of skeletal muscles. Once it binds to ACh receptors, the drug causes muscle relaxation like ACh does. Because succinylcholine is not destroyed by AChE, it causes a lengthy, continuous depolarization of muscle cells. With no repolarization, calcium returns, and muscles relax. Succinylcholine does not enter the CNS or produce loss of consciousness or anesthesia. The patient can still feel pain and is fully aware of the environment. It is used as one part of balanced anesthesia. It is also the only example of an ultrashort-acting neuromuscular blocker.

The other nondepolarizing neuromuscular blockers are more numerous and have short, intermediate, and long actions. They produce muscle paralysis during surgical procedures that require an extended period. All of the neuromuscular blockers are summarized in **Table 21.2**.

TABLE 21.2 The neuromuscular blockers

Generic name	Trade name	Primary use
Ultrashort acting		
succinylcholine	Anectine	Muscle relaxation during surgery or while on a ventilator/respirator
Short acting		
mivacurium	(generic only)	Same
rocuronium	(generic only)	Same
Intermediate acting		
atracurium	Tracrium	Same
cisatracurium	Nimbex	Same
vecuronium	Norcuron	Same
Long acting		
pancuronium	Pavulon	Same

Pharmacokinetics

These drugs affect the body by causing muscle weakness and spasms, followed by paralysis. *Succinylcholine* is given IM or IV, with good absorption via the IM route. It is widely distributed and crosses the placenta. The drug is metabolized in the blood plasma by plasma cholinesterase, also known as **pseudocholinesterase**. It is mainly excreted in the urine. Succinylcholine has an onset of action of 2–3 minutes when given IM. Its IV duration of action is 2–3 minutes, and its IM duration is 10–30 minutes. The short-acting *mivacurium* and *rocuronium* have durations of action lasting about 15–20 minutes, so a continuous infusion may be needed to maintain the neuromuscular block for longer. The intermediate-acting *atracurium, cisatracurium,* and *vecuronium* have durations of action of 30–45 minutes. The kidneys or liver does not eliminate atracurium and cisatracurium, so they are better choices for patients with diseases of these organs. Vecuronium is advantageous because it causes no release of histamine. The long-acting *pancuronium* has a duration of action of 60–90 minutes.

Mechanism of action

Succinylcholine binds to cholinergic receptor sites at neuromuscular junctions, causing depolarization. The skeletal muscle membranes cannot repolarize while the drug is present, and total muscle relaxation or paralysis occurs. The nondepolarizing neuromuscular blockers compete with ACh to bind the receptors on the motor end plate. This blockage prevents depolarization. However, these nondepolarizing blockers do not cause sustained depolarization as succinylcholine does. Instead, they inhibit the action of ACh without activating the muscle.

Clinical indications

The primary indication for the prototype drug, succinylcholine, as an adjunct to surgical anesthesia is to achieve complete skeletal muscle relaxation of the abdominal muscles. This and the other agents are also used to allow for better insertion of endotracheal tubes and to assist with mechanical ventilation. Succinylcholine reduces the amount of general anesthesia that will be needed for surgery. Given intravenously, muscle relaxation starts in under 60 seconds. Once discontinued, muscle control returns within several minutes because plasma cholinesterase quickly destroys the drug. Succinylcholine is perfect for short procedures such as electroconvulsive shock therapy or intubation. The other medications in this group have identical clinical indications.

Contraindications

Succinylcholine is contraindicated with a personal or family history of **malignant hyperthermia**, acute phases of injury after multiple trauma, significant burns, denervation of skeletal muscle, skeletal muscle myopathies, or hypersensitivity to succinylcholine. It should be used with caution in patients with electrolyte imbalances, kidney disease, fractures or muscle spasms, or heart failure. Monitoring for pulmonary or metabolic disorders is done carefully

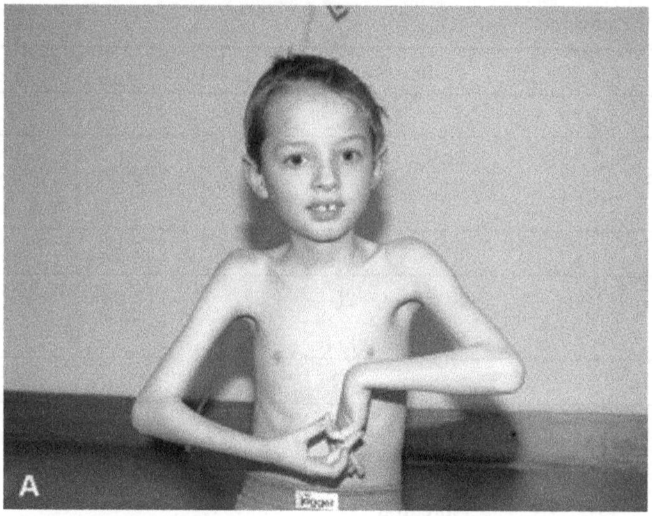

FIG. 21.5 A patient with Duchenne's muscular dystrophy.

to avoid respiratory depression and acidosis. Use is not recommended in patients with narrow-angle glaucoma, penetrating eye injuries, chronic abdominal infection, subarachnoid hemorrhage, or conditions causing degeneration of central or peripheral nervous systems. *Mivacurium, rocuronium, vecuronium*, and *pancuronium* are contraindicated with known hypersensitivity. *Atracurium* and *cisatracurium* are contraindicated with known hypersensitivity or hypersensitivity to benzyl alcohol with the multidose vial; single-dose vials do not contain benzyl alcohol and may be used. Caution is advised for these agents in patients with hepatic or renal impairment, myasthenia gravis, or electrolyte imbalances.

Adverse effects

The adverse effects of depolarizing and nondepolarizing neuromuscular blockers include increased salivation, rash, weakness, and transient flushing of the face, neck, or chest. The serious adverse effects include anaphylaxis, respiratory depression, cardiac arrest, prolonged apnea, bradycardia, dysrhythmias, hypotension, changes in heart rate, malignant hyperthermia, and muscle paralysis. In some patients, succinylcholine has induced hyperkalemia, resulting in many potentially life-threatening effects. A black box warning against succinylcholine is used in children with **Duchenne muscular dystrophy** and other congenital musculoskeletal diseases because they are at increased risk for cardiac arrest (see **Fig. 21.5**).

Toxicity

Succinylcholine toxicity can cause severe or fatal respiratory depression. *Mivacurium* and *rocuronium* toxicity primarily cause decreases in BP or other hemodynamic effects. *Atracurium, cisatracurium, vecuronium*, and *pancuronium* have no significant toxicities.

You should remember

The first neuromuscular blocker was *curare*, extracted from South American plants. The substance was cooked and then rubbed on the tips of arrows for use in hunting animals. Curare was later used during operations because it reduced muscle spasms and caused skeletal muscle paralysis. The active chemical in curare is *tubocurarine*, which is no longer used for medical procedures today.

Key Terms

Adynamic ileus
Allergic conjunctivitis

Candidiasis
Cholinergic antagonists
Cholinergic crisis
Choreiform movement
Cyclic adenosine monophosphate is a second messenger, or cellular signal occurring within cells, that is important in many biological processes
Cycloplegia
Duchenne muscular dystrophy
Ganglionic blockers
Gastroesophageal reflux disease
Glaucoma
Malignant hyperthermia
Muscarinic antagonists
Neuromuscular blockers
Paralytic ileus
Photophobia
Pseudocholinesterase
Ulcerative colitis
Uremia

Clinical Case Studies

Clinical Case Study 1

A 24-year-old male college student bought the illegal drug known as "magic mushrooms" from his roommate and consumed them in an attempt to experience hallucinations. What he finished, however, was not what he thought. Instead, it was the species of muscarinic mushroom known as *Clitocybe dealbata*, also known as "ivory funnel," which contains potentially deadly levels of muscarine. The student was hospitalized with diarrhea, nausea, vomiting, abdominal pain, and dehydration symptoms. Gastric lavage was performed, and a nasogastric tube was put in place. Activated charcoal was administered, and atropine was carefully administered IV as an antidote. His aspartate transaminase levels increased dramatically, peaking 3 days after consuming the mushrooms. Though he recovered, the patient's liver was somewhat damaged by toxins from the mushrooms.

Critical Thinking Questions

1. Why has the general use of muscarinic antagonists declined over time?
2. What are the pharmacokinetics of atropine?
3. What are the absolute contraindications of atropine?

Clinical Case Study 2

A 67-year-old male was hospitalized after his physician diagnosed him with COPD. The patient has had hypertension for 1 year and is currently taking amlodipine. He has been a chronic smoker for the past 48 years. He has a productive cough and has endured a recent respiratory tract infection. Examination revealed him to have a respiratory rate of 28 breaths per minute, but no cyanosis was present. He was given nebulized ipratropium, salbutamol, and normal saline. Symptoms soon improved. After discharge, he was prescribed a metered dose inhaler of ipratropium and another containing salbutamol. At 1 month follow-up, his symptoms were significantly reduced in severity.

Critical Thinking Questions

1. How do muscarinic antagonists such as ipratropium work?
2. What are the other indications of the muscarinic antagonists?
3. What are the adverse effects of ipratropium?

Further Reading

[1] G.J. Blokdijk, Mecamylamine Hydrochloride; Complete Self-Assessment Guide, CreateSpace Independent Publishing Platform, 2018.
[2] G.J. Blokdijk, Succinylcholine Chloride, third ed., CreateSpace Independent Publishing Platform, 2018.
[3] G.J. Blokdijk, Ipratropium Bromide, second ed., CreateSpace Independent Publishing Platform, 2018.
[4] E.A. Dauncey, S. Larsson, Plants that Kill: A Natural History of the World's Most Poisonous Plants, Princeton University Press, 2018.
[5] S. Elisa, J.J. Nagelhout, J.S. Heiner, Current Anesthesia Practice: Evaluation & Certification Review, Elsevier, 2020.
[6] A. Fung, Ophthalmic Clinical Examination – the Sydney Eye Hospital Registrars' Manual, Fung, 2010.

[7] Icon Group International, Anticholinergics: Webster's Facts and Phrases, Icon Group International, Inc, 2010.
[8] Icon Group International, Anticholinergics: Webster's Timeline History 1953 to 2007, Icon Group International, Inc, 2010.
[9] K.B. Johnson, Clinical Pharmacology for Anesthesiology, McGraw Hill Education/Medical, 2014.
[10] D. Joseph, Peptic Ulcer Disease: Clinical Perspectives, Foster Academics, 2019.
[11] K.J. Knoop, L.B. Stack, A.B. Storrow, R.J. Thurman, Atlas of Emergency Medicine, fifth ed., McGraw Hill/Medical, 2020.
[12] M. Knouff, Historical Use of Belladonna in Medicine, Knouff, 2017.
[13] S.M. Marcus, Medical Toxicology: Antidotes and Anecdotes, Springer, 2017.
[14] A. Martinez-Rubio, J. Tamargo, G.A. Dan, Antiarrhythmic Drugs (Current Cardiovascular Therapy), Springer, 2020.
[15] S.T. Ohnishi, T. Ohnishi, Malignant Hyperthermia: A Genetic Membrane Disease, CRC Press, 2021.
[16] R. Watts, D. Standaert, J. Obeso, Movement Disorder, third ed., McGraw Hill/Medical, 2011.

UNIT IV

Mental and behavioral health drugs

CHAPTER

22

Anxiety and insomnia drugs

OUTLINE

LEARNING OUTCOMES

After study of the chapter, readers should be able to:

1. Describe the signs and symptoms of anxiety disorders.
2. Explain the most common anxiety disorders.
3. Describe the consequence of insufficient sleep.
4. Describe the primary medications for anxiety and sleep disorders.
5. Compare the sedative hypnotics and anxiolytics.
6. Discuss the pharmacokinetics of benzodiazepines.
7. Describe the contraindications to benzodiazepines.

The Science of Pharmacology
https://doi.org/10.1016/B978-0-443-29038-1.00022-1

8. Explain the pharmacokinetics of barbiturates.
9. Describe common adverse effects of barbiturates.
10. Explain the classifications of atypical drugs for anxiety and sleep disorders.

Overview

Anxiety is a distressing and unpleasant emotional state of nervousness and uneasiness often related to uncertain causes. It is not always closely tied to the exact timing of a threat and may be anticipatory before a danger, persist afterward, or occur without an identifiable threat. Anxiety can manifest as physical changes and behaviors similar to those caused by fear. Some degree of anxiety can be adaptive, helping to prepare and improve functioning and promote being effectively cautious. However, when anxiety exceeds a certain level, it causes dysfunction and excessive distress, becoming maladaptive until it is considered a disorder. Anxiety disorders are the most common class of psychiatric disorders. They often are not recognized and consequently not treated. Chronic maladaptive anxiety can contribute to or interfere with treating general medical disorders. Sleep disorders are usually related to anxiety disorders, including insomnia. A sleep disorder may affect overall health, safety, and quality of life. Sleep deprivation affects the ability to drive safely and increases risks for other health problems.

Some ways to manage anxiety disorders include learning about anxiety, mindfulness, relaxation techniques, correct breathing techniques, dietary adjustments, exercise, assertiveness, self-esteem, cognitive therapy, exposure therapy, structured problem solving, medication, and support groups. Benzodiazepines reduce anxiety at low doses and induce sleep at higher doses.

Epidemiology

Anxiety disorders are widespread, with lifetime prevalence rates between 13.6% and 28.8% in Western countries. Comorbidity among individuals with an anxiety disorder is high: three out of four people with a lifetime anxiety disorder experience at least one other mental illness. There is a solid association between anxiety disorders and affective disorders and a considerably lower but still substantial relation between anxiety disorders and substance use disorders. In general, anxiety disorders develop relatively early in life. In 80%–90% of cases, the disease manifests before age 35, and the time between 10 and 25 years seems to be a high-risk period for developing anxiety disorders. However, there are significant differences between the anxiety disorders concerning age of onset. Females have a higher prevalence of anxiety disorders.

Anxiety disorders

Anxiety disorders are the most common mental health illnesses, often causing many signs and symptoms, including physical, somatic, cognitive, and behavioral. The experience of anxiety triggers the sympathetic nervous system. Physical symptoms of the fight-or-flight response may include tachycardia, shortness of breath, hypertension, dry mouth, and excessive sweating. The most common anxiety disorders are *generalized anxiety disorder, social anxiety disorder, panic disorder,* obsessive-compulsive disorder (OCD), and posttraumatic stress disorder (PTSD).

Excessive, irrational worry about events or circumstances characterizes **generalized anxiety disorder**. It often interferes with daily functioning, causing anxiety about health, money, life and death, family, friends, interpersonal relationships, and work. Social anxiety disorder is also known as **social phobia**. It is characterized by fear and anxiety in social situations, causing extreme distress and impaired ability to function in daily living. **Panic disorder** is recurrent panic attacks usually accompanied by concerns about future episodes or behavioral changes to avoid any situation that could instigate an attack. **OCD** causes the affected individual to have specific recurrent thoughts, called *obsessions*, and a need to perform certain behaviors repeatedly, called *compulsions*, often to attempt to control the obsessive thoughts.

Usually, *OCD* develops gradually, with insidious onset. The patient may experience worries or fears that they will be harmed, perhaps by being exposed to and forming a deadly disease, self-harm, or hurting another person. Compulsions are deliberate acts that are usually done to neutralize or offset obsessions. They include repeated checking of things such as door locks, excessive washing of hands, excessing counting, or excessive arranging and ordering of certain items. For some individuals, obsessions and compulsions have logical connections, such as fearing contamination and engaging in extreme protective and sanitary behaviors to prevent disease.

PTSD is a mental health condition that develops in some individuals who have experienced shocking, frightening, or dangerous events. It is common following certain traumatic events such as car accidents, fires, earthquakes, sexual assault, physical violence, and military combat. Intense memories of the causative event, hypervigilance, and reactivity to possible threats, recurrent nightmares, and mood disturbances characterize the disorder. The patient often reports feeling anxious or frightened, even in the absence of danger. The medications used to treat PTSD consist of selective serotonin reuptake inhibitors and antianxiety drugs.

You should remember

Panic attacks, phobias, OCD, social anxiety, and PTSD affect more than 40 million adults in the United States alone. Famous people who have battled panic attacks include Selena Gomez, Emma Stone, Carson Daly, Prince Harry, Jennifer Lopez, Sarah Silverman, and Hugh Grant.

Sleep disorders and insomnia

Sleep disorders may involve problems falling asleep, staying asleep at the wrong times, excessive sleep, and abnormal sleeping behaviors. **Insomnia**, acute or chronic, includes trouble falling or staying asleep. Excessive nighttime sleepiness often results in individuals being tired throughout the day. Sleep disorders are among the most common conditions in medicine and psychiatry, with the potential to significantly impair the quality of life. They can also result from a variety of medical and psychiatric disorders. Insufficient sleep prevents the brain from clearing away **beta-amyloid**. This leads to toxic accumulation levels, increasing the risks of developing **Alzheimer disease (AD)** or other dementias. People who sleep less than 6 hours per night in their 50s and 60s are more likely to develop **dementia**.

Clinical manifestations of sleep disorders include **sleep apnea**, **restless legs syndrome**, and disturbances of the circadian rhythms. Psychiatric manifestations of sleep disorders often include anxiety and depression as well as **cognitive** difficulties. It is important to distinguish primary sleep disorders from secondary sleep disorders, and there is usually difficulty in determining if depression and anxiety are causing problems with sleep or whether sleep problems are causing these psychiatric conditions.

Insomnia is signified by difficulty falling asleep or staying asleep, awakening too early, or feeling unrefreshed after sleep. It may involve symptoms related to a primary medical illness, a mental illness, other sleep disorders, stressors, or use and exposure to certain substances.

You should remember

Normal sleep contributes to tissue repair, thermoregulation, homeostatic restoration, memory consolidation, and preservation of neuroimmune-endocrine integrity. Sleep allows the brain to remove toxins and self-protect against accumulating peptides and proteins linked to AD. Therefore insomnia and other sleep disorders are directly related to higher levels of the precursors of AD, increasing the risks for its development.

TABLE 22.1 Benzodiazepines and nonbenzodiazepine anxiolytics

Generic name	Trade name	Average dosage range (mg/day)	Dosage forms (in mg)
Benzodiazepines for anxiety			
alprazolam	Xanax	0.25–4	0.25, 0.5, 1, 2
chlordiazepoxide	Librium	5–100	5, 10, 25, 100
clonazepam	Klonopin	0.25–4	0.125, 0.25, 0.5, 1, 2
clorazepate	Tranxene	15–60	3.75, 7.5, 15
diazepam	Valium	2–40	2, 2.5, 5, 10, 15, 20, 5 mg/mL, 5 mg/5 mL
lorazepam	Ativan	2–9	0.5, 1, 2
oxazepam	Serax	10–60	10, 15, 30
Benzodiazepines for insomnia			
estazolam	Prosom	1–2	1, 2
flurazepam	Dalmane	15–30	15, 30
quazepam	Doral	7.5–15	15
temazepam	Restoril	7.5–30	7.5, 15, 22.5, 30
triazolam	Halcion	0.125–0.5	0.125, 0.25
Nonbenzodiazepine anxiolytics			
buspirone	BuSpar	5 - 60	5, 7.5, 10, 15, 30
eszopiclone	Lunesta	1–3	1, 2, 3
meprobamate	Miltown	1200–1600	200, 400
ramelteon	Rozerem	8	8
suvorexant	Belsomra	5–20	5, 10, 15, 20
tasimelteon	Hetlioz	20	20, 4 mg/mL
zaleplon	Sonata	5–20	5, 10
zolpidem	Ambien	1.75–12.5	1.75, 3.5, 5, 10, mg/oral spray, extended release: 6.25, 12.5 tablets
zopiclone	Zimovane	3.75–7.5	3.75, 5, 7.5

You should remember

Chronic insomnia can result in a variety of severe conditions. These include asthma, irregular heartbeat, coronary heart disease, heart failure, excessive stress levels, depression, anxiety, suicidal thoughts, hypertension, stroke, obesity, lowered immunity and related conditions, diabetes mellitus, complications during pregnancy, sexual problems, substance abuse, and memory loss.

Pharmacotherapy of anxiety and sleep disorders

The most prominent antianxiety drugs for immediate relief are those known as benzodiazepines. Sleep disorders are mainly treated with benzodiazepines, antidepressants, *doxepin, eszopiclone, lemborexant, ramelteon, suvorexant, zaleplon, zolpidem,* and OTC antihistamines. Antidepressants are discussed in **Chapter 23**. **Table 22.1** summarizes the benzodiazepines and nonbenzodiazepine anxiolytics used for anxiety and insomnia.

Benzodiazepines

Benzodiazepines are primary medications for anxiety and sleep disorders. Newer and safer benzodiazepines have been developed, with *chlordiazepoxide (Librium)* being identified in 1955. Miscellaneous drugs followed, which were also called *nonbenzodiazepines*. They may have various durations of action. Benzodiazepines were the most commonly prescribed type of sedative hypnotics. Today, they are less often used than nonbenzodiazepine drugs. Even so, when benzodiazepines are used correctly, they have minimal adverse effects and significant effectiveness and safety. Benzodiazepines have two classifications: *sedative hypnotics* and *anxiolytics*. This is based on their primary uses. While sedative hypnotics are used to induce sleep and calmness, anxiolytics are used to relieve anxiety. Benzodiazepines are also classified as psychoactive drugs and are commonly referred to as minor tranquilizers. Regardless, these drugs have sedative, hypnotic, and anxiolytic properties. The short-acting, intermediate-acting, and long-acting benzodiazepines are summarized in **Table 22.2**.

Pharmacokinetics

Benzodiazepines are lipid soluble, well absorbed from the GI tract, and have significant distribution to the brain. Rapid redistribution of these drugs from the brain to the skeletal muscles and other highly perfused tissues stops the CNS effects. Mainly, liver enzymes metabolize benzodiazepines before being eliminated from the body. Each drug has different metabolic rates and pathways. Many benzodiazepines are first converted to active metabolites, which have long half-lives. After several days of use, accumulation of active metabolites may lead to extreme sedation. Examples of benzodiazepines that undergo extrahepatic **conjugation** and do not form active metabolites include *lorazepam* and *oxazepam*.

The liver metabolizes flurazepam, and its elimination half-life is 40–250 hours via the kidneys. *Alprazolam* has 80%–100% bioavailability and 80% protein binding. Its onset of action is less than 60 minutes. The immediate-release form has an elimination half-life of 11–13 hours, while the extended-release state has an elimination half-life of 11–16 hours.

TABLE 22.2 Benzodiazepines

Generic name	Trade name
Short acting	
midazolam	Versed
oxazepam	Serax
triazolam	Halcion
Intermediate acting	
alprazolam	Xanax
lorazepam	Ativan
temazepam	Restoril
Long-acting	
clonazepam	Klonopin
diazepam	Valium
flurazepam	Dalmane

Mechanism of action

The action of benzodiazepines is linked to how they depress CNS activity. The hypothalamus, thalamus, and limbic system may be affected (see **Fig. 22.1**). There are specific brain receptors for benzodiazepines. Benzodiazepines **potentiate** the action of the gamma-aminobutyric acid (GABA) receptors. They bind onto receptors on chloride ion channels, enhancing the effects of GABA and facilitating the opening of these channels. This allows negatively charged chloride ions to flow into the neurons, decreasing their excitability, dampening the limbic alert system, and calming overall brain excitation. They are capable of causing entire CNS depression, from relaxation to the induction of sleep to coma.

Clinical indications

Benzodiazepines are regularly used for sedation, to relieve anxiety and agitation, to treat depression related to stress, to induce sleep, to relax the skeletal muscles, and to treat acute seizures. Benzodiazepines are commonly used with analgesics, anesthetics, and neuromuscular blockers as part of balanced anesthesia and moderate sedation. The amnesic properties of benzodiazepines reduce memories of painful procedures. Benzodiazepines are also used to treat and prevent alcohol withdrawal symptoms.

Benzodiazepines are preferred in the treatment of acute anxiety and panic attacks. They are also used for primary insomnia. Lower doses are used for older patients because they are more sensitive to CNS depressive effects. *Triazolam* is often used for short-term treatment of acute insomnia and circadian rhythm sleep disorders such as jet lag. It is important to note that short-term use of benzodiazepines is preferred because prolonged use over 6 months may lead to tolerance and dependence.

Contraindications

Contraindications to benzodiazepines include known drug allergies, **narrow-angle glaucoma**, **chronic obstructive pulmonary disease** (COPD), psychosis, and pregnancy because they may cause fetal malformations. Benzodiazepines are also contraindicated in lactating females.

Adverse effects

The most common adverse effects of benzodiazepines include drowsiness, confusion, lightheadedness, dizziness, muscle weakness, slurred speech, constipation, memory problems, nausea, blurred vision, and dry mouth. In older people, unsteadiness is a significant problem, which may result in falls and injuries. It is essential to avoid tolerance, dependence, and potential for abuse and cognitive impairment.

FIG. 22.1 The hypothalamus, thalamus, and limbic system.

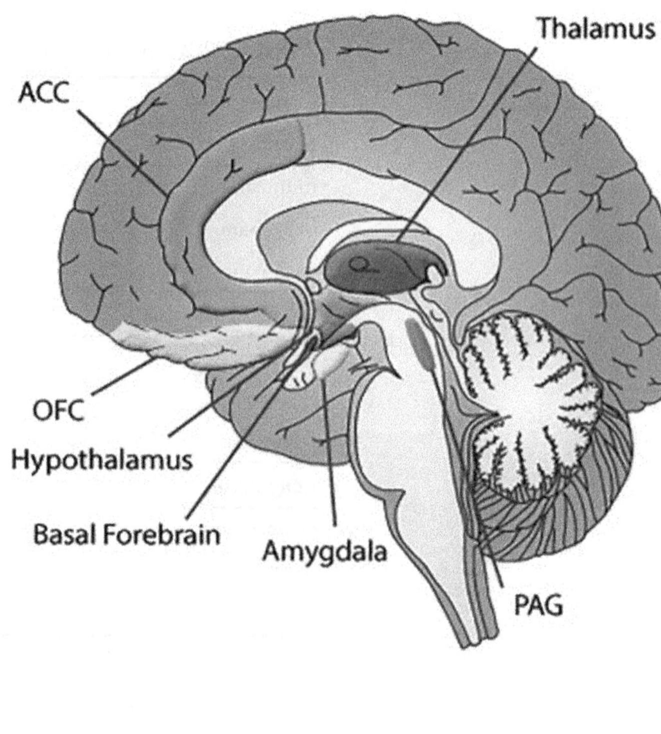

TABLE 22.3 Barbiturates

Generic name	Trade name
Ultrashort acting	
methohexital	Brevital
thiopental	Pentothal
Short acting	
pentobarbital	Nembutal
secobarbital	Seconal
Intermediate acting	
butabarbital	Butisol
Long acting	
phenobarbital	(generic only)
mephobarbital	Mebaral

You should remember

The FDA issued a black box warning in 2016 for all benzodiazepines and opioids concerning the risk of combined use. This combination should only occur when there are no other alternatives available. Chances of this combination include extreme sleepiness, respiratory depression, coma, and death.

Toxicities

Some benzodiazepines can cause psychomotor dysfunction, including cognitive impairment, reduced psychomotor skills, and unwanted daytime sedation. These conditions are dangerous when driving an automobile or operating other types of machinery. Older adults are more susceptible to drugs that cause psychomotor dysfunction and increase risks of falling and fractures. At high dosages, **anterograde amnesia** can occur—making these drugs commonly used in cases of date rape. Additive depression can arise if benzodiazepines are combined with alcohol, antihistamines, antipsychotic drugs, opioid analgesics, and tricyclic antidepressants. Overdosage causes extreme cardiovascular and respiratory depression. For intoxication, a patent airway must be established along with ventilatory support.

Barbiturates

Barbiturates are sedative-hypnotic medications, meaning they cause people to feel relaxed or sleepy. For over a century, they have treated many conditions, including seizures, migraines, insomnia, and more. They are less common today because of the risk of misuse and specific side effects. However, they can be a backup treatment when others do not work. They are classified into ultrashort acting, short acting, intermediate acting, and long acting (see **Table 22.3**). It is essential to understand that barbiturates are not used for anxiety much anymore due to the risks involved.

Pharmacokinetics

Barbiturates have a bioavailability of more than 95% and protein binding. They are extensively metabolized in the liver, except for phenobarbital, a weak acid partly excreted unchanged in the urine. The CNS effects of most barbiturates are based on the dose. The effects of barbiturates, as well as benzodiazepines, range from sedation and **anxiolysis** to **hypnosis**, anesthesia, and coma. There are additive depressant effects when two or more drugs are administered together. The dose-response curve varies between different drugs. The barbiturates have a "steeper curve" than the benzodiazepines, meaning that barbiturates must be used much more carefully in comparison.

Mechanism of action

Barbiturates primarily act upon the **reticular formation** of the **brainstem**. They prolong the inhibitor effects of both GABA and glycine. *Phenobarbital* is an **allosteric modulator** that extends the length of chloride ion channels open by interacting with GABA-A receptor subunits. This decreases the excitability of the postsynaptic neuron. *Secobarbital* decreases presynaptic and postsynaptic membrane excitability by facilitating the actions of GABA. Barbiturates increase the length of time that GABA-mediated chloride ion channels remain open. They also have the potential to block glutamic acid, an excitatory neurotransmitter. At high concentrations, barbiturates can block sodium channels.

Clinical indications

Phenobarbital is used for all types of seizures except absence seizures, and it is the first-line choice for neonatal seizures. It is sometimes used for alcohol or benzodiazepine detoxification and insomnia and anxiety. *Secobarbital* is indicated to treat epilepsy, temporary treatment of insomnia, and as a preoperative medication to produce anesthesia and anxiolysis in short-term surgical, diagnostic, or therapeutic procedures that are only minimally painful. *Thiopental* is used in anesthesia, for medically induced coma, in refractory status epilepticus, for euthanasia, for lethal injection, and in psychiatry to desensitize patients with phobias or help recall repressed memories. *Butabarbital* is used for the short-term treatment of sleep and anxiety disorders and as a presurgical sedative. *Mephobarbital* is primarily used as an anticonvulsant and as a sedative and anxiolytic. *Pentobarbital* is used as a sedative, short-term hypnotic and anesthetic to treat insomnia and control convulsions in emergencies. It is also used to reduce intracranial pressure in **Reye syndrome** and traumatic brain injury and to induce coma in cerebral ischemia patients or those with acute liver failure refractory to mannitol. Barbiturates are no longer as widely used due to their addiction potential and low therapeutic index.

Contraindications

Contraindications to barbiturates include known drug allergies, pregnancy, severe kidney or liver disease, and significant respiratory difficulties. Barbiturates must be used cautiously in older adults because of their sedative properties and the likelihood of increasing the risk of falling. *Phenobarbital* is also contraindicated with acute intermittent porphyria, prior dependence upon the drug, and during breastfeeding.

Adverse effects

Common adverse effects of barbiturates include drowsiness, headache, hypotension, nausea, sedation, and skin rash. Serious adverse effects include abnormally slow breathing, confusion, fainting, hallucinations, **hypopnea**, and coma. *Phenobarbital* may also cause dizziness, nystagmus, and ataxia. In elderly patients, it can cause extreme excitement and, in children, **paradoxical hyperactivity**.

Toxicities

Barbiturates may be toxic to some people, and large doses can cause death. The symptoms of toxicity include depressed breathing, **Cheyne-Stokes respirations**, blurred vision, pupillary constriction, hypotension, tachycardia, CNS depression, **areflexia**, loss of consciousness or coma, and circulatory collapse. The other symptoms of toxicities include **cyanosis**, shivering, slurred speech, and sweating.

You should remember

Death from overdose is the most significant risk factor related to using barbiturates. These drugs can be hazardous because the correct dose is difficult to predict. Just a slight overdose can cause a coma or be fatal. Deaths have occurred with amounts ranging between 2 and 10 g. Barbiturates are also addictive and can cause a life-threatening withdrawal syndrome.

TABLE 22.4 Atypical sedative hypnotics

Generic name	Trade name
Melatonin agonists	
agomelatine	Valdoxan
ramelteon	Rozerem
tasimelteon	Hetlioz
Orexin antagonists	
lemborexant	Dayvigo
suvorexant	Belsomra

Atypical drugs

The latest medications for anxiety and sleep disorders are **atypical drugs**, including **melatonin** agonists and **orexin** antagonists. As of 2014 three melatonin agonists were on the market, including ramelteon (also classified as a miscellaneous sedative hypnotic earlier), agomelatine, and *tasimelteon*. The currently available orexin antagonists include *lemborexant* and *suvorexant*. Suvorexant is also classified as a miscellaneous sedative hypnotic. Orexins are neuropeptides that control wakefulness. They are also known as hypocretins. The atypical sedative hypnotics are summarized in **Table 22.4.**

Pharmacokinetics

Ramelteon has a bioavailability of 1.8% and protein binding of about 82%. It is metabolized in the liver and has an elimination half-life of 1–2.6 hours. Excretion is in the urine and the feces. *Tasimelteon* has an oral bioavailability of 38%, with peak concentrations occurring 0.5–3 hours after fasted oral administration. The drug is about 90% bound to proteins and extensively metabolizes via the liver. The elimination half-life is 0.9–1.7 hours, and the medicine is mainly excreted via the urine and small amounts via the feces. *Lemborexant* has 94% protein binding and is metabolized in the liver. The elimination half-life is 17–19 hours. The drug is mainly excreted in the feces and only 29% in the urine. *Suvorexant* has 82% bioavailability and nearly 100% protein binding. It is also metabolized in the liver. Its elimination half-life is about 12 hours, primarily eliminated in the feces and 23% in the urine.

Mechanism of action

Ramelteon is a receptor agonist with a high affinity for the melatonin receptors. *Tasimelteon* is a selective agonist for the same melatonin receptors. *Lemborexant* is a dual antagonist of the orexin receptors.

Clinical indications

Atypical drugs are indicated for treating non-24-hour sleep-wake disorder and insomnia characterized by sleep onset or maintenance difficulties. *Ramelteon* is approved for insomnia characterized by problems with sleep onset. *Tasimelteon* is indicated for non-24-hour sleep-wake disorder in adults and nighttime sleep disturbances in Smith-Magenis syndrome in people aged 16 and older. *Lemborexant* is used in the treatment of various types of insomnia.

Contraindications

Ramelteon is contraindicated with high prolactin levels, suicidal thoughts, alcoholism, depression, liver disease, sleep apnea, and complex sleep behaviors such as eating or driving while asleep. There are no proven contraindications with *tasimelteon*. Atypical drugs are contraindicated in patients with narcolepsy and pregnancy (category C).

Adverse effects

The common adverse effects of the atypical drugs include agitation, anxiety, confusion, depression, abnormal dreams or nightmares, disturbed sleep, drowsiness, hallucinations, memory problems, thoughts of self-harm, trouble moving or talking on awakening, unusual thoughts or behaviors, headache, elevated liver enzymes, upper respiratory tract infections, urinary tract infections, and a weak feeling in the legs. Older adults may have an increased risk of falling because of excessive drowsiness. Overweight adults may be more likely to experience various adverse effects. Serious adverse effects of the atypical drugs include signs of hypersensitivity, sleepwalking, sleep driving, sleep eating, and having sexual intercourse while asleep.

Toxicities

Ramelteon may be toxic in patients with impaired hepatic function. *In animal studies, tasimelteon* has caused the development of tumors and adverse events during pregnancy. *Lemborexant* may cause depression or suicidal thoughts. In animal studies, this drug has caused abnormalities during the period of organogenesis and can also pass through breast milk to potentially harm an infant. *Suvorexant* may be hepatotoxic and, based on animal testing, may cause fetal harm during pregnancy. There is inconclusive evidence about whether this drug is harmful to breast-feeding infants.

You should remember

Melatonin receptor agonists such as ramelteon may have an advantage over benzodiazepines and nonbenzodiazepines because they specifically target the brain structures responsible for the sleep-wake cycle. It has shown no evidence of abuse, dependence, or withdrawal and has been approved for long-term use in adults. Ramelteon is also safe for older adults with COPD and sleep apnea.

Miscellaneous drugs

Miscellaneous drugs used as sedative hypnotics include *eszopiclone, ramelteon, zaleplon,* and *zolpidem*. Eszopiclone, ramelteon, and zolpidem are also referred to as *nonbenzodiazepines*. Even with this named classification, these medications are still benzodiazepine-like in their actions, binding to and activating the benzodiazepine receptor in the brain. Other nonbenzodiazepines, such as buspirone, a 5-HT1A agonist, work differently. Eszopiclone, zaleplon, and zolpidem have a rapid onset of CNS action. It should be noted that buspirone, an anxiolytic, and hypnotics (eszopiclone, ramelteon, zaleplon, and zolpidem) are sometimes also atypical drugs. The term "miscellaneous drugs" is that these agents are unique in their action and not comparable to other anxiolytics, sedatives, or hypnotics. However, their adverse effects may be similar. They are not structurally identical to benzodiazepines or barbiturates. Miscellaneous drugs used as sedative hypnotics include eszopiclone (Lunesta), zaleplon (Sonata), and zolpidem (Ambien).

Pharmacokinetics

Eszopiclone was the first FDA-approved hypnotic for long-term use to provide 8 hours of sleep. It should only be used when the patient has 8 hours of sleep before performing any regular activities. Cytochrome P450 metabolizes eszopiclone and has a 6-hour half-life. *Zaleplon* has an even faster liver metabolism via *aldehyde oxidase* and *cytochrome P450*. *Zolpidem* has a short duration of action due to rapid metabolism by hepatic enzymes. Kidneys and small amounts of bile and feces primarily excrete these drugs.

Mechanism of action

Eszopiclone appears to create CNS effects by interacting with the benzodiazepine receptor subtypes. It has more selective binding than the benzodiazepines. It interacts with the GABA receptor. The onset of action of eszopiclone is 30–60 minutes, the half-life of elimination is 6 hours, and the duration of action is about 8 hours. *Zaleplon* interacts with the GABA-benzodiazepine receptor complex. It also binds selectively to the brain omega-1 receptor. *Zolpidem* has high intrinsic activity at the omega-1 subtype. This may account for the drug's relative lack of anticonvulsants, muscle relaxants, and anxiolytic effects at therapeutic doses. The onset of action is 30 minutes, the half-life of elimination is 1–6 hours, and the duration of action is 6–8 hours.

Clinical indications

Eszopiclone is an efficient treatment for insomnia when nonpharmacological treatments have been unsuccessful. *Zaleplon* is used for the short-term treatment of insomnia, which generally means not for longer than 30 days. *Zolpidem* is also used to treat insomnia and has immediate-release and extended-release forms. The immediate-release form is used for those with difficulty falling asleep, while the extended-release form is used for patients with difficulty remaining asleep.

Contraindications

Eszopiclone is contraindicated if the patient regularly uses alcohol or any of the following conditions are present: confusion, depression, suicidal thoughts, decreased lung function, worsening of coexisting COPD, overall weakness, severe liver disease, and complex sleep behaviors such as eating or driving while asleep. *Zaleplon* is contraindicated if the patient has depression, mental problems, severe liver disease, COPD, sleep apnea, or complex sleep behaviors such as eating or driving while asleep. *Zolpidem* has the most contraindications out of all the miscellaneous sedative hypnotics. These include confusion, alcoholism, suicidal thoughts, depression, drug abuse, aggression, myasthenia gravis, liver disease, hallucinations, memory loss, and sleep apnea.

Adverse effects

The common adverse effects of miscellaneous drugs include dizziness, headache, drowsiness, nausea, vomiting, dry mouth, fatigue, dream disturbances, decreased testosterone, increased prolactin levels, and unpleasant taste sensations. However, these drugs result in less cognitive impairment and reduced risk of dependency in comparison to the traditional benzodiazepines. The serious adverse effects of the miscellaneous drugs include blurred vision, confusion, mood changes, **myalgia**, paradoxical excitation, and **tachycardia**. The "Z" drugs—eszopiclone, zaleplon, and zolpidem—can cause sleep-related, complex behaviors, including sleepwalking and sleep driving. They have been involved in some legal cases.

Toxicities

Eszopiclone may cause a rash, swelling, wheezing, chest or throat tightness, difficulty breathing or swallowing, depression, suicidal thoughts, **hallucinations**, memory problems, dizziness, confusion, fatigue, weakness, nausea, vomiting, fever, and chills. *Zaleplon* may cause a blue or green discoloration of the mouth, lips, and urine and has also caused vomiting, confusion, sinus tachycardia, hallucinations, and muscle tremors. *Zolpidem* may cause respiratory or cardiovascular depression, pinpoint pupils, slurred speech, vomiting, delusions, loss of consciousness, coma, and death.

You should remember

Miscellaneous sedatives and hypnotics work in the brain to reduce anxiety and induce a feeling of calmness. The newer drugs in this class are less toxic than their older counterparts. A subset called the "Z-drugs" (zolpidem, eszopiclone, and zaleplon) are among the newer drugs and are highly effective for insomnia because of their quick onset and short duration of action.

Key Terms

Allosteric modulator
Alzheimer disease
Anterograde amnesia
Anxiety disorders
Anxiolysis
Areflexia
Atypical drugs
Beta-amyloid
Brainstem
Cheyne-Stokes
Chronic obstructive pulmonary disease
Cognitive
Conjugation
Cyanosis
Dementia
Generalized anxiety disorder

Hallucinations
Hypervigilance
Hypnosis
Hypopnea
Insomnia
Melatonin
Myalgia
Narrow-angle glaucoma
Obsessive-compulsive disorder
Orexin
Panic disorder
Paradoxical hyperactivity
Posttraumatic stress disorder
Potentiate
Reticular formation
Restless legs syndrome
Reye syndrome
Sleep apnea
Social phobia
Tachycardia

Clinical Case Studies

Clinical Case Study 1

A 30-year-old female has struggled with anxiety and depression since age 18. She has attended a variety of therapists, and one of them prescribed her citalopram, an selective serotonin reuptake inhibitor. It gradually improved her mood and reduced her anxiety, and the patient admits to having no panic attacks. It has helped her focus on work and daily living activities to a large degree.

Critical Thinking Questions

1. What are the most common anxiety disorders?
2. What is the description of generalized anxiety disorder?
3. What are the characteristics of social anxiety disorder?

Clinical Case Study 2

A 39-year-old male visited his primary care physician complaining of insomnia. He has difficulty falling asleep nearly every night but can usually remain asleep afterward. The patient admits to regularly feeling tired during the day, affecting his ability to work. He prescribed zolpidem, a short-acting nonbenzodiazepine. After only a short time of taking the drug, the patient's ability to fall asleep improves significantly.

Critical Thinking Questions

1. What is the description of insomnia?
2. What symptoms may be involved in insomnia?
3. What are the trade name, average dosage range, and zolpidem dosage forms?

Further Reading

[1] C. Adamec, Barbiturates and Other Depressants (Understanding Drugs), Chelsea House Publishing Library, 2011.
[2] K. Brown, Diazepam: What No One will Tell you About (Pocket Pharmacy)—Books on Demand, 2019.
[3] E. Bui, M.E. Charney, A.W. Baker, Clinical Handbook of Anxiety Disorders: From Theory to Practice (Current Clinical Psychiatry), Humana Press, 2020.
[4] J. Chamberlin, P. Lehmann, P. Lahti, L.R. Mosher, Coming off Psychiatric Drugs: Successful Withdrawal from Neuroleptics, Antidepressants, Mood Stabilizers, Ritalin and Tranquilizers, Peter Lehmann Publishing, 2015.
[5] L.D. Chowdhury, O.P. Singh, Psychiatric Drug Handbook, Jaypee Brothers Medical Publishers Ltd, 2017.
[6] V. Dhikav, K. Singh Anand, Clinical Neuropsychopharmacology: Desk Reference for Physicians, Springer, 2019.
[7] J.M. Gorman, Essential Guide to Psychiatric Drugs, fourth ed., Griffin, 2007.
[8] D. Herzberg, Happy Pills in America: From Miltown to Prozac, JHUP, 2010.
[9] P.K. Jjemba, Pharma-Ecology: The Occurrence and Fate of Pharmaceuticals and Personal Care Products in the Environment, second ed., Wiley, 2018.
[10] H. Ketha, U. Garg, Toxicology Cases for the Clinical and Forensic Laboratory, Academic Press, 2020.

[11] B. Kramer, Medications for Anxiety & Depression–A No-nonsense, Comprehensive Guide to the Most Common (And Not so Common) Antidepressants and Anti-anxiety Drugs Available, BK Publications, 2014.
[12] D. Martins, Alprazolam & Benzodiazepine: A Reference Guide, CreateSpace Independent Publishing Platform, 2015.
[13] W.H. McGlothlin, Amphetamines, Barbiturates, and Hallucinogens: An Analysis of Use, Distribution, and Control (Volume 1), University of California Libraries, 2012.
[14] M. Mohan Varshney, A. Husain, A Textbook of Medicinal Chemistry. I.K, International Publishing House, 2015.
[15] T.L. Pazdernik, L. Kerecsen, Rapid Review Pharmacology, third ed., Mosby, 2010.
[16] J. Peppin, J.V. Pergolizzi, R.B. Raffa, S.L. Wright, The Benzodiazepines Crisis: The Ramifications of an Over-used Drug Class, Oxford University Press, 2020.
[17] N. Pramod, G.M. Basha, Structural Classification of Drugs: A Quick Reference Guide, BSP Books, 2020.
[18] W.S. Root, F.G. Hofmann, The Nervous System: Central Nervous System Drugs, Academic Press, 2017.
[19] C. Scott, Dangerous Depressants & Sedatives, Mason Crest, 2014.
[20] C. Small, Valium and Other Antianxiety Drugs (Dangerous Drugs), Cavendish Square Publishing, 2015.
[21] E. Spina, G. Trifiro, Pharmacovigilance in Psychiatry, Adis, 2016.
[22] A. Tone, The Age of Anxiety: A History of America's Turbulent Affair with Tranquilizers, Basic Books, 2008.
[23] I. Walker, Sedatives & Hypnotics: Deadly Downers (Illicit and Misused Drugs), Mason Crest, 2014.

CHAPTER

23

Antidepressants

OUTLINE

LEARNING OUTCOMES

After study of the chapter, readers should be able to:

1. Describe the causes of major depressive disorder.
2. Explain the effectiveness of cognitive behavioral therapy for major depressive disorder.
3. Identify the most common treatments for major depression.
4. Explain the classifications of antidepressants.

The Science of Pharmacology
https://doi.org/10.1016/B978-0-443-29038-1.00023-3

5. Discuss the indications of the selective serotonin reuptake inhibitors.
6. Describe the mechanism of action for serotonin modulators.
7. Explain the characteristics of the norepinephrine-dopamine reuptake inhibitors.
8. Describe the features of the monoamine oxidase inhibitors.

Overview

Major depressive disorder (MDD) is a common and serious medical illness that negatively affects feelings, thoughts, and actions. There is usually a profound and constant sense of hopelessness and despair. Major depression is marked by combined symptoms that interfere with the ability to eat, sleep, study, work, and enjoy previously pleasurable activities. A major depressive episode may occur only once but usually happens several times in a lifetime. Depression can lead to many emotional and physical problems with long-term consequences. MDD is believed to be caused by genetic, environmental, and psychological factors, with about 40% of cases being genetic. Risk factors include a family history of the condition, life changes, medications, chronic health problems, and substance use disorders. MDD affects approximately 16.1 million people in the United States annually. Globally, it affects about 163 million people annually.

Major depressive disorder

MDD, also known simply as depression, is a mental disorder characterized by at least 2 weeks of low mood in most situations. It is often accompanied by low self-esteem, loss of interest or pleasure in previously enjoyed activities, low energy, and pain of no identifiable cause. Depressive disorders occur at all ages but most often initially develop during the midteenage years, 20s, or 30s. Depressive disorders are more common in urban populations than rural ones and are more prevalent among people from lower socioeconomic classes. The exact cause of depressive disorders is not always known. However, it is believed to be related to heredity, abnormal levels of neurotransmitters, changes in neuroendocrine function, psychosocial factors, or combinations of all of these. Low mood or sadness often is due to disappointments. These may come from financial problems, illnesses, natural disasters, or deaths of family members and friends.

A recent example is the COVID-19 pandemic, affecting millions of people worldwide physically, mentally, and emotionally. Fear of the pandemic resulted in many low or discouraged moods because of the requirements of isolation for weeks or months, loss of social activities, and general anxiety produced by news reports of deaths, serious illness, rapid spread of infection, and hospitalizations. The inability to continue working and loss of finances complicated the situation even further, even for those already receiving treatment or on antidepressant therapy. For some people, the pandemic added another contributing factor to depression.

People who have experienced significant *depression* have a higher risk of recurrent episodes. MDD runs in families, and those diagnosed have a three times greater chance of having a first-degree relative with the disease. People with anxiety are more likely to develop depression because they may not have developed sufficient coping or social skills to adjust to life pressures. Depression also develops in people with other mental disorders. Females are at higher risk than males for depressive disorders.

Changes in neurotransmitter levels are most likely involved with depression. These include abnormal catecholaminergic, cholinergic, glutamatergic, and serotonergic neurotransmission regulation.

For a depressive disorder to be diagnosed, the symptoms must be present for 2 weeks or more. All types of depression feature symptoms that vary in number, severity, and persistence. For *MDD*, diagnosis requires five or more signs and symptoms of the disease to be present nearly every day over 2 weeks, with one being a depressed mood or loss of pleasure or interest. Symptoms of depression that are more commonly associated with an underlying biological etiology are often neurovegetative. They may include anhedonia, sleep disturbance, fatigue, decreased libido, appetite disturbance, concentration problems, and psychomotor retardation. When these symptoms are present or predominant, an underlying dysregulation of neurotransmitters in the brain is suggested, and thus antidepressant medications are often more effective.

Psychotherapy

For MDD, the most common treatments include psychotherapy, medication, and electroconvulsive therapy. Psychotherapy is the treatment of choice for patients under age 18. Exercise is also effective and equivalent to most patients using drugs or psychological medicines. The activity also appears to decrease depression in older adults, so it may be recommended to those willing, motivated, and healthy enough to participate in appropriate physical activity. The most effective psychotherapeutic approach to treating depression is **cognitive behavioral therapy** (CBT).

In some cases, CBT has been proven more effective than antidepressants for major depression. It is also highly beneficial in preventing relapse. Variants of CBT include **rational emotive behavior therapy** and **mindfulness-based cognitive therapy. In contrast,** alternative approaches might consist of acceptance and commitment therapy, which focuses on accepting thoughts and feelings while making changes to improve, and interpersonal psychotherapy, which centers on improving interpersonal functioning and relationships. Psychotherapy treats acute symptoms as well as decreases the likelihood of relapses.

Talk therapy is available individually, in the form of group therapy, or family therapy. With more complex and chronic conditions of depression, psychotherapy is usually combined with medications, and in more severe cases or when depression is associated with suicidality, intensive inpatient treatment may be recommended. Psychodynamic and humanistic therapies may focus less on practical behavioral considerations and more on deep relational and underlying psychoemotional dynamics, often outside conscious awareness. These therapies contribute to patients' interpersonal history and a more profound sense of identity.

Pharmacotherapy

Several classes of medications are used to treat depressive disorders (see **Table 23.1**). The choice of drugs is often guided by a patient's past responses to certain antidepressants. However, treatment-naive patients' symptoms might be targeted using a medication's side effect profile. For example, a drug known to cause weight gain might be avoided for an overweight patient experiencing increased appetite. Still, it might be more aptly considered for an underweight patient experiencing decreased appetite and further weight loss.

While psychotherapy has demonstrated effectiveness in treating depression, evidence suggests that more "biological" forms of depression might respond better to antidepressant medication. Some patients experience depression about identifiable life stressors, while others might develop depressive symptoms for no apparent reason. Biological forms of depression may also be related to certain medical conditions, changes in sex hormones, use of medications or illicit substances, or other endogenous factors. For most classes of antidepressants, a therapeutic response usually occurs in 2–3 weeks, but sometimes as early as 4 days after starting them and as late as 8 weeks. When mild to moderate depression has occurred once, an antidepressant is usually given for 6 months, assuming a therapeutic response has been achieved, and then tapered off over 2 months. For severe depression, recurrence, or risks of suicide, the medication's dose that will produce complete remission may be continued indefinitely as maintenance therapy to prevent relapse. For depression that occurs alongside psychosis, an antidepressant is usually combined with an antipsychotic because this generally leads to better effectiveness. A patient who has recovered from a psychotic depression is at higher risk of relapse than those with nonpsychotic depression. Therefore prophylactic treatment is critical.

To prevent relapse, continued antidepressant therapy is usually maintained for 6–12 months and up to 2 years if the patient is 50 or older. Decreasing doses by about 25% per week must be done to taper off most antidepressants—especially the selective serotonin reuptake inhibitors (SSRIs). Stopping antidepressants abruptly is not advised, and SSRIs may cause discontinuation syndrome: anxiety, chills, dizziness, fatigue, insomnia, irritability, muscle aches, and nausea. The half-life of the SSRI determines the likelihood and severity of withdrawal symptoms.

You should remember

Depressive disorders are pervasive, with about 5% of adults suffering from some form globally. It is a leading cause of disability and a significant contributor to global disease. More females are affected than males. It also affects 5.7% of adults older than age 60. At its worst, depression leads to suicide. There are more than 700,000 people who take their own lives every year.

TABLE 23.1 Antidepressants and their classifications.

Generic name	Trade name	Average dosage range (mg/day)	Dosage forms (in mg)
Selective serotonin	Celexa	20–40	20
reuptake inhibitors	Lexapro	10–20	10
citalopram	Prozac	20–60	10
escitalopram	Luvox	100–200	50
fluoxetine	Paxil	20–62.5	20, 25
fluvoxamine	Zoloft	50–200	50
paroxetine	Viibryd	10–40	10, 20
sertraline	Trintellix	10–20	5, 10, 20
vilazodone			
vortioxetine			
Serotonin modulators	BuSpar	5–60	5, 7.5, 10, 15, 30
buspirone	Remeron	15–45	15
mirtazapine	Serzone	100–600	50, 100, 140, 200, 250
nefazodone	Desyrel	150–300	50
trazodone			
Serotonin-	Pristiq	50–100	50
norepinephrine	Cymbalta	60–120	20
reuptake inhibitors	Fetzima	40–120	20, 40
desvenlafaxine	Effexor	72–375	25, 37.5
duloxetine	Trintellix	10–20	5, 10
levomilnacipran			
venlafaxine			
vortioxetine			
Norepinephrine-	Wellbutrin	200–450	100, 150
dopamine reuptake	Focalin	2.5–20	2.5, 5, 10
inhibitors	Ritalin	5–60	5, 10, 20
bupropion			
dexmethylphenidate			
methylphenidate			
Heterocyclic	Elavil	150–300	50
antidepressants	Asendin	150–400	50
amitriptyline	Anafranil	100–250	25
amoxapine	Norpramin	150–300	25
clomipramine	(generic only)	150–300	25
desipramine	Tofranil	150–300	25
doxepin	Ludiomil	150–225	75
imipramine	Pamelor	50–150	25
maprotiline	Vivactil	15–60	5
nortriptyline	Surmontil	150–300	50
protriptyline			
trimipramine			
Monoamine oxidase	Marplan	30–60	10
inhibitors	Nardil	45–90	15
isocarboxazid	Eldepryl	6–12	6
phenelzine	Parnate	30–60	10
selegiline			
tranylcypromine			

Selective serotonin reuptake inhibitors

SSRIs are often prescribed as the initial medications for depressive disorders. They are usually first-line drugs because their safety, efficacy, and tolerability are high. Still, it is often advised to begin with a very low dose and slowly increase over weeks to minimize potential side effects. When an SSRI is ineffective following an adequate trial, another one can be substituted, or a different type of antidepressant may be used. SSRIs such as Prozac can stimulate patients with depression, so they should be administered in the morning and might benefit patients experiencing fatigue. Meanwhile, other SSRIs such as Paxil can be somewhat sedating and thus should be administered at night but may help patients experiencing insomnia. As such, a medication's side effect profile can occasionally be used to the prescriber's advantage, depending on the specific symptoms a patient exhibits.

Pharmacokinetics

While the SSRIs have similar antidepressant effectiveness and mostly similar adverse effects, their pharmacokinetic properties are different. Half-lives range between 1 and 4 days for fluoxetine, 21 hours for paroxetine, and 36 hours for citalopram. Sertraline and citalopram have linear pharmacokinetics, but fluoxetine, fluvoxamine, and paroxetine have nonlinear pharmacokinetics. The SSRIs have an extensive metabolism rate but high individual variability, in which the cytochrome P450 isoenzymes play a significant role. The resulting blood concentrations are widely variable between patients. The SSRIs are eliminated from the kidneys. Summarizes the half-lives of escitalopram (in two doses), sertraline, and paroxetine.

Mechanism of Action

The SSRIs inhibit serotonin reuptake, so it remains in the synaptic gap longer than usual. It may repeatedly stimulate the receptors of the recipient cell. This leads to increased signaling across synapses, with serotonin being the primary neurotransmitter. With chronic SSRI doses, the presynaptic neurons synthesize and release less serotonin. Ultimately, there is downregulation of postsynaptic serotonin receptors. There is no widely accepted theory of how these changes result in mood-elevating and antianxiety effects; however, clinical improvement in depressive symptoms appears to coincide with the nerve circuit's adaptation to an increased presence of serotonin over weeks. Although SSRIs inhibit serotonin reuptake reasonably immediately, the therapeutic benefit is delayed. It thus appears to be related to subsequent changes in neuronal functioning such as downregulation of postsynaptic receptors, changes in second messengers within nerve cells, and alterations in DNA transcription within nuclei.

Some SSRIs are also ligands of the **sigma receptors**. Their use has also shown reduced production of inflammatory cytokines, leading to decreased inflammation and a decrease in the activation level of the immune response. Research is ongoing about using genetic markers that predict if a patient will respond to SSRIs or have adverse effects requiring discontinuation of these drugs. The SSRIs are described as *selective* because they only affect reuptake pumps responsible for serotonin, while earlier antidepressants affected other monoamine neurotransmitters as well.

Clinical indications

The primary indication for SSRIs is an MDD. However, they are often prescribed for anxiety disorders, including social anxiety disorder, generalized anxiety disorder, panic disorder, obsessive-compulsive disorder, posttraumatic stress disorder, and eating disorders.

Contraindications

The contraindications with the SSRIs include known hypersensitivity, suicidal thoughts, unusual changes in behavior, bradycardia, hypokalemia, hypomagnesemia, recent acute myocardial infarction, seizure disorders, mania, abnormal bleeding, and heart failure.

Adverse effects

Insomnia is a common adverse effect of SSRIs. It is treated by dose reduction or by adding a low dose of sedating antidepressants such as trazodone. At first, there may be gastrointestinal symptoms such as nausea and loose stools, which usually disappear over time. Sexual side effects are also somewhat common, particularly with paroxetine (Paxil). A severe and throbbing headache may develop less frequently, which does not always dissipate, requiring medication changes. Ways to manage some of the most common adverse effects include the following:

- Nausea: take with a meal.
- Insomnia: take stimulating medications such as fluoxetine (Prozac) only in the morning.
- Hypersomnia: take sedating medications such as paroxetine at bedtime.
- Increased anxiety: avoid taking caffeine and oral decongestants.
- Sexual dysfunction: consider adjunctive medications such as sildenafil (Viagra) or bupropion (Wellbutrin).

Toxicities

The SSRIs should be stopped if they cause the patient to become agitated. If **anorgasmia**, decreased libido, or impotence develops, dose reductions or changing medications to serotonin modulators or norepinephrine-dopamine reuptake inhibitors (NDRIs) may be helpful. The SSRIs may sometimes cause serotonin syndrome, a potentially severe condition.

You should remember

The last line of intervention for MDD is electroconvulsive therapy in which seizures are electrically induced. This is effective for about 50% of treatment-resistant MDD, but about half of those who respond well will relapse within 1 year. The FDA-approved **transcranial magnetic stimulation** as a noninvasive method to stimulate small brain regions for treatment-resistant MDD.

You should remember

Symptoms of serotonin syndrome include abdominal pain, diarrhea, sweating, tachycardia, hypertension, myoclonus, rigidity, delirium, eventual hyperpyrexia (>106.7°F), cardiovascular shock, and death. It can occur with a serotonergic drug alone, intentional overdose of serotonergic drugs, or, more commonly, from drug interactions between two or more serotonergic agents. Two weeks must pass before switching from an SSRI to a monoamine oxidase inhibitor (MAOI) to avoid the syndrome when changing medications. The exception to this is fluoxetine (Prozac), which requires a 5-week waiting period due to its long half-life.

Serotonin modulators

The serotonin modulators, 5-hydroxytryptamine$_2$ blockers, have multimodal actions specific to the serotonin neurotransmitter system. They modulate one or more serotonin receptors while inhibiting the reuptake of serotonin. These medications were developed because there are many different subtypes of serotonin receptors, and not all are involved in the antidepressant effects of serotonin reuptake inhibitors.

Pharmacokinetics

The serotonin modulators have 50% bioavailability and 85% protein binding. They are metabolized in the liver. The elimination half-life is between 10 and 40 hours, and they are primarily excreted in the urine and remain in the feces.

Mechanism of action

The serotonin modulators inhibit presynaptic alpha$_2$-adrenergic receptors, causing increased release of serotonin and norepinephrine. They activate the sympathetic nervous system and act as a potent antagonist of the H1 histamine receptors. *Trazodone* has a multifunctional mechanism of action. In lower doses, it has hypnotic movements, but higher doses recruit the blockade of the serotonin transporter, resulting in antidepressant effects. Its controlled-release formulation improves the tolerability of higher doses.

Clinical indications

Mirtazapine is used in the treatment of major depression. It is also used off label for insomnia and to increase appetite. *Trazodone* is only indicated for the treatment of MDD.

Contraindications

The serotonin modulators are contraindicated with known hypersensitivity, high cholesterol, high blood triglycerides, hyponatremia, dehydration, being overweight or having gained weight unintentionally, manic behaviors or bipolar disorder, neuroleptic malignant syndrome, angina, stroke, hypotension, liver abnormalities or abnormal liver function tests, seizures, extreme restlessness, brain blood vessel disorders, decreased blood volume, kidney impairment, low neutrophil counts, and muscle pain or tenderness with increased creatine kinase. They are also contraindicated in patients with suicidal thoughts and a risk of angle-closure glaucoma.

Adverse effects

The serotonin modulators may cause severe allergic reactions, including skin reactions, decreased need for sleep, extreme happiness or sadness, being more talkative than usual, severe eye abnormalities, lightheadedness, seizures, low white blood cell counts, fever, chills, sore throat, coughing, sores in the mouth or nose, flulike symptoms, increased appetite, and weight gain. They may cause difficulty breathing, mood or behavior changes, anxiety, panic attacks, insomnia, impulsivity, irritability, agitation, aggressiveness, hostility, restlessness, hyperactivity, increased depression, suicidal thoughts or thoughts of self-harm, unusual thoughts or behaviors, hyponatremia, headaches, confusion, slurred speech, severe weakness, vomiting, loss of coordination, unsteadiness, serotonin syndrome, drowsiness, and dizziness.

Drug interactions

The serotonin modulators have moderate drug interactions with metoprolol and quetiapine. They have significant drug interactions with duloxetine and moderate drug interactions with aripiprazole, pregabalin, and alprazolam. *Buspirone, mirtazapine,* and *trazodone* also have major drug interactions with escitalopram and sertraline. Buspirone also has substantial drug interactions with acetaminophen/hydrocodone and fluoxetine. Trazodone has moderate drug interactions with lamotrigine. *Nefazodone* also has significant drug interactions with suvorexant, quetiapine, and vortioxetine.

Toxicities

The serotonin modulator toxicity causes tachycardia, mild hypertension, and mild CNS depression. Doses less than 1000 mg are not likely to cause any significant toxicity. Signs of dangerous toxicity include respiratory arrest, angina, arrhythmias, lack of coordination, tremors, seizures, vomiting, potentially life-threatening serotonin syndrome, and coma.

You should remember

Serotonin modulators have multimodal actions specific to the serotonin neurotransmitter system. They simultaneously module one or more serotonin receptors and inhibit serotonin reuptake. These drugs are effective in increasing serotonin to treat depression symptoms. The exact mechanism of action is unknown.

Serotonin-Norepinephrine Reuptake Inhibitors

The *serotonin-norepinephrine reuptake inhibitors* (SNRIs) are antidepressant drugs for many conditions other than depression. They inhibit serotonin and norepinephrine reuptake and are believed to be essential in regulating mood. The human serotonin transporter and norepinephrine transporter are membrane transport proteins responsible for reuptake neurotransmitters from the synaptic cleft back into the presynaptic nerve terminal. Along with the SSRIs, the SNRIs are considered second-generation antidepressants, which have, in recent years, widely replaced first-generation antidepressants. They have improved tolerability and a better safety profile. The SNRIs include *desvenlafaxine, duloxetine, levomilnacipran, venlafaxine,* and *vortioxetine.*

Pharmacokinetics

The *SNRIs* have an 80% bioavailability but only 30%–95% protein binding. They metabolize in the liver and have an elimination half-life of 11 hours. The drug is 70% excreted in the urine and 20% in the feces. *Vortioxetine* has 75% bioavailability that peaks in 7–11 hours.

Mechanism of action

Venlafaxine works similarly to the other SNRIs but weakly inhibits dopamine reuptake when high doses are administered. It also indirectly affects opioid receptors and the alpha$_2$-adrenergic receptor. The exact mechanism of action of *desvenlafaxine* is not fully understood, but the drug appears to be associated with potentiation of serotonergic and noradrenergic activity in the CNS. *Duloxetine* increases dopamine mainly in the prefrontal cortex, where few dopamine reuptake pumps inhibit norepinephrine reuptake pumps. *Levomilnacipran* has an unknown mechanism of action but is believed to be similar to the other SNRIs. *Vortioxetine* also has a similar mechanism of action and is often used when other antidepressants have failed, and it is associated with the lowest remission rates for generalized anxiety disorder.

Clinical indications

The *SNRIs* are used for MDD in adults. *Duloxetine* is also used for MDD, generalized anxiety disorder in adults or children (over age 7), fibromyalgia, diabetic neuropathy, and chronic muscle or joint pain. *Venlafaxine* is used for MDD, anxiety, and panic disorder.

Contraindications

The *SNRIs* are contraindicated with known hypersensitivity to the drug and any ingredient. These drugs cannot be used with MAO inhibitors or within 2 weeks of stopping an MAO inhibitor. Venlafaxine is also contraindicated with seizure disorders, glaucoma, pregnancy, and during breastfeeding. *Duloxetine* is contraindicated with known hypersensitivity, MAOIs, or CNS-acting drugs if uncontrolled narrow-angle glaucoma is present. *Levomilnacipran* is contraindicated with syndrome of inappropriate antidiuretic hormone, hyponatremia, increased risk of bleeding, bipolar disorder, suicidal behavior, alcoholism, serotonin syndrome, hypertension, urinary tract blockage, seizures, abnormal liver function tests, risk of angle-closure glaucoma due to a narrow-angle of the anterior chamber of the eye, kidney disease, and tachycardia. *Vortioxetine* is contraindicated with known hypersensitivity, seizure disorders in children or adolescents with suicidal thoughts, bipolar disorder, liver disease, increased risk of bleeding, hyponatremia, hypovolemia during pregnancy and breastfeeding, closed-angle glaucoma or increased intraocular pressure, and in any geriatric patient with a high risk of developing hyponatremia.

Adverse effects

The *SNRIs* often cause sexual side effects, constipation, decreased appetite, dizziness, drowsiness, tiredness, hyperhidrosis, nausea, and xerostomia. Other adverse effects include abnormal dreams, blurred vision, chills, mydriasis, tremors, vertigo, vomiting, and excessive yawning. They may cause allergic reactions or severe skin reactions, worsened depression, panic attacks, impulsivity, irritability, agitation, hostility, aggressiveness, restlessness, increased energy or talkativeness, suicidal thoughts, thoughts about self-harm, anxiety, and insomnia.

Drug interactions

Desvenlafaxine interacts significantly with escitalopram, lisdexamfetamine, bupropion, and sertraline. It has moderate drug interactions with aripiprazole, lamotrigine, lurasidone, and quetiapine. Desvenlafaxine, *duloxetine, levomilnacipran, venlafaxine,* and *vortioxetine* have significant drug interactions with amphetamine/dextroamphetamine. Desvenlafaxine and duloxetine have moderate drug interactions with diphenhydramine, pregabalin, alprazolam, and cetirizine. Duloxetine also has moderate drug interactions with aspirin, apixaban, metoprolol, acetaminophen/hydrocodone, albuterol, and budesonide/formoterol. Levomilnacipran has significant drug interactions with citalopram, duloxetine, cyclobenzaprine, escitalopram, paroxetine, lisdexamfetamine, bupropion, and sertraline. It has moderate drug interactions with aripiprazole, aspirin, and acetaminophen/oxycodone. Venlafaxine has similar moderate drug interactions to the previously listed SNRIs. Vortioxetine also has significant drug interactions with duloxetine, escitalopram, lithium, desvenlafaxine, fluoxetine, lisdexamfetamine, bupropion, and sertraline.

Toxicities

The *SNRIs* toxicities usually occur along with the use of alcohol and other drugs, resulting in tachycardia or bradycardia, somnolence, mydriases, seizures, vomiting, diarrhea, abdominal cramps, hypotension, rhabdomyolysis, liver necrosis, vertigo, serotonin syndrome, coma, and death.

You should remember

There needs to be more clarity about whether the SNRIs have improved efficacy compared to the SSRIs. Also, the SSRIs do have a slightly longer list of adverse effects than the SNRIs.

Norepinephrine-dopamine reuptake inhibitors

The *NDRIs* are agents used for the second-line treatment of clinical depression but more commonly for attention-deficit/hyperactivity disorder (ADHD) and narcolepsy. They act as reuptake inhibitors by blocking the actions of the norepinephrine and dopamine transporters. This leads to increased extracellular neurotransmitter concentrations and adrenergic and dopaminergic neurotransmission. The most commonly used NDRI is *bupropion,* with *dexmethylphenidate* and *methylphenidate* being less common options.

Pharmacokinetics

NDRIs have 84% protein binding. They are metabolized in the liver and have an elimination half-life of 11–21 hours. NDRIs are 87% excreted in the urine, with 0.5% unchanged. They are also 10% excreted in the feces. NDRIs have very different bioavailability based on each patient, between 11% and 52%.

Mechanism of action

The mechanism of action for NDRIs is varied. For example, *bupropion* has an unclear mechanism of action, which is believed to be related to its antagonism of nicotinic acetylcholine receptors. The tool of *dexmethylphenidate* and *methylphenidate* is the inhibition of dopamine and norepinephrine reuptake transporters in synapses, primarily in the thalamus and striatum. There are changes to the blood flow of various brain regions, including the striatum, supplementary motor area, and posterior parietal cortex.

Clinical indications

Bupropion is indicated for depressive disorders, seasonal affective disorder, bipolar disorder, smoking cessation, and obesity. It is also used to treat ADHD, often in cases where traditional stimulant use is contraindicated. *Dexmethylphenidate* is mainly used for ADHD but is also used similarly to *methylphenidate* on an off-label basis to treat depressive disorders. Use of these medications for depression is usually reserved for severe cases or if extreme psychomotor retardation is present.

Contraindications

Bupropion is contraindicated with epilepsy or other conditions that lower the seizure threshold. These include alcohol withdrawal, anorexia nervosa, bulimia nervosa, and benzodiazepine withdrawal. Bupropion should not be used along with MAOIs, and there should be at least 2 weeks between stopping either type of medication before starting the other. Bupropion must be used with caution if there is liver damage, severe kidney disease, or severe hypertension and in children, adolescents, or young adults because of an increased risk of suicidal thoughts. *Dexmethylphenidate* and *methylphenidate* are contraindicated with agitation, glaucoma, tics, or known hypersensitivity. They are not proven to cause fetal defects but are only to be used by pregnant females if the benefits outweigh the potential risks.

Adverse effects

NDRIs may cause dry mouth, constipation, insomnia, anxiety, nausea, excessive sweating, and tremor. In rare cases, they may have serious adverse effects, including seizures and Stevens-Johnson syndrome. NDRIs should be avoided in the first trimester of pregnancy because they are linked to increased congenital heart defects. They may also cause loss of appetite, abdominal pain, weight loss, **akathisia**, irritability, dyskinesia, **oromandibular dystonia**, lethargy, dizziness, palpitations, blurred vision, diplopia, mydriasis, worsening of psychotic states, skin rash, urticaria, and fever. It is important to note that these medications have potential for abuse and addiction.

Drug interactions

Bupropion interacts significantly with aripiprazole, duloxetine, escitalopram, amphetamine/dextroamphetamine, and lisdexamfetamine. It has moderate drug interactions with metoprolol, alprazolam, and cetirizine. *Dexmethylphenidate* only has moderate drug interactions with escitalopram, fluoxetine, vortioxetine, and sertraline. *Methylphenidate* has a significant drug interaction with the extended-release form of bupropion. Methylphenidate also has the same moderate drug interactions as dexmethylphenidate, except not with vortioxetine.

Toxicities

Bupropion has an increased likelihood of causing liver toxicity that can lead to transplantation or death. It can also trigger an angle-closure glaucoma attack. *Dexmethylphenidate* and *methylphenidate* toxicity may cause nausea, vomiting, agitation, tremor, hyperreflexia, muscle twitching, confusion, euphoria, delirium, hallucinations, hyperthermia, sweating, flushing, headache, palpitations, tachycardia, arrhythmias, hypertension, dryness of mucous membranes, and mydriasis. Severe toxicity may cause hyperpyrexia, sympathomimetic toxidrome, convulsions, paranoia, repetitive movements, rhabdomyolysis, circulatory collapse, and coma.

You should remember

The NDRIs offer the advantage of not usually causing adverse effects caused by other antidepressants. These include weight gain and reduced libido. Bupropion (Wellbutrin) is primarily used to treat major depression and is the only currently approved drug. Other brand names include Zyban and Alpezin. The different medications classified as NDRIs are methylphenidate and dexmethylphenidate, but these are first and foremost used for ADHD and less often for depression.

Heterocyclic antidepressants

The *heterocyclic antidepressants* are not used today as much as in the past. They include tricyclic antidepressants (TCAs), tetracyclic antidepressants, and *tiazesim*, an older drug with tricyclic and heterocyclic properties. Today, TCAs are second-line agents because of more significant adverse effects. The tetracyclic antidepressants differ little from the TCAs except that their chemical structure contains four rings of atoms instead of three. Tiazesim has been discontinued and is no longer marketed. Giving the entire dose of a heterocyclic antidepressant at bedtime usually means that a sedative will not be needed. It also minimizes daytime adverse effects and improves patient adherence.

Pharmacokinetics

All of the heterocyclic antidepressants are totally or partially metabolized in the liver. The elimination half-life is 21 hours, and they are excreted in the urine after 48 hours. The drug's elimination half-life is 8 hours. They have 90% protein binding.

Mechanism of action

The heterocyclic antidepressants inhibit serotonin and norepinephrine transporters. Inhibition of norepinephrine leads to increased neurotransmitter concentrations in the posterior gray column of the spinal cord, providing analgesia. The blocking effect of heterocyclic antidepressants on sodium channels may contribute to their effectiveness.

Clinical indications

TCAs are indicated for depression, ADHD, and chronic pain. The TCAs are primarily meant for MDD.

Contraindications

A general contraindication for these drugs is that they should not be used during the recovery period from a myocardial infarction. *Amitriptyline* is contraindicated with a history of arrhythmias and any degree of heart block. It is also contraindicated with coronary artery disease, porphyria, severe liver disease, and a patient younger than 6 years. *Amoxapine* is contraindicated with suicidal thoughts, known hypersensitivity, severe cardiovascular disorders, and uncorrected narrow-angle glaucoma. *Clomipramine* is contraindicated with known hypersensitivity, recent myocardial infarction, any degree of heart block or other arrhythmias, mania, severe liver disease, narrow-angle glaucoma, and urinary retention and should only be used with caution during pregnancy or lactation. *Desipramine* is also contraindicated in acute recovery after myocardial infarction, with known hypersensitivity, and in patients with suicidal thoughts. *Doxepin* is contraindicated with known hypersensitivity, glaucoma, benign prostatic hyperplasia, and urinary retention and should only be used with caution during pregnancy and lactation.

Imipramine may be unsafe to use during pregnancy. *Maprotiline* is contraindicated with known hypersensitivity, hypertrophy of the prostate gland with urine hesitancy, and closed-angle glaucoma. It must be used with caution if severe liver or kidney impairment, epilepsy, brain tumors, alcohol withdrawal, arrhythmias, heart insufficiency, after a myocardial infarction, or in patients under age 18. *Nortriptyline* is contraindicated in the recovery period after a myocardial infarction. It must be closely monitored if used in a patient with a history of cardiovascular disease, stroke, glaucoma, seizures, hyperthyroidism, or if thyroid hormones are being administered. *Protriptyline* is contraindicated in the recovery period after a myocardial infarction, with schizophrenia or manic-depressive psychosis, and in patients with paranoid delusions. *Trimipramine* is contraindicated with recent myocardial infarction, any degree of heart block or other cardiac arrhythmias, mania, severe liver disease, known hypersensitivity, and during lactation.

Adverse effects

The TCAs have a range of anticholinergic, adrenergic, and antihistaminic side effects and often cause dry mouth or nose, blurred vision, lowered GI motility, constipation, urinary retention, sedation, cognitive or memory impairment, and increased body temperature. They may also cause drowsiness, anxiety, apathy or anhedonia, sexual dysfunction, confusion, restlessness, dizziness, akathisia, hypersensitivity, changes in appetite, weight gain or loss, sweating, muscle twitching, weakness, nausea, vomiting, hypotension, tachycardia, and, in rare cases, arrhythmias.

Drug interactions

These antidepressants have significant drug interactions with duloxetine, and most have major drug interactions with escitalopram and sertraline. *Amitriptyline* has substantial drug interactions with cyclobenzaprine and topiramate. *Amoxapine* interacts significantly with citalopram, vortioxetine, vilazodone, and bupropion. *Clomipramine* has significant drug interactions with fluoxetine. *Desipramine* has major drug interactions with citalopram. *Doxepin* has substantial drug interactions with cyclobenzaprine and topiramate. *Imipramine* has important drug interactions with cyclobenzaprine, fluoxetine, and topiramate. *Maprotiline* has powerful drug interactions with clozapine. *Nortriptyline* has substantial drug interactions with cyclobenzaprine, topiramate, and ondansetron. *Protriptyline* has meaningful drug interactions with vortioxetine. *Trimipramine* has significant drug interactions with paroxetine, desvenlafaxine, and bupropion.

Toxicities

TCA toxicity may cause severe muscle twitching, hallucinations, delirium, rhabdomyolysis, muscle breakdown, and coma. It may also cause disorientation, extreme drowsiness, memory impairment, tachycardia or bradycardia, arrhythmias, restlessness, agitation, seizures, loss of muscle coordination, stupor, shortness of breath, hypotension, vomiting, sweating, urinary problems, and coma.

You should remember

The heterocyclic antidepressants are older drugs that increase the availability of noradrenaline and, to a lesser degree, serotonin by blocking their reuptake in the synaptic cleft (also called the synaptic gap). Tricyclic and tetracyclic antidepressants are sometimes used for patients who do not respond well to the newer drugs. The TCAs are the oldest subtype, discovered in the 1950s.

Monoamine oxidase inhibitors

MAOIs were the first type of antidepressant developed. MAOIs elevate norepinephrine, serotonin, and dopamine levels by inhibiting an enzyme called monoamine oxidase. They also treat Parkinson disease, tuberculosis, and several other disorders. Currently, they are typically only used when other antidepressant medications have failed, in part due to the increased risk of hypertensive reaction with tyramine-rich foods (e.g., cured meats, alcohol, cheese, smoked fish) and increased risk of serotonin syndrome when taken with other medications that increase serotonin. Therefore developing efficient analytical methods for monitoring and management is very important.

Pharmacokinetics

Isocarboxazid has low bioavailability, with peak actions at 1–2 hours. It is metabolized in the liver into carboxylesterase. Its metabolite is hippuric acid, and the elimination half-life is 1.5–4 hours. Isocarboxazid is excreted in the urine. *Phenelzine* is metabolized in the liver but has a longer elimination half-life of 11.6 hours. It is also excreted in the urine. *Selegiline* has 73% bioavailability in its transdermal patch form but only 10% oral bioavailability. Its protein binding is 94%, metabolized in the intestines and liver. The metabolites are *N*-desmethylselegiline, levoamphetamine, and levomethamphetamine. The transdermal elimination half-life is 18–25 hours, and the oral elimination half-life is 1.5–3.5 hours. The drug is excreted in the urine. *Tranylcypromine* has 50% bioavailability. It is metabolized in the liver and has an elimination half-life of 2.5 hours. It is excreted in the urine and feces.

Mechanism of action

The irreversible MAOIs, such as *isocarboxazid* and *phenelzine,* bind MAO-A and MAO-B to transform them into reactive metabolites. *Selegiline* is irreversibly selective for MAO-B, but larger doses also inhibit MAO-A. *Tranylcypromine* has a slight preference for MAO-B over MAO-A.

Clinical indications

Isocarboxazid is mainly used to treat mood and anxiety disorders and has been investigated to treat schizophrenia, Parkinson disease, and other dementia-related conditions. *Phenelzine* is mainly used for MDD and is also helpful if a patient does not respond well to first- or second-line medications for depression. It is also effective for dysthymia, bipolar depression, panic disorder, social anxiety disorder, bulimia, posttraumatic stress disorder, and obsessive-compulsive disorder. *Selegiline* is used to treat MDD and Parkinson disease. *Tranylcypromine* is used for MDD, including atypical depression (usually when anxiety is a component), mainly as a second-line treatment. It is also used for depressive disorders that do not respond to reuptake inhibitor antidepressants such as SSRIs, TCAs, or bupropion.

Contraindications

Isocarboxazid is contraindicated with known hypersensitivity, cardiovascular disease, hypertension, cerebrovascular defects, history of headaches, liver disease or abnormal liver function tests, pheochromocytoma, and severe kidney impairment. *Phenelzine* is contraindicated with known hypersensitivity, pheochromocytoma, congestive heart failure, severe kidney impairment or disease, history of liver disease, and abnormal liver function tests. *Selegiline* is contraindicated with known hypersensitivity. *Tranylcypromine* is contraindicated with porphyria, cardiovascular or cerebrovascular disease, pheochromocytoma, and tyramine-containing foods.

Adverse effects

Isocarboxazid has common adverse effects, including headaches, dizziness, drowsiness, tremors, insomnia, constipation, nausea, and dry mouth. *Phenelzine* may cause chills, cold sweats, confusion, faintness or lightheadedness, overactive reflexes, tremors, muscle twitching, and inflammation. *Selegiline* commonly causes muscle twitching and twisting motions of the tongue, lips, face, arms, or legs. *Tranylcypromine* often causes dizziness secondary to orthostatic tachycardia, hypomania, paresthesia, weight loss, confusion, dry mouth, sexual dysfunction, hypertension, rash, and urinary retention.

Drug interactions

Isocarboxazid interacts significantly with citalopram, duloxetine, trazodone, venlafaxine, amitriptyline, and escitalopram. *Phenelzine interacts substantially* with amphetamine/dextroamphetamine, citalopram, duloxetine, fentanyl, escitalopram, and vortioxetine. *Selegiline* has significant drug interactions with escitalopram and moderate interactions with pramipexole and carbidopa/levodopa. *Tranylcypromine substantially interacts* with vortioxetine and has mild interactions with aripiprazole, suvorexant, lurasidone, pregabalin, metoprolol, and quetiapine.

Toxicities

Tachycardia, hypotension, convulsions, respiratory depression, slow reflexes, pyrexia, sweating, and coma signify isocarboxazid toxicity. *Phenelzine* toxicity causes drowsiness, dizziness, severe headaches, neck pain or stiffness, hallucinations, shallow breathing, fast and uneven heart rate, cold sweats, lightheadedness, and convulsions. *Selegiline* toxicity is signified by severe headaches, hallucinations, vision problems, sweating, cool or clammy skin, tachycardia, palpitations, lightheadedness, fainting, and convulsions. *Tranylcypromine* toxicity causes restlessness, anxiousness, insomnia, agitation, confusion, weakness, severe headache, neck pain or stiffness, pounding heartbeats, and unconsciousness.

You should remember

The MAOIs were the first antidepressants ever developed. While still effective, they have generally been replaced by newer antidepressants that are safer and cause fewer adverse effects. MAOIs usually require diet restrictions (foods containing tyramine) and avoiding certain medications (prescription and OTC) because dangerously high blood pressure can occur.

Key Terms

Akathisia
Anorgasmia
Bipolar disorder
Cognitive behavioral therapy
Humanistic therapies
Major depressive disorder
Mindfulness-based cognitive therapy
Monoaminergic systems
Oromandibular dystonia
Psychodynamic therapies
Rational emotive behavior therapy
Sigma receptors
Tetracyclic antidepressants
Transcranial magnetic stimulation
Tricyclic antidepressants

Clinical Case Studies

Clinical Case Study 1

A 33-year-old female visited her psychiatrist along with her husband. She described constant neck and shoulder tightness, weakness of her muscles, inability to concentrate on work, being disturbed by loud voices of other people, sleep problems, and crying that she could not control. The patient admitted that a couple of close relatives had struggled with depression. After her physician assessed the patient during interviews, she was diagnosed with MDD and scheduled for CBT.

Critical Thinking Questions

1. What is the clinical description of MDD?
2. How significant is a family history of MDD?
3. What is the most effective therapeutic approach?

Clinical Case Study 2

A 28-year-old male visited his physician for a psychotherapy evaluation because he constantly felt sad for no apparent reason. The physician noted he came with his head down and avoided eye contact with others. His mood was dysphoric, with some features of anxiety, depression, and anger. Over multiple appointments, his attitude became less dysphoric. He described a lack of support from his family and became distressed while discussing this. While discussing the patient's past, his physician found out that he had a history of physical and emotional abuse, problems in high school that ended with him dropping out, and participation in a street gang. Several times during each appointment, his eyes would tear up as he spoke or break down and cry. The diagnosis was MDD, and the patient was scheduled for rational emotive behavior therapy before any medications were started.

Critical Thinking Questions

1. Which type of antidepressant would be the most likely to be used first?
2. What are the contraindications of these agents?
3. Is there a direct cause of depressive disorders?

Further Reading

[1] J.K. Aronson, Meyler's Side Effects of Psychiatric Drugs, Elsevier, 2008.
[2] A. Balax, Medication for Depression: Best Advice for Relieving Depression, Stress, Fears. Balax, 2017.
[3] Y. Fang, Depressive Disorders: Mechanisms, Measurement and Management (Advances in Experimental Medicine and Biology, 1180, Springer, 2019.
[4] F.K. Goodwin, K. Redfield Jamison, Manic-Depressive Illness: Bipolar Disorders and Recurrent Depression, second ed., Oxford University Press, 2007.
[5] D.J. Hales, M. Hyman Rapaport, K. Moeller, Focus: Major Depressive Disorder, American Psychiatric Publishing, 2012.
[6] A. Jordan, Antidepressants: History, Science, and Issues (The Story of a Drug), Greenwood, 2018.
[7] S.H. Kennedy, R.W. Lam, D.J. Nutt, M.E. Thase, Treating Depression Effectively: Applying Clinical Guidelines, 2007, CRC Press, 2007.
[8] Y.K. Kim, Major Depressive Disorder: Rethinking and Understanding Recent Discoveries (Advances in Experimental Medicine and Biology, 1305), Springer, 2021.
[9] B. Kramer, Medications for Anxiety & Depression: A no-nonsense, Comprehensive Guide to the Most Common (And Not so Common) Antidepressants and Anti-anxiety Drugs Available, fourth ed., CreateSpace Independent Publishing Platform, 2014.
[10] J. Luciano de Quevedo, P. Riva-Posse, W.V. Bobo, Managing Treatment-Resistant Depression: Road to Novel Therapeutics, Academic Press, 2021.
[11] R.S. McIntyre, D.S. Cha, J.K. Soczynska, Cognition in Major Depressive Disorder (Psychiatry Library), Oxford University Press, 2014.
[12] R.S. McIntyre, C. Rong, M. Subramaniapillai, Y. Lee, Major Depressive Disorder, Elsevier, 2019.
[13] M. Palfreyman, Enzymes as Targets for Drug Design, Academic Press, 2012.
[14] J.K. Penberthy, Persistent Depressive Disorders–Advances in Psychotherapy–Evidence-Based Practice, Hogrefe, 2019.
[15] R. Sabri, The Addictive Potential of Selective Serotonin Reuptake Inhibitors, Lap Lambert Academic Publishing, 2011.
[16] S.K. Sharma, Monoamine Oxidase Inhibitors: Clinical Pharmacology, Benefits, and Potential Health Risks, Nova Science Publishing Inc, 2016.
[17] S.M. Stahl, Stahl's Illustrated Antidepressants, Cambridge University Press, 2009.
[18] S. Strakowski, E. Nelson, Major Depressive Disorder (American Psychiatry Library), Oxford University Press, 2015.
[19] J.L. Sullivan, P. DeRemer Sullivan, Biomedical Psychiatric Therapeutics, Butterworth-Heinemann, 2013.
[20] J. Wegmann, Psychopharmacology: Straight Talk on Mental Health Medications, fourth ed., PESI, 2021.
[21] M. Widdowson, Transactional Analysis for Depression: A Step-by-Step Treatment Manual, Routledge, 2015.
[22] M. Youdim, Monoamine Oxidases and Their Inhibitors, Academic Press, 2013.

CHAPTER

24

Antipsychotic drugs

OUTLINE

LEARNING OUTCOMES

After studying the chapter, readers should be able to:

1. Describe the classifications of bipolar disorder.
2. Identify neurochemical alterations in bipolar disorder.
3. Explain the pharmacotherapy used to treat bipolar disorder.
4. Discuss the specific mechanism of action of lithium.
5. Explain the signs and symptoms of lithium toxicity.
6. Identify typical antipsychotics used for bipolar disorder.
7. Discuss the mechanism of action of the atypical antipsychotics.
8. Explain the toxicities of the atypical antipsychotics.

Overview

Bipolar disorder is a severe mental illness that causes unusual shifts in mood, ranging from extreme highs (mania or "manic" episodes) to lows (depression or "depressive" episodes). A person who has bipolar disorder also

https://doi.org/10.1016/B978-0-443-29038-1.00024-5

experiences changes in their energy, thinking, behavior, and sleep. Affected individuals alternate between periods in which they feel delighted and energized and periods of feeling hopeless, sad, and sluggish. The average age of onset is about 25, but the disorder can occur in the teens or, less often, in childhood. Bipolar disorders are linked to heredity, abnormal levels of brain neurotransmitters, and psychosocial factors. Without treatment, bipolar disorder usually becomes worse over time. However, many people live well with the condition with appropriate early identification of symptoms, psychotherapy, medications, lifestyle, and a regular schedule. According to the National Institute of Mental Health, bipolar disorder affects approximately 5.7 million adults or about 2.6% of the United States aged 18 and older every year. An equal number of males and females develop bipolar disease at all ages, races, ethnic groups, and social classes. More than two-thirds of people with bipolar disorder have at least one close relative with the illness or **unipolar** major depression, indicating that the disease has a heritable component. Bipolar disorder results in a 9.2-year reduction in expected lifespan, and as many as one in five patients with bipolar disorder completes suicide.

Bipolar disorder

Bipolar disorder is characterized by one or more manic episodes, with or without mixed or psychotic features. A **hypomanic stage** occurs before progression to full mania. Generally, acute symptoms happen initially, followed by repeated courses of remission and relapse. The remissions are often complete, but many patients have residual symptoms such as manic, depressive, hypomanic, or mixtures of manic and depressive features. The residual symptoms persist for several weeks to 6 months, with depressive episodes usually lasting longer than manic episodes. In a manic phase, the patient may have intense energy and excessively and impulsively seek pleasurable activities of high risk. These include gambling, **sexual promiscuity**, excessive spending sprees, or dangerous sporting activities.

The ability to consider any possible self-harm may be impaired. Scientists believe the factors that may cause bipolar disorders include genetics, stress, and brain structure or function. Severe bipolar episodes may consist of psychotic symptoms such as hallucinations, agitation, racing thoughts, unusual talkativeness, insomnia, euphoria, and delusions. These psychotic symptoms can be wrongly diagnosed as schizophrenia.

Classifications

There are four different types of bipolar disorders, which include:

- *Bipolar I disorder:* an illness involving one or more episodes of mania. Most people diagnosed with bipolar I disorder will have episodes of mania and depression, though a bout of depression is not necessary for a diagnosis. To be diagnosed, a person's manic episodes must last at least 7 days or be so severe that hospitalization is required.
- *Bipolar II disorder:* In this form, depressive episodes shift back and forth with hypomanic episodes, but a "full" manic episode never occurs.
- *Cyclothymic disorder or cyclothymia:* a chronically unstable mood state in which hypomania and mild depression are present for at least 2 years. There may be brief periods of everyday mood, but they last less than 8 weeks.
- *Unspecified disorder:* the criteria for bipolar I, II, or **cyclothymia** are not present, but experienced periods of clinically significant symptoms still occur.

You should remember

Bipolar disorder often runs in families because people with specific genes are more likely to develop it than others. No single gene causes this disorder. The older terms for bipolar disorder were *manic-depressive disorder* and *manic depression*. The affected individual is experiencing the manic phase when they are extremely happy or irritable. In the depressive phase, the individual is sad, indifferent, or hopeless. Bipolar disorder usually develops during late adolescence or early adulthood.

Pharmacotherapy

Drug treatment for bipolar disorder usually involves mood stabilizers such as lithium plus certain anticonvulsants (see **Chapter 10**), a second-generation antipsychotic, or both; see **Table 24.1**. Support and psychotherapy are also necessary. Choices of drugs can be difficult because they all have significant adverse effects, and interactions are shared. There is no single drug that is universally effective for bipolar disorder. For severe manic psychosis, there is a need for urgent control of behavior. This usually requires a sedating second-generation antipsychotic that may be initially administered along with a benzodiazepine, such as clonazepam or lorazepam, intramuscularly or orally.

Lithium

Lithium was approved in the 1970s by the FDA as a mood stabilizer and a treatment for mania. Lithium is a powerful medication that has antimanic properties. Most patients with uncomplicated bipolar disorder respond to lithium, which is started orally and titrated based on steady-state blood levels and the ability of the patient to tolerate the drug. Blood levels of the drug are checked after 5 days of a stable dose and 12 hours after the last dose. Target drug levels for maintenance are lower. Higher levels give better protection against manic, not depressive, episodes.

Pharmacokinetics

Lithium is wholly absorbed but is not metabolized. The drug is distributed to all tissues and body fluids. It crosses the blood-brain barrier and the placenta, is secreted in the breast milk, and is not bound to plasma proteins. Lithium is primarily excreted in the urine. Peak levels for the oral tablet form are reached in 4–12 hours and, in the oral solution form, within 15–60 minutes. The overall duration of action is unknown.

TABLE 24.1 Common medications used for bipolar disorder.

Generic name	Trade name	Average dosage range (mg/day)	Dosage forms (in mg)
lithium (lithium carbonate)	Lithobid, Eskalith	600–2400	Oral tablet: 300, 600, 900 Oral solution: 15 mL, 20 mL
Atypical antipsychotics			
aripiprazole	Abilify	15–30	15, 30
asenapine	Saphris	5–20	5, 10
brexpiprazole	Rexulti	0.5–3	0.5, 1, 2, 3
cariprazine	Vraylar	1–6	1.5, 3, 4.5, 6
clozapine	Clozaril	12.5–900	12.5, 25, 50, 100, 150, 200, 50 mg/mL
iloperidone	Fanapt	6–12	1, 2, 4, 6, 8, 10, 12
lurasidone	Latuda	20–120	20, 40, 60, 80, 120
olanzapine	Zyprexa	2.5–20	2.5, 5, 7.5, 10, 15, 20
olanzapine-fluoxetine	Symbyax	6/25–12/50	3/25, 6/25, 6/50, 12/50
paliperidone	Invega	3–12	1.5, 3, 6, 9
quetiapine	Seroquel	25–800	25, 50, 100, 200, 300, 400
risperidone	Risperdal, Rykindo	2–6	2, 3
ziprasidone	Geodon	20–100	20, 40, 60, 80

Mechanism of action

The specific mechanism of action of *lithium* is unknown. It is widely distributed in the CNS and interacts with many neurotransmitters and receptors, decreasing the release of norepinephrine and increasing serotonin synthesis.

Clinical indications

Lithium is a mood stabilizer used to treat or control the manic episodes of bipolar disorder. It also helps prevent or lessen the intensity of manic episodes and is used in adults and children (over age 7). For bipolar disorder in children and adolescents, treatment is with mood stabilizers, antidepressants, or psychotherapy, and most often a combination of these approaches. Mood stabilizers treat manic or agitated episodes. Psychotherapy and antidepressants are usually used to address depressive episodes. However, psychotherapy can help manage all aspects of the disorder. Mood stabilizers include anticonvulsants, antipsychotics, and lithium. Antidepressants can cause a switch from depression to mania, so they are usually used with a mood stabilizer.

Contraindications

Lithium is contraindicated with significant renal or cardiovascular disease, dehydration, severe debilitation, and sodium depletion. There is a very high risk of toxicity under these conditions. Lithium is only used in patients with these conditions if the psychiatric indication is life-threatening or if there are other failed treatments. If lithium is used, there must be extreme caution, including daily serum lithium determinations and adjustments to lower, more tolerable doses.

Adverse effects

The adverse effects of lithium include dry mouth, nausea or vomiting, dizziness, headache, diarrhea, lack of appetite, hair loss, polydipsia, and polyuria. Lithium can cause direct or indirect cognitive impairment and sedation due to the development of hypothyroidism. It often worsens acne and psoriasis. The most common acute and mild adverse effects include **fasciculation** and fine tremor. Sometimes kidney damage occurs. Blood urea nitrogen and creatinine are measured at the start of treatment, two to three times in the first 6 months and then once every 6 or 12 months. Cumulative doses are risk factors for kidney damage. Therefore the minimal effective dose is used for prevention.

Toxicities

Lithium can become dangerous when taken in high doses. When excessive amounts are taken intentionally or accidentally, it can cause acute or chronic overdose symptoms. Lithium toxicity first causes gross tremors, more deep tendon reflexes, continuing headaches, confusion, and vomiting. It may evolve to cause arrhythmias, seizures, and **stupor**. Toxicity is more likely in elderly patients with reduced creatinine clearance or sodium loss from diuretics, diarrhea, fever, or vomiting. Angiotensin-converting enzyme inhibitors, NSAIDs, and thiazide diuretics may worsen hyperlithemia. Lithium blood levels are measured every 6 months, and doses are changed at any time.

You should remember

Lithium use is associated with a higher risk of cardiovascular malformations in the unborn child during pregnancy. The drug appears to increase the chances of congenital abnormalities by about two times. Discussing the risks and benefits of treatment with all females of childbearing age is very important.

Atypical antipsychotics

Atypical antipsychotics are also known as *second-generation antipsychotics* or *serotonin-dopamine antagonists*. They have now become the primary drugs used for psychosis, mostly because of their fewer adverse effects. The atypical antipsychotics include aripiprazole, asenapine, brexpiprazole, cariprazine, clozapine, iloperidone, luradisone, olanzapine, paliperidone, quetiapine, risperidone, and ziprasidone.

Pharmacokinetics

The atypical antipsychotics have 87% bioavailability and more than 99% protein binding. They are metabolized in the liver by CYP3A4 and CYP2D6 and eliminated by the kidneys.

Mechanism of action

Atypical antipsychotics block specific dopamine and serotonin receptors. Unlike first-generation antipsychotics, they also activate other dopamine and serotonin receptors. Their ability to block some receptors while activating others is why they work differently than first-generation antipsychotics.

Clinical indications

Atypical antipsychotics are used to decrease mood swings, psychosis, mania, severe aggression, depression, agitation, or tics. They are prescribed to treat schizophrenia, obsessive-compulsive disorder, and treatment-resistant mania. Off-label uses include Tourette syndrome.

Contraindications

Contraindications for using atypical antipsychotics include a history of severe allergy, use of CNS depressants, use of scopolamine or phencyclidine, severe cardiac abnormalities, history of seizure disorders, narrow-angle glaucoma, prostatic hypertrophy, and history of or continuing dyskinesia. Atypical antipsychotics carry an FDA black box warning of increased incidence of stroke in elderly patients with dementia.

Adverse effects

Atypical antipsychotics are associated with significant weight gain and the development of metabolic syndrome. Patients should monitor their personal and family history of diabetes mellitus, dyslipidemia, weight, waist circumference, BP, fasting plasma glucose, and fasting lipid profiles. *Risperidone* may cause dizziness, anxiety, sedation, and extrapyramidal side effects. *Paliperidone* can cause sensitivity to hot or cold temperatures and QTc prolongation. *Olanzapine* is most often associated with weight gain, increased appetite, and somnolence. *Quetiapine* has the fewest extrapyramidal side effects, which include drowsiness, orthostatic hypotension, and dizziness. *Aripiprazole* mainly causes agitation, headache, and akathisia-like restlessness.

Toxicities

The primary signs of toxicity from atypical antipsychotics include sedation, respiratory depression, loss of airway reflexes, seizures, and sometimes coma. The combination drug *olanzapine/fluoxetine* has minimal toxicities, but these did result in unconsciousness in three test patients and one coma. Before their loss of consciousness, signs of toxicity included ataxia, confusion, convulsions, **dysarthria**, arrhythmias, tremor, lethargy, acute psychosis, agitation, hypotension and hypertension, and aggression.

You should remember

Atypical antipsychotics have several significant benefits over typical antipsychotics. They significantly improve negative symptoms, cognitive function, prevention of deterioration, and quality of life. These drugs also cause fever and extrapyramidal symptoms. If the patient has acute psychosis, the atypical antipsychotics can take effect within hours to days. However, they may take up to 6 weeks to reach their full effect.

Key Terms

Autism
Atypical antipsychotics
Bipolar disorder
Creatinine clearance
Cyclothymia
Dysarthria
Decompensated heart failure

Fasciculation
Galactosemia
Gynecomastia
Homeostatic downregulation
Hyperintensities
Hypomanic stage
Leukopenia
Locus ceruleus
Phenylketonuria
Sexual promiscuity
Stupor
Unipolar

Clinical Case Studies

Clinical Case Study 1

A 59-year-old male had a past medical history of hypertension, type II diabetes mellitus, and bipolar disorder (which was controlled by escitalopram, risperidone, and valproic acid). His chief complaints included shortness of breath, cough, and confusion. He was sent to the local emergency department for evaluation. A chest X-ray showed a significant consolidation in the base of his right lung. The patient was started on broad-spectrum antibiotics. The patient was positive for *Streptococcus pneumoniae*. By the fourth day of treatment, his fever had increased, and the lung consolidation was beginning to improve. The patient's fever was suspected to be due to neuroleptic malignant syndrome, so risperidone, valproic acid, and escitalopram were stopped. By the ninth day, the patient had significantly improved but was kept in the ICU until he normalized utterly.

Critical Thinking Questions

1. What is risperidone classified as?
2. How do the atypical antipsychotics work?
3. What are the adverse effects of risperidone?

Clinical Case Study 2

A 19-year-old college student withdrew from his university after an episode of manic behavior that resulted in him damaging school property. He had repeatedly changed his primary field of study, began to sleep much less than usual, and often told his friends that his knowledge had surpassed that of his instructors. He would be angry at anyone who disagreed with him about anything. He began drinking alcohol excessively and had multiple sexual relationships with females he barely knew. A diagnosis of bipolar disorder was made. In early childhood, he had a history of problems with anxiety, withdrawal, and depression. The patient was started on lithium, monitored for a few weeks, and then began psychotherapy.

Critical Thinking Questions

1. What are the characterizations of bipolar disorder?
2. What can severe bipolar episodes include?
3. What are the most severe adverse effects of lithium?

Further Reading

[1] F. Andrasik, Comprehensive Handbook of Personality and Psychopathology (Volume 2), Wiley, 2008.
[2] S. Bahn, P. Guest, Biomarkers of Neurological and Psychiatric Disease Volume 101 (International Review of Neurobiology), Academic Press, 2011.
[3] M. Bauer, P. Grof, B. Muller-Oerlinghausen, Lithium in Neuropsychiatry: The Comprehensive Guide, CRC Press, 2006.
[4] J.C. Csernansky, J. Lauriello, Atypical Antipsychotics: From Bench to Bedside, CRC Press, 2004.
[5] G. De Girolamo, P.D. McGorry, N. Sartorius, Age of Onset of Mental Disorders: Etiopathogenetic and Treatment Implications, Springer, 2019.
[6] J. DiPiro, R.L. Talbert, G.C. Yee, G.R. Matzke, B.G. Wells, L.M. Posey, Pharmacotherapy: A Pathophysiologic Approach, tenth ed., McGraw-Hill Education/Medical, 2016.
[7] F. Goodwin, K. Redfield Jamison, Manic-Depressive Illness: Bipolar Disorders and Recurrent Depression, Volume II, second ed., Oxford University Press, 2007.
[8] K. Leonhard, H. Beckmann, C.H. Cahn, Classification of Endogenous Psychoses and Their Differentiated Etiology, second ed., Springer-Verlag, 2012.
[9] G.S. Malhi, M. Masson, The Science and Practice of Lithium Therapy, Springer, 2016.
[10] S. Marie, The Art and Science of Psychopharmacology: Essential Tools for Treating Anxiety, Depression, Bipolar Disorder & Psychosis, PESI Publishing & Media, 2020.

[11] D.J. Miklowitz, M.J. Gitlin, Clinician's Guide to Bipolar Disorder, The Guilford Press, 2015.
[12] P. Morrison, D.M. Taylor, P. McGuire, The Maudsley Guidelines on Advanced Prescribing in Psychosis, Wiley-Blackwell, 2020.
[13] R.J. Muller, P.R. McHugh, The Four Domains of Mental Illness (FDMI): An Alternative to the DSM-5, Routledge, 2017.
[14] V. Poole Arcangelo, A.M. Peterson, V. Wilbur, T.M. Kang, Pharmacotherapeutics for Advanced Practice: A Practical Approach, fifth ed., Wolters Kluwer, 2021.
[15] W.H. Reid, M.G. Wise, DSM-IV Training Guide, Routledge, 2014.
[16] S. Sadiq, N. Ahmed, Atypical Antipsychotics: Road to Metabolic Toxicity, Lap Lambert Academic Publishing, 2018.
[17] J. Schnittker, The Diagnostic System: Why the Classification of Psychiatric Disorders is Necessary, Difficult, and Never Settled, Columbia University Press, 2017.
[18] J. Wegmann, Psychopharmacology: Straight Talk on Mental Health Medications, fourth ed., 2021. PESI.
[19] A.H. Young, M.F. Juruena, Bipolar Disorder: From Neuroscience to Treatment (Current Topics in Behavioral Neurosciences, 48), Springer, 2021.
[20] Zero to Three, Diagnostic Classification of Mental Health and Developmental Disorders of Infancy and Early Childhood: DC: 0-5, Zero to Three–The National Center, 2016.

CHAPTER

25

Schizophrenia drugs

OUTLINE

LEARNING OUTCOMES

After study of this chapter, readers should be able to:

1. Define the various phases of schizophrenia.
2. Identify the four symptoms involved in schizophrenia.
3. Explain the positive and negative symptoms of schizophrenia.
4. Describe the risk factors for schizophrenia.
5. Discuss the pathophysiology of schizophrenia.
6. Identify various options used for psychotherapy to treat patients with schizophrenia.
7. Compare the advantages of first-generation with second-generation antipsychotics.
8. Describe the mechanism of action of the second-generation antipsychotics.
9. Explain the primary adverse effects of medications used for schizophrenia.
10. Discuss the indications of anesthesia adjuncts.

The Science of Pharmacology
https://doi.org/10.1016/B978-0-443-29038-1.00025-7

Overview

Schizophrenia is a severe mental illness affecting slightly less than 1% of the US population. People with schizophrenia often seem to have lost touch with reality, which causes significant distress for the individual and their family members and friends. Positive symptoms include delusions and hallucinations, while negative symptoms include blunted affect and lack of motivation. Individuals with schizophrenia also often exhibit elements of a thought disorder such as disorganized speech, distractibility, and trouble with thinking. While there is no cure, research is leading to improved treatments. With treatment, most symptoms of schizophrenia significantly improve, and the likelihood of psychotic episode recurrence can be diminished. If untreated, the symptoms of schizophrenia can be persistent and disabling. When delivered early and sustained adequately, treatment can help affected individuals to engage in school or work, achieve independence, and enjoy personal relationships. Schizophrenia does not mean split personalities or multiple personalities. Most people with schizophrenia are no more dangerous or violent than the general population. While limited mental health resources may lead to homelessness and frequent hospitalizations, it is a misconception that most people with schizophrenia are homeless or living in hospitals. Many patients with schizophrenia live with their families, in group homes, or independently. However, one of the significant problems with individuals who have schizophrenia is insufficient adherence to their medication regimens, which is a frequent precursor to the reemergence of psychotic symptoms.

Phases of schizophrenia

The clinical symptoms of schizophrenia can be described in multiple phases. Schizophrenia typically develops in late adolescence and lasts throughout life, usually with poor psychosocial functioning. It is a chronic condition, progressing through several stages with varied duration and phasic patterns. Schizophrenia involves psychosis, hallucinations, **delusions**, flattened affect, cognitive deficits, and occupational and social dysfunction. There are five phases of schizophrenia, as follows:

- *Prodromal phase:* No symptoms, impaired social skills, slight cognitive disorganization or distortions of perception, anhedonia, and general inability to cope with life. In this phase, symptoms may not be recognizable or can be realized due to impaired social, school, and work functions.
- *Advanced prodromal phase: Subclinical symptoms may appear,* including isolation, withdrawal, irritability, suspicion of others, distortions of perception, unusual thoughts, and disorganization. Delusions and hallucinations can occur over days, weeks, or sometimes years.
- *Early psychosis phase:* Symptoms become active and sometimes are at their worst out of all stages.
- *Middle phase:* There may be episodes of symptoms that have identified exacerbations and remissions, or symptoms may be continuous, with functional deficits usually worsening.
- *Late phase:* the pattern of illness may be well established yet still widely varying; it can stabilize, diminish, or worsen.

Also, other experts list just three phases of schizophrenia, which are as follows:

- Prodromal: Occurs before noticeable psychotic symptoms appear, but there are behavioral and cognitive changes that may progress to psychosis. Symptoms may include social isolation, anxiety, lack of motivation, difficulty concentrating, irritability, changes to regular routines, neglecting personal hygiene, sleep problems, erratic behaviors, and mild or poorly formed hallucinations. Up to 73% of patients experience the prodromal stage before developing the characteristic symptoms of schizophrenia.
- Active: Symptoms appear, including hallucinations, delusions, and paranoia. There may be confusion, disorganized thoughts, disordered or jumbled speech, excessive or useless movements, wandering, mumbling, laughing to "internalized" jokes, and apathy towards others.
- Residual: Though no longer recognized by the *DSM-5* for diagnostic purposes, this phase is still used to describe symptoms that are fewer or less severe than in the active stage. Usually hallucinations and delusions no longer occur. Negative symptoms such as lack of motivation, low energy, or depressed mood are typically present. Other symptoms include social withdrawal, difficulty concentrating, problems planning or participating in activities, reduced or absent facial expressions, a flat or monotone voice, and general disinterest in life.

Four symptom categories are involved in schizophrenia: *positive, negative, disorganized,* and *cognitive*. The positive symptoms are merely distortions of standard functions. They include delusions and hallucinations. Delusions are mistaken beliefs that the individual maintains despite clear evidence to the contrary. Delusions are often extraordinary, not real, and do not come from everyday experiences. Hallucinations are sensory perceptions that the person with schizophrenia experiences. They can be auditory, visual, **gustatory**, olfactory (smell), or **tactile**, but auditory hallucinations are the most commonly reported. The patient may "hear" voices that abuse, criticize, or comment on their behaviors.

Negative symptoms often lead to very little motivation and a reduced sense of goals and purpose in life. If symptoms become disorganized, the individual has thought disorders and bizarre behaviors. These may be considered positive symptoms. The thinking needs to be more organized. There are rambling speech patterns that shift between topics quickly and seem to have no "goals" in their direction. The individual's speech may be slightly disorganized, incomprehensible, and incoherent. Behaviors may involve agitation, almost childlike silliness, and inappropriateness in appearance, conduct, or hygiene. **Catatonia** may develop, including a rigid posture, resisting efforts to move, or unstimulated motor activities with no purpose. Cognitive symptoms include problems with attention, concentration, and memory. For some individuals, the mental symptoms of schizophrenia are subtle, but for others, they are more prominent and interfere with activities such as following conversations, learning new things, or remembering appointments.

Schizophrenic patients are usually unable to perform well on cognitive tasks because of disturbances in cortical information processing, which can be seen as abnormalities in EEG signals. In one study of depressed, schizophrenic, and normal control subjects, EEG results appeared quite different when each group of patients was resting or attempting to perform tricky arithmetic tasks. Another method of evaluating the degree of schizophrenia is a *clock drawing test*. **Fig. 25.1** shows six different clock scores drawn by patients with schizophrenia.

You should remember

A patient with schizophrenia describes seeing, hearing, smelling, or feeling things no one else is experiencing. Many individuals with schizophrenia hear voices that command them to perform tasks or warn them of danger and risks. Moreover, people with schizophrenia sometimes hear multiple voices that may even at times talk to one another. Other types of hallucinations include seeing objects or people not evident to anyone else and the sensation of being touched when, in fact, no one is touching them.

You should remember

The actual cause of schizophrenia is unknown. However, it is widely understood as involving alterations in brain structure, changes in neurochemistry, and genetics. The primary neurochemical alterations involve activity in dopamine and glutamate transmission markers. Aside from genetics, childhood factors that influence its development include complications in the intrauterine period or during or after birth. Also, viral infections and trauma of the CNS are implicated.

You should remember

There is no cure for schizophrenia, so treatments are focused on managing the symptoms. Prognosis is best for people who are diagnosed early and treated effectively. A good support team is essential, and patients with close family or friends who can assist them do much better than those on their own. Within 10 years of diagnosis, about 25% of patients are completely recovered, 25% are vastly improved and relatively independent, 25% are somewhat improved but require support, 15% are unimproved and must be hospitalized, and 10% are dead, primarily by suicide.

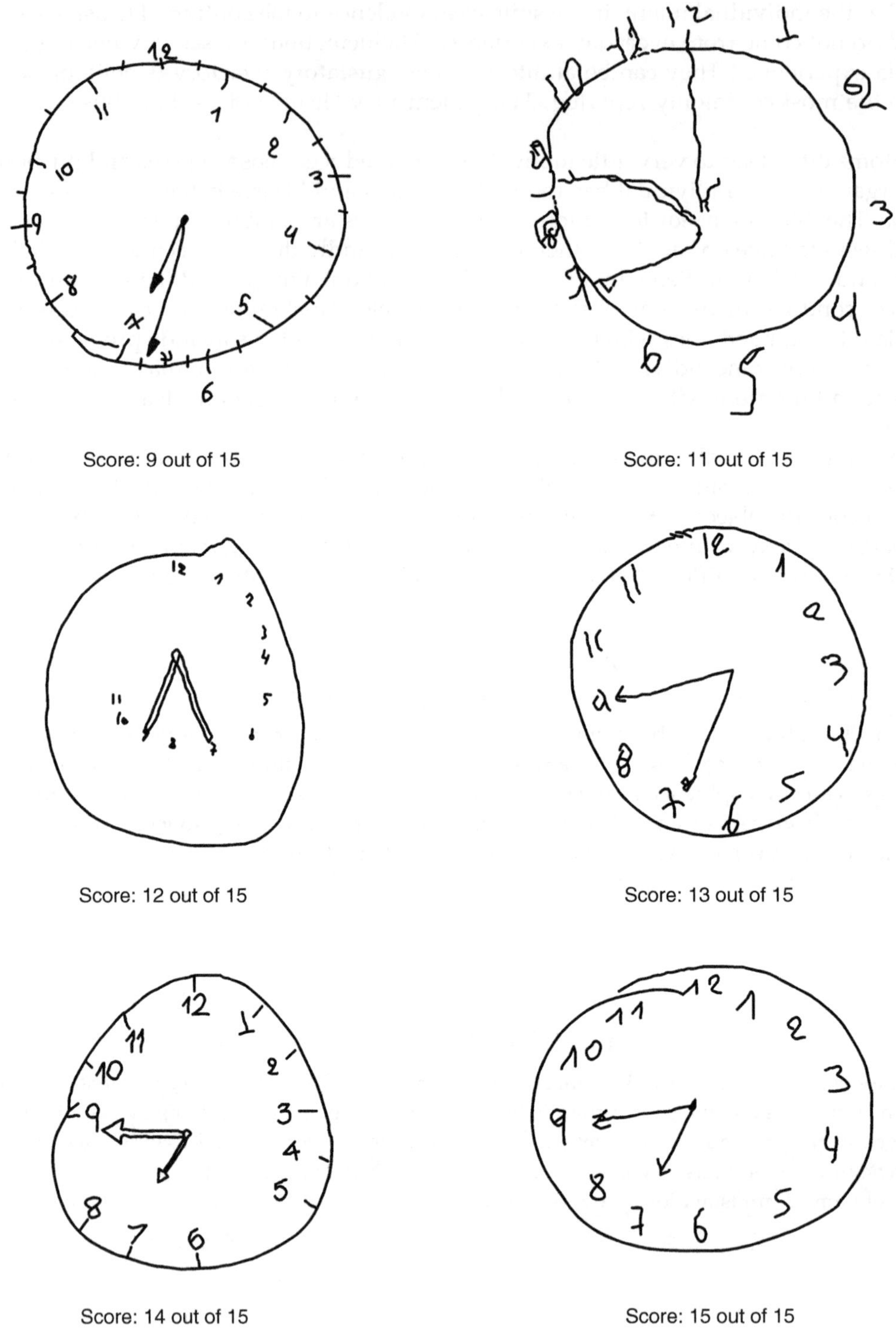

FIG. 25.1 Clock drawing test results: a different schizophrenic patient completed each drawing.

Pharmacotherapy

Medications have been the mainstay of treatment for schizophrenia and other psychoses since they were introduced more than 50 years ago. Pharmacotherapy is essential in managing acute psychotic symptoms, remission induction, and relapse prevention. Schizophrenia requires lifelong treatment, even when symptoms have subsided.

Treatment with medications and psychosocial therapy can help manage the condition. In some cases, temporary or permanent hospitalization may be needed. Medications are the cornerstone of schizophrenia treatment, and antipsychotic medications are the most commonly prescribed drugs. They are thought to control symptoms by affecting dopamine and generally seem to have a more significant therapeutic effect on positive and negative symptoms. The psychiatrist may try different drugs, doses, or combinations over time to achieve the desired result. Other medications also may help, such as antidepressants or antianxiety drugs. It can take several weeks to notice an improvement in symptoms.

First-generation drugs

The *first-generation antipsychotics* were the initial drugs used for schizophrenia. Still, they have frequent and potentially significant neurological side effects, including the possibility of developing extrapyramidal symptoms such as parkinsonism or an involuntary movement disorder called tardive dyskinesia, which may or may not be reversible. However, they are cheaper than second-generation antipsychotics, especially the generic versions, which can be an essential consideration when long-term treatment is necessary. The first-generation antipsychotics include the following, subdivided into *phenothiazines* and nonphenothiazines:

- Phenothiazines:
  - chlorpromazine (Thorazine)
  - fluphenazine (Prolixin)
  - mesoridazine (Serentil)
  - perphenazine (Trilafon)
  - prochlorperazine (Compazine, Compro)
  - thioridazine (Mellaril)
  - trifluoperazine (Stelazine)
- Nonphenothiazines:
  - droperidol (Inapsine) (though primarily used for nausea and vomiting in the United States)
  - haloperidol (Haldol)
  - loxapine (Loxitane)
  - molindone (Moban)
  - pimozide (Orap)
  - thiothixene (Navane)
- New agents:
  - asenapine (Saphris)
  - iloperidone (Fanapt)
  - lurasidone (Latuda)

Pharmacokinetics

The first-generation antipsychotics are generally well absorbed via oral or parenteral administration. Plasma concentrations usually peak within 1–4 hours (orally) or 30–60 minutes (intramuscularly). These drugs typically reach a steady state in approximately three to five half-lives, meaning about 3–5 days because the half-lives are about 24 hours. Most of these drugs are highly protein bound. They are primarily metabolized in the liver by the cytochrome P450 subfamilies.

Mechanism of action

The primary mechanism of action of first-generation antipsychotics is the postsynaptic blockade of the dopamine receptor (D2). They reduce dopaminergic neurotransmission in dopamine pathways.

Clinical indications

Aside from schizophrenia, first-generation antipsychotics are indicated for schizoaffective disorders, acute mania, major depressive disorder with psychotic features, delusional disorder, severe agitation, Tourette syndrome, borderline personality disorder, dementia, delirium, and substance-induced psychotic disorder. These drugs are also used for childhood (early-onset) schizophrenia.

Contraindications

The first-generation antipsychotics are contraindicated for those with a history of severe allergy, severe cardiac abnormalities, seizure disorder, narrow-angle glaucoma, prostatic hypertrophy, opioids, and ongoing tardive dyskinesia.

Adverse effects

Of the first-generation drugs, the phenothiazines commonly cause drowsiness, sedation, dizziness, constipation, photosensitivity, anticholinergic effects, orthostatic hypotension, and seizures. Serious adverse effects include agranulocytosis, **pancytopenia**, anaphylaxis, tardive dyskinesia, **neuroleptic malignant syndrome**, hypothermia, and **adynamic ileus**. Nonphenothiazines commonly cause akathisia, sedation, drowsiness, orthostatic hypotension, tremor, anticholinergic effects, and weight changes. Serious adverse effects of the nonphenothiazines include acute kidney failure, respiratory depression, hepatotoxicity, laryngospasm, agranulocytosis, and sudden death.

Toxicities

Overall, the chance of developing toxicity from the first-generation antipsychotics is low. Death by overdose is rare. This is because the therapeutic index is usually extensive. For *chlorpromazine*, for example, it is about 200, meaning the lethal dose is 200 times the therapeutic dose. Signs of toxicity from first-generation antipsychotics include **extrapyramidal reactions**, CNS depression, hypotension, and neuroleptic malignant syndrome.

You should remember

Treating older adult patients with antipsychotic agents poses several challenges for healthcare providers. Due to physiologic changes associated with aging, older adults can have variable and unpredictable responses to medications. For example, organ function declines as a process of aging. The kidneys and liver are the common pathways that break down and eliminate drugs. As a result of these changes, antipsychotics can be retained and accumulate in the older adult patient. Elderly patients are also more sensitive to medications' effects and side effects.

You should remember

The first-generation antipsychotics have been around since the 1950s, but because of their sometimes extreme adverse effects, the development of the second-generation antipsychotics was needed. There is controversy over the dangerousness of the original drugs. Some experts believe that first-generation medications such as haloperidol can cause apoptosis of cells, necrosis, decreased cell viability, inhibited cell growth, increased caspase activity, impaired glutamate transport, and mitochondrial damage.

Second-generation drugs

The second-generation medications are generally preferred because they pose a lower risk of severe side effects than the first-generation antipsychotics. The second-generation antipsychotics are listed in **Table 25.1**.

Pharmacokinetics

Second-generation antipsychotics have an 87% bioavailability and more than 99% protein binding. They metabolize in the liver, and their elimination half-life is about 75 hours. These agents are excreted mainly in the feces and urine.

Mechanism of action

The mechanism of action of most of the second-generation antipsychotics is primarily believed to be postsynaptic blockage of dopamine D2 receptors in the brain. There are several exceptions. *Aripiprazole* and *brexpiprazole* are D2 receptor partial agonists. *Cariprazine* is a D3-preferred D3/D2 receptor partial agonist. Many atypical

TABLE 25.1 Second-generation antipsychotics

Generic name	Trade name	Average dosage range (mg/day)	Dosage forms (in mg)
aripiprazole[a]	Abilify	2–30	2, 5, 10, 15, 20, 30
asenapine	Saphris	5–20	5, 10
brexpiprazole	Rexulti	1–4	0.25, 0.5, 1, 2, 3, 4
cariprazine	Vraylar	1.5–6	1.5, 3, 4.5, 6
clozapine	Clozaril, Versacloz	12.5–900	Oral tablet: 25, 50, 100, 200 Oral suspension: 50 mg/mL
iloperidone	Fanapt	1–24	1, 2, 4, 6, 8, 10, 12
lurasidone	Latuda	40–160	20, 40, 60, 80, 120
olanzapine	Zyprexa	5–20	2.5, 5, 7.5, 10, 15, 20
paliperidone[a]	Invega	6–12	1.5, 3, 6, 9
quetiapine	Seroquel	25–750	Standard release: 25, 50, 100, 200, 300, 400 Extended release: 50, 150, 200, 300, 400
risperidone[a]	Risperdal	2–16	Oral tablet: 0.25, 0.5, 1, 2, 3, 4 Oral solution: 1 mg/mL
ziprasidone	Geodon	20–100	20, 40, 60, 80

[a]Available in long-acting injectable forms used widely in the patient population.

antipsychotics are also serotonin antagonists, primarily blocking 5-HT2A receptors, which seems to account for a relatively better reduction of negative symptoms than typical antipsychotics. Some of them, such as cariprazine, also antagonize the 5-HT2B receptors.

Clinical indications

Aside from being indicated for schizophrenia, there are other uses for some of these drugs. *For example*, they treat Tourette syndrome, autism, bipolar disorder, and major depressive disorder.

Contraindications

Second-generation antipsychotics are contraindicated in patients with diabetes mellitus, suicidal thoughts, Alzheimer disease, neuroleptic malignant syndrome, heart failure, seizures, and metabolic syndrome X. They are also contraindicated with known hypersensitivity to the active ingredient and severe hepatic impairment. *Brexpiprazole* and cariprazine have a black box warning stating they cannot be used for patients with dementia-related psychosis. The drug has caused rash, facial swelling, **urticaria**, and **angioedema**. *Clozapine* also has black box warnings because of outcomes that include neutropenia, agranulocytosis, seizures, myocarditis, cardiomyopathy, orthostatic hypotension, bradycardia, syncope, and increased mortality in elderly patients with dementia-related psychosis. *Iloperidone* is contraindicated with hypersensitivity to the active ingredient.

Adverse effects

The primary adverse effects of second-generation antipsychotics include tardive dyskinesia (although much less risky compared to first-generation antipsychotics), drowsiness, sedation, restlessness, muscle spasms, dry mouth, blurred vision, tremors, constipation, hypotension, weight gain, and diabetes mellitus.

Toxicities

Second-generation antipsychotics may have the potential toxicity levels to cause life-threatening cardiac events. The most common and dangerous cardiac effects include sinus tachycardia, QT prolongation, sudden cardiac death, myocarditis, and cardiomyopathy. Of all the medications, *clozapine* is the most harmful to the heart. The least damaging is *asenapine*.

You should remember

The primary predictor for nonadherence to treatment for schizophrenia is the adverse effects that many patients cannot accept. Healthcare providers need to understand the negative impact of these medications and why patients often choose to stop taking them. Generally, adverse effects are dose related. Extrapyramidal symptoms from antipsychotic drugs include dystonia, akathisia, pseudoparkinsonism, and tardive dyskinesia.

You should remember

The *long-acting injectable antipsychotics* may be given intramuscularly or subcutaneously. They are usually given every 2–4 weeks, depending on the medication. This may be an option if someone prefers fewer pills, and it may help with adherence. Common drugs available as an injection include aripiprazole, fluphenazine, haloperidol, paliperidone, and risperidone.

Psychotherapy

Various psychotherapy options are used to treat and manage patients with schizophrenia. They include individual, cognitive-behavioral (CBT), and cognitive enhancement therapy (CET). *Individual therapy* involves a therapist or psychiatrist teaching patients how to deal with their thoughts and behaviors. The patient learns more about the illness and its effects and how to differentiate between what is real and what is not. This helps them manage their daily living skills.

In *CBT*, the patient learns to change thoughts and behaviors. The therapist shows the patient how to handle voices and hallucinations. By combining CBT with medications, the patient eventually learns to identify factors that trigger psychotic episodes and how to reduce or stop them. In *CET*, also known as *cognitive remediation*, the patient learns how to recognize triggers (social cues) to improve attention, memory, and organization of thoughts. Methods used in CET include computer-based brain training and group sessions.

Additionally, psychosocial therapy helps schizophrenic patients learn how to become part of their community and better interact with others. Psychosocial treatment includes social skills training, rehabilitation, family education, self-help groups, coordinated specialty care, assertive community treatment, and social recovery therapy.

You should remember

CBT has been proven to be the best form of psychotherapy for patients with schizophrenia. The patient works with a facilitator to discuss negative thoughts, behaviors, and ideas. This helps the patient cope with symptoms, accept the diagnosis, and follow a broader treatment plan, often involving medications. CBT usually takes place in sessions that last 1 hour every week over 12–16 weeks. The therapist teaches the patient how to test the reality of thoughts and perceptions, ignore voices, and manage symptoms.

Key Terms

Adynamic ileus
Angioedema
Anhedonia
Brain circuits
Catatonia
Delusions
Extrapyramidal reactions
Gustatory
Hallucinations
Neuroleptic malignant syndrome
Pancytopenia
Tactile
Urticaria

Clinical Case Studies

Clinical Case Study 1

A 25-year-old male with schizophrenia has been taking quetiapine since his diagnosis 2 years previously. The patient visits his physician and admits to not following his dosage regimen exactly due to dizziness, vomiting, and excessive weight gain occurring whenever he takes the quetiapine. His medication is switched to risperidone because this drug is better for patients experiencing these adverse effects. His medication use is carefully monitored over time, which appears successful over the first few months.

Critical Thinking Questions

1. What are the phases of schizophrenia?
2. Is patient noncompliance with medication regimens a severe concern with schizophrenia?
3. When treatment regimens are followed, what is the usual outcome?

Clinical Case Study 2

A 32-year-old male was evaluated at a psychiatric unit after he was found roaming around the town. On evaluation, he admitted to hearing voices talking to him at all hours of the day, feelings that others wanted to harm him, and a severe loss of appetite. Past medical history included a history of paranoid delusions but no family history of mental illness. He would not return to his parents' home, where he temporarily lived due to losing his job, because he said he was not safe because of the people who "wanted to get him." After being hospitalized, the patient repeatedly expressed his desire to leave, saying that the problems he was experiencing were all due to other (evil) people. Haloperidol was administered first but was not well tolerated, so olanzapine was substituted. Over a few days, the patient began to behave much more typically. He was discharged but, like so many people with schizophrenia, vanished. He never reported back for any psychiatric follow-ups.

Critical Thinking Questions

1. What type of hallucinations may occur with schizophrenia?
2. How are auditory hallucinations commonly perceived?
3. What are the risk factors that contribute to the development of schizophrenia?

Further Reading

[1] A.T. Beck, N.A. Rector, N. Stolar, P. Grant, Schizophrenia: Cognitive Theory, Research, and Therapy, The Guilford Press, 2011.
[2] C.M. Doran, Prescribing Mental Health Medication: The Practitioner's Guide, second ed., Routledge, 2013.
[3] D. Durham, R. Thirumaran, Psychiatric Pharmacogenetics: From Concepts to Cases (One), Fortis Caliga Academic Press, 2017.
[4] E.L. Granholm, J.R. McQuaid, J.L. Holden, Cognitive-Behavioral Social Skills Training for Schizophrenia: A Practical Treatment Guide, The Guilford Press, 2016.
[5] J.P. Heldt, Memorable Psychopharmacology, CreateSpace Independent Publishing Platform, 2017.
[6] J.A. Lieberman, Textbook of Schizophrenia, second ed., American Psychiatric Association Publishing, 2020.
[7] C.W. Pratt, K.J. Gill, N.M. Barrett, M.M. Roberts, Psychiatric Rehabilitation, third ed., Academic Press, 2016.
[8] J.D. Preston, J.H. O'Neal, M.C. Talaga, B.A. Moore, Handbook of Clinical Psychopharmacology for Therapists, ninth ed., New Harbinger Publications, 2021.
[9] J. Rose, Schizophrenia: A Guide to the Symptoms, Management, and Treatment of Schizophrenia, Ingram Publishing, 2020.
[10] A.J. Rothschild, The Evidence-based Guide to Antipsychotic Medications, American Psychiatric Publishing, 2009.

[11] B. Sadock, V.A. Sadock, N. Sussman, Kaplan & Sadock's Pocket Handbook of Psychiatric Drug Treatment, seventh ed., Lippincott, Williams, and Wilkins, 2018.
[12] K. Shivakumar, S. Amanullah, Complex Clinical Conundrums in Psychiatry–From Theory to Clinical Management, Springer, 2018.
[13] W.D. Spaulding, S.M. Silverstein, A.A. Menditto, The Schizophrenia Spectrum, second ed., Hogrefe Publishing, 2017.
[14] S.M. Stahl, Stahl's Illustrated Antipsychotics: Treating Psychosis, Mania and Depression, second ed., Cambridge University Press, 2010.
[15] D.M. Taylor, T.R.E. Barnes, A.H. Young, The Maudsley Prescribing Guidelines in Psychiatry, thirteenth ed., Wiley-Blackwell, 2018.
[16] R. Vitelli, What You Need to Know About Schizophrenia (Inside Diseases and Disorders), Greenwood, 2021.

CHAPTER

26

Attention-deficit/hyperactivity disorder drugs

OUTLINE

LEARNING OUTCOMES

After study of the chapter, readers should be able to:

1. Describe the signs and symptoms of attention-deficit/hyperactivity disorder.
2. Identify the causes of attention-deficit/hyperactivity disorder.
3. Explain the pathophysiology of attention-deficit/hyperactivity disorder.
4. Compare central nervous system stimulants with nonstimulant drugs.
5. Discuss behavioral therapy for attention-deficit/hyperactivity disorder.
6. Explain the mechanism of action of amphetamines and amphetamine-like drugs and how they affect the CNS and autonomic nervous system.
7. Describe the adverse effects of amphetamines and amphetamine-like drugs.
8. Discuss nonstimulant drugs used for attention-deficit/hyperactivity disorder.

The Science of Pharmacology
https://doi.org/10.1016/B978-0-443-29038-1.00026-9

Overview

Attention-deficit/hyperactivity disorder is a complex disorder that lasts a person's lifetime. It develops in the preschool years, and symptoms often continue into adulthood. The condition is a common childhood psychiatric disorder with genetic solid, neurobiological, and neurochemical bases. According to the *DSM-5*, It is characterized by symptoms of inattention with or without impulsivity and hyperactivity, which can significantly impact many aspects of behavior and performance, both at school and home. The relative prevalence of the disorder is high, affecting approximately 4% of all children, although estimates range from 5%–15%. The disorder is characterized by excessive activity, even when developmental level and limited behavioral control are considered.

Attention-deficit/hyperactivity disorder

ADHD involves attention, language, memory, perception, problem-solving, and social interaction dysfunction. It is a syndrome of hyperactivity, impulsivity, and inattention, ranked as childhood's most common neuropsychiatric disorder. The disorder affects an estimated 5%–15% of school-age children, with boys affected two to three times more often than girls. Most affected children have moderate dysfunction, followed by significant dysfunction. Symptoms usually begin between ages 3 and 7 and most commonly persist into the teenage years. Although some children with ADHD may experience a decrease in hyperactivity as they become teenagers, many of the core symptoms of impulsivity, attention difficulties, and lack of intrinsic motivation often continue into adulthood.

It is believed that ongoing maturation of the frontal lobes throughout the teenage years and into the 20s contributes to a reduction in symptom severity among some individuals. ADHD tends to run in families. It has no specific cause but is linked to a deficiency in the neurotransmitter *dopamine*. Often a child's behavior at school results in a teacher alerting parents that evaluation may be required. Potential causes of ADHD include behavioral, biochemical, genetic, physiologic, and sensorimotor factors. Risk factors include birth weight less than 1000 grams, head trauma, lead exposure, and potential exposure to alcohol, cocaine, and tobacco during the prenatal period.

Exposure to environmental toxins explicitly may be a causal factor for ADHD. Many toxins in the modern environment harm the CNS, ranging from severe organic destruction to subtle brain dysfunction. Toxic metals, including fumigants, herbicides, pesticides, and a wide range of aromatic and aliphatic solvents, are common in the contemporary setting. These environmental pollutants have been linked to abnormalities in behavior, cognition, motor ability, and perception that can be subtle during early childhood but disabling over the long term. Children exposed to lead, aluminum, arsenic, cadmium, or mercury often have permanent neurological sequelae, including attentional deficits, emotional lability, and behavioral reactivity.

A child with ADHD cannot concentrate, acts out impulsively, makes excessive **fidgety movements**, and has trouble finishing tasks before moving on to others. Diagnosis of ADHD is clinical and based on comprehensive developmental, medical, educational, and psychological evaluations. A detailed clinical history is critical to establish the precise nature and onset of behavioral symptoms, characterizing current symptoms and how they manifest across different environments or situations. The diagnosis of ADHD must be carefully handled because similar symptoms may be caused by anxiety and depression, abuse or neglect, and significant situational or family stressors. ADHD is classified as *predominately inattentive, predominately hyperactive impulsive,* or *combined* types. Symptoms mimic mood disorders in adults, including anxiety, mania, depression, and restlessness. In adulthood, ADHD is signified by constantly feeling overwhelmed, being disorganized, having difficulty with self-control, being a workaholic, excessive talking, having poor tolerance for frustration, a short temper, chronic boredom, quitting jobs abruptly, continual driving infractions, and relationship problems. Adults with ADHD are more likely to have addictions and habits such as smoking tobacco products and using illegal substances. Treatments for ADHD are the same regardless of the age of the patient.

Boys with ADHD generally have more trouble learning to read and write, while girls with ADHD have more difficulty with numbers and arithmetic. Two groups of overactive children can be identified early in life. In the first group, infants are overactive from birth, feeding poorly and sleeping less than usual. They may also cry a lot and have difficulty being soothed. By age 2, the syndrome is seen. In the second group, the inability to behave quietly without getting up to expend energy becomes apparent during preschool, between 4 and 6 years. These children usually cannot remain in one position for more than several seconds, regardless of which activity they are undertaking. They constantly move and often find it hard to restrain themselves in public places. Their abnormal impulsivity is obvious, and they usually cannot tolerate restraint. There are three clinical subgroups of ADHD, as follows:

- *Hyperactivity, impulsivity, and inattention:* this subgroup makes up 80% of all affected children.
- *Predominantly inattention*
- *Only hyperactivity*

You should remember

Girls and boys tend to show different signs of ADHD disorder. Boys are more likely to be hyperactive and have problems with self-control. Girls tend to adapt better to school and are less likely to have sudden, impulsive behaviors in the classroom. Instead, girls with hyperactivity may be emotional, sensitive, distracted, and prone to daydreaming.

A syndrome with most ADHD features can be accompanied by different forms of cognitive and developmental delay, including **autism**. In school, the child with ADHD has difficulty sitting still, watching and listening to the teacher, and not reacting to distracting stimuli. Their impulsivity is out of control. Teachers and schools often must insist that parents take their child for a medical consultation. Some children are so highly hyperactive that they cannot attend regular classes. In about 50% of affected children, hyperactivity resolves slowly by puberty or soon afterward, but the rest of the symptoms continue in a modified form into adulthood.

Many children have symptoms that do not directly indicate an attention deficit or hyperactivity but still have problems concentrating. These children have a similar core deficit and are called **hyperkinetic** children. This is a crucial issue in adults who do not have obvious signs of ADHD yet have always had difficulty concentrating. Children with these difficulties are generally clumsy, uncoordinated, and defective in communication.

Up to 20% of children with ADHD also have depression, and some antidepressant medications may be beneficial in treating the core symptoms of ADHD, mainly if they promote the availability of dopamine or norepinephrine. Among children, depression is more often characterized by irritability and **anhedonia** rather than feelings of sadness. They may also experience low self-esteem, social withdrawal, and sleep disturbances. Children who develop depression at a young age are at greater risk of frequently recurrent depressive episodes. Although the development of bipolar disorder in childhood is uncommon, many symptoms of ADHD can appear similar to symptoms of mania. However, children with ADHD are less likely to experience a decreased need for sleep. In contrast, children with bipolar disorder are more likely to experience prolonged intense anger and rage episodes. Significant symptoms in children and teenagers include the following:

- Having a short attention span
- Being easily distracted
- Making careless mistakes, such as in schoolwork
- Appearing to be forgetful
- Losing things
- Being unable to focus on tasks that are tedious or time consuming
- Being unable to listen to or carry out instructions

You should remember

ADHD is not caused by poor parenting or teaching, family problems, too much television or video games, food allergies, or excess sugar. It is believed to be caused by biological factors that influence neurotransmitter activity in specific brain parts. There is a strong genetic link because studies on twins have shown that an identical twin has a 92% likelihood of having ADHD if the other twin has the disorder. Also, about 25% of family members diagnosed with the disease have other relatives with ADHD. This is much higher than the 5% prevalence within the general population.

You should remember

It is believed that about 8 million people in the United States have adult attention-deficit disorder (ADD). Many adults eventually realize that they have had a lifelong problem with motor restlessness and poor attention after learning about the diagnoses of ADHD in their children. Many affected adults are of above-average intelligence and highly successful because they have learned strategies that combat their restlessness and lack of attention. However, they may still struggle to focus while completing tedious or mundane tasks.

Diagnosis

There is not a specific single test that diagnoses ADHD. Other conditions such as sleep disorders, anxiety, depression, and learning disabilities have similar symptoms. Clinical diagnosis of ADHD can be made by a mental health professional or a primary care provider. The American Academy of Pediatrics (AAP) recommends that providers ask parents, teachers, and other caregivers about the child's behavior in different settings. Often, symptoms of ADHD are first identified in preschool, where children encounter their first sustained contact with other children their age and are expected to adhere to social standards of behavior, such as following rules and staying on task.

The diagnosis of ADHD in adults and adolescents aged 17 is based on five required symptoms that may appear differently with aging. In adults, for example, hyperactivity may appear as significant restlessness or energy levels that tire other people out just by being around them.

Behavioral therapy

For ADHD, behavioral therapy helps children learn and strengthen positive behaviors while reducing unwanted or problematic behaviors. The AAP recommends that behavioral therapy be used as the first treatment for children under 6. A combination of behavioral therapy and medications should be used for children aged 6 or older. Interestingly, much behavioral therapy focuses on training parents in over 8 to 16 sessions for preschool- and elementary school–aged children. Parents learn how to encourage positive behaviors while addressing negative behaviors. They know how to improve communication and strengthen their relationship with their child. Parents trained in behavioral therapy can help the child succeed in all parts of their life. Though training takes time, it can have long-lasting benefits for children with ADHD.

Pharmacotherapy

Pharmacotherapy is more effective when used along with behavioral therapy for ADHD. Drug therapy allows participation in activities the patient could not previously participate in due to poor attention and impulsivity. The most widely used drugs for ADHD are CNS stimulants such as methylphenidate and dextroamphetamine. The dosage is adjusted until an optimal response is achieved. Additional medications include amphetamine, dexmethylphenidate, and lisdexamfetamine, all CNS stimulants. Untreated ADD or ADHD in adults is linked to low self-esteem, criminal or violent behaviors, and diminished social success. The CNS stimulants and other drugs used for ADHD are summarized in **Table 26.1**.

Central nervous system stimulants

The CNS stimulants are pharmacologically diverse agents that increase alertness, enhance concentration, and delay fatigue. They range from easily accessible agents such as *caffeine* to Schedule I controlled substances such as *ecstasy*. Every CNS stimulant raises the brain's general alertness. There is increased wakefulness and the ability to concentrate or focus. The CNS stimulants often elevate mood, and there may be temporary unawareness of physical fatigue. For some controlled substances with CNS stimulant activities, mood elevation may increase to **euphoria**,

TABLE 26.1 CNS stimulants and other drugs used for ADHD in children.

Generic name	Trade name	Average dosage range (mg/day)	Dosage forms (in mg)
Amphetamines and amphetamine-like drugs.			
amphetamine/ dextroamphetamine	Adderall	2.5–40	1.25/1.25 (extended-release form: 5, 7.5, 10)
dexmethylphenidate	Focalin	2.5–20	2.5, 5, 10; (extended-release and multiple dosage forms: 5, 10, 15)
dextroamphetamine	Dexedrine	5–60	5, 10, 15
lisdexamfetamine	Vyvanse	10–70	10, 20, 30, 40, 50, 60, 70
methylphenidate	Ritalin, Concerta, Daytrana (many others)	5–60	5, 10, 15, 20, 30, 40; (long-acting form: 60)
viloxazine	Quelbree, Vivalan	100–400	100, 150, 200
Nonstimulants			
atomoxetine	Strattera	40–100	10, 18, 25, 40, 60, 80, 100
bupropion	Wellbutrin	37.5–250	75, 100, 150, 200, 300
clonidine	Kapvay	0.1–4	0.1, 0.2, 0.3
guanfacine	Intuniv	1–4	1, 2, 3, 4 (regular and extended-release forms)

an extreme sense of well-being and happiness. Because CNS stimulation is generally desirable because of its good feelings, many people reuse CNS stimulants to achieve the same "high." Over time, physical and psychological dependence occurs. This is why many CNS stimulants are rigidly regulated as scheduled drugs; see **Table 26.2**.

In past decades, amphetamines were often used for asthma, the common cold, and hay fever. They became more popular during World War II because they helped soldiers remain alert for extended periods and delayed combat fatigue. Amphetamines did not become scheduled substances until 1970. Amphetamine sulfate is used illegally to manufacture drugs such as *methamphetamine* and *ecstasy*—the medications derived from amphetamine sulfate work "in reverse" in people with ADHD. Instead of stimulating the brain, they increase attention and improve the individual's ability to focus on tasks and learn. When used correctly, they do not cause euphoria. Childhood use of these medications does not result in a higher incidence of alcohol, tobacco, or illicit drug use later in life. These **psychostimulants** reduce symptoms in 70%–80% of treated children. For many with ADHD, ongoing medication treatment will be necessary into adolescence and perhaps adulthood.

TABLE 26.2 CNS stimulants that are also scheduled drugs

Drug schedule	Examples
I	3,4-Methylenedioxymethamphetamine (ecstasy, MDMA), aminorex, cathinone, fenethylline, mephedrone, methcathinone, methylaminorex
II	Amphetamine (Adderall), cocaine, lisdexamfetamine (Vyvanse), methamphetamine (Desoxyn), methylphenidate (Daytrana, Ritalin), phenmetrazine (Preludin)
III	Benzphetamine (Didrex), chlorphentermine, dronabinol (Marinol), phendimetrazine (Plegine)
IV	Diethylpropion (Tenuate), mazindol (Sanorex), modafinil (Provigil), phentermine (Adipex)
V	Pyrovalerone

You should remember

Though CNS stimulants do not cure ADHD, they help control symptoms and assist patients in staying focused and paying attention. These medications work by stimulating networks of nerve cells in the brain to work more effectively with each other—primarily by stimulating the dopamine system. If symptoms persist, a change in the dose or the actual medication may be required.

Nonstimulants

Stimulants make up 75% of the medications taken for ADHD. The nonstimulant drugs are newer, developed in 2003, and offer fewer adverse effects plus more prolonged duration of action.

Pharmacokinetics

The *amphetamines and amphetamine-like drugs* are rapidly absorbed orally and widely distributed to all body tissues, including the CNS. They are primarily metabolized in the liver and excreted in the urine. Their onset of action is 30–60 minutes. These drugs have an elimination half-life of 4 hours. They have 96% bioavailability. Extended-release versions of many stimulants are also available and often ultimately preferred. *Nonstimulant drugs* are rapidly absorbed orally and distributed to most body tissues. They are 98% bound to protein and metabolized in the liver. Nonstimulant drugs are primarily excreted in the urine, with a lesser amount in the feces. Their onset of action is over 2–4 weeks. Their half-life is 5 hours.

Mechanism of action

The amphetamines and amphetamine-like drugs affect the CNS and autonomic nervous system. Their primary mechanism of action is to inhibit dopamine reuptake while also increasing dopamine release from presynaptic neurons. They also activate alpha-and beta-adrenergic receptors by promoting the release of norepinephrine in the autonomic nervous system.

The mechanism of action of the nonstimulant drugs is also based on the attenuation of dopamine and norepinephrine neurotransmission. *Atomoxetine* is a norepinephrine reuptake inhibitor. *Clonidine* is understood to work by stimulating alpha receptors throughout the CNS and many other organs to prevent the release of norepinephrine. *Wellbutrin* inhibits the reuptake of norepinephrine and dopamine.

Clinical indications

There are a variety of indications for CNS stimulants. These include ADHD, migraines, narcolepsy, stimulation of respiration, and weight management. In the past, CNS stimulants were used to treat major depressive disorder because they are nonselective and they affect all brain parts. *Amphetamine/dextroamphetamine*, aside from ADHD, is also used to treat narcolepsy. *Dexmethylphenidate* and *atomoxetine* are only clinically indicated for ADHD. *Lisdexamfetamine* is also indicated for severe binge eating disorder in adults. *Methylphenidate* is also indicated for *ADD* and narcolepsy. *Clonidine* and *guanfacine* are also used to treat hypertension.

Contraindications

Amphetamine/dextroamphetamine is contraindicated with known hypersensitivity of idiosyncrasy to sympathomimetic amines, symptomatic cardiovascular disease, hyperthyroidism, hypertension, glaucoma, advanced arteriosclerosis, and in agitated patients. *Dexmethylphenidate* and *methylphenidate* are contraindicated with known hypersensitivity, severe anxiety, tension, agitation, glaucoma, motor tics, and a family history of Tourette syndrome. *Atomoxetine* is contraindicated with known hypersensitivity or angle-closure glaucoma. *Clonidine* is contraindicated if bleeding, **diathesis**, an injection site infection, severe cardiovascular disease, hemodynamic instability, or known hypersensitivity. *Guanfacine* and *lisdexamfetamine* are only contraindicated if there is known hypersensitivity.

Adverse effects

CNS stimulants can cause unpleasant effects. Excessive excitation can lead to a variety of adverse effects. At higher doses, convulsions may occur. Most CNS stimulants also affect the cardiovascular system, with increased heart rate and dysrhythmias occurring. The amphetamines and amphetamine-like drugs have common adverse effects, including dizziness, irritability, euphoria, palpitations, insomnia, tachycardia, stomachache, and weight loss. There is also a transdermal patch form of methylphenidate called Daytrana, which can cause application site reactions. The serious adverse effects of these drugs include dependence, psychosis, seizures, and sudden death. It is also of note that the appearance of unusual "side effects" might suggest a misdiagnosis of ADHD. For example, a child with an anxiety disorder may experience increased anxiety when taking a stimulant, while a child developing bipolar disorder may experience manic symptoms or mood cycle accelerations with stimulant use.

The nonstimulants used for ADHD each have adverse effects, but they all may cause constipation. *Atomoxetine* has common adverse effects, including headache, palpitations, decreased appetite, insomnia, fatigue, irritability, dry mouth, drowsiness, upper abdominal pain, nausea, vomiting, cough, and urinary retention. Its serious adverse effects include severe liver injury and suicidal ideation. *Clonidine* has common adverse effects, including fatigue, tiredness, irritability, upper respiratory tract infection, insomnia, sore throat, emotional disorders, nightmares, and increased body temperature. Its serious adverse effects are the same as with the drug *guanfacine*: bradycardia, profound sedation, severe hypotension, and syncope. The common adverse effects of guanfacine include abdominal pain, dizziness, mild hypotension, and dry mouth.

Toxicities

Restlessness, tremors, muscle twitching, rapid breathing, confusion, hallucinations, panic, aggressiveness, muscle pain or weakness, dark-colored urine, depression, and tiredness signify amphetamine/dextroamphetamine toxicity. Severe toxicity can be fatal. *Dexmethylphenidate* toxicity causes similar symptoms: dry mouth, vomiting, agitation, dilated pupils, fever, sweating, headaches, pounding in the neck or ears, fast or pounding heartbeats, convulsions, or coma. *Lisdexamfetamine* may additionally cause hostility and violence. *Methylphenidate* may also cause euphoria, delirium, flushing, and permanent brain damage. *Atomoxetine* can also cause dizziness, GI upset, arrhythmias, hypertension, hyperactivity, and disorientation. *Clonidine* may also cause reduced sensations, hypotension, and bradycardia. *Guanfacine* may cause severe dizziness, and toxicity has been fatal.

You should remember

Amphetamines are Schedule II drugs with a high potential for abuse and were first discovered in 1887. Unauthorized possession of these drugs and distribution are tightly controlled due to significant health risks associated with their recreational use. However, it is noteworthy that the risk of abuse is relatively low among individuals with true ADHD.

Key Terms

Aliphatic
Anhedonia
Autism
Diathesis
Dyslexia
Euphoria
Fidgety movements
Hyperkinetic
Psychostimulants
Striatum

Clinical case studies

Clinical case study 1

An 8-year-old boy was diagnosed with ADHD because of severe outbursts, disruptions, and lack of attention while in school. His pediatrician, discussing with a child psychiatrist, decided to start the boy on a course of methylphenidate. It took some time to find the perfect dosage for the boy, but by the time he was 9 years of age, his schoolwork had greatly improved, and he seldom got into any trouble from disruptive behaviors in the classroom. His parents told the pediatrician that their son had much better attention at home and could complete his chores regularly. Before, he had never been able to focus before taking the medication.

Critical thinking questions

1. How common is ADHD in children?
2. What are the potential causes and risk factors for ADHD?
3. What are the most widely used drugs to treat ADHD?

Clinical case study 2

A 24-year-old male went to his physician's office because of his distress. He was constantly moving and fidgeting around and became upset as he told the physician about losing his job and fighting with his girlfriend regularly. He could not manage his schedule, was disorganized, was late, and lost common everyday objects regularly. The patient has missed essential deadlines at work and made careless errors. The physician refers the patient to a psychiatrist, who conducts structured assessments in great detail, resulting in a diagnosis of adult ADHD. The patient is started on atomoxetine along with CBT.

Critical thinking questions

1. How is ADHD signified in adulthood?
2. How common is ADHD during adulthood?
3. Why are nonstimulants such as atomoxetine becoming more popular for ADHD?

Further reading

[1] D.G. Amen, Healing ADD–The Breakthrough Program that Allows You to See and Heal the 7 Types of ADD, Berkley, 2013.
[2] R.A. Barkley, C.M. Benton, Taking Charge of Adult ADHD, Proven Strategies to Succeed at Work, Home, and Relationships, second ed., The Guilford Press, 2021.
[3] R.A. Barkley, Attention-Deficit Hyperactivity Disorder–A Handbook for Diagnosis & Treatment, fourth ed., The Guilford Press, 2018.
[4] T.E. Brown, Outside the Box: Rethinking ADD/ADHD in Children and Adults–A Practical Guide, American Psychiatric Publishing, 2017.
[5] T.E. Brown, A New Understanding of ADHD in Children and Adults–Executive Function Impairments, Routledge, 2013.
[6] G. Carroccia, Treating ADHD/ADD in Children and Adolescents, Charles C. Thomas Publishing Ltd, 2019.
[7] A. Chronis-Tuscano, K. O'Brien, C.M. Danko, Supporting Caregivers of Children with ADHD–An Integrated Parenting Program, Therapist Guide, Oxford University Press, 2020.
[8] C. Goldrich, C. Goldrich, ADHD, Executive Function & Behavioral Challenges in the Classroom: Managing the Impact on Learning, Motivation, and Stress, PESI Publishing & Media, 2019.
[9] E.M. Hallowell, J.J. Ratey, Delivered from Distraction: Getting the Most out of Life with Attention Deficit Disorder, Ballantine Books, 2005.
[10] A. Kalali, S. Preskorn, J. Kwentus, S.M. Stahl, Essential CNS Drug Development, Cambridge University Press/Medicine, 2012.
[11] R. Merki, ADHD Pro: Sustainable Productivity for People with ADHD, Merki, 2021.
[12] G.J. Sherrod, Adulting with ADHD: Navigating Adult Life with Attention Deficit Hyperactivity Disorder, Sherrod, 2020.
[13] S. Solden, Females with Attention Deficit Disorder–Embrace Your Differences and Transform Your Life, second ed., Introspect Press, 2012.
[14] E.P. Sparrow, D. Erhardt, Essentials of ADHD Assessment for Children and Adolescents, 2014.
[15] P.H. Wender, D.A. Tomb, ADHD: A Guide to Understanding Symptoms, Causes, Diagnosis, Treatment, and Changes over Time in Children, Adolescents, and Adults, fifth ed., Oxford University Press, 2016.

UNIT V

Cardiovascular drugs

CHAPTER

27

Antihyperlipidemic drugs

OUTLINE

LEARNING OUTCOMES

After study of the chapter, readers should be able to:

1. Describe the classifications of lipids and lipoproteins.
2. Explain the role of cholesterol in the human body.
3. Compare the function of LDL with HDL.
4. Explain the relationship between high cholesterol and atherosclerosis.
5. Identify the most common treatments for hyperlipidemia.
6. Explain the classifications of antidepressants.

The Science of Pharmacology
https://doi.org/10.1016/B978-0-443-29038-1.00027-0

7. Discuss the adverse effects of statins.
8. Describe the mechanism of action for the bile acid sequestrants.
9. Explain the significant adverse effects of niacin.
10. Describe the newest cholesterol-lowering drugs on the market and their mechanisms of action.

Overview

Hyperlipidemia is characterized by elevated fats or lipids in the blood. "Lipids" generally refers to cholesterol and triglycerides found in the blood. An elevation in low-density lipoproteins (LDLs), one of the three main subclasses of cholesterol, has been linked to the development of atherosclerosis and the most common type of heart disease, coronary heart disease. Atherosclerosis is the accumulation of plaque, which narrows and stiffens the arteries. This contributes to heart disease, the leading cause of death in the United States. Approximately every 34 seconds, one American adult has a coronary event, and roughly every minute, an American adult will die of one type of cardiovascular disease (CVD). This represents a financial burden to society, with the total direct and indirect costs of CVD in 2021 estimated to be $407 billion. For comparison, the estimated cost of all cancers was $201.5 billion. CVD costs more than any other disease state. Because avoiding CVDs is desired, hyperlipidemia treatments exist, and these include diet, exercise, and drugs such as statins, bile acid sequestrants (BASs), niacin, fibrates, and selective cholesterol absorption inhibitors. Statins are the mainstay of hyperlipidemia treatment.

Classifications of lipids and lipoproteins

Lipids are a group of organic compounds that are insoluble in water but soluble in organic solvents. They are mainly classified into simple, complex, and derived lipids. Simple lipids are **triglycerides**, esters of fatty acids, and wax esters. The hydrolysis of these lipids gives glycerol and fatty acids. Complex lipids are heterogeneous compounds of steroids, fats, waxes, oils, and other substances. These chemical features are present in many molecules such as **fatty acids**, **phospholipids**, **sterols**, **sphingolipids**, and **terpenes**.

A lipoprotein's **density** is determined by its protein and lipid content (**Table 27.1**). LDL carries 60%–70% of the total blood **cholesterol**. High-density lipoprotein (HDL) is about 20%–30% of total blood cholesterol. Very-low-density lipoprotein (VLDL) carries approximately 10%–15% of total blood cholesterol and most triglycerides in a fasting state.

Elevated HDL has been linked to removing extra VLDL or LDL from the blood and returning it to the liver or bile for elimination. This process accounts for some of the beneficial effects of high HDL, often called "good cholesterol."

TABLE 27.1 Classification of cholesterol levels

Total cholesterol	
Less than 200 mg/dL	Desirable
200 to 239 mg/dL	Borderline high
240 mg/dL or higher	High

LDL cholesterol	
Less than 100 mg/dL	Optimal
100 to 129 mg/dL	Above optimal
130 to 159 mg/dL	Borderline high
160 to 189 mg/dL	High
190 mg/dL or higher	Very high

When triglycerides are 400 mg/dL, a more complex, specialized laboratory technique is required for accuracy. A fasting lipid panel should be measured in all adults 20 years or older at least once every 5 years. The optimal cholesterol laboratory values for each of the four standard tests in a lipid panel are as follows:

- Total cholesterol: below 200 mg/dL (borderline high: 200–239 mg/dL)
- HDL cholesterol: above 40 mg/dL (60 mg/dL or above is protective against heart disease)
- LDL cholesterol: below 100 mg/dL (for people with diabetes: below 70 mg/dL)
- Triglycerides: Below 150 mg/dL (borderline high: 150 to 199 mg/dL and high: 200 to 499 mg/dL)

Functions of cholesterol and lipoproteins

Cholesterol and triglycerides are the major blood lipids. They are essential for forming cell membranes and hormone production and provide an energy source of free fatty acids. Because lipids are not water soluble, they do not circulate in the blood in free form but instead are bound to proteins in a macromolecule called a lipoprotein.

The structure of a lipoprotein consists of a lipid core and a surface coat. The lipid core, the interior of a lipoprotein, contains triglycerides and cholesterol esters, both of which are insoluble in water. Cholesterol esters are cholesterol molecules that have been attached to a fatty acid. The surface coat of lipoproteins comprises water-soluble components (see **Fig. 27.1**). They include **apolipoprotein B** (Apo-B), phospholipids, and unesterified cholesterol. The phospholipids are oriented so that their water-soluble heads face outward and their fat-soluble tails face inward. Additionally, Apo-B also interacts with external water.

Lipids, including triglycerides in food, are broken down into fatty acids and cholesterol by enzymes found in the gut. Fatty acids are then converted to triglycerides and brought back together with cholesterol to make chylomicrons that eventually enter the bloodstream. Intestinal cholesterol absorption is assisted by Niemann-Pick C1-like 1 protein, which targets the cholesterol-lowering drug ezetimibe. After gaining entry into the circulation, chylomicrons are broken down in muscle and fat cells, which are stored as energy or used as free fatty acids.

An enzyme breaks down VLDLs into intermediate-density lipoproteins (IDLs). The liver either removes IDLs or is further processed into cholesterol-rich LDLs. LDL particles last longer in circulation than VLDLs and contain about two-thirds of all blood cholesterol. Lastly, LDLs are recycled into the liver or other peripheral cells via LDL receptors (see **Fig. 27.2**). Cellular cholesterol requirements ultimately regulate this process. When fasting or on low fat intake, most cholesterol is created in organs other than the liver. Individual abnormalities may develop in the gene that destroys LDL receptors, proprotein convertase subtilisin-kexin type 9 (*PCSK9*). This abnormality can cause blood elevations in LDL by increasing the destruction of LDL receptors and decreasing the uptake of LDL into the liver. Lastly, LDL may be excreted into small intestine fluid and out of the body through the stool.

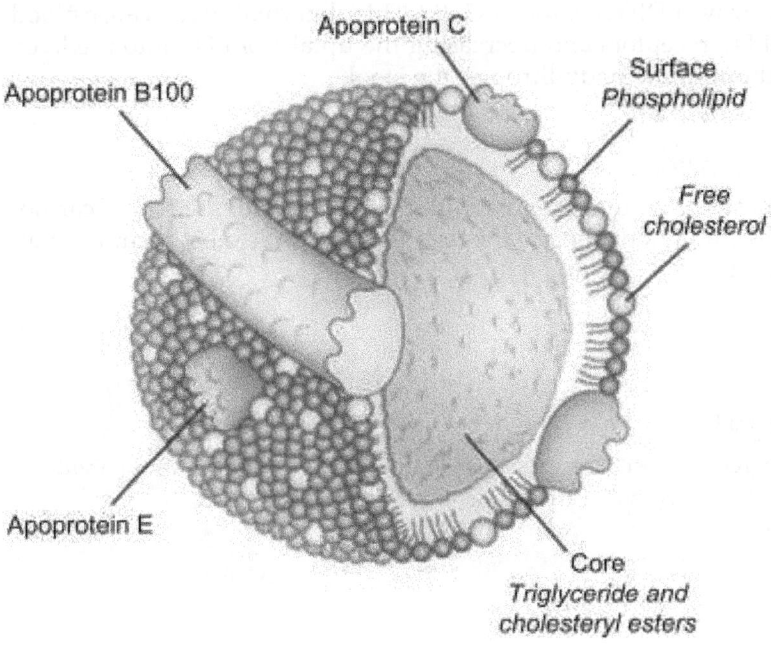

FIG. 27.1 Structure of a lipoprotein.

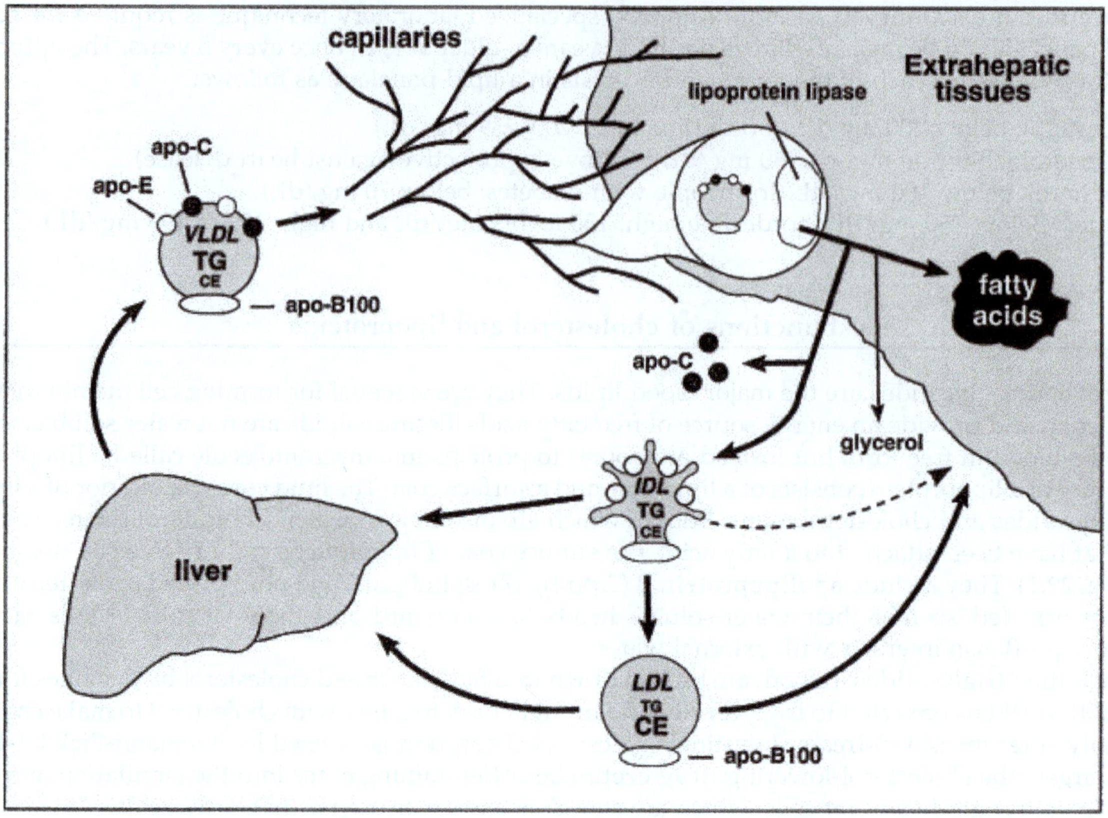

FIG. 27.2 Recycling of LDL.

The liver is primarily responsible for the regulation of cholesterol in the body. The endogenous pathway begins in the liver with the creation of VLDLs. VLDL production is stimulated in the liver when there is an increase in the number of free fatty acids. An enzyme breaks down VLDLs into IDLs. Cellular cholesterol requirements ultimately regulate this process. When fasting or on a low-fat diet, most cholesterol is created in organs other than the liver. Of note, the rate-limiting enzyme for intracellular creation of cholesterol is 3-hydroxy-3-methylglutaryl coenzyme A (HMG-CoA) reductase, the target of the statin drug class, which includes simvastatin or atorvastatin. A person's genetics may create abnormalities in the gene that destroys LDL receptors, *PCSK9*. This abnormality can cause blood elevations in LDL by increasing the destruction of LDL receptors and decreasing the uptake of LDL into the liver. Lastly, LDL may be excreted into stomach fluid and out of the body through the stool.

Blood lipid profiles

A **lipid profile** is a standard blood test that healthcare providers use to monitor and screen for the risk of cardiovascular disease. A blood lipid profile is used to measure 14 hours before the test. This gives the most accurate evaluation of the cholesterol and triglycerides in the blood.

You should remember

Children can also have high cholesterol to the degree that they may need a lipid profile blood test. High cholesterol in children is linked to heredity, diet, and obesity. In most cases, children with high cholesterol have a parent with elevated cholesterol.

Biosynthesis of cholesterol and excretion

Large amounts of cholesterol can be found in the brain, nervous tissues, liver, kidneys, spleen, and skin. The total cholesterol for a male weighing 70 kg is about 140 g. The more significant part of the body's cholesterol is synthesized (about 1 gram daily) de novo, whereas the average diet provides approximately 0.3 g daily. Because cholesterol is not synthesized in plants, dietary cholesterol is obtained from animal sources such as skeletal muscle, the liver, the brain, and egg yolks.

Slightly less than half of the cholesterol in the body is derived de novo: the liver accounts for ~10%; the intestines make ~15%. The cholesterol biosynthesis pathway involves enzymes in the cytoplasm, **endoplasmic reticulum**, and **peroxisomes**. Because the majority of cholesterol synthesis in the body occurs in extrahepatic tissues and the only quantitatively significant site for excretion and **catabolism** of cholesterol is the liver, some 600–800 mg of cholesterol each day must be transported from peripheral tissues through the plasma compartment to the liver.

Once in the liver, cholesterol is converted into bile salts or secreted as unesterified cholesterol into the **bile**. From there, cholesterol enters the small intestine, is partially reabsorbed, and then is excreted via the feces. Biliary cholesterol secretion is essential for two major disease complexes: atherosclerotic CVD and cholesterol **gallstone** disease.

You should remember

Cholesterol homeostasis is associated with multiple human diseases, including CVD, cancer, and neurodegenerative and hepatic diseases.

Cholesterol and atherosclerosis

Atherosclerosis is the most common form of **arteriosclerosis**. Atherosclerotic plaques are either stable or unstable. *Stable plaques* can grow slowly over several decades until stenosis or occlusion occurs. *Unstable plaques* are weaker and more likely to erode, develop fissures, or rupture. They can cause acute **thrombosis**, occlusion, and infarction for a long time before causing extreme stenosis. Unstable plaques cause the majority of signs and symptoms. They do not appear to be severe during **angiography**. Therefore stabilization of unstable plaques may help reduce disease and death. The rupture of plaques is based on activated **macrophages** inside that secrete **cathepsins** and **collagenases**.

Pharmacotherapy

Various medications can lower blood cholesterol. Statins are recommended for most patients and have been directly associated with reducing the risk of heart attack or stroke. Statins continue to provide the most effective lipid-lowering treatment in most cases. Other drugs include BASs, *PCSK9* inhibitors, fibrates, niacin, cholesterol absorption inhibitors, and omega-3. They are discussed in this chapter.

Statins

Statins can help lower the LDL and total cholesterol in the blood. They are the most common cholesterol-lowering drugs. Also known as **HMG-CoA reductase inhibitors**, they reduce illness and mortality in those at high risk of CVD. There are various types of statins. Statins are prescribed primarily for their LDL-lowering capabilities, but they can lower triglycerides and raise HDL. There are seven types of statins (see Table 27.2). Based on their metabolic fates, they all differ in their LDL-lowering efficacy and potential for drug and disease interactions. All statins are classified as category X in pregnancy and should be used cautiously in females of childbearing potential because category X drugs are known to cause fetal congenital disabilities.

TABLE 27.2 Properties of statins.

Statin	Dose range	% LDL lowering
Atorvastatin (Lipitor)	10–80	38–54
Fluvastatin (Lescol)	20–80	17–33
Lovastatin (Mevacor)	10–80	29–48
Pitavastatin (Livalo)	1–4	31–41
Pravastatin (Pravachol)	10–80	19–40
Rosuvastatin (Crestor)	5–40	52–63
Simvastatin (Zocor)	5–80	28–41

Pharmacokinetics

Statins are dosed orally and enter the systemic circulation through intestinal cells. The significant organs of metabolism and elimination include the liver and, to a lesser extent, the kidneys. Short-acting statins include pravastatin, simvastatin, lovastatin, and fluvastatin with 2–5 hours of half-lives. Long-acting statins include rosuvastatin and atorvastatin with half-lives of 14–19 hours.

Mechanism of action

Statins inhibit the enzyme HMG-CoA. This inhibition occurs early in the hepatic pathway, producing cholesterol and other vital metabolic products. Cholesterol is an intermediate product in pathways with corticosteroids, sex steroids, vitamin D, and bile acids—metabolic pathways influenced by statins and *PCSK9* inhibitors. Decreased cholesterol synthesis results in upregulation of LDL cholesterol receptors and greater clearance of LDL cholesterol. When *PCSK9* is bound to the LDL cholesterol receptor, the internalized receptor is more likely to be degraded. With lower *PCSK9* activity due to *PCSK9* inhibitors, LDL receptors are more likely to be recycled to the cell surface to clear plasma LDL cholesterol.

Clinical indications

Statins are the mainstay for the treatment of hyperlipidemia and **mixed dyslipidemia**.

They are also used for hypertriglyceridemia, atherosclerosis, and primary prevention of atherosclerotic CVD. They are used for adults aged 40–75 years with one or more cardiovascular risk factors such as dyslipidemia, diabetes, hypertension, or smoking.

Contraindications

Statins are contraindicated in individuals who have hypersensitivity to medication.

They are also contraindicated in acute liver failure or decompensated cirrhosis, pregnancy, and lactation.

Adverse effects

While statins are highly effective and safe for most people, they have been linked to muscle pain, digestive problems, and mental fuzziness in some people. Rarely, they may cause liver damage. **Rhabdomyolysis** is the most severe adverse effect of statin use, though it seldom occurs (less than 0.1%). The most common risk factors for statin-related myopathy include hypothyroidism, polypharmacy, and alcohol abuse. Headache, tiredness, dizziness, and insomnia are also common.

Toxicities

Statin intolerance occurs when a person develops side effects from statin use. There are different symptoms a patient may experience. The most common is muscle pains or cramps. Statins can also cause liver and muscle toxicity.

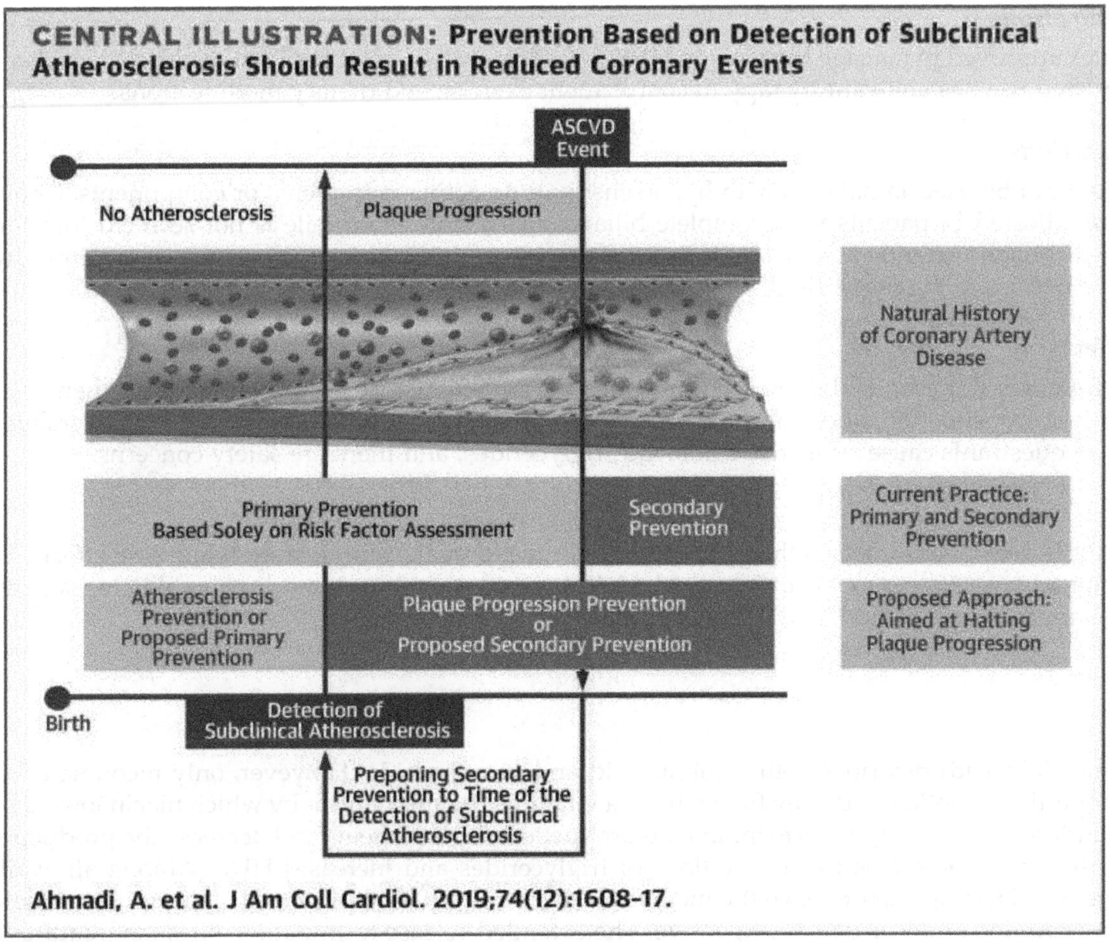

FIG. 27.3 Recycling of LDL.

Bile acid sequestrants

BASs are also called anion-exchange resins because they bind bile acid through an anion-exchange reaction. Typically bile acids emulsify dietary fats to help them be absorbed in the small intestine. Due to a decreased absorption of bile acids, the liver increases the production of bile acids from blood cholesterol and thus increases the removal of cholesterol from the circulation. As a class, their main effect is to decrease LDL. There are three BASs available for use: cholestyramine (Questran), colestipol (Colestid), and colesevelam (Welchol). Because BAS's site of action is in the intestines, they can decrease the absorption of multiple drugs when administered simultaneously. It is generally recommended that the coadministration of BAS with other medications should be separated by 1 hour before or 4 hours after other medicines.

Pharmacokinetics

BAS are large polymeric structures not significantly absorbed from the gut into the bloodstream. Thus BAS and any bile acids bound to the drug are excreted via the feces after passage through the gastrointestinal tract.

Mechanism of action

The BASs are highly positively charged molecules that bind to the negatively charged bile acids in the intestine, inhibiting their lipid-solubilizing activity and thus blocking cholesterol absorption.

Clinical indications

BAS is FDA approved to manage hypercholesterolemia. They can be combined with statins or used as monotherapy. BAS is often used as adjuvant therapy to complement exercise and dietary modifications.

Contraindications

BAS should not be used in patients with hypersensitivity to active ingredients or components. Cholestyramine use is contraindicated in patients with complete biliary obstruction where bile is not secreted into the intestine. The only medications currently acceptable during pregnancy are BASs because they are not systemically absorbed and therefore not felt to pose fetal risk.

Adverse effects

Because BASs are not absorbed, they lack systemic toxicity. Still, GI side effects often limit their use, including nausea, bloating, constipation, and cramping. Colesevelam has been reported to have better tolerability than the other BASs. Sequestrants cause an increase in blood triglycerides, and there are safety concerns.

Toxicities

Because BASs are not absorbed in the gastrointestinal tract, they have limited systemic side effects. Some of the most common adverse effects are gastrointestinal, including constipation, stomach pain, bloating, vomiting, heartburn, loss of appetite, indigestion, and upset stomach.

Niacin

Niacin (nicotinic acid) describes both nicotinic acid and nicotinamide. However, only nicotinic acid has lipid-lowering properties. Nicotinamide only functions as a vitamin. The mechanism by which niacin lowers blood lipids is not fully understood, but it appears to inhibit the production of lipoproteins and decrease the production of VLDL in the liver. It also reduces blood concentrations of triglycerides and increases HDL. Among all available lipid-lowering agents, niacin appears to have the most favorable effect on the lipid profile. Niacin is available with and without a prescription and is usually inexpensive. The extended-release formulation, Niaspan, requires a prescription. Niacin is typically administered in two to three doses per day except for Niaspan, which is taken as a single dose at bedtime. Because some niacin preparations are available over the counter, it is essential to counsel patients that their use is associated with many side effects.

Niacin has multiple side effects that limit its long-term use. The most common side effect is flushing (redness) of the skin, often described as a "hot flash." This usually leads to discontinuation of the drug. Most people develop tolerance after prolonged use. Slowly increasing the niacin dose over weeks is essential to reduce the frequency and severity of these skin reactions. Other strategies include taking niacin with food or premedicating with one dose of aspirin, 325 mg, 30 minutes before administration. Niaspan is associated with less flushing. Niacin is also associated with gastrointestinal symptoms such as nausea, diarrhea, flatulence, vomiting, and peptic ulcer disease. Other side effects include liver toxicity, **hyperglycemia**, and **hyperuricemia**. Significant liver toxicity is more common with high doses of the short-acting formulation of niacin.

Pharmacokinetics

When administered orally, niacin is rapidly and extensively absorbed (at least 60%–76% of the dose). To maximize bioavailability and reduce the risk of GI upset, niacin should be administered with a low-fat meal or snack.

Mechanism of action

Niacin influences lipoprotein metabolism by decreasing triglyceride synthesis via multiple pathways. In adipocytes, it inhibits the lipolysis of triglycerides and retards the mobilization of free fatty acids to the plasma.

Clinical indications

Niacin oral tablets are indicated as monotherapy or in combination with simvastatin or lovastatin to treat primary hyperlipidemia and mixed dyslipidemia. They can also reduce the risk of nonfatal myocardial infarctions in patients with a history of hyperlipidemia. However, a new analysis featured in *JAMA Network Open*, published by the *Journal of the American Medical Association*, suggests this old drug offers no benefit for most people.

Contraindications

Niacin should be avoided in patients with hypersensitivity, active peptic ulcer disease, active liver disease, or those presenting with unexplained and persistent elevations in hepatic transaminases.

Adverse effects

A significant number of different types of severe side effects have been associated with niacin therapy. They include skin rashes, gastrointestinal problems, complications with managing preexisting diabetes, and an increased risk of developing diabetes.

Toxicities

Toxicity when eating foods containing niacin is rare but can occur from long-term use of high-dose supplements. A reddened skin flush with itchiness or tingling on the face, arms, and chest is a common sign.

Fibrates

Fibrates or fibric-acid derivatives have a complex mechanism of action and may vary among the drugs in their class. It is thought that fibrates work in the liver to reduce the formation of VLDL triglycerides. Fibrates are primarily used to decrease triglycerides up to 35%–50% in people with hypertriglyceridemia but have very modest LDL-lowering effects. Sometimes LDL rises during this therapy. Elevated triglycerides increase the risk of pancreatitis (inflammation of the pancreas). Two fibrates are currently on the market: gemfibrozil (Lopid) and fenofibrate (Tricor). They are administered once to twice daily and come in tablet and capsule formulations. Fibrates are highly bound to blood albumin (which means they may interact with other medications) and can cause displacement of other protein-bound drugs when administered together.

Pharmacokinetics

Fibrates are metabolized by the hepatic cytochrome P450 3A4. All members of this class are primarily excreted via the kidneys and display some increase in plasma half-life in individuals with severe renal impairment. Plasma half-life is variable among fibrates (2–80 hours). Recently it has been shown that fibrates produce plasma lipid changes mainly by stimulating peroxisome-proliferation activation receptor alpha.

Mechanism of action

Fibrates reduce hepatic triglycerides by inhibiting hepatic extraction of free fatty acids and thus hepatic triglyceride production. These drugs may also lower cholesterol by increasing endothelial lipoprotein lipase activity. They also promote receptor-mediated clearance of LDL after stimulating its secretion, causing this catabolism to occur 20% faster than in an untreated patient. This action results in an overall decrease in VLDL.

Clinical indications

Fibrates help to reduce serum LDL, total cholesterol, triglycerides, and Apo-B and increase HDL. They are to be used as an adjunct to dietary modifications in adults with severe hypertriglyceridemia.

Contraindications

Fibrates are contraindicated with known hypersensitivity to the drug class and active liver disease, as fibrates are shown to be hepatotoxic if preexisting liver inflammatory states exist. They are also contraindicated if creatinine clearance is less than 30 mL/min or the patient has severe renal dysfunction.

Adverse effects

Fibrates are generally well tolerated, but GI complaints are the most common adverse effect of their use. They also increase the risk of gallstone formation and may increase the risk of muscle toxicity when given together with statins. Of note, the risk of muscle toxicity is lessened with fenofibrate.

Toxicities

Fenofibrates can be toxic to the liver. Mild liver enzyme elevations to rare cases of liver failure have been reported. Liver enzymes should be measured before starting therapy and periodically after that. Fenofibrate should be discontinued if liver injury symptoms develop or persistent liver enzyme elevations occur. Treatment should also be terminated if an elevated bilirubin accompanies any enzyme elevation.

Cholesterol absorption inhibitors

Ezetimibe (Zetia) is the only drug in the class of cholesterol absorption inhibitors. It works by preventing a protein that decreases cholesterol absorption in the gut. This inhibition is only for cholesterol, and there is no impact on the absorption of other drugs or fat-soluble vitamins. A decrease in the cholesterol delivery to the liver results in an increase in the uptake of cholesterol in the bloodstream by the liver and decreased systemic cholesterol. Ezetimibe has modest effects on LDL and other cholesterol parameters and is FDA approved only as an add-on therapy to statins or fibrates. Ezetimibe is primarily used for high-risk patients such as those with a history of prior myocardial infarction or diabetes, as well as those who cannot tolerate high-intensity statin therapy and do not meet cholesterol goals on lower doses alone. Ezetimibe was studied in the IMPROVE-IT trial, which showed that it improved cardiac outcomes in patients who had a past heart attack. Ezetimibe is administered as a tablet taken once daily. Ezetimibe is typically well tolerated and takes on the side effect profile of statins when used as combination therapy. Myopathy is rarely reported when ezetimibe is used alone.

Proprotein convertase subtilisin-kexin type 9

PCSK9 inhibitors are the newest cholesterol-lowering drugs on the market. This new drug class includes evolocumab (Repatha) and alirocumab (Praluent). Both drugs are monoclonal antibodies that bind to and inhibit the PCSK9 enzyme responsible for the degradation of LDL receptors in the liver. By increasing LDL receptors in the liver, there is an increase in the removal of cholesterol from the bloodstream. This novel mechanism leads to significantly decreased LDL (up to 70%), more than any other lipid-lowering therapy currently available. Because of their potent LDL-lowering effects, their target population is those who have CVD and need additional lowering of LDL or have a genetic predisposition to high cholesterol. While PCSK9 inhibitors are undoubtedly very effective in lowering LDL levels, it is unknown if they improve long-term cardiovascular outcomes.

Omega-3

Omega-3 fatty acid ethyl esters are derived from chemically changed and purified fish oils. They are used with dietary changes to help reduce triglycerides. Omega-3 drugs available in the United States include omega-3-acid ethyl esters (Lovaza), icosapent ethyl (Vascepa), *omega-3 carboxylic acids* (Epanova), and *omega-3-acid ethyl esters A* (Omtryg).

Nonmedication therapy

The backbone of treating hyperlipidemia is lifestyle changes. This includes dietary therapy with low total and saturated fat and reduced cholesterol intake. A registered dietitian may be consulted to help patients change their diet. In addition to making healthy food choices, patients must be encouraged to exercise. A reasonable goal is at least 30 minutes of moderate-intensity exercise at least 5 days a week. All patients should be encouraged to diet and exercise to maintain a healthy weight, limit alcohol use, and avoid tobacco use.

Key Terms

Apolipoprotein B
Catabolism
Endoplasmic reticulum
Fatty acids
Gallstone
HMG-CoA reductase inhibitors
Hyperglycemia
Hyperuricemia
Lipid profile
Mixed dyslipidemia

Niacin
Oxidation
Peroxisomes
Phospholipids
Rhabdomyolysis
Sphingolipids
Statins
Sterols
Terpenes
Triglycerides

Clinical Case Studies

Clinical Case Study 1

A 36-year-old female developed angina while she was breastfeeding her daughter. Cardiac catheterization revealed a partial blockage of three vessels, which led to coronary artery bypass grafting. The patient's father had previously had the same procedure after he had a myocardial infarction. Therefore the woman was diagnosed with familial hypercholesterolemia. During follow-up, she was treated with rosuvastatin and ezetimibe daily. She received six coronary stents as well.

Critical Thinking Questions

1. Which types of drugs are FDA approved to manage hypercholesterolemia?
2. What are the adverse effects of statins?
3. What is the classification of ezetimibe?

Clinical Case Study 2

A 57-year-old male is assessed because of untreated hypertension and is also found to have hyperlipidemia. He has persistently elevated triglycerides and a possible family history of atherosclerotic CVD. Additionally, he has recently quit smoking after many years and is prediabetic. Pitavastatin, a moderate-intensity statin, is initiated. Over time, as the patient's condition begins to improve, ezetimibe is added to provide additional LDL cholesterol reduction.

Critical Thinking Questions

1. What is the description of atherosclerosis?
2. What are the ideal and high ranges of triglycerides?
3. What are the dose range and percentage of LDL-lowering capacity of pitavastatin?

Clinical Case Study 3

A 76-year-old female with a history of phenotypic heterozygous familial hypercholesterolemia and subclinical coronary artery disease is assessed by her cardiologist. Her mother had experienced a myocardial infarction when she was in her late 40s. The patient initially was taking rosuvastatin but developed thigh pain, headache, and malaise, resulting in her stopping the medication. She changed her diet and began exercising regularly, improving her condition. The patient was given ezetimibe, and her cholesterol dropped dramatically. Encouraged, she increased her exercise regimen under her physician's direction and improved her dietary choices even more. Her most recent bloodwork revealed that she is no longer in the "danger zone" regarding cholesterol.

Critical Thinking Questions

1. What are the nonmedication therapies for hyperlipidemia?
2. What laboratory values of total cholesterol are considered desirable or high?
3. For LDL cholesterol, what is considered optimal or high?

Further Reading

[1] L. Arpilor, Health Benefits of Omega 3. Explore the Potential Health Benefits of Omega-3 Fatty Acids Found in Certain Foods and Supplements. Learn About their Advantages for Heart and Brain Health, Arpilor, 2023.
[2] M. Banach, Combination Therapy in Dyslipidemia, Adis, 2015.
[3] X. Cheng Jiang, Lipid Transfer in Lipoprotein Metabolism and Cardiovascular Disease (Advances in Experimental Medicine and Biology, 1276), Springer, 2020.
[4] J.M. Keenan, K.M. Dunn, The Niacin Breakthrough – the Keenan Protocol for Heart Health and Healthy Aging, Keenan, 2022.
[5] D. Kritchevky, Lipids, Lipoproteins, and Drugs (Advances in Experimental Medicine and Biology, 63), Springer, 2012.
[6] NetCE, A.J. Lanca, Hyperlipidemias and Atherosclerotic Cardiovascular Disease, NetCE, 2022.

[7] M. Ollero, D. Touboul, Bioactive Lipids and Lipidomics 2018 (International Journal of Molecular Sciences), MDPI, 2020.
[8] B.V. Reamy, Hyperlipidemia Management for Primary Care: An Evidence-Based Approach, Springer, 2010.
[9] N.D. Ridgway, R.S. McLeod, Biochemistry of Lipids, Lipoproteins and Membranes, seventh ed., Elsevier Science, 2021.
[10] W. Sears, J. Sears, The Omega-3 Effect, Little Brown Spark, 2012.
[11] G. Singh, Role of Fibrates in Abrogated Potentials of Ischemic Preconditioning, Scholars' Press, 2017.
[12] A. Sniderman, P. Durrington, Fast Facts: Hyperlipidemia: Bringing Clarity to Lipid Management, sixth ed., S. Karger, 2021.
[13] M.J. Sorrentino, Hyperlipidemia in Primary Care – A Practical Guide to Risk Reduction. (Current Clinical Practice), Humana Press, 2011.
[14] H. Yassine, Lipid Management – from Basics to Clinic, Springer, 2015.

CHAPTER

28

Drug effects on angina pectoris and myocardial infarction

OUTLINE

LEARNING OUTCOMES

After study of the chapter, readers should be able to:

1. Describe the three layers of the heart's wall.
2. Explain the branches of coronary arteries.
3. Describe the stroke volume, heart rate, and cardiac output.
4. Describe the four types of angina pectoris.
5. Discuss the classification of drugs for angina pectoris.
6. Explain the pharmacokinetics of organic nitrates.

https://doi.org/10.1016/B978-0-443-29038-1.00028-2

7. Describe the indications of beta-blockers.
8. Describe the mechanism of action of calcium channel blockers.
9. Explain the signs and symptoms of myocardial infarction.
10. Describe the goals of pharmacotherapy for myocardial infarction.

Overview

Cardiovascular disorders are those that affect the heart and blood vessels, and they are often related to atherosclerosis and arteriosclerosis. As plaque builds up in the arterial walls, it narrows, making it more difficult for blood to flow normally. Angina is chest pain or discomfort when insufficient blood flows to the heart muscle. The discomfort may not always be in the chest, but it may be felt in the jaw or arm when a blood clot forms, and blood flow can be blocked entirely, resulting in myocardial infarction (MI) or stroke. Other chronic cardiovascular disorders include hypertension and heart failure. MI, commonly known as a "heart attack," is caused by decreased or complete cessation of blood flow to a portion of the myocardium. MI may be "silent" and go undetected, or it could be a catastrophic event leading to hemodynamic deterioration and sudden death.

Structure and function of the heart

The heart is a muscle that pumps blood throughout the body. The core of the organ consists of four valves. They open and close to let blood flow from one area of the heart to another and into and out of the heart. The valves are unidirectional to help ensure blood moves at the right time and in the correct direction. As the valves open and close, they create the two sounds that make up the *heartbeat*. Heart valves include the mitral, aortic, tricuspid, and pulmonary valves.

The heart wall comprises three layers: the outer **epicardium**, middle **myocardium**, and **endocardium**. The myocardium consists of cardiac muscle fibers and is responsible for the contraction and relaxation that result in heart pumping. The two atria have a thinner myocardium layer than the ventricles, as the force required for atrial contractions is much less than that needed for ventricular contractions. The walls of the right ventricle pump blood to the lungs. Comparatively, the left ventricle, which has much thicker walls, must generate enough force to pump oxygenated blood throughout the rest of the body (see **Fig. 28.1**).

When the proper ventricle contracts, deoxygenated blood flows through the **pulmonary valve** into the lungs through the pulmonary trunk. The **pulmonary trunk** splits into the left and right **pulmonary arteries,** the only arteries in the body to carry deoxygenated blood. However, during pregnancy, the umbilical artery takes deoxygenated blood from the fetus to the placenta to reoxygenate the fetal blood supply. The left ventricle receives oxygenated blood from the left atrium through the **mitral valve**. The aortic valve remains closed to allow the left ventricle to fill with blood. The ventricles contract when complete, causing the mitral valves to close and the aortic valves to open. Oxygenated blood is pumped through the aortic valve into the aorta when the left ventricle contracts. The aortic valve carries blood to the rest of the body.

The coronary arteries

The myocardium requires constant oxygen and nutrients to maintain the contractions and relaxations that keep the heart pumping. This blood supply is maintained through **coronary arteries** and veins in the myocardium. The right and left coronary arteries, which branch off the first section of the aorta, known as the ascending aorta, between the left ventricle and the aortic arch, supply blood to a network of capillaries in the myocardium. Deoxygenated blood from the myocardium is carried through **cardiac veins** to the right atrium and drained through the **coronary sinus**. The coronary arteries run along the **coronary sulcus** of the myocardium of the heart. Their primary function is to supply blood to the heart. This is a crucial function for myocardial function and body homeostasis. The four coronary arteries include the left and right coronary arteries. The left coronary artery extends along the coronary sulcus

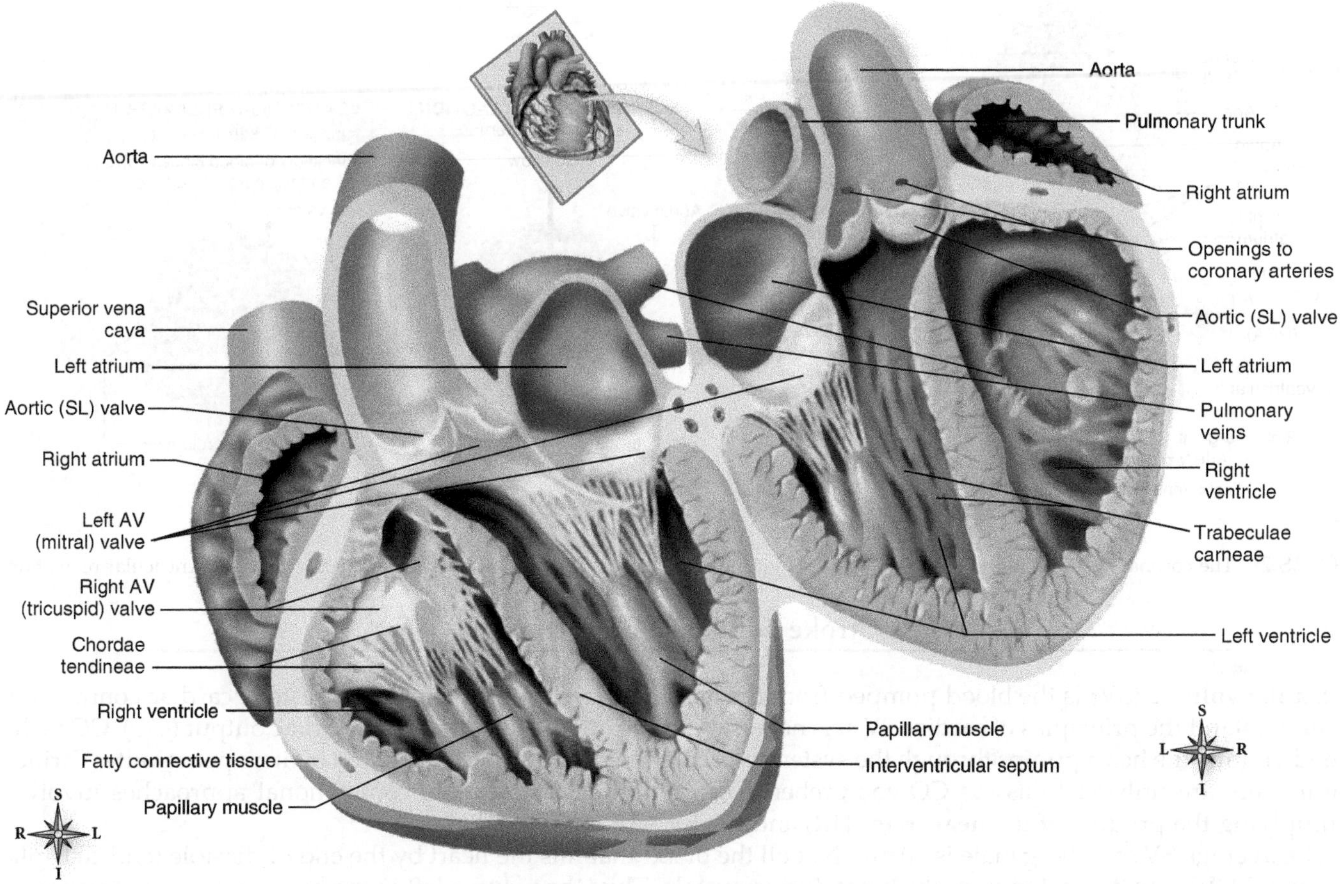

FIG. 28.1 The structure of the heart.

and supplies the left portion of the heart. It further branches into the **circumflex artery** and the left anterior descending artery.

The right coronary artery supplies blood to the right ventricle, the right atrium, and the sinoatrial (SA) and atrioventricular (AV) nodes, which regulate the heart rhythm. The right coronary artery divides into smaller branches, including the right posterior descending artery and the acute marginal artery (see **Fig. 28.2**).

The cardiac conduction system

The specialized **cardiomyocytes** that constitute the conduction system in the human heart initiate the electric impulse and result in rhythmic and synchronized contraction of the atria and ventricles. An electrical stimulus is generated by the SA node, tissue located in the right upper atrium. The sinus node generates electrical stimulation regularly, 60 to 100 times per minute under normal conditions. The atria are then activated. The electrical stimulus travels down through the conduction pathways and causes the heart's ventricles to contract and pump blood (see **Fig. 28.3**). The atria are stimulated first and contract briefly before the ventricles.

The electrical impulse travels from the SA node to the AV node. The impulses are slowed down for a very short period and then continue down the conduction pathway via the **bundle of His** into the ventricles. The bundle of His divides into right and left pathways, called bundle branches, to stimulate the right and left ventricles. Typically at rest, as the electrical impulse moves through the heart, the heart contracts about 60 to 100 times a minute, depending on a person's age. Each contraction of the ventricles represents one heartbeat. The atria contract a fraction of a second before the ventricles, so their blood empties into the ventricles before the ventricles contract.

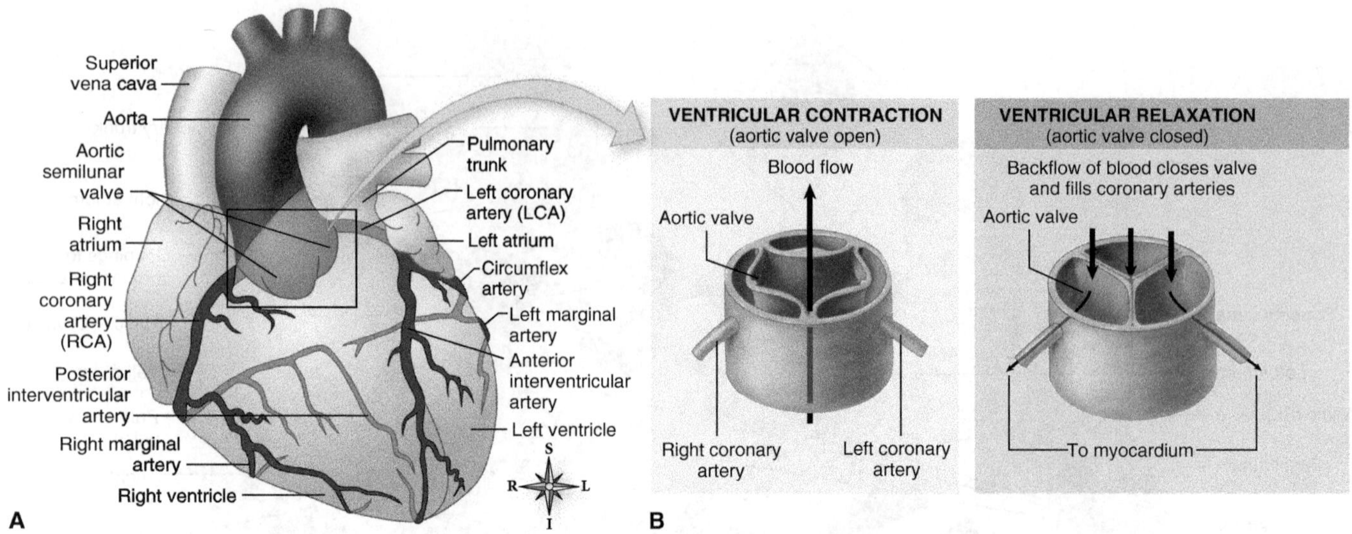

FIG. 28.2 The coronary arteries of the heart. (A) The anatomy of the coronary arteries. (B) Ventricular contraction. (C) Ventricular relaxation.

Stroke volume and heart rate

Stroke volume (SV) is the blood pumped from the heart's left ventricle during each systolic cardiac contraction. To understand the principles of cardiac SV, it is necessary first to define the concept of cardiac output (CO). **CO** is the blood volume the heart pumps through the systemic circulation over a period measured in liters per minute. Various parameters are utilized to assess CO comprehensively. Still, one of the more conventional approaches involves multiplying the product of the **heart rate** (HR) and the SV, $CO = SV \times HR$.

The average SV of a 70-kg male is 70 mL. Not all the blood that fills the heart by the end of diastole (end-diastolic volume [EDV]) can be ejected from the heart during systole. Thus the volume left in the heart at the end of systole is the end-systolic volume (ESV). The SV volume may be calculated as the difference between the left ventricular EDV and left ventricular ESVs. Therefore this formula is used: $SV = EDV - ESV$.

According to the American Heart Association (AHA), the average resting HR is between 60 and 100 beats per minute. However, some people may have a slower rate than 60, which is still expected. The average resting HR is about 70 beats per minute. The HR naturally falls during sleep (sometimes as low as 30 beats per minute in young people), and this increases with exercise and emotion. The average human heart beats about 100,000 times per day.

Angina pectoris

Angina pectoris is a clinical syndrome of precordial discomfort or pressure because of transient myocardial ischemia without infarction. It is often precipitated by exertion or psychological stress. There are four types of angina pectoris:

- **Stable angina:** Pain is predictable in frequency and duration. It is relieved by rest and nitroglycerin.
- **Unstable angina:** Pain increases in frequency and duration. It is induced more quickly than stable angina. This indicates a worsening coronary artery disease that may progress to MI.
- **Prinzmetal angina:** Also referred to as *variant angina*. Spasms of the coronary arteries cause pain. It may occur spontaneously and is unrelated to physical exercise or emotional stress.
- **Microvascular angina:** Caused by impairment of vasodilator reserve, resulting in angina-like chest pain in a person with normal coronary arteries.

Etiology of angina pectoris

The cause of angina is usually insufficient coronary blood flow, resulting in a decreased oxygen supply to meet an increased myocardial demand for oxygen in response to physical exertion or emotional stress.

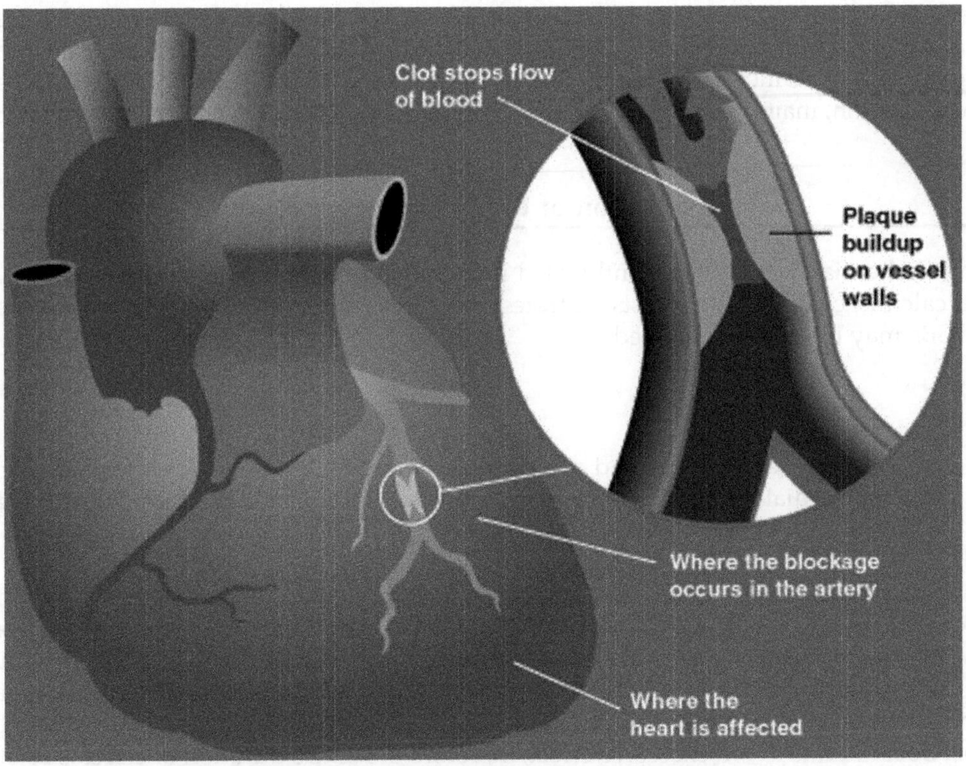

FIG. 28.3 The conduction system of the heart.

Pathophysiology of angina pectoris

Coronary atherosclerosis usually occurs at points of turbulence known as vessel bifurcations. If an atherosclerotic plaque ruptures, an acute thrombus may result, leading to ischemia, which can trigger angina pectoris. The consequences of acute ischemia are collectively referred to as acute coronary syndromes (ACSs). A transient, focal increase in vascular tone is known as coronary artery spasm. This markedly narrows the lumen and reduces blood flow, possibly resulting in symptomatic ischemia or variant angina. Thrombi may form as a consequence, causing infarction or life-threatening arrhythmia. In arteries without atheroma, the basal coronary artery tone is probably increased. Response to vasoconstricting stimuli may then be exaggerated. In arteries with atheromas, local hypercontractility may occur. Causes of coronary artery spasms include abnormalities of nitric oxide production, decreased sensitivity to intrinsic vasodilators, increased production of vasoconstrictors, use of vasoconstricting drugs, and emotional stress.

You should remember

Coronary heart disease is the major component of cardiovascular morbidity and mortality in the United States. This is because the initial coronary event is often quickly fatal.

Pharmacotherapy for angina pectoris

Treatment of CAD includes drugs and procedures to reduce ischemia and restore or improve coronary blood flow. Nitrates such as nitroglycerin are commonly used (given sublingually, orally, transdermally, or topically in ointment form). Isosorbide may reduce myocardial oxygen consumption. Beta-adrenergic blockers (β-blockers) may reduce the heart's workload and oxygen demands by lowering HR and peripheral resistance to blood flow. Calcium channel blockers (CCBs) may prevent coronary artery spasms. Antiplatelet drugs minimize platelet aggregation and the risk of coronary occlusion. Antilipemic drugs are also given to reduce serum cholesterol or triglycerides.

Coronary artery bypass graft (CABG) surgery restores blood flow. It bypasses an occluded artery using another vessel and is an option for certain patients. For patients with partial occlusion and without calcification, angioplasty may relieve occlusion. Lifestyle modifications are indicated to reduce the progression of CAD. These include regular exercise, smoking cessation, maintaining an ideal body weight, stress management, and a low-fat, low-sodium diet.

Classification of drugs for angina pectoris

Three major antiischemia drugs are currently used in managing angina pectoris: β-blockers, nitrates (short and long acting), and calcium channel antagonists. Nitrates or β-blockers are usually preferred for the initial treatment of angina, and CCBs may be added if needed.

Organic nitrates

Organic nitrates are potent vasodilators and are the most widely used antianginal agents during acute events. They selectively dilate epicardial coronaries, enhancing collateral flow and inhibiting platelet aggregation.

Pharmacokinetics

The liver contains a high-capacity organic nitrate reductase that removes nitrate groups and ultimately inactivates the drug. Therefore oral bioavailability of the traditional organic nitrates (e.g., nitroglycerin and isosorbide dinitrate) is low (typically less than 10%–20%). For this reason, the sublingual route, which avoids the first-pass effect, is preferred for rapidly achieving a therapeutic blood level. Nitroglycerin and isosorbide dinitrate are absorbed efficiently by this route and reach therapeutic blood levels within a few minutes. However, the total dose administered by this route must be limited to avoid excessive effect; therefore the entire duration of effect is brief (15–30 minutes). Other ways of administering nitroglycerin include transdermal and buccal absorption from slow-release preparations. Amyl nitrite and related nitrites are highly volatile liquids. The inhalation route provides very rapid absorption. Once absorbed, the unchanged nitrate compounds have a half-life of only 2–8 minutes. The kidney mainly does excretion.

Mechanism of action

Organic nitrate esters have a direct relaxant effect on vascular smooth muscles. Dilation of coronary vessels improves oxygen supply to the myocardium. Dilation of peripheral veins and, in higher doses, peripheral arteries reduces preload and afterload, lowering myocardial oxygen consumption.

Clinical indications

Nitroglycerin and long-acting nitrates are widely used in all anginal syndromes and have proven effective in relieving or preventing myocardial ischemia. They are also used to manage BP through vasodilation. Nitroglycerin can be administered through various methods, including sublingual and transdermal routes, rectal ointment, and IV infusion.

Contraindications

Nitroglycerin and long-acting nitrates must be avoided in patients with known sensitivity to nitrate medications, those who are hypotensive, and children younger than 12 years of age. Patients with severe anemia or alcohol intoxication must also avoid nitroglycerin.

Adverse effects

Headache, skin flushing, and orthostatic hypotension with reflex tachycardia are the most common adverse effects of nitrates and nitrites, and they occur frequently, even with therapeutic doses of organic nitrates.

Toxicity

Signs of acute nitrate toxicity result from severe inhibition of oxygen transfer and are undeniable. Symptoms include a bluish color of mucous membranes, rapid and complex breathing, a fast pulse (>150 beats/minute), tremors, staggering, collapse, and death.

You should remember

Sublingual nitroglycerin is administered before acute attacks or to prevent an attack before exertion. Relief usually occurs within 1.5–3 minutes. Patients should always carry nitroglycerin tablets or aerosol spray in case of angina attacks. If symptoms persist after maximizing a β-blocker dose, long-acting oral or transdermal nitrates are used. Oral nitrates include isosorbide dinitrate and mononitrate, effective within 1–2 hours.

Beta-adrenergic blockers

β-Blockers are an essential class of drugs for treating various heart diseases, including angina pectoris, hypertension, **arrhythmias**, hypertrophic cardiomyopathy, and heart failure. β-Blockers can also be used to treat **migraine headaches** and **glaucoma**. Norepinephrine and epinephrine stimulate adrenergic receptors. Catecholamines are released from nerve endings of the sympathetic nervous system, an involuntary nerve network that enables the body to withstand stress, anxiety, and exercise. β-Adrenergic receptors are found in the heart, blood vessels, and lungs and are stimulated by catecholamine binding, thus increasing the activity of cells in the body. β-Adrenergic receptor stimulation causes an increase in HR, heart muscle contraction, blood pressure, and relaxation of smooth muscle in the bronchial tubes in the lung, making it easier to exercise and expand the lungs. Several β-blockers are available (**see Table 28.1**).

Pharmacokinetics

All beta-adrenoreceptor–blocking drugs are fairly wholly and rapidly absorbed from the GI tract. Absorption, however, appears to be less in elderly patients and possibly in patients with renal failure than in younger patients. The extent of bioavailability varies considerably among different β-blockers, and these drugs are relatively rapidly eliminated from the body. Most have an elimination half-life between 2 and 4 hours.

Mechanism of action

β-Blockers reduce nerve impulses to the heart and blood vessels and reduce the effect of norepinephrine throughout the body. They cause the heart to beat more slowly and with less force. As CO decreases, blood pressure is lowered.

Clinical indications

β-Blockers are not recommended as a first treatment if a patient only has high blood pressure. They are usually used only if other medicines, such as diuretics, have not worked well. A β-blocker may be one of several medicines used to lower blood pressure. They effectively treat systolic heart failure, atrial fibrillation, and angina by preventing the cardiac muscle from changing shape after heart attacks.

Contraindications

Traditional contraindications to β-blockers are peripheral vascular diseases, diabetes mellitus, chronic obstructive pulmonary disease, and asthma. They are also contraindicated in Raynaud phenomenon, certain arrhythmias, and hypoglycemia.

Adverse effects

Common adverse effects of β-blockers can include cold hands or feet, extreme tiredness, and dizziness. They also exacerbate signs and symptoms of chronic obstructive pulmonary disease and asthma. Other side effects include fatigue, bradycardia, and fluid retention in the extremities.

Toxicity

β-Blocker toxicity can produce bradycardia, hypotension, arrhythmias, hypothermia, hypoglycemia, and seizures.

TABLE 28-1 Beta-adrenergic blockers.

Generic name	Trade name
acebutolol	Generic only
atenolol	Tenormin
bisoprolol	Zebeta
carvedilol	Coreg
esmolol, injectable	Brevibloc
labetalol	Normodyne
metoprolol	Toprol XL, Lopressor
nadolol	Corgard
nebivolol	Bystolic
propranolol	Inderal

Calcium channel blockers

CCBs prevent calcium from entering cardiac and peripheral cells, which prevents the blood vessels from constricting. The two main subclasses are dihydropyridine and nondihydropyridine CCBs (see **Table 28.2**). The two categories differ in their pharmacological action. The dihydropyridine CCBs are amlodipine, felodipine, nifedipine, and nicardipine.

Pharmacokinetics

CCBs are absorbed well orally. However, many have low bioavailability due to hepatic first-pass metabolism, primarily by CYP3A4. They are highly protein bound, and many have high distribution volumes. Calcium channel antagonists are mainly excreted renally after metabolism. There are potential drug-drug interactions because CCBs are metabolized by CYP3A4, which is responsible for the metabolism of many other xenobiotics.

Mechanism of action

CCBs block the inward movement of calcium by binding to the long-acting voltage-gated calcium channels in the heart and vascular smooth muscle. There are two significant categories of calcium channel antagonists based on their primary physiologic effects. The nondihydropyridines inhibit the SA and AV nodes, slowing cardiac conduction and contractility. This allows for the treatment of hypertension, reduces oxygen demand, and helps to control the rate of tachydysrhythmias. In therapeutic dosing, dihydropyridines have little direct effect on the myocardium and instead are more often peripheral vasodilators, which is why they are helpful for hypertension, postintracranial hemorrhage–associated vasospasm, and migraines.

Clinical indications

CCBs are used for coronary spasms, angina pectoris, hypertension, supraventricular dysrhythmias, hypertrophic cardiomyopathy, and **pulmonary hypertension**. In addition to these, they are also prescribed for Raynaud phenomenon, **subarachnoid hemorrhage**, and migraine headaches.

Contraindications

Nondihydropyridines are contraindicated in those with heart failure with reduced ejection fraction, second- or third-degree AV blockade, and sick sinus syndrome because of the possibility of causing bradycardia and worsening CO. CCBs are also contraindicated in patients with known hypersensitivity to the drug or its components. Other contraindications include sick sinus syndrome (except in patients with an artificial pacemaker), severe hypotension, acute MI, and pulmonary congestion. CCBs may cause AV blockade or sinus bradycardia, especially if taken with agents known to slow cardiac conduction. There are reports of dermatologic reactions and hypotension with or without syncope with calcium channel antagonist use. Peripheral edema may occur within 2–3 weeks of initiating CCB therapy. These drugs should be used with caution in the presence of renal or hepatic impairment, and a dose adjustment to a lower dose may be required.

TABLE 28.2 Calcium channel blockers.

Generic name	Trade name
Dihydropyridines	
amlodipine	Norvasc
clevidipine, injectable	Cleviprex
felodipine	Plendil
nicardipine, injectable	Cardene
nifedipine	Adalat, Procardia
nimodipine	Nimotop
nisoldipine	Sular
Nondihydropyridines	
diltiazem	Cardizem
verapamil	Calan, Isoptin

Adverse effects

Nondihydropyridines may cause constipation, worsening CO, and bradycardia. Dihydropyridines may lead to lightheadedness, flushing, headaches, and peripheral edema. Peripheral edema is likely related to the redistribution of fluid from the intravascular space to the interstitium. There have also been reports of **gingival hyperplasia**.

Toxicity

Hypotension and bradycardia are the primary features seen with CCB poisoning. Hypotension may be life-threatening, as it results from peripheral vasodilation, bradycardia, and decreased **inotropy**. Cardiac conduction may also cause impairment of AV conduction abnormalities, complete heart block, or idioventricular rhythms.

Patients may present with lightheadedness, fatigue, or syncope. Coma and sudden death can occur too. Noncardiac symptoms may include nausea and vomiting, metabolic acidosis secondary to hypoperfusion, and hyperglycemia from the blockade of insulin release in the pancreas. The insulin blockade also impairs glucose uptake by myocardial cells, which further contributes to the reduction of cardiac contractility and worsens hypotension. Severe poisoning can lead to pulmonary edema, presumably due to precapillary vasodilation and increased transcapillary pressure. Dihydropyridines in mild to moderate overdose may cause reflex tachycardia; however, receptor selectivity may be lost in severe overdose, leading to bradycardia.

Myocardial infarction

MI involves necrosis of the myocardium, which results from an occlusion of a coronary artery. According to the Centers for Disease Control and Prevention (CDC), as of 2021 approximately 805,000 people have MIs in the United States annually, and MIs are fatal in 30%–40% of cases. Because of people's awareness about methods of preventing heart disease and better diagnostic and treatment techniques, MIs are decreasing in prevalence. *Chronic MI* occurs more than 1 year after the initial presentation of a patient with ACS. *Subacute MI* occurs between 30 days and 1 year after this presentation, while *acute MI* occurs less than 30 days after the presentation.

The signs and symptoms of an MI usually begin with unstable angina, shortness of breath, and fatigue. The symptoms start with pain or pressure below the sternum that radiates outward. It is more severe and longer lasting than angina pectoris. There is often dyspnea, fainting, sweating, nausea, and vomiting. Symptoms differ between males and females; therefore many females do not realize they are experiencing heart attacks. Diagnosis of MI is via serial ECGs, serial cardiac markers, and immediate coronary angiography. Prehospital treatments include oxygen, aspirin, nitrates, and triage to an appropriate medical facility. Medications include antiplatelet drugs, antianginal drugs, and anticoagulants. After hospitalization and treatment for CAD, the patient must be rehabilitated and undergo ongoing medical management.

Pathophysiology

The result of ACSs varies based on the obstruction's size, location, and duration. Occlusion can stem from atherosclerosis, thrombosis, platelet aggregation, and coronary artery stenosis or spasm. If prolonged ischemia is caused by coronary artery occlusion and lasts longer than 30–45 minutes, it can cause irreversible myocardial cell damage and muscle death or infarction. Ischemic tissue has impaired contractility that results in hypokinetic or akinetic segments. The segments may expand or bulge during systole, called paradoxical motion.

Clinical manifestations

Although the first symptom of acute MI is usually sudden and severe chest pain, **dyspnea**, fatigue, **diaphoresis**, nausea, vomiting, and syncope, pain may radiate to the back, jaw, and left arm. The signs and symptoms of ACSs are widely varied. Aside from reinfarction, the possible complications of acute MI include various types of arrhythmias, heart failure, cardiac arrest, angina, infarct extension, **cardiogenic shock**, mitral valve dysfunctions, aneurysms, cardiac rupture, sinus or AV node dysfunction, embolization, pericarditis, and death. The most common and severe complication of MI is arrhythmia. Arrhythmia begins soon after acute MIs, with most deaths occurring due to ventricular fibrillation. Deaths from ventricular fibrillation can be avoided if cardiopulmonary resuscitation is started within 5 minutes of the onset of the fibrillation.

Pharmacotherapy for myocardial infarction

The goals of pharmacotherapy for MI are to reduce morbidity and to prevent complications. The main objectives of emergency department medical therapy are rapid intravenous thrombolysis and rapid referral for percutaneous coronary intervention, optimization of oxygenation, reduction of cardiac workload, and pain control.

Thrombolytics or fibrinolytics are a group of medications used to dissolve intravascular clots. They are used in the emergency treatment of a stroke caused by a blood clot, MI, or a massive pulmonary embolism. Some people who have heart attacks, receive stents in their coronary arteries, or undergo CABG are treated with two types of antiplatelet agents simultaneously to prevent blood clotting. This is dual antiplatelet therapy. One antiplatelet agent is aspirin. Many people with coronary artery disease, including those who have had a heart attack, a stent, or CABG, are treated with aspirin for the rest of their lives. A second type of antiplatelet agent, a P2Y inhibitor, is usually prescribed for months or years in addition to aspirin therapy. The type of medication and the duration of the treatment will vary based on the patient's condition and other risk factors. Examples of thrombolytics include streptokinase (Streptase), tenecteplase (TNKase), reteplase (Retavase Half-Kit), urokinase (Kinlytic), alteplase (Cathflo Activase), and urokinase (Abbokinase)

Key Terms

Arrhythmias
Bundle of His
Cardiac output
Cardiac veins
Cardiogenic shock
Cardiomyocytes
Circumflex artery
Coronary arteries
Coronary sinus
Coronary sulcus
Diaphoresis
Dyspnea
Endocardium
Epicardium
Gingival hyperplasia
Glaucoma
Heart rate
Inotropy
Microvascular angina
Migraine headaches

Mitral valve
Myocardium
Prinzmetal angina
Pulmonary arteries
Pulmonary hypertension
Pulmonary trunk
Pulmonary valve
Raynaud phenomenon
Stable angina
Stroke volume
Subarachnoid hemorrhage
Unstable angina

Clinical case studies

Clinical case study 1

A 59-year-old male goes to his physician complaining of chest pain after playing golf. He has had similar episodes during the past 6 months. He describes the pain as being under his breastbone and that it does not radiate. None of the attacks ever lasted for more than a few minutes. The patient admits that his father died at 53 years of age of a heart condition of which he is unsure. The patient also states that he smokes up to one pack of cigarettes daily and drinks two or three alcoholic beverages every night. His blood pressure is measured at 162/94 mm Hg.

Critical thinking questions

1. What are the four types of angina pectoris?
2. What is the common cause of angina pectoris?
3. What is the pharmacotherapy for angina pectoris?

Clinical case study 2

A 38-year-old female was hospitalized because of severe chest pain that had awakened her from sleep, which radiated to her right shoulder and arm. She was also nauseous on the way to the hospital. The episode lasted about 50 minutes. Her family had no significant atherosclerotic coronary artery disease history, but her mother had hypertension and diabetes mellitus. The patient admitted smoking up to five cigarettes daily for 6 months but did not drink alcohol. The next night in the hospital, the patient experienced additional retrosternal chest tightness for 15 minutes, with more inversions readable on the electrocardiogram. After a diagnostic cardiac catheterization, the cause of her unstable angina was found to be the dissection of the left anterior descending coronary artery.

Critical thinking questions

1. What is the description of unstable angina?
2. Where does coronary atherosclerosis usually occur?
3. What are the classifications of drugs for angina pectoris?

Clinical case study 3

A 67-year-old male went to the hospital for severe chest pain that persisted for more than 24 hours. He had previously been diagnosed with hypertension and was a smoker. At the hospital, his BP was 110/70 mm Hg, and there was a systolic murmur in the lower left sternal border and mitral area. An electrocardiogram revealed an HR of 100 bpm, sinus rhythm, AV block, and various electrical heart abnormalities. Coronary angiography disclosed anterior interventricular branch occlusion and a 70% blockage of the circumflex artery, plus additional arterial blockages. Angioplasty with a stent implant was performed, but distal blood flow was not restored. The patient experienced cardiac arrest, did not respond to treatment, and died.

Critical thinking questions

1. How is the pain of angina described?
2. How is a MI diagnosed?
3. Aside from reinfarction, what are the possible complications of acute MI?

Further Reading

[1] B. Allen, Diagnosis, Pathophysiology and Treatment of Angina Pectoris, Foster Academics, 2015.

[2] C. Arampalzis, E.P. McFadden, L.K. Michalis, R. Virmani, P.W. Serruys, Coronary Atherosclerosis: Current Management and Treatment, Informa Healthcare, 2012.

[3] P. Avanzas, J.C. Kaski, Pharmacological Treatment of Chronic Stable Angina Pectoris (Current Cardiovascular Therapy), Springer, 2015.

[4] R.R. Baliga, K.A. Eagle, Practical Cardiology: Evaluation and Treatment of Common Cardiovascular Disorders, third ed., Springer, 2020.

[5] D.L. Brown, D. Warriner, Manual of Cardiac Intensive Care, Elsevier, 2022.

[6] B.P. Griffin, Manual of Cardiovascular Medicine, fifth ed., Lippincott, Williams, and Wilkins, 2018.

[7] E.B. Hanna, Practical Cardiovascular Medicine, second ed., Wily Blackwell, 2022.

[8] M.C. Hawkey, S.B. Lauck, Valvular Heart Disease – A Guide for Cardiovascular Nurses and Allied Health Professionals, Springer, 2022.

[9] N. Herring, D.J. Paterson, Levick's Introduction to Cardiovascular Physiology, sixth ed., CRC Press, 2018.

[10] P. Jevon, Angina and Heart Attack (The Facts). all the Information you Need Straight from the Experts, Oxford University Press, 2012.

[11] P. Libby, R.O. Bonow, D.L. Mann, G.F. Tomaselli, D.L. Bhatt, S.D. Solomon, Braunwald's Heart Disease – A Textbook of Cardiovascular Medicine, twelfth ed., Elsevier, 2022.

[12] L.S. Lilly, Pathophysiology of Heart Disease – an Introduction to Cardiovascular Medicine, seventh ed., Lippincott, Williams, and Wilkins, 2020.

[13] D.V. Miller, M.P. Revelo, Diagnostic Pathology – Cardiovascular, third ed., Elsevier, 2023.

[14] U.S. Department of Health and Human Services, Agency for Healthcare Research and Quality, Antiplatelet and Anticoagulant Treatments for Unstable Angina / Non-ST Elevation Myocardial Infarction, AHRC, 2013.

CHAPTER

29

Antihypertensive drugs

OUTLINE

LEARNING OUTCOMES

After studying this chapter, readers should be able to:

1. Describe the classifications of hypertension.
2. Explain the causes of primary and secondary hypertension.
3. Describe the main organs affected by hypertension.
4. Discuss the main goal in treating hypertension.
5. Explain the first-line drugs for the treatment of hypertension.
6. Describe the contraindications of both ACE-Is and ARBs.
7. Identify the two direct vasodilators.
8. Explain prehypertension.
9. Describe resistant hypertension.
10. Explain hypertensive crisis.

The Science of Pharmacology
https://doi.org/10.1016/B978-0-443-29038-1.00029-4

Overview

Hypertension is the most common disease affecting humans; its prevalence includes both sexes, and it extends to industrialized as well as developing countries. Compared with normotensive individuals, those with high blood pressure (BP) are at greater risk for stroke, coronary heart disease, heart or renal failure, and peripheral artery disease and have a substantially higher risk of developing atrial fibrillation, deterioration of cognitive function, and dementia. In 2021 hypertension was a primary or contributing cause of 691,095 deaths in the United States. Mexican Americans and Native Americans have the lowest incidence of low HP. An estimated 1.28 billion adults aged 30–79 worldwide have hypertension, most living in low- and middle-income countries. An estimated 46% of adults with hypertension are unaware that they have the condition.

Hypertension

Hypertension is chronically elevated pressure in the vasculature. People with high BP may be asymptomatic, so measuring BP is used to confirm hypertension, which is clinically defined as a systolic pressure of 130 mm Hg or more and a diastolic pressure exceeding 80 mm Hg. The definition of hypertension and its categories have evolved over the years. Still, there is a consensus that persistent BP readings of 140/90 mm Hg or more should be treated with the usual therapeutic target of 130/80 mm Hg or less. A patient's BP varies throughout the day and is influenced by various factors such as cigarette smoking, caffeine, and medications.

Classifications

The two main types of hypertension **are primary and secondary hypertension. Primary hypertension is multifactorial high BP and does not have one distinct cause. It is also known as idiopathic or essential hypertension. Secondary hypertension is caused by another medical condition, such as one involving the kidneys, arteries, heart, or endocrine system**. The American College of Cardiology and the American Heart Association divide BP into four categories (see **Table 29.1**).

BP exceeding 180/120 mm Hg is considered a **hypertensive crisis** (emergency). Untreated, high BP increases the risk of heart attack, stroke, and other serious health problems. It is essential to monitor BP at least every 2 years, starting at age 18, but some people will require more frequent monitoring.

Etiology

Primary hypertension means that the causes are unknown and are likely considered genetic. Ninety percent of hypertensive patients are diagnosed with primary hypertension. The remaining 10% of cases are diagnosed with *secondary hypertension*, with identifiable causes or other conditions triggering the hypertension. Obstructive sleep apnea and chronic kidney disease are common conditions that can cause secondary hypertension. Rare conditions that cause secondary hypertension include **aldosteronism**, **pheochromocytoma**, **hyperthyroidism**, **preeclampsia**, **eclampsia**, and specific medications that may trigger hypertension.

TABLE 29.1 Blood pressure classifications.

Classification	Systolic BP (mm Hg)	Diastolic BP (mm Hg)
Normal	Less than 120	Less than 80
Prehypertension	120–139	Less than 80
Stage 1 hypertension	140–159	80–89
Stage 2 hypertension	160 or higher	90 or higher

The effect of drugs on BP varies with the individual. This may explain why many patients taking antihypertensive drugs and a medicine that can increase BP can still have adequately controlled BP. Nonsteroidal antiinflammatory drugs such as ibuprofen, naproxen, and diclofenac are associated with modest increases in BP. On the opposite spectrum, some medications can trigger sudden increases in BP when abruptly stopped, such as beta-blockers (e.g., metoprolol, atenolol) or $alpha_2$ antagonists such as clonidine. For this reason, these medications need to be slowly tapered over some time, even weeks, instead of suddenly discontinued. Illegal drugs such as cocaine and amphetamines also are causative of hypertension.

The risk of an MI or stroke increases for every 20-mm Hg rise in systolic BP and 10-mm Hg rise in diastolic pressure. Hypertension accelerates atherosclerosis, a condition in which fatty substances such as cholesterol accumulate in the artery walls. This accumulation can lead to plaque deposits, which cause hardening and scarring of the vessels. This damage narrows and stiffens the artery walls, which may lead to blockages of blood flow and increase total peripheral resistance. These conditions may lead to cardiac events such as unstable angina and MI.

Pathophysiology

There is still much unknown about the pathophysiology of hypertension. A small number of patients (2%–5%) have an underlying renal or adrenal disease as the cause for the hypertension. Several physiological mechanisms are involved in maintaining normal BP, and their alterations may play a part in developing essential hypertension.

The renin-angiotensin system is the most critical endocrine system that affects BP control. Renin is secreted from the **juxtaglomerular apparatus** of the kidney in response to glomerular underperfusion or reduced salt intake. It is also released in response to stimulation from the sympathetic nervous system. Renin converts **angiotensinogen** to angiotensin I (ATI), a physiologically inactive substance rapidly converted to angiotensin II (ATII) in the lungs by angiotensin-converting enzyme (ACE). ATII is a potent **vasoconstrictor** and increases BP. In addition, it stimulates the release of **aldosterone** from the adrenal gland, which further increases BP related to sodium and water retention.

The circulating renin-angiotensin system is not thought to cause BP to increase essential hypertension directly. Many hypertensive patients have low renin and ATII (especially the elderly and Black people), and drugs that block the renin-angiotensin system are ineffective.

The **autonomic nervous system** maintains normal BP. **Sympathetic nervous system** stimulation can cause arteriolar constriction and dilatation. Thus it is also necessary to mediate short-term changes in BP in response to stress and physical exercise.

The **atrial natriuretic peptide** is a hormone secreted from the heart's atria in response to increased blood volume. It increases sodium and water excretion from the kidneys as a natural diuretic. A defect in this system may cause fluid retention and hypertension.

You should remember

Genetic factors account for approximately 30% of the differences in BP in various populations. Therefore genetic factors have been linked to the development of essential hypertension; multiple genes are most likely to contribute to the development of the disorder in a particular individual.

Clinical manifestations

Hypertension is known as the "silent killer" because most patients lack symptoms. As hypertension progresses, target organs may become damaged. The main organs affected are the heart, brain, kidneys, peripheral blood vessels, and eye (see **Fig. 29.1**). Patients with very high BP (usually 180/120 mm Hg or higher) can experience severe headaches, blurred vision, **epistaxis**, dizziness, anxiety, dyspnea, chest pain, nausea, and vomiting.

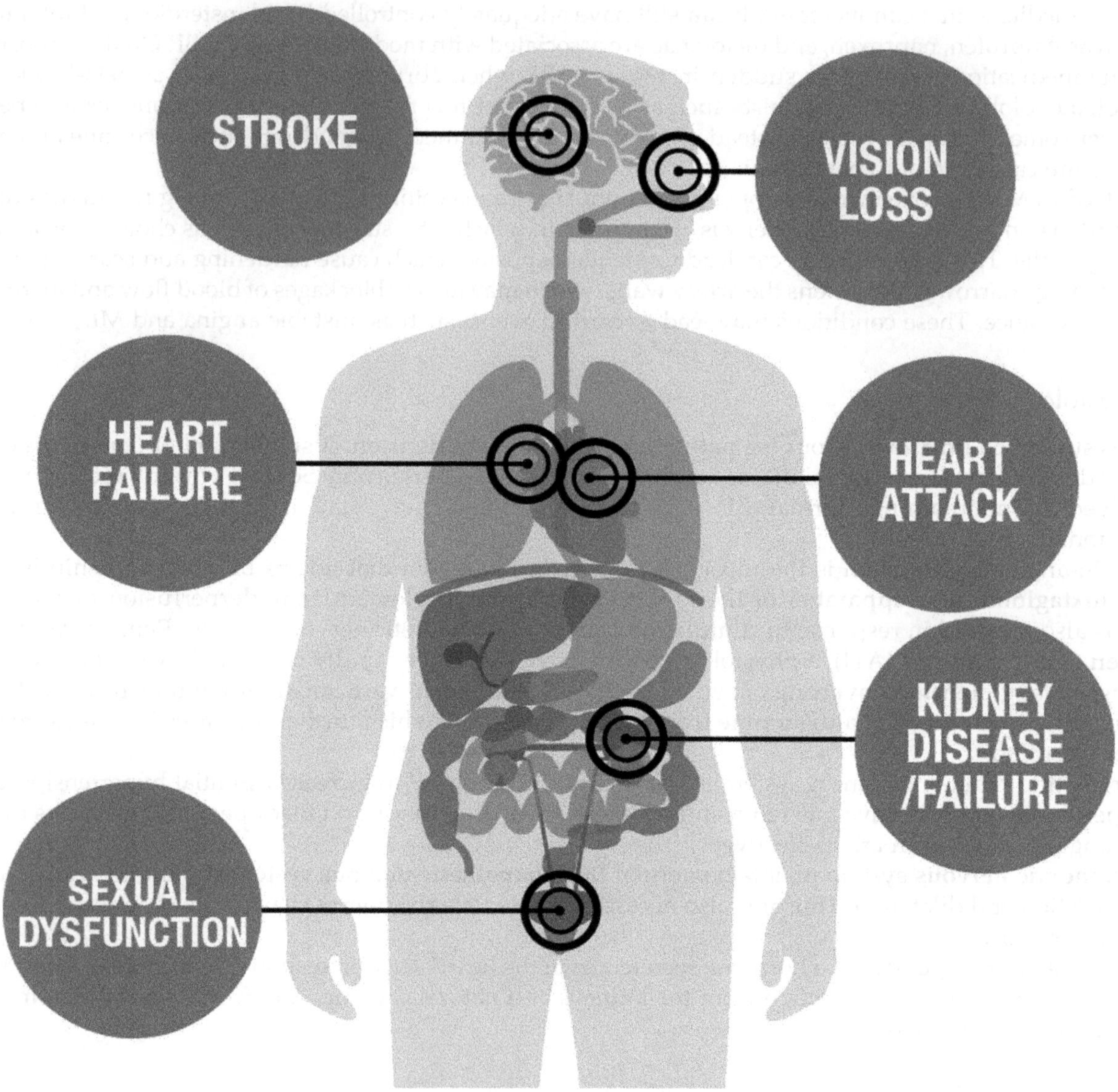

FIG. 29.1 The effects of hypertension on various body systems.

You should remember

A pheochromocytoma is a tumor in the adrenal gland. It causes the gland to make too many epinephrine and norepinephrine hormones. It usually occurs in people in their 30s, 40s, or 50s. It happens to both males and females, with unknown causes. However, it might be familial. The most common sign is hypertension. Most of these tumors are benign.

Pharmacotherapy

The main goal in treating hypertension is to decrease the risk of morbidity or mortality from target organ damage. BP goals are individualized based on the patient's preexisting conditions. Lower targets are generally desired if the patient is at higher risk for end-organ damage or if the damage is already present.

Lifestyle changes are well documented to lower BP effectively; they can reduce or even eliminate the need for drug therapy. Lifestyle changes include consuming a healthy diet, reducing sodium intake (table salt), exercising adequately, and moderating alcohol, which are thought to influence BP positively. On average, increased salt in the diet corresponds with increased BP. Greater than 75% of salt is derived from processed foods, so plans to reduce salt intake must include less restaurant dining and fewer manufactured foods. A diet of less than 2.3 grams of sodium daily can prevent and treat hypertension. Naturally, the human body needs about 1.5 grams/day of salt to function correctly. Increasing potassium intake may also improve BP, although the effect is more significant when the salt intake is higher. Natural potassium sources found in fruits and vegetables are recommended. If increasing dietary potassium is the goal, the patient should note any drugs that can inhibit potassium excretion and thus elevate the potassium levels: nonsteroidal antiinflammatory drugs, ACE inhibitors (ACE-Is), angiotensin receptor blockers (ARBs), and potassium-sparing diuretics. Chronic kidney disease can also increase potassium in later stages.

Angiotensin-converting enzyme inhibitors

ACE-Is are medications used to treat and manage hypertension, a significant risk factor for coronary disease, heart failure, stroke, and other cardiovascular conditions. Commonly used ACE-Is are listed in **Table 29.2**.

Common examples of ACE-Is include lisinopril, enalapril, and benazepril.

Pharmacokinetics

The predominant elimination pathway of ACE-Is is excretion via the kidneys. Therefore renal insufficiency is associated with reduced elimination of most ACE-Is and thus altered pharmacokinetic properties. Both the liver and kidneys metabolize these drugs.

Mechanism of action

ACE is involved in the renin-angiotensin-aldosterone system and stimulates the conversion of ATI to ATII (see **Fig. 29.2**). ACE-Is are competitive inhibitors of ACE that prevent the conversion of ATI to ATII. ATII acts as a potent vasoconstrictor that, when inhibited, can reduce BP by dilating vessels and decreasing aldosterone secretion.

TABLE 29.2 Classifications of commonly used antihypertensive agents.

Generic name	Trade name
Angiotensin-converting enzyme inhibitors	
benazepril	Lotensin
captopril	Capoten
enalapril	Vasotec
fosinopril	Monopril
lisinopril	Zestril
perindopril	Aceon
quinapril	Accupril
ramipril	Altace
Angiotensin receptor blockers	
candesartan	Atacand
irbesartan	Avapro
losartan	Cozaar
telmisartan	Micardis
valsartan	Diovan
Direct renin inhibitor	
aliskiren	Tekturna

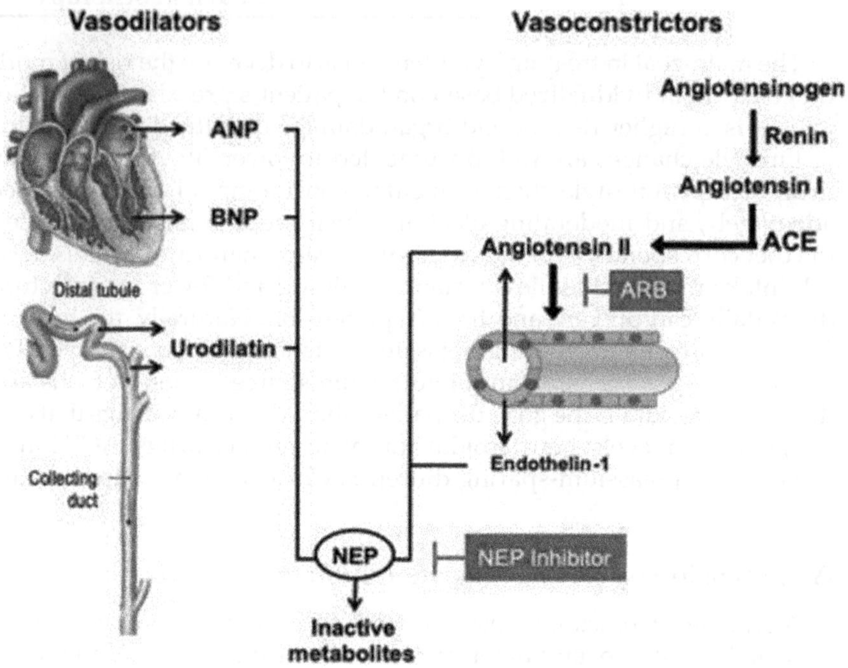

FIG. 29.2 The renin-angiotensin-aldosterone system.

Therefore inhibiting the production of ATII is a target for pharmacological intervention. ACE-I is a first-line treatment for hypertension.

Clinical manifestations

ACE-Is are a medication class used to treat and manage hypertension, a significant risk factor for coronary disease, heart failure, stroke, and other cardiovascular conditions. Most cases are primary and not attributable to any specific etiology. They also are helpful as adjunctive therapy in heart failure and in patients following a heart attack.

Contraindications

ACE-Is are contraindicated for conditions such as bilateral **renal artery stenosis**, when the major artery supplying blood to the kidney is narrowed by atherosclerosis or another cause. ACE-Is may slightly increase **creatinine** in some patients, but the effect is minor and passes with time. If the increase in creatinine becomes significant, the drug can be discontinued.

Adverse effects

ACE-Is are well tolerated, but side effects can occur. One unique side effect is a dry, persistent cough in up to 20% of patients. The cough is not harmful but may be annoying. Once the drug is discontinued, the cough will also stop. Other side effects include hyperkalemia, hypermagnesemia, and acute renal failure. ACE-Is decrease the production of aldosterone, which increases potassium. Usually, the increase in potassium is insignificant, but patients with chronic kidney dysfunction or taking concomitant medicines that can also increase potassium need to be monitored closely. One potentially profound side effect that can occur in less than 1% of patients is **angioedema**. African American patients and smokers are at higher risk for this reaction. Angioedema occurs less frequently with ARBs. If swelling of the larynx occurs or there is difficulty breathing, the condition is considered a medical emergency. Once patients have experienced angioedema with ACE-Is, they should discontinue them indefinitely. ACE-Is should be initiated at a low dose to avoid the risk of causing hypotension as the patient sits up from a prone position.

Toxicity

Overdose with ACE-Is may cause hypotension, tachycardia, hyperkalemia, and acute renal failure. However, most overdoses are asymptomatic, and severe morbidity is exceptionally rare. Activated charcoal, adequate fluids, and a short observation period are generally required.

You should remember

The main mechanisms contributing to hyperkalemia with ACE-Is include decreased aldosterone concentrations, reduced sodium delivery to the distal nephron, abnormal collecting tubule function, and excessive potassium intake.

Angiotensin-receptor blocking agents

ARB agents are also first-line drugs for treating hypertension. ARBs are often reserved for use in patients who are intolerant to the side effects of ACE-Is because ARBs have fewer side effects. They are unlikely to cause a cough or angioedema. Patients may be given an ARB when the benefits outweigh the risks.

Pharmacokinetics

ARBs are well absorbed after oral administration. Most have long half-lives to allow once-a-day dosing, except for twice-daily valsartan. They are highly plasma bound and have a large volume of distribution (except candesartan). Losartan undergoes first-pass metabolism and has active metabolites. All other ARBs have inactive metabolites. They are excreted through urine and feces.

Mechanism of action

ARBs block receptors for angiotensin, specifically ATI receptors in the heart, blood vessels, and kidneys. Blocking the action of ATII helps to lower BP and prevent damage to the heart and kidneys. Renin secreted from the juxtaglomerular cells of the kidneys catalyzes the conversion of angiotensinogen to ATI in the liver. ATI is converted to ATII by ACE and other non-ACE pathways.

Clinical manifestations

ARBs are similar in efficacy to ACE-Is for treating hypertension, heart failure, and kidney disease and lowering the risk of heart attacks and strokes. The ARBs are also more expensive than ACE-I because generic substitutes are unavailable. The routine use of ACE-Is and ARBs for hypertension is not recommended. ARBs include losartan, valsartan, and telmisartan.

Contraindications

ARBs are contraindicated in all trimesters of pregnancy. They also are contraindicated in patients with severe bilateral renal artery stenosis, aortic stenosis, and coarctation of the aorta.

Adverse effects

ARBs have excellent safety profiles alone and in combination with other antihypertensive drugs. They have a better tolerability profile than ACE-Is. Common side effects include headache, dizziness, drowsiness, GI disturbances, rash, and fatigue. It also causes first-dose hypotension and orthostatic hypotension. In patients with renal insufficiency, it may cause hyperkalemia, so potassium levels should be continuously monitored. It can precipitate renal failure in patients with bilateral renal artery stenosis and low, fixed renal blood flow. Cough and angioedema are rare (less than ACE-Is).

Toxicity

Overdoses have been widely reported, and mild toxicity may be produced with a single, supratherapeutic dose; however, severe toxic effects and deaths rarely occur. There are reports of children 6 years of age and younger who have ingested up to 8 mg/kg captopril or up to 2 mg/kg enalapril or lisinopril and remained asymptomatic. Most pediatric ingestions may be managed at home.

You should remember

ARBs differ from ACE inhibitors in that they are pharmacologically distinct but have similar hypotensive efficacy. They have other mechanisms of action. ACE-Is inhibit only one enzyme responsible for the production of ATII, whereas ARBs cause complete blockade of ATII activity. ARBs do not affect bradykinin concentrations as do ACE-Is, so cough and angioedema are more likely to occur late. The choice between ARBs and ACE-Is depends upon familiarity and cost.

Beta-adrenergic blockers

Beta-adrenergic blockers are medicines that lower BP. The drugs block the effects of the hormone epinephrine, causing hypotension and bradycardia. Beta-blockers also help widen veins and arteries to improve blood flow. Beta-blockers mainly affect the heart, while others affect the heart and blood vessels. **Chapter 28** discussed beta-adrenergic blockers.

Calcium channel blockers

Calcium channel blockers are medicines used to lower BP. They stop calcium from entering the cells of the heart and arteries, which causes them to squeeze more strongly. By blocking calcium, calcium channel blockers allow blood vessels to relax and open. Chapter 28 also discussed calcium channel blockers.

Central alpha$_2$ agonists

When the first-line agents are insufficient or cannot be used, alternative agents can be added. Clonidine and methyldopa are central alpha$_2$ agonists that reduce sympathetic outflow from the brain. Reduced sympathetic activity reduces cardiac output and total peripheral resistance. Chronic use causes sodium and water retention and depression at higher doses. Reserpine is rarely used as an antihypertensive agent.

Alpha$_1$-blockers

Alpha$_1$-receptors are found on the peripheral vasculature; when these receptors are blocked, the arterioles relax. The alpha$_1$-blockers are prazosin, terazosin, and doxazosin (see **Table 29.3**). Doxazosin is dosed 1–16 mg once daily, prazosin 2–20 mg divided two to three times daily, and terazosin 1–20 mg administered in one or two divided doses daily. Because these agents block alpha$_1$-receptors on the prostate, improving urinary flow, these agents are approved for benign prostatic hyperplasia. They can be used for patients with both benign prostatic hyperplasia and hypertension. These agents are known for the "first-dose" phenomenon: dizziness, lightheadedness, and low BP when rising from lying down or sitting within 1–3 hours of taking the dose. Patients are advised to take medicine at bedtime. In the morning, they should slowly and cautiously dangle their legs over the side of the bed before slowly sitting up. This "first-dose" effect can occur when the dose is increased or if the drug is discontinued and later restarted. Elderly patients are particularly susceptible to these effects, which may persist with chronic use.

Direct vasodilators

Hydralazine and minoxidil are **vasodilators**. They relax blood vessels so blood can flow more quickly through the body. Hydralazine and minoxidil directly relax arterioles and lower BP. The exact mechanism of how hydralazine causes arterial smooth muscle relaxation is unknown. It affects calcium movement within blood vessels. Calcium is required for muscle contraction, so disturbances in calcium movement may cause smooth muscle relaxation in the blood vessels. Hydralazine is selective for **arterioles**. Minoxidil can reduce BP in most patients with resistant

TABLE 29.3 Direct vasodilators, combined alpha-beta-blockers, $alpha_2$ and $alpha_1$ antagonists, and other related drugs.

Generic name	Trade name
Direct vasodilator	
Hydralazine	Generic only
Combined alpha-beta-blockers	
carvedilol	Coreg
labetalol	Normodyne
$Alpha_2$ agonists and $alpha_1$ antagonists	
clonidine	Catapres
doxazosin	Cardura
prazosin	Minipres
terazosin	Hytrin
Other related drugs	
fenoldopam, injectable	Corlopam
nitroglycerin, injectable	Generic only
sodium nitroprusside, injectable	Generic only

hypertension, where therapy has failed with multidrug regimens. However, these medications are not used as first-line agents due to unique side effects.

Diuretics

Diuretics are medicines that help reduce fluid buildup in the body. They are sometimes called "water pills." Most diuretics help the kidneys remove salt and water from the urine, lowering fluid flow through the veins and arteries. As a result, BP goes down. Diuretics are among the most commonly used drugs for hypertension and treating edema or fluid retention. They will be discussed in detail in **Chapter 34**.

Prehypertension

When BP is slightly higher than usual, it is prehypertension. A regular reading is 120/80 mm Hg. With prehypertension, systolic values can be as high as 139 mm Hg, or the diastolic pressure can be as high as 89 mm Hg. About 70 million people 20 years of age and older have prehypertension, and males are nearly twice as likely to have prehypertension compared to females. This category was added because studies showed patients with borderline BP had more risk factors for cardiac disease than nonhypertensive patients. Prehypertension increases the risk of MI by 3.5-fold, but not stroke.

Resistant hypertension

Resistant hypertension is defined as chronically high BP that does not meet the goal despite being on three or more medications from different classes. These medications are given at optimal doses, and one of these medications includes a diuretic. Factors associated with resistant hypertension are chronic kidney disease, older age, left ventricular hypertrophy, African American race, female sex, and residence in the southeastern United States. Chronic kidney disease may be the most significant factor affecting resistant hypertension. Other factors are modifiable: obesity, excessive dietary salt, and heavy alcohol intake. Excessive salt or alcohol intake increases the risk of hypertension and interferes with treatment efficacy. Excessive nutritional salt has a particularly harmful impact on patients who are African American, are elderly, or have chronic kidney disease.

Drugs can also induce resistant hypertension. Before confirming the diagnosis of resistant hypertension, factors such as inappropriate BP technique and lack of medication adherence need to be ruled out. BP should be measured after the patients have had an opportunity to sit quietly, and the cuff size should not be too small. Both mistakes can lead to falsely elevated BP readings. Medication adherence also contributes significantly to a lack of BP control. These patients do not have true resistant hypertension. Healthcare providers may inquire about patients' consistency in taking their medications and any barriers such as cost and adverse effects. However, if the patient's self-report is insufficient, reviewing the pharmacy's prescription refill histories or the patient's pillbox use may provide additional insight. Once these causes of nonadherence or inaccurate BP monitoring have been ruled out, medical reasons can be investigated. These disease states are the same conditions that cause secondary hypertension: obstructive sleep apnea, elevated aldosterone, Cushing syndrome, or pheochromocytoma.

Multiple risk factors usually contribute to the development of resistant hypertension. Modifying risk factors is similar to lifestyle modifications for standard hypertension. Patients should be encouraged to achieve desired weight loss, restrict salt intake, and reduce alcohol intake to a moderate level. They are encouraged to increase regular physical exercise and ingest a high-fiber, low-fat diet. If adherence to a prescribed antihypertensive regimen is complex, the healthcare provider can simplify the regimen by prescribing once-daily, long-acting drugs and fixed-dose combination drugs. The patient can be encouraged to take a more active role in documenting home BP measurements in a diary and increasing the frequency of clinical appointments. Furthermore, a multidisciplinary healthcare team, including pharmacists, can improve treatment results.

Hypertensive crisis

Hypertensive crisis is a frequent cause of admission to the emergency department and may require subsequent access to the hospital. The hypertensive crisis will develop in about 1% of patients with underlying hypertension. Because chronic hypertension is a highly prevalent condition, acute hypertensive crisis accounts for many emergency room cases. From the period of 1983–1990, the rate of admissions for hypertensive emergencies more than tripled. Common causes for crisis are nonadherence to antihypertensive medication, lack of a primary care provider, or administration of illicit drugs such as cocaine.

Key Terms

Aldosterone
Aldosteronism
Angioedema
Angiotensinogen
Arterioles
Atrial natriuretic peptide
Autonomic nervous system
Bradycardia
Creatinine
Eclampsia
Epistaxis
Hypertensive crisis
Hyperthyroidism
Juxtaglomerular apparatus
Pheochromocytoma
Preeclampsia
Primary hypertension
Raynaud phenomenon
Renal artery stenosis

Resistant hypertension
Secondary hypertension
Sympathetic nervous system
Vasoconstrictor
Vasodilators

Clinical Case Studies

Clinical Case Study 1

A 46-year-old female with a family history of heart disease comes in for a standard checkup. Her father had a myocardial infarction at 61 years of age. The patient does not smoke, exercises only occasionally, and regularly has two glasses of wine after dinner each night. Her BP is 138/87 mm Hg, her body mass index is above average, and her LDL cholesterol is high.

Critical Thinking Questions

1. What are the two main types of hypertension?
2. How common is each type?
3. How significantly can changes in BP influence an MI or stroke?

Clinical Case Study 2

A 47-year-old male with treatment-resistant hypertension has been taking antihypertensive medications since he was 43 years of age. His hypertension is difficult to control, and his BP is consistently above 140/90 mm Hg. He is currently taking valsartan, extended-release metoprolol, and amlodipine. The patient is on a low-sodium diet, rarely drinks alcohol, never smokes, and rides a stationary bicycle for 1 hour daily. Medical history includes obesity, hyperlipidemia, impaired fasting glucose, hypothyroidism, gout, and obstructive sleep apnea.

Critical Thinking Questions

1. What factors are associated with resistant hypertension?
2. What must be ruled out before confirming the diagnosis of resistant hypertension?
3. What should patients with resistant hypertension be encouraged to do?

Clinical Case Study 3

A 69-year-old female in a hypertensive crisis is being treated in the intensive care unit with intravenous nitroprusside. The patient's BP was eventually normalized, but she complained of a burning sensation in her throat. This was followed by nausea, vomiting, sweating, agitation, and dyspnea. Her breath had a sweet, "almond-like" smell, and an arterial blood gas test revealed significant metabolic acidosis. A serum test indicated that a metabolite of nitroprusside, thiocyanate, was at toxic concentrations.

Critical Thinking Questions

1. What is the clinical definition of a hypertensive crisis?
2. How severe is a hypertensive crisis regarding hospitalization?
3. What are the common causes of this type of crisis?

Further Reading

[1] N. Aeddula, P. Gupta, I. Ahmed, Certified Hypertension Specialist: Board and Certification Review, StatPearls, 2023.
[2] G.L. Bakris, M.J. Sorrentino, K.J. Laffin, Hypertension: A Companion to Braunwald's Heart Disease, fourth ed., Elsevier, 2023.
[3] J. Berberian, W. Brady, A. Mattu, Emergency ECGs—Case-Based Revie and Interpretations, Emergency Medicine Residents Association, 2022.
[4] E.B. Hanna, Practical Cardiovascular Medicine, second ed., Wiley Blackwell, 2022.
[5] G. Heller, R.C. Hendel, Nuclear Cardiology—Practical Applications, fourth ed., McGraw Hill, 2022.
[6] N. Herring, D.J. Paterson, Levick's Introduction to Cardiovascular Physiology, sixth ed., CRC Press, 2018.
[7] M.C. Houston, L. Bell, Controlling High Blood Pressure Through Nutrition, Nutritional Supplements, Lifestyle, and Drugs, CRC Press, 2021.
[8] N.M. Kaplan, R.G. Victor, Kaplan's Central Hypertension, eleventh ed., Lippincott, Williams, and Wilkins, 2014.
[9] E.V. Lerma, J.S. Berns, A.R. Nissenson, Current Essentials: Nephrology & Hypertension, McGraw Hill-Lange, 2012.
[10] E.V. Lerma, J.M. Luther, S. Hiremath, Hypertension Secrets, second ed., Elsevier, 2022.
[11] P. Libby, R.O. Bonow, D.L. Mann, G.F. Tomaselli, D.L. Bhatt, S.D. Solomon, Braunwald's Heart Disease—A Textbook of Cardiovascular Medicine, twelfth ed., Elsevier, 2020.
[12] L.S. Lilly, Pathophysiology of Heart Disease—An Introduction to Cardiovascular Medicine, seventh ed., Lippincott, Williams, and Wilkins, 2020.

[13] S. Nadar, G.H. Lip, Hypertension, third ed., Oxford University Press, 2023.
[14] K. Rodriguez, Pulmonary Hypertension: Navigating the Path to Wellness with a Comprehensive Guide to Understanding, Treating, and Overcoming Pulmonary Hypertension for Improved Respiratory Health and Quality of Life, Rodriguez, 2023.
[15] M. Salvetti, Resistant Hypertension—Practical Case Studies in Hypertension Management, Springer, 2016.

CHAPTER

30

Antiarrhythmic drugs

OUTLINE

LEARNING OUTCOMES

After study of the chapter, readers should be able to:

1. Explain the action potential and cardiac conducting system.
2. Describe the various types of arrhythmias.
3. Discuss the four classes of drugs for treating arrhythmias.
4. Describe the indications of procainamide.
5. Identify various drugs in sodium channel blockers.
6. Describe the adverse effects of lidocaine.
7. Explain the indications of propranolol and common adverse effects.
8. Describe the mechanism of action for amiodarone.
9. Identify the two medications used for treating dysrhythmias as calcium channel blockers.
10. Explain the mechanism of actions of adenosine.

The Science of Pharmacology
https://doi.org/10.1016/B978-0-443-29038-1.00030-0

Overview

Various conditions, such as endocarditis or myocardial infarction, can damage the heart's conduction system and disturb the heart's regular rhythmic beating. These events can result in arrhythmia, which may also be called dysrhythmia. These are abnormal heart rhythms, as the only normal rhythm of the heart is a normal sinus rhythm. With this rhythm, an impulse is generated in the sinoatrial (SA) node, which is conducted through and slowed while passing through the atrioventricular (AV) node. Arrhythmias can be classified as bradycardias or tachycardias. Bradycardias are further divided into sinus bradycardia and heart block. Tachycardias can be supraventricular or ventricular. Antiarrhythmics prevent and can be used to treat an irregular heart rhythm. They can reduce symptoms and help avoid life-threatening complications. Their mechanism of action classifies them. The four primary classes of antiarrhythmic medications include class Ia, Ib, Ic, and sodium blockers. Class II drugs are beta blockers; class III drugs are potassium channel blockers; and class IV drugs include calcium channel blockers (CCBs).

Action potential

An **action potential** is a sudden and transient **depolarization** of the membrane. The membrane potential is determined at any time by the relative ratio of ions, extracellular to intracellular, and the permeability of each ion. The rapid rise in potential depolarization in myocytes is an all-or-nothing event initiated by opening sodium ion channels within the plasma membrane. Then, return to resting potential, **repolarization**, is mediated by the opening of potassium ion channels. An ATP-driven pump (Na/K-ATPase) induces the movement of sodium ions out of the cell and potassium ions into the cell to reestablish the appropriate balance of ions. Action potentials trigger myocardial contractions, which must be coordinated carefully for the heart to pump effectively. This requires a system for generating rhythmic impulses and distributing them quickly to the different regions of the myocardium along impulse-conducting pathways. Without such a system, other areas of the myocardium would be contracting too slowly and at slightly different rates. Thus the heart's electrical conduction system includes the **SA node**, **AV node**, the AV bundle (**bundle of His**), and **Purkinje fibers**.

The conduction of cardiac impulses generates tiny electrical currents in the heart that can be read from beyond the heart. This fact has significant clinical importance and allows visible records of the heart's electrical activity to be made with an electrocardiograph taken from electrodes placed on this skin. The electrocardiogram (ECG or EKG) is a graphic record of the heart's electrical activity and its conduction of impulses (see **Fig. 30.1**). To produce an ECG, electrodes of a recording electrocardiograph are attached to the limbs and chest. Changes in voltage within the cardiac tissue, representing changes in the heart's electrical activity, are observed as deflections of a line drawn on paper or traced on a video monitor.

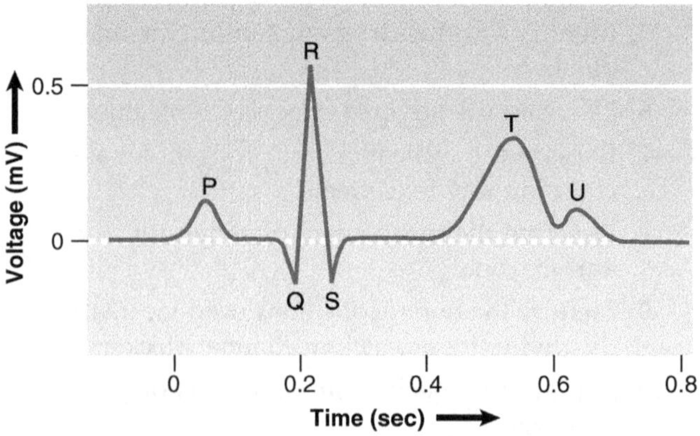

FIG. 30.1 An electrocardiogram.

Arrhythmia classifications

Certain types of arrhythmia occur in patients with severe heart diseases, and these can cause sudden cardiac death. The prevalence of arrhythmias is expected to be 1.5%–5% in the general population, with atrial fibrillation being the most common cardiac abnormality. Arrhythmias may be asymptomatic, paroxysmal, or irregular, making it difficult to estimate their true prevalence. Such arrhythmias may range from a minor inconvenience or discomfort to a potentially fatal problem. Arrhythmia is classified according to its origin, means of transmission, and associated symptoms. The various types include the following:

- **Bradycardia** is a slow heart rhythm—less than 60 beats per minute. Slight bradycardia is normal during sleep and in conditioned athletes while at rest. Abnormal bradycardia can result from improper autonomic nervous control of the heart or a damaged SA node. If the problem is severe, artificial pacemakers can increase the heart rate by replacing the SA node.
- **Tachycardia** is a rapid heart rhythm—more than 100 beats per minute. Tachycardia is expected during and just after exercise and during the stress response. Abnormal tachycardia can result from improper autonomic control of the heart, blood loss or shock, the action of drugs and toxicants, fever, and other factors.
- **Sinus dysrhythmia** is a variation in heart rate during the breathing cycle. Typically the rate increases during inspiration and decreases during expiration. The causes of sinus dysrhythmia are not clear. This phenomenon is common in young people and usually does not require treatment.
- **Atrial fibrillation** is a condition characterized by irregular and rapid heart rhythm. It is the most common type of treated heart arrhythmia. The symptoms include angina, dyspnea, palpitations, and fatigue. It is the leading cardiac cause of stroke and death. Risk factors for atrial fibrillation include advanced age, hypertension, underlying heart and lung disease, congenital heart disease, **rheumatic heart disease**, mitral stenosis, infarction of the atrial myocardium, and increased alcohol consumption. This condition can be treated with a beta blocker (esmolol, atenolol) or a CCB (verapamil or diltiazem). Each drug may be offered depending on patients' symptoms and general health. Digoxin can also be prescribed if other medications are not suitable. Sometimes **cardioversion** can also be used. The complications of atrial fibrillation include stroke, heart failure, cognitive impairment, hypertension, and syncope.
- **Extrasystoles** occur before the next expected contraction in a series of **cardiac cycles**. They often occur due to lack of sleep, too much caffeine or nicotine, alcoholism, or heart damage. Ventricular depolarizations that appear earlier than expected are called **premature ventricular contractions** (PVCs). They occur as early, vast QRS complexes without a preceding related P wave on the ECG. PVCs can result in a variety of conditions that include hypoxemia, electrolyte imbalance, acidosis, stress, ventricular hypertrophy, and drug reactions. Occasional PVCs are not clinically significant in otherwise healthy individuals. However, in patients with heart disease, **cardiac output** may be reduced.
- **Ventricular fibrillation** is a malfunction of the heart's typical pumping sequence. It is the most common deadly arrhythmia. Without treatment, the condition is fatal within minutes. The most common causes include angina, MI, family history of sudden cardiac death, heart surgery, use of certain medications, electrical shock, electrolyte imbalances, and other arrhythmias. The condition is a life-threatening medical emergency, and every minute counts. All patients with cardiac arrest should have an initial assessment while receiving quality CPR. Complications of ventricular fibrillation include hypoxia of the brain, injuries from CPR, long-term disabilities, postdefibrillation arrhythmias, and death. Ventricular fibrillation can be treated with **defibrillation** and medications. The drugs used for treating ventricular fibrillation include amiodarone, lidocaine, sotalol, and mexiletine.
- **Ventricular flutter** is a potentially lethal cardiac arrhythmia characterized by extremely rapid, hemodynamically unstable ventricular tachycardia (150–300 beats/minute). If untreated, ventricular flutter can progress to ventricular fibrillation. **Fig. 30.2** illustrates various types of arrhythmia.

Drugs for arrhythmia

Antiarrhythmics can prevent and treat a heart rhythm that is too fast or irregular. These drugs are also referred to as antidysrhythmics. These medications can reduce symptoms and help avoid life-threatening complications. Some of these drugs stop irregular, extra electrical impulses. Others block abnormally fast impulses from traveling along heart tissues. Most antiarrhythmics are intended for long-term use. The medications for treating arrhythmias include

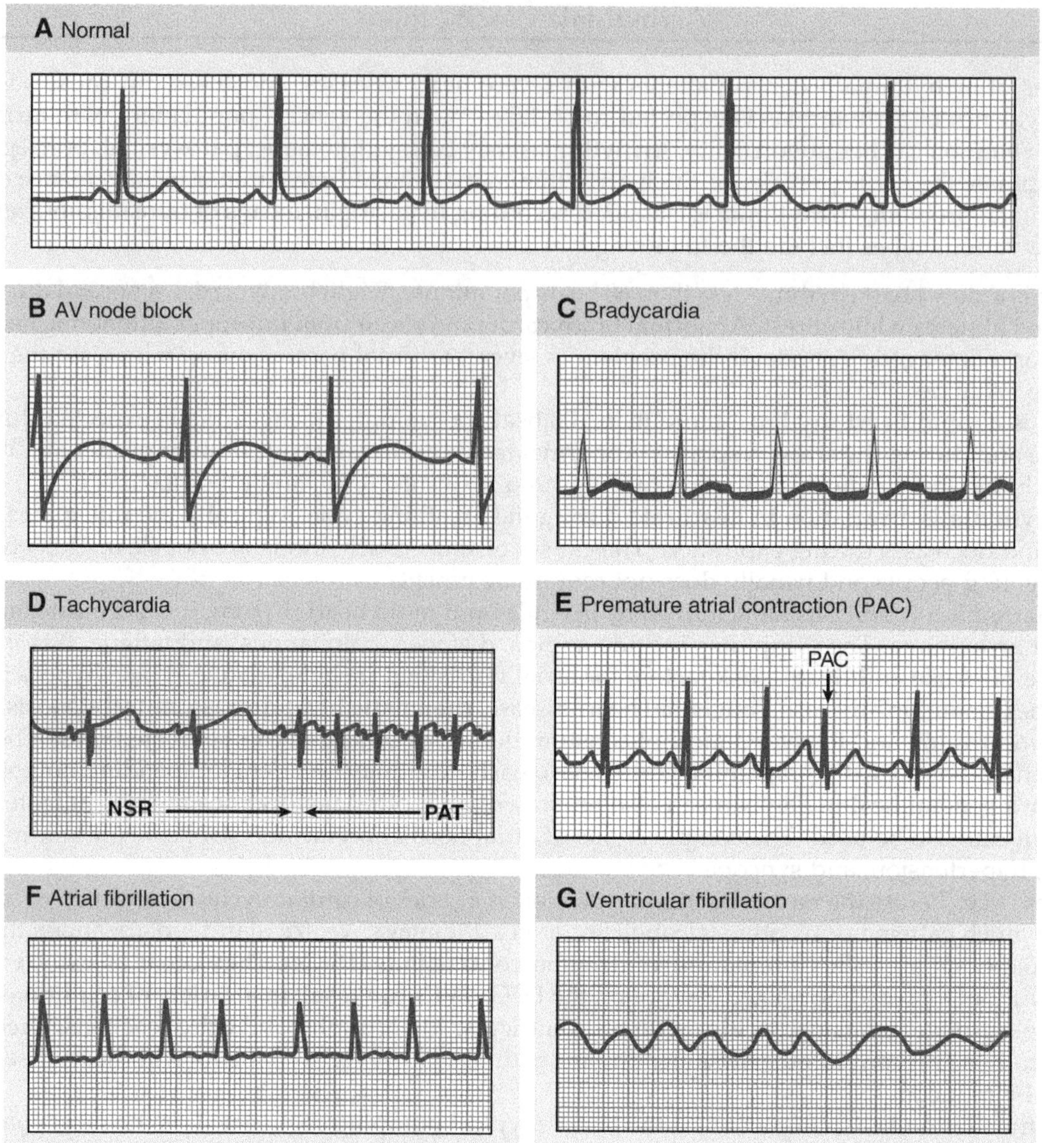

FIG. 30.2 Various types of arrhythmia.

sodium channel blockers, beta-blocker antagonists, potassium channel blockers, and calcium channel blockers (see **Table 30.**).

Class I: Sodium channel blockers

Sodium channel blockers inhibit the fast sodium channels, thereby slowing electrical conduction in the heart. They were among the first drugs used for several decades and are divided into three groups according to their cellular electrophysiologic effects. Sodium channel blockers therefore prolong conduction time and refractoriness of the atria, ventricle, and Purkinje fibers. These agents are effective against many arrhythmias, such as atrial fibrillation.

The three subgroups of sodium channel blockers include those in class IA, which slow conduction and prolong repolarization (procainamide, disopyramide); those in class IB, which slow conduction and shorten repolarization (lidocaine, mexiletine, phenytoin); and those in class IC, which prolong conduction with little to no effect on repolarization (flecainide, propafenone).

TABLE 30.1 Drugs for treating arrhythmias.

Generic names	Trade names	Route of drug administration
Class IA: Sodium channel blockers		
disopyramide	Norpace	PO
procainamide	Pronestyl	PO, IV
Class IB: Sodium channel blockers		
Lidocaine	Xylocaine	IV
Mexiletine	Mexitil	PO
Phenytoin	Dilantin	IV
Class IC: Sodium channel blockers		
Flecainide	Tambocor	PO
propafenone	Rythmol	PO
Class II: Beta-adrenergic blockers		
Acebutolol	Sectral	PO
Esmolol	Brevibloc	IV
Propranolol	Inderal, InnoPran XL	PO, IV
Class III: Potassium channel blockers		
amiodarone	Pacerone, Cordarone	PO
dofetilide	Tikosyn	PO
ibutilide	Corvert	IV
Sotalol	Betapace, Betapace AF, Sorine	PO
Class IV: Calcium channel blockers		
diltiazem	Cardizem, Dilacor, Taztia XR	IV
verapamil	Calan, Isoptin SR, Verelan	
Miscellaneous		
adenosine	Adenocard, Adenoscan	IV
digoxin	Lanoxin, Lanoxicaps	

Procainamide

Procainamide is a class IA antiarrhythmic agent. It has been used for more than 60 years. Long-term procainamide therapy can induce hypersensitivity reactions, autoantibody formation, and a lupus-like syndrome.

Pharmacokinetics

Procainamide is readily absorbed after oral administration and crosses the placenta. It is secreted in breast milk. Procainamide binds only 15% to plasma protein and is metabolized in the liver. It is about 50%–70% unchanged in the urine. The peak plasma concentrations generally reach within 1–2 hours. A rapid initial distribution phase is completed about 30 minutes after intravenous administration. The half-life of procainamide is 2.5–5 hours, and the maximum dose is 17 mg/kg.

Mechanism of action

Procainamide can bind to fast sodium channels by inhibiting recovery after repolarization. It can also prolong the action potential and reduce the speed of impulse conduction. Therefore it inhibits the ionic fluxes required to initiate and conduct impulses, affecting local anesthetic action.

Clinical indications

Procainamide is indicated for treating ventricular arrhythmias, supraventricular arrhythmias, atrial flutter, atrial fibrillation, AV nodal reentrant tachycardia, and **Wolf-Parkinson-White syndrome**.

Contraindications

Procainamide is contraindicated in patients with complete heart block because of its effects in suppressing ventricular pacemakers and may cause **asystole**. It should be avoided in patients with severe heart failure, **myasthenia gravis**, and peripheral neuropathy.

Adverse effects

The adverse effects of procainamide include bradycardia, hypotension, cardiac toxicity, and blood dyscrasias. PR prolongation and QRS are procainamide's most potentially harmful cardiac side effects and may worsen when serum procainamide concentrations rise.

Toxicities

Toxicities associated with procainamide are uncommon, but overdose may cause increased ventricular extrasystoles, ventricular tachycardia, or fibrillation. Widening of the QRS complex, prolonged QT and PR intervals, and lowering of the R and T waves may occur.

Lidocaine

Lidocaine is a local anesthetic agent commonly used for local and topical anesthesia. Still, it also has antiarrhythmic and analgesic uses and can be used as an adjunct to tracheal intubation. It is a tertiary amine class IB antiarrhythmic drug. Lidocaine is most commonly used in the treatment of ventricular arrhythmias, particularly those associated with acute myocardial infarction, such as ventricular tachycardia, ventricular fibrillation, and multiple ventricular extrasystoles. It is often effective in atrial arrhythmias. Lidocaine blocks cardiac sodium channels, shortening the action potential, and is used intravenously only for arrhythmia. It is not recommended for prophylactic administration to suppress PVCs or prevent ventricular tachycardia or ventricular fibrillation after acute coronary syndrome. The adverse effects of lidocaine include QRS widening, hypotension, shock, and asystole. Lidocaine toxicity is usually dose dependent, and the risk is increased in individuals with renal and hepatic impairments.

You should remember

Lidocaine, a class IB sodium channel blocker, was used in the 1940s as a local anesthetic and is still used for this purpose. It was later discovered to have antiarrhythmic properties as well. Some cardiologists still use lidocaine to treat acute ventricular arrhythmias. It slows conduction velocity and decreases action potential amplitude.

Mexiletine

Mexiletine is a local anesthetic, antiarrhythmic drug classified as a class IB antiarrhythmic. Structurally similar to lidocaine, mexiletine is orally active and has a fast onset and more significant effects at faster heart rates. It inhibits the inward sodium current required for the conduction of impulses, thus reducing the rate of the action potential; it is primarily used to suppress ventricular arrhythmias. It is also used in peripheral neuropathy and chronic pain. Symptoms of overdose include nausea, hypotension, sinus bradycardia, paresthesia, seizures, bundle branch block, AV heart block, asystole, ventricular fibrillation, cardiovascular collapse, and coma.

Propafenone is classified as a class IC antiarrhythmic agent; its sodium channel b extends the effective refractory period. Propafenone directly slows cardiac nerve impulses. It can be used in combination with a beta-blocker or a CCB for pharmacologic cardioversion of recent-onset atrial fibrillation in patients without structural heart disease.

Propafenone should be administered after administering a beta-blocker or a CCB to prevent the conversion from atrial fibrillation to atrial flutter with a rapid ventricular rate. However, this combination carries the potential risk of cardiogenic shock. Adverse effects of propafenone include unusual taste, nausea, vomiting, headache, blurred vision, fatigue, dyspnea, and bradycardia.

Class II: Beta-adrenergic antagonists

Class II antidysrhythmics or beta-blockers block sympathetic nervous system stimulation and the heart's conduction system. By doing so, beta-blockers prevent catecholamine-mediated actions on the heart. This is a cardioprotective effect. The resulting cardiovascular effects include a reduced heart rate, delayed AV node conduction, reduced myocardial contractility, and decreased myocardial automaticity. The pharmacologic effects of beta-blockers are especially beneficial after an MI, when many catecholamines are released that make the heart hyperirritable and predisposed to many types of dysrhythmias. Beta-blockers protect against dangerous complications and sudden cardiac death after MI in patients. Although several beta-blockers exist, only a few are commonly used as antidysrhythmics. Those currently approved by the FDA for this purpose are acebutolol, esmolol, propranolol, and sotalol (which have class II and III properties); however, other beta-blockers are commonly used. Selected drugs are described here. The beta-adrenergic blockers were reviewed in **Chapter 28** in more detail.

Acebutolol

Acebutolol is a cardioselective beta-blocker used to treat cardiac dysrhythmias, hypertension, and angina pectoris. It blocks specific beta-receptors in the blood vessels and the heart, preventing adrenaline activation. Acebutolol's common adverse effects include headache, dizziness, bradycardia, dyspnea, fatigue, muscle aches, diarrhea, or constipation. This drug is contraindicated in patients with AV block degree (second or third degree), heart failure, or bradycardia.

Propranolol is a short-acting, cardioselective beta-blocker, a class II antiarrhythmic agent. It is used alone or with other medications to treat hypertension, dysrhythmia, and pheochromocytoma. Propranolol is also used to prevent angina and migraine headaches. It works by relaxing blood vessels and slowing the heart rate to improve blood flow and decrease blood pressure. The most common adverse effects of propranolol are headaches, dizziness, fatigue, cold fingers or toes, stomach pain, nausea, vomiting, diarrhea, insomnia, and nightmares.

Class III: Potassium channel blockers

Potassium channel blockers such as dronedarone, dofetilide, sotalol, and ibutilide treat life-threatening dysrhythmias such as ventricular fibrillation and ventricular tachycardia. They decrease potassium efflux out of the cell and prolong the QT interval.

Amiodarone

Amiodarone is a class III antiarrhythmic drug. It blocks potassium currents that cause repolarization of the cardiac muscle during the third phase of the cardiac action potential.

Pharmacokinetics

Amiodarone's oral absorption ranges from 25%–85%. It is metabolized in the liver via cytochrome 450 enzymes. Amiodarone is eliminated from the body through the bile, with less than 1% being excreted unchanged in the urine. The half-life can be several weeks. In addition, after discontinuing amiodarone treatment, its pharmacological effects could persist for 1–3 months.

Mechanism of action

Amiodarone's mechanism of action includes inhibiting potassium's ability to repolarize the heart during phase III of the cardiac action potential. This potassium channel–blocking effect increases action potential duration and a prolonged effective refractory period in cardiac muscle, reducing excitability.

Clinical indications

Amiodarone is explicitly used for the management of life-threatening ventricular fibrillation and pulseless ventricular tachycardia. However, this drug is also used to treat atrial fibrillation.

Contraindications

Amiodarone should be avoided in individuals with second- or third-degree heart blockage who do not have pacemakers. It is also contraindicated in patients with Wolff-Parkinson-White syndrome when concurrent atrial fibrillation is present.

Adverse effects

Adverse effects include photophobia, optic neuropathy, blurred or double vision, fatigue, chest pain, dyspnea, headache, dizziness, and chills. A baseline ophthalmological assessment is recommended for patients initiating amiodarone therapy. When thyroid dysfunction, visual disturbances, pulmonary infiltrates, ataxia, cardiac conduction abnormalities, and drug interactions occur, amiodarone must be used.

Toxicities

The overdose toxicity of amiodarone includes hypotension, bradycardia, and ventricular tachycardia.

Dofetilide

Dofetilide is a class III antiarrhythmic for treating acute atrial fibrillation or flutter and preventing atrial fibrillation or flutter recurrence. It is also used to treat paroxysmal supraventricular tachycardias (PSVTs). Dofetilide inhibits potassium channels in phase 3 of the action potential and slows the efflux of potassium cations back out of the myocyte, slowing the repolarization rate of the cell. The **refractory periods** of atrial, ventricular, and Purkinje cells are increased, leading to lengthening of the QT interval. Oral absorption is approximately 100%. The half-life of dofetilide was reported to be 4.8–13.5 hours. Fifty percent of dofetilide metabolism into inactive metabolites is in the liver. Dofetilide is metabolized to a small extent by CYP3A4. Dofetilide may induce or worsen ventricular dysrhythmias with therapeutic use, producing life-threatening polymorphic ventricular tachycardia. The adverse effects of dofetilide include dizziness, rash, sweating, loss of appetite, vomiting, and diarrhea. It is classified as category C during pregnancy.

Sotalol

Sotalol is a beta-blocker with antiarrhythmic properties that affect the atrium and ventricles. It is used to treat life-threatening ventricular arrhythmia or atrial fibrillation. Sotalol is a competitive inhibitor of the rapid potassium channel. This inhibition lengthens the duration of action potentials and the refractory period in the atria and ventricles. The inhibition of rapid potassium channels increases as the heart rate decreases. Approximately 80%–90% of sotalol is excreted in the urine as unchanged, and a small amount is excreted in the feces as unchanged. The adverse effects of sotalol include chest pain, headache, blurred vision, confusion, fatigue, sweating, skin rash, anxiety, bleeding gums, and edema.

Overdose of sotalol may cause hypotension, bradycardia, congestive heart failure, bronchospasm, and hypoglycemia. Such intentional toxicity may result in a prolonged QT interval, bradycardia, hypotension, cardiac asystole, ventricular tachycardia, and premature ventricular complexes.

Class IV: Calcium channel blockers

Class IV antidysrhythmic drugs are CCBs. The two medications that are commonly used for treating dysrhythmias are verapamil and diltiazem. The CCBs were reviewed in **Chapter 28** in more detail.

Diltiazem

Diltiazem is a CCB that moves calcium into the myocardial cells. It increases the supply of blood and oxygen to the heart while reducing its workload. Diltiazem is primarily used to treat hypertension and control angina. It is also used as an antiarrhythmic. The FDA has approved indications for atrial arrhythmia and PSVT. The adverse effects of diltiazem include headaches, bradycardia, flushing, edema of the legs, dizziness, blurred vision, and stomach pain.

Verapamil

Verapamil is a CCB that is used alone or in combination with other medicines to treat dysrhythmia, hypertension, and severe angina. It is indicated for PSVT and supraventricular tachycardia. CCBs inhibit the influx of calcium ions into the myocardium and vascular smooth muscle during depolarization. This inhibition will relax coronary vascular smooth muscle and cause coronary vasodilation, which is helpful for patients with hypertension. Verapamil also increases myocardial oxygen delivery, which helps patients with vasospastic angina. This medication can be administered either orally or intravenously. The adverse effects of verapamil include **gingival hyperplasia,** hypotension, dyspepsia, constipation, and peripheral edema.

Miscellaneous drugs

The miscellaneous drugs do not belong to a traditional class of antiarrhythmics. They have varied mechanisms of action and uses. The medications in this class include adenosine and digoxin.

Adenosine

Adenosine (Adenocard, Adenoscan) is a naturally occurring substance that relaxes and dilates blood vessels. It also affects the electrical activity of the myocardium. This agent is used to help restore normal heartbeats in patients with specific dysrhythmias. It is also used during a stress test of the heart. Adenosine slows conduction time through the AV node and can restore normal sinus rhythm in patients with PSVT. Adenosine has a rapid onset of action with a very short half-life. Adenosine is administered intravenously. The contraindications include known hypersensitivity to adenosine, heart block, asthma, or COPD.

Digoxin

Digoxin is used to improve the myocardium's strength or regulate the rate and rhythm of the heartbeat. Therefore it is mainly used for congestive heart failure, atrial fibrillation, or flutter. It has a very narrow therapeutic window for the medication. Digoxin is a toxic substance with a well-known cardiotoxic effect. See **Chapter 33** for more detail.

You should remember

Digoxin is an agreeable therapeutic option for elderly patients with atrial fibrillation. Unlike other rate-control strategies, digoxin does not cause hypotension or have adverse inotropic effects. However, caution is advised regarding potential drug interactions with digoxin use in older people.

Key Terms

Action potentials
Asystole
Atrial fibrillation
Atrioventricular node
Bradycardia
Bundle of His
Cardiac cycles
Cardioversion
Defibrillation
Depolarization
Extrasystoles
Gingival hyperplasia
Myasthenia gravis
Premature ventricular contractions
Purkinje fibers

Refractory periods
Repolarization
Rheumatic heart disease
Sinoatrial node
Sinus dysrhythmia
Tachycardia
Ventricular fibrillation
Ventricular flutter
Wolf-Parkinson-White syndrome

Clinical Case Studies

Clinical Case Study 1

A 78-year-old male comes to a medical clinic to get vaccines for the flu and whooping cough because he is expecting a new granddaughter in the next 2 months. His blood pressure is 127/85 mm Hg, and his pulse is 115 bpm. The patient was diagnosed with hyperlipidemia 12 years ago and hypertension 4 years ago. He currently takes medication for these two conditions. He has never smoked or consumed alcoholic beverages. His age and history of hypertension suggest he might be at risk for atrial fibrillation. His heart rate was 120 bpm during the physical exam, and he had an irregular rhythm. He denies experiencing dyspnea, fatigue, dizziness, palpitations, or chest pains. The EKG is performed and shows atrial fibrillation with a rapid ventricular response.

Critical Thinking Questions

1. What are the risk factors of atrial fibrillation?
2. What medication can be used for treating atrial fibrillation?
3. What are the complications of atrial fibrillation?

Clinical Case Study 2

A 45-year-old female was brought to the emergency department with a past medical history of coronary artery disease, hypertension, hypothyroidism, asthma, and tobacco use. The patient complained of chest pain that started at rest and radiation to the jaw and left arm with dyspnea. Although previously effective, nitroglycerin tablets did not relieve her pain. She became unresponsive and pulseless. Cardiopulmonary resuscitation was initiated, and she had a heart rhythm of ventricular fibrillation. The defibrillator was used, and the patient returned to spontaneous circulation. The ECG showed ST elevations in anterolateral and inferior leads.

Critical Thinking Questions

1. What are the most common causes of ventricular fibrillation?
2. What are the complications of ventricular fibrillation?
3. What are the treatments for ventricular fibrillation?

Further Reading

[1] D.H. Bennett, Bennett's Cardiac Arrhythmias – Practical Notes on Interpretation and Treatment, eighth ed., Wiley-Blackwell, 2013.
[2] G.E. Billman, Novel Therapeutic Targets for Antiarrhythmic Drugs, Wiley, 2010.
[3] G. Breithardt, M. Borggrefe, J.A. Camm, M. Shenasa, Antiarrhythmic Drugs – Mechanisms of Antiarrhythmic and Proarrhythmic Actions, Springer, 2012.
[4] T.B. Garcia, D.J. Garcia, Arrhythmia Recognition – the Art of Interpretation, second ed., Jones & Bartlett Learning, 2019.
[5] R.T. Ho, Electrophysiology of Arrhythmias – Practical Images for Diagnosis and Ablation, second ed., Wolters Kluwer, 2022.
[6] J. Huff, ECG Workout – Exercises in Arrhythmia Interpretation, eighth ed., Wolters Kluwer, 2022.
[7] R.E. Kass, C.E. Clancy, Basis and Treatment of Cardiac Arrhythmias (Handbook of Experimental Pharmacology, 171), Springer, 2010.
[8] P.R. Kowey, G.V. Naccarelli, Advances in Antiarrhythmic Drug Therapy – an Issue of Cardiac Electrophysiology Clinics (Volumes 2-3) (The Clinics – Internal Medicine), Saunders, 2010.
[9] P. Kowey, J.P. Piccini, G. Naccarelli, J.A. Reiffel, Cardiac Arrhythmias, Pacing and Sudden Death, Springer, 2017.
[10] A. Martinez-Rubio, J. Tamargo, G.A. Dan, Antiarrhythmic Drugs (Current Cardiovascular Therapy), Springer, 2020.
[11] D. Murray, A Clinical Approach to Antiarrhythmic Drugs, American Medical Publishers, 2023.
[12] NEDU, EKG / ECG Interpretation Made Easy – an Illustrated Study Guide for Students to Easily Learn How to Read and Interpret ECG Strips, NEDU LLC, 2021.

[13] B. Stone, Critical Care Medications – Pharmacology of Common Anti-arrhythmic Medications Used in Critical Care – A Study Guide and Resource Book for Nurses, Physicians and More, Stone, 2023.

[14] G. Walraven, Basic Arrhythmias with 12-lead EKGs, eighth ed., Pearson, 2016.

[15] P. Wang, A. Al-Ahmad, Advances in Antiarrhythmic Drug Therapy – an Issue of Cardiac Electrophysiology (The Clinics – Internal Medicine Book 3), Saunders, 2011.

CHAPTER

31

Antianemia drugs

OUTLINE

LEARNING OUTCOMES

After study of the chapter, readers should be able to:

1. Describe the hemopoiesis and hematopoietic growth factors.
2. Explain the mechanism of action of epoetin alfa.
3. Describe the adverse effects of epoetin alfa.
4. Discuss various types of anemia.
5. Explain the pharmacokinetics of ferrous sulfate.
6. Describe the symptoms of iron deficiency anemia.
7. Explain the overdose of iron.
8. Describe the causes of pernicious anemia.
9. Discuss the clinical indications of cyanocobalamin.
10. Describe common adverse effects of cyanocobalamin.

The Science of Pharmacology
https://doi.org/10.1016/B978-0-443-29038-1.00031-2

Overview

Anemia is a common blood disorder ultimately characterized by abnormally low red blood cells (RBCs), which are critical to health, as they contain the protein hemoglobin (Hb), which carries oxygen from the lungs to all body tissues. Several types of anemia exist, each with a cause and a treatment. These anemia types include iron deficiency anemia, vitamin B_{12} deficiency anemia, anemia of folate deficiency, hemolytic anemia, sickle cell anemia, and aplastic anemia. Anemia is commonly a symptom of another disease, and it can occur with bleeding or significant blood loss, destruction of RBCs, poor nutrition, certain drugs, and other specific diseases. Anemia caused by nutritional deficiency can be prevented by eating an iron- and vitamin B_{12}-rich diet or supplementing with either minerals or vitamins when dietary intake is insufficient. Most other types of anemia cannot be prevented, and treatment depends on the severity and cause of the anemia. Severe anemia may require a blood transfusion. Anemia caused by drug therapy can be treated by stopping the medication. In contrast, inherited hemolytic anemia may require splenectomy.

Physiology of hemopoiesis

Hematopoiesis is blood cell production. The body continually makes new blood cells to replace old ones, ensuring a steady blood supply. This production chiefly occurs in the **bone marrow**, especially before birth, with the liver and spleen being minor contributors to this process after we are born. Three types of hematopoiesis include erythropoiesis, leukopoiesis, and thrombopoiesis, which create erythrocytes, leukocytes, and platelets, respectively.

Erythrocytes made via erythropoiesis contain the protein Hb, which carries oxygen from the lungs to all body tissues. RBCs also carry carbon dioxide to the lungs for removal from the body. Due to their importance in oxygenating the tissues, blood contains more erythrocytes than any other type of blood cell.

Leukopoiesis creates **leukocytes,** which fight infection and protect the body from pathogens. Five types of leukocytes include neutrophils, basophils, eosinophils, monocytes, and lymphocytes. **Thrombocytes**, made via thrombopoiesis, are blood cell fragments that clump together to form a clot after injury. They seal damaged tissue, preventing blood loss (Fig. 31.1).

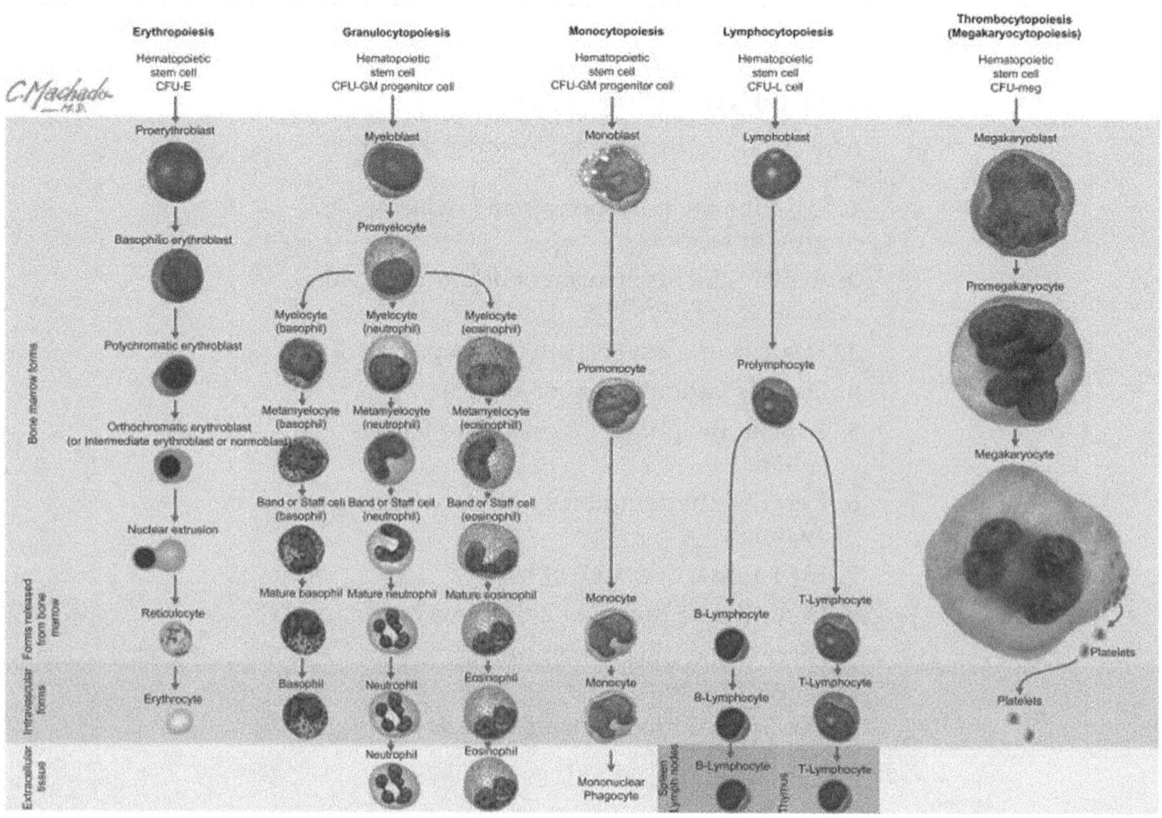

FIG. 31.1 Blood cell formation from stem cells.

Hematopoietic growth factors

Hematopoietic growth factors are a family of glycoproteins with critical regulatory functions in the **proliferation**, differentiation, and functional activation of hematopoietic progenitors and mature blood cells. They produce blood cells in the bone marrow, making them useful in various clinical conditions. Myeloid growth factors, or colony-stimulating factors when used as drugs, are used to support patients after chemotherapy and bone marrow transplantation, and they have potential applications in treating infectious diseases. Erythropoietin (EPO) is widely used for patients with anemia due to failure of marrow production, having established its effectiveness in chronic renal failure. Thrombopoietin (TPO) is a thrombocyte growth factor, and drugs that mimic its effects are called platelet enhancers.

T lymphocytes, monocytes/macrophages, **fibroblasts**, and **endothelial cells** are the essential cellular sources of most hematopoietic growth factors, excluding EPO and TPO. EPO is produced primarily by the adult kidney, and TPO is made in the liver and kidney. **Table 31.1** summarizes hematopoietic growth factors.

Epoetin alfa is a drug used to manage anemia secondary to bone marrow failure. It is one of the erythropoiesis-stimulating classes of drugs and is available in single-dose, preservative-free, and multidose preserved vials. Epoetin can be administered via the intravenous or subcutaneous route, which is preferred except for patients with kidney disease who are on maintenance hemodialysis.

Pharmacokinetics

Subcutaneously injected epoetin alfa is absorbed slowly and reaches its peak concentration at 5–24 hours after dosing. The bioavailability is about 20%–30%, and its plasma half-life is more than 24 hours. About 3%–10% of epoetin is excreted unchanged in the urine.

Mechanism of action

Epoetin alfa is recombinant human EPO, closely identical to the endogenous EPO hormone. It interacts directly with the EPO receptor on the RBC surface, activating several signal transduction pathways and increasing and dividing RBC precursors. Therefore it increases the number of erythrocytes.

Clinical indications

Epoetin treats severe anemia in kidney dialysis patients or those with renal diseases. It may also be given to prevent or treat anemia caused by surgery or medicines such as zidovudine.

TABLE 31.1 Hematopoietic Growth Factors.

Generic name	Trade name	Route of administration
Erythropoietic growth factors darbepoetin alfa epoetin alfa (synthetic EPO)	Aranesp Epogen, Procrit	Subcutaneous, IV Subcutaneous, IV
Colony-stimulating factors filgrastim pegfilgrastim sargramostim	Granix, Neupogen, Zarxio Neulasta Leukine	Subcutaneous, IV Subcutaneous IV
Platelet enhancers eltrombopag oprelvekin romiplostim	Promacta Neumega Nplate	PO Subcutaneous Subcutaneous

EPO, Erythropoietin.

Contraindications

Epoetin alfa is contraindicated in patients with known hypersensitivity, uncontrolled hypertension, and a history of seizures.

Adverse effects

The adverse effects of epoetin alfa may include severe headaches, myocardial infarction, stroke, thrombosis, seizures, fatigue, hyperglycemia, hypokalemia, and hypertension. Common adverse effects include nausea, vomiting, fever, chills, cough, dyspnea, itching, weight loss, and insomnia.

Toxicities

Overdose of epoetin alfa is very rare, and there is no antidote. However, it may increase the risk of serious cardiovascular events.

Classification of anemias

Anemia is a reduced Hb, hematocrit, or RBC count. It is an underlying condition and can be subdivided into **macrocytic**, **microcytic**, or **normocytic**. Patients with anemia typically present with vague symptoms such as lethargy, weakness, and fatigue. Many people are at risk for anemia because of infections, poor diet, intestinal disorders, chronic diseases, and other conditions. Females who are menstruating or pregnant, children, older adults, and people with chronic medical conditions are most at risk. The risk of anemia increases as people grow older. Various types of anemia include iron, vitamin B_{12}, or folate deficiencies or aplastic, hemolytic, and sickle cell anemias.

Iron deficiency anemia

Iron is crucial in maintaining many bodily functions, including Hb production, to carry oxygen. Iron is also necessary to maintain healthy cells, skin, hair, and nails. Iron metabolism is illustrated in **Fig. 31.2**. Iron deficiency anemia is the most common anemia, characterized by low iron concentrations. This is usually due to blood loss but may occasionally be caused by poor dietary iron absorption. Pregnancy and childbirth require a great deal of iron. Deficiency can also occur in individuals who have peptic ulcers or have had gastric bypass surgery for weight loss, vegetarians, vegans, and those whose diets do not include iron-rich foods. Iron deficiency anemia can be diagnosed by measuring a complete blood count. Additional tests may be ordered to evaluate serum ferritin, iron, total iron-binding capacity, and transferrin. For patients with iron deficiency, blood tests may reveal low Hb and hematocrit, low mean cellular volume, low ferritin, low serum iron, and low iron saturation. There are several ways to increase iron intake, which include dietary sources, medicinal iron (ferrous sulfate), and blood transfusions.

Ferrous sulfate is an iron supplement used to treat iron deficiency anemia. It may be needed if the diet does not supply enough iron. Ferrous sulfate is available as a tablet and as a liquid.

Pharmacokinetics

When taken on an empty stomach, ferrous sulfate is best absorbed with water or fruit juice. However, iron may be taken with food or immediately after meals to lessen the possibility of stomach upset. Iron is absorbed mainly in the duodenum and upper jejunum, but food and achlorhydria may decrease absorption. Once absorbed, iron binds to transferrin and is transported to the bone marrow, and the half-life is approximately 2 hours. How iron is excreted from the body has yet to be established, and it may be done via multiple processes, including exfoliation of dead skin, blood loss, and turnover of the intestinal epithelium.

Mechanism of action

The primary mechanism of action of ferrous sulfate is to combine with porphyrin and globin chains to form Hb, which is needed for oxygen delivery from the lungs to other tissues. In an iron-deficient state, Hb cannot be synthesized, resulting in *microcytic anemia* due to the formation of small RBCs with insufficient Hb.

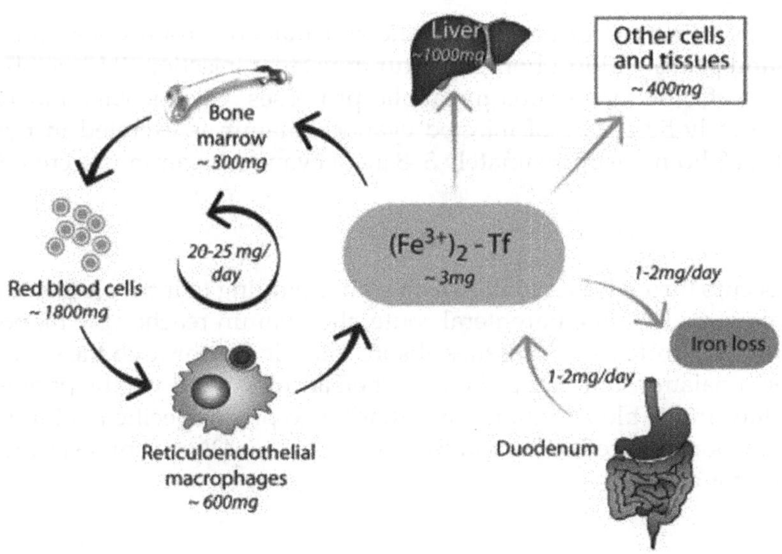

FIG. 31.2 Iron metabolism.

Clinical indications

Ferrous sulfate is used for iron deficiency anemia, blood loss, nutritional deficiency, iron malabsorption, or an increase in the body's need for iron, such as during pregnancy. Iron is essential for general health. Reducing iron stores may result in decreased production of Hb and circulating erythrocytes, leading to anemia. Symptoms of iron deficiency can present as dyspnea, hypothermia, fatigue, tachycardia, altered mental status, and increased risk of infection.

Contraindications

Ferrous sulfate is contraindicated in patients with hereditary hemochromatosis or hemosiderosis or for those with a history of hemolytic anemia.

Adverse effects

The adverse effects of ferrous sulfate include nausea, vomiting, stomach discomfort, heartburn, loss of appetite, constipation, diarrhea, darkening of the stool, and dark-colored tooth staining.

Toxicities

Iron toxicity often occurs with high doses and can manifest as hepatic, cardiovascular, and central nervous damage. Symptoms of overdose include initial GI upset that slowly develops into acute **metabolic encephalopathy**, seizures, **metabolic acidosis**, hypoxia, and tachycardia.

Pernicious anemia

Pernicious anemia is a rare condition affecting people of all ages worldwide, but it is mainly a concern for those older than 60. It is a complex disease with a clear autoimmune basis. Pernicious anemia is characterized by megaloblastic or giant red cells caused by vitamin B_{12} deficiency secondary to **intrinsic factor** deficiency. Parietal cells produce and secrete intrinsic factors that bind B_{12} and facilitate its transport to the terminal ileum for absorption. Vitamin B_{12} is essential for erythropoiesis and nerve myelination. Dietary B_{12} from food in the acidic gastric environment binds to intrinsic factors and then, in the terminal ileum, is released in the bloodstream and delivered to the liver for metabolism (see **Fig. 31.3**).

The progression of pernicious anemia is typically slow, and it may be challenging to recognize the symptoms. Common symptoms include headaches, fatigue, weight loss, pale skin, depression, dementia, and peripheral neuropathy. Cyanocobalamin is used to treat and prevent vitamin B_{12} deficiencies.

Pharmacokinetics

Cyanocobalamin can be given via intranasal, oral, sublingual, intramuscular, and subcutaneous routes of administration. It is rapidly absorbed from injection sites and peaks within 1 hour after intramuscular injection. It is metabolized in the liver and converted in tissues into a cofactor for various metabolic processes. Cyanocobalamin is primarily excreted from the kidneys, and approximately 50%–98% of injected cyanocobalamin is excreted in the urine. A significant portion is excreted within the first 8 hours. Approximately 3–8 μg of cyanocobalamin is secreted via the bile, and most is reabsorbed.

Mechanism of action

When taken orally, cyanocobalamin absorption occurs through the small intestine after binding to intrinsic factors and other cobalamin-binding proteins. When administered via the parenteral route, the vitamin reaches the blood immediately. In the blood, vitamin B_{12} attaches to plasma proteins, and tissues absorb vitamin B_{12} through the small intestine after binding to intrinsic factors and other cobalamin-binding proteins. When administered via the parenteral route, the vitamin reaches the blood immediately. In the blood, vitamin B_{12} attaches to pl via specific B_{12}-binding proteins, transcobalamin I and II, facilitating transport into cells. Vitamin B_{12} is essential for DNA synthesis and energy production, particularly in erythroid progenitor cells.

Clinical indications

Cyanocobalamin is a synthetic vitamin B_{12} compound used to treat pernicious anemia, impairment of B_{12} absorption, *Helicobacter pylori* infection, gastric atrophy, total or partial gastrectomy, small bowel bacteria overgrowth, pancreatic insufficiency, bowel or pancreatic cancers, and malnutrition.

Contraindications

Cyanocobalamin is contraindicated in patients with allergies, optic neuropathy, gout, and hypokalemia.

Adverse effects

The adverse effects of cyanocobalamin include dyspnea, peripheral vascular thrombosis, weight gain, **pulmonary edema**, and congestive heart failure. Other adverse effects include leg cramps, irregular heartbeats, tingling/numbness, hypokalemia, fatigue, numbness, and joint pain.

Toxicities

Vitamin B_{12} toxicity does not occur; the typical therapeutic dose of cyanocobalamin cannot be overdosed.

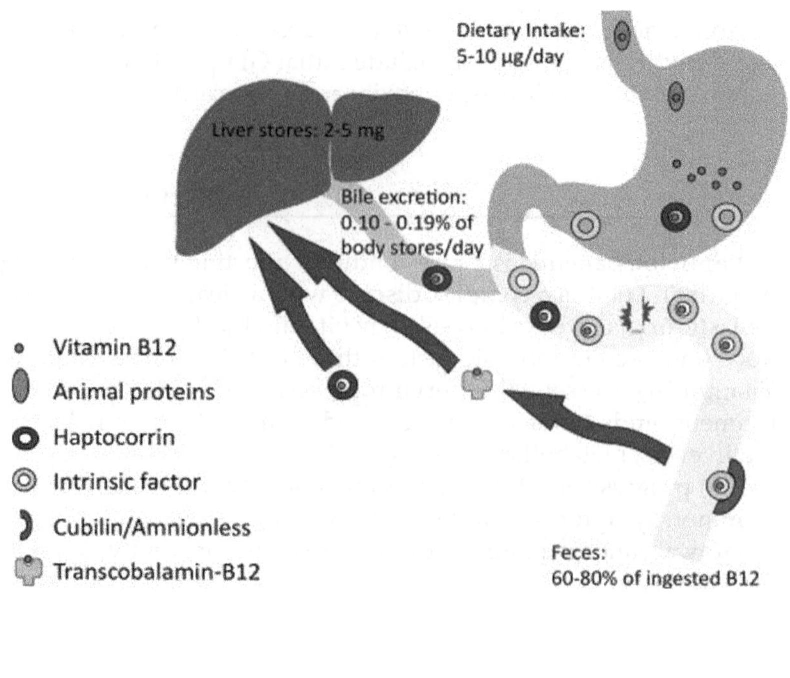

FIG. 31.3 Metabolism and malabsorption of vitamin B_{12}.

You should remember

Vitamin B_{12} deficiency can cause paresthesia and subacute combined nerve degeneration. It can also cause glossitis, hair and nail changes, and skin hyperpigmentation.

You should remember

Lifelong treatment for patients with confirmed pernicious anemia begins with an intramuscular injection of 1000 μg of B_{12} daily or every other day for 1–2 weeks, followed by weekly injections for 1–2 months, and then a monthly injection (cyanocobalamin) or every 2–3 months.

Key Terms

Bone marrow
Endothelial cells
Erythrocytes
Fibroblasts
Hematopoiesis
Hematopoietic growth factors
Hemosiderosis
Intrinsic factor
Leukocytes
Macrocytic
Metabolic acidosis
Metabolic encephalopathy
Microcytic
Normocytic
Pernicious anemia
Pulmonary edema
Proliferation
Thrombocytes

Clinical Case Studies

Clinical Case Study 1

A 36-year-old male was evaluated for microcytic anemia, a subtype of iron deficiency anemia. He was given oral iron supplementation. However, after 2 months, no significant improvement was shown, so intravenous iron supplementation was given, and the improvement was substantial. The patient has two cousins with iron deficiency anemia that was diagnosed early in their lives, and they also benefited from intermittent IV infusions of iron.

Critical Thinking Questions

1. How does iron deficiency anemia occur?
2. How can iron deficiency anemia be diagnosed?
3. What is the primary mechanism of action of ferrous sulfate?

Clinical Case Study 2

A 21-year-old female on a vegetarian diet visited her physician with severe macrocytic anemia, low Hb, leukopenia, thrombocytopenia, and splenomegaly. Laboratory data revealed severe vitamin B_{12} deficiency. The patient reported increased well-being following cobalamin replacement therapy, including restored appetite and weight gain.

Critical Thinking Questions

1. What are the causes and symptoms of pernicious anemia?
2. What are the clinical indications of cyanocobalamin?
3. What are the adverse effects of cyanocobalamin?

Further Reading

[1] A. Al Mosawi, Hypoparathyroidism, Vitiligo, Poliosis, and Macrocytic Anemia Syndrome, Lap Lambert Academic Publishing, 2019.
[2] L. Arpilor, Pernicious Anemia Symptoms—Learn About the Symptoms of Pernicious Anemia, from Fatigue to Pale Skin. Discover Potential Signs and the Implications of Vitamin B12 Deficiency, Arpilor, 2023.
[3] H.F. Bunn, J.C. Aster, Pathophysiology of Blood Disorders, second ed., McGraw-Hill / Medical, 2016.
[4] S. Eugenia, Iron Deficiency Anemia—Comprehensive Insights, Interventions, and Future Frontiers (Medical Care and Health), Eugenia, 2023.
[5] T. Grayson, Understanding Iron Deficiency Anemia—A Unique Guide to Understanding the Symptoms, Diagnosis, Treatment of Iron Deficiency Anemia with Medical and Alternative Forms of Treatment, Grayson, 2021.
[6] M. Hooper, What you Need to Know About Pernicious Anemia and Vitamin B_{12} Deficiency, Hammersmith Health Books, 2015.
[7] M. Hooper, Pernicious Anemia—The Forgotten Disease—The Causes and Consequences of Vitamin B_{12} Deficiency, Hammersmith Health Books, 2012.
[8] R. Jean, Blood Disorders—the complete guide on blood disorders causes, symptoms, Treatment and Remedies for your Complete Wellness, Jean, 2022.
[9] K.W. Jeon, International Review of Cell and Molecular Biology, Academic Press, 2011.
[10] N. Maheshwari, Clinical Pathology Hematology and Blood Banking, third ed., Jaypee, 2018.
[11] D.W. McCandless, Metabolic Encephalopathy, Springer, 2010.
[12] A. Meselson, The Complete Guide on Anemia—Learn Anemia Symptoms, Causes, and Treatments, Meselson, 2013.
[13] M. Pratt, Anemia—Clinical Aspects, American Medical Publishers, 2022.

CHAPTER

32

Drugs used in coagulation disorders

OUTLINE

LEARNING OUTCOMES

After study of the chapter, readers should be able to:

1. Explain the various coagulation disorders.
2. Identify the most common cause of pulmonary embolism.
3. Explain the complications of atrial fibrillation.

https://doi.org/10.1016/B978-0-443-29038-1.00032-4

4. Describe the mechanism of action of warfarin.
5. Explain the newest direct thrombin inhibitors and their contraindications.
6. Describe the clinical indications of low-molecular-weight heparins.
7. Explain the adverse effects of factor Xa inhibitors.
8. Describe the indications of antiplatelet drugs.
9. Identify the modifiable risk factors for intermittent claudication.
10. List thrombolytic agents available in the market.

Overview

A blood clotting disorder causes blood to form clots too quickly or inappropriately. This condition is also referred to as a hypercoagulable state or thrombophilia. Anticoagulation therapy prevents and treats blood clots associated with many disease states, surgeries, and medical conditions that perturb blood coagulation. Thrombolytics, or clot-dissolving drugs, can break up clots, reestablish blood flow to the heart, brain, lungs, and other organs, and prevent organ damage. Thrombolytics can be used acutely to stop a heart attack or stroke that would otherwise be potentially deadly if the clot were to remain, blocking blood flow. The ultimate goal of anticoagulant use is to prevent venous thromboembolic events or blood clots. In the United States, as many as 300,000–600,000 people are diagnosed annually with deep vein thrombosis (DVT) or a pulmonary embolism (PE). Within that population, it is estimated that as many as 100,000 may die as a result of a coagulation problem. Atrial fibrillation (AF) is the most common heart arrhythmia associated with coagulopathies, and it has been identified as the most significant independent risk factor for stroke. Stroke, the leading cause of death in the United States, costs an estimated 38.6 billion dollars per year in healthcare services, medications, and missed days from work.

Coagulation disorders

Coagulation disorders are conditions that affect the blood's ability to clot. These disorders include **hemophilia**, clotting factor deficiencies, **von Willebrand disease**, hypercoagulable states, and deep venous thrombosis (VTE). The complications of **thrombosis** may include PE, stroke, AF, and heart damage that necessitates heart valve replacements. Hypercoagulable states are genetic or acquired conditions. For congenital forms, there is a greater tendency for an individual to form blood clots. Acquired coagulation conditions are usually a result of surgery, trauma, medications, or a medical condition that increases the risk of developing clots. Blood clots can form in arteries (arterial clots) or veins (venous clots).

Deep vein thrombosis

DVT occurs when a **thrombus** forms in the body's deep veins. These clots usually develop in the lower leg, thigh, or pelvis but can also occur in the arm. DVT can happen to any individual and can cause serious illness, disability, and death. The good news is that DVT is preventable and treatable if discovered early. When the blood clot breaks off within the vein wall, it may travel through the circulation and settle in a lung, resulting in a PE. Approximately 50% of patients who have a DVT will have long-term complications caused by the damage the clot does to the valves in the vein, called **postthrombotic syndrome**. People with **postthrombotic syndrome** have symptoms such as swelling, pain, discoloration, and ulcers in the affected part of the body.

In some cases, the DVT symptoms can be so severe that the patient becomes physically disabled. About half of the people with DVT are asymptomatic, however. The most common symptoms of DVT include localized swelling, pain, and redness of the skin.

Pulmonary embolism

An embolus is a blood clot that forms in a blood vessel, breaks away, and travels to another location, such as the lung, in which case, this is a **PE**. An embolus can block the blood supply to a particular organ or create an **embolism**. Blood clots that cause pulmonary emboli may be due to slowed blood flow, an abnormality in coagulation, or an injury to the blood vessel wall. However, DVT is the most common cause of PE. Other less frequent sources of pulmonary emboli are a **fat embolus,** amniotic fluid embolus, air bubbles, and DVT in the upper body. Clots may also form on the end of an indwelling intravenous (IV) catheter, break off, and travel to the lungs.

Risk factors for PE include a family history of blood clotting disorders, surgery or injury (especially to the legs), extended bed rest, flying or riding long distances, paralysis, older age, obesity, cigarette smoking, cancer therapy, and oral contraceptives. Along with a complete medical history and physical exam, tests for a PE may include chest X-ray, CT scan, electrocardiogram, duplex ultrasound, and pulmonary angiogram, which must be done to diagnose PE. Treatment for PE includes anticoagulants, fibrinolytic therapy, **vena cava filter, pulmonary embolectomy,** and percutaneous thrombectomy.

Stroke

An **ischemic stroke** is caused by a blockage cutting off the blood supply to the brain. A **hemorrhagic stroke** is caused by bleeding in or around the brain. A transient ischemic attack (TIA) is also known as a ministroke. The bleeding can result in pressure on brain cells and damage them. About 90% of strokes involve ischemic stroke. A stroke or cerebrovascular accident is a medical emergency. Fewer Americans die now from stroke than they did even several years ago, possibly due to increased awareness and better control of certain risk factors. Age is the most critical risk factor. While males have a higher age-adjusted incidence of stroke overall, women have a higher lifetime risk. Because females live longer, they are older at the time of onset. Consequently, 55,000 more females suffer strokes in the US each year.

The risk factors for stroke include hypertension, obesity, poor diet, physical inactivity, and smoking. Other risk factors are based on lifestyle, genetics, and environment, including age, sex, race and ethnicity, stress, family history, sleep apnea, unhealthy lifestyle habits, **rheumatoid arthritis**, and lupus erythematosus.

Atrial fibrillation

AF is characterized by rapid, disorganized contraction of the atria. The term fibrillation means contracting very fast and irregularly. Normally blood empties from the atria into the ventricles. AF can lead to blood clots in the heart, which increases the risk of stroke, heart failure, and other heart-related complications. It is estimated that about 12 million people in the United States will have AF by 2030. People of European descent are more likely to have AF than African Americans. Because the number of AF cases increases with age and females generally live longer than males, more females than males experience AF. The risk factors for AF include advancing age, obesity, hypertension, diabetes, heart failure, ischemic heart disease, chronic kidney disease, smoking, and hyperthyroidism.

Heart valve replacements

The mitral and tricuspid valves move blood from the atria to the ventricles. The other two valves, the aortic and pulmonary valves, carry blood to the lungs and the rest of the body through the ventricles. A valve replacement is required if it becomes narrowed or leaks. The aortic and mitral valves are the most commonly replaced. Pulmonary and tricuspid valve replacements are relatively uncommon. However, the risk of developing a blood clot is possible after replacing the aortic or mitral valve.

Anticoagulants

Anticoagulants come in many dosage forms, including injections, IV drugs, or oral medications. They are used to treat DVT, PE, AF, angina, and heart attack and to reduce the risks of stroke. They may be divided into four main groups: heparins, warfarin, direct thrombin inhibitors, and **factor Xa inhibitors**. The three main anticoagulant medications are vitamin K antagonists, direct oral anticoagulants, and low-molecular-weight heparins (LMWHs). **Table 32.1** summarizes the anticoagulants used in the United States.

Warfarin

Warfarin (Coumadin) is an oral anticoagulant commonly used to treat and prevent blood clots. It is the most widely prescribed outpatient anticoagulant. For over 50 years, this agent was the only available oral anticoagulant on the market. Warfarin limits the body's ability to form blood clots by inhibiting the production of vitamin K–dependent clotting factors.

Pharmacokinetics

Warfarin is easily and wholly absorbed, reaching a maximum plasma concentration between 2 and 6 hours. The onset of action is typically 24–72 h. A peak therapeutic effect is seen 5–7 days after initiation, and the drug is hepatically metabolized, primarily through the CYP2C9 enzyme. The half-life of warfarin is generally 20–60 hours. However, it is highly variable among individuals. Warfarin is eliminated mainly as metabolites by glomerular filtration in the kidney (92% via urine).

Mechanism of action

Warfarin competitively inhibits the vitamin K epoxide reductase complex 1, an essential enzyme for activating the vitamin K available in the body. This mechanism can deplete functional vitamin K reserves, thereby reducing the synthesis of active clotting factors. The hepatic synthesis of coagulation factors II, VII, IX, and X, as well as coagulation regulatory factors protein C and protein S, requires the presence of vitamin K.

Clinical indications

Warfarin is used to prevent and treat VTE arising from pulmonary emboli. It is also indicated for the prevention and treatment of thromboembolic complications from AF or cardiac valve replacement.

Contraindications

Warfarin is contraindicated for patients with hypersensitivity to the drug, hemorrhagic tendencies, and recent or contemplated surgery of the eye, central nervous system, or traumatic surgery resulting in large open surfaces. Elderly patients are at an increased risk of bleeding complications secondary to falls, concomitant drug interactions, cognitive status, and living situations.

TABLE 32.1 Common anticoagulants used in the United States.

Generic name	Brand name	Route of administration	Dosage forms
warfarin	Coumadin, Jantoven	Oral	Tablet
dabigatran	Pradaxa	Oral	Capsules
rivaroxaban	Xarelto	Oral	Tablet
apixaban	Eliquis	Oral	Tablet
enoxaparin	Lovenox	Subcutaneous, intravenous	Injectable solution
dalteparin	Fragmin	Subcutaneous, intravenous	Injectable solution
tinzaparin	Innohep	Subcutaneous, intravenous	Injectable solution
fondaparinux	Arixtra	Subcutaneous	Injectable solution
heparin	Hep Flush-10	Subcutaneous, intravenous	Injectable solution
bivalirudin	Angiomax	Intravenous	Injectable solution (once reconstituted)
desirudin	Iprivask	Subcutaneous	Injectable solution
argatroban	Argatroban, Acova	Intravenous	Injectable solution

Adverse effects

Serious adverse effects of warfarin include bleeding. A significant hemorrhage (e.g., intracranial hemorrhage), GI bleeding, hematemesis, intraocular bleeding, and **hemarthrosis** can occur. The risk of bleeding and hemorrhage is dependent on multiple variables, including the intensity of anticoagulation and patient susceptibility. Other adverse effects include nausea, vomiting, abdominal pain, bloating, flatulence, and an altered sense of taste.

Toxicities

Warfarin toxicity is assessable through signs and symptoms of bleeding. The initial step would be to discontinue warfarin and then administer vitamin K (phytonadione). Vitamin K may be administered via the oral, IV, or subcutaneous route. However, the initial administration of oral vitamin K is often preferable in patients without significant bleeding. Administering agents such as prothrombin complex concentrate, fresh frozen plasma, and activated factor VII may be considered for cases of significant bleeding.

You should remember

Warfarin has two different pregnancy categories depending on the presence of a mechanical heart valve. Warfarin was listed as a category D drug for pregnant females with an automatic heart valve and category X for all other indications in pregnant females. Warfarin crosses the placental barrier, reaching fetal plasma concentrations similar to maternal values. Warfarin can cause bleeding in the fetus, and use during pregnancy is commonly associated with spontaneous abortion, **stillbirth**, preterm birth, and neonatal death. It should be avoided during the first trimester and close to delivery.

Direct thrombin inhibitors

Dabigatran, rivaroxaban, and apixaban are the newest anticoagulants approved by the FDA in the United States. Each drug prevents blood clots by inhibiting one clotting factor. These new agents offer several advantages over warfarin. They produce a predictable effect: when given in fixed doses, drug interactions are significantly less common, dietary interactions are nonexistent, and routine laboratory monitoring is unnecessary. Rivaroxaban was the first oral factor Xa inhibitor in the US market. This agent has multiple approved indications: reducing the risk of stroke in AF patients, DVT and PE treatment and secondary preventions, and specifically, preventing VTE events in patients recently having knee and hip replacements. Apixaban has been classified as an oral factor Xa inhibitor and is approved for patients with AF to prevent stroke and systemic VTE events.

Pharmacokinetics

Dabigatran reversibly inhibits thrombin, the critical enzyme in the coagulation cascade. Peak plasma concentrations of dabigatran are reached approximately 2 hours after oral administration. Excretion is predominantly via the renal route as an unchanged drug. CYP450 isoenzymes do not metabolize dabigatran. The minor differences in dabigatran pharmacokinetics associated with age and gender are attributed to variations in renal function. The peak plasma concentrations of dabigatran are reached approximately 2 hours after oral administration. The elimination half-life is 12–14 hours, with clearance predominantly occurring via renal excretion of unchanged drug.

Mechanism of action

Dabigatran reversibly binds to the active site on the thrombin molecule, preventing thrombin-mediated activation of coagulation factors. It may have less of an antagonistic effect on thrombin-mediated platelet aggregation. Furthermore, dabigatran can inactivate thrombin even when fibrin bound; it reduces thrombin-mediated inhibition of fibrinolysis and may even enhance fibrinolysis.

Clinical indications

Direct thrombin inhibitors are used for treatment or prevention of acute coronary syndrome, blood clots in the heart due to AF, heparin-induced thrombocytopenia (HIT), and VTE. They are a novel class of drugs that have been developed as an effective alternative mode of anticoagulation, especially in patients who suffer from HIT or who require dialysis or cardiopulmonary bypass and for the management of thromboembolic disorders.

Contraindications

Direct thrombin inhibitors are contraindicated in severe renal impairment or hemodialysis, hypersensitivity, impairment of hemostasis, active pathologic bleeding, and mechanical prosthetic heart valves.

Adverse effects

Common adverse effects of dabigatran include life-threatening bleeding, bruising, indigestion, abdominal pain, diarrhea, and hypersensitivity. Some other side effects include swelling, headache, dizziness, pain in the arms and legs, and itching.

Toxicities

Accidental or intentional overdose or accumulation of dabigatran due to renal impairment may lead to hemorrhagic complications. There is no antidote for dabigatran, unlike warfarin and heparin.

Heparin

Unfractionated heparin (UH) is a naturally occurring anticoagulant released from mast cells. It binds reversibly to antithrombin III (ATIII) and greatly accelerates the rate at which ATIII inactivates coagulation enzymes thrombin (factor IIa) and factor Xa. UH is different from LMWH in the following ways: the average molecular weight of LMWH is about 4.5 kDa, whereas it is 15 kDa for UH; UH requires continuous infusions; activated **partial prothrombin time** monitoring is required when using UH; and UH has a higher risk of bleeding and osteoporosis in long-term use. UH is more specific than LMWH for thrombin. Furthermore, the effects of UH can typically be reversed using protamine sulfate. Several examples include heparin, bivalirudin, desirudin, and argatroban.

Low-molecular-weight heparins

LMWHs comprise a class of antithrombotic medications headed by UH. They have moved to the forefront and replaced the routine use of heparin to prevent and treat VTE events, mainly due to improved drug properties and ease of use. As with all forms of anticoagulant therapy, correct dosing of LMWHs is essential for achieving the optimal balance between effectiveness and bleeding risk. However, due to the differences among LMWHs, equivalent doses within the class have yet to be established; thus substituting one product for another is not recommended. Some examples of LMWHs include enoxaparin, dalteparin, tinzaparin, and fondaparinux.

Enoxaparin has the broadest range of FDA-approved indications and is used most often. The advantage of enoxaparin over other LMWHs is that this medication has been studied in two additional populations: pediatric and pregnant patients. Dosing adjustments are recommended for patients with kidney impairment and obese patients. This drug is administered IV and subcutaneously. Patients can be taught how to give subcutaneous injections of enoxaparin at home. This is usually done before and after surgical procedures. Some possible side effects associated with enoxaparin use include confusion, nausea, diarrhea, and fever. In addition, injection site reactions such as irritation and pain.

Dalteparin has been approved for the long-term secondary prevention of VTE in patients with prior VTE and a history of cancer. It also has fixed dosing for specific indications for DVT prophylaxis and dosing recommendations considering the patient's body weight subcutaneously daily for VTE extended treatment in cancer patients. Dalteparin should not be used in certain patients with kidney or liver disease. Some possible side effects associated with dalteparin use include injection-site reactions such as irritation, pain, and bruising. Tinzaparin has the fewest FDA-approved indications. A labeling revision in 2008 created an age criterion. Patients 90 years or older are not to use this agent under any circumstance. The smaller number of indications and the maximum age criteria outlined by the drug manufacturer may explain why it is used infrequently in the United States today. However, when used, tinzaparin can be given IV or subcutaneously. Also, dosing may be fixed or variable depending on patient-specific characteristics. Some of the reported side effects of this medication include chest pain and rashes.

Pharmacokinetics

LMWH administration is via subcutaneous injection. Compared to heparin, LMWHs have a longer half-life, so dosing is more predictable and can be less frequent.

Mechanism of action

LMWHs are anticoagulants acting by inhibition of the final common pathway of the coagulation cascade. The last common pathway is the conversion of fibrinogen into fibrin by thrombin activity (see **Fig. 32.1**). They inhibit coagulation by activating ATIII. ATIII binds to and inhibits factor Xa. Heparin works similarly by binding ATIII and activating it. Heparin also has a binding site for thrombin so that thrombin can interact with ATIII and heparin, thus inhibiting coagulation. Heparin has a faster onset of anticoagulant action, as it will hinder factor Xa and thrombin, while LMWH inhibits only factor Xa.

Clinical indications

LMWHs are used in the prophylaxis of VTE on acute or elective admission to the hospital, and they are employed in the treatment of DVT and PE.

Contraindications

LMWHs are contraindicated in patients who have peptic ulcer disease, severe hypertension, recent stroke, and recent eye surgery. As LMWHs are self-administered, it is essential to consider dosing in cases of chronic kidney disease, where there is a risk of accumulation and thus higher chances of problematic bleeding.

Adverse effects

LMWH is an anticoagulant, so its main risk is bleeding. Treatment of bleeding associated with LMWH involves stopping the drug and administering protamine sulfate. This vital half-life protein forms a solid bond with the heparin, producing an inactive complex. Other less common adverse effects include HIT, osteoporosis, spontaneous fractures, hypoaldosteronism, and hypersensitivity reactions. In assessing the need for anticoagulant medication, a risk-benefit analysis must be performed to determine the risks posed by bleeding versus the risks of clotting.

Toxicities

Overdose is unpredictable and may develop insidiously in deep tissues such as retroperitoneal and intramuscular spaces. Protamine sulfate partially reverses the anticoagulant effect of LMWH and may prevent bleeding from an LMWH overdose.

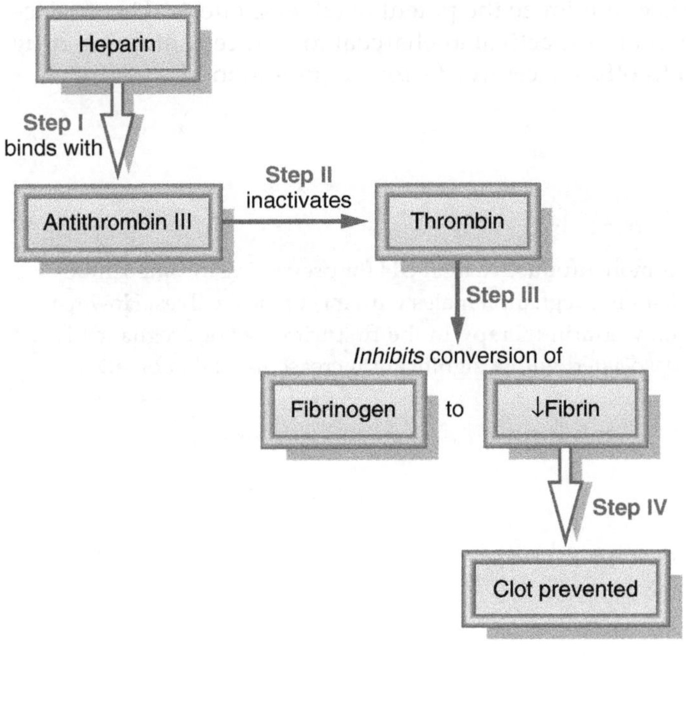

FIG. 32.1 Mechanism of action of the anticoagulant heparin.

Factor Xa inhibitors

Fondaparinux is the only injectable factor Xa inhibitor available and is used for many FDA-approved indications. However, fondaparinux's unique use is for patients allergic to heparin, LMWH, or HIT. This, however, is not an FDA-approved indication. Patients can use this product at home to prevent or treat VTE. Possible side effects of fondaparinux are fever, swelling, rash, insomnia, dyspepsia, and injection site reactions such as pain, bruising, and redness.

Pharmacokinetics

Apixaban is rapidly absorbed, with maximum concentration occurring 3–4 hours after oral administration, and has a half-life of approximately 12 hours. Elimination occurs via multiple pathways, including metabolism, biliary excretion, and direct intestinal excretion, with about 27% of total apixaban clearance occurring via renal excretion. The pharmacokinetics of apixaban are consistent across a broad range of patients, and apixaban has limited clinically relevant interactions with most commonly prescribed medications, allowing for fixed doses without the need for therapeutic drug monitoring.

Mechanism of Action

Fondaparinux exhibits antithrombotic activity resulting from ATIII-mediated selective inhibition of factor Xa. By selectively binding to ATIII, fondaparinux activates ATIII's innate neutralization of factor Xa. This neutralization interrupts the blood coagulation cascade and thus inhibits thrombin formation and thrombus development.

Clinical Indications

Fondaparinux is an anticoagulant to prevent venous thromboembolism, treat DVT, and improve survival following myocardial infarction. It is a synthetic, short molecule shaped like heparin. Apixaban is used in several thromboembolic disorders, including reduction of stroke risk in nonvalvular AF, thromboprophylaxis following hip or knee replacement surgery, the treatment of DVT or PE, and prevention of recurrent DVT and PE.

Contraindications

Direct Xa inhibitors are contraindicated in patients who have an allergy to these medications or are at high risk of bleeding.

Adverse effects

The adverse effects of fondaparinux include mild injection site reactions, anemia, skin rash, edema, nausea, vomiting, insomnia, constipation, skin rash, and fever.

Toxicities

The immediate response to an accidental drug overdose is to minimize the potential adverse effects. The absence of an approved rivaroxaban antidote left two possible interventions: activated charcoal to reduce continuing drug absorption and prothrombin complex concentrate infusion to offset excessive factor Xa inhibition.

You should remember

Anticoagulants are indicated in pregnancy for the treatment of acute VTE, valvular heart disease, and pregnancy-related complications in females with antiphospholipid antibody syndrome, antithrombin deficiency, or other thrombophilias when there has been a prior VTE. Warfarin is more productive than UH for preventing thromboembolism in pregnant females with mechanical valves. However, warfarin therapy in the first trimester of pregnancy is associated with a significant increase in fetal anomalies.

You should remember

Heparin is the anticoagulant of choice for pediatric patients. Dosing differs in children compared to adults, as pediatric patients have different physiological characteristics that influence the activity of heparin. When selecting a product for this population, preservative-free products are essential for neonates and infants.

You should remember

When protamine is given to reverse the effects of heparin, the neutralization begins about 5 minutes after administration. The protamine dose is determined by the amount of heparin received. One milligram of protamine is needed for every ~100 units of heparin received, with a maximum dose of 50 mg of protamine.

Antiplatelet drugs

Platelets, or **thrombocytes**, are small, colorless cell fragments in the blood that form clots and stop or prevent bleeding. Antiplatelet drugs are medications that prevent blood clots from developing. They work by blocking the platelets from sticking together. A platelet count that falls below the lower limit of normal, 150,000/μL (for adults), is called thrombocytopenia—the risks associated with thrombocytopenia range from no risk to bleeding risks and thrombosis. Spontaneous bleeding can occur with a platelet count under 10,000/μL and surgical bleeding with counts below 50,000/μL. Aspirin was the first antiplatelet medication and is a cyclooxygenase inhibitor. Other oral antiplatelet include clopidogrel (Plavix), ticagrelor (Brilinta), prasugrel (Effient), dipyridamole/aspirin (Aggrenox), and eptifibatide (Integrilin).

Pharmacokinetics

Aspirin is rapidly absorbed in the stomach and upper intestine. Plasma levels peak 30–40 minutes after aspirin ingestion, and inhibition of platelet function is evident within 1 hour. The oral bioavailability of regular aspirin tablets is about 40%–50% over a wide range of doses. A considerably lower bioavailability for enteric-coated tablets and sustained-release, microencapsulated preparations has been reported.

Mechanism of action

Antiplatelet drugs inhibit thrombus formation, which is believed to be how they exert their cardiovascular protective effect. Clopidogrel, a thienopyridine derivative, binds specifically and irreversibly to the platelet P2RY12 purinergic receptor, inhibiting adenosine diphosphate (ADP)–mediated platelet activation and aggregation. Similar to clopidogrel, ticagrelor also inhibits ADP receptors of subtype P2Y12. However, ticagrelor acts differently because it has a binding site unique to ADP, making its inhibition reversible.

Clinical indications

Antiplatelet drugs are used to reduce the risk of MI, stroke, or blood clots. Clopidogrel is superior to aspirin in reducing cardiovascular outcomes in patients with cardiovascular disease and provides additional benefits to patients with acute coronary syndromes already taking aspirin.

Contraindications

Antiplatelet drugs are contraindicated in patients with active pathological bleeding such as peptic ulcer or intracranial hemorrhage. The primary concern of ticagrelor plus aspirin is the higher risk of all bleeding events and severe to moderate bleeding events.

Adverse effects

Hematologic complications and bleeding have been the most feared outcome of antithrombotic and antiplatelet agents. Clopidogrel is considered to be a safer alternative to ticlopidine due to its decreased incidence of hematologic adverse effects. However, thrombotic thrombocytopenia purpura is the most reported hematologic adverse effect of clopidogrel, **neutropenia**, acquired hemophilia, isolated thrombocytopenia, and idiopathic immune thrombocytopenia.

Toxicities

Symptoms of overdose include vomiting, dyspnea, and GI bleeding. Clopidogrel is irreversibly bound to platelets for their lifetime, approximately 11 days. The toxicity of clopidogrel can be treated with platelet transfusions to restore clotting ability.

Drugs for intermittent claudication

Intermittent claudication (IC) typically refers to lower extremity skeletal muscle pain during exercise. IC presents when there is insufficient oxygen delivery to meet the metabolic requirements of the skeletal muscles. IC is a common manifestation of peripheral arterial disease, including atherosclerotic stenosis of the extremities' arteries. IC is commonly localized to the thigh, hip, buttock, and calf muscles. Pain within these muscle groups is reproducibly induced by walking and relieved with rest. However, IC is a symptom rather than a specific health condition. Modifiable risk factors include smoking, hypertension, dyslipidemia, obesity, metabolic syndrome, and diabetes mellitus. Nonmodifiable risk factors include age, male gender, family history, and congenital predisposition. Treatments focus on lowering the risks of vascular disease, reducing pain, increasing mobility, and preventing tissue damage. Two drugs (cilostazol and pentoxifylline) are approved for the treatment of IC. These medications improve the flow of blood through the blood vessels. They reduce leg pain caused by poor circulation.

Thrombolytics

Thrombolytics or fibrinolytics are medications in the plasminogen activator class used to manage and treat dissolving intravascular clots.

Currently, available thrombolytic agents include the following:

- **Alteplase (tPA):** This is often the top choice for strokes, PEs, and cardiovascular cases. It rarely causes allergic reactions.
- **Anistreplase:** It can work throughout the body because it targets all plasminogens, not just those attached to fibrin.
- **Prourokinase:** Researchers are testing this new drug. It has to be converted to urokinase to work.
- **Reteplase:** This works faster than other thrombolytics.
- **Streptokinase:** This is used the most globally but less frequently in the United States. It is cheaper than others, but many people have allergic reactions. Similar to anistreplase, it can affect the entire body.
- **Tenecteplase:** This works efficiently and is a frequent choice of many providers in North America and Europe. It also has a more negligible bleeding risk.
- **Urokinase:** Healthcare providers may choose this for peripheral vascular clots (in the legs) and catheters with clots. Many providers outside the United States prefer this because it is cheaper than other thrombolytic drugs.

Pharmacokinetics

tPA and saruplase have relatively short half-lives and are high-clearance compounds. Their clearance is dependent upon hepatic blood flow. This is relevant, as myocardial function strongly influences liver blood flow and the clearance of tPA and saruplase. The clearance of reteplase is less dependent upon liver blood flow and is partly reliant on renal excretion.

Mechanism of action

Thrombolytic agents actively dissolve fibrin clots that have already formed. Exogenous plasminogen activators such as streptokinase and urokinase dissolve a thrombus and affect circulating plasminogen, leading to decreased plasminogen and fibrin.

Clinical indications

Thrombolytic therapy can include medications to destroy or prevent new blood clots from forming. They are used for acute myocardial infarction, DVT, PE, acute ischemic stroke, acute peripheral arterial occlusion, occlusion of indwelling catheters, and intracardiac thrombus formation.

Contraindications

Thrombolytic agents are contraindicated in patients with recent intracranial hemorrhage, aortic dissection, intracranial neoplasm, bleeding **diathesis**, recent surgery, and significant head injury.

Adverse effects

The adverse effects of thrombolytic drugs include major bleeding in the brain, severe hypertension, kidney disease, internal bleeding, and damage to the blood vessels. The main risk of thrombolytic therapy is internal bleeding. About 5% of people who have thrombolytic therapy have significant bleeds, and approximately 1% have brain bleeds that cause a stroke.

Hemophilia

Hemophilia is an inherited bleeding disorder in which the blood does not clot properly. This can lead to spontaneous bleeding as well as bleeding after injuries or surgery. Hemophilia occurs when a clotting factor is missing or when the abundance of the clotting factor is low. Reduced clotting factors are congenital hemophilia, most commonly hemophilia A, associated with low factor VIII. The next most common type, hemophilia B, is associated with low factor IX. Some people develop hemophilia with no family history of the disorder, and they acquire hemophilia. During acquired hemophilia, the immune system attacks clotting factor VIII or IX in the blood. This can be associated with autoimmune conditions, pregnancy, cancer, or due to drug reactions.

Hemophilia almost always occurs in boys and is genetically passed from mother to son. Most females with defective coagulation factor genes are carriers who have no signs or symptoms of hemophilia. However, some carriers can have bleeding symptoms if their clotting factors decrease moderately.

Signs and symptoms of hemophilia vary, depending on clotting factors. For instance, a patient might bleed only after surgery or trauma if clotting factors are mildly reduced. The best way to treat hemophilia is to replace the missing blood clotting factor so the blood can clot properly. This is typically done IV by injecting treatment products or clotting factor concentrates. Replacements for clotting factors can be sourced from donated blood. Similar products, recombinant clotting factors, are made in a laboratory and not from human blood. Other therapies include **desmopressin,** emicizumab (Hemlibra), fibrin sealants, and antifibrinolytics.

You should remember

For people with a family history of hemophilia, genetic testing might be used to identify carriers to help people make informed decisions about becoming pregnant.

Key Terms

Atrial fibrillation
Diathesis
Embolism
Factor Xa inhibitors

Fat embolus
Hemarthrosis
Hemophilia
Hemorrhagic stroke
Intermittent claudication
Ischemic stroke
Partial prothrombin time
Pulmonary embolectomy
Pulmonary embolism
Rheumatoid arthritis
Thrombolytics
Thrombosis
Thrombus
Vena cava filter
Von Willebrand disease

Clinical Case Studies

Clinical Case Study 1

A 32-year-old African-American male with no significant past medical history presented to the emergency department with severe left leg pain and swelling of a 2-week duration and a nonproductive cough with dyspnea for the past 3 days. At the time of admission, vital signs were remarkable for mild tachycardia. The left calf was swollen and tender compared with the right calf. A duplex scan was positive for acute DVT in the left proximal femoral and posterior tibial veins. CT pulmonary angiography was performed immediately, showing bilateral extensive pulmonary emboli.

Critical Thinking Questions

1. What are the causes and risk factors of PE?
2. What is the diagnosis of PE?
3. What are the treatments for PE?

Clinical Case Study 2

An 86-year-old male presented with fatigue and weakness along with a 3-week history of dark brown–colored stools. He was recently admitted to the hospital, where he was found to be in AF and diagnosed with nonischemic cardiomyopathy. He was placed on rivaroxaban (Xarelto), one of the newer anticoagulants, as a preventative measure due to his AF. His past medical history included hypertension, type 2 diabetes mellitus, mild aortic stenosis, hematuria, and arteriovenous malformations in the GI tract.

Critical Thinking Questions

1. Which newer drugs are classified as direct thrombin inhibitors?
2. What are the clinical indications of direct thrombin inhibitors?
3. What are the contraindications of direct thrombin inhibitors?

Further Reading

[1] J.P. Antovic, M. Blomback, Essential Guide to Blood Coagulation, second ed., Wiley-Blackwell, 2013.
[2] T.G. DeLoughery, Hemostasis and Thrombosis, fourth ed., Springer, 2019.
[3] A. Dorgalaleh, Congenital Bleeding Disorders – Diagnosis and Management, second ed., Springer, 2023.
[4] E.J. Favaloro, G. Lippi, Hemostasis and Thrombosis – Methods and Protocols (Methods in Molecular Biology, 1646), Humana Press, 2017.
[5] S.H. Goodnight Jr., W.E. Hathway, Disorders of Hemostasis and Thrombosis: A Clinical Guide, second ed., McGraw-Hill / Medical, 2000.
[6] D. Green, H.C. Kwaan, Coagulation in Cancer (Cancer Treatment and Research, 148), Springer, 2009.
[7] V. Hach-Wunderle, P.P. Nawroth, Life-Threatening Coagulation Disorders in Critical Care Medicine, Springer, 2012.
[8] S.D. Hudnall, Hematology – A Pathophysiologic Approach (Physiology Series / Physiology Monograph), second ed., Mosby / Elsevier, 2023.
[9] A. Ibrahim, H. El-Sanhoty, S. El-Sayed, Coagulopathy in Chronic Liver Diseases – Impact of Liver Diseases in Coagulation Disorders, Lap Lambert Academic Publishing, 2012.
[10] D.M. Kamat, M. Frei-Jones, Benign Hematologic Disorders in Children – A Clinical Guide, Springer, 2021.
[11] K. Kaushansky, M. Levi, Williams Hematology – Hemostasis and Thrombosis, McGraw-Hill, 2017.
[12] S. Kitchen, J.D. Olson, F.E. Preston, Quality in Laboratory Hemostasis and Thrombosis, second ed., Wiley-Blackwell, 2013.
[13] M. Laposata, Coagulation Disorders: Quality in Laboratory Diagnosis (Diagnostic Standards of Care), Demos Medical, 2011.
[14] A. Lichtin, J. Bartholomew, The Coagulation Consult – A Case-based Guide, Springer, 2014.

[15] V.J. Marder, W.C. Aird, J.S. Bennett, S. Schulman, G.C. White III, Hemostasis and Thrombosis – Basic Principles and Clinical Practice, Wolters Kluwer / Lippincott, Williams, and Wilkins, 2012.
[16] A. Saleh, Drugs for Coagulation Disorders, Saleh, 2020.
[17] A.M. Taloyan, D.S. Bankiewicz, Coagulation: Kinetics, Structure Formation and Disorders (Recent Advances in Hematology Research), Nova Biomedical, 2012.
[18] A. Wahed, A. Quesada, A. Dasgupta, Hematology and Coagulation: A Comprehensive Review for Board Preparation, Certification and Clinical Practice, second ed., Elsevier, 2019.
[19] M.A. Weiner, D.J. Yamashiro, P. Satwani, M. Bhatia, C. Neunert, Pediatric Hematology and Oncology Secrets, second ed., Elsevier, 2023.

CHAPTER

33

Drugs used in heart failure

OUTLINE

LEARNING OUTCOMES

After study of the chapter, readers should be able to:

1. Describe the etiology and risk factors of heart failure.
2. Explain the pathophysiology of heart failure.
3. Describe the clinical manifestations of heart failure.
4. Describe the cornerstone medications to treat heart failure.
5. Explain the four heart failure stages.
6. Describe the side effects of ACE inhibitors.
7. Explain the medication therapy for heart failure.
8. Discuss the pharmacokinetics of digoxin.
9. Describe common adverse effects of digoxin.
10. Explain the toxicity of digoxin.

Overview

Heart failure (HF) is a common disease affecting more than 5.7 million Americans older than 21 years of age. The prevalence of HF is increasing and is estimated to affect more than 8 million people older than 18 years of age by 2030. There are currently 870,000 new patients diagnosed with HF every year. At 40 years of age, males and females

https://doi.org/10.1016/B978-0-443-29038-1.00033-6

have a one in five risk of developing HF over their lifetime. The risk of HF increases with age and is more common after the age of 65 years. Gender plays a role in the time of HF onset, and HF is more common in males under the age of 80 years, but after the age of 80 years, more females have HF. The increasing number of HF patients makes it likely that pharmacy technicians will come into contact with these patients regardless of their practice setting (hospital, retail, or specialty). Seven groups of drugs indicated for HF will be discussed in this chapter.

Etiology and risk factors

Unhealthy diets, smoking, using cocaine or other illegal drugs, heavy alcohol use, and lack of physical activity increase the risk of HF. Heart or blood vessel conditions, severe lung disease, or infections such as HIV or SARS-CoV-2 raise the risks. Cardiomyopathy, coronary artery disease, hypertension, myocardial infarction (MI), arrhythmia, diabetes, kidney disease, obesity, or valve abnormalities are also risk factors for HF.

Pathophysiology

When HF starts, there is initially a drop in the blood volume pumped by the heart (specifically the left ventricle), which can be caused by damage (such as a heart attack) or decreased heart filling. The blood pumped by the heart is measured in liters/minute, which is cardiac output (CO). Cardiac standard production is between 5 and 6 L/minute and is higher for males than females. Another critical measure of heart function is the **ejection fraction** (EF). The EF is determined by dividing the amount of blood pumped out during contraction ("ejected" from the left ventricle) by the amount at the beginning of the heartbeat. A typical EF is more significant than 60% and is considered abnormal when below 40%.

As a patient's heart function declines, there is a complex interplay of the sympathetic nervous system (SNS) and multiple neurotransmitters. The SNS increases CO (makes the heart beat harder and faster), constricts blood vessels to increase blood pressure, and opens the lungs to take in more oxygen. Initially, this change is suitable for patients with HF, but over time, overstimulation of the SNS leads to worsening heart function and may cause dangerous heart rhythms and death. Neurotransmitters norepinephrine and epinephrine bind to beta-receptors in the heart, increasing heart rate and myocardium power. Over time, higher epinephrine and norepinephrine damage the heart muscle, worsening heart function. Also, overstimulation of the beta-receptors contributes to an abnormal heart rhythm, ventricular fibrillation, or sudden cardiac death, which is fatal. Thankfully, medications are available that inhibit the overactivation of the SNS and protect patients from these bad outcomes. The pathophysiology of HF is shown in **Fig. 33.1**.

You should remember

Age is a significant determinant of HF. Regardless of the cause or the definition used to classify patients with HF, the prevalence of HF increases steeply with age. The incidence of HF for males doubles with each 10-year age increase after the age of 65. HF has a 25% greater prevalence in Black patients compared to Caucasians, and metabolic risk factors and a sedentary lifestyle increase the risk of HF.

Clinical manifestations

Signs and symptoms of HF differ depending on the affected ventricle. Severe left ventricular failure may cause **pulmonary edema or cardiogenic shock**. The most common symptoms are dyspnea, **rales**, fatigue, and reflecting pulmonary congestion due to low CO. Dyspnea usually occurs during exertion and is relieved with rest. Worsening HF causes dyspnea at night, sometimes with a **nocturnal cough**. As the condition advances, orthopnea is common.

Right ventricular failure's most common symptoms are **pitting edema** and fatigue. There may be a sensation of fullness in the abdomen or neck. Jugular vein distention occurs as a later symptom of HF. **Hepatic congestion** can cause hepatomegaly and splenomegaly with **ascites**. Older people's symptoms may be atypical, including confusion, delirium, falls, incontinence, and sleep disturbances. General examination may detect systemic disorders that aggravate HF, such as anemia, alcoholism, **hemochromatosis**, and hyperthyroidism. Patients may appear dyspneic, **cyanoses**, hypotensive, confused, or agitated. Four HF stages are depicted below: A, B, C, and D.

Stage A
Stage A (pre-HF) means patients are at a high risk of developing HF because they have a family history of **congestive HF** or have one or more of these medical conditions, such as hypertension, diabetes, coronary artery disease, history of alcohol-use disorder, or history of rheumatic fever.
Stage B
Stage B (pre-HF) means the left ventricle is not working well and is structurally abnormal, but a patient has never had symptoms of HF.
Stage C
Patients with stage C HF have a congestive HF diagnosis and currently have or previously had signs and symptoms of the condition.
Stage D
Stage D (reduced EF) features advanced symptoms that do not improve with treatment. This is the final stage of HF.

You should remember

A comprehensive assessment is required when evaluating a patient with HF. This includes a complete blood analysis with iron measurements and a renal and liver panel. Patients may require further investigations after the basic serum biochemistries are completed, depending on the etiology and clinical stage.

Pharmacotherapy

HF is a complex chronic disease, and patients may be taking as many as seven different medications to control this disease. Thus it is essential to understand therapy goals to ensure the treatment achieves them. Medication therapy is the cornerstone of treatment for HF. Drugs known to improve HF but not overall survival include diuretics and digoxin.

HF treatment includes diet and lifestyle changes and pharmacotherapy to address the cause. Numerous classes of drugs, multidisciplinary care, and sometimes devices such as biventricular pacing or implantable cardioverter-defibrillators can be used. Treatment must be immediate for those with acute or worsening HF caused by disorders such as acute MI, atrial fibrillation with a very rapid ventricular rate, acute valvular regurgitation, severe hypertension, and pulmonary edema. Treatment is individualized based on the patient's short-term and long-term goals for existing symptoms.

Angiotensin-Converting Enzyme Inhibitors

The renin-angiotensin-aldosterone system plays a vital role in the disease process of HF. Increased angiotensin II and aldosterone cause elevations in blood pressure and "cardiac remodeling" long term. Angiotensin-converting enzyme (ACE) inhibitors block the formation of angiotensin II, which results in lower blood pressure and slows the progression of HF. In many different clinical studies, ACE inhibitors have been shown to increase survival and decrease hospitalizations for patients with New York Heart Association (NYHA)-FC II (mild), III (moderate), or IV (severe) HF symptoms. ACE inhibitors should be given to most patients early in the disease. These medications are started at low doses and titrated up at 2- to 4-week intervals to the "maximum tolerated dose" or the highest dose the patient can take without having side effects. Patients should not take ACE inhibitors if they have a severe side effect, **angioedema,** are pregnant, or plan to become pregnant. Other significant side effects include hypotension or dizziness (ACE inhibitors should be used cautiously if a patient's systolic blood pressure is less than 90 mm Hg). This medication class has also been shown to lower mortality .

Beta-adrenergic blockers

Many different beta-blockers are available, but only three of them have been shown to benefit patients with HF. These beta-adrenergic blockers are bisoprolol, carvedilol, and metoprolol succinate. Clinical trials have shown that these medications lower the risk of death and hospitalization and improve symptoms in patients with HF (see **Chapter 29**).

Vasodilators

Vasodilators dilate the blood vessels to allow better blood flow and can be used to manage HF, hypertension, angina, MI, and other conditions. Each vasodilator class has different actions on the coronary and peripheral arteries and veins. Vasodilators primarily affect the arteries, but some, such as nitroglycerin, primarily affect the veins.

TABLE 33.1 Medication therapy for heart failure

Generic name	Trade name
Angiotensin-converting enzyme	
Enalapril	Vasotec
Fosinopril	Monopril
Lisinopril	Prinivil, Zestril
Quinapril	Accupril
Angiotensin receptor blockers	
candesartan	Atacand
losartan	Cozaar
valsartan	Diovan
Beta-adrenergic blockers	
bisoprolol	Zebeta
carvedilol	Coreg, Coreg CR
metoprolol succinate	Toprol XL
Aldosterone antagonists/potassium-sparing diuretics	
eplerenone	Inspra
spironolactone	Aldactone
Vasodilator/nitrate combination drugs	
Hydralazine/isosorbide dinitrate	Bidil
Loop diuretics	
Bumetanide	Bumex
Furosemide	Lasix
Torsemide	Demadex
Thiazide diuretics	
Chlorothiazide	Diuril
Hydrochlorothiazide	Microzide, HCTZ
Metolazone	Zaroxolyn
Cardiac glycoside	
digoxin	Lanoxin, Cardoxin

Vasodilators can also prevent blood vessel constriction. ACE inhibitors and angiotensin receptor blockers also have vasodilator activity (see **Chapter 29**).

Vasodilator/nitrate combination drugs

The fixed-dose combination of hydralazine and nitrate was the first treatment to improve the survival of patients with HF with reduced left ventricular EF. Hydralazine and isosorbide dinitrate relax blood vessels, decreasing the heart's work (see **Chapter 28**).

Diuretics

Diuretics promote sodium and water excretion by inhibiting sodium reabsorption in the renal tubules. They are most commonly used to treat hypertension and conditions that involve volume overload, such as HF and liver cirrhosis. Different classes of diuretics have unique pharmacokinetic and pharmacodynamic properties and varying mechanisms of action. They will be discussed in detail in **Chapter 34**.

Cardiac glycosides

Cardiac glycosides are medications derived from *foxglove* plants such as *Digitalis lantana* or *Digitalis purpura*. The most commonly used cardiac glycoside is digoxin. Digoxin increases the force of the heart's contractions. These medicines are a common cause of toxicity and include digitalis and digitoxin.

Pharmacokinetics

The pharmacokinetics of different cardiac glycosides are altered by renal dysfunction in other ways, depending on their basic pharmacokinetic properties. The renal clearance of digoxin is reduced in renal dysfunction and is closely associated with **creatinine clearance**. The bioavailability of digitoxin is unaffected by renal dysfunction. Protein binding is probably significantly reduced, but the clinical significance of this effect is unclear because the apparent volume of distribution and total body clearance of digitoxin appear unchanged. Decreased renal function can increase serum digoxin concentrations because the drug is mainly excreted through the kidneys.

Mechanism of action

Digoxin reversibly binds to and inhibits the sodium/potassium/ATPase, or the sodium-potassium pump, preventing sodium and potassium exchange across the membrane. Sodium builds up inside heart cells, decreasing the ability of the sodium-calcium exchanger to push calcium out of them. Therefore calcium builds up in the sarcoplasmic reticulum. Increased intracellular calcium has a positive inotropic effect, which increases the force of the heart's contractions.

Clinical indications

Cardiac glycosides are used for congestive HF (when other medications fail), atrial fibrillation, and atrial flutter. Because of the potential for severe adverse effects and toxicity, cardiac glycosides are used less often than safer options such as ACE inhibitors and beta-blockers.

Contraindications

Digoxin is contraindicated in patients with acute MI, hypersensitivity to the drug, ventricular fibrillation, myocarditis, hypomagnesemia, hypokalemia, and **Wolf-Parkinson-White syndrome**. Cautious use is required in cases of hypercalcemia, hypocalcemia, renal impairment, disease of the sinoatrial node, bradycardia, atrioventricular block, restrictive cardiomyopathy, constrictive pericarditis, and thyroid disease.

Adverse effects

Adverse effects of digoxin include unusual tiredness, fatigue, anxiety, and hallucinations. The drug can cause poisoning and toxicity, resulting in arrhythmias, electrolyte imbalances (sodium, potassium, calcium, and magnesium), nausea, vomiting, and visual disturbances. Toxicity can be worsened by using digoxin with other medications such as diuretics, calcium channel blockers, amiodarone, cyclosporine, quinidine, and nonsteroidal antiinflammatory drugs. Adverse effects can often be reversed by reducing the dose of digoxin. Patients with cardiac arrhythmias must be monitored with blood tests to measure serum digoxin and electrolytes, and an electrocardiogram should be used to assess the heart.

Toxicities

The predominant features of acute toxicity of digoxin include nausea, vomiting, abdominal pain, diarrhea, hyperkalemia, generalized weakness, drowsiness, and cardiotoxicities such as bradycardia, heart block, and dysrhythmias.

You should remember

Many commonly used drugs interact with digoxin. The class IA antiarrhythmic quinidine competes with digoxin for binding sites and depresses renal clearance of digoxin. These effects increase serum digoxin concentrations and can produce toxicity. Similar interactions occur with non-steroidal antiinflammatory drugs and calcium channel blockers.

Key Terms

Angioedema
Ascites
Cardiogenic shock
Congestive heart failure
Creatinine clearance
Cyanoses
Ejection fraction
Hemochromatosis
Hepatic congestion
Nocturnal cough
Pitting edema
Pulmonary edema
Wolf-Parkinson-White syndrome

Clinical Case Studies

Clinical Case Study 1

An 80-year-old male was hospitalized due to decompensated HF. He previously had progressive dyspnea triggered by light activities, lower leg edema, and ascites. The patient had smoked from his teenage years up until he was 40 years old. He also had alcoholism but stopped drinking a year before his hospitalization. His medications were enalapril, spironolactone, furosemide, omeprazole, and ferrous sulfate. An X-ray revealed cardiomegaly.

Critical Thinking Questions

1. What lifestyle factors increase the risk of HF?
2. What are the risk factors for HF?
3. What are the links between dyspnea and HF?

Clinical Case Study 2

A 55-year-old female presented to the hospital with shortness of breath that had worsened to affect her ability to perform daily activities. Her history included hypertension, dyslipidemia, diabetes mellitus, and triple bypass surgery. Current medications include aspirin, atorvastatin, amlodipine, and metformin. Physical examination revealed bilateral diffuse rales in her lungs, elevated jugular venous pressure, and lower leg edema. A chest X-ray showed vascular congestion. An echocardiogram revealed systolic dysfunction, a dilated left atrium, and a low EF.

Critical Thinking Questions

1. What are the "rules" that often accompany HF?

2. In HF, when do changes to the jugular vein occur?
3. How is EF determined?

Clinical Case Study 3

A 64-year-old male had a history of two MIs, hypertension, non–insulin-dependent diabetes, and left leg stasis dermatitis. He had a coronary bypass in the previous year. His current symptoms include progressive shortness of breath that is worsened by exertion. The patient complains of constant fatigue and anorexia. His lips have a bluish discoloration. His jugular veins are prominent and distended to the mandible while sitting upright. The patient's liver is palpable and tender. Examination of the extremities shows diminished peripheral pulses. There is pitting edema in both lower legs. The patient is hospitalized for further evaluation.

Critical Thinking Questions

1. What are the most common symptoms of HF?
2. What is pitting edema?
3. When must treatment for HF be immediate?

Further Reading

[1] G. Bestman, Congestive Heart Failure—Identifying Early Symptoms and Treatment of Heart Failure, Bestman, 2023.
[2] T. Bryon, Heart Failure—The Ultimate Guide on Heart Failure Treatment, Management, and Strategies for Surviving and Coping with Heart Failure, Bryon, 2021.
[3] A.L. Clark, R.S. Gardner, T.A. McDonaugh, Textbook of Heart Failure, second ed., Oxford University Press, 2022.
[4] H. Eisen, Heart Failure: A Comprehensive Guide to Pathophysiology and Clinical Care, Springer, 2017.
[5] G.M. Felker, D.L. Mann, Heart Failure: A Companion to Braunwald's Heart Disease, fourth ed., Elsevier, 2019.
[6] R.S. Harris, Congestive Heart Failure—Understanding Your Heart Disease—Simple and Compact, Harris, 2016.
[7] B. Jaski, The 4 Stages of Heart Failure, CardioText Publishing, 2015.
[8] A.P. Kalogeropoulos, H. Skopicki, J. Butler, S. Murali, Heart Failure: An Essential Clinical Guide, CRC Press, 2022.
[9] S. Katz, R. Baliga, Heart Failure. Oxford American Cardiology Library, Oxford University Press, 2013.
[10] M.C. Konerman, S.L. Hummel, Heart Failure with Preserved Ejection Fraction (Clinics Review Articles, Cardiology Clinics), Elsevier, 2022.
[11] L.S. Lilly, Pathophysiology of Heart Disease—An Introduction to Cardiovascular Medicine, seventh ed., Lippincott, Williams, and Wilkins, 2022.
[12] K.M. Smith Hayes, N.R. Dellise, Managing Heart Failure in Primary Care: A Case-Study Approach, Springer, 2023.

CHAPTER

34

Diuretics

OUTLINE

LEARNING OUTCOMES

After study of this chapter, readers should be able to

1. Describe the components of the nephron.
2. Explain the pathophysiology of chronic kidney disease.
3. Discuss the classifications of diuretics.
4. Explain the pharmacokinetics of thiazides and loop diuretics.
5. Discuss the clinical indications of all subclasses of diuretics.
6. Describe the adverse effects of loop diuretics.

The Science of Pharmacology
https://doi.org/10.1016/B978-0-443-29038-1.00034-8

7. Discuss the mechanism of action of potassium-sparing diuretics.
8. Describe the indications of osmotic diuretics.
9. Explain the mechanism of action of carbonic anhydrase inhibitors.
10. Discuss the contraindications of carbonic anhydrase inhibitors.

Overview

Diuretics are drugs that increase the rate of urine flow and sodium excretion to adjust the volume and composition of body fluids. They are the most commonly prescribed drugs for hypertension in the United States. They are also widely used to treat heart failure, water poisoning, cirrhosis of the liver, and edema. Diuretics are sometimes called "water pills." This drug class has several significant categories, and the compounds vary in structure and physicochemical properties. They affect urinary organization, renal hemodynamics, and site and mechanism of action. Typically, the pharmacological group consists of five categories: thiazide diuretics, loop diuretics, potassium-sparing diuretics, osmotic diuretics, and carbonic anhydrase inhibitors (CALs). Diuretics promote sodium and water excretion by inhibiting sodium reabsorption in renal tubules. Each class of diuretic can affect different parts of the nephron.

Renal physiology and structure of a nephron

The renal system comprises the kidney, ureters, urinary bladder, and the urethra. One kidney contains over 1 million functioning units called **nephrons**. The main components of the nephron are the glomerulus, the Bowman capsule, the proximal convoluted tubule, the loop of Henle, the distal convoluted tubule (DCT), and the collecting duct (see **Fig. 34.1**). Approximately 200 L of fluid filter from renal blood flow daily, allowing metabolic waste products, toxins, and excess ions to be removed while keeping essential substances in the blood. The kidney regulates **plasma osmolarity** by controlling the blood's water, solutes, and electrolytes. It ensures long-term acid-base balance and produces **erythropoietin**. It also produces **renin** for blood pressure regulation and converts vitamin D to its active form.

The **renal corpuscle** consists of the **glomerulus** and the **Bowman capsule.** The glomerulus filters the blood free of cells and large proteins. From the **proximal convoluted tubule** (PCT), the nonreabsorbed filtrates move on to the **loop of Henle** to reabsorb water via **osmosis**. The loop is divided into a descending and an ascending limb. Sodium, potassium, and chloride are reabsorbed in the thick segment of the ascending limb, and calcium and magnesium ions are reabsorbed in the ascending limb. There is no water reabsorption in the ascending limb.

The **DCT** is a short nephron segment between the **macula densa** and the collecting duct. Even though it is short in length, it plays a crucial role in regulating extracellular fluid volume and electrolyte homeostasis.

The **collecting tubule** is where the final reabsorption stage occurs and plays an essential role in fluid-electrolyte balance. In response to antidiuretic hormone (ADH), the collecting duct reabsorbs water, and the hormone aldosterone stimulates the collecting duct to reabsorb sodium.

The kidneys regulate plasma osmolarity by modulating the water concentration in relationship to solutes and electrolytes in the blood. Erythropoietin from the kidneys stimulates the production of red blood cells and renin for blood pressure regulation. The kidneys also convert vitamin D to its active form. There are three steps for urine formation: glomerular filtration, tubular reabsorption, and **tubular secretion**.

Urine formation begins with filtration, which takes place in the renal corpuscle. The glomerular capillaries contain blood that enters the kidney through the renal artery. Glomerular filtration is a passive process in which **hydrostatic pressure** pushes fluid and solute through a membrane without an energy requirement, and this pressure is the main filtration force. Another potential filtration force is the capsular space colloid **osmotic pressure**, which plays a significant role in the **glomerular filtration rate** (GFR).

The process of **tubular reabsorption** occurs primarily in the PCT. The kidneys reabsorb glucose, amino acids, and electrolytes. The PCT reabsorbs water by osmosis, which is operated by solute reabsorption. It also reabsorbs

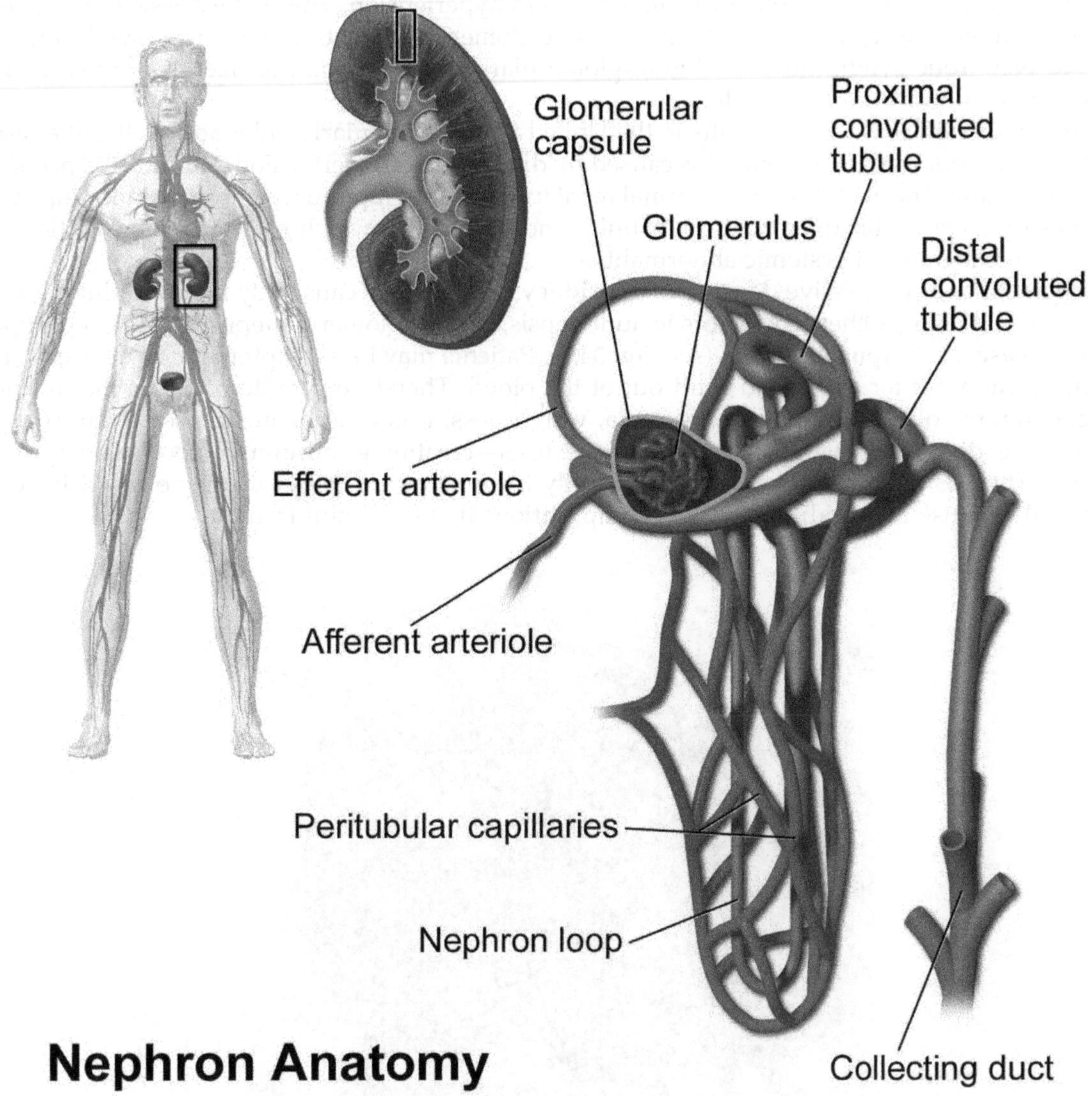

FIG. 34.1 The structure of a nephron.

lipid-soluble solutes via passive diffusion caused by the concentration gradient created by water reabsorption. Urea reabsorption also occurs in the PCT by passive paracellular diffusion driven by a chemical gradient.

From the PCT, the nonreabsorbed filtrates move on to the loop of Henle, which has a descending and an ascending limb. The descending limb can reabsorb water via osmosis, but solutes are not reabsorbed here. However, sodium, calcium, magnesium, potassium, and chloride are reabsorbed in the ascending limb. There is no water reabsorption in the ascending limb. The DCT reabsorbs sodium chloride by regulation of aldosterone. Calcium reabsorption is also via passive uptake controlled by **parathyroid hormone**. The collecting duct plays an essential role in fluid-electrolyte balance, specifically reabsorbing sodium and water in response to ADH and aldosterone.

Pathophysiology of chronic kidney disease

Acute kidney injury occurs in more than 2 million people worldwide and is a significant risk factor for the development of chronic kidney disease (CKD). However, the availability of dialysis and the success of renal transplantation have improved the prognosis for patients. **Nephritic syndrome** is a clinical syndrome caused by glomerular disease that presents as **hematuria**, proteinuria, **oliguria**, and hypertension. This is the classic presentation of acute poststreptococcal **glomerulonephritis**. Rapidly progressive glomerulonephritis is a nephritic syndrome with a rapid decline in GFR. Nephrotic syndrome, also due to glomerular disease, is characterized by proteinuria, lipiduria, hyperlipidemia, hypoalbuminemia, and edema.

CKD is estimated to affect 11% of all adults in the United States, particularly older adults. It is the result of a variety of renal diseases, but most commonly it is caused by diabetes and hypertension, and it is the primary cause of death from renal disease. The evolution from normal renal function to symptomatic chronic kidney injury progresses through a series of stages defined by serum creatinine measures from which estimates of reduction in GFR are derived. CKD causes significant systemic abnormalities.

CKD is permanent and progressive damage to the kidneys that may be caused by kidney failure, diabetes mellitus, hypertension, and aging. Other risk factors include sepsis, chronic glomerulonephritis, HIV nephropathy, **polycystic kidney disease**, and **lupus nephritis** (see **Fig. 34.2**). Patients may be asymptomatic in the early stages. Over time, the kidneys cannot filter waste and fluid out of the blood. Therefore symptoms occur that include itching, edema, muscle cramps, oliguria, dyspnea, insomnia, weight loss, loss of appetite, nausea, vomiting, and foamy urine. CKD can be diagnosed using blood and urine tests—creatinine, **albumin**, blood electrolyte tests, and measuring GFR. There is no cure or medicine specifically for treating CKD, but medicine can help control many of the problems that cause the condition and the complications that can result from it.

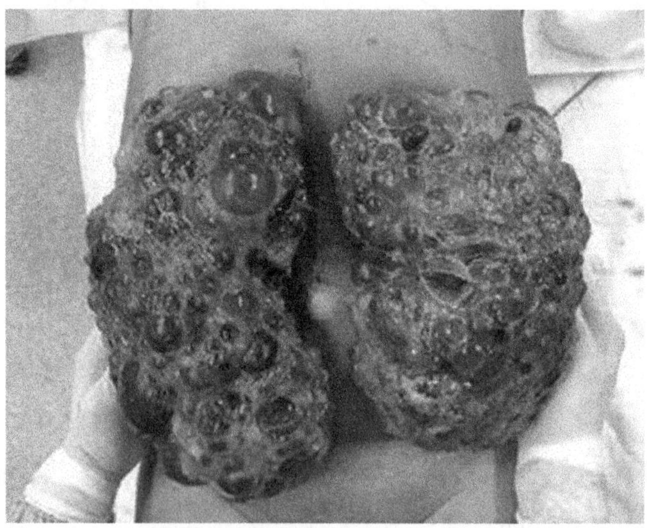

FIG. 34.2 Polycystic kidney disease.

Pharmacotherapy of diuretics

Diuretics are medicines that help reduce fluid buildup in the body. They are sometimes called water pills. Most diuretics help the kidneys remove salt and water from the urine. This lowers the fluid flow through the veins and arteries, reducing blood pressure. Diuretics are classified according to their sites of action within the nephron, chemical structure, and diuretic potency. The sites of action of the various diuretics are determined by how they affect the electrolyte and water transport systems along the nephron. The most valuable diuretics are the loop diuretics, mannitol, metolazone, and potassium-sparing diuretics. The potency of diuretics is a function of where they work in the nephron to inhibit sodium and water resorption. The more sodium and water they inhibit from resorption, the greater the amount of diuresis and the greater the potency.

Diuretics can be divided into five subclasses: thiazide and thiazide-like, loop, potassium sparing, osmotic diuretics, and CALs. Diuretics combined with another antihypertensive agent are more effective in lowering blood pressure than each agent alone. For this reason, they are commonly mixed with other antihypertensive agents.

You should remember

Diuretics are often abused by athletes to excrete water for rapid weight loss and to mask the presence of other banned substances. Because of their abuse by athletes, diuretics have been included on the World Anti-Doping Agency's list of prohibited substances; diuretics are banned both in and out of competition, and antidoping laboratories routinely screen for diuretics.

Thiazide and thiazide-like diuretics

Thiazide and thiazide-like diuretics are traditionally known as first-line therapy for hypertension uncomplicated by other disease states. Thiazide diuretics, like several of the loop diuretics, are benzothiadiazine, which are chemical derivatives of sulfonamide antibiotics. Three thiazide diuretics are commonly used: hydrochlorothiazide (HCTZ), chlorthalidone, and indapamide. HCTZ and chlorthalidone are FDA approved for clinical use in managing primary hypertension.

Pharmacokinetics

Thiazides are well absorbed orally and are widely distributed. The GI absorption ranges between 60%–80%, most of which occurs in the duodenum and the upper jejunum. Thiazides are subject to various degrees of metabolism by the liver. They are eliminated mainly from the kidneys, with no significant biliary excretion. Most thiazides have a half-life of about 8–12 hours, allowing effective once-daily administration. HCTZ is not metabolized in the liver but is eliminated rapidly by the kidneys.

Mechanism of action

The mechanism of action for thiazide and thiazide-like diuretics inhibits the sodium/chloride channel in the DCT to reduce extracellular fluid and cardiac output. Thiazide diuretics significantly reduce cardiovascular events and death without causing severe side effects. In specific hypertensive patient populations, such as patients with salt sensitivity, obesity, and diabetes, thiazide diuretics are more efficacious than other antihypertensive drugs.

Clinical indications

Thiazide and thiazide-like diuretics are the first-line therapies for hypertension. For hypertensive patients with diabetes, the American Diabetes Association prefers thiazide-like diuretics (chlorthalidone and indapamide) because they are longer-acting diuretics that have a proven effect on cardiovascular event reduction. Thiazide-like diuretics are superior to thiazide-type diuretics in reducing blood pressure without increasing the occurrence of hyponatremia and hypokalemia and without altering serum total cholesterol and blood glucose. Thiazide and thiazide-like diuretics are also indicated for treating edema and heart failure, idiopathic hypercalciuria, diabetes insipidus, and hepatic cirrhosis.

TABLE 34.1 Thiazide and thiazide-like diuretics

Generic names	Brand names	Route of administration
chlorothiazide	Thalitone	PO
hydrochlorothiazide	HCTZ, Hydrodiuril	PO
chlorthalidone	Hygroton	PO
indapamide	Lozol	PO
metolazone	Zaroxolyn	PO

Contraindications

Thiazide and thiazide-like diuretics are contraindicated in patients with kidney failure, hypotension, gout, hepatic coma, and sulfonamide allergies. They should also be avoided in hyponatremia, hypokalemia, and Addison disease.

Adverse effects

In the past, thiazides were given at high doses, predisposing patients to many side effects. Current guidelines recommend the maximum dose of HCTZ to be 12.5–25 mg orally once daily, which is considered a low dose. As a result, the side effects of thiazide diuretics are less common and can be easily detected with routine monitoring before they become significant problems. Thiazide diuretics can cause electrolyte abnormalities such as hypercalcemia, hypokalemia, hyperuricemia, hyperlipidemia, hyperglycemia, and hypomagnesemia. Hyponatremia may occur within the first 2 weeks of thiazide therapy.

Toxicity

The most common toxicity associated with thiazide and thiazide-like diuretics includes skin rashes, pancreatitis, hypertriglyceridemia, hypercholesterolemia, hypomagnesemia, gout, hypokalemia, hyperglycemia in diabetics, interstitial nephritis, and azotemia.

Loop diuretics

Loop diuretics are chemically related to the sulfonamide antibiotics. Because of this, they are listed as contraindicated for sulfa-allergic patients. Loop diuretics are potent and widely used agents to treat edematous states and congestive heart failure, and they are less commonly used for hypertension. Clinically apparent acute liver injury due to the loop diuretics is exceedingly rare if it occurs at all. **Table 34.2** summarizes loop diuretics.

Pharmacokinetics

Loop diuretics have a rapid onset of action and are particularly useful when rapid diuresis is needed. Furosemide has an average bioavailability of 50%; torsemide provides the most extended duration of action and can give even more significant diuretic effects in patients with hepatic dysfunction or heart failure. Furosemide's half-life is prolonged in patients with renal insufficiency. The other two loop diuretics, bumetanide and torsemide, are metabolized by the liver, so they are unaffected by renal insufficiency. Furosemide may need to be dosed several times a day, whereas the other two loop diuretics have a longer duration of action.

Mechanism of action

Loop diuretics reduce sodium chloride reabsorption in the thick ascending limb of the loop of Henle by blocking chloride and, secondarily, sodium resorption. There, luminal sodium and chloride entry into the cell is minimized. This is achieved by inhibiting the Na-K-2Cl carrier in the luminal membrane in this segment, thereby minimizing the entry of luminal sodium and chloride into the cell. Loop diuretics also activate renal prostaglandins, which dilate the blood vessels of the kidneys, the lungs, and other body parts. Loop diuretics are highly bound to plasma protein, mainly albumin.

Clinical indications

Loop diuretics are usually the first choice for treating pulmonary edema, heart failure, nephrotic syndrome, and hepatic cirrhosis; they are also used for hypertension. In patients with heart failure resistant to loop diuretics, a

TABLE 34.2 Loop diuretics.

Generic names	Brand names	Route of administrations
furosemide	Lasix	PO, IM, IV
bumetanide	Bumex	PO, IV
ethacrynic acid	Edecrin	PO, IM, IV
torsemide	Demadex	PO, IV

thiazide, amiloride, or triamterene may be added to increase the response. Loop diuretics in high doses may cause toxicity in the ears in the form of edema and hearing loss, which is usually transient. Loop diuretics may deplete a significant amount of potassium and magnesium, so oral supplements are necessary.

Contraindications

Loop diuretics are contraindicated in patients with severe hypersensitivity, hypokalemia, severe hyponatremia, hypotension, azotemia, oliguria, and hepatic coma. They are also contraindicated when fluid depletion is foreseen, such as surgery.

Adverse effects

Loop diuretics may cause electrolyte imbalances due to diuresis and include hypokalemia, hyponatremia, hypochloremia, hypomagnesemia, azotemia, metabolic alkalosis, dehydration, hyperuricemia, **gout**, headache, dizziness, vertigo, restlessness, **orthotic hypotension**, and syncope. Other adverse reactions include skin photosensitivity, **interstitial nephritis**, tinnitus, ototoxicity, and deafness. Thrombocytopenia, **aplastic anemia**, hemolytic anemia, leukopenia, **agranulocytosis**, pneumonitis, pulmonary edema, blurred vision, abdominal cramping, anorexia, diarrhea, constipation, **urticaria**, anaphylaxis, **exfoliative dermatitis**, jaundice, pancreatitis, hepatic coma, fever, and **impotence** also may occur.

Toxicity

Loop diuretics in high doses may cause toxicity in the ears, which is usually transient. They may deplete a significant amount of potassium and magnesium, so oral supplements are necessary. Loop diuretics can also result in hyponatremia, hypocalcemia, and dehydration secondary to excessive diuresis.

You should remember

Chlorthalidone is the preferred option for treating hypertension. This is because its effects last longer in the body than other diuretics, and it lowers the risk of cardiovascular disease.

Potassium-sparing diuretics

Potassium-sparing diuretics can increase urination without causing potassium loss. Because aldosterone promotes the retention of sodium and water, if potassium-sparing diuretics are used to block this effect, more sodium and water can pass into the collecting ducts of the kidneys, increasing diuresis. These diuretics are not as potent as the thiazides or the loops and are often combined with a thiazide diuretic to minimize potassium loss in susceptible patients. **Table 34.3** summarizes potassium-sparing diuretics.

Pharmacokinetics

Potassium-sparing diuretics are taken orally. Spironolactone is metabolized in the liver to **canrenone**, which has a much longer half-life and is probably responsible for most of the diuretic effect. The potassium-sparing diuretics prevent sodium reabsorption in the collecting tubule or inhibit aldosterone receptors (spironolactone, eplerenone). This prevents excessive excretion of potassium ions in urine, decreases water retention, and prevents hypokalemia.

TABLE 34.3 Potassium-sparing diuretics.

Generic names	Brand names	Route of administration
amiloride	Midamor	PO
eplerenone	Inspra	PO
spironolactone	Aldactone, Carospir	PO
triamterene	Dyrenium	PO

Mechanism of action

Potassium-sparing diuretics are usually weak and work by interfering with the sodium-potassium exchange in the DCT of the kidneys or as an antagonist at the aldosterone receptor, promoting sodium and water retention. Therefore blocking this effect can cause more sodium and water to pass into the collecting ducts of the kidneys and increase urination.

Clinical indications

Potassium-sparing diuretics are most often used to correct potassium deficiencies in patients with hypertension, heart failure, hypokalemia, **primary hyperaldosteronism**, cirrhosis of the liver, ascites, edema, and **hirsutism**. Spironolactone is recommended for patients with advanced heart failure due to compelling evidence that this agent can reduce morbidity by 35% and mortality by 30%. It also effectively treats patients with fluid retention from liver failure or ascites.

Contraindications

Potassium-sparing diuretics are contraindicated for patients with hyperkalemia, advanced renal failure, or CKD who are at risk of hyperkalemia. Spironolactone is a pregnancy category C drug, and along with triamterene, it should be avoided in pregnant patients. Eplerenone is a category B medication. It should also be avoided when using oral vitamin K.

Adverse effects

The main adverse effect is hyperkalemia, especially in patients with impaired renal function. Spironolactone may cause **gynecomastia**, menstrual abnormalities, diarrhea, gastritis, **peptic ulcers**, bleeding, and dysrhythmia. Central nervous system effects include headache, drowsiness, lethargy, and confusion. Eplerenone, a derivative of spironolactone, cannot significantly affect **androgen receptors**. However, the risk of hyperkalemia is similar to or even more significant than spironolactone.

Toxicity

The most toxic effects of potassium-sparing diuretics are hyperkalemia, kidney impairment, and electrolyte imbalance. Triamterene is potentially harmful to the kidneys and can be associated with the formation of kidney stones and acute kidney failure. Amiloride is better tolerated. For this reason, the drug should be avoided in patients with kidney disease. Eplerenone is effective in preserving left ventricular function and has been found effective in heart failure patients. The initial dose of eplerenone is 25 mg once daily, with a target dose of 50 mg once daily.

You should remember

Because diuretics flush excess water, they are sometimes described to patients as water pills. Patients are advised to take these agents at the beginning of the day or in the late afternoon, a few hours before bedtime, to avoid having to rise at night to urinate.

Osmotic diuretics

Osmotic diuretics mainly inhibit water absorption in the PCT, the thin descending loop of Henle, and the collecting duct. These areas of the kidney are highly permeable to water. As sodium is reabsorbed in the proximal tubule, water usually follows and is reabsorbed via passive diffusion. Osmotic diuretics are the first choice for **cerebral edema**. These drugs promote sodium ion and water loss through the nephron by excretion of nonreabsorbable filtrate. **Table 34.4** summarizes osmotic diuretics.

Pharmacokinetics

Osmotic diuretics are freely filtered at the glomerulus but are poorly reabsorbed. Mannitol is the prototype osmotic diuretic. It produces diuresis by increasing osmotic pressure in the lumen of the proximal tubule and loop of Henle. The half-life is 0.5–2.5 hours with normal renal function and 6–36 hours in those with renal failure.

TABLE 34.4 Osmotic diuretics.

Generic names	Brand names	Route of administration
mannitol	Osmitrol	IV infusion
glycerin	None	PO
isosorbide	Imdur	Sublingual

TABLE 34.5 Carbonic anhydrase inhibitors.

Generic names	Brand names	Route of administration
acetazolamide	Diamox	IM, IV, ophthalmic
methazolamide	Neptazane	PO
dorzolamide	Trusopt	Ophthalmic
brinzolamide	Azopt	Ophthalmic
diclofenamide	Cambia, Voltaren	PO
ethoxzolamide	Cardrase	PO
zonisamide	Zonegran	PO

Mechanism of action

Osmotic diuretics mainly inhibit water and sodium chloride reabsorption in the PCT, the thin descending loop of Henle, and the collecting duct. This causes resorption of urea and uric acid. Mannitol reduces tubular reabsorption of water and enhances sodium and chloride excretion by increasing the glomerular filtrate's osmolarity.

Clinical indications

Osmotic diuretics are used when increased water excretion with minimal sodium excretion is required. They are indicated to treat conditions associated with impaired renal hemodynamics or to maintain urine volume and prevent **anuria**, which can occur during **hemolysis**. The primary indication for mannitol is the treatment of acute angle-closure glaucoma. Glycerin lowers intraocular pressure and reduces superficial corneal edema. These drugs can also treat congenital glaucoma and keratoplasty after retinal detachment repair.

Contraindications

Osmotic diuretics are avoided in patients with anuria, kidney, or heart failure. Mannitol and urea should not be used in patients with active cranial bleeding. Glycerin is contraindicated in patients with known hypersensitivity to this drug and diabetic patients. It should be administered with caution to patients with hypervolemia and cardiac failure.

Adverse effects

Common adverse effects of osmotic diuretics include fever, headache, dizziness, convulsions, chest pain, hypotension, phlebitis, chills, acidosis, fluid or electrolyte imbalances, polydipsia, nausea, vomiting, blurred vision, urinary retention, rhinorrhea, skin rashes, and hives.

Toxicity

The toxicity of osmotic diuretics can cause acute closed-angle glaucoma, mild headache, neck pain, nausea, vomiting, heart failure, pulmonary congestion, and pulmonary edema.

Carbonic anhydrase inhibitors

Carbonic anhydrases are responsible for the reversible hydration of carbon dioxide to bicarbonate, a significant reaction involved in various physiological and pathological processes. CALs are considered essential drugs for pathologies such as glaucoma, epilepsy, and cancer. CALs that are currently available are summarized in **Table 34.5**.

Pharmacokinetics

CALs are well absorbed when taken orally. They do not undergo biotransformation, and urine pH increases due to bicarbonate. Their plasma half-life is about 6–9 hours, and renal excretion is the primary route of elimination via secretion in the proximal tubule segment.

Mechanism of action

CALs block calcium in the proximal tubule of the nephron. Inhibition of calcium causes a decrease in the secretion of hydrogen ions to exchange sodium. This prevents sodium and water from being resorbed into the blood and lowers blood pH. Increased carbonic acid can be reversibly converted to bicarbonate and a hydrogen ion.

Clinical indications

CALs are indicated to treat **open-angle glaucoma**, congestive heart failure, edema, periodic **paralysis idiopathic**, intracranial hypertension, **high-altitude sickness**, and epilepsy (see **Fig. 34.3**). Acetazolamide is also indicated for treating edema secondary to heart failure that has become resistant to other diuretics. However, as a class, CALs are much less potent diuretics than loop diuretics or thiazides because of the metabolic acidosis they can induce.

Contraindications

CALs are contraindicated in patients with known drug allergies, renal impairment, liver disease, pregnancy, and breastfeeding. Acetazolamide should be avoided in people with hypokalemia or hyponatremia. Patients with hyperchloremic acidosis should not use acetazolamide.

Adverse effects

The common adverse effects of CALs include fatigue, nausea, vomiting, diarrhea, and abdominal pain. Some patients may have black stools, tinnitus, decreased libido, **paresthesia**, and taste alterations. Less commonly, there is a risk of forming kidney stones and acquiring hyponatremia, hypokalemia, and metabolic acidosis. Occasionally, patients may develop toxic epidermal necrolysis, Stevens-Johnson syndrome, agranulocytosis, aplastic anemia, or severe hepatic necrosis.

Toxicity

CALs can cause CNS toxicity with coma. In addition, hyperchloremic metabolic acidosis and electrolyte disturbances are usually seen in acetazolamide overdose. There is no specific antidote to acetazolamide toxicity, and treatment is generally supportive. Bicarbonate administration can usually correct metabolic acidosis. Dialysis may be especially valuable in treating acetazolamide overdose and complicated acute kidney injury.

You should remember

There are also drugs known as vasopressin receptor antagonists, or *vaptans,* which are classified as aquaretics because they do not affect sodium reabsorption. These drugs promote water excretion by inhibiting ADH-mediated water reabsorption in the collecting duct.

Key Terms

Addison disease
Agranulocytosis
Albumin
Androgen receptors
Anuria
Aplastic anemia
Bowman capsule
Canrenone
Cerebral edema
Collecting tubule
Distal convoluted tubule

Erythropoietin
Exfoliative dermatitis
Glomerular filtration rate
Glomerulonephritis
Glomerulus
Gout
Gynecomastia
Hematuria
Hemolysis
High-altitude sickness
Hirsutism
Hives
Hydrostatic pressure
Impotence
Interstitial nephritis
Loop of Henle
Lupus nephritis
Macula densa
Nephritic syndrome
Nephrons
Oliguria
Open-angle glaucoma
Orthotic hypotension
Osmosis
Osmotic pressure
Paralysis idiopathic
Parathyroid hormone
Paresthesia
Peptic ulcers
Phlebitis
Plasma osmolarity
Polycystic kidney disease
Primary hyperaldosteronism
Proximal convoluted tubule
Renal corpuscle
Renin
Rhinorrhea
Tubular reabsorption
Tubular secretion
Urticaria

Clinical Case Studies

Clinical Case Study 1

A 66-year-old male with a history of diabetes and CKD takes five antihypertensive drugs. Even so, his blood pressure is 176/92 mm Hg. The patient has mild dyspnea on exertion as well as edema. He has been taking furosemide twice a day for the past year. At his visit, HCTZ is added for better BP control and to treat signs and symptoms of fluid overload. Two weeks later, his wife took him to the emergency department with symptoms of anorexia, general malaise, and weakness. His BP upon arrival was 91/58 mm Hg, and he had lost 15 pounds in the last 2 weeks. His laboratory tests are significant for high serum creatinine, indicating acute kidney damage.

Critical Thinking Questions

1. What is the trade name and classification of furosemide?
2. When are thiazide diuretics such as HCTZ used?
3. Why are diuretics often combined with other antihypertensive agents?

Clinical Case Study 2

A 58-year-old male with diabetes had undergone coronary artery bypass grafting. After a month, he was brought back to the hospital because of nausea, altered taste sensations, and malaise. The patient had been taking furosemide, a loop diuretic, and spironolactone. Tests revealed that he had hyponatremia. The patient was prescribed ondansetron to treat his nausea, but symptoms persisted. His serum sodium was 124 mEq/dL, indicating profound hyponatremia. The patient was given sodium chloride as a slow intravenous infusion plus tablets of tolvaptan, a vasopressin receptor antagonist. His symptoms quickly improved, and the patient was discharged in 3 days.

Critical Thinking Questions

1. What is the trade name and classification of spironolactone?
2. Which types of diuretics are avoided in patients with hyponatremia?
3. What is the mechanism of action of loop diuretics?

Clinical Case Study 3

An 81-year-old female has taken spironolactone for about 7 years to control moderate hypertension and mild heart failure. She is brought to the emergency department with rales in the lower and middle lung lobes. Her BP is 190/120 mm Hg. She has dyspnea, anxiety, sweating, and a heart rate of 134 beats per minute. Her family members state that her condition has worsened over the last 2 weeks because she has asked friends to bring her some favorite lunch foods, including hot dogs and potato chips, nearly daily. The patient is diagnosed with pulmonary edema. She is given an immediate IV push of furosemide and morphine sulfate. She is also given oxygen and electrolytes via nasal cannula. A complete blood count and an indwelling urinary catheter are placed.

Critical Thinking Questions

1. Which diuretics are usually the first choice for pulmonary edema?
2. Where is spironolactone metabolized?
3. What are the contraindications of potassium-sparing diuretics?

Further Reading

[1] R. Aiden, Diuretics Complete Guide—Ultimate Guide: Understanding the Purpose, Benefits, Downsides, Interactions, Dosages & Many More, Aiden, 2022.

[2] W.R. Chegwidden, N.D. Carter, The Carbonic Anhydrases—Current and Emerging Therapeutic Targets, Springer, 2021.

[3] F. Earlstein, Glaucoma Explained-Glaucoma Facts, Diagnosis, Symptoms, Treatment, Causes, Effects, Alternative Medicines, Therapeutic Methods, History, Home Remedies, and More! Pack & Post Plus, LLC.

[4] D.C. Eaton, J.P. Pooler, Vander's Renal Physiology, tenth ed., McGraw Hill / Lange, 2023.

[5] S.Z. Fadem, Staying Healthy with Kidney Disease—A Complete Guide for Patients, Springer, 2022.

[6] S.J. Gilbert, D.E. Weiner, A.S. Bomback, M.A. Perazella, D.E. Rifkin, National Kidney Foundation's Primer on Kidney Diseases, eighth ed., Elsevier, 2022.

[7] J. Hewitt, M. Gabata, Nephrotic Syndrome—Causes, Tests, and Treatments, CreateSpace Independent Publishing Platform, 2011.

[8] R.J. Johnson, J. Floege, M. Tonelli, Comprehensive Clinical Nephrology, seventh ed., Elsevier, 2023.

[9] A.P. Kalogeropoulos, H. Skopicki, J. Butler, S. Murali, Heart Failure - An Essential Clinical Guide, CRC Press, 2022.

[10] B.M. Koeppen, B.A. Stanton, Renal Physiology—Physiology Series, sixth ed., Mosby / Elsevier, 2018.

[11] J.L. Koyner, J.M. Topf, E.V. Lerma, Handbook of Critical Care Nephrology, Wolters Kluwer, 2021.

[12] G. Landoni, A. Pisano, A. Zangrillo, R. Bellomo, Reducing Mortality in Acute Kidney Injury, Springer, 2016.

[13] A. Saleh, Diuretic Therapy and Drugs for Kidney Failure, Saleh, 2020.

[14] C.S. Wilcox, M. Choi, M.S. Segal, L. Chen, W.W. Williams, Handbook of Nephrology and Hypertension, seventh ed., Wolters Kluwer, 2022.

[15] L. Wouters, Diuretics—Pharmacology, Therapeutic Uses and Adverse Side Effects, Nova Medical, 2013.

[16] J.E. Zuther, It's Not Just a Swelling! Lymphedema-Causes, Prevention, Treatment, Self-Management, Prolymph Consultants.

CHAPTER

35

Drugs affecting the renin-angiotensin-aldosterone system

OUTLINE

LEARNING OUTCOMES

After study of this chapter, readers should be able to

1. Describe the components of the renin-angiotensin-aldosterone system.
2. Explain the role of renin in the kidneys.
3. Discuss the precursors to angiotensin II.

The Science of Pharmacology
https://doi.org/10.1016/B978-0-443-29038-1.00035-X

4. Explain the angiotensin-converting enzyme inhibitors.
5. Describe the adverse effects of captopril.
6. Discuss the mechanism of action of lisinopril.
7. Describe angiotensin II receptor inhibitors.
8. Explain the mechanism of action of azilsartan.
9. Describe the indication of losartan.
10. Explain the adverse effects of aldosterone.

Overview

The renin-angiotensin-aldosterone (ALD) system (RAAS) is a vital regulator of blood volume, electrolyte balance, and systemic vascular resistance. It comprises three significant compounds: renin, angiotensin II, and aldosterone. They elevate arterial pressure in response to decreased renal blood pressure (BP), salt delivery to the distal convoluted tubule, and beta-agonism. The RAAS involves several organ systems such as the kidneys, lungs, systemic vasculature, adrenal cortex, and brain. Angiotensin-converting enzyme (ACE) inhibitors and angiotensin II receptor blockers (ARBs) are used primarily to treat hypertension. Lisinopril (Zestril), enalapril (Vasotec), and benazepril (Lotensin) are popular options for ACE inhibitors. Losartan is the most commonly used angiotensin receptor blocker (ARB). However, other options may be better in some situations, including olmesartan, telmisartan, and valsartan.

Physiology

The RAAS is regulated by three significant compounds: renin, angiotensin II, and ALD. As the kidneys' incoming BP drops below 100 mm Hg or lower, tissue near the vessels known as the **juxtaglomerular (JG) apparatus** secretes renin into the blood. **Renin** is an enzyme that causes a standard blood component known as **angiotensinogen** to be converted into *angiotensin I.* Angiotensin I moves through the bloodstream, where ACE in the blood capillaries in the lungs splits the molecule to form *angiotensin II.* Angiotensin II moves to the adrenal cortex, stimulating ALD secretion; also, some ALD is synthesized in the blood vessels and heart. **ALD** causes more sodium reabsorption, increasing water retention and blood volume; this increased blood volume raises the BP, and the RAAS stops. **Fig. 35.1** illustrates the RAAS pathway.

The RAAS is a negative feedback mechanism that helps maintain BP homeostasis. One method involves increasing the overall blood volume, a function of ALD. Another method is angiotensin II, which improves smooth muscle tone in the artery walls and arterial BP. *ACE inhibitors* reduce abnormally high BP by blocking the formation of angiotensin II, reducing both BP-enhancing actions.

Renin

Renin is an enzyme synthesized, stored, and secreted by **JG cells**. These cells are also known as *granular cells.* These cells are in the afferent arteriole that supplies blood to the **glomerulus** and are specialized smooth muscle cells that function as pressure sensors. As BP falls, there is reduced pressure on the JG cells, so they respond by releasing renin into the blood circulation. The increased renin eventually leads to more circulating angiotensin II, returning BP to normal. Renin release is due to factors that reduce BP, such as blood volume loss because of bleeding or dehydration. Through negative feedback, higher BP is sensed by the JG cells, which then stop renin secretion.

Other factors influence the release of renin as well. Near the JG cells in the **distal convoluted tubule** of the nephron is a specialized cell cluster called the **macula densa**. It is in an ideal location to monitor the flow rate and concentration of sodium ions (known as **osmolality**) in the urinary filtrate. As BP falls, blood flow through the kidney reduces as renal tubular filtrate flow slows. The macula densa recognizes the reduced flow rate and lowered sodium, sending a chemical message to the JG cells to release more renin. Renin release causes more angiotensin II to be formed, and BP rises. The JG cells and macula densa are near (see **Fig. 35.2**). They are sometimes referred to as a single anatomic unit, known as the JG complex.

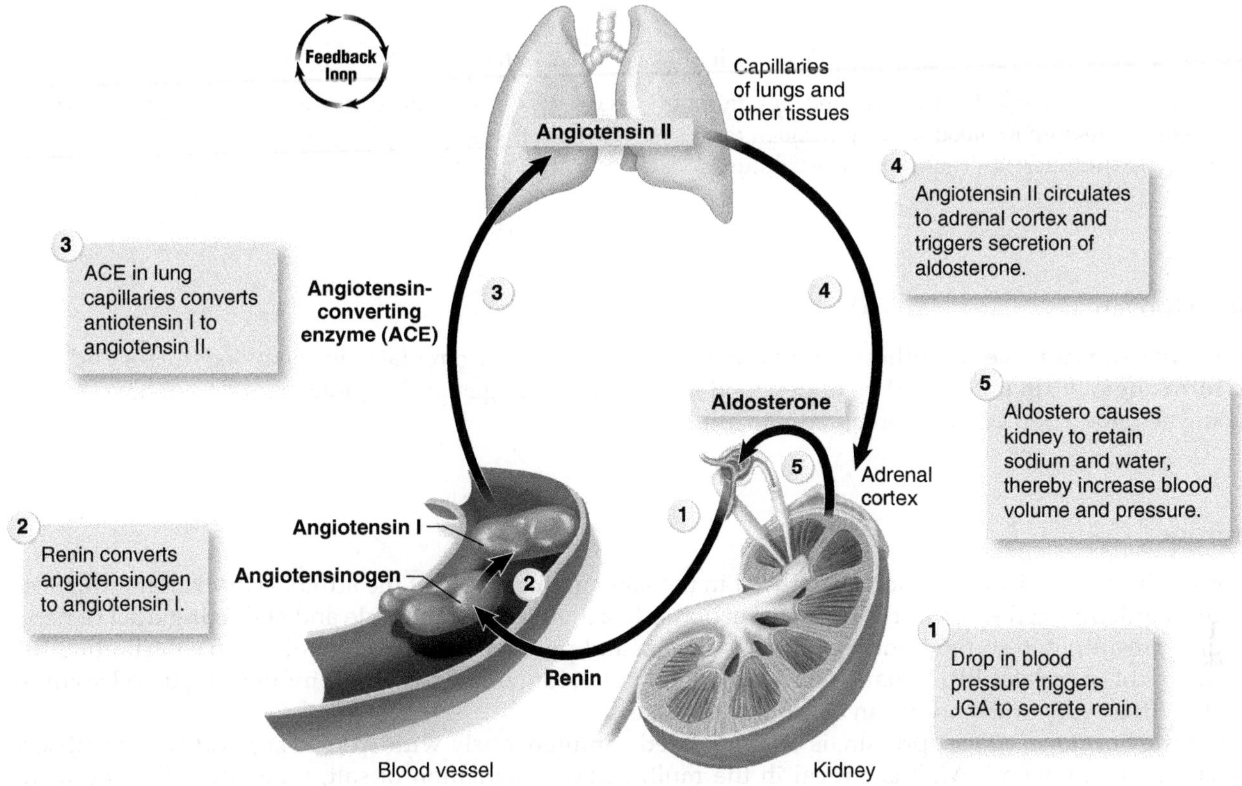

FIG. 35.1 The renin-angiotensin-aldosterone system pathway.

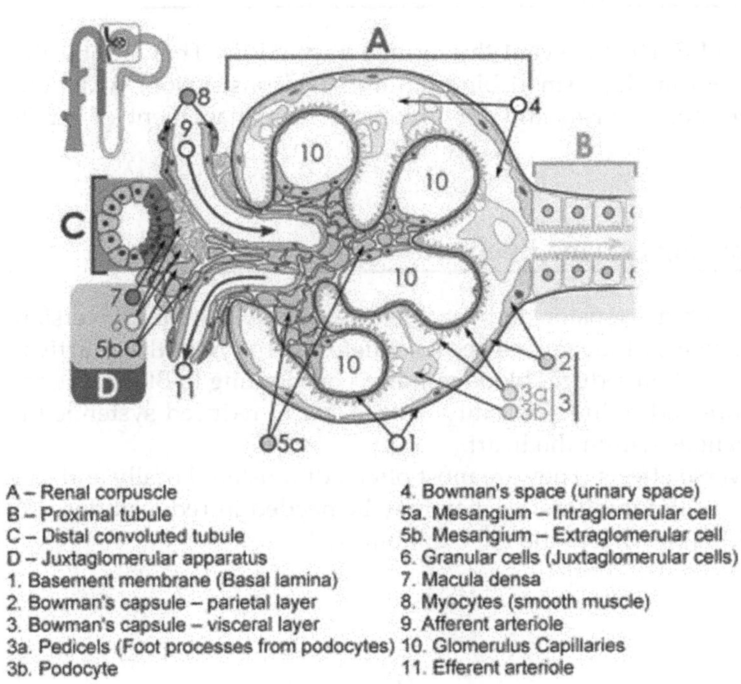

FIG. 35.2 Juxtaglomerular structure.

A third way that renin release is controlled is by activating the sympathetic nervous system. JG cells have beta$_1$-adrenergic receptors activated by the sympathetic nervous system's fight-or-flight response. Renin release helps increase BP in stressful or harmful situations.

You should remember

The three main factors that cause an increase in renin are decreased pressure in blood flowing through the kidney, decreased tubular flow rate or fewer sodium ions sensed by the macula densa, and activation of the sympathetic nervous system.

Angiotensinogen

Angiotensinogen is a protein synthesized by the liver. It continuously circulates in the bloodstream and splits by renin to form angiotensin I. It should be understood that angiotensinogen and angiotensin I do not have any critical physiologic actions. They are only precursors to angiotensin II.

Aldosterone

ALD is a mineralocorticoid hormone produced in the **zona glomerulosa** of the adrenal cortex that influences water and salt regulation in the body. Its primary function is to act on the distal tubule and **collecting duct** of nephrons in the kidney, resulting in sodium and water reabsorption and potassium excretion while also contributing to acid-base balance. ALD regulates BP by managing sodium and potassium in the blood and influencing blood volume. Too much or too little ALD in the body can cause health issues.

Antidiuretic hormone, or vasopressin, is often released simultaneously with ALD to support water reabsorption into the circulation. Overall, ALD is critical in the multifactorial regulation of salt, potassium, BP, and acid-base balance.

Pharmacotherapy

ACE inhibitors can relax the blood vessels to lower BP. They prevent the formation of ARBs. They inhibit the angiotensin II type-1 receptor (AT_1) receptor to prevent angiotensin II binding and vasoconstriction. ARBs are used as the treatment of choice in idiopathic hyperaldosteronism and for preoperative management of ALD-producing adenoma.

Angiotensin-converting enzyme inhibitors

ACE inhibitors are first-line drugs for the treatment of hypertension and heart failure. They block the conversion of angiotensin I to angiotensin II. As angiotensin II declines, BP decreases because there is less sympathetic activation and lower peripheral resistance. Decreased ALD secretion reduces blood volume, contributing to BP reduction. ACE inhibitors can slow the progression of heart failure and reduce mortality. This is due to reduced systemic BP and a reversal of angiotensin II-induced structural changes within the heart.

All ACE inhibitors have similar indications and adverse effects. They are most often administered orally and can usually be taken once daily. The kidneys excrete most ACE inhibitors, so they may be needed in reduced doses if advanced chronic kidney disease is present. **Table 35.1** summarizes the ACE inhibitors.

Captopril

Captopril is an ACE inhibitor used to treat high BP, heart failure, and heart attacks. The initial dose is 25 mg orally two to three times daily, 1 hour before meals. It may be increased every 1–2 weeks up to 50 mg orally thrice daily. If BP remains uncontrolled after 1–2 weeks at this dose, a thiazide diuretic can be added.

TABLE 35.1 ACE inhibitors.

Generic name	Trade name	Route of administration
benazepril	Lotensin	PO
captopril	Capoten	PO
enalapril	Vasotec	PO
fosinopril	Monopril	PO
lisinopril	Prinivil, Zestril	PO
moexipril	Univasc	PO
perindopril	Aceon	PO
quinapril	Accupril	PO
ramipril	Altace	PO
trandolapril	Mavik	PO

Pharmacokinetics

Captopril is well absorbed orally, with peak plasma concentration achieved within 1 hour of administration. Food decreases captopril's bioavailability, so it should be administered 1 hour before meals. Plasma protein binding is approximately 30%, and it can cross the blood-brain barrier. Captopril is metabolized in the liver.

Mechanism of action

Captopril inhibits ACE, converting angiotensin I to angiotensin II. Angiotensin II binds to AT_1 receptors on smooth muscles to produce vasoconstriction of precapillary arterioles and postcapillary venules, inhibiting norepinephrine reuptake and releasing catecholamines from the adrenal medulla, which all increase BP. Angiotensin II also stimulates the adrenal cortex to secrete ALD. ALD causes the distal tubules and collecting ducts of the kidneys to reabsorb water and sodium in exchange for potassium, which results in an expansion in extracellular volume and an increase in BP.

Clinical indications

Captopril is used alone or together with other medicines to treat hypertension. Lowering BP can reduce the risk of strokes and heart attacks. It is also used to treat heart failure, a condition in which the heart is less efficient at pumping blood. Captopril may be started within the first few days after a heart attack to increase survival. Captopril is also used to treat nephropathy caused by diabetes.

Contraindications

Captopril is contraindicated in patients with hypersensitivity to this agent, diabetes, a history of **angioedema**, bilateral renal artery stenosis, pregnancy, and kidney impairment.

Adverse effects

The adverse effects of captopril include dry cough, angioedema, rash with pruritus, angina pectoris, myocardial infarction, hypotension, **Raynaud syndrome**, proteinuria, and loss of taste.

Toxicities

Acute captopril toxicity may cause severe hypotension, acute kidney damage, and altered mental status. ACE inhibitors rarely cause cholestatic jaundice, severe hepatic necrosis, and sometimes death.

You should remember

Captopril is fetotoxic; using ACE inhibitors in pregnancy can lead to fetal lung hypoplasia, skull hypoplasia, renal agenesis, and oligohydramnios. ACE inhibitors are associated with congenital malformations and miscarriages.

Benazepril

Benazepril is used alone or in combination with other antihypertensive medicines to treat hypertension. It can be combined with thiazide diuretics. Benazepril lowers BP, reducing the risk of a stroke, heart failure, or kidney failure. It is available as oral tablets in 10-, 20-, and 40-mg strengths. The adverse effects of benazepril include dry cough, hypotension, renal impairment, and hyperkalemia. This agent is contraindicated in patients with a history of hypersensitivity to any ACE inhibitor. It should be avoided during pregnancy because the use of benazepril in the second and third trimesters is associated with fetal and neonatal injury, including neonatal skull hypoplasia, hypotension, anuria, and death.

Enalapril

Enalapril maleate is an ACE inhibitor used to treat chronic hypertension and heart failure. It inhibits ACE, reducing angiotensin-II and decreasing peripheral resistance without increasing cardiac oxygen demand. Enalapril is absorbed quickly when taken orally, with peak concentration achieved in about 1 hour. It poorly crosses the blood-brain barrier and is metabolized in the liver. Approximately two-thirds of enalapril is eliminated unchanged in the urine as enalaprilat. Enalapril is contraindicated in patients with idiopathic angioedema or a previous history of angioedema associated with ACE inhibitor use. It should be avoided in patients with myocardial infarction, stroke, renal impairment, and bilateral renal artery stenosis.

Fosinopril

Fosinopril inhibits ACE to prevent the conversion of angiotensin I to angiotensin II. It differs from other ACE inhibitors by its long half-life, hydrophilicity, and resistance to liver breakdown. Fosinopril is absorbed in the duodenum and jejunum. Fosinopril is highly plasma protein binding bound (about 99%) and can cross the blood-brain barrier. It is metabolized in the liver and eliminated by the liver and kidneys.

Lisinopril

Lisinopril is an older ACE inhibitor that has been available for the past three decades. It relaxes blood vessels, lowering BP while increasing blood and oxygen supply to the heart.

Pharmacokinetics

Lisinopril absorption is unchanged by food and is excreted unchanged in the urine. It has poor bioavailability after oral intake, ranging from 10%–30%. The time to peak concentration can vary from 6–8 hours. The drug does not bind to albumin, and its distribution in patients with heart failure is poor.

Mechanism of action

Lisinopril prevents the conversion of angiotensin I to angiotensin II, a potent vasoconstrictor. A decrease in angiotensin II subsequently causes a reduction in ALD secretion.

Clinical indications

The FDA has approved lisinopril for the management of hypertension in adults and children 6 years of age and older. It is also used as adjunctive therapy in the treatment of heart failure.

Contraindications

Lisinopril should be avoided in patients with a history of angioedema, renal failure, bilateral renal artery stenosis, or hyperkalemia. It is contraindicated in pregnant females and is a category class D drug due to its teratogenic effects.

Adverse effects

The primary adverse effects of ACE inhibitors include dry cough, angioedema, hypotension, dizziness, headache, hyperkalemia, and renal insufficiency. These effects may be more common in patients with renal, autoimmune, or collagen vascular diseases. The specific adverse effects of lisinopril include headache, allergic reactions, chest pain, cough (which may or may not be dry), hypotension, nausea, dizziness, blurred vision, sore throat, weakness, decreased sexual ability, fainting, hyperkalemia, indigestion, decreased urination, shortness of breath, erectile dysfunction, fatigue, heartburn, sneezing, abdominal pain, and confusion.

Toxicities

Lisinopril's toxicity can result in severe headaches, dizziness, sleepiness, hypotension, blurred vision, rash, itching, hoarseness, dyspnea, or swelling of the hands, face, and mouth.

You should remember

Lisinopril blocks ALD secretion, relaxing the blood vessels to lower BP while increasing blood and oxygen supplies to the heart. It is used to treat acute myocardial infarction, hypertension, and heart failure.

Moexipril

Moexipril, a prodrug, is used to treat hypertension. It relaxes blood vessels, lowering BP and preventing strokes, heart attacks, and kidney damage. Moexipril is incompletely absorbed, with a bioavailability of about 13% compared to intravenous formulations. The common adverse effects include cough, runny or stuffy nose, headache, dizziness, fatigue, diarrhea, skin rash, and polyurea. It is contraindicated in pregnancy and patients with diabetes, kidney disease, or liver impairment.

Perindopril

Perindopril is an ACE inhibitor used alone or in combination with other agents to treat hypertension. It blocks the ACE from forming angiotensin II, allowing blood vessels to relax and lower BP. The adverse effects of perindopril include chest pain, cough, headache, dizziness, nausea, and **oliguria**.

Quinapril

Quinapril is an ACE inhibitor developed in the 1980s. It is indicated to manage hypertension and reduce the risk factor for coronary heart disease. Quinapril is also used to treat chronic heart failure and slow the progression of renal disease in patients with diabetes. It inhibits the conversion of angiotensin I to angiotensin II. Quinapril is converted to its active metabolite quinaprilat, which has a short elimination half-life. It is contraindicated in patients with hepatic and renal impairments. Quinapril is considered a pregnancy category D drug. Adverse effects of quinapril include dry cough, hyperkalemia, angioedema, dizziness, hypotension, and renal dysfunction. Less common adverse effects include skin rash and dysgeusia.

Ramipril

Ramipril is an ACE inhibitor used to treat hypertension and heart failure. It is available in tablet and capsule form for oral administration. The maximum plasma concentration is 1 hour, and the bioavailability is about 60%. Ramipril is metabolized in the liver and primarily excreted through urine (60%) and feces (40%). The adverse effects include postural hypotension, dry cough, angioedema, hyperkalemia, increase in serum creatinine, and anxiety.

Angiotensin II receptor inhibitors

ARBs inhibit the AT_1 receptor. They are also used for hypertension and heart failure. Unlike ACE inhibitors, these inhibitors do not prevent the formation of angiotensin II but effectively block it from activating its target receptors. **Table 35.2** summarizes the ARBs.

Azilsartan

Azilsartan is an ARB agent used to treat hypertension. It increases the supply of blood and oxygen to the heart. The FDA approved it in 2011 as an antihypertensive drug.

Pharmacokinetics

Azilsartan is rapidly absorbed in the small intestine and metabolized in the liver by the enzyme CYP2C9. It is 60% bioavailable, with an elimination half-life of about 10 hours. The time to peak concentrations in the plasma ranges between 1.5 and 3 hours, and steady-state concentrations are reached after 5 days. This drug is excreted primarily in the feces (60%) and 40% via urine.

Mechanism of action

Azilsartan selectively inhibits angiotensin II from binding to the AT_1. This receptor inhibition provides azilsartan's antihypertensive activity because it blocks the pressor effects of angiotensin II.

Clinical indications

Azilsartan is used to treat hypertension as monotherapy or in combination therapy. In patients with diabetes mellitus and hypertension, azilsartan is effective in lowering BP.

Contraindications

Azilsartan is a teratogenic antihypertensive agent that can substantially cause congenital abnormalities. It is also considered fetotoxic during the second and third trimesters. As with other ARBs, azilsartan should be avoided in patients with a history of angioedema.

TABLE 35.2 Angiotensin II receptor inhibitors (blockers).

Generic name	Trade name	Route of administration
azilsartan	Edarbi	PO
candesartan	Atacand	PO
eprosartan	Teveten	PO
irbesartan	Avapro	PO
losartan	Cozaar	PO
olmesartan medoxomil	Benicar	PO
telmisartan	Micardis	PO
valsartan	Diovan	PO

Adverse effects

Overall, azilsartan is well tolerated in most patients. The primary adverse effect is orthostatic hypotension, which results in the discontinuation of the drug. Other adverse effects include hyperkalemia, nausea, diarrhea, fatigue, muscle spasms, confusion, dizziness, oliguria, and cough.

Toxicities

No maximum toxic doses have been established yet for azilsartan. Patients on azilsartan with volume depletion, severe heart failure, or renal stenosis are at risk for oliguria or progressive azotemia.

You should remember

Azilsartan is an ARB used to manage and treat hypertension. It is administered as an oral tablet and targets a critical element of the RAAS.

Candesartan

Candesartan is an ARB used alone or in combination with other medicines to treat hypertension in adults and children from 1–16 years of age. Lowering BP can reduce the risk of strokes and heart attacks. This agent is also indicated for treating heart failure and inhibits angiotensin II. The FDA approved it in 1998, and in October 2009 it also approved its use to treat hypertension in adolescents and children 12 months of age and older. The adverse effects include severe allergic reactions, hypotension, kidney damage, liver impairment, and hyperkalemia. Candesartan is considered a teratogen and has a boxed warning for fetal toxicity. Medications that interfere with the RAAS diminish fetal renal function if used in the second or third trimesters of pregnancy. There is an increased risk of morbidity and death secondary to **oligohydramnios** resulting from decreased renal function. The neonates may develop **skull hypoplasia**, lung hypoplasia, hypotension, renal failure, and fetal mortality. Candesartan should be avoided in children younger than 12 months of age due to adverse effects on the development of immature kidneys. Candesartan overdose causes hypotension, dizziness, and tachycardia.

Eprosartan

Eprosartan is an ARB. This agent and hydrochlorothiazide combination is used alone or together with other medicines to treat high hypertension and heart failure. Eprosartan is a tablet usually taken once or twice a day with or without food. The adverse effects include headache, sinusitis, diarrhea, bronchitis, **myalgia**, dizziness, edema, **dyspepsia**, and chest pain.

Irbesartan

Irbesartan is an angiotensin receptor blocker drug widely used to treat hypertension. It also helps prevent stroke and diabetic kidney disease. The main adverse effects of irbesartan are chills, dizziness, cold sweats, headaches, confusion, chest pain, and hypotension. It should be avoided during pregnancy and for individuals who have a history of allergic reactions to it. Irbesartan is also contraindicated in patients with diabetes and kidney impairment.

Losartan

Losartan is an ARB. Losartan is first-line therapy for stage 1 hypertension, along with thiazide diuretics, calcium channel blockers, and ACE inhibitors. For patients with type 2 diabetes and hypertension, it can be used to treat diabetic nephropathy.

Pharmacokinetics

Losartan is well absorbed orally but undergoes extensive first-pass metabolism. Its systemic bioavailability is approximately 35%. The onset of action is 6 hours, and the effect lasts approximately 24 hours. The plasma protein binding is high (99%). It is metabolized in the liver, and its half-life is 2 hours.

Mechanism of action

Losartan inhibits angiotensin II-induced vasopressin and adrenal catecholamine release. It also inhibits angiotensin II-induced vasoconstriction and the effects of ALD, thereby lowering BP.

Clinical indications

Losartan is used to treat hypertension and diabetic nephropathy, consequently reducing the risk of stroke in these patients.

Contraindications

Losartan is contraindicated with hypersensitivity to this drug or any of its components. It should be avoided during pregnancy, as it causes oligohydramnios, resulting in fetal lung and skull hypoplasia and skeletal deformities. Additional potential neonatal adverse effects include hypotension, renal failure, anuria, and death. Therefore therapy with the drug should be discontinued when pregnancy is detected.

Adverse effects

The primary adverse effects of losartan include angioedema, hypotension, hyperkalemia, and renal damage. Other adverse effects are chest pain, anemia, dizziness, fatigue, hypoglycemia, urinary tract infection, nausea, diarrhea, and cough.

Toxicities

Losartan overdose manifests as hypotension, dizziness, tachycardia, or loss of consciousness. It also causes hepatotoxicity and acute kidney injury.

Telmisartan

Telmisartan is an angiotensin II receptor antagonist that is widely used to treat hypertension. The adverse effects of telmisartan include allergic reactions, hyperkalemia, hypotension, renal impairment, headache, back pain, and diarrhea.

Aldosterone antagonists

ALD antagonists are crucial in managing primarily the cardiovascular and renal systems. They are vital for patients suffering from hypertension, heart failure, and certain kidney conditions. They block ALD's action, causing more sodium and water release via the kidneys. Examples of ALD antagonists are spironolactone (Aldactone) and eplerenone (Inspra). Spironolactone specifically competitively inhibits ALD receptor–mediated activity. The effect of the blockade is that sodium reabsorption with water retention does not occur, and there is increased potassium retention. It is available as a tablet in 25-mg, 50-mg, or 100-mg doses. Spironolactone has adverse effects such as **gynecomastia, impotence,** and menstrual irregularities. ALD antagonists are contraindicated in patients with anuria, acute renal insufficiency, marked renal impairment, and hyperkalemia. Rarely, spironolactone can cause liver toxicity that is manifested as elevations in serum aminotransferases and alkaline phosphatase in a hepatocellular mixed pattern after nearly 1 month of taking spironolactone, and this resolves over time after discontinuation of the drug.

Eplerenone is the first agent in a new class of drugs known as selective ALD receptor antagonists, which provide practical and well-tolerated BP reduction. Because eplerenone has little affinity for androgen and progesterone receptors, it produces fewer steroid-like effects (such as gynecomastia in males) than spironolactone. In addition to lowering BP, eplerenone protects the heart and kidneys. Hyperkalemia is a dose-related adverse effect.

Key Terms

Aldosterone
Angioedema
Angiotensinogen
Collecting duct
Distal convoluted tubule
Dyspepsia
Glomerulus
Gynecomastia
Impotence
Juxtaglomerular apparatus
Juxtaglomerular cells
Macula densa
Myalgia
Oligohydramnios
Oliguria
Osmolality
Raynaud syndrome
Renin
Skull hypoplasia
Vasopressin
Zona glomerulosa

Clinical Case Studies

Clinical Case Study 1

A 59-year-old male has a medical history of elevated low-density lipoprotein and well-controlled chronic stable angina secondary to coronary artery disease. After an episode of hypertension (165/94 mm Hg), a follow-up visit was scheduled, and the hypertension was still present (166/93 mm Hg). The patient is currently on atorvastatin (a 3-hydroxy3-methylglutaryl coenzyme A reductase inhibitor) and metoprolol (a beta-blocker) with no adverse effects. His resting heart rate is 65–70 beats per minute. The patient is then started on lisinopril (an ACE inhibitor).

Critical Thinking Questions

1. What is the mechanism of action of lisinopril?
2. What are the clinical indications of lisinopril?
3. What are the contraindications of lisinopril?

Clinical Case Study 2

A 46-year-old female has a medical history of hypertension for 6 years and diabetic nephropathy. Her physical examination reveals her BP is 155/110 mm Hg with edema in her legs. After evaluation of laboratory tests, she begins with losartan (angiotensin II receptor inhibitors).

Critical Thinking Questions

1. What is the mechanism of action of losartan?
2. What are the contraindications for losartan?
3. What are the adverse effects of losartan?

Further Reading

[1] M. Amechi Onuigbo, ACE Inhibitors—Medical Uses, Mechanisms of Action, Potential Adverse Effects and Related Topics (Pharmacology—Research, Safety Testing and Regulation), Nova Science Publishers, Inc., 2013.
[2] M. Burnier, Drug Adherence in Hypertension and Cardiovascular Protection (Updates Series), Springer, 2018.
[3] M.C. Houston, L. Bell, Controlling High Blood Pressure Through Nutrition, Supplements, Lifestyle and Drugs, CRC Press, 2021.
[4] M. Houston, Handbook of Hypertension, Wiley-Blackwell, 2011.
[5] P. Mainkar, S. Sawant, P. Pandit, Angiotensin Receptor Blockers and ACE Inhibitors—Role as Anti-inflammatory Agents, Lap Lambert Academic Publishing, 2013.
[6] S.J. Mann, Hypertension and You—Old Drugs, New Drugs, and the Right Drugs for your High Blood Pressure, Rowman and Littlefield Publishers, 2012.

[7] S.I. McFarlane, Renin-Angiotensin-Aldosterone System, InTechOpen, 2021.
[8] A. Saleh, Drugs for Hypertension, Saleh, 2020.
[9] M. Salvetti, Resistant Hypertension (Practical Case Studies in Hypertension Management), Springer, 2016.
[10] A.K. Singh, G.H. Williams, Textbook of Nephro-Endocrinology, second ed., Academic Press, 2017.
[11] G. Strube, ACE Inhibitors in Hypertension—A Guide for General Practitioners, Springer, 2012.
[12] T. Taniguchi, S.S. Lee, Cardio-Hepatology—Connections Between Hepatic and Cardiovascular Disease, Academic Press, 2022.
[13] S.E. Thatcher, The Renin-Angiotensin-Aldosterone System—Methods and Protocols (Methods in Molecular Biology, 1614), Human Press, 2017.
[14] R.M. Touyz, E.L. Schiffin, Hypertension—Methods and Protocols (Methods in Molecular Biology, 1527), Humana Press, 2017.
[15] T. Unger, B.A. Scholkens, Angiotensin Volume 1 (Handbook of Experimental Pharmacology 163), Springer, 2012.
[16] C.S. Wilcox, M. Choi, L. Chen, M.S. Segal, W.W. Williams, Handbook of Nephrology and Hypertension, seventh ed., Wolters Kluwer, 2022.

UNIT VI

Endocrine drugs

CHAPTER

36

Review of hypothalamic and pituitary drugs

OUTLINE

LEARNING OUTCOMES

After studying this chapter, readers should be able to:

1. Describe the primary function of the hypothalamus.
2. Explain the location of the pituitary gland and the hypothalamus.
3. Describe the neurohormones and their effects on the body.
4. Discuss the main hormones that are secreted from the anterior pituitary lobe.
5. Describe the pituitary-hypothalamic relationships.
6. Identify hormones that are released from the supraoptic and paraventricular nuclei.
7. Explain the effects of growth hormones in the body.
8. Explain hormones that are stored in the posterior lobe of the pituitary gland.

The Science of Pharmacology
https://doi.org/10.1016/B978-0-443-29038-1.00036-1

Overview

The hypothalamus is the ventral brain region, coordinating the endocrine system. It receives many signals from the various areas of the brain. It releases and inhibits hormones, which then act on the pituitary gland to direct the functions of the thyroid gland, adrenal glands, and reproductive organs, influencing growth, fluid balance, and milk production. It is also involved in the nonendocrine functions of temperature regulation, autonomic nervous system regulation, and appetite control. The pituitary is a pea-sized gland in the skull's sphenoid bone at the brain's base. The pituitary controls the function of most other endocrine glands and is sometimes called the master gland. The hypothalamus primarily controls it. By detecting the levels of hormones produced by glands under the pituitary's control (target glands), the hypothalamus or the pituitary can determine how much stimulation the target glands need. The pituitary gland malfunctions in several ways, usually due to developing adenoma. The tumor may overproduce one or more pituitary hormones or press on the normal pituitary cells, causing the underproduction of one or more pituitary hormones. This chapter discusses the pharmacotherapy for growth hormone (GH) conditions and antidiuretic hormone (ADH) disorder.

Physiology of the hypothalamus

The **hypothalamus, which includes many masses of gray matter and lies below the thalamus, represents a link between the nervous and endocrine systems**. Its primary function is to relay signals from the limbic system to the thalamus. The hypothalamus controls the center of the autonomic nervous system and endocrine system. It plays an essential role in the homeostatic regulation of nearly all body organs.

Physiology of the pituitary gland

The **pituitary gland** (hypophysis) is tiny and is found inside the **sphenoid bone** of the skull. It is only about the size of a pea, yet it secretes several hormones. The pituitary is connected to the hypothalamus by the infundibulum. The pituitary has two significant lobes, one consisting of neural tissue and one of glandular tissue.

The *posterior pituitary lobe* releases neurohormones from the hypothalamus. Therefore this lobe stores two hormones secreted by the hypothalamus. Together, the posterior pituitary and **infundibulum** make up the **neurohypophysis**. The *anterior pituitary lobe* is also known as the **adenohypophysis**. It is composed of glandular tissue and manufactures and releases several hormones. **Table 36.1** illustrates the hormones secreted from the pituitary gland lobes.

Pituitary-hypothalamic relationships

The posterior lobe is the part of the brain derived from a downward growth of hypothalamic tissue. It maintains its neural connection with the hypothalamus via a group of nerves called the *hypothalamic-hypophyseal tract*, linked through the infundibulum. The tract arises from neurons in the *supraoptic* and *paraventricular nuclei* of the hypothalamus. Oxytocin is synthesized mainly by the **paraventricular neurons**. ADH is also secreted chiefly by the **supraoptic neurons**.

You should remember

Through direct attachment to the pituitary gland, the hypothalamus influences water balance and milk production during pregnancy and lactation and also affects the sensation of both pain and pleasure.

Anterior lobe of the pituitary gland

The anterior lobe is called the "master gland" because many of its hormones regulate the activity of other endocrine glands. However, it is now understood that the hypothalamus controls the action of the anterior pituitary. There are six distinct anterior pituitary hormones, and they are all proteins. The hypothalamus stimulates the

TABLE 36.1 Pituitary gland hormones.

Lobe	Hormone	How it is regulated	Targeted effects
Anterior pituitary	ACTH	CRH from the hypothalamus	Controls secretion of certain hormones from the adrenal cortex
	FSH	Gonadotropin-releasing hormone from the hypothalamus	In females, it is responsible for the development of egg-containing follicles in ovaries and stimulates follicular cells to secrete estrogen; in males, it stimulates production of sperm cells
	GH	GH-releasing hormone and GH release-inhibiting hormone from the hypothalamus	Stimulates an increase in the size and division rate of body cells; enhances movement of amino acids across membranes
	LH	Gonadotropin-releasing hormone from the hypothalamus	Promotes secretion of sex hormones; it plays a role in releasing an egg cell in females
	PRL	Secretion restrained by PRL release–inhibiting hormone and stimulated by PRL-releasing factor from the hypothalamus	Sustains milk production after birth
	TSH	TRH from the hypothalamus	Controls secretion of hormones from the thyroid gland
Posterior Pituitary	ADH, or vasopressin	Hypothalamus in response to changes in water concentration in body fluids	Causes kidneys to conserve water; in high concentration, increases blood pressure
	OXT	Hypothalamus in response to stretching of uterine and vaginal walls and stimulation of breasts	Contracts muscles in the uterine wall; contracts muscles associated with milk-secreting glands

ACTH, Adrenocorticotropic hormone; *ADH*, antidiuretic hormone; *CRH*, corticotropin-releasing hormone; *FSH*, follicle-stimulating hormone; *GH*, growth hormone; *LH*, luteinizing hormone; *OXT*, oxytocin; *PRL*, prolactin; *TRH*, thyrotropin-releasing hormone; *TSH*, thyroid-stimulating hormone.

anterior lobe to release specific hormones. Four of the six anterior pituitary hormones are *tropins*, also called **trophic hormones**. Trophic hormones regulate the secretory action of other endocrine glands (see **Fig. 36.1**). The anterior pituitary hormones include:

- **GH:** also known as **somatotropin**, primarily targets bones and skeletal muscles. Most effects of GH are controlled by **insulin-like growth factors** produced by the liver, skeletal muscle, bone, and other tissues. GH stimulates the breakdown of stored triglycerides by adipocytes, releasing fatty acids into the blood. GHs in the liver produce the breakdown of **glycogen** reserves by liver cells, releasing glucose into the bloodstream.
- **Thyroid-stimulating hormone**, or **thyrotropin**, is a trophic hormone that simulates normal development and secretion from the thyroid gland. It is released following the hypothalamic-pituitary-target endocrine organ

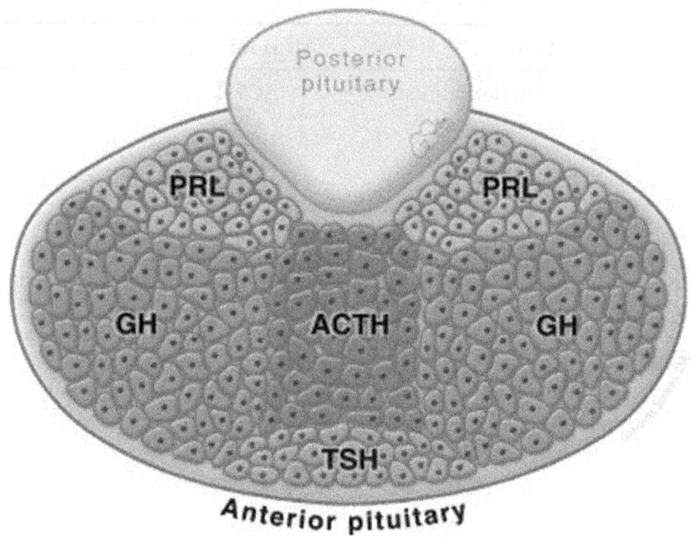

FIG. 36.1 The anterior pituitary hormones.

feedback loop—thyrotrophs of the anterior pituitary release thyroid-stimulating hormone, triggered by **thyrotropin-releasing hormone**.

- **Adrenocorticotropic hormone** (ACTH): also known as **corticotropin**, is secreted by the *corticotrophs* of the anterior pituitary. It stimulates the adrenal cortex to release corticosteroid hormones. ACTH release has a daily rhythm, peaking in the morning shortly before awakening. ACTH specifically targets the cells that secrete corticosteroids, which affect glucose metabolism.
- **Follicle-stimulating hormone** (FSH) and **luteinizing hormone** (LH): also known as **gonadotropins**, regulate functions of the ovaries in females and testes in males. Follicle-stimulating hormone stimulates sperm and egg production, while LH promotes the production of gonadal hormones. In females, they help the ovarian follicle to mature. LH then triggers **ovulation** and the release of ovarian hormones. In males, this gonadotropin is also called **interstitial cell–stimulating hormone** because it stimulates testosterone production. Testosterone is also classified as an **androgen**.
- **Prolactin** (PRL): lactotrophs produce this hormone. In humans, PRL stimulates milk production in females, but its role in males is not understood. It is controlled by the **PRL-inhibiting hormone**, which is now understood to be **dopamine**. In females, PRL levels change along with estrogen blood levels. PRL is also called **mammotropin.** PRL, estrogens, progesterone, glucocorticoids, and pancreatic hormones prepare the mammary glands for secreting milk.

The posterior lobe of the pituitary gland

The posterior pituitary gland is made mainly of axons of the hypothalamic neurons. It stores *ADH* and *oxytocin* after they have been sent from the hypothalamus. It then releases them on an "as-needed" basis. ADH and oxytocin are almost identical and composed of amino acids. ADH influences body water balance, while oxytocin stimulates smooth muscle contraction, mainly in the uterus and breasts of females.

- **ADH**: also known as **vasopressin**, controls water balance, helping to avoid dehydration and water overload. Therefore the primary function of ADH is to decrease the amount of water lost by the kidneys. Antidiuretic means "inhibiting or preventing urine formation" (*diuresis* is urine production). **Osmoreceptors** monitor solute and water concentrations in the blood. They transmit impulses to the hypothalamus to synthesize and release ADH. When blood concentrations of ADH are high, ADH causes vasoconstriction of most visceral blood vessels. When there is severe blood loss, enormous amounts of ADH are released, causing a rise in blood pressure (hence its alternate name, vasopressin).
- **Oxytocin**: a potent stimulant of uterine contraction, is released chiefly during childbirth and lactation. Stretching of the uterus and cervix triggers its release. Oxytocin also triggers milk ejection (the "letdown" reflex), which results from positive feedback mechanisms such as uterine contractions. It has also been discovered that oxytocin also plays a role in **sexual arousal** and **orgasm**. The functions of oxytocin in sexual activity are not certain, but levels of oxytocin rise during sexual arousal, peaking at orgasm (in both sexes). In males, it stimulates smooth

muscle contractions in the ductus deferens and prostate gland, which may be required for producing reproductive secretions. In females, oxytocin may stimulate smooth muscle contractions in the uterus and vagina, helping to transport sperm toward the uterine tubes.

You should remember

Drinking alcoholic beverages inhibits ADH secretion and causes increased urine output. Its release is also inhibited by drinking excessive amounts of water.

You should remember

Until the final stages of pregnancy, the uterine smooth muscles are relatively insensitive to oxytocin. They become more sensitive as delivery approaches. Oxytocin secretion and milk ejection are part of a neuroendocrine reflex called the *milk letdown reflex*.

Growth hormone disorders

GH deficiency (GHD), also known as **dwarfism** or pituitary dwarfism, is caused by insufficient amounts of GH in the body. Children with GHD have abnormally short stature with normal body proportions. Congenital GHD can occur at birth or can develop later. In adults, lack of GH is usually caused by damage to the pituitary gland or the hypothalamus. The damage may be due to a tumor, surgery, radiation used to treat the cancer, or problems with the blood supply to the pituitary gland.

Even after we stop growing, adults still need GHs. GH is a protein made by the pituitary gland and released into the blood. GHs play a role in healthy muscle, how our bodies collect fat (especially around the stomach area), and the ratio of high-density to low-density lipoproteins in our cholesterol levels and bone density. In addition, GHs are needed for normal brain function. A person who has too little adult GH will have symptoms that include:

- A higher level of body fat, especially around the waist
- Anxiety and depression
- Changes in the makeup of the blood cholesterol
- Greater sensitivity to heat and cold
- Less muscle (lean body mass)
- Decreased sexual function and interest
- Fatigue
- Feelings of being isolated from other people
- Reduced bone density and a tendency to have more bone fractures as they get older

A lack of GH is usually caused by damage to the pituitary gland or the hypothalamus, a part of the brain that controls the pituitary gland. The damage may be due to a tumor, surgery or radiation used to treat the cancer, or problems with the blood supply to the pituitary gland. A lack of GH can appear either in childhood or in adulthood.

Pharmacotherapy of growth hormone disorders

For patients with dwarfism due to GHD, treatment with (vosoritide [Voxzogo]) synthetic hormone injections may increase final height. In most cases, children receive daily injections for several years until they reach a maximum adult height—often within the average adult range for their family. GH therapy should not be given to people who have active cancer or tumors. It also should not be given to people who are seriously ill as a result of complications from open heart or abdominal surgery, have multiple injuries from a major accident, or have breathing problems. Taking GHs will not cause an adult to begin growing again.

Pharmacokinetics

Vosoritide is absorbed within 15 minutes. The metabolism of vosoritide is expected to occur via catabolic pathways and be degraded into small peptide fragments and amino acids.

Mechanism of action

Vosoritide works by binding to a target receptor called *natriuretic peptide receptor type B*, which reduces the activity of fibroblast growth factor receptor 3. It then increases cartilage cell growth, thereby increasing bone growth.

Clinical indications

Vosoritide is indicated to increase linear growth in pediatric patients with achondroplasia who are 5 years of age or older and have open epiphyses. This indication is approved under accelerated approval based on an improvement in annualized growth velocity.

Contraindications

There are no contraindications for vosoritide except hypersensitivity to the active substance.

Adverse effects

The most common side effects of vosoritide include injection site reactions, vomiting, and hypotension. Vosoritide's labeling lists decreased blood pressure as a warning and precaution, a potentially severe side effect. To reduce the risk of hypotension and associated symptoms such as dizziness, fatigue, blurred vision, headache, muscle pain, shivering, and nausea, instruct patients to be well hydrated and have adequate food intake before administration of vosoritide.

Toxicity

Vosoritide is an effective treatment to increase growth in children with achondroplasia. It is unknown what the harms of long-term therapy might be. Therefore toxicity is rare.

Antidiuretic hormone disorders

Diabetes insipidus (DI) is caused by a lack of ADH, which causes the body to make too much urine. It is rare when the kidneys cannot conserve water while filtering blood. ADH enables the kidneys to retain water in the body. Diabetes insipidus is also called **arginine vasopressin deficiency** and arginine vasopressin resistance. The primary symptoms of DI are **polydipsia** and polyuria, sometimes as often as every 15 minutes. This is caused by the lack of ADH or the inability of the kidneys to respond to ADH. Adults typically urinate an average of about 1–3 L a day. People who have DI and who drink a lot of fluids may make as much as 20 L of urine a day. Damage to the pituitary gland or hypothalamus from surgery, a tumor, a head injury, or an illness can cause central DI. That damage affects the production, storage, and release of ADH. An inherited disorder may cause this condition too. The risk factors include a family history of the disorder and certain medicines, such as diuretics, hypercalcemia, and hypokalemia. Blood and urine tests must be done to diagnose DI. In some cases, an MRI is also required.

Pharmacotherapy of antidiuretic hormone disorders

There is no cure for DI. However, a treatment that can ease its symptoms is available. That includes relieving thirst, lowering the amount of urine the body makes, and preventing dehydration. Desmopressin (DDAVP, Nocturne) is used for treatment. This medication replaces the missing ADH and lowers the amount of urine the body makes. Desmopressin is available as a pill, a nasal spray, and an injection.

Pharmacokinetics

The mean time to reach maximum plasma desmopressin levels is about 1.1 hours after administration. Increasing oral doses produces dose-dependent increases in the drug's plasma levels. The plasma half-life of desmopressin has been estimated to be between 1 and 2 hours, whereas the antidiuretic effect lasts 7–10 hours.

Mechanism of action

The agonist activity of desmopressin raises intracellular concentrations of cyclic adenosine monophosphate, inducing exocytosis from its storage sites.

Clinical indications

Desmopressin is used for DI for ADH replacement therapy and management of temporary polyuria and polydipsia following head trauma or surgery.

Contraindications

Desmopressin is contraindicated in patients with moderate to severe renal impairment. It is also contraindicated in patients with hyponatremia or a history of hyponatremia.

Adverse effects

Though adverse effects from desmopressin are rare, they include confusion; convulsions; decreased urine output; dizziness; arrhythmia; headache; increased thirst; muscle pain or cramps; nausea or vomiting; shortness of breath; edema on face, hands, or ankles; fatigue; weight gain; delusions; dementia; and diarrhea.

Toxicity

The only reported toxic effects are convulsions or altered consciousness resulting from water intoxication.

Key Terms

Adenohypophysis
Androgen
Arginine vasopressin deficiency
Corticotropin
Dopamine
Dwarfism
Glycogen
Gonadotropin
Hypothalamus
Infundibulum
Insulin-like growth factors
Interstitial cell–stimulating hormone
Mammotropin
Neurohypophysis
Orgasm
Osmoreceptors
Ovulation
Paraventricular neurons
Pituitary gland
Polydipsia
Prolactin-inhibiting hormone
Sexual arousal
Somatotropin
Sphenoid bone
Supraoptic neurons
Thalamus
Thyrotropin
Trophic hormones
Vasopressin

Clinical Case Studies

Clinical Case Study 1

A 9-year-old girl was brought to a pediatrician for slowed growth. Previous growth velocity had been average—no history of headaches, vomiting, or vision changes. No fatigue, cold intolerance, constipation, or skin or hair changes were found. Her appetite and weight were normal. Breast development began at eight with scant pubic hair that developed shortly after. The patient was premenarchal. Examination revealed a nondysmorphic, proportionate child who appeared much younger than her chronological age. After several blood tests and imaging, she was diagnosed with GHD.

Critical Thinking Questions

1. What are the causes of pituitary dwarfism?
2. What are the symptoms of GHD?
3. What is the mechanism of action for vosoritide (synthetic GH)?

Clinical Case Study 2

A 27-year-old professional footballer was admitted to a polyclinic with symptoms of polyuria and polydipsia. He was complaining about excessive thirst in the past 2 days and continuous water drinking, with constant urination throughout the day, reaching up to 14 L a day. The patient had no other medical history or history of medication use. The patient had no known medical history or history of taking medications. He said that after the strike, he had a blackout and was taken to the emergency department. After laboratory tests and imaging, DI was diagnosed.

Critical Thinking Questions

1. What are the signs and symptoms of DI?
2. What are the causes of DI?
3. How can it be treated, DI?

Further Reading

[1] M.J. Alfred, The Human Growth Hormone and its Corresponding Effects on Your Body, Alfred, 2022.
[2] P. Beck-Peccoz, Syndromes of Hormone Resistance on the Hypothalamic-Pituitary-Thyroid Axis (Endocrine Updates, Book 22), Springer, 2004.
[3] F.F. Casaneuva, E. Ghigo, Hypothalamic-Pituitary Diseases (Endocrinology), Springer, 2018.
[4] R.C. Gaillard, The ACTH Axis – Pathogenesis, Diagnosis and Treatment (Endocrine Updates Book 21), Springer, 2012.
[5] V. Grinevich, A. Dobolyi, Neuroanatomy of Neuroendocrine Systems (Masterclass in Neuroendocrinology, Book 12), Springer, 2022.
[6] J.L. Jameson, L.J. De Groot, Endocrinology: Adult and Pediatric, Expert Consult Premium Edition, sixth ed., Saunders / Elsevier, 2010.
[7] E.R. Laws, S. Ezzat, S.L. Asa, L.M. Rio, L. Michel, R. Knutzen, Pituitary Disorders – Diagnosis and Management, Wiley-Blackwell, 2013.
[8] G. Leng, The Heart of the Brain – the Hypothalamus and Its Hormones, The MIT Press, 2018.
[9] G. Litwack, Hormones, fourth ed., Academic Press, 2022.
[10] G. Litwack, Hormonal Signaling in Biology and Medicine (Comprehensive Modern Endocrinology), Academic Press, 2019.
[11] S. Melmed, The Pituitary, fifth ed., Academic Press, 2022.
[12] P. Molina, Endocrine Physiology, sixth ed., McGraw-Hill / Lange, 2023.
[13] A.W. Norman, H.L. Henry, Hormones, third ed., Academic Press, 2014.
[14] J. Porter, Hypothalamic Peptide Hormones and Pituitary Regulation (Advances in Experimental Medicine and Biology, 87), Springer, 2012.
[15] J.,J.T. Potts, J.L. Jameson, L.J. De Groot, Endocrinology Adult and Pediatric – the Parathyroid Gland and Bone Metabolism, Elsevier, 2013.
[16] S. Radovick, M. Misra, Pediatric Endocrinology – A Practical Clinical Guide, third ed., Springer, 2018.
[17] S.L. Samson, A.G. Ioachimescu, Pituitary Disorders Throughout the Life Cycle – A Case-based Guide, Springer, 2022.
[18] G.I. Uwaifo, The Human Hypothalamus – Anatomy, Dysfunction and Disease Management (Contemporary Endocrinology), Humana Press, 2021.
[19] E. Van Cauter, G. Copinschi, Human Pituitary Hormones – Circadian and Episodic Variations (Developments in Endocrinology, 1), Martinus Nijhoff Publishers, 2011.

CHAPTER

37

Pharmacotherapy of thyroid disorders

OUTLINE

LEARNING OUTCOMES

After studying this chapter, readers should be able to:

1. Describe the structure and functions of the thyroid gland.
2. Explain the mechanism of negative feedback in controlling thyroid hormones.
3. Describe the effects of thyroid hormones on body systems.
4. Discuss the pathophysiology of hypothyroidism.
5. Explain the first-line drugs for the treatment of hypothyroidism.
6. Discuss the contraindications of levothyroxine.
7. Describe the adverse effects of levothyroxine.
8. Identify the differences between hyperthyroidism and thyrotoxicosis.
9. Explain the mechanism of action of propylthiouracil.

https://doi.org/10.1016/B978-0-443-29038-1.00037-3

10. Describe the contraindications of propylthiouracil.

Overview

The thyroid gland produces, stores, and secretes thyroxine (T_4) and triiodothyronine (T_3) hormones through a negative feedback process involving the hypothalamus and pituitary gland. Thyroid dysfunction can result when any part of this process is affected and is usually characterized by high or low levels of thyroid-stimulating hormone (TSH) secreted by the pituitary gland and free thyroid hormones. There are two main types of thyroid disease: hyperthyroidism and hypothyroidism. Both conditions can be caused by other diseases that impact the functions of the thyroid glands. All kinds of hyperthyroidism are due to an overproduction of thyroid hormones; hypothyroidism responds highly to thyroid hormones. For example, levothyroxine (LT_4) is nearly always used. The pathophysiology of hypothyroidism and hyperthyroidism is essential to understanding pharmacotherapy.

Physiology of the thyroid gland

The thyroid gland is the largest purely endocrine gland in the body. It is located in the anterior neck and has a butterfly-like shape. It curves across the anterior surface of the trachea and is slightly inferior to the larynx. It consists of two lateral lobes connected by a median tissue mass called the isthmus. The average weight is approximately 34 grams. The thyroid gland regulates body metabolism via the various hormones that it releases. The thyroid is also involved in **gluconeogenesis**, protein synthesis, **glycogenolysis**, **lipogenesis**, and thermogenesis. The parathyroid glands are embedded in the posterior surface of the thyroid gland's lateral lobes, aiding in calcium homeostasis.

The thyroid gland is controlled by hypophyseal **TSH**—the secretion of TSH results in **endocytosis** of colloid droplets at the luminal epithelium. TSH is released from the anterior pituitary gland. The hypothalamus, via **negative feedback**, detects low plasma concentrations of thyroid hormone and releases **thyrotropin-releasing hormone** (TRH) into the hypophyseal portal system. The TRH binds to receptors on thyrotrophic cells of the anterior pituitary gland and causes them to release TSH into the systemic circulation (see **Fig. 37.1**). This liberates the hormones T_3 and T_4, which move to the base of the cell and are released. They move out from the thyroid mainly through the capillaries and the lymphatics. When circulating TSH is prolonged and at high levels, hypertrophy of the follicular cells occurs. There is also continued resorption of colloid, increased vascularity of the stroma, and often thyroid enlargement.

The thyroid also contains other endocrine cells such as C or **parafollicular cells**. They are located between the cuboidal follicle cells and their basement membrane. The C cells are more significant than the follicular epithelium cells. They produce **calcitonin** (CT) in the form of *thyrocalcitonin*, the peptide hormone that lowers blood calcium via inhibition of bone resorption and calcium recovery from the ultrafiltrate of the renal tubules. The C cells fill the middle third portion of each lateral thyroid lobe. Sometimes they cluster in the interfollicular stroma. This is why they are also called parafollicular cells. The thyroid gland is essential for many body regulatory states.

The inside of the thyroid gland is composed of hollow, round *follicles*. The thyroid follicles produce **thyroglobulin**—the central cavity of the thyroid stores *colloid*, which is sticky and amber colored. Thyroid hormone is derived from thyroglobulin, which contains the amino acid **tyrosine**, the building block of thyroid hormones. The **parafollicular cells** of the thyroid produce **CT**. The thyroid gland is unique because it can store large amounts of its hormone extracellularly—enough to provide expected levels of hormone release for 2–3 months. There are two responses after TSH binds to receptors on follicle cells. The first is the secretion of stored thyroid hormone, and the second is the synthesis of more colloids to produce additional hormones. Levels of TSH are usually highest just before sleep. Follicle cells synthesize thyroid hormone as follows:

- Thyroglobulin is synthesized and moved into the follicle lumen.
- The digestive tract absorbs iodide ions from the diet, and the bloodstream transports them to the thyroid gland.
- Iodide is oxidized to iodine.
- Iodine is attached to tyrosine.
- Iodinated tyrosine link to form T_3 and T_4.
- Thyroglobulin colloid is endocytosed.
- Lysosomal enzymes split T_3 and T_4 from thyroglobulin, and the hormones diffuse into the bloodstream.

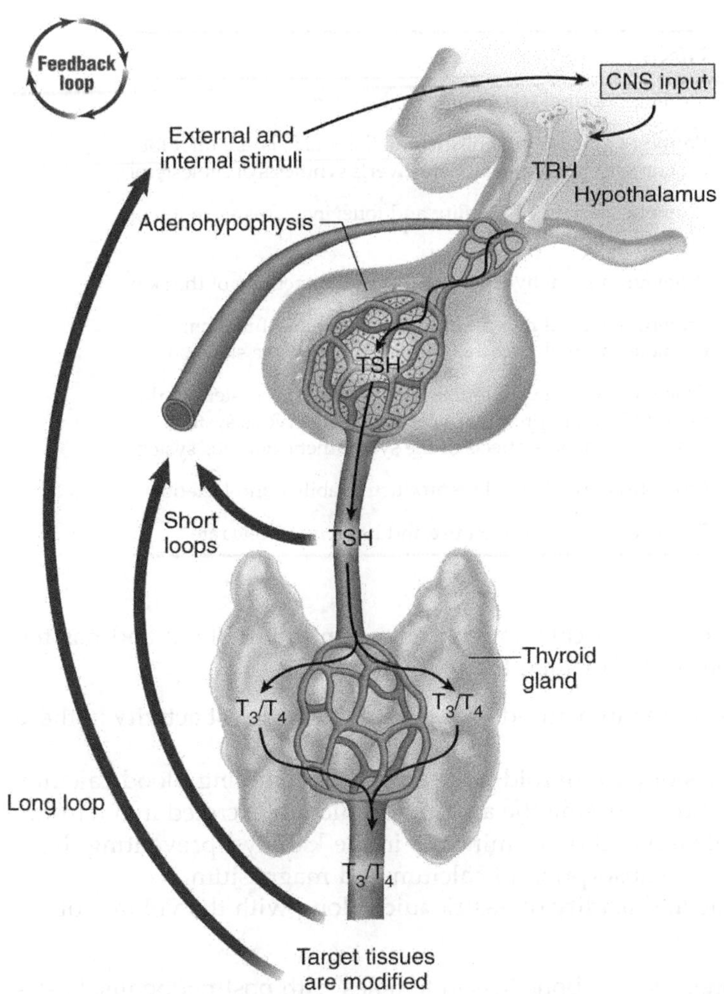

FIG. 37.1 Feedback mechanism of the thyroid gland.

Most thyroid hormones bind quickly to T_4-binding globulins produced by the liver. Decreasing thyroid hormone blood levels causes the release of TSH, and then more thyroid hormone is produced. The hypothalamus secretes the TRH in response to extreme conditions such as pregnancy and severe temperature changes. This triggers TSH release as well. The release of TSH is inhibited by GH inhibitors and dopamine and is raised by glucocorticoid levels. Excessive concentrations of blood iodide inhibit thyroid hormone release. **Table 37.1** lists the significant effects of thyroid hormone throughout the body.

You should remember

People who take thyroid hormones may need to continue them for the rest of their lives. This is especially true following thyroid surgery or radioactive iodine treatment.

Calcitonin hormone

CT is a hormone produced by the parafollicular thyroid gland cells, called C cells or **clear cells**. They are larger than the follicular epithelium cells and do not stain as clearly. CT regulates calcium ion concentration in the blood. It inhibits **osteoclasts**, decreasing the rate of calcium ion release from bone. CT also stimulates calcium ion excretion by

TABLE 37.1 Effects of thyroid hormone.

Body system	Effects
Cardiovascular	Promotes normal functioning of the heart
Digestive	Promotes glucose catabolism; mobilizes fats; is essential for protein synthesis; enhances the liver's synthesis of cholesterol
Gastrointestinal	Promotes normal GI motility and tone; increases secretion of digestive juices
Integumentary	Promotes normal hydration and secretory activity of the skin
Musculoskeletal	Promotes normal muscular development and function; promotes normal growth and maturation of the skeleton
Nervous	Promotes normal development of the nervous system in the fetus and infant; promotes normal adult nervous system function; enhances effects of the sympathetic nervous system
Reproductive	Promotes normal female reproductive ability and lactation
Respiratory	Promotes normal oxygen use and basal metabolic rate

the kidneys, therefore having bone-sparing effects. CT lowers the calcium concentration in the blood and has the opposite effect of parathyroid hormone. The main actions of CT include the following:

1. In postmenopausal females with osteoporosis: The use of manufactured CT can inhibit osteoclast activity in these patients.
2. Maintenance of calcium balance: CT opposes the effects of parathyroid hormone while lowering blood calcium levels by suppressing osteoclast activity in the bones and increasing the amount of calcium excreted in the urine.
3. Effects upon the kidneys: CT regulates the level of calcium and other minerals in the kidneys, preventing the reabsorption of phosphates and increasing the kidneys' reabsorption of calcium and magnesium.
4. Affecting hunger and appetite: CT reduces the volume and acidity of gastric juice along with the volume of pancreatic juice and its trypsin and amylase content.

CT injections are used to treat Paget disease of the bone, prevent bone loss in females with postmenopausal osteoporosis, and treat hypercalcemia.

Pathophysiology of hypothyroidism

Hypothyroidism is a clinical state mainly identified by reduced thyroid hormone production and decreased free thyroid hormone circulating levels. Resistance to hormone action may also cause it. The thyroid gland can be permanently lost or destroyed. Hypothyroidism is a common disorder. It occurs at all ages but is most common in older people and in females. Although it is usually easy to diagnose in younger adults, hypothyroidism can be subtle, manifesting atypically in older adults.

Cretinism occurs when congenital hypothyroidism is untreated for long periods and is a form of severe hypothyroidism. Cretinism occurs in areas of the world with a severe deficiency of iodine. **Myxedema** is acquired hypothyroidism in adults. It affects females much more often than males, and most affected patients are middle aged. In all patients with myxedema, there are destructive changes to the thyroid gland. Usually, delicate fibrous tissue replaces the typical thyroid gland structures. This fibrous development also often occurs in the skin and less frequently in the visceral organs, suggesting an irritative or inflammatory process. There is slowed mental and physical activity, and the patient becomes apathetic. Mental sluggishness may resemble depression. Speech and intellectual functions are slower, and the effect is flat. Other signs and symptoms include hair and tooth loss; alterations in speech, movement, sensation, consciousness, and intellect plus extensive collections of mucin in the skin, fibrous tissues, blood, and salivary glands. Deficiency of thyroid hormone affects almost all body tissue, causing multiple symptoms.

You should remember

Characteristic signs and symptoms of hypothyroidism in older adults can be challenging to recognize, and changes in mental status are sometimes attributed to dementia or just advancing age. The American Thyroid Association estimates that one in four nursing home patients have undiagnosed hypothyroidism. Diagnosis is based on laboratory criteria.

Pharmacotherapy

Hypothyroidism usually responds exceptionally well to thyroid hormones. LT_4 is nearly always used. Popular brand names for LT_4 in the United States include Synthroid, Levoxyl, Unithyroid, and Tirosint. Another medication used to treat hypothyroidism is liothyronine (Cytomel, Triostat).

Levothyroxine

LT_4 is generally considered the treatment of choice for patients with hypothyroidism. In those with secondary hypothyroidism, free T_4 should be measured with the goal of normal free T_4 levels, as TSH is not an accurate measure of efficacious thyroid hormone dose.

Pharmacokinetics

LT_4 is taken on an empty stomach because bioavailability is best in this state. Absorption is also markedly decreased when it is consumed with iron, calcium, and dietary fiber. LT_4 is usually given once per day orally, based on age, body mass index, and absorption. It starts with low doses and is adjusted every 6 weeks until a maintenance dose is achieved. Pregnant females should increase their daily dose of LT_4 by 30% once pregnancy is diagnosed, and they should have thyroid function checked every trimester, as pregnancy results in increased binding globulins, resulting in less free T_4. The dose may also be increased if the patient takes medications that decrease LT_4 absorption or increase biliary excretion. The individual patient dose should be the lowest one that restores serum TSH levels to normal.

Mechanism of action

T_3 and LT_4 diffuse into the cell nucleus and bind to thyroid receptor proteins attached to DNA. This hormone nuclear receptor complex activates gene transcription and synthesis of messenger RNA and cytoplasmic proteins.

Clinical indications

Oral LT_4 is primarily indicated for treating primary, secondary, and tertiary hypothyroidism. There is also an injectable form, usually used to load patients until they can start oral therapy. Primary hypothyroidism is when the problem occurs in the thyroid gland. Liothyronine is more rapidly metabolized and has a more rapid effect than LT_4.

Contraindications

LT_4 is contraindicated in patients with thyrotoxic heart disease and uncorrected *adrenocorticoid* insufficiency.

Adverse effects

Common side effects of LT_4 include heat intolerance, tachycardia, and diarrhea. More serious LT_4 side effects, such as tremors or mood changes, are also possible. LT_4 can also raise the risk of bone loss and fractures.

Toxicity

Massive amounts of LT_4 may be ingested intentionally or accidentally. The most common intentional reasons include weight loss and suicidal ideation. A potentially toxic dose includes acute ingestion of more than 5 mg of LT_4 or 0.75 mg of T_3. Symptoms of LT_4 overdose include tachycardia, chest pain, headache, anxiety, agitation, nervousness, insomnia, anxiety, shaking, sweating, fatigue, confusion, and disorientation.

You should remember

Because thyroid hormones can increase the body's metabolism and promote weight loss, there has been interest in using them as a diet aid. Some people use prescription thyroid medications for this reason, but thyroid hormones are sometimes found as illicit additives in over-the-counter weight loss supplements. Unlike prescription medications, which are tightly regulated, over-the-counter weight loss products may contain several different hormone preparations of variable potency. Because over-the-counter weight loss products are dietary supplements, they should not have prescription medications such as thyroid hormones.

Hyperthyroidism

The various manifestations of excessive amounts of thyroid hormones are described as either *hyperthyroidism* or *thyrotoxicosis*. However, these two terms are not synonymous. The difference is that **thyrotoxicosis** is a state of excessive thyroid hormone, while hyperthyroidism results from excessive thyroid function. Hyperthyroidism, however, is just one cause of thyrotoxicosis. Primary hyperthyroidism may arise from an intrinsic thyroid abnormality. Graves disease is an autoimmune disorder that can cause hyperthyroidism. The immune system attacks the thyroid gland, causing it to manufacture more thyroid hormones than are needed, making many body functions more active. About four out of five cases of hyperthyroidism are caused by Graves disease. Secondary hyperthyroidism may arise from processes outside the thyroid, such as a TSH-secreting pituitary tumor.

Pharmacotherapy

Treatment of hyperthyroidism is based on the cause. Pharmacologic doses of iodine inhibit the release of TH and the organification of iodine within hours. This transitory effect lasts a few days to a week, with inhibition usually stopping. Iodine helps in the emergency management of thyroid storms for hyperthyroid individuals having emergency nonthyroid surgery. Because it decreases thyroid vascularity, it is helpful for preoperative preparation before subtotal thyroidectomy. Iodine is not usually used for routine hyperthyroidism treatment.

Propylthiouracil and methimazole

The antihyperthyroidism drugs are called thionamides. These include propylthiouracil (PTU) and methimazole (Tapazole). They function by inhibiting thyroid peroxidase (TPO) to reduce oxidation and organification of iodide. They also reduce thyroid antibody levels by unclear mechanisms, enhancing remission rates. PTU inhibits the deiodination of T_4 to T_3. Except for the most severe cases of thyrotoxicosis, this minor effect is offset by the extremely short half-life of the drug—only 90 minutes—compared to the 6-hour half-life of methimazole.

Pharmacokinetics

PTU absorption via the GI tract is 75%, and almost 85% is bound to plasma proteins. The therapeutic effect is 24–36 hours, and the half-life elimination is approximately 1 hour. PTU primarily undergoes metabolism in the liver to glucuronides or inorganic sulfate and is excreted from urine.

Mechanism of action

PTU inhibits the production of new thyroid hormones in the thyroid gland. It acts by inhibiting the enzyme TPO, which usually converts iodide to an iodine molecule and incorporates the iodine molecule into the amino acid tyrosine. Therefore it inhibits the conversion of T_4 to T_3.

Clinical indications

PTU is commonly used in patients with hyperthyroidism before thyroidectomy or radioactive iodine therapy. It is also indicated for the treatment of thyroid storm and thyrotoxicosis crises.

Contraindications

PTU is contraindicated in patients with a previous history of hypersensitivity to the drug or any of its drug components. Caution is advised in patients with hepatic impairment or myelosuppression and pediatric patients.

Adverse effects

PTU can cause significant hepatotoxicity and acute liver failure. However, the FDA has approved its use in pregnant women and children.

Toxicity

There is no information regarding the lethal dose, serum-level concentration of PTU associated with overdose symptoms, or the amount of single drug dose assumed to be causing overdose symptoms.

Beta-blockers

Propranolol or a longer-acting selective beta$_1$-receptor blocker such as atenolol may effectively control adrenergic symptoms, mainly in the early stages before antithyroid drugs can take effect. Beta-blockers are also effective for those with thyrotoxic periodic paralysis as long as thyrotoxicosis is corrected. Beta-blockers were discussed in **Chapter 18**.

You should remember

Anticoagulation with warfarin must be considered for those with cardiovascular conditions if the patient has atrial fibrillation. These patients often spontaneously revert to sinus rhythm when hyperthyroidism is controlled. If the patient is thyrotoxic, decreased doses of warfarin are required. If digoxin is being used, increased amounts are often needed.

You should remember

Newer injectable treatments have also become available. They include teprotumumab-trbw, a monoclonal antibody used to treat thyroid eye disease. It works by blocking the action of proteins that cause eye inflammation. Other new treatments include biologics and immunomodulators such as rituximab and intravenous glucocorticoids.

Key Terms

Calcitonin
Clear cells
Cretinism
Endocytosis
Gluconeogenesis
Glycogenolysis
Lipogenesis
Myxedema
Negative feedback
Parafollicular cells
Thyroid-stimulating hormone
Thyroglobulin
Thyrotropin-releasing hormone
Thyrotoxicosis
Tyrosine

Clinical Case Studies

Clinical Case 1

A baby boy was diagnosed with congenital hypothyroidism early in childhood. He was relatively inactive and growing slower than the average rate for his age. When participating in outdoor activities with other children, he always required more clothing than the others due to his inability to keep warm. However, with daily medication, the boy could live a nearly normal life.

Critical Thinking Questions

1. How is congenital hypothyroidism usually diagnosed?
2. What medications will be required to manage this condition?
3. Can congenital hypothyroidism affect a patient's offspring?

Clinical Case 2

A 38-year-old female had been previously diagnosed with an underactive thyroid gland. She visits her physician, complaining of increasing fatigue, fluid retention, weight gain, and constipation. Tests reveal that her anti-thyroglobulin and anti-TPO antibodies were extremely high, as was her TSH level.

Critical Thinking Questions

1. What is the likely diagnosis for this patient?
2. What should this patient's TSH level be maintained?
3. Is this condition related to other autoimmune diseases?

Clinical Case 3

A 35-year-old female complained of nervousness, weakness, and palpitations with exertion. These symptoms have existed for about 6 months. She recently noticed excessive sweating. Her weight is the same as over the past year, yet she can eat much more. Her menstrual periods were regular but have involved less bleeding than before. Examination revealed warm, moist skin, fine tremors, bounding cardiac apical impulses, and three thyroid nodules.

Critical Thinking Questions

1. What is the most likely cause of this patient's illness?
2. What tests are needed to confirm the cause?
3. What are the treatment options?

Further Reading

[1] D. Edison, Understanding Hyperthyroidism – A Unique Guide to Understanding the Symptoms, Diagnosis, Treatment of Hyperthyroidism with Medical and Alternative Forms of Treatment, Edison, 2021.
[2] H.A. Hamilton, Impaired Sensitivity to Thyroid Hormone (Thyroid Hormone Resistance), third ed., Hamilton, 2016.
[3] R. Jatwa, A. Kar, Chronic Medication and Thyroid Functions – an Experimental Approach, Lap Lambert Academic Publishing, 2016.
[4] F.S. Kuehn, M.P. Lozada, Thyroid Hormones – Functions, Related Diseases and Uses (Endocrinology Research and Clinical Development), Nova Science Publishers, Inc., 2010.
[5] G. Litwack, Thyroid Hormone (Vitamins and Hormones – Volume 106), Academic Press, 2018.
[6] M. Mcgarvey, A Guide on Thyroid Disease – How to Reduce the Intense Pressure Behind your Eyes, Mcgarvey, 2021.
[7] E. Moore, The Thyroid Eye Disease Book – Understanding Graves' Ophthalmopathy, Your Health Press, 2013.
[8] R. Pitt-Rivers, J.R. Tata, R.K. Callow, P.N. Campbell, S.P. Datta, The Thyroid Hormones, Pergamon Press, 2013.
[9] G.W. Randolph, Surgery of the Thyroid and Parathyroid Glands – Expert Consult Premium Edition, second ed., Elsevier / Saunders, 2012.
[10] J. Rosai, R.A. DeLellis, M.L. Carcangiu, W.J. Frable, G. Tallini, Tumors of the Thyroid and Parathyroid Glands (Atlas of Tumor Pathology, Series 4), American Registry of Pathology, 2015.
[11] R.A. Sofferman, A.T. Ahuja, Ultrasound of the Thyroid and Parathyroid Glands, Springer, 2012.
[12] J. Somsuzen, Myxedema Symptoms – Understand Hypothyroidism and Support Thyroid Function, Somsuzen, 2023.
[13] M. Woodward, Hashimoto Thyroiditis Guide – A Healing Plan for Managing Symptoms, Diagnosis & Treatment. Woodward, 2023.
[14] S. Zaidi, Graves' Disease and Hyperthyroidism – what you must Know Before they Zap your Thyroid with Radioactive Iodine, CreateSpace Independent Publishing Platform, 2013.

CHAPTER

38

Adrenocorticosteroids and aldosterone antagonists

OUTLINE

LEARNING OUTCOMES

After studying this chapter, readers should be able to:

1. Describe the structure of the adrenal gland.
2. Explain the primary functions of the three layers of the adrenal cortex.
3. Describe the adrenal medulla hormones.
4. Discuss the clinical indications of corticosteroids.
5. Explain the adverse effects of corticosteroids.
6. Describe the various types of aldosterone antagonists.
7. Identify the contraindications of spironolactone.
8. Explain the adverse effects of spironolactone.
9. Describe the features of Cushing syndrome.
10. Explain the treatment of Addison disease.

The Science of Pharmacology
https://doi.org/10.1016/B978-0-443-29038-1.00038-5

Overview

The adrenal glands secret several hormones. The primary hormones of the adrenal cortex are corticosteroids and mineralocorticoids. Cortisol, cortisone, and corticosterone are all glucocorticoids used by the body in many conditions and disorders. They are among the most widely prescribed drug classes worldwide, with an estimated market of more than 10 billion prescriptions per day. They have both endocrine and nonendocrine indications. Corticosteroids affect almost all body tissues, and disorders include contact dermatitis, asthma, anaphylaxis, urticaria and angioedema, allergic rhinitis, rheumatoid arthritis, sarcoidosis, systemic lupus erythematosus, adrenal insufficiency, ulcerative colitis, cerebral edema, and nephrotic syndrome. Aldosterone, a steroid hormone, regulates the salt and water balance of the body by increasing the retention of sodium and water and the excretion of potassium by the kidneys.

Physiology of adrenal glands

The adrenal glands are located on the top of the kidneys. Each has an *adrenal cortex* and *adrenal medulla*, which have separate and unique functions. The outer portion of the gland is called the adrenal cortex, and the inner portion is called the adrenal medulla. Even though the adrenal cortex and adrenal medulla are part of the same organ, they have different embryological origins. They are structurally and functionally so different that they are often spoken of as separate glands. The adrenal cortex comprises regular endocrine tissue, but the adrenal medulla comprises neurosecretory tissue. As you might guess, each of these tissues synthesizes and secretes different hormones. Glandular function occurs in the outer adrenal cortex—and the inner medulla functions as part of the sympathetic nervous system (see **Fig. 38.1**).

Adrenal cortex

The adrenal cortex has three distinct zones: the zona glomerulosa, the zona fasciculata, and the zona reticularis. Cells of the outer zone secrete mineralocorticoids. Cells of the middle zone secrete glucocorticoids. The inner zone secretes small amounts of glucocorticoids and **gonadocorticoids**. All these cortical hormones are steroids, which are known as corticosteroids. These include the following:

- An outer **zona glomerulosa**: an area of clustered cells that produces **mineralocorticoids** that help balance minerals and water in the blood; **aldosterone** is the most potent mineralocorticoid, which reduces the excretion of

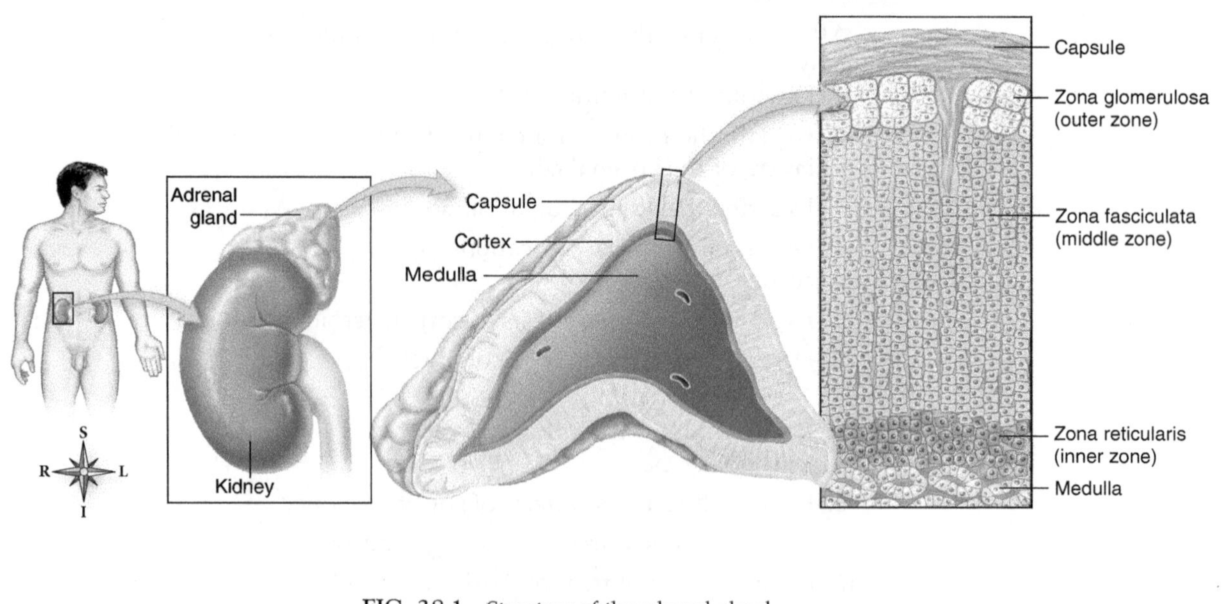

FIG. 38.1 Structure of the adrenal gland.

sodium and the elimination of potassium ions from the body, mainly targeting the distal kidney tubules. Aldosterone secretion is primarily controlled by the renin-angiotensin-aldosterone system (RAAS) and blood potassium concentration. Aldosterone secretion is controlled mainly by the RAAS and blood potassium concentrations. **Renin** is an enzyme that converts angiotensinogen to angiotensin I. Angiotensin II circulates to the adrenal cortex, which stimulates aldosterone secretion. A middle **zona fasciculata**, which mainly produces steroid hormones collectively called **glucocorticoids,** is vital for glucose metabolism in most body cells and helps the body resist stress. They keep blood glucose levels under control and maintain blood pressure. When severe stress occurs, many released glucocorticoids allow the body to react. It causes the release of glucose, fatty acids, and amino acids. *Cortisol (hydrocortisone), cortisone,* and *corticosterone* are all glucocorticoids, with cortisol being the most abundant. A negative feedback loop regulates glucocorticoid secretion. When cortisol is excessive, it is related to antiinflammatory and antiimmune effects.

- An inner **zona reticularis** forms a gonadocorticoid, which refers to sex hormones released from the zona reticularis of the adrenal cortex rather than the gonads. The normal adrenal cortex secretes small amounts of male hormones (androgens). Usually, not enough androgen is produced to give females masculine characteristics, but it is sufficient to influence the appearance of pubic and axillary hair in both boys and girls. **Table 38.1** summarizes the adrenal cortex hormones.

You should remember

Glucocorticoids regulate the conversion of fats, proteins, and carbohydrates to energy. They also regulate the immune response and suppress inflammatory reactions.

You should remember

Excessive levels of glucocorticoids cause depression of cartilage and bone formation, inhibition of inflammation, depressed immune system function, and changes in neural, cardiovascular, and gastrointestinal function.

Adrenal medulla

The adrenal medulla is located in the inner part of the adrenal gland. It contains many cells similar to those in the sympathetic ganglia, which are stimulated by preganglionic sympathetic fibers. The adrenal medulla synthesizes the catecholamines **epinephrine** (Epi) and **norepinephrine** (NE or NR). They play essential roles in handling both short-term and more prolonged stress. Epi is a potent stimulator of metabolic activities, bronchial dilation, and increased blood flow to the heart and skeletal muscles. NE has a strong influence on blood pressure and peripheral vasoconstriction.

The chief glucocorticoids secreted by the zona fasciculata of the adrenal cortex are cortisol (also called hydrocortisone), cortisone, and corticosterone. Of these, only cortisol is secreted in significant quantities in humans. Glucocorticoids affect every cell in the body. Although much remains to be discovered about their precise mechanisms of action, we do know enough to make some generalizations.

Glucocorticoids are essential for maintaining normal blood pressure. Without adequate amounts of glucocorticoids in the blood, the hormones NE and Epi cannot produce vasoconstricting effects on blood vessels, and blood pressure falls. In other words, glucocorticoids exhibit permissiveness by permitting NE and Epi to have full effects. When glucocorticoids are at high concentrations for a prolonged time, they may elevate blood pressure beyond normal (hypertension).

TABLE 38.1 Hormones of the adrenal cortex.

Zone	Hormone	Main target	Effect of hormone	Regulation
Zona glomerulosa (adrenal cortex)	Mineralocorticoids (mostly aldosterone)	Kidneys	Increase renal absorption of sodium ions and water; accelerate urinary loss of potassium ions	Angiotensin II, elevated plasma potassium ions, or decreased plasma sodium ions; inhibited by ANP and BNP
Zona fasciculate (adrenal cortex)	Glucocorticoids (cortisol and corticosterone)	Most cells	Release of amino acids from skeletal muscles and lipids from adipose tissues; promote liver formation of glycogen and glucose; promote peripheral use of lipids; antiinflammatory effects	Stimulated by ACTH from the anterior lobe of the pituitary gland
Zona reticularis (adrenal cortex)	Androgens	Most cells	Encourages bone and muscle growth and blood formation in children and females; not important in adult males	Stimulated by ACTH from anterior lobe of pituitary gland
Adrenal medulla	Epinephrine and norepinephrine	Most cells	Releases lipids by adipose tissue; increases cardiac activity, blood pressure, breakdown of glycogen, blood glucose levels	Stimulated by sympathetic preganglionic fiber during sympathetic activation

ACTH, Adrenocorticotropic hormone; *ANP,* atrial natriuretic peptide; *BNP,* brain natriuretic peptide.

Corticosteroid pharmacotherapy

Corticosteroids, commonly referred to as steroids, are antiinflammatory drugs typically used to treat rheumatologic diseases such as rheumatoid arthritis, lupus, or vasculitis. Specific corticosteroids include the medications cortisone and prednisone.

Corticosteroids are synthetic drugs that closely resemble cortisol, a hormone that the adrenal cortex produces naturally. Synthetic hormones have varying degrees of glucocorticoid and mineralocorticoid properties. Glucocorticoids are predominantly involved in metabolism and have immunosuppressive, antiinflammatory, and vasoconstrictive effects. Mineralocorticoids regulate electrolytes and water balance by affecting ion transport in the renal tubules. Some corticosteroid medicines include cortisone, prednisone, and methylprednisolone. Prednisone is the most commonly used type of steroid to treat certain rheumatologic diseases. Steroids might be given locally or systemically to the precise place where a problem exists. Examples of local steroid treatments include joint injections, eye drops, ear drops, and skin creams. Systemic steroid treatments include oral, IV, or IM routes of medication administration. **Table 38.2** summarizes various types of corticosteroids.

Pharmacokinetics

Glucocorticoids have good oral bioavailability and rapid absorption. The liver and renal excretion mainly metabolizes the metabolites. Cortisone and cortisol are short- acting, with a biological half-life of under 12 hours. Prednisone, prednisolone, methylprednisolone, and triamcinolone are intermediate acting, with a biological half-life of 18–36 hours.

Mechanism of action

The mechanism of action of corticosteroids has both genomic and nongenomic effects. The glucocorticoid receptor mediates the genomic action, leading to most antiinflammatory and immunosuppressive effects. The glucocorticoid receptor is located in the cell nucleus and causes inhibition of gene expression and translation for inflammatory leukocytes and epithelium.

Clinical indications

Corticosteroids are among the most widely prescribed drug classes worldwide, with an estimated market of more than 10 billion prescriptions per year. They have both endocrine and nonendocrine indications. Their endocrine role is often in the diagnosis of **Cushing syndrome** or the management of adrenal insufficiency and congenital adrenal **hyperplasia**. Their nonendocrine role regularly uses their potent antiinflammatory and immunosuppressive effects to treat patients with various immunologic and inflammatory disorders. Corticosteroids are used at physiologic doses as replacement therapy in cases of adrenal insufficiency and supraphysiologic doses in treatments for antiinflammatory and immunosuppressive effects. Common indications for corticosteroids, by field, include:

- Rheumatology: rheumatoid arthritis, systemic lupus erythematosus, **polymyositis**, dermatomyositis, **polymyalgia rheumatica**
- Ophthalmology: **uveitis**, keratoconjunctivitis

TABLE 38.2 Corticosteroids.

Generic name	Trade name	Route of administration
betamethasone	Celestone, Diprolene	PO, IM, topical
budesonide	Entocort EC, Rhinocort	PO, intranasal
dexamethasone	Baycadron Elixer, Decadron	PO, IM, IV
hydrocortisone	Cortef, Solu-Cortef, Hydrocort	PO, inhaled, topical, IM, IV, rectal
methylprednisolone	Depo-Medrol	PO, IM, IV
prednisone	Deltasone	PO, nasal, rectal, IV, topical
triamcinolone	Aristospan, Kenalog	PO, topical
prednisolone	Orapred, Prelone	PO, nasal, rectal, IM, IV

- Allergy and Pulmonology: asthma exacerbations, COPD exacerbations, anaphylaxis, urticaria and angioedema, rhinitis, pneumonitis, sarcoidosis, and interstitial lung disease
- Dermatology: contact dermatitis, pemphigus vulgaris
- Endocrinology: adrenal insufficiency, congenital adrenal hyperplasia
- Gastroenterology: inflammatory bowel disease, autoimmune hepatitis
- Hematology: **hemolytic anemia**, lymphoma, leukemia, idiopathic thrombocytopenic purpura
- Other: organ transplantation, multiple sclerosis, cerebral edema, nephrotic syndrome

Contraindications

Corticosteroids should be avoided in patients with hypersensitivity to any component of the formulation, concurrent administration of live or live-attenuated vaccines, diabetes mellitus, systemic fungal infection, uncontrolled hyperglycemia, osteoporosis, glaucoma, uncontrolled hypertension, herpes simplex keratitis, varicella infection, and joint infection. Additional relative contraindications include peptic ulcer disease, congestive heart failure, and viral or bacterial infections not controlled by antiinfectives.

Adverse effects

The chance of adverse effects depends on the dose, type of steroid, and length of treatment. Adverse effects are more common at higher dosages and with chronic use, though they are not limited to these cases. These effects are seen in up to 90% of patients who take them for more than 60 days. The common adverse effects include weight gain, increased appetite, fatigue, edema, a "puffy" face, acne, and mood changes. Other adverse effects might be osteoporosis, hypertension, gastritis, insomnia, cataracts, glaucoma, diabetes, and agitation.

Toxicities

The toxicity of corticosteroids includes hypertension, hyperglycemia, and infection. Rapid and complete withdrawal can lead to adrenocorticotropic hormone suppression and the cause of the underlying disease. Courses over 3 weeks should quickly reduce to physiologic doses, and then slow stopping should follow while evaluating the adrenal function. Long-term, high-dose suppressive therapy can lead to suppression of the hypothalamic-pituitary-adrenal axis for as long as 9–12 months following withdrawal.

You should remember

The route of corticosteroid administration depends on many factors, primarily the disorder treated. The route can be parenteral, oral, inhaled, topical, injected (intramuscular, intraarticular, intralesional, intradermal), or rectal. The clinician must consider many factors upon deciding to initiate corticosteroid therapy, including the route of administration, preparation, dosing, frequency, and duration of treatment.

Aldosterone antagonists

Aldosterone regulates the body's salt and water balance by increasing sodium and water retention and the excretion of potassium by the kidneys. Its primary function is to control the blood pressure. Aldosterone secretion is regulated mainly by the RAAS and blood potassium concentration. Aldosterone antagonists include eplerenone, finerenone, and spironolactone. **Table 38.3** summarizes various types of aldosterone antagonists.

Spironolactone

Spironolactone is a potassium-sparing diuretic. It prevents the kidney from absorbing too much salt and prevents hypokalemia.

TABLE 38.3 Aldosterone antagonists.

Generic name	Trade name	Route of administration
eplerenone	Inspra	PO
finerenone	Kerendia	PO
spironolactone	Aldactone	PO

Pharmacokinetics

Spironolactone is absorbed from the GI tract, and its bioavailability is over 90%. It has high protein binding (98%) to human plasma proteins. It is wholly and rapidly metabolized to a large number of metabolites. Elimination is primarily in the urine (50%) and bile (5%). The mean half-life of spironolactone is 1.4 hours.

Mechanism of action

Spironolactone specifically works by competitively blocking aldosterone receptor–mediated action. The effect of the blockade is that sodium reabsorption with water retention does not occur, and there is increased potassium retention.

Clinical indications

Spironolactone is used in combination with other medicines to treat hypertension and heart failure. Lowering blood pressure can reduce the risk of strokes and heart attacks. Spironolactone is also used to decrease the hospitalization of patients for heart failure.

It is also used to diagnose and treat hyperaldosteronism. This medicine may also be used to treat edema in patients with congestive heart failure, liver cirrhosis, or nephrotic syndrome.

Contraindications

Spironolactone is contraindicated in patients with hyperkalemia, hyponatremia, renal impairment, acute renal failure, anuria, Addison disease, and hypersensitivity to spironolactone.

Adverse effects

The adverse effects of spironolactone may include headache, chest pain, cough, dyspnea, bleeding gums, loss of appetite, vomiting, diarrhea, hyperkalemia, dehydration, hyponatremia, dizziness, loss of consciousness, seizures, arrhythmias, hematuria, and tarry stools. Spironolactone may also cause loss of libido, menstrual irregularities, **gynecomastia**, and impotence.

Toxicities

Drowsiness, mental confusion, maculopapular rashes, nausea, vomiting, dizziness, or diarrhea may manifest in acute overdosage of spironolactone. Rarely, severe hyponatremia, hyperkalemia, or hepatic coma may occur in patients with liver disease, but these are unlikely due to acute overdosage.

Hyperadrenalism (Cushing syndrome)

Hyperadrenalism may be seen in patients taking corticosteroids through all routes of administration. It can be divided into endogenous and exogenous causes. The vast majority of cases of Cushing syndrome are the result of the administration of exogenous glucocorticoids. The endogenous form may be caused by excessive secretion of ACTH from a pituitary adenoma or primary adrenal adenoma. The features include weight gain, a buffalo hump, a moon-shaped face, severe muscle weakness, hypertension, hirsutism, decreased libido, menstrual irregularity, thin skin, and **truncal obesity**. These features may develop within the first 2 months of corticosteroid treatment. The risk is higher in patients with a higher body mass index at baseline, younger patients, and those with higher caloric intake. Treatment depends on what is causing Cushing syndrome. The patients may need surgery to remove tumors or the adrenal glands, radiation, chemotherapy, and certain hormone-inhibiting drugs.

Hypoadrenalism (Addison disease)

Hypoadrenalism may be a primary or secondary adrenal disease. Primary acute adrenocortical insufficiency is called *adrenal crisis*, and primary chronic adrenocortical insufficiency is called **Addison disease**. Secondary adrenocortical insufficiency is due to a deficiency of ACTH. Addison disease is an uncommon disorder resulting from the progressive destruction of the adrenal cortex. The clinical manifestations of Addison disease do not appear until at least 90% of the adrenal cortex has been compromised. Addison disease symptoms usually occur slowly, often over months, and include extreme fatigue, hypotension, weight loss, salt craving, depression, irritability, skin pigmentations, nausea, diarrhea, and vomiting.

The causes of this condition may be autoimmune adrenalitis, genetics, tuberculosis, low cortisol levels, or metastatic cancers. Addison disease is treated with medication to replace the missing hormones. Treatment usually involves steroid replacement therapy for life. Corticosteroid medicines are used to replace the hormones cortisol and aldosterone.

Hyperaldosteronism (Conn syndrome)

Hyperaldosteronism is a chronic excess aldosterone secretion. Hyperaldosteronism may be primary or secondary. Primary hyperaldosteronism (**Conn syndrome**) may be caused by overproduction of aldosterone, with resultant suppression of the renin-angiotensin system and decreased plasma renin activity. Conn syndrome may be caused by hyperplasia or tumors. Blood pressure elevation is the most common manifestation of primary hyperaldosteronism. Hypersecretion of aldosterone leads to increased water retention and muscle weakness, resulting in potassium loss. In secondary hyperaldosteronism, in contrast, aldosterone release occurs in response to activation of the renin-angiotensin system. The signs and symptoms associated with Conn syndrome include hypertension, hypokalemia, headache, fatigue, muscle cramps, palpitations, anxiety, depression, and memory difficulties. The treatment of hyperaldosteronism depends on the cause. If a tumor causes it, adrenalectomy is needed. However, the main goal is to manage hypertension. The most common medications to treat Conn syndrome are aldosterone antagonists.

Hypersecretion of androgens can result from tumors of the adrenal cortex, called virilizing tumors. Adrenal **virilism** is a syndrome in which excessive adrenal androgens cause virilization. Diagnosis is clinical and confirmed by elevated androgen levels. Symptoms of virilization include excess facial and body hair, baldness, acne, deepening of the voice, and increased muscularity and sex drive.

Hyposecretion of aldosterone

Hypoaldosteronism is a condition marked by the diminished release of aldosterone from the adrenal cortex. Symptoms include hyponatremia, hyperkalemia, and metabolic acidosis. These symptoms may cause nausea, fatigue, heart palpitations, arrhythmia, and hypotension. Most patients with hypoaldosteronism respond well to a low-potassium diet and a loop or thiazide diuretic to enhance potassium excretion. Fludrocortisone may be needed for hormone deficiency.

You should remember

Sometimes, the symptoms of Addison disease appear suddenly. Acute adrenal failure can lead to life-threatening shock. This condition is called Addison crisis. The symptoms include confusion, delirium, hypotension, severe weakness, vomiting, diarrhea, and dehydration.

Key Terms

Addison disease
Aldosterone
Angioedema

Angiotensinogen
Catecholamines
Conn syndrome
Cushing syndrome
Epinephrine
Glucocorticoids
Hemolytic anemia
Hyperadrenalism
Hyperaldosteronism
Hyperplasia
Hypoadrenalism
Mineralocorticoids
Norepinephrine
Polymyalgia rheumatica
Polymyositis
Renin
Sarcoidosis
Truncal obesity
Urticaria
Virilism
Zona fasciculata
Zona glomerulosa
Zona reticularis

Clinical Case Studies

Clinical Case Study 1

A 35-year-old female presented with menstrual irregularity, severe muscle weakness, and significant weight gain over the last year. Cortisol and ACTH levels indicated a diagnosis of Cushing syndrome. The patient was found to have a tuberculum sellae meningioma within the sellae region. The tumor was successfully resected. The patient was placed on hydrocortisone treatments for 11 months, and her condition had nearly totally resolved.

Critical Thinking Questions

1. What are the clinical indications of corticosteroids?
2. What are the contraindications of corticosteroids?
3. What are the adverse effects of corticosteroids?

Clinical Case Study 2

A 59-year-old female presented with symptoms of lethargy, low mood, and exertional dyspnea. She also had facial hyperpigmentation. The patient was weak and had proximal myopathy, with difficulty standing up from a seated position. Laboratory tests revealed hyponatremia with hyperkalemia. A preliminary diagnosis of Addison disease was made. Hydrocortisone treatment was initiated, and 6 weeks later, the patient's symptoms had generally resolved.

Critical Thinking Questions

1. What are the clinical manifestations of Addison disease?
2. What are the causes of Addison disease?
3. What are the precibal of treatments for Addison disease?

Clinical Case Study 3

A 68-year-old hypertensive male was evaluated for ways to optimize his blood pressure therapy. His aldosterone and renin levels were measured, which eventually led to an abdominal imaging study, revealing an adrenal cortex tumor. A diagnosis of Conn syndrome was made. An adrenalectomy was scheduled to remove the adrenal tumor, which was successful, and the patient made a full recovery.

Critical Thinking Questions

1. What are the clinical manifestations of Conn syndrome?
2. What are the causes of Conn syndrome?
3. What are the principal treatments for Conn syndrome?

Further Reading

[1] U. Ahmed, Introduction to Adrenocorticosteroids – Pharmacokinetics, Physiological and Pharmacological Effects (Medical School – Lectures in Detail), Adrenal Alternatives Foundation, 2023.
[2] M.D. Bronstein, Cushing's Syndrome – Pathophysiology, Diagnosis and Treatment (Contemporary Endocrinology), Humana Press, 2011.
[3] E. Dean, Beyond the Diagnoses – Thriving with Addison's Disease, Dean, 2024.
[4] W.E. Dixon, Adrenal Alternatives Foundation, Adrenal Insufficiency 101 – A Patient's Guide to Managing Adrenal Insufficiency, Adrenal Alternatives Foundation, 2020.
[5] J. Ebuch, A Comprehensive Guide to Hormone Replacement Therapy – Unlock the Power Within, Restore Balance, and Transform your Life, Ebuch, 2023.
[6] E.D. Frohlich, R.N. Re, The Local Cardiac Renin-Angiotensin Aldosterone System, second ed., Springer, 2010.
[7] A.B. Grossman, J.L. Jameson, L.J. De Groot, Endocrinology Adult and Pediatric – the Adrenal Gland, sixth ed., Elsevier / Saunders, 2013.
[8] J. Lamorgese, Adrenal Glands – Discover the Biology of Adrenal Glands, Lamorgese, 2022.
[9] National Comprehensive Cancer Network, NCCN Guidelines for Patients' Adrenal Tumors, NCCN, 2022.
[10] T. Quinn, Endocrine Disorders – an Issue of the Endocrinology Clinics, Foster Academics, 2019.
[11] M. Radenokovic, Updates on Corticosteroids, InTechOpen, 2023.
[12] J.W. Rankin, Curable Hypertension – Primary Aldosteronism, Rankin, 2015.
[13] J. Reeds, Cushing Syndrome – Overview of the Treatment, Reeds, 2023.

CHAPTER

39

Gonadal hormones and inhibitors

OUTLINE

LEARNING OUTCOMES

After study of the chapter, readers should be able to:

1. Explain the characteristics of the menstrual cycle.
2. Identify the pharmacologic estrogens.
3. Explain the indications for estrogens.
4. Identify the pharmacokinetics of progestins.
5. Describe the drugs used for menopause.
6. Explain the clinical indications for oxytocin.
7. Describe the adverse effects of oxytocin.

The Science of Pharmacology
https://doi.org/10.1016/B978-0-443-29038-1.00039-7

8. Explain the clinical indications of clomiphene.
9. Discuss hormonal regulation of male reproductive function.
10. Describe the contraindications of testosterone.

Overview

The gonads are endocrine glands whose functions support the development and maturation of the male and female germ cells. The female gonads, the ovaries, are responsible for the development and maturation of the ova and the synthesis and secretion of the female sex steroid hormones, estrogen, and progesterone. The testes are responsible for synthesizing and secreting the male sex steroid hormone. The role of this hormone is the development and maturation of sperm and sexual differentiation of the gonads, internal genital tract, and external genitalia. Estrogen and progesterone replacement therapy is often used to manage and treat menopausal symptoms, especially vasomotor symptoms and urogenital atrophy, which is usually associated with a significantly decreased quality of life. Testosterone is the treatment of choice for testosterone deficiency and hypogonadism.

Hormonal regulation of female reproductive function

Controlling the hypothalamic-pituitary-gonadal axis is complex and occurs at several levels, including peripheral hormonal regulation and the extensive network of neuronal function. The regulation of the **gonadotropin-releasing hormone** (GnRH) depends on the precise coordination of internal and external signals. The increased release of GnRH is triggered by a positive feedback loop involving the rapid increase in plasma estradiol concentration. Estradiol and progesterone stimulate an increase in **luteinizing hormone** (LH). In the early stages of the estrus cycle, estradiol levels are low, and the release of GnRH is inhibited. As estradiol levels surge at proestrus, GnRH is released and causes the release of LH, which stimulates progesterone production in the ovaries. Hormone secretion must be turned on and off as needed. The feedback mechanisms may adjust the secretory rates of these hormones. **Table 39.1** summarizes selected estrogens and progestins regulating female reproductive function.

TABLE 39.1 Estrogens and progestins.

Generic name	Trade name	Route of administration
Estrogens	Alora, Estrace,	PO, transdermal patch,
estradiol	Estraderm,	topical gel, vaginal
estradiol valerate	Delestrogen	cream, vaginal ring
estrogen, conjugated	Cenestin, Enjuvia,	IM
estropipate	Premarin	PO
	Ogen	PO, vaginal cream
Progestins	Depo-Provera, Provera,	PO, IM, subcutaneous
medroxyprogesterone	MPA, Depo-subQ	IM, IV, PO, vaginal gel,
progesterone	Crinone, Endometrin,	vaginal tablets
	Prochieve, Progestin	
Estrogen-progestin	Premphase, Prempro	PO, vaginal cream
combinations	MonoNessa, Ortho-	PO
conjugated estrogens	Cyclen-28	PO, transdermal patch
with	Activella	
medroxyprogesterone		
estradiol with		
norgestimate		
ethinyl estradiol with		
norethindrone acetate		

Functions of estrogens and progestins

Estrogen is one of the two ovarian steroid hormones. Their functions are coordinated to support the reproductive activity of the female, including the development of the ovum, the development and maintenance of the **corpus luteum** to sustain a fertilized **ovum**, the maintenance of pregnancy, and the preparation of the breasts for lactation. Estrogen also involves functions that include the neuroendocrine, skeletal, vascular, and immune systems. This hormone may be involved in many various diseases and conditions, such as endometriosis, osteoporosis, infertility, obesity, and some cancers. Progesterone plays a vital role in the maintenance of the uterus during pregnancy. As such, an important issue of concern regarding the loss of this steroid hormone correlates with **miscarriage** and preterm labor. It also influences the production of inflammatory processes such as human T cells within the uterine cavity. Thus a loss of progesterone leads to an increase in myometrial contractility coupled with a decrease in fighting off immunologic threats, which can lead to a miscarriage and early delivery of the fetus. Loss of progesterone is also associated with decreased **fertility**, increased endometrial hyperplasia, and *endometrial cancers*.

Without estrogen and its upregulatory action, progesterone has little biological activity. Conversely, progesterone downregulates estrogen receptors in some target tissues, decreasing their responsiveness to estrogen. At puberty, the ovaries, driven by pulsatile secretion of **follicular stimulating hormone** (FSH) and LH, begin to secrete estrogen. In turn, estrogen promotes the growth and development of the female reproductive tract: the uterus, **fallopian tubes**, cervix, and vagina. Progesterone is also active in these tissues, usually increasing their secretory activity. Thus, in the uterus, estrogen causes **cell proliferation**, cell growth, and increased contractility; progesterone increases secretory activity and decreases contractility.

In the fallopian tubes, estrogen stimulates ciliary activity and contractility, aiding in the movement of sperm toward the uterus; progesterone increases secretory activity and decreases contractility. In the vagina, estrogen stimulates proliferation of epithelial cells; progesterone stimulates differentiation but inhibits proliferation of epithelial cells.

You should remember

Problems with the chromosomes of the fetus often cause first-trimester miscarriages. The risk factors include age, obesity, smoking, consumption of too much coffee, and alcohol.

Menstrual cycle

For the **menstrual cycle**, estrogen and progesterone are responsible for the changes that occur in the **endometrium**, cervix, and vagina and are accountable for feedback regulation of FSH and LH secretion by the anterior pituitary. Based on a "typical" 28-day cycle, the follicular phase of the menstrual cycle is the 14 days preceding **ovulation**. This phase, also called the proliferative phase, is dominated by estrogen. 17β-Estradiol, whose secretion increases markedly during this phase, has significant effects on the endometrial lining of the uterus, preparing it for the possibility of accepting a fertilized ovum. Estradiol stimulates the growth of the endometrium, growth of glands and **stroma**, and elongation of the spiral arteries, which supply the endometrium. Estradiol also causes the cervical mucus to become **copious**, watery, and elastic.

The luteal phase of a 28-day menstrual cycle is the 14 days following ovulation. This phase, also called the secretory phase, is dominated by progesterone. The endometrium slows in proliferation and decreases in thickness. The menstrual cycle includes the development of an ovarian follicle and its **oocyte**, ovulation, preparation of the reproductive tract to receive the fertilized ovum, and shedding of the endometrial lining if **fertilization** does not occur. The cycle length can vary from 21 to 35 days, but the average length is 28 days. The variability in cycle length is attributable to variability in the duration of the follicular phase; the luteal phase is constant. The hormonal changes and events of a 28-day menstrual cycle are shown in **Fig. 39.1**.

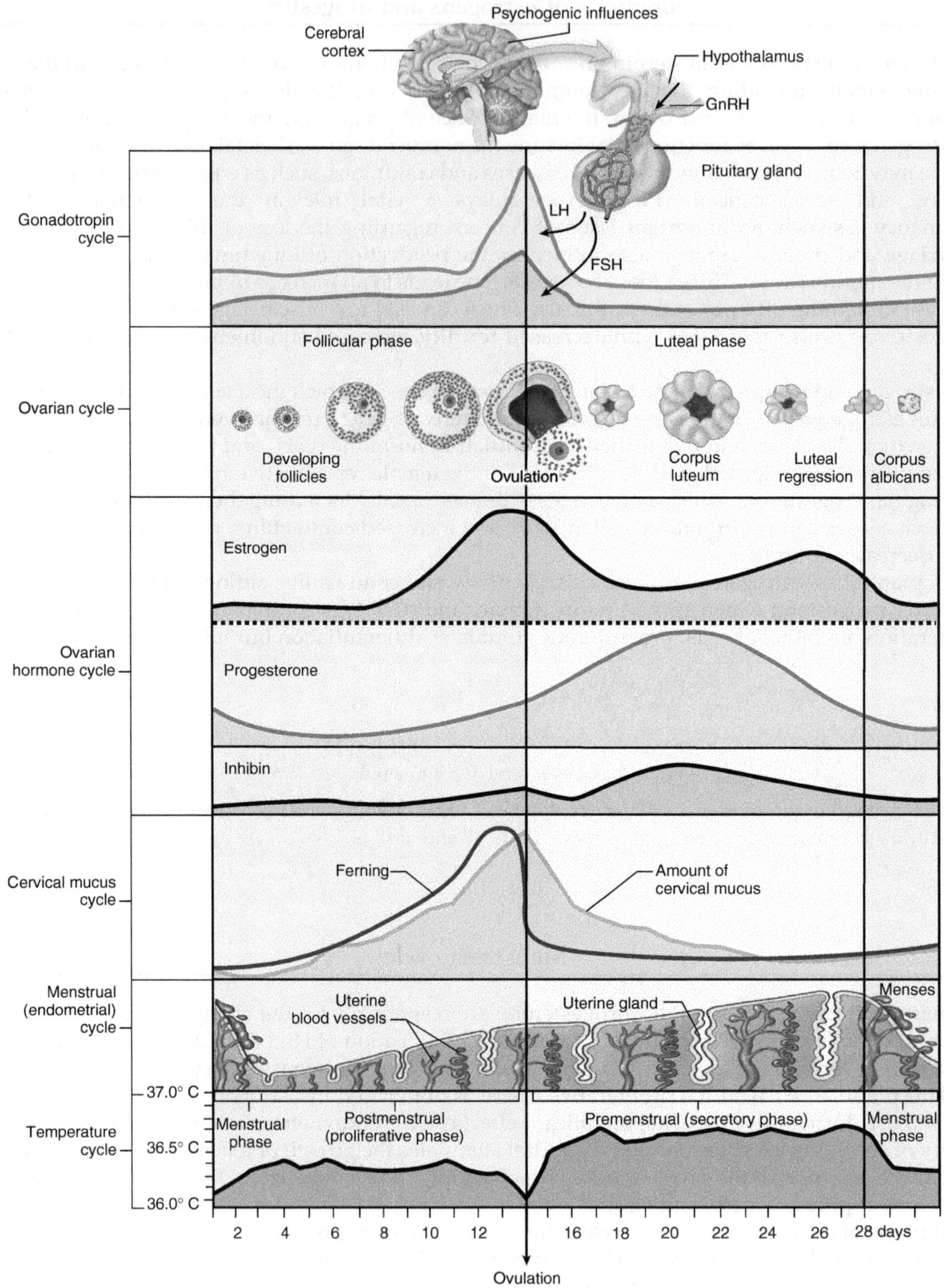

FIG. 39.1 Events of the menstrual cycle.

Pharmacologic estrogens

Estrogen is involved in both the male and female reproductive systems. It contributes to reproductive and breast health in females, among other functions. The primary source of estrogen, ovarian 17β-estradiol, is usually converted to estrone and estriol. In postmenopausal females, the primary sources of estrogen are nonovarian, including the production of hormones from the adrenal cortex, adipose tissue, skeletal muscle, kidney, brain, and hair follicles. Estrogen circulates bound to sex hormone–binding globulin and albumin.

Pharmacokinetics

Due to the complex nature of endogenous and exogenous hormone concentrations, formation, metabolism, and assay complexity, the pharmacokinetics of estrogens are challenging to study. Oral estrogens have minimal systemic bioavailability due to the metabolism of the gut and liver (first-pass effect). High concentrations of estrone are achieved with oral administration, whereas higher concentrations of estradiol are generally achieved after percutaneous absorption. Exogenously administered estrogens are metabolized in the same fashion as endogenous estrogens. Metabolic transformation occurs primarily in the liver and intestines. Estradiol is metabolized to estrone, and both are converted to estriol, which is later excreted in the urine. Biliary secretion of metabolic conjugates is released into the intestine. The CYP3A4 hepatic cytochrome enzyme is heavily involved in the metabolism of estradiol. Therefore estrogen is excreted in the urine and feces.

Mechanism of action

More than 95% of estradiol is bound loosely to albumin or tightly to sex hormone–binding globulin, the major binding protein. The terminal half-lives for the different estrogen compounds (after oral or intravenous administration) vary from 1–12 hours.

Clinical indications

The clinical indications of estrogen are primary ovarian insufficiency and female hypogonadism. Hormone replacement therapy is often used to manage and treat menopausal symptoms. The form of administration varies with estrogen therapy and depends on the specific symptoms the treatment is targeting. Essentially, certain symptoms, such as the vasomotor symptoms experienced during **menopause**, would best be controlled with estrogen therapy that acts systemically. Conversely, symptoms involving the vaginal lumen, such as **dyspareunia**, vaginal itching, and vaginal dryness, experience more control with locally acting estrogen therapy. Typically, females with an intact uterus receive a combination of estrogen and progesterone therapy. Females who have had hysterectomies receive estrogen alone.

Contraindications

Hormone replacement therapy is contraindicated and correlates with the adverse effects and relative toxicity of estrogen-based formulations. It must be avoided in patients who have a history of any form of breast or uterine cancer, a history of deep vein thrombosis or **pulmonary embolism**, a history of myocardial infarction and stroke, and a history of blood clotting disorders. These contraindications do not apply to estrogen taken transvaginally, as in the form of creams or suppositories, as the serum level of estrogen via this route is too low to cause any effect.

Adverse effects

Females rarely have severe side effects from taking estrogens to replace estrogen. The prolonged use of estrogens may increase the risk of endometrial cancer in females after menopause. This risk seems to increase as the dose and length of use increase. There is less risk when estrogens are used in low doses for less than 1 year. The risk is also reduced if progestin is added to or replaces part of the estrogen dose. If there is a total hysterectomy, there is no risk of endometrial cancer. However, some general adverse effects of estrogen include headache, breast pain, diarrhea, vaginal discharge, chills, dizziness, chest pain, fatigue, and dark urine.

Toxicity

The toxicity of estrogen is dose dependent. In high doses, estrogen therapy can potentially cause severe effects, including excessive fluid retention, vaginal bleeding, and mental status changes. High doses of estrogen affect the heart but negatively impact renal function.

You should remember

For postmenopausal females generally, the benefits of estrogen therapy are preventing osteoporotic fractures, reducing heart disease, decreasing mortality, and possibly reducing the risk of Alzheimer disease, outweighing the risks of endometrial and breast cancers. A female must be fully informed of the risks and benefits of hormone therapy.

Pharmacologic progestins

Pharmaceutical progesterone is made from a plant source as a starting material and is chemically identical to progesterone of human ovarian origin. It is available in tablet form, gelatinized capsule form, vaginal gel form, vaginal insert form, and injection form, which are all used for various purposes. Progestin is a synthetic progestogen used most commonly in hormonal birth control and menopausal hormone therapy. They can also be used in the treatment of gynecological conditions, to support fertility and pregnancy, and to lower sex hormone levels for various purposes, in addition to other uses.

Pharmacokinetics

The concentration of the progestin available to elicit biological actions in target tissues depends on several factors such as route of administration, metabolism, bioavailability, half-life, and availability after binding to steroid-binding proteins. Progesterone is 96%–99% bound to serum albumin. The liver mainly metabolizes it. After oral administration, the primary plasma metabolites are found. Some progesterone metabolites are found excreted in the bile, and they may be deconjugated and subsequently metabolized in the gut by reduction. The significant plasma and urinary metabolites are comparable to those found during the physiological progesterone secretion of the corpus luteum. The metabolites are excreted mainly by the kidneys and bile. Progesterone metabolites, excreted in the bile, may undergo enterohepatic recycling or may be found excreted in the feces.

Mechanism of action

Progesterone binds and activates its nuclear receptor, integral in signaling stimuli that maintain the endometrium during pregnancy preparation. It may prevent pregnancy by inhibiting FSH, which generally causes ovulation.

Clinical indications

Hormone replacement therapy helps treat symptoms of menopause, such as hot flashes and vaginal dryness. The age, personal medical history, and severity of the symptoms are indicated by hormone therapy.

Contraindications

The progesterone contraceptive should not be used during pregnancy, unexplained vaginal bleeding, breast cancer, endometrial cancer, migraines with auras, hypertension, ischemic heart disease, cirrhosis, malignant hepatoma, and hepatocellular adenoma.

Adverse effects

The most common adverse effect of oral progesterone pills is bleeding. Most females may complain of headaches, abdominal cramping, nausea, breast tenderness, and increased vaginal discharge or decreased libido. Nausea can be avoided by taking the medication at night before sleep. Smoking cigarettes while using oral contraceptives can significantly increase the risk of severe adverse effects. Cigarette smoking also increases the risk of serious cardiovascular adverse effects from oral contraceptive use. The risk increases with age and with heavy smoking.

Toxicity

Toxicity to progesterone can activate genes that trigger inflammation in the mammary gland, which may be a critical factor in increasing the risk of breast cancer. Progesterone at high doses is also considered an antifertility drug.

You should remember

Progesterone has been detected in nursing mothers' milk. No adverse effects have been found on breastfeeding ability or the growing infant's health, growth, or development.

You should remember

Progestin plus estrogen therapy should not be used for the prevention of cardiovascular disease. Increased risks of myocardial infarction, stroke, pulmonary emboli, deep vein thrombosis, and breast cancer in postmenopausal females have been reported with treatment. An increased risk of developing dementia in postmenopausal females has also been reported. Progestins with estrogens should be prescribed at the lowest effective doses and for the shortest duration possible.

Menopause

Menopause is the cessation of menstrual cycles in females. It occurs at approximately 50 years of age. For several years preceding menopause, **anovulatory cycles** become more common. Accordingly, estrogen secretion gradually declines and eventually ceases. Because of the decreased estrogen level, there is reduced negative feedback on the anterior pituitary and increased secretion and pulsatility of FSH and LH at menopause. The causes of menopause may include naturally declining reproductive hormones and oophorectomy, chemotherapy, and radiotherapy. The signs and symptoms of menopause include the decrease of ovarian estrogen and atrophy of the vaginal epithelium, decreased vaginal secretions, decreased breast mass, bone loss, hot flashes, night sweats, dry skin, weight gain, insomnia, sexual dysfunction, urinary incontinence, and mood changes. Estrogen replacement therapy is aimed at replacing the ovarian source of estrogen, thus minimizing or preventing the symptoms of menopause.

Uterine stimulants

Uterine stimulants are medications used to induce contractions of the uterus. They increase the tone of the **myometrium**. They're mainly used to induce labor, reduce postpartum bleeding, and induce abortion. Oxytocin, prostaglandin, and their synthetic derivatives are the most commonly used uterine stimulants. They speed up labor, **stem bleeding**, termination, and labor induction but have the risk of uterine hyperstimulation and rupture. Oxytocin is a natural hormone produced in the hypothalamus and released into the bloodstream by the pituitary gland. Its primary function is to facilitate childbirth. It manages critical aspects of the female and male reproductive systems, including labor, delivery, lactation, and human behavior.

Pharmacokinetics

Oxytocin has a duration of action of 2–3 hours intramuscularly and 1 hour intravenously. The volume of distribution is 0.3 L/kg. It is rapidly metabolized in the liver and plasma and excreted in small amounts in the urine. The half-life is 1–6 minutes, which is decreased in late pregnancy and lactation.

Mechanism of action

Oxytocin is released explicitly from the hypothalamus into the posterior pituitary gland for later use. This part of the posterior pituitary gland that stores oxytocin is called the pars nervosa, also known as the neural or posterior lobe. Most hormones create negative feedback loops after they are released. Still, oxytocin is one of the few that exhibit positive feedback loops. Exogenous oxytocin causes the same response in the female reproductive system as endogenous oxytocin. Both stimulate uterine contractions in the myometrium by causing G-protein–coupled receptors to increase intracellular calcium in uterine myofibrils. Oxytocin receptor activation causes many signals that stimulate uterine contraction by increasing intracellular calcium levels, which is where positive feedback comes into play.

Clinical indications

Oxytocin is indicated in antepartum and postpartum. In the **antepartum** period, exogenous oxytocin is for strengthening uterine contractions with the aim of successful vaginal delivery of the fetus. In the postpartum period, oxytocin may be used to induce contractions in the third stage of labor for controlling postpartum bleeding. Oxytocin is also indicated for mothers who have **preeclampsia**, maternal diabetes, and premature rupture of the membranes.

Contraindications

Oxytocin should be avoided in conditions such as prematurity, **partial placenta previa**, fetal distress, **hydramnios**, prematurity, borderline cephalopelvic disproportion, previous caesarean section, and any condition in which there is a predisposition for uterine rupture.

Adverse effects

The adverse effects of oxytocin include nausea, vomiting, severe allergic reactions, bleeding after labor, dysrhythmia, hypertension, and rupture of the uterus.

Toxicity

An inappropriate dosage of oxytocin may result in arrhythmias, tachycardia, and myocardial ischemia. High dosages of oxytocin can cause uterine rupture, hypertonicity, and spasms. When oxytocin is given to females in the first or second stages of labor or to females to cause induction of labor, uterine rupture, maternal death, and even fetal death can result. If oxytocin is given in doses too large or even slowly for 24 hours, the medication can exhibit an antidiuretic effect, resulting in extreme water intoxication. This excessive dosing can cause seizures, coma, and even death in the mother.

You should remember

Preeclampsia is a potentially life-threatening form of hypertension that can occur during the second half of pregnancy. In addition to high blood pressure, a pregnant female with this condition also has albumin in the urine. Without treatment, it can lead to severe complications such as seizures (eclampsia), stroke, and maternal or fetal death.

Uterine relaxants

Uterine relaxants may be needed to inhibit uterine contractions and decrease the activity of the uterine muscles. The term tocolytics contains the word parts toco—(referring to childbirth) and—lytic, meaning "to terminate." They are used to stop premature labor to allow time for the fetal lungs to mature. **Table 39.2** summarizes various uterine stimulants and relaxants.

Infertility

Infertility is when a male or female cannot **conceive** due to a problem with the reproductive system of either partner. It can be primary or secondary. Primary infertility is when someone is not able to conceive at all. Secondary infertility is when someone is unable to conceive or carry a pregnancy to term after having given birth before. In males, the causes of infertility might be problems with semen or sperm, a testicular infection, cancer or surgery, mumps, **cryptorchidism**, or testosterone deficiency. The causes of infertility in females may include ovulation disorders, hyper- or hypothyroidism, **polycystic ovary syndrome**, endometriosis, tubal ligation, and **submucosal fibroids**.

TABLE 39.2 Uterine stimulants and relaxants.

Generic name	Trade name	Route of administration
Stimulants (oxytocics) oxytocin	Pitocin	IV
Ergot alkaloid methylergonovine	Methergine	PO
Prostaglandins carboprost dinoprostone	Hemabate Cervidil, Prepidil, Prostin E2	IM Intravaginal insert, intravaginal gel, intravaginal suppository
Relaxants (tocolytics) magnesium sulfate nifedipine terbutaline	(generic only) Adalat, Procardia Brethine	IV PO, IV, ointment IV, PO

Clomiphene is a selective estrogen receptor modulator indicated to treat anovulatory or **oligo-ovulatory** infertility to induce ovulation for patients desiring to conceive. It may also improve semen quality by stimulating hormone synthesis and **spermatogenesis**.

Pharmacokinetics

Clomiphene is readily absorbed orally. It is metabolized in the liver and eliminated in urine and feces.

Mechanism of action

Clomiphene is a selective estrogen receptor modulator with both estrogenic and antiestrogenic properties. It is an antagonist at hypothalamic estrogen receptors and inhibits the negative feedback of estrogen on gonadotropin release. It is used to stimulate ovulation in anovulatory infertility.

Clinical indications

Clinical indications of clomiphene include ovulatory dysfunction in females desiring pregnancy as well as male infertility. It is also used in patients diagnosed with polycystic ovarian syndrome, amenorrhea-galactorrhea syndrome, post–oral contraceptive amenorrhea, and psychogenic amenorrhea. Patients indicated for clomiphene therapy must not have an ovarian cyst, vaginal bleeding, or hepatic impairment.

Contraindications

Clomiphene should not be used if a female is pregnant, has liver disease, unexplained abnormal vaginal bleeding, ovarian cysts, or untreated thyroid/adrenal disorders. It is also contraindicated in patients with pituitary tumors or hypersensitivity to the drug.

Adverse effects

The adverse effects of clomiphene may be allergic reactions, headaches, hot flashes, vision changes, irregular menstrual cycles, **ovarian hyperstimulation syndrome**, pancreatitis, and breast tenderness. The other adverse effects include gynecomastia, testicular tumor, gastrointestinal disturbance, blurred vision, **scotoma**, pelvic pain, abnormal uterine bleeding, hypertriglyceridemia, and **mastalgia**.

Toxicity

The toxic effects after the acute use of clomiphene citrate are rare. However, the signs and symptoms of clomiphene overdose may include nausea, vomiting, scotoma, visual disturbance, hot flashes, ovarian enlargement, and abdominal pain.

Hormonal regulation of male reproductive function

The hypothalamic-pituitary-gonadal axis plays a significant role in sexual maturity, sperm production, and the development of secondary sex characteristics (see **Fig. 39.2**). It maintains spermatogenesis and sexual function

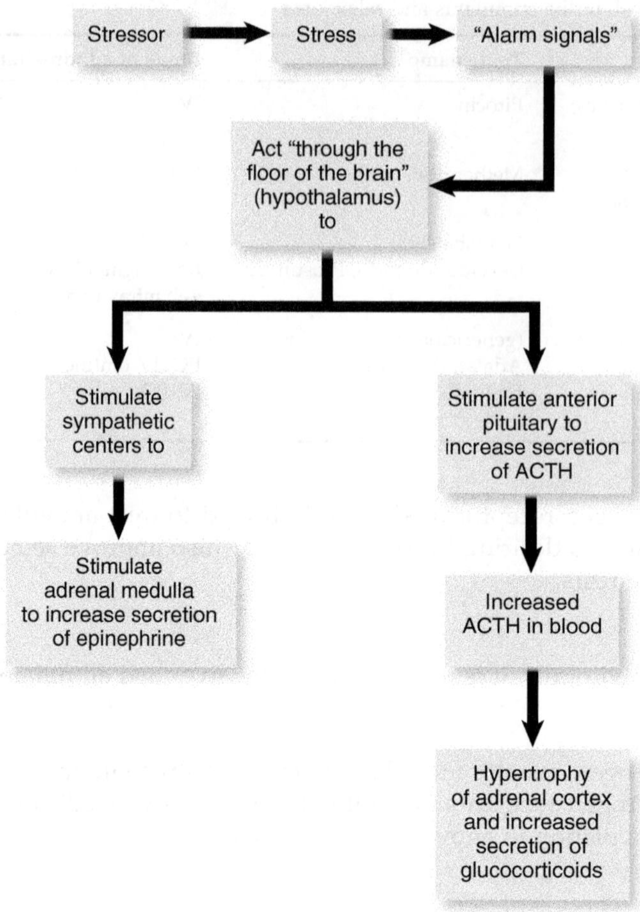

FIG. 39.2 The hypothalamic-pituitary-gonadal axis.

throughout the male's lifetime. The hypothalamus secretes GnRH into the hypothalamic-hypophyseal portal system to stimulate the anterior pituitary. In response, the anterior pituitary secretes LH and FSH into the blood. These gonadotropic hormones act on membrane receptors in the Leydig and Sertoli cells of the testes, respectively.

Before puberty, the levels of androgens and gonadotropins typically remain low and constant. Once puberty occurs, the hypothalamus releases GnRH in a pulsatile fashion every 1–2 hours to maintain amounts of FSH, LH, and plasma testosterone, all of which regulate each other to maintain hormonal balance. In the third decade of life, testosterone levels are found to decline.

Testosterone, the primary androgenic hormone, is synthesized and secreted by the testes' Leydig cells. The steroidogenic pathways in the testes are similar to those in the adrenal cortex. The hypothalamic-pituitary axis controls both testes' functions, spermatogenesis, and testosterone secretion. The hypothalamic hormone is GnRH, and the anterior pituitary hormones are FSH and LH.

Pharmacologic testosterone

Testosterone is a hormone produced primarily in the testicles. It helps maintain male sperm production, sex drive, muscle strength and mass, bone density, fat distribution, facial and body hair, and red blood cell production. Testosterone therapy can help reverse the effects of hypogonadism. Pharmacologic testosterone is used to treat male hypogonadism, gender dysphoria, and some types of breast cancer. In the form of *anabolic steroids*, it can also be used to increase athletic ability. **Table 39.3** summarizes various forms of testosterone (as androgens and anabolic steroids).

TABLE 39.3 Various forms of testosterone.

Generic name	Trade name	Route of administration
fluoxymesterone	(generic only)	PO
methyltestosterone	Android, Methitest, Testred	PO, buccal
nandrolone	(generic only)	IM
oxandrolone	Oxandrin	PO
oxymetholone	Anadrol-50	PO
testosterone	Striant, Androderm, AndroGel, others	Buccal, transdermal, gel, pellets, nasal spray
testosterone cypionate	Depo-Testosterone	IM
testosterone enanthate	Delatestryl, Xyosted	IM
testosterone undecanoate	Aveed, Jatenzo	PO, IM

Pharmacokinetics

The pharmacokinetics of testosterone differ by route of administration, as do its potency and local effects in specific tissues. For example, the liver differs by route of administration as well. In particular, the oral route is subject to a high first-pass effect, which results in high levels of testosterone in the liver and consequent hepatic androgenic effects as well as low potency due to first-pass metabolism in the intestines and liver into a metabolite. The half-life of testosterone cypionate is one of the longest, being approximately 8 days. It presents a lower clearance rate after intramuscular administration compared to other analogs of testosterone.

Mechanism of action

The mechanism of action includes binding to the androgen receptor and indirectly through the aromatization of testosterone to estradiol, which allows action via binding to the estrogen receptor.

Clinical indications

Testosterone replacement therapy is indicated for the treatment of patients with **hypogonadism**, sexual dysfunction in males, and hot flashes in females. Potential benefits include increased libido and energy levels, bone density, strength, and muscle and cardioprotective effects. Both males and females use a low dose of testosterone, which can be administered through various routes of administration. Testosterone therapy is often used to treat symptoms of hormone deficiency in pre- and postmenopausal females. It can be used as oral, buccal, sublingual, intranasal, and transdermal, vaginal, and rectal. It can also be given through intramuscular or subcutaneous injections or implants.

Contraindications

Testosterone is contraindicated in patients with breast or prostate cancers, myocardial infarction, stroke, and untreated obstructive sleep apnea.

Adverse effects

The adverse effects of testosterone in males include **polycythemia**, peripheral edema, and cardiac and hepatic dysfunction. Other adverse effects may include hesitation, erectile dysfunction, depression, chest pain, and breast swelling. However, adverse effects of testosterone in females are uncommon if levels are maintained within the female physiological range. The most common are weight gain, **hirsutism,** and acne and are usually reversible with a reduction in dosage or discontinuation.

Toxicity

Toxicity of testosterone can result in altered mental status with psychosis, dry skin, hypertension, arrhythmia, depression, nausea or vomiting, insomnia, and seizures.

You should remember

Testosterone levels fluctuate throughout the day, typically highest in the morning. Its production declines with age, leading to reduced muscle mass, increased body fat, change in body composition, and decreased sex drive.

You should remember

Regularly taking anabolic steroids can lead to physical and psychological changes in both males and females, as well as potentially dangerous medical conditions.

Key Terms

Anovulatory cycles
Antepartum
Cell proliferation
Copious
Corpus luteum
Cryptorchidism
Dyspareunia
Endometriosis
Endometrium
Fallopian tubes
Fertilization
Fertility
Follicular stimulating hormone
Gonadotropin-releasing hormone
Hirsutism
Hydramnios
Hypogonadism
Lutein hormone
Mastalgia
Menopause
Menstrual cycle
Miscarriage
Myometrium
Oligo-ovulatory
Oocyte
Ovarian hyperstimulation syndrome
Ovulation
Ovum
Partial placenta previa
Polycystic ovary syndrome
Polycythemia
Preeclampsia
Scotoma
Spermatogenesis
Stem bleeding
Stroma
Submucosal fibroids

Clinical Case Studies

Clinical Case Study 1

A 47-year-old female began experiencing symptoms of menopause, which included depression, joint pain, dry eyes, hair loss, low self-esteem, and extreme fatigue. She was started on hormone replacement therapy. Within several weeks, the patient's symptoms began to resolve.

Critical Thinking Questions

1. Why does menopause occur in females?
2. What are the causes of menopause?
3. What are the signs and symptoms of menopause?

Clinical Case Study 2

A 38-year-old female had been trying to have a baby with her husband for nearly 2 years. Since stopping birth control, her periods have occurred every 5–7 weeks. After testing both the patient and her husband, it was discovered that the patient had endometriosis. The patient is started on a fertility medication called clomiphene.

Critical Thinking Questions

1. What are the causes of infertility?
2. What are the indications of clomiphene?
3. What are the contraindications of clomiphene?

Clinical Case Study 3

A 56-year-old male presented with a 5-year history of lethargy, low libido, and poor results from exercise. His testosterone levels were low, and he was placed on a trial of testosterone replacement therapy. His symptoms dramatically improved after 2 months. The patient began to lose weight and gain lean muscle. In combination with an improved diet and more exercise, his overall health significantly improved.

Critical Thinking Questions

1. What are the indications of testosterone in males and females?
2. What are the contraindications of testosterone?
3. What are the adverse effects of testosterone?

Further Reading

[1] A. Bennie, K. MacLaren, C. O'Keeffe, Our Guide to Understanding Premature Ovarian Insufficiency, Daisy Network / Grosvenor House Publishing Limited, 2021.
[2] B.J. Cohlen, E. Van Santbrink, J.S.E. Laven, Ovulation Induction – Evidence-based Guidelines for Daily Practice – Reproductive Medicine and Assisted Reproductive Techniques Series, CRC Press, 2016.
[3] M.R. Doster, I.R. Petrock, E.R. Petrock, Muscle Through Menopause – Kinda Vintage, Kinda Savage – Real Conversation, Facts and Solutions to Take Control of the Menopause Dilemma Through Muscular Strength and Nutrition, Doster Petrock, 2024.
[4] O. Elliott, Achieving Hormone Balance – A Science-Backed Blueprint to Unlock Natural Remedies, Manage Menopause, and Thrive with More Energy and Joy, Shuo Luo, 2023.
[5] M.A. Fritz, L. Speroff, Clinical Gynecologic Endocrinology and Infertility, eighth ed., Wolters Kluwer / Lippincott, Williams, and Wilkins, 2010.
[6] A.C. Hacknew, Sex Hormones, Exercise and Woman – Scientific and Clinical Aspects, second ed., Springer, 2023.
[7] A.B. Hoffman, Sex Hormones – Development, Regulation and Disorders (Endocrinology Research and Clinical Developments), Nova Biomedical, 2013.
[8] E.H. Holt, B. Lupsa, G.S. Leo, H. Bassyouri, H.E. Peery, Goodman's Basic Medical Endocrinology, fifth ed., Elsevier, 2021.
[9] M. Hohner, A Practical Treatise on Disorders of the Sexual Function in the Male and Female, Legare Street Press, 2023.
[10] N. Keay, Hormones, Health, and Human Potential – A Guide to Understanding your Hormones to Optimize your Health and Performance, Sequoia Books, 2022.
[11] G. Litwack, Hormones, fourth ed., Academic Press, 2022.
[12] H. Lofqvist, Modern Menopausal Hormone Treatment – Facts and Myths About Sex Hormones, Springer, 2022.
[13] K.W. McKerns, Z. Naor, Hormonal Control of the hypothalamo-pituitary-gonadal Axis, Springer, 2012.
[14] H.S. Taylor, L. Pal, E. Seli, Speroff's Clinical Gynecologic Endocrinology and Infertility, ninth ed., Wolters Kluwer, 2023.

CHAPTER

40

Diabetes mellitus and antidiabetic drugs

OUTLINE

The Science of Pharmacology
https://doi.org/10.1016/B978-0-443-29038-1.00040-3

LEARNING OUTCOMES

After studying this chapter, readers should be able to:

1. Describe the regulation of blood glucose.
2. Compare the pathophysiology of type 1, type 2, and gestational diabetes.
3. Describe the significant acute complications of diabetes.
4. Discuss the major chronic complications of diabetes.
5. Explain the contraindication of glucagon administration.
6. Describe the various types of insulin.
7. Identify the adverse effects of Humulin R U-500.
8. Explain oral diabetes medications and their classifications.
9. Discuss the contraindications of thiazolidinediones.
10. Describe the adverse effects of metformin.

Overview

Diabetes is a disease in which the body cannot regulate blood sugar levels and is the seventh leading cause of death in the United States. The most common types of diabetes are type 1 (T1D), which includes 5%–10% of total cases, and type 2 (T2D), which accounts for 90%–95%. People with T1D generally do not make enough insulin, while people with T2D cannot use their insulin correctly. Almost 75% of all cases of T1D are diagnosed in individuals under 18, although adults can also be diagnosed with T1D. People are at greater risk of developing T2D if they are overweight or obese, inactive, and have a family history of diabetes. It is the seventh leading cause of death in the United States. T2D is the most common form of diabetes and accounts for at least 90% of all cases, while approximately 5%–10% of cases are T1D. People with T1D generally do not make enough insulin, while people with T2D are unable to use their insulin correctly.

Regulation of blood glucose

Glucose is essential to fuel both aerobic and anaerobic cellular respiration. It often enters the body as galactose and fructose (monosaccharides), lactose and sucrose (disaccharides), or starch (polysaccharides). The body stores excess glucose as **glycogen**, which becomes liberated during fasting. Glucose is also derived from fat and protein breakdown products through gluconeogenesis. The regulation of glycogen, and thus glucose, is controlled primarily through the peptide hormones insulin and glucagon. Both hormones are produced in the pancreatic **Islet of Langerhans**—glucagon from alpha-cells and insulin from beta-cells. A balance exists between these two hormones, depending on the body's metabolic state, with insulin in higher concentrations during energy-rich states and glucagon during fasting. Insulin and glucagon, with other hormones, also control glucose transport in and out of cells.

Glucose has a vital role in every organ system. However, there are select organs that play a crucial role in glucose regulation. The pancreas releases the hormones primarily responsible for controlling blood glucose levels. When blood glucose concentration is increased, the beta-cell releases insulin to lower blood glucose. If blood glucose levels are low, alpha-cells of the pancreas will release glucagon, which raises blood glucose. **Somatostatin** is also removed from delta cells of the pancreas, decreasing blood glucose levels.

The liver is an essential organ for maintaining appropriate blood glucose levels. Glycogen is primarily found in the liver and skeletal muscle. Glucose is liberated from glycogen under the influence of glucagon and fasting conditions, raising blood glucose. Glucose is added to glycogen under the control of insulin and energy-rich conditions, lowering blood glucose. The adrenal cortex releases glucocorticoids, which will raise blood glucose levels, the most potent and abundant being cortisol. Thyroxine also increases blood glucose levels.

Diabetes mellitus

Diabetes mellitus (DM) is a condition in which the body cannot regulate blood sugar levels. It is the seventh leading cause of death in the United States. Approximately 38.4 million people in the United States have diabetes, which is 9.4% of the population, and 8.7 million (22.8%) are undiagnosed. About 97.6 million people aged 18 years or older have prediabetes (38.0% of the adult US population). There are two main types of diabetes: T1D and T2D. T2D is the most common form of diabetes and accounts for at least 90% of all cases, while approximately 5%–10% of cases are T1D. People with T1D generally do not make enough insulin, while people with T2D cannot use their insulin correctly. Without enough of this key, too much glucose is in the bloodstream, which can be damaged. T1D is usually caused by an autoimmune attack against the cells that produce insulin, which leads to a lack of insulin. Another less common type is **gestational diabetes** (GDM)—females who develop diabetes during pregnancy.

Pathophysiology of diabetes mellitus

Autoimmunity is considered the primary factor in the pathophysiology of T1D. In a genetically susceptible individual, viral infection may stimulate the production of antibodies against a viral protein that triggers an autoimmune response against antigenically similar beta-cell molecules. Patients with T1D require lifelong insulin replacement with multiple daily insulin injections, insulin pump therapy, or an automated insulin delivery system.

T2D is often associated with genetic predispositions, environmental factors, lifestyle choices, and the dynamic interactions between these aspects. This ailment is a disease state that involves the dysfunction of insulin-producing pancreatic beta-cells, insulin hormone resistance in body cells, or a combination of both. T2D typically begins with a body cell's resistance to insulin, which worsens over time. This resistance and the compensating insulin production by pancreatic beta-cells may eventually lead to beta-cell failure.

GDM can result from beta-cell dysfunction and chronic insulin resistance during pregnancy. Thus both beta-cell impairment and tissue insulin resistance represent critical components of the pathophysiology of GDM. In most cases, these impairments exist before pregnancy and can be progressive—meaning an increased risk of T2D postpregnancy.

Clinical manifestations

T1D, especially in children, classically presents with hyperglycemic symptoms, which can be sudden and include polydipsia, polyuria, polyphagia, **nocturnal enuresis**, blurred vision, unintentional weight loss, fatigue, and weakness. If not evaluated and treated promptly, it can become a medical emergency. In addition to hyperglycemia, electrolyte abnormalities may be present. In adult-onset diabetes, the onset of symptoms is more variable than in youth. It can be challenging to distinguish between T1D and T2D.

Diagnosis

Diagnosis is often based on clinical manifestations and is generally not complicated. Laboratory tests to diagnose diabetes include a fasting blood sugar test, glucose tolerance test, hemoglobin A1c test, random blood sugar test, and urine test. In 90% of T1D cases, one of these autoantibodies is positive. However, the longer the time that has passed since diagnosis, the more likely the present autoantibodies will have diminished.

Glucose in the blood plasma attaches itself to the hemoglobin components of red blood cells. This is known as *glycosylation*. Because most red blood cells live 90–120 days, it can be measured as hemoglobin A1c. When tested, it is expressed as a percentage of glycated hemoglobin. The level reflects the average blood glucose concentration over that period. The ways that A1c levels correlate to average blood glucose are shown in **Table 40.1**.

Complications

The major acute complication of diabetes mellitus is severe hyperglycemia, including **diabetic ketoacidosis**. The major chronic complications include nephropathy, retinopathy, macular edema, neuropathy, coronary artery disease, heart failure, cardiomyopathy, stroke, foot ulcers and amputations, and hearing loss. Diabetic macular edema is shown in **Fig.** 40.1.

TABLE 40.1 Hemoglobin A1c levels with estimated average blood glucose.

Hemoglobin A1c percentage	Blood glucose in mg/dL
5	97
6	111
7	154
8	183
9	212
10	240
11	269
12	298

Glucagon therapy

Glucagon is a hormone that raises blood glucose levels and is used to manage and treat severe hypoglycemia. It is sprayed into the nose as a solution. It also comes as a powder to be mixed with a provided liquid and is injected subcutaneously, intramuscularly, or intravenously.

Pharmacokinetics

Glucagon is administered intranasally and parenterally. Like other polypeptides, parenteral administration avoids rapid and complete degradation in the GI tract. The time to maximum hyperglycaemic activity is dependent upon the route of administration. The onset and duration of GI smooth muscle effects depend on the dose and route of administration. The glucagon metabolism has yet to be clearly defined, but the liver, kidneys, and plasma extensively degrade it. The plasma half-life of IV glucagon is approximately 8–18 minutes. The half-life of intranasal glucagon is 35 minutes and 45 minutes for intramuscular injection.

Mechanism of action

Glucagon binds G-coupled surface receptors in the liver, GI tract, heart, pancreas, fat, adrenal glands, and kidneys to activate adenylate cyclase, which raises cyclic adenosine monophosphate levels. The cyclic adenosine monophosphate stimulates glycogenolysis and glucogenesis, resulting in the release of glucose, primarily from liver glycogen stores. The extrahepatic effects of glucagon are also mediated by adenylate cyclase, including relaxation of GI smooth muscle and positive **inotropic** effects.

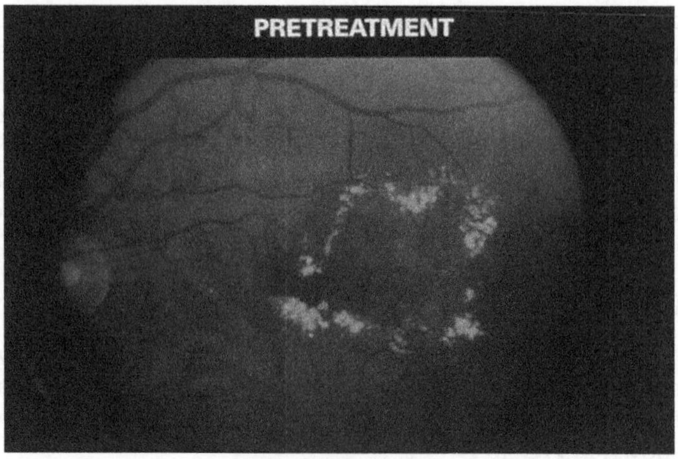

FIG. 40.1 Diabetic macular edema.

Clinical indications

Glucagon injection is an emergency medicine used to treat severe hypoglycemia in patients with diabetes treated with insulin who are unconscious or cannot take some form of sugar by mouth.

Contraindications

The only absolute contraindication to glucagon administration is known hypersensitivity to the medication. Most hypersensitivity reactions occur in GI imaging patients. Other contraindications include use in neonates or children, which may not have sufficient glycogen stores, patients with known insulinoma, glucagon-secreting tumors, and known lactose allergy.

Adverse effects

The adverse effects of glucagon administration include nausea and hypertension. Less common adverse reactions include rebound hypoglycemia in the setting of insulinoma and worsening hyperglycemia in the setting of pancreatic glucagon–secreting tumor. Additionally, the positive inotropic effects of glucagon can precipitate severe hypertension when administered to patients with pheochromocytoma.

Toxicity

Glucagon overdose may result in adverse reactions, but toxicity should not be treated with insulin in most circumstances. The transient hyperglycemia associated with glucagon administration is rarely life-threatening, and iatrogenic rebound hypoglycemia has a substantial risk of harm. Treatment should focus on mitigating the hypertensive response to glucagon with alpha-blocking agents and vasodilators.

Insulin therapy

Insulin therapy replaces the insulin that the body would usually make. People with T1D must administer insulin every day. It is often an essential part of diabetes treatment. Insulin therapy helps keep blood sugar under control and prevents diabetes complications. It works like the hormone insulin that the body usually makes. Patients with T2D must take insulin when other treatments and medicines fail to control blood sugar levels. The main types of insulin therapy include long-acting, ultra–long-acting, and intermediate-acting insulins. The other types are rapid-acting and short-acting insulins. The different types of insulin are described in **Table 40.1**.

Long-acting insulins

Long-acting insulins include insulin glargine U-100 (Lantus, Basaglar), insulin glargine U-300 (Toujeo), insulin detemir (Levemir), and insulin degludec U-100, U-200 (Tresiba). In general, most long-acting insulins can be dosed once daily. The exceptions are that insulin glargine U-100 and insulin detemir have shorter durations of action than the others; in some patients, they act less than 24 hours, giving twice-daily dosing better glucose control. **Table 40.2** summarizes the different types of long-acting insulins.

Rapid-acting insulin

Rapid and short-acting insulins are used to provide coverage at mealtimes. In T1D, they are often matched to cover a specific amount of carbohydrates to offer patients flexibility with eating. Some patients, however, may be on set doses and eat consistent meals from day to day. These insulins are generally injected 5–10 minutes before the meal or at the start to provide coverage with the meal to prevent the blood glucose from spiking too high. Insulin aspart (Novolog), insulin lispro U-100 (Humalog, Admelog), and insulin glulisine (Apidra) are considered rapid-acting insulins and are available in vials and disposable pens. Admelog is the first rapid-acting follow-up on biological insulin. The pens may be dosed up to 60 units in a single injection. There are also options for reusable pens that use pen cartridges. The reusable pens can often be divided into half units, benefiting patients on very low insulin doses. Insulin lispro recently added a disposable insulin pen option for half units. All three of these insulins are commonly used in insulin pumps. Insulin lispro also has a U-200 formulation (Humalog U-200). It is only available as a pen, but because it is more concentrated, it contains 600 units instead of the traditional 300 units that the other rapid-acting insulin pens hold (see **Table 40.3**).

TABLE 40.1 Insulin classification.

Basal		Bolus
Long acting	**Intermediate acting**	**Short acting and rapid, ultra rapid**
insulin degludec U-100 (Tresiba) or U-200 (Tresiba)	human insulin NPH (Humulin N, Novolin N)	insulin aspart U-100 (Novolog, Fiasp)
insulin detemir (Levemir)	human insulin regular (Humulin R U-500)	insulin glulisine U-100 (Apidra)
insulin glargine U-100 (Lantus, Basaglar) or U-300 (Toujeo)		human insulin regular (Humulin R U-100, Novolin R U-100)
		inhaled insulin (Afrezza)
		insulin lispro U-100 (Humalog, Admelog) or U-200 (Humalog)

Ultra–rapid-acting insulin

The newest insulin on the market is aspart (Fiasp), an ultra–rapid-acting insulin. This provides a quicker onset of 2.5 minutes compared to the 15 minutes seen with the rapid-acting insulins, including the other formulation of insulin aspart (NovoLog). This may offer patients more flexibility to inject immediately after meals if they still determine how much they will eat. Fiasp is available in an insulin pen and vial. This type of insulin may become preferred in insulin pumps and is ideal for quickly lowering high blood glucose.

Intermediate-acting insulins

The older types of insulin include *regular insulin (Humulin R* and *Novolin R)* and *neutral protamine Hagedorn* (or *NPH*) insulin, also known as *isophane insulin*. These types have mostly been replaced by the newer long-acting and rapid-acting insulins, which offer effects closer to the functions of a normal human pancreas. Regular insulins are used as *bolus insulin* but have largely been replaced by rapid-acting insulins due to their faster coverage and offset, which helps reduce the chances of hypoglycemia. Regular insulins take longer to become effective and should be given 30 minutes before meals.

Situations in which older insulins are required include during pregnancy and in individuals taking steroids such as prednisone. In such situations, the "peak" of NPH may be beneficial. Because NPH insulin has been available for a long time, there are more accumulated pregnancy safety data. The longer duration of regular insulin may also be better for patients with slowed stomach emptying or *gastroparesis*. Also, NPH can be mixed in a syringe with regular insulin or rapid-acting insulin. This is not commonly done today but allows for two daily injections instead of multiple injections. This method usually does not offer close control of blood glucose, but it may help patients who cannot or are unwilling to administer more than two injections daily. Additionally, NPH and regular insulins are available in over-the-counter, inexpensive vials. The older, intermediate-acting insulins are compared in **Table 40.4**.

Inhaled insulin

Afrezza is the only FDA-approved inhaled insulin drug on the market used to treat high blood glucose in adults with T1D and T2D. In 2014 Afrezza became available for patient use. It provides an option for patients to reduce the injection burden. This drug can be inhaled at the beginning of a meal to lower blood sugar levels in as little as 12 minutes without injections. Afrezza uses a small, disposable inhaler and cartridges of 4, 8, and 12 units in blister packs. The dosing is less exact than other insulins because patients must round to the nearest four units.

The onset and offset are quicker than the injectable rapid-acting insulins. Afrezza is contraindicated in patients with COPD or in patients who smoke. Before initiation, a detailed medical history, physical exam, and spirometry are required to identify potential lung diseases. A spirometry test is needed again in 6 months and annually after that. Afrezza blister packs should be stored in the refrigerator until ready to use. Once opened, cartridges must be utilized within 3 days. Sealed cartridges should be used within 10 days at room temperature. The inhaler should be replaced every 15 days. The same inhaler can be used for different-sized cartridges.

TABLE 40.2 Long-acting insulins.

Property	degludec U-100 (Tresiba)	degludec U-200 (Tresiba)	detemir U-100 (Levemir)	glargine U-100 (Lantus)	glargine U-300 (Toujeo)
Concentration	100 units/mL	200 units/mL	100 units/mL	100 units/mL	300 units/mL
Onset	30–90 minutes	30–90 minutes	1.1–2 hours	1.1 hours	6 hours
Duration of Action	42 hours	42 hours	7.6–24 hours	10.8–24 hours	24–36 hours
Max units injected per dose	80 units	160 units	80 units	80 units	80 units
Formulation	Pen/vial	Pen	Pen/vial	Pen/vial	Pen
Pen dial	1 unit	2 units	1 unit	1 unit	1 unit
Units per pen	300 units in 3 mL	600 units in 3 mL	300 units in 3 mL	300 unit in 3 mL	450 units in 1.5 mL

TABLE 40.3 Rapid-/short-acting insulins.

Property	Insulin aspart (Novolog)	Insulin aspart (Fiasp)	Insulin glulisine (Apidra)	Insulin lispro (Humalog) U-100, U-200	Inhaled insulin (Afrezza)	Human insulin regular (Novolin R, Humulin R)
Onset	10–20 minutes	2.5 minutes	25 minutes	15–30 minutes	12–30 minutes	30 minutes
Duration of action	3–5 hours	3–5 hours	4–5.3 hours	3–6.5 hours	160 minutes	8 hours
Meal timing	SC 5–10 minutes before meals	SC at start of meal or 20 minutes after meal	SC within 15 minutes before or 20 minutes after starting meal	SC up to 15 minutes before or immediately after meal	Inhaled at beginning of meal	SC 30 minutes before meal
Dosage form	Vial/pen	Vial/pen	Vial/pen	U-100: Vial/pen U-200: pen only	Inhaled	Vial
Units per pen	300 units in 3 mL	300 units in 3 mL	300 units in 3 mL	U-100: 300 units in 3 mL U-200: 600 units in 3 mL	N/A	300 units in 3 mL
Max units injected per dose	60 units	60 units	80 units	60 units	4-, 8-, or 12-unit cartridges	60 units

SC, Subcutaneous.

TABLE 40.4 Intermediate-acting insulins.

Property	Humulin N, Novolin N	Humulin R, U-500
Onset	1–2 hours	30 min
Duration of action	16–24 hours	12–24 hours
Concentration	100 units per mL	500 units per mL
Dosage form	Vial or Kwikpen	Vial or Kwikpen
Pen dial	1 unit	5 units
Meal timing	Taken without regard to meals	30 minutes before meals
Typical dosing	One to two times per day alone, or mixed with rapid- or short-acting insulin	Three to four times per day before meals or snacks

Premixed insulins

Premixed insulins are also available in various formulations. *Novolog mix 70/30*, for example, contains 70% insulin aspart protamine and 30% insulin aspart. Twice-daily dosing is offered instead of the usual four-per-day injections used in basal or bolus regimens, with one long-acting and three mealtime injections. Most often, these are not given at lunch because the peak from the protamine helps cover the lunchtime meal. Such insulin formulations are not as flexible. When a dose is adjusted because it was premixed, the intermediate-acting and mealtime insulin must be adjusted simultaneously. Tight glycemic control is usually hard to achieve without significant hypoglycemia occurring.

Other premixed insulins include *Humalog mix 75/25*, *Humulin 70/30*, *Humalog mix 50/50*, and *Humulin 50/50*. They all have an intermediate-acting protamine component that allows the insulin to last longer. This is mixed with either regular insulin (Humulin or Novolin) or rapid-acting insulin (Novolog or Humalog). Overall, premixed insulins are suitable for patients needing a more straightforward regimen or who have problems adhering to their injections. With these formulations, patients must eat regularly and avoid skipping meals or snacks to reduce hypoglycemia.

U-500 insulin

The *Humulin U-500* is used only for patients with serious insulin resistance who take more than 200 units of insulin daily. When the body can no longer respond to insulin and glucose storage at safe levels, higher blood glucose results, and insulin resistance occurs. Therefore U-500 insulin is commonly used for T2D. It is also possible for patients with T1D to develop insulin resistance, primarily if they are obese. U-500 insulin is dosed twice to four times daily before meals. It functions closely to the intermediate-acting insulins and should be administered 30 minutes before meals or snacks. Because U-500 insulin is five times more potent than other forms, there is a long history of dosing errors. Over time, patients often used U-100 syringes, resulting in much confusion because just 5 units in a U-100 syringe is 25 units of U-500 insulin. Today there are dedicated U-500 syringes and insulin pens. They have significantly reduced dosing errors of this type of insulin.

Pharmacokinetics

The high concentration of U-500 results in delayed absorption and is responsible for a slow delivery rate. Single doses of U-500 are generally active for 8 hours, although activity can last up to 24 hours. The range is due to variability in blood flow at the injection site and sensitivity of insulin receptors. Initial effects of U-500 are similar to regular insulin, with an onset of 30 minutes and peak effects seen within 1–3 hours. Based on its unique pharmacokinetic properties, U-500 is dosed similarly to NPH, with two to three daily injections.

Mechanism of action

Humulin U-500 lowers blood glucose by stimulating peripheral blood glucose uptake by skeletal muscle and fat and inhibiting hepatic glucose production.

Clinical indications

Humulin R U-500 is an insulin used to control high blood sugar in adults and children with diabetes mellitus who need more than 200 units of insulin a day. Humulin R U-500 is highly concentrated and contains five times as much insulin in 1 mL as standard U-100 (100 units/mL).

Contraindications

Humulin R U-500 is contraindicated during episodes of hypoglycemia and in patients hypersensitive to it or any of its excipients. Any change of insulin should be made cautiously and only under medical supervision.

Adverse effects

The adverse effects of Humulin R U-500 include hypoglycemia, allergic reaction, **lipodystrophy**, rash, and injection site reaction. Other adverse effects are chills, sweating, chest tightness, headache, cough, flushing, anxiety, blurred vision, dizziness, tachycardia, dysphagia, polyphagia, polydipsia, oliguria, weight gain, and seizures.

You should remember

Long-acting insulins are preferred over intermediate-acting insulins because they are more likely to provide consistent 24-hour coverage with a once-daily injection. Intermediate-acting insulins often need twice-daily dosing to get full 24-hour coverage. Regular insulin needs to be injected 30 minutes before meals, while the rapid-acting (aspart, lispro, glulisine) and ultra–rapid-acting (inhaled, ultra-rapid aspart) insulins are injected closer to the start of the meal.

You should remember

Brain cells are unique because they do not need insulin for glucose entry. Most other cells do require insulin for this purpose. Brain cells also do not use free fatty acids or amino acids for energy. Instead they only use glucose or glycogen to meet energy demands and power cellular functions. Therefore gluconeogenesis in the liver is very important. Between meals, if the liver did not produce glucose, the brain would not have a usable energy source.

Antidiabetic drugs for type 2 diabetes

Oral diabetes medications help patients with T2D manage blood sugar levels. There are several different types. The patients may need to take more than one kind or may have to take insulin and pills. They have other characteristics when adding insulin, including onset of action, duration, and concentration. The noninsulin medication classes are listed in **Table 40.5**.

Biguanides

Metformin is the only medication in the biguanides class that reduces the amount of glucose that the liver produces. Patients with T2D produce more glucose from their liver than is needed. Metformin helps to turn this off and significantly lowers the fasting blood glucose. This medication is considered the first-line therapy for T2D. Metformin is one of the older oral medications and has demonstrated safety and effectiveness over time. It is also inexpensive, especially compared to many newer diabetes medications.

TABLE 40.5 Noninsulin medication classes.

Class	Generic name	Brand name
Biguanide	metformin	Glucophage, Riomet
TZDs	pioglitazone rosiglitazone	Actos Avandia
Sulfonylureas	glimepiride glipizide glyburide	Amaryl Glucotrol Micronase, Glynase
Meglitinides	nateglinide repaglinide	Starlix Prandin
Alpha-glucosidase inhibitors	acarbose miglitol	Precose Glyset

TZDs, Thiazolidinediones.

Pharmacokinetics

Food reduces the absorption of metformin, as demonstrated by about a 40% lower mean peak plasma concentration and a 35-minute increase in time to peak plasma concentration after ingestion of an 850-mg tablet of metformin taken with food, compared to the same dose administered during fasting. Metformin is bound to plasma proteins, excreted as an unchanged drug in the urine, and does not undergo hepatic metabolism (no metabolites have been identified in humans) or biliary excretion. The kidney substantially excretes this drug. The plasma elimination half-life of metformin is 6.2 hours in the plasma. The elimination half-life in the blood is approximately 17.6 hours.

Mechanism of action

The mechanisms of action for metformin are complex and still need to be fully understood. Early evidence highlighted the liver as the central organ in reducing blood glucose levels. However, increasing evidence points toward other sites of action that might also have an important role, including the GI tract and its microbiota interactions that contribute to metformin's therapeutic effects. At the molecular level, the mechanisms of action seem to vary depending on the metformin dose and the treatment duration.

However, metformin decreases blood glucose levels by reducing hepatic glucose production, lowering the intestinal absorption of glucose, and increasing insulin sensitivity by increasing peripheral glucose uptake and utilization.

Clinical indications

Metformin is used to treat T2D and GDM. It is also used to help prevent T2D in people at high risk of developing it.

Contraindications

Metformin is contraindicated in patients with congestive heart failure, renal impairment, acute or chronic metabolic acidosis, hypersensitivity to the drug, and dysfunction of the liver.

Adverse effects

Metformin should be avoided in patients with chronic kidney disease and lactic acidosis.

Common adverse effects of metformin include diarrhea and stomach upset. A metallic taste or vitamin B_{12} deficiency can often occur, leading to anemia or peripheral neuropathy. Therefore periodic monitoring of vitamin B_{12} levels is recommended. Metformin is usually not given when a person is hospitalized because of the interaction with iodinated contrast media.

Toxicity

Metformin rarely causes hypoglycemia, but it can generate profound lactic acidosis in overdose and patients with renal failure.

Thiazolidinediones

Thiazolidinediones (TZDs), also termed "glitazones," are used as antidiabetic agents for treating T2D. They increase insulin sensitivity in the muscle and adipose cells. Drugs in this class include pioglitazone and rosiglitazone, which are dosed once daily. In 2013 the FDA lifted its earlier restrictions on rosiglitazone after reviewing the results of a 2009 trial that failed to show increased heart attack risk. However, they remained banned in markets overseas.

Pharmacokinetics

Pioglitazone is well absorbed, with a mean absolute bioavailability of 83%, and reaches maximum concentrations in about 1.5 hours. The hepatic cytochrome P450 enzyme system metabolizes it. The half-life is about 9 hours, but two active metabolites mainly contribute to the extended glucose-lowering effects. It is administered once daily without regard to meals. The pharmacokinetics are not significantly altered in T2D, renal or hepatic insufficiency, or older adults. Pioglitazone also had a beneficial effect on the abnormal lipid profile seen in T2D.

Mechanism of action

TZDs do not stimulate insulin secretion. They act by improving insulin sensitivity via activation of the nuclear receptor. There is an increase in glucose utilization by skeletal muscle and fat cells, increased uptake of free fatty acids, reduced lipolysis by fat cells, and decreased hepatic gluconeogenesis. The ratio of adipogenesis to apoptosis is also differentially altered for fat cells, favoring **apoptosis** of more giant insulin-resistant cells and the proliferation of smaller insulin-sensitive adipocytes. This is accompanied by a shift in fat distribution from central to peripheral depots.

Clinical indications

Lifestyle changes, including weight loss and increased activity, are the primary recommendations for treating T2D. However, because of the progressive nature of the disease, the treatment of T2D usually requires the stepwise introduction of oral hypoglycemic drugs followed by insulin.

Contraindications

The use of TZDs is contraindicated in people with active liver disease, congestive heart failure, and T1D.

Adverse effects

TZDs have a black box warning for congestive heart failure. They may cause fluid retention, which can worsen heart failure. There is also a risk of bone fractures and weight gain. Some studies have shown an association with pioglitazone and bladder cancer. TZDs can cause elevated liver enzymes.

Toxicity

The toxicity of TZDs during chronic therapy can cause hepatic failure. The patient may develop jaundice, anorexia, nausea, abdominal discomfort, fatigue, and dyspnea. TZDs may also cause hypotension, bradycardia, and coma.

Sulfonylureas

Drugs in this class include glimepiride, glyburide, and glipizide. Glyburide is the longest acting and is not recommended for use in people with impaired kidney function or older adults. These drugs work by causing the pancreas to release more insulin. They are generally dosed once or twice daily before mealtimes. They are inexpensive but can induce hypoglycemia, especially if meals are skipped. This low-cost option could be considered second line if drug cost is an issue. Caution should be used if combined with insulin, as the risk of hypoglycemia would be even more significant, especially with mealtime insulins. These tend to become less effective over time, as the pancreatic beta-cell may lose its ability to produce insulin. There is some concern that these medications may speed up this process. They can also cause weight gain.

Pharmacokinetics

The sulfonylureas are well absorbed after oral administration, though absorption of glipizide is delayed by food. All sulfonylureas are highly bound (90%–99%) to plasma protein.

Mechanism of action

The sulfonylureas exert hypoglycemic effects by stimulating insulin secretion from pancreatic beta-cells. Their primary mechanism of action is to close the ATP-sensitive potassium channels in the beta-cell plasma membrane, initiating a chain of events that results in insulin release.

Clinical indications

Sulfonylureas are used to control hyperglycemia in people with T2D who cannot achieve appropriate control with changes in diet and exercise alone.

Contraindications

Contraindications to the use of sulfonylureas include hypersensitivity to them or drugs with similar structures. Another contraindication is pregnancy. Caution must be used in cases of reduced renal or hepatic function. Patients with ketoacidosis should receive insulin instead of an oral antihyperglycemic agent.

Adverse effects

The most common adverse effect associated with sulfonylureas is hypoglycemia. This condition can be severe and prolonged, resulting in neurologic sequelae and death. Signs and symptoms of **neuroglycopenia** include headache, confusion, drowsiness, dizziness, weakness, seizures, and coma. Other adverse effects comprise nausea, palpitations, shaking, and diaphoresis. Hypoglycemia-related dysrhythmias and **acute coronary syndrome** have been reported and are associated with electrolyte abnormalities and increased release of catecholamines. Electrolyte abnormalities include hypokalemia and hypomagnesemia.

Toxicity

In overdose, sulfonylureas cause profound and prolonged hypoglycemia, usually apparent within 8 hours postingestion of a standard preparation.

Meglitinides

Meglitinides drugs include repaglinide and nateglinide. These medications are similar to sulfonylureas in that they cause the pancreas to release more insulin. They are shorter than sulfonylureas and should be dosed up to three times daily before meals. They are also relatively inexpensive, although less effective compared to sulfonylureas. They are dosed 1–30 minutes before meals and have more of an impact on the postmeal glucose levels. They should not be combined with sulfonylureas. Similar to sulfonylureas, caution should be used in combination with insulin. The two examples of meglitinides include prandin and starlix.

Pharmacokinetics

Repaglinide is rapidly absorbed from the GI tract, approximately 97% bound to plasma proteins. It is extensively metabolized in the liver by the CYP3A4 isoform of cytochrome P450 and excreted about 90% in the bile. Repaglinide has a short plasma half-life.

Mechanism of action

Repaglinide binds to receptors on beta-cells of the pancreas and stimulates insulin release. It also binds to an ATP-dependent potassium channel on beta-cells. Because they promote insulin secretion, they are helpful only in patients with some beta-cell function.

Clinical indications

Meglitinides, diet, and exercise improve blood glucose control in adults with T2D. These medications have been approved by the FDA since 1997. The first drug in this class, repaglinide, was approved in 1997, and a second, nateglinide, was approved in 2000. Patients with allergies to meglitinides should not use them. Meglitinides are taken about 30 minutes before mealtime.

Contraindications

Meglitinides are contraindicated in patients with T1D, diabetic ketoacidosis, and severe liver dysfunction.

Adverse effects

Meglitinides are well tolerated by most patients, including older adults who need help lowering their mealtime blood sugar. Hypoglycemia is the most common adverse effect of meglitinides. Symptoms of hypoglycemia include confusion, shakiness, sweating, and lightheadedness.

Toxicity

Overdose of meglitinides includes diaphoresis, restlessness, altered mental status, aggressive behavior, tremors, confusion, or coma.

Alpha-glucosidase inhibitors

The drugs in this class include acarbose and miglitol. They are relatively inexpensive and can be taken up to three times daily with the first bite of the meal. Still, patients must use pure glucose and not table sugar such as sucrose to treat hypoglycemia.

Pharmacokinetics

Acarbose acts locally in the GI tract on the surface of enterocytes. About 2% of an oral acarbose dose is systemically absorbed, with a plasma half-life of 2 hours. The intestinal microbial flora and digestive enzymes metabolize acarbose, which is excreted in the stool.

Mechanism of action

Acarbose slows glucose absorption by delaying the digestion of carbohydrates and reducing postprandial glucose blood concentrations. It is also a competitive inhibitor of alpha-glucosidase enzymes in the brush border of the intestine.

Clinical indications

Acarbose is indicated as an adjunct to diet and exercise to improve glycemic control in adults with T2D. It is usually taken three times a day, and it is essential to take each dose with the first bite of each main meal.

Contraindications

Alpha-glucosidase inhibitors should not be used in patients with obstructive bowel disorders, inflammatory bowel disease, or **gastroparesis**.

Adverse effects

The adverse effects of acarbose include abdominal pain, mild diarrhea, gas, bloating, and skin rash or itching, worse with meals containing more carbohydrates. It is recommended to start at a lower dose and slowly increase. If hypoglycemia is not treated, severe symptoms may include seizures, confusion, and unconsciousness.

Toxicity

Overdose with acarbose will not cause hypoglycemia but may increase GI symptoms. Patients should not have food or beverages that contain carbohydrates for 4–6 hours if an overdose occurs.

Key Terms

Acute coronary syndrome
Apoptosis
Diabetic ketoacidosis
Diabetes mellitus
Enterocytes
Gastroparesis
Gestational diabetes
Glycogen
Islet of Langerhans
Lipodystrophy
Neuroglycopenia
Nocturnal enuresis

Clinical case studies

Clinical case study 1

A previously healthy 4-year-old girl was brought to the emergency room due to being almost unconscious. She was well up to 5 days before her admission. After that, she presented with dysuria and loss of appetite and then developed polyuria, polydipsia, and weight loss. There was no history of diabetes in her family. A serum glucose test was performed, and her glucose level was very high. After various blood and urine tests, she was diagnosed with T1D mellitus.

Critical thinking questions

1. What is the pathophysiology of T1D?
2. What are the laboratory tests to diagnose diabetes mellitus?
3. What are the various types of insulin?

Clinical case study 2

A 74-year-old male has a 7-year history of T2D. His weight is 207 pounds, and his A1C has never been less than 8%. He was advised to lose at least 15 pounds at the initial diagnosis. His BP was 160/100. The patient had never undergone surgeries or hospitalizations; his immunizations were current. In general, he remained remarkably healthy for many years.

Critical thinking questions

1. What are the causes and risk factors for T2D?
2. What are the classifications of antidiabetic drugs for T2D?
3. What are the various types of sulfonylureas and their contraindications?

Further Reading

[1] R. Chawla, S. Jaggi, Novel Insights on SGLT-2 Inhibitors, Jaypee Brothers Medical Publishers, Ltd, 2019.
[2] R.A. DeFronzo, E. Ferrannini, P. Zimmet, G. Alberti, International Textbook of Diabetes Mellitus, 2 Volume Set, 4th Edition, Wiley-Blackwell, 2015.
[3] U. Ghani, Alpha-Glucosidase Inhibitors – Clinically Promising Candidates for Anti-diabetic Drug Discovery, Elsevier, 2019.
[4] M. Grau, Pathological Mechanisms in Diabetes, Mdpi AG, 2023.
[5] R. Khardori, V.V. Gossain, Drugs in Diabetes, Jaypee Brothers Medical Publishers, Ltd, 2021.
[6] J.L. Leahy, W.T. Cefalu, Insulin Therapy – an Issue of Endocrinology and Metabolism Clinics (Internal Medicine Book 41), Saunders, 2013.
[7] V. Mohan, R. Unnikrishnan, World Clinics – Diabetology – Type 2 Diabetes Mellitus, Jaypee Brothers Medical Publishers, Ltd, 2012.
[8] R. Nandaniya, P. Ram, R. Pada, Anti-Diabetic Drugs, Lap Lambert Academic Publishing, 2015.
[9] L. Poretsky, Principles of Diabetes Mellitus, third ed., Springer Reference, 2017.
[10] M.W.J. Strachan, B.M. Frier, Insulin Therapy – A Pocket Guide, Springer, 2013.
[11] N. Thomas, A Practical Guide to Diabetes Mellitus, eighth ed., Jaypee Brothers Medical Publishers Ltd, 2018.
[12] A. Todkar, D. Thite, S. Suryawanshi, Diabetes Mellitus – Pathophysiology of Diabetes, Lap Lambert Academic Publishing, 2023.
[13] G.E. Umpierrez, Therapy for Diabetes Mellitus and Related Disorders, sixth ed., American Diabetes Association, 2014.
[14] J.R. White, The 2022-2023 Guide to Medications for the Treatment of Diabetes Mellitus, American Diabetes Association, 2023.

UNIT VII

Gastrointestinal drugs

CHAPTER

41

Review of the digestive system

OUTLINE

LEARNING OUTCOMES

After study of the chapter, readers should be able to:

1. Describe the structure and function of the upper digestive tract.
2. Explain the functions of the mouth, larynx, and esophagus in the digestive tract.
3. Identify the layers of the stomach and its cells in the gastric mucosa.
4. Explain the functions of enteroendocrine cells in the stomach.
5. Describe the physiology of the small intestine.
6. Explain the role of cholecystokinin, secretin, and motilin in digestion.
7. Discuss the structure and function of the large intestine.
8. Describe the accessory organs of the digestive system.
9. Explain the functions of the liver.
10. Describe the drug absorption in the lower rectum.

Overview

The gastrointestinal (GI) system begins in the mouth and ends in the anus. The primary function of the GI system is the digestion and absorption of food and many potentially harmful ingested substances. Food breakdown begins in the mouth with chewing and continues in the stomach, where food is mixed with acid, mucus, enzymes, and other substances. From the stomach, the fluid and partially digested food pass into the small intestine, where biochemicals and enzymes secreted by the liver, exocrine pancreas, and small intestinal epithelium break it down into absorbable

https://doi.org/10.1016/B978-0-443-29038-1.00041-5

components of proteins, carbohydrates, and fats. These nutrients pass through the small intestinal epithelium into underlying blood vessels and lymphatics that carry them to the liver via the hepatic portal circulation for further processing and storage. The GI system also includes the exocrine pancreas, which secretes protein enzymes into the duodenum and facilitates the digestion of sugars, proteins, and fats. Bile released by the liver also plays a critical role in absorbing fats and fat-soluble vitamins. The liver is considered an essential part of the GI tract but has a broad range of metabolic functions. One of the liver's vital functions is drug metabolism and detoxification, which have a specific role in pharmacokinetics.

The upper digestive tract

The digestive system breaks down ingested food, prepares it for uptake by the body's cells, provides body water, and eliminates waste. This system consists of the GI tract and accessory organs of digestion: the liver, gallbladder, and exocrine pancreas (see **Fig. 41.1**).

The upper digestive tract begins from the mouth through the stomach. The mouth is also called the oral cavity. It receives food by ingestion, breaking it into small particles. The digestive process begins in the mouth while chewing. The salivary glands secret saliva, which moistens food to move a **bolus** more quickly through the esophagus into the stomach. Saliva also has an enzyme that begins to break down starches in the food. The surface of the oral mucosa is covered by the **squamous stratified epithelium**. This is an avascular and semipermeable tissue whose thickness and degree of keratinization vary according to the location in the oral cavity and the area's functional and mechanical requirements. Sublingual or buccal drugs are absorbed quickly and are essential during emergencies. The pharynx and esophagus allow for the passage of material from the mouth and throat to the stomach. The drugs cannot be absorbed in these two areas. Delivery routes for the esophagus are being investigated directly concerning passive absorption.

The stomach has three layers of smooth muscle: an outer, longitudinal layer, a middle, circular layer, and an inner, oblique layer (see **Fig. 41.2**). These layers become progressively thicker in the body and **antrum**, where food is mixed, churned, and pushed into the duodenum. The gastric mucosa contains glands and several cells in the stomach's inner layer. The stomach cells include the parietal, chief, endocrine, and enteroendocrine. **Parietal cells** within the stomach secrete hydrochloric acid and **intrinsic factors**. Hydrochloric acid lowers the stomach's pH and activates **pepsin**. These cells are located in the gastric glands found in the lining of the fundus and body regions of the

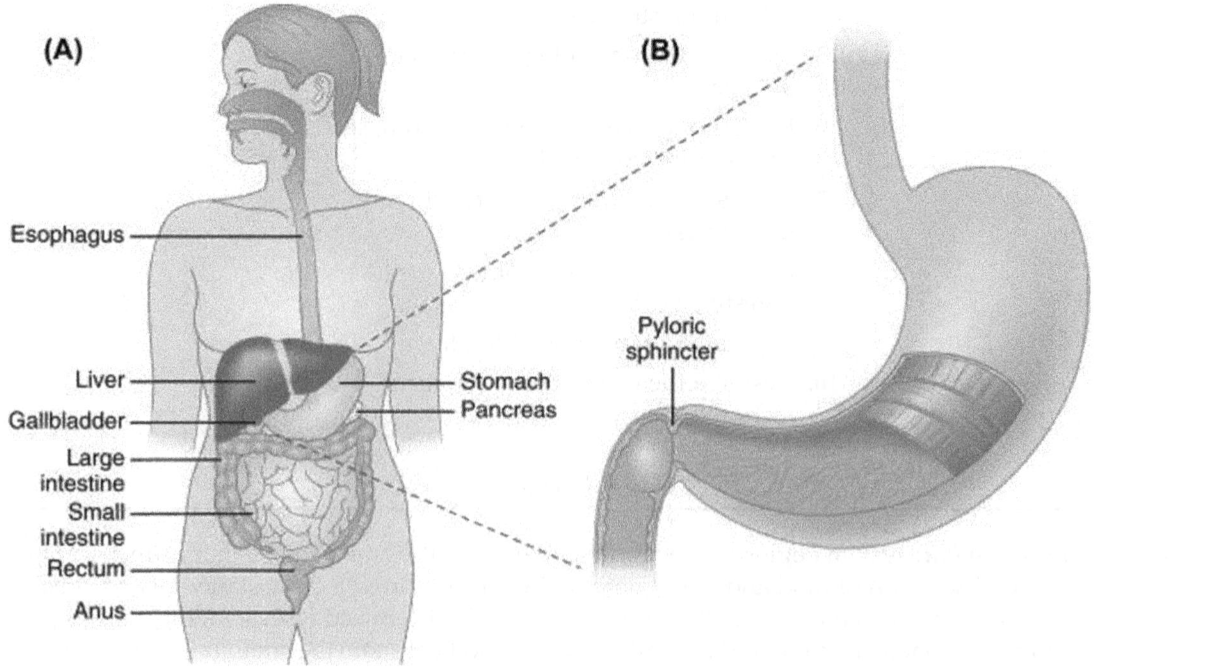

FIG. 41.1 Structures of the digestive system.

stomach. Chief cells release the zymogen **pepsinogen** when stimulated by various factors, including cholinergic activity from the vagus nerve and acidic conditions in the stomach.

Gastric enteroendocrine cells are found in the gastric glands: the G cells of the stomach and upper small intestine secrete **gastrin** into the blood circulation. During a meal, this hormone stimulates the stomach to release gastric acid, which enhances gastric mucosal growth, motility, and hydrochloric acid. **Enteroendocrine cells** are specialized in the stomach and pancreas. **Ghrelin** is another hormone secreted by the stomach. It is known as the "hunger hormone." The stomach can absorb most acidic and weak alkaline drugs such as salicylic acid, aspirin, thiopental, secobarbital, and antipyrine. The postganglionic fibers of the vagus nerve can release gastrin-releasing peptides during parasympathetic stimulation to stimulate secretion.

Gastric motility is essential for the proper processing and gastric emptying of an ingested meal. It is a response to an ingested meal that involves the actions of several different stomach regions. These include fundus relaxation meal accommodation and subsequent tonic fundus contractions. Then, the onset of antral phasic contractions breaks down foods into tiny particles, allowing minor, solid particles to be emptied into the small intestines. This event can influence neurohormonal and contractile activity.

You should remember

A motility disorder is a condition that causes food and waste to move through the digestive tract in an atypical way. It may move slower or faster than it should, allowing food to move backward. The motility disorders of the upper digestive tract include gastroesophageal reflux disease, gastroparesis, analysis, and dumping syndrome.

You should remember

By aging increases, gastric volume and motility secretion decreaised, and gastric mucus in most older people—gastric atrophy results in hypochlorhydria, delayed gastric emptying, and compromise of the gastric mucosal barrier. Decreased production of intrinsic factors leads to absorption of vitamin B_{12} and pernicious anemia. Aging changes in the intestinal microflora and increased susceptibility to infectious and gut-associated diseases. Intestinal absorption, motility, and blood flow decrease. Carbohydrates, proteins, fats, iron, calcium, and vitamins are absorbed more slowly. Constipation often occurs in old age, but it is probably caused by lifestyle factors such as diet and lack of fluid intake rather than physiological decline.

Lower digestive tract

The lower digestive tract, or the alimentary canal, includes the small and large intestines. The small intestine is a tube measuring about 1 inch in diameter and 20–26 feet long. It has three portions: the duodenum, the jejunum, and the ileum. The duodenum is the uppermost part to which the pyloric end of the stomach attaches. It is about 10 inches long and roughly shaped like the letter C. The jejunal portion continues for approximately 8 feet. The ileum is about 12 feet long and is the last part of the small intestine.

From the stomach, the fluid and partially digested food pass into the small intestine, where biochemicals and enzymes secreted by the liver, exocrine pancreas, and small intestinal epithelium break it down into absorbable components of proteins, carbohydrates, and fats. These nutrients pass through the small intestinal epithelium into underlying blood vessels and lymphatics that carry them to the liver via the **hepatic portal circulation** for further processing and storage.

Absorptive epithelial cells on the surface of **villi** are called **enterocytes**. Intestinal digestive enzymes are embedded in the brush border of these cells. The presence of villi and microvilli increases the surface area of the small intestine hundreds of times, thus making this organ the primary site of digestion and absorption.

Mucus-secreting goblet cells are found in large numbers on villi. Enteroendocrine cells produce intestinal hormones. The duodenum and jejunum handle the secretion of **cholecystokinin** (CCK), secretin, gastric inhibitory peptide, and motilin. The physiological actions of CCK include stimulation of pancreatic secretion and gallbladder contraction, gastric emptying regulation, and satiety induction. Therefore in a highly coordinated manner, CCK regulates the ingestion, digestion, and absorption of nutrients.

Secretin is the intestinal peptide hormone, the primary regulator of pancreatic fluid and bicarbonate secretion. Gastric inhibitory peptide is found in the duodenum and jejunum's K cells and is stimulated by glucose and lipids in the duodenum. It promotes insulin secretion to transport and metabolize nutrients and inhibits gastric secretion and motility. **Motilin** stimulates gastric and small intestine motility to move into the large intestine.

Hormones and the autonomic nervous system control the activities of the digestive system. As ingested substances move through the GI tract, they trigger the release of hormones that stimulate or inhibit the muscular contractions (motility) that mix and propel food from the esophagus to the anus and the timely secretion of substances that aid in digestion. The autonomic innervation, sympathetic and parasympathetic, is controlled by brain centers and local stimuli mediated by **neural plexuses** within the GI walls.

The primary absorption of almost all drugs occurs in the small intestine via oral administration because drugs last longer and have a larger surface area. Drug absorption in the small intestine can occur in three ways: active transport of larger molecules by transport proteins, passive diffusion of lipophilic drugs through the membrane, and passive diffusion of hydrophilic drugs through **gap junctions**.

The large intestine is divided into the cecum, colon, and rectum (**Fig. 41.3**). The length is about 5 or 6 feet. Its average diameter is approximately 2½ inches. The first portion of the large intestine is the cecum. The colon includes ascending, transverse, descending, and sigmoid. The ileum joins the large intestine at the junction of the cecum and ascending colon. The **ileocecal valve** permits material to pass from the ileum into the large intestine, but sometimes in the reverse direction. The rectum holds the feces in place until defecation occurs. The large intestine absorbs water and electrolytes, produces and absorbs vitamins, and forms and propels feces toward the rectum for elimination. Drug absorption in the lower rectum is transported directly to the systemic blood circulation. However, drug absorption in the upper part of the rectum is transported to the liver via the portal system and thus undergoes first-pass metabolism. The drug is readily absorbed because the rectum's wall is thin and blood supply rich. A suppository is administered for patients who cannot take a drug orally because they have nausea, difficulty swallowing, or restrictions on eating, as is required before and after many surgical operations.

You should remember

Motility disorders affecting the lower digestive tract include intestinal pseudo-obstruction, small intestinal bacterial overgrowth, and Hirschsprung disease. Small intestinal bacterial overgrowth occurs when the microbes that usually live in the large intestine begin growing in large numbers in the small intestine and producing gases that they cannot quickly expel. Hirschsprung disease is a congenital condition that causes blockage of the large intestine due to abnormal ganglion nerve development in the colon. It occurs five times more frequently in males than in females and results in severe constipation.

Accessory organs of the digestive system

The accessory organs of the digestive system include teeth, tongue, salivary glands, liver, gallbladder, and pancreas. The organs that have an essential pharmacology are the liver and pancreas. The liver is the largest gland in the body and occupies most of the right **diaphragm**. It is one of the body's most vital organs, performing functions critical to a healthy life. The metabolic functions of the liver require a large amount of blood. The liver receives blood from both arterial and venous sources. The **hepatic artery** branches from the **celiac artery** and provides oxygenated blood. The hepatic portal vein receives deoxygenated blood from the inferior and superior mesenteric and splenic veins. The hepatic portal vein, which carries 70% of the blood supply to the liver, is rich in nutrients absorbed from the digestive tract (**Fig. 41.2**).

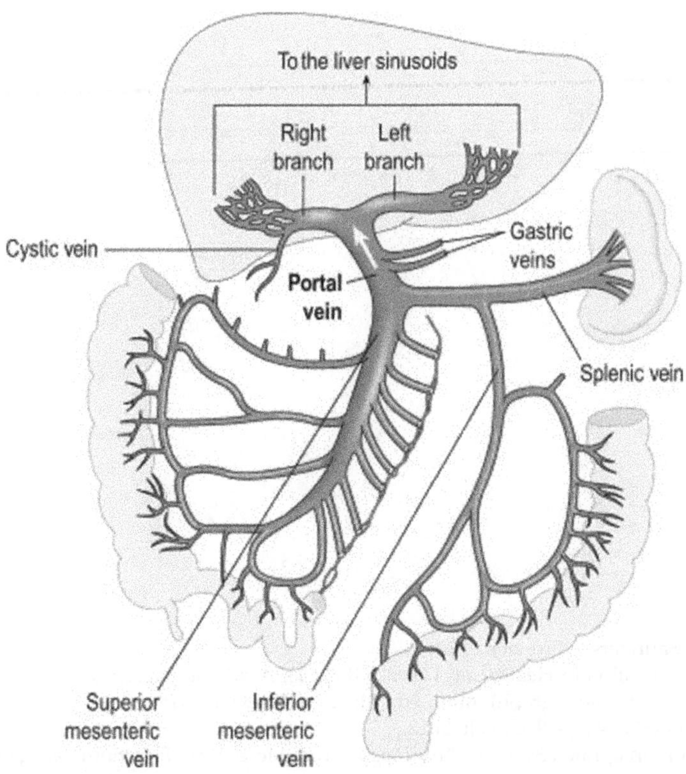

FIG. 41.2 The hepatic portal circulation.

The liver's primary functions include detoxifying various substances, secreting bile, breaking down and removing old red blood cells, recycling the iron from hemoglobin, metabolizing foods and drugs, storing fat-soluble vitamins, and producing clotting factors and albumin.

Bile is formed by **hepatocytes** and is required for the intestinal emulsification and absorption of fats. The common bile duct and pancreatic duct join at the **ampulla of Vater**, which empties into the duodenum. The liver alters exogenous and endogenous chemicals such as drugs, foreign molecules, and hormones to make them less toxic or less biologically active. This process, called biotransformation, diminishes intestinal or renal tubular reabsorption of potentially poisonous substances and facilitates intestinal and renal excretion. In this way, alcohol, barbiturates, amphetamines, steroids, and hormones (including estrogens, aldosterone, antidiuretic hormone, and testosterone) are metabolized or detoxified, preventing excessive accumulation and adverse effects.

Cytochrome P450 enzymes are essential for the metabolism of many medications. They are involved in more than 90% of enzymatic reactions. Cytochrome P450 enzymes can be inhibited or induced by drugs, resulting in clinically significant drug-drug interactions that can cause unanticipated adverse reactions or therapeutic failures. Interactions with warfarin, antiepileptic and antidepressant medicines, and statins often involve the cytochrome P450 enzymes. Knowledge of the essential medications metabolized by cytochrome P450 enzymes and the most potent inhibiting and inducing drugs can help minimize the possibility of adverse drug effects and interactions. Biliary excretion is essential for eliminating some drugs and metabolites in patients.

The pancreas comprises acinar cells that secrete enzymes and networks of ducts that secrete alkaline fluids with critical digestive functions. The acinar units that constitute most of the pancreatic tissue secrete pancreatic juice. The digestive juice is mostly water but contains sodium bicarbonate and various digestive enzymes. Hence, the exocrine part of the pancreas plays an essential role in digestion. The endocrine functions of the pancreas were discussed in **Chapter 40**. Recall that beta-cells of the pancreatic islets secrete insulin, a hormone that significantly controls carbohydrate metabolism. Alpha-cells secrete glucagon.

Key Terms

Ampulla of Vater
Antrum
Celiac artery

Cholecystokinin
Cytochrome P450
Diaphragm
Enterocytes
Enteroendocrine cells
Gap junctions
Gastrin
Ghrelin
Hepatic artery
Hepatic portal circulation
Hepatocytes
Ileocecal valve
Intrinsic factors
Motilin
Neural plexuses
Parietal cells
Pepsin
Pepsinogen
Secretin
Squamous stratified epithelium
Villi

Further Reading

[1] G.W. Boland, Gastrointestinal Imaging – the Requisites, fourth ed., Saunders / Elsevier, 2013.
[2] A. El-Hashash, E.A. Meguid, The Intestine – Volume 2 (Stem Cell Innovation in Health and Disease Book 1), Academic Press, 2021.
[3] L.R. Johnson, Gastrointestinal Physiology – Physiology Series (Physiology Monograph), ninth ed., Mosby / Elsevier, 2018.
[4] S. Keshav, A. Bailey, The Gastrointestinal System at a Glance, second ed., Wiley-Blackwell, 2012.
[5] P.R. Kvietys, D.N. Granger, J. Granger, The Gastrointestinal Circulation (Integrated Systems Physiology – from Molecule to Function), Morgan and Claypool Life Sciences, 2010.
[6] K. Moore, Human Gastrointestinal System – Anatomy and Physiology of the Human Gastrointestinal System, Moore, 2022.
[7] J.C. Reynolds, The Netter Collection of Medical Illustrations – Digestive System – Part I – the Upper Digestive Tract (Netter Green Book Collection 9), second ed., Elsevier, 2016.
[8] J.C. Reynolds, The Netter Collection of Medical Illustrations – Digestive System – Part II – the Lower Digestive Tract (Netter Green Book Collection 9), second ed., Elsevier, 2016.
[9] P. Sing Leung, The Gastrointestinal System – Gastrointestinal, Nutritional, and Hepatobiliary Physiology, Springer, 2014.
[10] M.E. Smith, D.G. Morton, The Digestive System – Systems of the Body Series, Churchill Livingstone, 2010.
[11] C. Tselepis, M.N. Quraishi, R. Horniblow, S.H. Hughes, The Digestive System – Systems of the Body Series, third ed., Elsevier, 2022.

CHAPTER

42

Drugs used for peptic ulcer disease

OUTLINE

LEARNING OUTCOMES

After study of the chapter, readers should be able to:

1. Describe the gastric pits and gastric glands.
2. Explain gastroesophageal reflux disease.
3. Describe the pathophysiology and etiology of peptic ulcer.
4. Explain the standard medications used to treat peptic ulcers.
5. Describe the symptoms of an omeprazole overdose.
6. Explain the H2 receptor antagonists.
7. Describe the clinical indications of H2 blockers.
8. Explain the mechanism of action of aluminum hydroxide.
9. Discuss the *Helicobacter pylori* infection and its signs and symptoms.
10. Describe the treatments of *H. pylori*.

The Science of Pharmacology
https://doi.org/10.1016/B978-0-443-29038-1.00042-7

Overview

Peptic ulcer disease (PUD) involves erosions in the gastrointestinal tract secondary to mucosal damage often caused by pepsin and gastric acid secretion. The erosions penetrate the muscularis mucosa in the stomach and duodenum. *Helicobacter pylori*–associated, nonsteroidal antiinflammatory drug (NSAID)–induced, and stress ulcers are the most common peptic ulcers. The stomach and duodenum are the most common sites for NSAID-induced and *H. pylori* ulcers to occur, while stress ulcers more often occur in the critically ill patient's abdomen. Medications and surgery are options in the treatment of PUD. Usually medications are the first line in treating ulcers. However, surgery may be indicated in certain patients with complications. Indications for surgery usually include complications of ulcers such as bleeding, perforation, gastric outlet obstruction, and untreated PUD. Pharmacotherapy of peptic ulcers includes proton pump inhibitors (PPIs), histamine type 2 (H2) receptor antagonists, and antacids.

Physiology of the upper gastrointestinal tract

The upper GI tract includes the mouth, pharynx, esophagus, and stomach, while the lower GI tract includes the small and large intestines (see **Fig. 42.1**). The esophagus is a muscular tube lined with mucosa that is about 10 inches in length, extending from the pharynx to the stomach. It continues through the **diaphragm** as it descends from the **thoracic cavity** to the abdominal cavity, lying posterior to the trachea and heart. The esophagus allows food to move downward to the stomach. It is subdivided into the cervical, thoracic, and abdominal portions. When in its resting state, the esophagus is nearly flattened. The **stratified squamous epithelium** of the esophageal mucosa provides an abrasion-resistant lining, which protects the esophagus from injury.

The stomach has several parts, including the **fundus**, body, and **pylorus**. The fundus is the enlarged portion to the left, located below where the esophagus opens into the organ. The body is the central part of the stomach, and the pylorus is its lower portion. The small margin of the stomach at its junction with the esophagus is called the cardia. The four layers of the stomach wall help its function, as summarized in **Table 42.1**.

The epithelial lining of the stomach is thrown into folds called rugae and marked by depressions called **gastric pits**. The gastric glands are found below the level of the pits, particularly in the fundus and body of the stomach. The glands secrete most gastric juice, a mucous fluid containing digestive enzymes, and hydrochloric acid.

The function of the upper digestive tract begins with digestion, and the process starts with **mastication**, where food is chewed and mixed with saliva, followed by **deglutition**. The food passes through the pharynx and esophagus before reaching the stomach, where gastric digestion transforms it into **chyme** through **peristalsis**. Chyme then travels through the small intestine. Simultaneously, the mucous membrane of the stomach is secreting gastric juice produced by both the sight of food and irritation on the mucous membrane due to the presence of food in the stomach. Gastric juice, a thin, colorless liquid with an average acidity level of two, contains hydrochloric acid, **pepsinogen**, **renin**, ammonium, calcium, potassium, sodium chloride, and water. **Pepsin** is present in an acidic medium and is made by the conversion of pepsinogen in hydrochloric acid. Endogenous chemicals such as acetylcholine, **gastrin**, and histamine stimulate gastric juice secretion. Acetylcholine is released on **vagal** stimulation by acid secretion when a person sees, smells, tastes, chews, or thinks about food. Gastrin is a hormone released by proteins in food, vagal stimulation, calcium, magnesium, aluminum, and alkalinization of the **antrum**.

Histamine, found in mast cells near the **parietal cells** of the stomach, causes acid secretion by acting on receptors in parietal cells. Hydrochloric acid and pepsin play significant roles in **PUD**. Endogenous prostaglandins utilize mucus, bicarbonate, mucosal blood, and cell renewal as possible defense mechanisms against aggressive factors that may cause damage to the mucosa, such as acid, pepsin, bile, and pancreatic enzymes. The respective roles of these defense mechanisms are to form a protective coat over mucosal cells, allow for a pH gradient between the acidic lumen environment and the mucosal surface, remove acid from the mucosa, and maintain mucosal integrity.

Gastroesophageal reflux disease

Gastroesophageal reflux disease (GERD) is a condition that develops when there is a retrograde flow of stomach contents back into the esophagus. It can present as nonerosive reflux disease or erosive esophagitis. It is one of the most commonly diagnosed digestive disorders in the United States. GERD is caused by multiple mechanisms that can be intrinsic, structural, or both, leading to the disruption of the esophagogastric junction barrier, resulting in

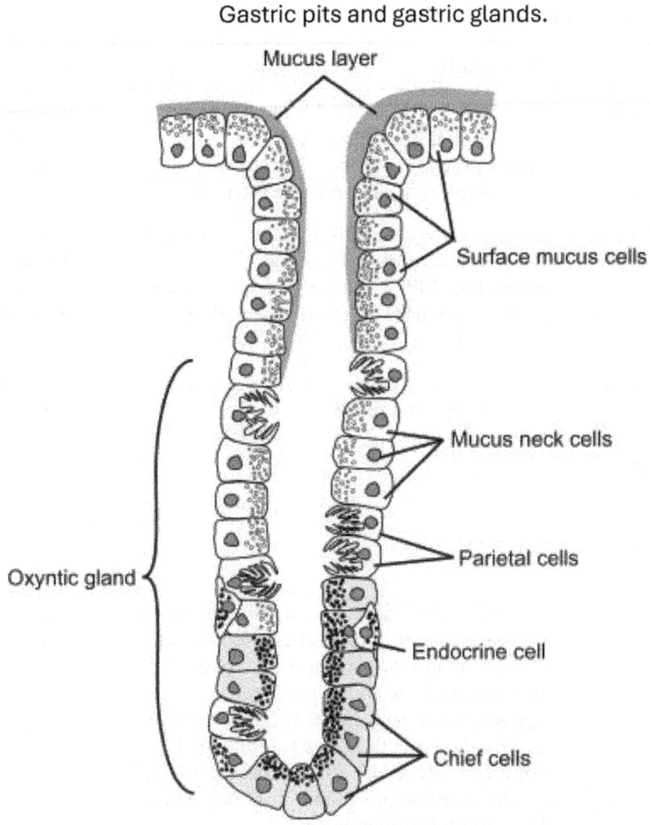

FIG. 42.1 Gastric pits and gastric glands.

exposure of the esophagus to acidic gastric contents. Clinically, GERD typically manifests with symptoms of heartburn and **regurgitation**. Based on endoscopic and histopathologic appearance, GERD is classified into three phenotypes: nonerosive reflux disease, erosive esophagitis, and **Barrett esophagus**. Over the years, the mainstay in the management of GERD has been lifestyle modifications and PPIs.

Pathophysiology and etiology of peptic ulcer disease

PUD is characterized by discontinuation in the inner lining of the GI tract caused by gastric acid secretion or pepsin. It extends into the muscularis layer of the gastric epithelium. PUD usually occurs in the stomach and proximal duodenum but may also involve the lower esophagus, distal duodenum, or jejunum.

PUDs include gastric and duodenal ulcers. Peptic refers to the fact that acid and pepsin are necessary to produce the break in the mucosa, which is called an ulcer. Patients whose parietal cells are continuously stimulated to secrete acid by gastrin from a **gastrinoma** develop ulcers. Those having the **achlorhydria** of **pernicious anemia** rarely develop ulcers.

The two most common causes of peptic ulcers are infection with the bacterium *H. pylori* and long-term use of NSAIDs such as ibuprofen (Advil, Motrin IB, others) and naproxen sodium (Aleve). Stress and spicy foods do not cause peptic ulcers. Acid secretion is higher in about 30%–40% of patients with duodenal ulcers. However, it is expected in most patients with gastric ulcers except those with **Zollinger-Ellison syndrome**. Additionally, bile and pancreatic juice reflux are thought to cause damage to the gastric mucosa by altering mucosal epithelial cells and disrupting the pH gradient formed, thus allowing the mucosa to become permeable to acid and pepsin. Also, ulcer patients may have reduced mucus, mucosal blood flow, and bicarbonate secretion. The risk factors for peptic ulcer include cigarette smoking, corticosteroid use, potassium chloride, chemotherapy, postgastric bypass, cocaine use, radiation therapy, and **sarcoidosis**.

Clinical symptoms include chronic discomfort, **bloating**, nausea, vomiting, significant weight loss, tarry stool, and burning pain in the epigastric region and chest that sometimes radiates toward the back.

TABLE 42.1 Layers of the digestive tract wall.

Organ and mucosa	Muscularis	Serosa
Esophagus (stratified squamous epithelium, which resists abrasion)	Two layers (inner: circular fibers, outer: longitudinal fibers); striated muscle in upper part; smooth muscle in lower esophagus and remainder of the tract	Fibrous outer layer (adventitia); serous around a portion of the esophagus in the thoracic cavity
Stomach (flexible longitudinal folds called rugae allow for distention; contains gastric pits with microscopic gastric glands)	Three layers (instead of usual two); circular, longitudinal, and oblique fibers; two sphincters: LES at entrance of stomach and pyloric sphincter at its exit, formed of circular fibers	Outer layer, visceral peritoneum; hangs in a double fold from lower edge of stomach over intestines; it forms an apron-like structure; greater omentum; lesser omentum connects stomach to liver
Small intestine (contains permanent circular folds called plicae circularis; microscopic fingerlike projections, villi with brush border; crypts of Lieberkühn; microscopic duodenal [Brunner] mucus glands; aggregated lymphoid nodules [Peyer patches]; many single lymphoid nodules [solitary nodules])	Inner layer has circular fibers; outer layer has longitudinal fibers	Outer layer, visceral peritoneum, continuous with mesentery
Large intestine (solitary lymph nodes, intestinal mucous glands, anal columns form in anal region)	Outer longitudinal layer forms three strips (taeniae coli), clumping of circular muscle creates small haustra (sacs) and give remainder of the wall a puckered appearance; internal anal sphincter formed by circular smooth fibers; external anal sphincter formed by striated fibers; visceral peritoneum (serous membrane) has small fatty epiploic appendages	Outer layer, visceral peritoneum, continuous with mesocolon

LES, Lower esophageal sphincter.

You should remember

Bleeding, perforation, and gastric outlet obstruction are complications that may occur with PUD. It occurs in about 25% of patients with PUD with upper gastrointestinal bleeding and is the most common cause of death because of the disease.

Pharmacotherapy of peptic ulcer

Medications and surgery are options in the treatment of PUD. Usually medications are the first line in treating ulcers. However, surgery may be indicated in certain patients with complications. Indications for surgery usually include complications of ulcers such as bleeding, perforation, gastric outlet obstruction, and untreated PUD.

Proton pump inhibitors

There are six PPIs on the market currently, and some are available without a prescription. Each PPI differs in the availability of dosage forms, strength, and dosing schedule (see **Table 42.2**).

Pharmacokinetics

Omeprazole is rapidly absorbed when taken orally. It is quickly eliminated from plasma. The half-life is less than 1 hour, and omeprazole is almost entirely cleared from plasma within 3–4 hours. Omeprazole is completely metabolized in the liver. About 80% of a given dose is excreted in the urine and the remainder via the feces. The absorption of the

TABLE 42.2 Proton pump inhibitors.

Generic name	Trade name	Route of administration
dexlansoprazole	Dexilant, Kapidex	PO
esomeprazole	Nexium	PO, IV
lansoprazole	Prevacid	PO
omeprazole	Prilosec	PO
pantoprazole	Protonix	PO, IV
rabeprazole	AcipHex	PO

coated granule formulation dispensed in hard gelatin capsules is slower, with peak concentrations 1–3 hours after the dose. Bioavailability after a single dose is about 35% and increases during repeated once-daily dosing to 60%.

Mechanism of action

The action of PPIs is to suppress gastric acid by inhibiting the proton pump in parietal cells. The PPIs irreversibly bind to the active $H+/K+$ATPase pumps, inhibiting hydrogen ions from flowing into the gastric lumen. PPIs inhibit basal and meal-stimulated acid production. Initially, there is only a limited amount of acid production inhibited by PPIs; however, more is inhibited once a steady state is reached after 5–7 days of therapy. Dosing PPIs twice daily allows for more pumps to be inhibited, leading to more rapid and complete gastric acid suppression.

Clinical indications

Omeprazole and esomeprazole are two of the most widely used drugs, with more than 20 million prescriptions filled yearly in the United States alone. Omeprazole is available in multiple forms, including 10-, 20-, and 40-mg standard and delayed-release capsules and powder for oral suspension in generic forms and under Prilosec. The typical dose of omeprazole is 20 mg once daily, with twice-daily doses for more severe cases of gastrointestinal reflux and PUD and doses of up to 120 mg daily for Zollinger-Ellison syndrome. A 10- to 14-day course of omeprazole in combination with antibiotics is effective and recommended for eradicating *H. pylori* infection. Omeprazole treats uncomplicated heartburn, PUD, gastrointestinal reflux disease, multiple endocrine adenomas, systemic **mastocytosis**, and erosive esophagitis.

Contraindications

Omeprazole is contraindicated in patients with a history of hypersensitivity to the drug or any excipients from the dosage form.

Adverse effects

The adverse effects are generally minimal. The most common ones include headache, abdominal pain, and diarrhea. It should be used with caution in patients with liver disease.

Toxicities

Symptoms of an omeprazole overdose include confusion, blurred vision, drowsiness, nausea, tachycardia, diaphoresis, flushing, dry mouth, and headache. The drug showed positive clastogenic effects in an in vitro human lymphocyte chromosomal aberration study, possibly leading to chromosomal mutations.

Histamine type 2 receptor antagonists

Selective H2 receptor antagonists are widely used in treating PUD, including duodenal and gastric ulcers, GERD, and common heartburn. The H2 blockers currently in use are available by prescription and over the counter and are some of the most widely used drugs in medicine. They are very well tolerated and include cimetidine, famotidine, and nizatidine (**Table 42.3**).

TABLE 42.3 H2 Receptor Antagonists

Generic name	Trade name	Route of administration
cimetidine	Tagamet	PO
famotidine	Pepcid	PO, IV
nizatidine	Axid	PO

Pharmacokinetics

All the H2 receptor antagonists are fairly rapidly absorbed orally. Peak plasma concentrations are usually attained within 1–3 hours after the dose, but a second peak after oral administration has been observed with each product. They are metabolized in the liver by the cytochrome P450 system. Cimetidine is distinctive among the agents because it potently inhibits the P450 system, which can result in significant drug interactions. All H2 antagonists are eliminated rapidly, with a terminal half-life of 1–3 hours and a total body clearance of 24–48 L/h. Elimination is mainly attributable to renal excretion.

Mechanism of action

The H2 receptor blockers bind to H2 receptors on the gastric parietal cells, interfering with gastric acid production and secretion pathways. They have little or no effect on the histamine type 1 receptors, are blocked by typical antihistamines that treat allergic reactions, and have little impact on gastric acid production.

Clinical indications

H2 receptor antagonists, or H2 blockers, treat duodenal ulcers and prevent their return. They are also used to treat gastric ulcers and some conditions such as Zollinger-Ellison disease, in which the stomach produces too much acid. Over the counter, they relieve and prevent heartburn and acid indigestion.

Contraindications

H2 receptor antagonists are contraindicated in patients with known allergies to the products. They should be used with caution in pregnancy or lactation, renal or liver impairments, and prolonged use.

Adverse effects

The adverse effects of H2 receptor antagonists are generally minimal. However, chest pain, diarrhea, constipation, fatigue, drowsiness, headache, and muscle aches have been reported.

Toxicities

H2 receptor antagonists have a broad therapeutic index, and therefore severe toxicity is rare. These drugs' toxicities may be associated with inhibiting H2 receptors in the myocardium and central nervous system.

You should remember

The FDA issued an immediate market withdrawal for ranitidine (Zantac) in April 2020, and there will be no more products with this drug in the United States because of the potential for increased cancer risk, such as pharyngeal, esophageal, stomach, liver, pancreatic, and colorectal.

Antacids

Antacids are a combination of various compounds, with multiple salts of calcium, magnesium, and aluminum as active ingredients. They neutralize the stomach's acid and inhibit pepsin, a proteolytic enzyme (**Table 42.4**).

Aluminum hydroxide is often used orally to relieve heartburn or gastroesophageal reflux temporarily.

TABLE 42.4 Antacids

Generic name	Trade name	Route of administration
aluminum hydroxide	AlternaGEL, others	PO
bismuth subsalicylate	Pepto-Bismol	PO
calcium carbonate	Titralac, Tums	PO
calcium carbonate and magnesium hydroxide	Mylanta Supreme, Rolaids	PO
magaldrate	Riopan	PO
magnesium hydroxide	Milk of magnesia	PO
magnesium trisilicate and aluminum hydroxide	Gaviscon	PO
magnesium hydroxide and aluminum hydroxide with simethicone	Mylanta, Maalox Plus, others	PO
sodium bicarbonate	Alka-Seltzer, baking soda	PO

Pharmacokinetics

Aluminum has extremely low bioavailability in the GI tract. Only about 0.1%–0.4% of ingested aluminum enters the systemic circulation. The remainder is not absorbed and is excreted in feces. Absorption is strongly influenced by GI pH, transport mechanisms, and co-ingested dietary compounds.

Mechanism of action

Aluminum hydroxide neutralizes gastric acid, inhibits pepsin, and binds bile acids. It also increases mucosal defense and suppresses *H. pylori*. Antacids usually contain aluminum or magnesium and cause more immediate relief for symptoms of **dyspepsia**. However, they have many drug interactions, which may decrease the absorption of certain medications.

Clinical indications

Although they may be used in patients with PUD, they are not considered first-line therapy.

Contraindications

Aluminum hydroxide is contraindicated for patients with known hypersensitivity to the drug. Prolonged administration should not be considered in a patient with renal impairment or a patient on dialysis, as impaired clearance of excess aluminum may precipitate the drug's adverse effects. Due to aluminum hydroxide's ability to bind phosphate, it should not be administered in patients with severe diarrhea, as **hypophosphatemia** may become exacerbated.

Adverse effects

The adverse effects of aluminum hydroxide include nausea, vomiting, aluminum intoxication, rebound hyperacidity, chalky taste, hypophosphatemia, constipation, fecal impaction, milk-alkali syndrome, osteomalacia, and stomach cramps.

Toxicities

The toxic effects of aluminum hydroxide include osteomalacia, seizures, and encephalopathy. Most reports of encephalopathy and osteomalacia came from a period when water purification standards for dialysis were not as strong as they are now, likely confounding the relationship of oral aluminum to toxicity. Reversal of aluminum hydroxide toxicity occurs with the cessation of the drug.

Pharmacotherapy of *Helicobacter pylori*

H. pylori infection occurs in the stomach and causes stomach ulcers. It may be present in more than half of the world's people. Most people do not realize they have *H. pylori* infection because they never get sick. When patients develop signs and symptoms of a peptic ulcer, a test may be done for *H. pylori* infection. Signs or symptoms of *H. pylori* infection are typically related to gastritis or a peptic ulcer. They may include nausea, loss of appetite, bloating, unintentional weight loss, and stomach pain that may be worse when the stomach is empty.

H. pylori infections are usually treated with two or more antibiotics simultaneously. This helps prevent the bacteria from developing a resistance to one of them. Treatment can also include medications to help the stomach heal. These medications include PPIs, bismuth subsalicylate, and H2 blockers. Repeat testing for *H. pylori* is done at least 4 weeks after treatment. If the tests reveal the infection is still present, additional treatment with a different combination of antibiotics may be required.

Key Terms

Achlorhydria
Antrum
Barrett esophagus
Bloating
Chyme
Deglutition
Diaphragm
Dyspepsia
Fundus
Gastric pits
Gastrin
Gastrinoma
Gastroesophageal reflux disease
Hypophosphatemia
Mastication
Mastocytosis
Parietal cells
Pepsin
Pepsinogen
Peptic ulcer disease
Peristalsis
Pernicious anemia
Pylorus
Regurgitation
Rennin
Rugae
Stratified squamous epithelium
Thoracic cavity
Vagal
Zollinger-Ellison syndrome

Clinical Case Studies

Clinical Case Study 1

A 62-year-old female was referred to a gastroenterology clinic due to chronic discomfort and significant weight loss. She had a tarry stool for the first time in the morning of the gastroenterology appointment. The patient described burning pain in the epigastric abdomen and chest that radiated toward her back. The pain was worse after taking aspirin or drinking coffee and was relieved by antacids. Her weight loss (10 pounds over 2 months) was from decreased food intake because of bloating, early fullness, and stomachaches between meals. The patient sometimes had nausea and vomiting. She had previously been diagnosed with gastritis, acute pancreatitis, and diabetes mellitus. Her mother died from gastric cancer at the age of 67. The patient was diagnosed with PUD.

Critical Thinking Questions

1. Which part of the GI tract does PUD usually occur?
2. What are the two most common causes of peptic ulcers?

3. What types of medications are used to treat peptic ulcers?

Clinical Case Study 2

A 43-year-old male presented with complaints of ribcage and abdominal pain. A gastric biopsy revealed that the patient was positive for *H. pylori* infection. He also had hypertension, GERD, epigastric pain, nausea, loss of appetite, bloating, unintentional weight loss, and fatigue. The patient had never been immunized with the HepB, Tdap, or Shingrix vaccines. He admits to being a chain smoker of cigarettes and occasionally consumes alcohol. His immediate relatives have histories of hypertension, type 2 diabetes mellitus, and cancer.

Critical Thinking Questions

1. How are *H. pylori* infections usually treated?
2. Which medications help the stomach heal from a *H. pylori* infection?
3. When is repeat testing for *H. pylori* done?

Further Reading

[1] Z. Anjum, Histamine H2-receptor Antagonist – Renal Clearance and Urinary Excretion of Famotidine in Females, Lap Lambert Academic Publishing, 2014.

[2] H. Donald, H. Pylori Treatment Manual – The Definitive Step-by-Step Guide on the Best Treatment and Cure for Helicobacter Pylori Infection, Donald, 2022.

[3] R.M. Feakins, Non-Neoplastic Pathology of the Gastrointestinal Tract – A Practical Guide to Biopsy Diagnosis, Cambridge University Press, 2020.

[4] I. Hall, Gastrointestinal Tract Disorders – A Clinician's Guide, States Academic Press, 2022.

[5] B.E. Lacy, M.D. Crowell, J.K. DiBaise, Functional and Motility Disorders of the Gastrointestinal Tract – A Case Study Approach, Springer, 2015.

[6] G. Maconi, G. Bianchi Porro, Ultrasound of the Gastrointestinal Tract (Medical Radiology), second ed., Springer, 2013.

[7] E.A. Montgomery, L. Voltaggio, Biopsy Interpretation of the Gastrointestinal Tract Mucosa – Volume 1 – Non-Neoplastic (Biopsy Interpretation Series), third ed., Wolters Kluwer, 2017.

[8] C.M. Morrison, Peptic Ulcer – A Book That Will Give You a Better Understanding of What Peptic Ulcer Is, Its Symptoms, Treatment, Management, Choice of Diet, Myths & Facts About It and More! Morrison, 2023.

[9] R. Natalie, Antacids – The Complete Guide on Everything You Need Know About Antacids, Natalie, 2022.

[10] R.D. Odze, J.R. Goldblum, Surgical Pathology of the GI Tract, Liver, Biliary Tract and Pancreas, fourth ed., Elsevier, 2022.

[11] B. Parker, Proton Pump Inhibitors (PPIs) – Prevalence of Use, Effectiveness and Implications for Clinicians (Pharmacology-Research, Safety Testing and Regulation), Nova Science Publishers, Inc., 2015.

[12] H.M. Said —physiology of the Gastrointestinal Tract, sixth ed., Academic Press, 2018.

[13] T. Wingate Todd, The Clinical Anatomy of the Gastrointestinal Tract, Legare Street Press, 2023.

CHAPTER

43

Drugs used for bowel disease and other GI conditions

OUTLINE

LEARNING OUTCOMES

After study of the chapter, readers should be able to:

1. Explain the physiology of the lower gastrointestinal tract.
2. Describe the description of inflammatory bowel disease.
3. Compare the characteristics of ulcerative colitis with Crohn disease.
4. List the medications that are used to treat inflammatory bowel disease.
5. Describe the mechanism of action of sulfasalazine.

The Science of Pharmacology
https://doi.org/10.1016/B978-0-443-29038-1.00043-9

6. Explain the causes of diarrhea and the drugs to treat it.
7. Describe the contraindications of diphenoxylate.
8. Explain the adverse effects of metoclopramide in treating nausea and vomiting.
9. Describe the drugs that might cause constipation.
10. Explain the mechanism of action of psyllium mucilloid for treating constipation.

Overview

The lower gastrointestinal tract, commonly referred to as the large intestine, begins at the cecum and also includes the appendix, colon, rectum, and anus. The primary function of the large intestine includes dehydrating and storing fecal material. Extensive reabsorption of water and electrolytes occurs in the right proximal colon and continues throughout. However, the lower GI tract also includes most of the small intestine (jejunum and ileum). Its primary function is to digest, absorb nutrients, and eliminate waste products. Irritable bowel syndrome (IBS), nausea, vomiting, constipation, and diarrhea are the most common conditions affecting the lower GI tract. IBS is a set of chronic, relapsing conditions of unknown origin, including ulcerative colitis and Crohn disease. Various drugs are used to treat IBS. Oral drugs are the most convenient application to target colonic diseases. Drugs used to treat digestive disorders of the lower GI tract include antidiarrheals, laxatives, and drugs used to treat IBS. Many drugs are also used to treat vomiting, constipation, and diarrhea.

Physiology of the lower gastrointestinal tract

The lower GI tract consists of the small and large intestines. Also contributing to the physiology of the tract are the vermiform appendix, **peritoneum**, liver, gallbladder, and pancreas. The small intestine is about 1 inch in diameter and between 20 and 26 feet long. It consists of **coiled loops** that fill up most of the abdominal cavity. The small intestine consists of the duodenum, jejunum, and ileum. The presence of villi and microvilli increases the surface area of the small intestine, making it the primary site of absorption. **Tuft cells** secrete prostaglandins and endorphins. **Paneth cells** produce enzymes and other molecules, inhibiting bacterial growth.

The large intestine is about 2½ inches in size, even though its length is 5 to 6 feet. It is divided into the cecum, colon, and rectum (see **Fig. 43.1**). The terminal of the rectum is known as the anal canal, and the opening is called the anus. Intestinal mucous glands produce lubricating mucus, coating the feces as they are formed. There are three primary physiological functions of the large intestine. These include water and electrolyte absorption, vitamin production and absorption, and the formation of feces to be propelled toward the rectum to be eliminated from the body.

Pathophysiology of inflammatory bowel disease

IBD is a set of chronic, relapsing conditions of unknown origin, including ulcerative colitis and Crohn disease. The incidence of inflammatory bowel diseases is increasing globally, affecting 3 to 300 people out of every 1000. Ulcerative colitis and Crohn disease are linked to genetic factors, changes in epithelial cell barrier functions, immunopathology related to abnormal T-cell reactions to **commensal**, luminal antigens, and different phenotypes.

Ulcerative colitis can causes ulceration of the colonic mucosa. It extends proximally from the rectum into the colon. Lesions appear in susceptible people between ages 20 and 40. Risk factors include a family history of ulcerative colitis and Jewish descent. The disease is more prevalent in Caucasian populations and northern Europeans. For unknown reasons, it is less common in people who smoke. Dietary, infectious, genetic, and immunologic factors may all be causative. The inflammation may be due to commensal or pathogenic enteric microorganisms, increased mucosal adherence and invasion, and persistent T-cell activation.

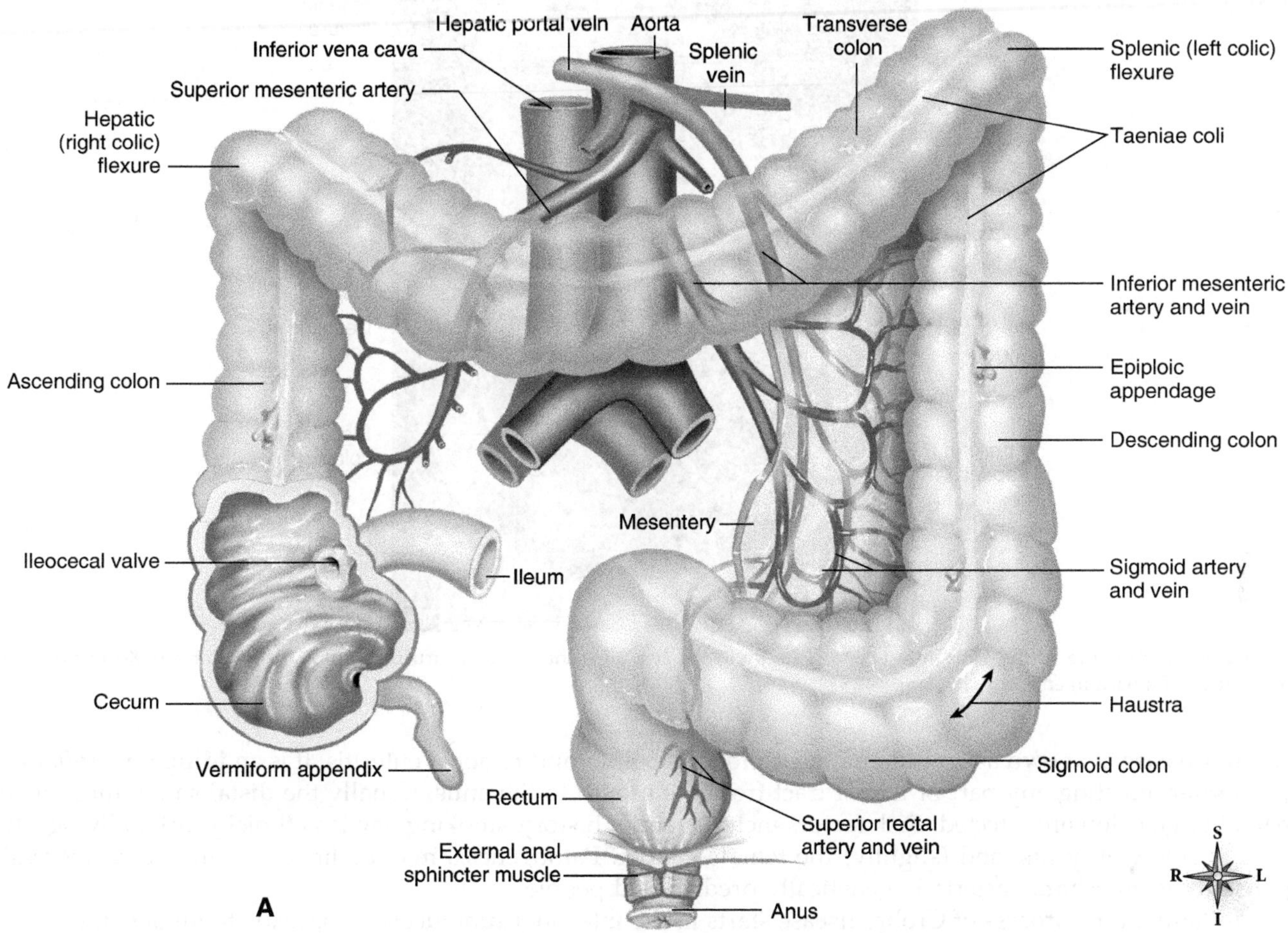

Hepatic portal vein
Aorta
Transverse colon
Inferior vena cava
Splenic vein
Splenic (left colic) flexure
Superior mesenteric artery
Hepatic (right colic) flexure
Taeniae coli
Inferior mesenteric artery and vein
Ascending colon
Epiploic appendage
Descending colon
Mesentery
Ileocecal valve
Ileum
Sigmoid artery and vein
Cecum
Haustra
Vermiform appendix
Sigmoid colon
Rectum
Superior rectal artery and vein
External anal sphincter muscle
Anus
A
S
R
L
I

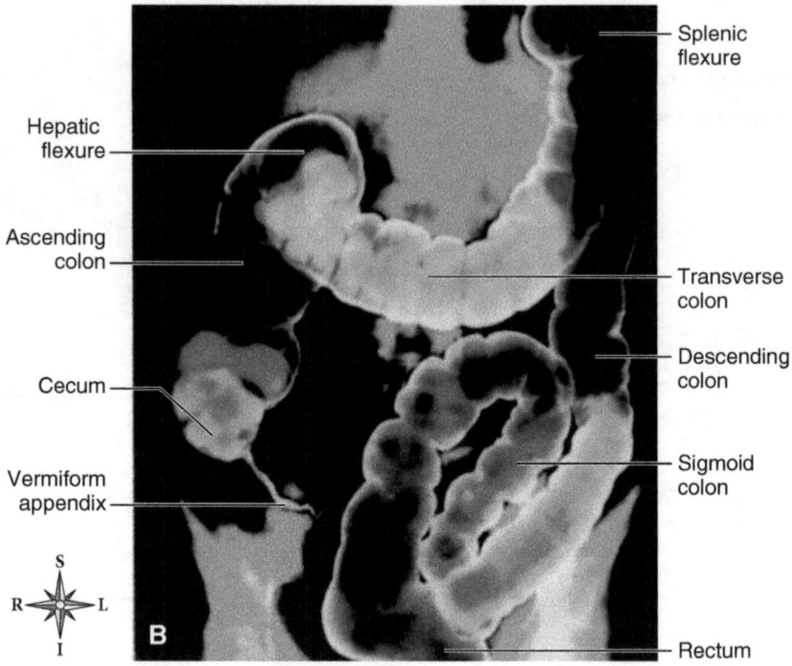

FIG. 43.1 The structure of the large intestine. (A) Its divisions and adjacent vascular structures, and (B) a colorized X-ray taken after administration of a barium enema.

Crohn disease is known as granulomatous colitis, ileocolitis, and regional enteritis. It is an **idiopathic** inflammatory disorder affecting any part of the GI tract from the mouth to the anus. Usually the distal small intestine and proximal large colon are affected. Risk factors include family history, smoking, Jewish ethnicity, urban living situations, age below 40 years, and (slightly) the female gender. Pathogenesis may be linked to an overly aggressive response to **normal flora** bacteria in genetically predisposed people.

The inflammatory process of Crohn disease starts in the intestinal submucosa. It spreads to involve the mucosa and serosa in areas that overlie lymphoid tissue. Progression involves neutrophil infiltration of the **crypts**, leading to abscesses and crypt destruction. The **ileocolon** is usually involved, though the large and small intestines can also be affected. The inflammation may affect specific **haustral segments**, creating skip lesions. One side of the intestinal wall may be affected, while the other is not. Ulcerations create longitudinal and transverse fissures that extend the inflammation into lymphoid tissues. Typical chronic lesions are granulomas, with projections of inflamed tissue surrounded by ulcerated areas.

Microscopic colitis often causes diarrhea and occurs mainly in females and older adults. It may be lymphocytic or collagenous. Symptoms of chronic daily watery diarrhea are the same for both types and may appear along with abdominal pain and weight loss. The etiology is unknown, but prevalence is increasing. It may be linked to various drugs as well as **celiac disease**. The colon mucosa appears normal during endoscopy, but a biopsy will reveal histopathologic descriptions.

You should remember

Inflammatory bowel disease comprises two idiopathic chronic relapsing and remitting GI disorders: ulcerative colitis and Crohn disease. In ulcerative colitis, abnormal immune system reactions cause inflammation and ulcers on the inner lining of the large intestine. In Crohn disease, there is chronic inflammation of the GI tract, primarily in the ilium of the small intestine—it involves all three layers of the tract's wall.

TABLE 43.1 Pharmacotherapy for inflammatory bowel disease.

Generic name	Trade name	Route of administration
balsalazide	Colazal, Giazo	PO
mesalamine	Asacol, Canasa, Lialda, others	PO
olsalazine	Dipentum	PO
sulfasalazine	Azulfidine	PO

Pharmacotherapy of inflammatory bowel disease

Inflammatory bowel disease treatments vary based on the particular subtype and symptoms. Medications that help control inflammation and prevent remission of IBS are summarized in **Table 43.1**.

Sulfasalazine reduces inflammation, pain, and swelling. It can be taken by adults and by children older than 6 years. It is usually given as an oral tablet that must be taken whole with a glass of water. The usual dose is two 500-mg tablets twice per day. The medication is also available as an oral liquid or as a rectal suppository.

You should remember

The drugs used to treat Crohn disease include antiinflammatories, corticosteroids, immunosuppressants, antibacterials, biologics, combination therapies, and OTC medications. The antiinflammatory drugs used for Crohn disease are aminosalicylates, which include sulfasalazine, balsalazide, mesalamine, and olsalazine. Sulfasalazine is taken orally and helps reduce irritation and swelling of the intestinal linings, usually becoming effective in 2–4 weeks. However, sulfasalazine should be combined with daily folic acid.

Pharmacokinetics

The absolute bioavailability of sulfasalazine is less than 15%. In the intestine, this drug is metabolized by intestinal bacteria, becoming sulfapyridine and 5-aminosalicylic acid. Sulfapyridine is relatively well absorbed and highly metabolized of these two metabolites, while 5-aminosalicylic acid is much less well absorbed.

Mechanism of action

The mechanism of action of sulfasalazine has yet to be fully understood, but it appears that this drug and its metabolites have immunosuppressive, antibacterial, and antiinflammatory effects. Sulfasalazine may also inhibit the cystine-glutamate antiporter and **sepiapterin reductase**.

Clinical indications

Sulfasalazine is used to treat a specific type of bowel disease, such as ulcerative colitis or Crohn disease.

Contraindications

Sulfasalazine must be avoided if the patient has a history of allergies, significant kidney or liver disease, porphyria, or a glucose-6-phosphate dehydrogenase deficiency.

Adverse effects

Common adverse effects of sulfasalazine include headache, nausea, vomiting, loss of appetite, stomach upset, diarrhea, **tinnitus**, fatigue, insomnia, and sores in the mouth. Serious adverse effects include sun sensitivity, hearing loss, mood changes, hematuria, cold sweat, blurred vision, and tachycardia.

Toxicities

Dose-related toxicity of sulfasalazine includes gastrointestinal upset, including nausea, vomiting, diarrhea, and anorexia. It also may cause central nervous system symptoms such as headaches and hematologic symptoms, including leukopenia, hemolytic anemia, macrocytosis, and megaloblastic anemia.

You should remember

Sulfasalazine treats and prevents acute attacks of mild to moderate ulcerative colitis by helping reduce inflammation and other disease symptoms. It helps stop the body from producing chemicals that cause GI redness and swelling.

Pathophysiology of diarrhea

Diarrhea is an abnormal increase in the fluidity and frequency of bowel movements. The small intestine receives about 9 L of fluid daily. Most of it is reabsorbed, and only about 1 L will reach the colon. More reabsorption occurs inside the colon so that about 100 mL remains to form the stool. If the small and large intestines do not reabsorb enough fluid, diarrhea may occur. Periodic diarrhea is self-limiting, and medications are not needed. Sometimes diarrhea signifies a body's defense to eliminate pathogens and toxins quickly. If prolonged or severe, diarrhea can cause a significant loss of body fluids, meaning pharmacotherapy is required. Prolonged diarrhea may result in fluid, acid-base, or electrolyte imbalances.

To determine the cause of diarrhea, assessing any recent traveling, dietary changes, immune system competence, and medication history is essential. Common causes include infections, medications, inflammation, foods, and malabsorption. Viral and bacterial infections are the most common causes. The most common organisms that cause diarrhea are *Campylobacter, Salmonella, Cryptosporidium, Giardia, Shigella, Escherichia coli, and Staphylococcus.* Antibiotics can cause diarrhea by killing normal intestinal flora. This allows for an overgrowth of opportunistic pathogenic organisms. Other common causes include laxatives, magnesium antacids, digoxin, orlistat, and NSAIDs. Inflammation of the bowel mucosa that leads to intense diarrhea may be caused by ulcerative colitis, Crohn disease, and **IBS**. Causative foods include dairy products, hot peppers, and the chronic use of alcohol. Diseases of the small intestine and pancreas can cause foods and fluids to be insufficiently absorbed, resulting in diarrhea.

You should remember

Diarrhea causes the body to lose fluids, which can lead to dehydration. Physicians often recommend drinking oral rehydration solutions, water, decaffeinated teas, low-sugar sports drinks, diluted fruit juices, and broths to treat diarrhea.

Pharmacotherapy of diarrhea

The drugs used to treat diarrhea include opiates and miscellaneous antidiarrheals. Also used are synthetic antidiarrheals; anticholinergics such as atropine and propantheline; adsorbents such as kaolin, pectin, and cholestyramine resin; and *Lactobacillus acidophilus.* **Table 43.2** summarizes various antidiarrheals.

Pharmacokinetics

Diphenoxylate has linear absorption, with a dose-dependent increase in peak plasma concentration and an area under the curve in the 2.5- to 10-mg dose range. The peak plasma concentration of its metabolite (diphenoxylic acid) is about 2 hours after being ingested. It is rapidly metabolized in the liver, and urinary excretion of the unchanged diphenoxylate accounts for less than 1% of the administered dose.

TABLE 43.2 Antidiarrheals.

Generic name	Trade name	Route of administration
Opioids	Motofen	PO
difenoxin with atropine	Lomotil	PO
diphenoxylate with atropine	Imodium	PO
loperamide	Paregoric	PO
opium tincture		
Miscellaneous antidiarrheals	Kaopectate, Pepto-Bismol	PO
bismuth subsalicylate	Sandostatin	Subcutaneous, IV
octreotide	Xermelo	PO
telotristat		

Mechanism of action

Diphenoxylate is an opioid agonist that mainly acts on the **presynaptic opioid receptors** (the *mu receptors*). By acting on presynaptic opioid receptors, the drug inhibits the release of acetylcholine in the synaptic cleft, inhibiting the motility and secretory actions of the enteric nervous system. This leads to decreased contractions of the GI tract. The drug reduces the epithelial secretion of fluid and electrolytes. Atropine is added in a fixed dose of 0.025 mg and is a competitive inhibitor of acetylcholine receptors, helping to prevent misuse of the diphenoxylate portion of the formulation.

Clinical indications

Diphenoxylate with atropine is used with fluid and electrolyte treatments for severe diarrhea.

Contraindications

Contraindications of diphenoxylate with atropine include patients with known hypersensitivity, **obstructive jaundice**, children under age 6 (due to a high risk of severe CNS and respiratory depression), and diarrhea associated with **pseudomembranous colitis** or enterotoxin-producing bacteria because of a risk of GI complications such as **sepsis** and prolonged or worsen diarrhea.

Adverse effects

The adverse effects of diphenoxylate with atropine include respiratory depression, anticholinergic adverse effects, electrolyte imbalance, GI complications, **toxic megacolon**, allergic reactions, and drug-drug interactions. Anticholinergic adverse effects include tachycardia, **hyperthermia**, urinary retention, skin and mucous membranes dryness, flushing, confusion, and headache. GI complications include prolonged diarrhea, pancreatitis, and, less often, **paralytic ileus**.

Toxicities

Overdose of diphenoxylate with atropine can be life-threatening. This can occur slowly, over up to 30 hours. Symptoms include respiratory depression, tachypnea, delirium, lethargy, hyperthermia, tachycardia, dryness of the mucous membranes, **mydriasis** or miosis, encephalopathy, seizures, and coma.

You should remember

Diphenoxylate with atropine is available in tablet form and as a liquid oral solution. The dose and regimen depend on the treatment and the severity of the diarrhea. It is essential to take the correct amount of medication every time and follow the schedule strictly.

Pathophysiology of nausea and vomiting

Nausea and vomiting develop because of **noxious** stimulation of the vomiting center. This may be direct or indirect via one or more of these sites: the GI tract, the **vestibular system**, the chemoreceptor trigger zone, and the higher centers of the cortex and thalamus. Nausea is the unpleasant feeling that causes the desire to vomit, while vomiting is the contraction of the abdominal and diaphragmatic muscles, triggering the expulsion of stomach contents. Common etiologies of nausea and vomiting in patients with serious illness include malignant bowel obstruction, infections, medications, intracranial issues, **vertigo**, vestibulitis, **schwannomas**, surgery, dehydration, migraine, pregnancy, cannabis hyperemesis syndrome, food poisoning, constipation, anxiety, and emotional distress.

Pharmacotherapy of nausea and vomiting

Nausea and vomiting are treated with antiemetics, which may be of several classifications. These include anticholinergics-antihistamines, benzodiazepines, cannabinoids, corticosteroids, **neurokinin receptor** antagonists, phenothiazine and phenothiazine-like drugs, and serotonin receptor antagonists. **Table 43.3** summarizes the various antiemetics.

The most commonly used antiemetics are phenothiazine and phenothiazine-like drugs (dopamine antagonists), of which metoclopramide is the prime example.

TABLE 43.3 Antiemetics

Generic name	Trade name	Route of administration
Anticholinergics-antihistamines	Dramamine	PO
dimenhydrinate	Benadryl	PO
diphenhydramine	Diclegis	PO
doxylamine and pyridoxine	Atarax, Vistaril	PO
hydroxyzine	Antivert, Bonine	PO
meclizine	Hyoscine, Transderm-Scop	Transdermal
scopolamine		
Benzodiazepines	Ativan	PO
lorazepam		
Cannabinoids	Marinol, Syndros	PO
dronabinol	Cesamet	PO
nabilone		
Corticosteroids	Decadron	PO
dexamethasone	Medrol, Solu-Medrol, others	PO
methylprednisolone		
Neurokinin receptor antagonists	Emend capsules	PO
aprepitant	Emend for injection	IV
fosaprepitant		
Phenothiazine and	Reglan	PO
phenothiazine-like drugs	(generic only)	PO
metoclopramide	Compazine, others	PO, rectal, IM, IV
perphenazine	Phenergan, others	PO
prochlorperazine	Tigan	PO, IM
promethazine		
trimethobenzamide		
Serotonin receptor antagonists	Anzemet	PO
dolasetron	Sancuso, Sustol	PO, IV, transdermal,
granisetron	Zofran, Zuplenz	subcutaneous
ondansetron	Aloxi	PO, IV
palonosetron		PO, IV

Pharmacokinetics

Metoclopramide is quickly absorbed in the GI tract, with an absorption rate of about 84%. The oral form's bioavailability is about 40.7%, but this can range between 30% and 100%. Nasal metoclopramide is 47% bioavailable. This drug undergoes first-pass metabolism, and its metabolism varies according to the patient. Metoclopramide is metabolized by cytochrome P450 enzymes in the liver. About 80% of the drug is excreted in the urine in the first 24 hours after administration.

Mechanism of action

Metoclopramide promotes GI motility in three ways: inhibition of presynaptic and postsynaptic D_2 receptors, stimulation of presynaptic excitatory 5-HT_4 receptors, and antagonism of presynaptic inhibition of muscarinic receptors.

Clinical indications

Metoclopramide treats nausea, vomiting, fullness after meals, and loss of appetite. It is also used for heartburn in gastroesophageal reflux patients.

Contraindications

Metoclopramide is contraindicated in patients with known hypersensitivity, GI bleeding, obstruction, or perforation.

Adverse effects

The adverse effects of metoclopramide include dizziness, changes in menstruation, drowsiness, anorexia, depression, fever, seizures, confusion, diarrhea, dark urine, hypertension, decreased sexual ability, breast pain, muscle pain or weakness, chills, and reduced libido.

Toxicities

Toxicities related to metoclopramide can result in tardive dyskinesia, which is unusual and uncontrollable movements of the muscles—primarily the facial muscles.

You should remember

Metoclopramide is relatively fast-acting and helps reduce nausea and vomiting within 30–60 minutes in most cases. It is also effective for the same conditions in patients who are on chemotherapy.

Pathophysiology of constipation

Constipation involves a complicated interplay of factors that affect the GI tract, nervous system, and pelvic muscles. Common risk factors include reduced colonic motility, delayed stool transit, impaired rectal sensation, and ineffective coordination of the pelvic floor muscles during defecation. Some drugs for pain, depression, hypertension, and Parkinson disease are linked to constipation. Also, calcium and iron supplements, especially when taken with any other medication that affects the stool, can result in constipation.

Pharmacotherapy of constipation

The pharmacotherapy of constipation includes laxatives and cathartics. Laxatives soften hard stools or stimulate the movement of the bowels. **Cathartics** accelerate defecation. Subtypes of these medications include bulk-forming agents, saline (osmotic) agents, stimulants, surfactants (stool softeners), herbal products, opioid antagonists, and miscellaneous laxatives. **Table 43.4** summarizes laxatives and cathartics.

TABLE 43.4 Laxatives and cathartics.

Generic name	Trade name	Route of administration
Bulk forming	Equalactin, FiberCon, others	PO
calcium polycarbophil	Citrucel	PO
methylcellulose	Metamucil, Naturacil, others	PO
psyllium mucilloid		
Saline (osmotic)	Milk of magnesia	PO
magnesium hydroxide	MiraLAX	PO
polyethylene glycol	Fleet Phospho-Soda	PO
sodium biphosphate		
Stimulants	Correctol, Dulcolax, others	PO
bisacodyl	Emulsoil, Neoloid	PO
castor oil		
Surfactants (stool softeners)	Colace, DulcoEase	PO
Docusate		
Herbal products	(generic only)	PO
Castor oil	Ex-Lax, Senokot, others	PO
Senna		
Opioid antagonists	Entereg	PO
Alvimopan	Relistor	Subcutaneous
Methylnaltrexone	Movantik	PO
Naloxegol		
Miscellaneous laxatives	(generic only)	PO
Mineral oil	Trulance	PO
Plecanatide		

Psyllium mucilloid is the most commonly used medication for constipation and is a bulk-forming laxative. It absorbs excess water while stimulating regular bowel elimination.

Pharmacokinetics

Psyllium mucilloid remains mainly in the gut as a "bulk" agent that passes predominantly unchanged throughout the GI tract. Therefore there is little opportunity for marked absorption into or metabolism by the body. Psyllium is usually excreted in the feces.

Mechanism of action

Psyllium mucilloid seeds are comprised of dietary fiber. When mixed with water, a gel-like mass forms, which works as a mild laxative. The gel-like mass moves down the digestive system and softens the stool by increasing water content.

Clinical indications

Psyllium mucilloid helps relieve constipation; treat IBS, hemorrhoids, and other GI problems; and regulate blood glucose levels in patients with diabetes mellitus.

Contraindications

Before taking psyllium mucilloid, it is essential to discuss with a physician any current or previous diabetes mellitus, heart disease, hypertension, kidney disease, rectal bleeding, intestinal blockage, or difficulty swallowing.

Adverse effects

The adverse effects of psyllium mucilloid may include difficulty breathing, abdominal pain, dysphasia, skin rash, itching, nausea, and vomiting.

Toxicities

Overdose of psyllium mucilloid can cause abdominal discomfort, flatulence, and intestinal obstruction.

You should remember

Many studies have shown the effectiveness of psyllium mucilloids for constipation. When combined with water, they swell and produce more bulk, stimulating the intestines to contract and speeding up the passage of the stool. This agent is widely used as a laxative in North America, Asia, and Europe.

Key Terms

Cathartics
Celiac disease
Coiled loops
Commensal
Crohn disease
Crypts
Haustral segments
Hyperthermia
Ileocolon
Irritable bowel syndrome
Microscopic colitis
Mydriasis
Neurokinin receptor
Normal flora
Noxious
Obstructive jaundice
Paneth cells
Paralytic ileus
Peritoneum
Presynaptic opioid receptors
Pseudomembranous colitis
Schwannomas
Sepiapterin reductase
Sepsis
Tinnitus
Toxic megacolon
Tuft cells
Ulcerative colitis
Vertigo
Vestibular system

Clinical Case Studies

Clinical Case Study 1

A 22-year-old female presented to the local hospital with right lower quadrant abdominal pain. A CT scan revealed a large mass surrounding the cecum. The patient had a chronic history of diarrhea. She was diagnosed with Crohn disease, a form of inflammatory bowel disease. The patient underwent surgery to remove the mass. Since then, she has regained 13 pounds of the total weight loss of 15 pounds that she experienced.

Critical Thinking Questions

1. What is the clinical description of Crohn disease?
2. How does the inflammatory process of Crohn disease start?
3. How is sulfasalazine used to treat Crohn disease?

Clinical Case Study 2

A 28-year-old female presented to the emergency department with abdominal pain, tiredness, persistent bloody diarrhea, and an unintentional weight loss of 19 pounds over 3 months. She was highly underweight for her height. She was given medication and told to consume a clear liquid diet for several days. Two days later, she developed epigastric tenderness, hand tremors, and back pain that was worse with physical activity. Then the vomiting worsened, and she became dehydrated. Testing revealed *Helicobacter pylori* infection, which may have initiated the patient's diagnosed condition of ulcerative colitis.

Critical Thinking Questions

1. What does ulcerative colitis cause?
2. How is sulfasalazine effective in treating ulcerative colitis?
3. What are the contraindications of sulfasalazine?

Clinical Case Study 3

A 76-year-old male had a long history of constipation refractory to years of using stool softeners and laxatives. Abdominal X-rays revealed a large amount of stool, and a CT scan showed a dilated colon with features of fecal impaction. Treatments with medications were not successful, so the decision was made to perform a subtotal colectomy. Over 2 weeks of follow-up, the patient reported improving symptoms with increased regularity and nearly normal stools. After 4 weeks, his stool had become regular, with average daily bowel movements.

Critical Thinking Questions

1. What are the common factors that influence the development of constipation?
2. What does the pharmacology of constipation involve?
3. What are the clinical indications of psyllium mucilloid?

Further Reading

[1] A.N. Ananthakrishnan, R.J. Xavier, D.K. Podolsky, Inflammatory Bowel Diseases – A Clinician's Guide, Wiley Blackwell, 2017.
[2] R. Bowen, Inflammatory Bowel Disease – Diagnosis and Therapeutics, American Medical Publishers, 2023.
[3] R.D. Cohen, Inflammatory Bowel Disease – Diagnosis and Therapeutics, third ed., Humana Press, 2017 (Clinical Gastroenterology).
[4] A. Ehret, J. Lust, Definite Cure of Chronic Constipation Also Overcoming Constipation Naturally, Benedict Lust Publications, 2021.
[5] F.A. Farraye, S.V. Kane, Mayo Clinic on Crohn's Disease and Ulcerative Colitis – Strategies to Manage IBD and Take Charge of your Life, Mayo Clinic Press, 2022.
[6] M. Feldman, L.S. Friedman, L.J. Brandt, Sleisenger and Fordtran's Gastrointestinal and Liver Disease – 2 Volume Set – Pathophysiology, Diagnosis, Management, eleventh ed., Elsevier, 2020.
[7] D.R. Fleisher, Management of Functional Gastrointestinal Disorders in Children – Biopsychosocial Concepts for Clinical Practice, Springer, 2014.
[8] P.H.R. Green, R. Jones, Celiac Disease – A Hidden Epidemic, William Morrow, 2011.
[9] B.E. Lacy, M.D. Crowell, J.K. DiBaise, Functional and Motility Disorders of the Gastrointestinal Tract – A Case Study Approach, Springer, 2015.
[10] E.A. Montgomery, L. Voltaggio, Biopsy Interpretation of the Gastrointestinal Tract Mucosa – Volume 1 – Non-neoplastic (Biopsy Interpretation Series), third ed., Wolters Kluwer, 2017.
[11] W. Persky, Microscopic Colitis. Persky Farms, 2012.
[12] R. Rajapakse, Inflammatory Bowel Disease – Pathogenesis, Diagnosis and Management (Clinical Gastroenterology), Humana Press, 2021.
[13] S. Sandberg-Lewis, Functional Gastroenterology – Assessing and Addressing the Causes of Functional Gastrointestinal Disorders, second ed., Sandberg-Lewis, 2017.
[14] S.R. Targan, F. Shanahan, L.C. Karp, Inflammatory Bowel Disease – Translating Basic Science into Clinical Practice, Wiley-Blackwell, 2011.
[15] Unigastro Profesor, Digestive Diseases 2019 to 2022 Edition, Editorial Edra, 2019.
[16] W.J. Wiersinga, C.W. Seymour, Handbook of Sepsis (European Sepsis Academy), Springer, 2018.
[17] Y. Yire, Stop Nausea and Vomiting – the Ultimate Remedy Guide for Patients on Understanding Everything about the Causes, Symptoms, Treatments, Preventions and How to Recover, Yire, 2021.

CHAPTER

44

Vitamins and minerals

OUTLINE

LEARNING OUTCOMES

After study of the chapter, readers should be able to:

1. Explain the classifications of fat-soluble vitamins.
2. Describe the effects of retinoids on the human body and contraindications.
3. Discuss the impact of vitamin D deficiency in children and older adults.
4. Identify good sources of vitamin E and its mechanism of action.
5. Describe classifications of vitamin K and its effects on the body
6. Explain the essential and trace minerals in the human body.

The Science of Pharmacology
https://doi.org/10.1016/B978-0-443-29038-1.00044-0

7. Describe the factors that decrease the bioavailability of minerals.
8. Discuss the effects of hyponatremia and hyperkalemia on the body.
9. Describe the signs and symptoms of magnesium deficiency.
10. List the microminerals and their requirements.

Overview

Vitamins are essential organic substances that do not provide energy but are required in small dietary amounts. They aid in energy metabolism, tissue growth, development, and maintenance. Vitamins A, D, E, and K dissolve in organic solvents and are termed "fat-soluble vitamins." The "water-soluble vitamins" include vitamin C and the vitamin B complex, which dissolve in the water inside the body. When vitamin intake is insufficient to meet the body's needs, a deficiency develops, with a significant decline in health. Initially, a deficiency and its signs and symptoms can be reversed by increasing intake of the particular vitamin. Vitamin toxicity is also called hypervitaminosis and usually occurs because of consuming megadoses of vitamins A or D. Minerals are nutrients needed in small amounts to keep the body healthy. Mineral nutrients include the elements calcium, magnesium, and iron. They occur naturally and are inorganic substances the human body cannot produce. A mineral is considered a nutrient when a biological function or overall health declines if not consumed sufficiently.

The effects of vitamins on health and disease

Vitamins are essential for bodily functions, including immune activities, wound healing, bone strengthening, and hormone regulation. They also help cells and organs function properly. Multivitamins are helpful for people who cannot reach their daily nutritional needs through diet alone, but they cannot replace a balanced diet. For most people, a healthy and varied diet that includes all five food groups is all that is needed for optimal health. It is best to get vitamins from eating various healthy, unrefined foods, though some can cause toxicity if consumed in large amounts. Vitamins and minerals are also called *micronutrients* because they are needed only in small quantities. Micronutrients do not provide energy but are involved in metabolic processes that allow the body to get energy from the *macronutrients* (carbohydrates, proteins, and fats). There are 13 vitamins, and eight of them come from the B group of vitamins.

Consuming too little of a vitamin can cause a nutritional disorder. However, individuals who eat various foods are unlikely to develop most vitamin deficiencies. A vitamin D deficiency is an exception, and it is common among certain groups of people (children and older people). A deficiency can develop for other vitamins if people follow a restrictive diet that does not contain enough of a particular vitamin. For example, vegans who consume no animal products may become deficient in vitamin B_{12}, which is available in animal products. Deficiency of the B vitamins biotin or pantothenic acid rarely occurs. People at high risk for vitamin deficiencies, including people who had bariatric surgery, are on hemodialysis, or consume heavy amounts of alcohol, may benefit from a daily multivitamin.

Vitamin regulation in the body

Vitamins regulate reactions that occur in metabolism. The absence of a vitamin blocks one or more specific metabolic reactions in cells and can eventually disrupt the metabolic balance inside cells and elsewhere. Except for vitamin C, all water-soluble vitamins have a catalytic function, meaning that they act as **coenzymes** of the enzymes that function in energy transfer or the metabolism of macronutrients. Fat-soluble vitamins are required for specific tasks in highly differentiated and specialized tissues. Some fat-soluble vitamins form part of the structure of biological membranes or aid in maintaining the membranes' integrity. They also may function at the genetic level by controlling enzyme synthesis.

Many people are unaware that taking too many vitamins or minerals can cause serious adverse effects and toxicities. In the United States, vitamin toxicities are more common than vitamin deficiencies. People should always consult their healthcare providers before taking vitamin or mineral supplements.

You should remember

The FDA regulates both finished dietary supplement products and dietary ingredients. By law, it is illegal to manufacture or market adulterated or misbranded dietary supplement products, and the FDA has regulatory authority to remove such products from the marketplace.

Fat-soluble vitamins

Fat-soluble vitamins include vitamins A, D, E, and K. They are soluble in organic solvents and are absorbed and transported like fats. Fat-soluble vitamins are integral to many physiological processes such as immune function, vision, bone health, and coagulation. The body stores fat-soluble vitamins, and they can often cause **keratomalacia** or potential toxicities.

Vitamin A

Vitamin A is naturally present in many foods and is essential for normal vision, the immune system, reproduction, growth, and development. More than 90% of vitamin A is stored in the liver, while lesser amounts are in the adipose tissue, eyes, bone marrow, kidneys, and testicles. **Retinoids** and provitamin A **carotenoids** are converted to active vitamin A. Retinoids are the biologically active forms of this vitamin. Three forms of retinoids include **retinol**, **retinal**, and retinoic acid. Retinoids are the biologically active forms of this vitamin. Retinoids promote growth, development, cell differentiation, vision, and immune function. They are essential in embryonic development. Vitamin A is part of the development of the eyes, cardiovascular, limb, and nervous systems. A lack of vitamin A in early gestation results in congenital disabilities and death of the fetus. **Retinoic acid** is required for the production, structure, and function of the lungs, trachea, skin, and epithelial cells in the GI tract. Vitamin A is highly important for maintaining normal differentiation of cells of the structural eye components, including the cornea and retina.

Pharmacokinetics

Vitamin A is mainly obtained orally from the diet. However, when used as a drug, additional routes of administration are available, including intramuscular and topical. The pharmacokinetic profile depends on each route of administration, the physicochemical characteristics of each vitamin form, and the pharmaceutical form used. Absorption differs significantly between animal vitamin A (retinol and its derivatives) and carotenoids. Its absorption is increased if consumed with fatty meals. Carotenoid intestinal absorption was initially believed to happen through passive diffusion. Retinyl esters reach the blood circulation, targeting tissues, mainly the liver, and are stored there. Vitamin A is eliminated from urine and feces.

Mechanism of action

Vitamin A's effects on cell proliferation, differentiation, and functioning might be due to its influence on **genome expression**, regulation of the transcription of specific genes, or changes in the membrane's structural-functional organization. Vitamin A can act in the biosynthesis of various proteins, including those involved in regulating development and cell functioning or determining cell sensitivity to hormones and hormone-like factors. Vitamin A can also influence the formation of secretory proteins, which play the role of hormones.

Clinical indications

Clinical indications for vitamin A include patients who suffer from deficiencies such as nutritional night blindness, **xerophthalmia**, and **keratomalacia**. The use of vitamin A in preventing these disorders is also well established.

Contraindications

Taking high doses of vitamin A may result in severe liver damage. Combining high doses of vitamin A supplements with other drugs that can damage the liver could increase the risk of liver failure.

Adverse effects

Consuming more than 3000 mcg daily of oral vitamin A supplements in the long term can cause headaches, nausea, diarrhea, bone thinning, pain in the joints and bones, congenital disabilities, liver damage, and skin irritation.

Toxicities

Hypervitaminosis A is uncommon and is usually caused by excessive supplementation or medication usage. The primary cause of toxicity is the consumption of substantial quantities of vitamin A through dietary supplements and foods. The signs and symptoms of vitamin A toxicity include vomiting, double vision, headache, congenital disabilities, bone and joint pain, dry mucous membranes, bleeding, liver damage, spontaneous abortion, and coma.

You should remember

Vitamin A deficiency diseases are not common in developed countries because the vitamin is abundant in the food supply. However, this is different in underdeveloped or developing countries. Globally, vitamin A deficiency is the primary cause of nonaccidental blindness.

You should remember

In North America, vitamin A deficiency is more commonly seen in low-income people, older adults, people with alcohol use disorder, cystic fibrosis, celiac disease, chronic diarrhea, Crohn disease, pancreatic insufficiency, and acquired immunodeficiency syndrome.

Vitamin D

Vitamin D is labeled the "sunshine vitamin," as it is produced in the skin during sun exposure. Vitamin D promotes calcium absorption in the gut and maintains adequate serum calcium concentrations for bone mineralization. Maintaining the serum calcium concentration within the normal physiologic range for musculoskeletal health is required. The Endocrine Society recommends a preferred serum vitamin D range of 40–60 ng/mL. To maintain this level, the Endocrine Society recommends an intake of 400–1000 international units (IU) daily for infants under 1 year, 600–1000 IU for children and adolescents from 1–18 years, and 1500–2000 IU for all adults. The two primary forms of vitamin D are D_2 and D_3. **Ergocalciferol** (vitamin D_2) is mostly humanmade and added to foods.

In contrast, **cholecalciferol** (vitamin D_3) is synthesized in humans' skin and consumed in the diet via animal-based foods. Therefore vitamin D is better classified as a hormone or **prohormone**. Without enough UV light exposure, adequate dietary intake of vitamin D is required. Most fortified foods and supplements that contain vitamin D have it in the form of ergocalciferol. This is also the form found naturally in food sources. Vitamin D deficiency may cause health problems such as brittle bones and muscle weakness.

Pharmacokinetics

The pharmacokinetics of vitamin D are more complex than those of a standard pharmacological agent because of the required stepwise **hydroxylation** into the active form, its endogenous skin synthesis, and the presence of vitamin D and its metabolites in the circulation and tissues. The liver and other tissues metabolize vitamin D from the skin or oral ingestion to 25OHD, the principal circulating vitamin D. Several enzymes have 25-hydroxylase activity, but

CYP2R1 is the most important. Vitamin D has a half-life of about 2–3 weeks in the body. Vitamin D metabolites are excreted through the bile into the feces, and very little is eliminated through the urine.

Mechanism of action

This vitamin D metabolite binds to endogenous receptors, including a hormone receptor at the cell's nucleus. This results in various regulatory roles, including maintaining calcium balance, regulating parathyroid hormone, promoting renal reabsorption, increasing intestinal absorption of calcium and phosphorus, and reducing inflammation.

Clinical indications

Vitamin D is essential for bones and teeth, the immune system, brain health, and inflammation regulation. It is also indicated for treating hypoparathyroidism, rickets in children, osteomalacia in adults, familial hypophosphatemia, and preventing osteoporosis.

Contraindications

The use of pharmacological or nutraceutical vitamin D or even excessive dietary intake of vitamin D is contraindicated in patients with hypercalcemia, malabsorption syndrome, abnormal sensitivity to the toxic effects of vitamin D, and hypervitaminosis. It should be used with caution in patients with liver disease, celiac disease, Crohn disease, cystic fibrosis, and ulcerative colitis.

Adverse effects

Children aged 9 years and older, adults, and pregnant and breastfeeding females who take more than 4000 IU a day of vitamin D might experience thirst, nausea, constipation, anorexia, fatigue, polyuria, and weight loss.

Toxicities

Vitamin D intoxication is extremely rare. Intoxication from sun exposure does not occur, as the skin destroys excess vitamin D. The only way an individual may get vitamin D toxicity is by ingesting high doses of vitamin D for a prolonged period. The main consequence of vitamin D toxicity is hypercalcemia, which can cause nausea and vomiting, weakness, constipation, polydipsia, polyuria, and confusion. Vitamin D toxicity might progress to bone pain, calcification of soft tissues, and kidney stones.

You should remember

Vitamin D has a physiologic function outside calcium metabolism. Its receptors are in the small intestine, colon, T and B lymphocytes, mononuclear cells, brain, and skin. Vitamin D stimulates insulin production, modulates the function of activated T and B lymphocytes, prevents inflammatory bowel diseases, and affects myocardial contractility.

Vitamin E

Vitamin E is essential for reproduction, blood, brain, vision, and skin. It also has antioxidant properties. Antioxidants might protect the cells against the effects of **free radicals**. Vitamin E deficiency is extremely rare in humans, as it is unlikely to be caused by a diet of low vitamin E. Rather, it tends to be caused by irregular dietary fat absorption or metabolism. The two types of vitamin E include **tocopherols** and **tocotrienols**. The most active form is *alpha-tocopherol*. It is found in foods and vitamin supplements. Good sources of vitamin E include canola, cottonseed, safflower, sunflower oils, avocado, wheat germ, almonds, peanuts, and sunflower seeds. Products from plant oils, including margarine, salad dressings, and shortenings, are also good sources.

Vitamin E is a potent chain-breaking antioxidant that inhibits the production of reactive oxygen species molecules when fat undergoes oxidation and during the propagation of free radical reactions.

Pharmacokinetics

Vitamin E is emulsified into lipid droplets at both gastric and duodenal levels. Over 70% of vitamin E is metabolized in the liver. The bioavailability of oral vitamin E is poor, especially for tocotrienols. Vitamin E is available as oral or topical formulations. The pharmacokinetic limitations of tocotrienols result from various factors, including their solubility, absorption, distribution, and elimination rate.

Mechanism of action

Vitamin E acts as an antioxidant, inhibiting the production of reactive oxygen species molecules when fat undergoes oxidation and during the propagation of free radical reactions.

Clinical indications

Supplementation with vitamin E is required in people with digestive disorders, including chronic bowel disease and cystic fibrosis, or those who have undergone gastrointestinal surgeries because their systems cannot absorb as many fat-soluble vitamins. Vitamin E may reduce atherosclerosis and lower rates of ischemic heart disease. Premature infants have low vitamin E reserves because vitamin E can only cross the placenta in small amounts. The early breakdown of red blood cells and hemolytic anemia signifies vitamin E deficiency. This is very serious in preterm infants, so they are given supplemental vitamin E and specialized infant formula containing it. Vitamin E deficiency can reduce immune function and cause neurological changes in the spinal cord and peripheral nervous system. These have occurred when the deficiency resulted from a genetic abnormality of lipoprotein synthesis that decreases vitamin E transport and distribution. Routine supplementation of vitamin E is not recommended for nondeficient children or adults.

Contraindications

Vitamin E supplements should be avoided by patients taking oral anticoagulants, those who are pregnant, those with iron deficiency anemia, and those with hyperthyroidism.

Adverse effects

Vitamin E may cause adverse effects when taken at high doses (400 units or more per day) or for an extended period. In these conditions, nausea, diarrhea, intestinal cramps, blurred vision, dizziness, fatigue, gonadal dysfunction, and headache may occur. The supplement might increase the risk of bleeding. If a person plans to have surgery, they should stop taking vitamin E 2 weeks beforehand.

Toxicities

The toxicity of vitamin E is rare, and it is the least toxic of the fat-soluble vitamins. For adults, the upper limits of vitamin E replacement are 1500–2200 IU, depending on whether the patient uses a natural or synthetic source. Daily limits for children rely on the child's age, starting at 200 IU at 1 year to 800 IU by 18 years old. Staying well below these levels, however, is recommended for daily supplementation.

You should remember

Vitamin E heavily depends on vitamins B_3, C, selenium, and glutathione. A diet high in vitamin E can only have an optimal effect if it is rich in foods that provide these other nutrients.

Vitamin K

Vitamin K is needed for blood clotting and the building of bones. **Prothrombin** is a vitamin-dependent protein involved with blood clotting. **Osteocalcin** is another protein that requires vitamin K to produce healthy bone tissue. There are two primary forms of vitamin K, also known as *quinones*. They include vitamin K_1 (**phylloquinone**) in plant foods such as leafy greens and vitamin K_2 (**menaquinone**) in animal and fermented foods. The most biologically active form is phylloquinone, the primary dietary form.

Pharmacokinetics

Phylloquinone is absorbed in the small intestine. Its process depends on the normal secretion of bile and pancreatic juice and is enhanced by dietary fat. After absorption, vitamin K is initially concentrated in the liver, but the concentration declines rapidly. Tiny amounts of vitamin K accumulate in tissues.

Mechanism of action

Vitamin K is required for the liver to synthesize blood clotting factors and for preprothrombin to be converted into prothrombin, an active blood clotting factor. The bacteria in the intestines can produce vitamin K.

Clinical indications

Vitamin K reduces the risk of bleeding in liver disease, conditions where the body cannot absorb enough vitamin K, or if patients take antibiotics for a long time. All newborns receive vitamin K injections to prevent the possibility of bleeding, particularly in the brain. Babies are born without any bacteria in their intestines and do not get enough vitamin K from breast milk to hold them over until their bodies can make it. Mothers on seizure medications are often given oral vitamin K for 2 weeks before delivery.

Contraindications

Vitamin K should be used with caution in patients with gallbladder stones or biliary disease, cystic fibrosis, celiac disease, and Crohn disease. It should also be avoided in patients taking blood thinners, those on long-term hemodialysis, and patients who experience a hypersensitivity reaction to vitamin K, which may exhibit an eczema-like skin rash. Vitamin K use requires caution in neonates, patients with hereditary hypoprothrombinemia, renal impairment, overanticoagulation due to heparin, and patients with hypersensitivity to vitamin K.

Adverse effects

The common adverse effects of vitamin K include allergic reactions, dysphagia, flushing, chest pain, and sweating. Vitamin K_1 may be associated with bronchospasm and cardiac arrest with IV administration. The oral form of vitamin K does not cause severe reactions.

Toxicities

Vitamin K toxicity is extremely rare. Its toxicity is thought to be associated with its water-soluble properties. When toxicity does occur, it manifests with signs of jaundice, hyperbilirubinemia, hemolytic anemia, and **kernicterus** in infants.

You should remember

The body needs vitamin K to use calcium to build bone. People with higher levels of vitamin K have greater bone density, while low levels of vitamin K have been found in those with osteoporosis. Similarly, some studies suggest that low vitamin K levels are associated with a higher risk of osteoarthritis.

Water-soluble vitamins

The water-soluble vitamins include the vitamin B complex and vitamin C. The vitamin B complex contains thiamine, riboflavin, niacin, pantothenic acid, pyridoxine, biotin, folate, and cobalamin. These vitamins form coenzymes that are effective in many body functions and have essential roles in the body (see **Table 44.1**).

Minerals

Minerals are nutrients needed in small amounts to keep the body healthy. A mineral is considered a nutrient when a biological function or overall health declines if not consumed sufficiently. A primary macromineral must

TABLE 44.1 Roles of the B vitamins.

B vitamin	Roles
Thiamine (B_1)	Energy metabolism
Riboflavin (B_2)	Energy metabolism, protein and amino acid metabolism, antioxidant defenses
Niacin (B_3)	Energy metabolism
Pantothenic acid (B_5)	Energy metabolism
Pyridoxine (B_6)	Energy metabolism, blood production, protein and amino acid metabolism, immune function, one-carbon metabolism, normal nerve function
Biotin (B_7)	Energy metabolism
Folic acid (B_9)	Blood formation, protein and amino acid metabolism, one-carbon metabolism
Cobalamin (B_{12})	Energy metabolism, blood formation, protein and amino acid metabolism, one-carbon metabolism

TABLE 44.2 Water-soluble vitamin deficiency symptoms.

Vitamin	Deficiency symptoms
B_1 (thiamine)	Beriberi (anorexia, peripheral neuropathy, weakness, weight loss), Wernicke-Korsakoff syndrome
B_2 (riboflavin)	Ariboflavinosis (cracks at the corner of the mouth, inflammation of the mouth and tongue)
B_3 (niacin)	Pellagra (dementia, dermatitis, diarrhea, and eventually, death)
B_5 (pantothenic acid)	Fatigue, GI tract disturbances, impaired muscle function, weakness
B_6 (pyridoxine)	Anemia, confusion, convulsions, depression, dermatitis
B_7 (biotin)	Conjunctivitis, dermatitis, hair loss, nervous system abnormalities
B_9 (folic acid)	Birth defects, megaloblastic (macrocytic) anemia
B_{12} (cobalamin)	Megaloblastic (macrocytic) anemia, paresthesia (tingling or numbness of extremities), pernicious anemia, difficulty concentrating, memory problems
C (ascorbic acid)	Scurvy (bleeding gums, pinpoint hemorrhages, poor wound healing)

be consumed in 100 mg or more daily. Examples of substantial minerals include calcium and phosphorus. A micromineral is needed in amounts less than 100 mg per day. Examples of minor minerals include iron, zinc, and copper. Minerals are required for many body functions and structures. For example, calcium and phosphorus provide rigidity and strength to the teeth and bones. Skeletal components also serve as a mineral storage area for other body needs. Minerals provide proper muscle contraction and nerve functions. Some minerals act as enzyme cofactors and maintain proper acid-base balance in body fluids. They are also required for blood clotting, tissue repair, and growth.

Macrominerals

Macrominerals are any mineral required in the diet in relatively large amounts, especially calcium, phosphorus, sodium, potassium, chloride, magnesium, and sulfur. They are essential for numerous body homeostatic functions across human life. Macrominerals are part of the biological structure of the human body, play a crucial role in metabolic processes, and participate in almost all processes that occur in the body. Macrominerals can be toxic if consumed in large quantities for an extended period. Many medical conditions could arise in cases of deficiency.

A deficiency of a macromineral refers to a lack of one or more of the essential minerals required in large amounts by humans. Macromineral deficiencies can lead to various health problems such as osteoporosis, muscle weakness, and electrolyte imbalances. The lack of macrominerals can result in many chronic diseases. Hormonal changes resulting from a deficiency of macrominerals have consequences that may lead to weight gain, obesity, and an increased risk of cancer in the future. It is essential to maintain a balanced diet to ensure adequate intake of macroelements.

Microminerals

Microminerals, also called trace minerals, are inorganic but essential substances. They are found in tiny amounts of less than 5 mg in the human body. Microminerals include iron, iodine, copper, manganese, fluoride, zinc, selenium, chromium, and molybdenum. They are required for normal development, function, and good health. Iron helps to build red blood cells. Copper, manganese, selenium, and zinc help protect from harm caused by **free radicals**. Iodine is required for the production of thyroid hormone and body metabolism.

Key Terms

Carotenoids
Cholecalciferol
Ergocalciferol
Free radicals
Genome expression
Hydroxylation
Keratomalacia
Menaquinone
Osteocalcin
Phylloquinone
Prothrombin
Retinal
Retinoic acid
Retinoids
Retinol
Tocopherols
Tocotrienols
Xerophthalmia

Clinical Case Studies

Clinical Case Study 1

Mrs. Johnson, a 72-year-old female, presented to her primary care physician with complaints of chronic fatigue, muscle weakness, and frequent falls. She also reported bone pain in her hips and lower back. Mrs. Johnson has a history of osteoporosis and spends most of her time indoors, rarely getting exposure to sunlight. Her blood work revealed a vitamin D deficiency.

Critical Thinking Questions

1. What are the common symptoms of vitamin D deficiency?
2. Why are older adults at higher risk for vitamin D deficiency?
3. What is recommended to treat vitamin D deficiency?

Clinical Case Study 2

Mr. Gomez, a 34-year-old vegan, presented to his primary care provider with fatigue, shortness of breath, and tingling in his hands and feet. He also reported having difficulty concentrating and experiencing memory problems. Mr. Smith has been following a strict vegan diet for 5 years. His blood tests revealed a vitamin B_{12} deficiency.

Critical Thinking Questions

1. What are the neurological symptoms associated with vitamin B_{12} deficiency?
2. Why might vegans be at risk for vitamin B_{12} deficiency?
3. How can vitamin B_{12} deficiency be prevented in individuals following a vegan diet?

Further Reading

[1] I.R. Ansari, Vitamin Deficiencies, Amazon Digital Services LLC - Kdp, 2023.

[2] L. Arpilor, Vitamin Deficiency Symptoms –Insight into the Signs and Symptoms of Various Vitamin Deficiencies and their Health Impacts, Arpilor, 2023.

[3] M. Davis, Eat Your Vitamins – your Guide to Using Natural Foods to Get the Vitamins, Minerals, and Nutrients your Body Needs, Adams Media, 2020.

[4] J. DiNicolantonio, S. Land, The Mineral Fix: How to Optimize your Mineral Intake for Energy, Longevity, Immunity, Sleep, and More, Amazon Digital Services LLC - Kdp, 2021.

[5] S.R. Gaines, The Mineral Deficiency Antidote – How to Boost up your Energy Consuming Ability, Amazon Digital Services LLC - Kdp, 2022.

[6] C. Gomes, M. Rautureau, Minerals *Latu Sensu* and Human Health – Benefits, Toxicity and Pathologies, Springer, 2021.

[7] A.F. Gualtieri, Mineral Fibres: Crystal Chemistry, Chemical-Physical Properties, Biological Interaction, and Toxicity (EMU Notes in Mineralogy 18), European Mineralogical Society, 2017.

[8] S. Liebermann, N. Bruning, The Real Vitamin and Mineral Book: The Definitive Guide to Designing Your Personal Supplement Program, fourth ed., Avery, 2007.

[9] R.J.S. Martin, Magnesium Deficiency – Weight Loss, Heart Disease and Depression – 13 Ways Curing Your Magnesium Deficiency can Rejuvenate your Body, Bright Ideas Editorial, 2015.

[10] M. Newman, F. Mason, Vitamin B12 Deficiency and Chronic Illness, Amazon Digital Services LLC - Kdp, 2016.

[11] P. Ochsenham, J. Vormann, The Magnesium Deficiency Crisis: Is this the World's Number 1 Mineral Deficiency? MadhouseMEDIA, 2015.

[12] W. Persky, Vitamin D and autoimmune disease – how vitamin D prevents autoimmune disease, Persky Farms, 2014.

[13] D. Purser, J. Larkin, Vitamin Deficiency Symptoms and Cures – Modern Deficiency Illness – using Intracellular Micronutrient Results, Amazon Digital Services LLC - Kdp, 2019.

[14] R. Rydon, Profiles of the Nutrients: 2. Minerals and Trace Elements, Rydon, 2017.

[15] J.J. Shatzel, Iron Deficiency – A Patient's Guide to the Most Common Nutrient Deficiency in the World, Amazon Digital Services LLC - Kdp, 2021.

[16] C. Walters, Minerals for the Genetic Code – an Exposition & Analysis of the Dr. Olree Standard Genetic Periodic Chart & the Physical, Chemical & Biological Connection, Acres U.S.A, 2013.

[17] P. Wartian Smith, What you must Know About Vitamins, Minerals, Herbs, and so Much More – Choosing the Nutrients that are Right for you, second ed., Square One, 2019.

UNIT VIII

Respiratory drugs

CHAPTER

45

Review of the respiratory system

OUTLINE

LEARNING OUTCOMES

After studying the chapter, readers should be able to:

1. Describe the structure and function of the upper respiratory tract.
2. Explain the role of paranasal sinuses.
3. Identify the lower respiratory tract.
4. Explain the types of bronchi and define the bronchial tree.
5. Describe the physiology of alveoli.
6. Explain the role of sympathetic and parasympathetic nerves in the airways.
7. Discuss the airway bronchoconstriction and bronchodilatation.
8. Describe the role of surfactant.

Overview

To sustain life, the body must provide sufficient energy. Energy is used by burning molecules in food. Oxidation combines carbon and hydrogen with oxygen to form carbon dioxide and water. The consumption of oxygen and carbon dioxide production are thus indispensable to life. The human body must have an organ system designed to remove carbon dioxide from the blood circulation and absorb oxygen from the atmosphere rapidly enough for the body's needs, even during peak exercise. The respiratory system may be divided into upper and lower tracts. The organs of the upper respiratory tract are located outside the thorax, whereas those in the lower tract are located almost entirely within the chest cavity. The lungs are the foundational organs of the respiratory system, whose most basic function is facilitating gas exchange from the environment into the bloodstream. Oxygen gets transported

https://doi.org/10.1016/B978-0-443-29038-1.00045-2

through the alveoli into the capillary network, where it can enter the arterial system. The alveoli are the primary location for gas exchange. This chapter will focus on the nasal cavity, bronchi, and alveoli and their relation to pharmacology.

The respiratory system

The respiratory system distributes a gas exchanger so that oxygen can be supplied and carbon dioxide removed from the body's cells. Because most of our trillions of cells lie too far from air to exchange gases directly with it, air must first exchange gases with blood, blood must circulate, and finally, blood and cells must exchange gases. These events require two functioning systems—the respiratory and circulatory systems, including all respiratory system parts—except the alveoli. Only the alveoli and the alveolar ducts serve as gas exchangers. In addition to air distribution and gas exchange, the respiratory system effectively filters, warms, and humidifies the air. When communicating oral language, respiratory organs also help produce sounds, including speech. Particular sensory epithelium in the respiratory tract makes **olfaction** possible. The respiratory system also plays an essential role in the body's regulation, or homeostasis, of pH.

Physiology of the nose

The upper respiratory tract comprises the nose, nasal cavities, nasopharynx, oropharynx, laryngopharynx, and larynx. Functionally, the respiratory system also includes several accessory structures such as the oral cavity, ribcage, respiratory muscles, and diaphragm. Together, these structures constitute the lifeline—the air supply line of the body. The nose has external and internal structures. Each nasal cavity is divided into three passageways, named the superior, middle, and inferior meatuses. The projection of the **conchae** forms incomplete tubes or turbinate curving from the lateral walls of the internal portion of the nose. The superior and middle conchae are processes of the **ethmoid bone**, whereas the inferior conchae are separate bones (see **Fig. 45.1**).

Once air enters the nasal cavity, it passes over the respiratory mucosa. The mucous membrane has a ciliated pseudostratified columnar epithelium rich in goblet cells. The respiratory mucosa has a rich blood supply, especially over the inferior turbinate, and is bright pink or red; the ciliated mucous membrane lines the rest of the respiratory tract as far as the smaller **bronchioles**.

Air enters the respiratory system through the nasal cavity, which is filtered of various substances, warmed, and moistened. The nasal hairs filter particulate from air entering the respiratory system. The respiratory membrane produces large quantities of mucus and maintains a rich blood supply, especially over the inferior conchae, which permits rapid warming and moistening of the dry inspired air. Mucous secretions trap some of the remaining particulate matter from the air and are removed as it travels through the nasal passages. Fluid from the **lacrimal glands** and additional mucus produced in the paranasal sinuses also trap particulate matter and moisten air passing through the nose.

Intranasal medications are used as an alternative route for the systemic availability of drugs restricted to intravenous administration. This is due to high total blood flow, the large surface area, the porous endothelial membrane, the avoidance of first-pass metabolism, and ready accessibility. Steroids; antiasthma medications such as salbutamol, ipratropium, and montelukast; and many inhalational anesthetic agents are commonly used. Intranasal administration vaccines can be used for children. Live attenuated influenza is a nasal spray vaccine that may be given to nonpregnant people aged 2 through 49.

The **paranasal sinuses** are air-containing spaces that lighten the weight of the skull and open into the nasal cavity. The paranasal sinuses include the frontal, maxillary, ethmoid, and sphenoid sinuses. Like the nasal cavity, each paranasal sinus is lined by respiratory mucosa. The mucous secretions provided in the sinuses are continually being swept into the nose by the ciliated surface of the respiratory membrane.

You should remember

The nasal concha comprises three thin, scroll-shaped bony elements forming the upper chambers of the nasal cavities. They increase the surface area of these cavities, thus providing rapid warming and humidification of air as it passes to the lungs.

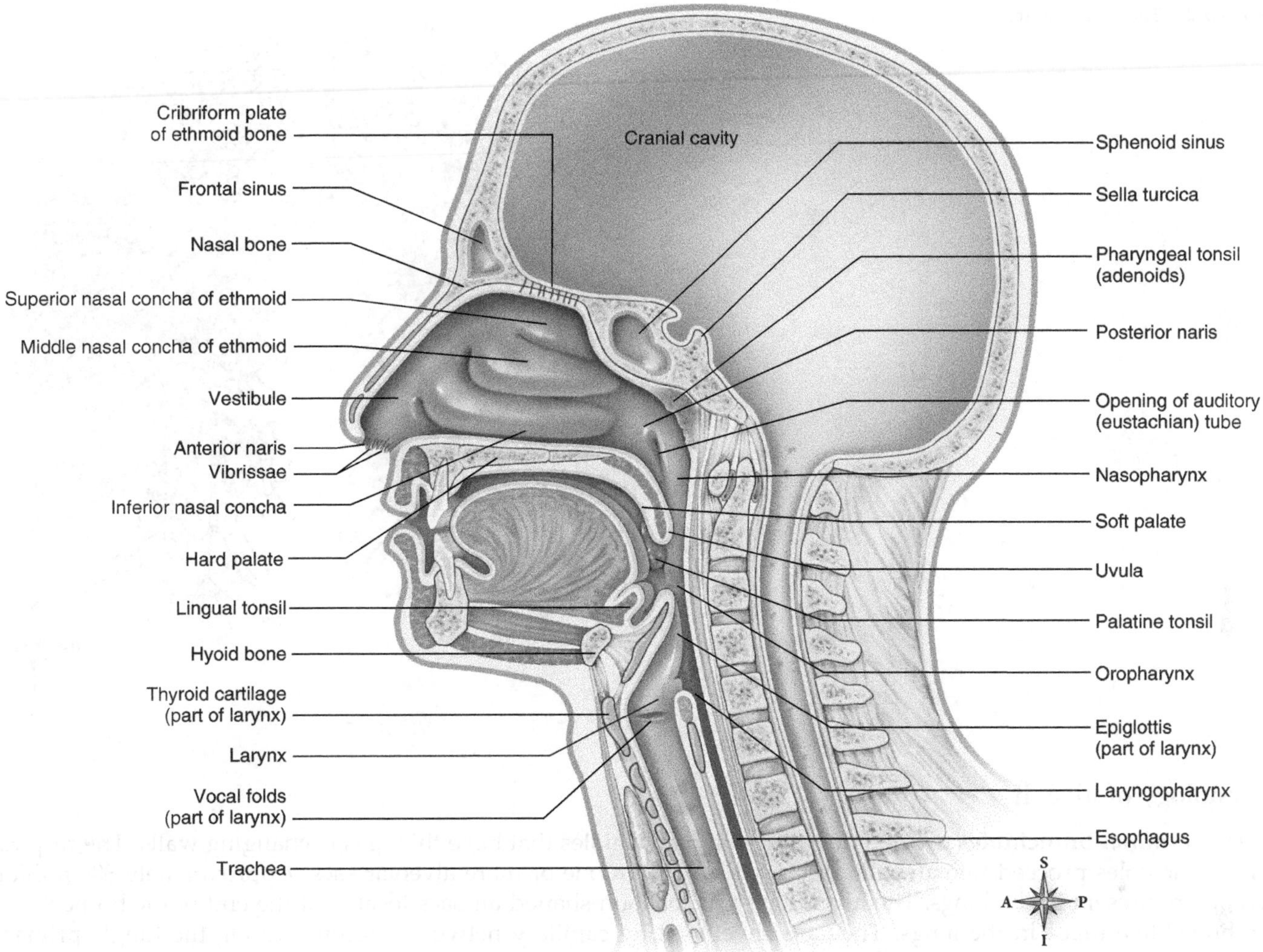

FIG. 45.1 The upper respiratory tract.

Physiology of bronchi and bronchial tree

The lower respiratory tract comprises the trachea, the bronchial tree, and the lungs.

The **trachea**, or windpipe, is about 4.5 inches long and extends from the **larynx** to the thoracic cavity's primary bronchi. The trachea is lined with respiratory mucosa. The mucosa is characterized by ciliated pseudostratified columnar epithelium and is typical of the respiratory tract. Mucous glands possessing many goblet cells help produce the blanket of mucus that continually moves upward toward the pharynx.

The trachea divides at its lower end into two **primary bronchi**, with the right bronchus wider, shorter, and more vertical in direction than the left, which explains why aspirated foreign objects often enter the right bronchus. In structure, the bronchi resemble the trachea. The bronchi walls have incomplete cartilaginous rings in the sections superior to the lungs but have complete rings in the sections within the lungs. Ciliated mucosa also lines the bronchi. Each primary bronchus enters the lung on its respective side and is immediately divided into smaller branches called **secondary bronchi**. The secondary bronchi continue to branch, forming **tertiary bronchi** and small bronchioles. The trachea, the two primary bronchi, and their many branches make the **bronchial tree** (see **Fig. 45.2**).

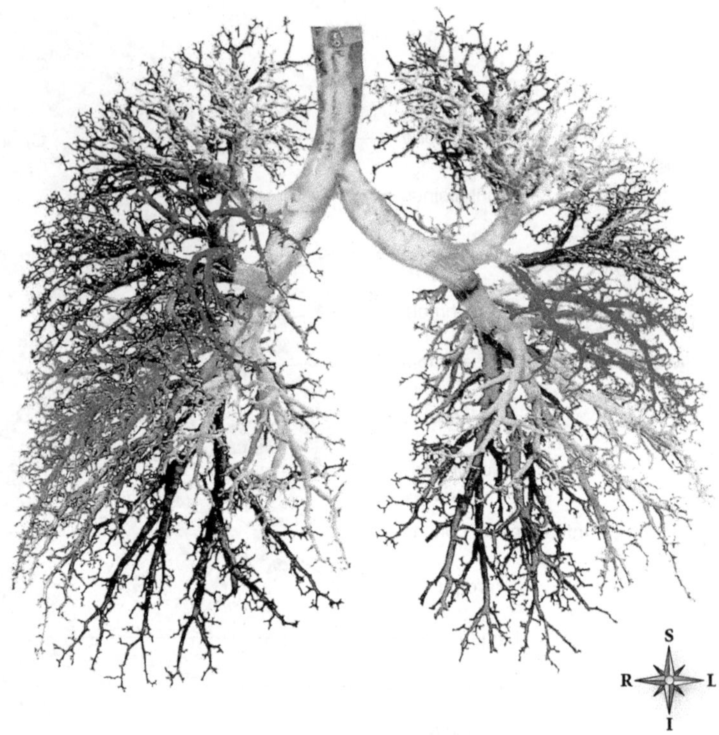

FIG. 45.2 The bronchial tree.

Physiology of alveoli

The **terminal bronchioles** divide into respiratory bronchioles that have thin, gas-exchanging walls. The respiratory bronchioles proceed into **alveolar ducts**, which end in one or more alveolar sacs. Approximately 300 million alveoli are present in the lungs. The **alveoli** are tiny, balloon-shaped air sacs located at the end of the bronchioles, the branchlike tubes in the lungs. They are enveloped by capillary networks, accomplishing the lung's primary and vital function, gas exchange between air and blood. They are the site of exchanging oxygen and carbon dioxide while breathing in and out. Oxygen breathed in from the air passes through the alveoli and into the blood and then travels to the tissues throughout the body. Carbon dioxide travels in the blood from the body's tissues and passes through the alveoli to be breathed out (see **Fig. 45.3**).

It is essential to consider that oxygen is necessary for normal metabolism, and carbon dioxide is a waste product of this metabolism. Gas exchange between the alveolar and blood occurs mainly within the pulmonary capillary bed, after which the blood flows into venules and arterioles. The movement of inspired gas into and exhaled gas out of the lung is called **ventilation**. The respiratory centers are located in the **pons** and **medulla oblongata** in the brain. They contain different inspiratory and expiratory neurons that stimulate during the respiratory cycle.

Both sympathetic and parasympathetic nerves innervate the airways and lungs. Cholinergic parasympathetic innervation is well conserved in the airways. Autonomic nerve function is regulated primarily through reflexes initiated upon bronchopulmonary **vagal nerves**. Autonomic excitatory cholinergic nerves secrete acetylcholine into the bronchial smooth muscle cells and submucosal glands to cause airway **bronchoconstriction** and mucus production. While the adrenergic system is essential in regulating airway blood flow and glandular secretion, it does not innervate smooth airway muscle. Inhibitory nonadrenergic and noncholinergic nerves lead to airway **bronchodilatation** via vasoactive intestinal peptide and neural nitric oxide.

Pulmonary vasoconstriction is a physiological phenomenon and mechanism in response to alveolar hypoxia or low oxygen partial pressures in the pulmonary arterioles and, to some extent, the pulmonary venules. Pulmonary vasoconstriction redirects blood flow within the vasculature away from poorly ventilated parts of the lungs toward better-ventilated portions. Bronchodilation reduces airway resistance caused by the relaxation of airway smooth muscle. It is the opposite of bronchoconstriction.

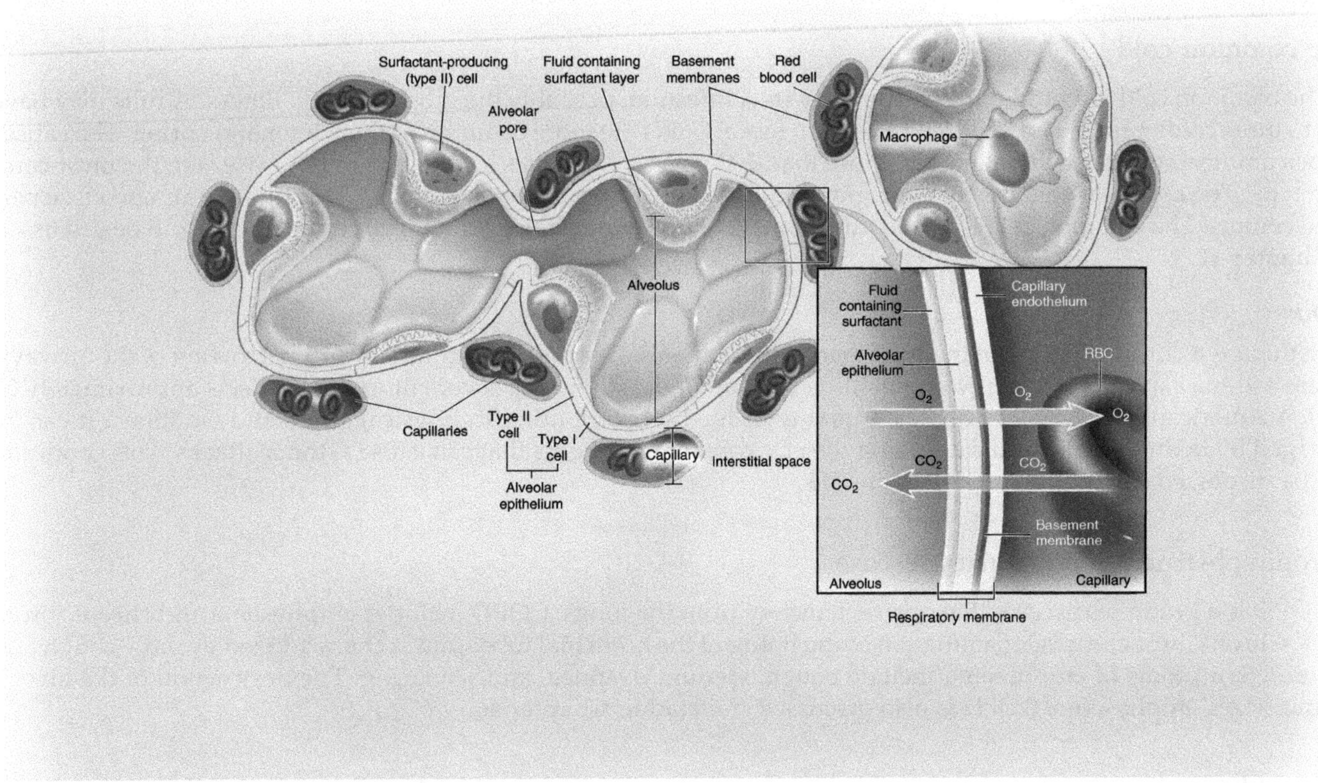

FIG. 45.3 Gas exchange between the alveolar gas and blood.

You should remember

Alveoli are lined by a fluid called surfactant, which maintains the shape of each air sac and helps keep it open so oxygen and carbon dioxide can pass through. Typically, type 1 alveolar cells comprise the major gas exchange surface of the alveolus and are integral to maintaining the permeability barrier function of the alveolar membrane. Type 2 pneumocytes are the progenitors of type 1 cells, responsible for surfactant production and homeostasis.

Specific chronic disorders of the respiratory system

Chronic respiratory disorders include allergic rhinitis, common cold, asthma, chronic obstructive pulmonary disease (COPD), and cystic fibrosis, which we will discuss in the following two chapters. If left untreated, lung disease can produce health complications, problematic symptoms, and sometimes life-threatening conditions.

Allergic rhinitis

Allergic rhinitis (hay fever) is an allergic reaction and inflammation of the inside of the nose caused by an **allergen**, such as mold, pollen, dust, or skin peeling from certain animals. Allergic rhinitis will be discussed in **Chapter 47**. Chronic sinusitis may occur as a consequence of allergic rhinitis. This condition may keep mucus from draining. It makes the nose stuffy, and breathing through the nose might be problematic. The area around the eyes might feel swollen or tender.

The common cold

The common cold is a mild upper respiratory tract infection, probably the most common illness. Adults may have two to three colds yearly, and children have even more. Colds are more common in the winter and spring. The causes of the common cold are generally viral. More than 200 viruses can cause a cold, but rhinoviruses are the most common type. The common cold is very contagious and can spread from person to person through the air and close personal contact. The common cold is a mild infection of the upper respiratory tract. The common cold will be discussed in **Chapter 47**.

Asthma

Asthma is a chronic disease of the bronchi and bronchioles. It causes inflammation and narrowing of the airways. Severe asthma can cause difficulty in breathing and talking. Asthma is a severe illness that affects approximately 25 million Americans. Asthma can decrease quality of life by contributing to physical stress and emotions. It can be managed by taking medicine and avoiding the environmental triggers that can cause asthma attacks. This condition will be discussed in more detail in **Chapter 46**.

Chronic obstructive pulmonary disease

COPD is a group of diseases that obstruct airflow from the lungs. COPD includes emphysema and chronic bronchitis. Chronic bronchitis is inflammation of the lining of the bronchial tubes and is characterized by daily cough and sputum. Symptoms of emphysema include cough, sputum dyspnea, and wheezing. The destruction of the alveoli characterizes emphysema. COPD is also discussed in detail in **Chapter 46**.

Cystic fibrosis

Cystic fibrosis is a progressive genetic disorder that damages the lungs and pancreas. It is caused by a defective gene that can be passed from parents. Cystic fibrosis causes sticky, thick mucus in the lungs and the pancreas. There is also a form of disease called **atypical cystic fibrosis**. It differs from classic CF because it is milder and may only affect one organ. CF is also discussed in detail in **Chapter 46**.

You should remember

Malnutrition occurs in up to one-third of individuals with COPD. It is a significant concern because these individuals have increased breathing and energy expenditure, decreased energy intake, and impaired oxygenation.

Key Terms

Allergen
Alveolar ducts
Alveoli
Atypical cystic fibrosis
Bronchial tree
Bronchioles
Bronchoconstriction
Bronchodilatation
Conchae
Epistaxis
Ethmoid bone
Lacrimal glands
Medulla oblongata

Olfaction
Paranasal sinuses
Pons
Primary bronchi
Secondary bronchi
Tertiary bronchi
Trachea
Vagal nerves
Ventilation

Further Reading

[1] R.D. Anbar, Functional Respiratory Disorders – when Respiratory Symptoms do Not Respond to Pulmonary Treatment (Respiratory Medicine), Humana Press, 2012.
[2] S. Duggins Davis, M. Rosenfeld, J. Chmiel, Cystic Fibrosis – A Multi-Organ System Approach (Respiratory Medicine), Humana Press, 2020.
[3] F. Earlstein, Asthma Explained – Facts & Information. (Asthma Facts, Diagnosis, Symptoms, Treatment, Causes, Effects, Alternative Medicines, Therapeutic Methods, History, Myths, and More! Pack & Post plus, , LLC, 2017.
[4] M. Grippi, D.E. Antin-Ozerkis, C.S. Dela Cruz, R. Kotloff, C.N. Kotton, A. Pack, Fishman's Pulmonary Diseases and Disorders, sixth ed., vol. 1, McGraw-Hill / Medical, 2022.
[5] A.L. Kau, J.M. Monroy, B.I. Polk, C.J. Rigell, Allergy, Asthma, and Immunology – Subspecialty Consult, third ed., Wolters Kluwer, 2021.
[6] D.A. Mahler, COPD: Answers to your Most Pressing Questions About Chronic Obstructive Pulmonary Disease, Johns Hopkins University Press, 2022.
[7] L.D. Thomson-Smith, Allergic Rhinitis – the Causes and Consequences, Facebook Publishing, 2013.
[8] J.P.T. Ward, J. Ward, R.M. Leach, The Respiratory System at a Glance, fourth ed., Wiley Blackwell, 2015.
[9] D.A. Mahler, COPD: Answers to your Most Pressing Questions About Chronic Obstructive Pulmonary Disease, Johns Hopkins University Press, 2022.
[10] Pegasus, Respiratory System—Human Body, B Jain Publishers Pvt Ltd., 2012.
[11] M. Penrod, L. Penrod, Respiratory System – Learn on the Go Quick and Easy Study Guide, Penrod, 2014.
[12] D. Petechuk, The Respiratory System (Human Body Systems), Greenwood, 2010.
[13] K.M. Surji, A Practical Guide to Respiratory System and its Related Disorders, CreateSpace Independent Publishing Platform, 2017.
[14] L.D. Thomson-Smith, Allergic Rhinitis – the Causes and Consequences, Facebook Publishing, 2013.
[15] J.P.T. Ward, J. Ward, R.M. Leach, The Respiratory System at a Glance, fourth ed., Wiley Blackwell, 2015.

CHAPTER

46

Asthma, chronic obstructive pulmonary disorder, and cystic fibrosis drugs

OUTLINE

LEARNING OUTCOMES

After study of the chapter, readers should be able to:

1. Identify the most critical factors for developing asthma.

The Science of Pharmacology
https://doi.org/10.1016/B978-0-443-29038-1.00046-4

2. Explain the common asthma medications used in the United States.
3. Identify the contraindications of steroid inhalers.
4. Explain the three most widely used bronchodilators.
5. Discuss the adverse effects of albuterol.
6. Describe mast cell stabilizers and their mechanism of action.
7. Explain the inhaler drugs and their classification.
8. Describe chronic obstructive pulmonary disorder and its causes.
9. Explain the characteristics of cystic fibrosis.
10. Describe the adverse effects of mucolytics.

Overview

Asthma is a chronic pulmonary disease that inflames and obstructs the airways, making it difficult for people to breathe. It is the most common childhood disorder but may affect people of all ages. Well-controlled asthma, defined as minimizing the risk of asthma attacks and related problems, is the primary goal of management. This is achievable by avoiding factors that worsen symptoms, using appropriate medications, and educating the patient. There is no cure for asthma. If not controlled with the proper maintenance therapy, it will progress. An asthma exacerbation, also known as an asthma attack or episode, develops in response to a trigger such as allergens, cigarette smoke, air pollution, exercise, drug therapy, emotions, or inappropriate diet. As the disease progresses, symptoms get worse or more intense. Chronic obstructive pulmonary disease (COPD) is a group of disorders that permanently impair lung function. It is caused mainly by inhaling toxic particles and cigarette smoking. Continuous exposure to similar molecules can lead to abnormal inflammatory responses, permanent damage to the respiratory system, and irreversible pathological changes. It is the third leading cause of death worldwide. Cystic fibrosis (CF) is a progressive genetic disease that affects the lungs, pancreas, and other organs.

Asthma

Asthma is a chronic pulmonary disease that inflames and obstructs the airways, making breathing difficult for patients. It is the most common childhood disorder but may affect individuals of all ages. To control asthma, minimizing the risk of asthma attacks and related problems is the primary goal of management. Other aspects of asthma management include optimizing maintenance medications and avoiding factors that worsen symptoms. This is achievable by avoiding factors that worsen symptoms, using appropriate medicines, and educating the patient.

Pathophysiology of asthma

Asthma is manifested by inflammation and obstruction of the airways. Inflammation is the central problem, making the airways swollen and reactive to various inhaled stimuli. Obstruction results from the tightening of the muscles around the airways. This leads to the main asthma symptoms, including **wheezing**, chest tightness, cough, and dyspnea. Increased mucus production may occur, which causes further narrowing of the airways. Dysfunction of the pulmonary system ultimately leads to **hypoxia**.

The most critical factors for developing asthma are a history of atopic diseases (**allergic rhinitis**, **conjunctivitis**, dermatitis) or viral respiratory infection during early childhood. Respiratory syncytial virus is the most common cause of **bronchiolitis** in children under 1 year of age. It is associated with wheezing in later childhood.

Asthma may affect anyone of any age, but it is not contagious. The disease affects more male children than females, but the gender differences change in adults to involve more females. African Americans and Puerto Ricans are at higher risk of asthma, possibly due to urbanization and lower socioeconomic status.

You should remember

Asthma is severe and a leading reason for emergency room visits, hospitalization, and lost days from school with subsequent lost work days for the caregiver. However, with appropriate medication therapy and environmental control, the frequency of missed school days, emergency department visits, and hospitalization and asthma deaths is reduced.

You should remember

Status asthmaticus is the most severe clinical form of asthma. It represents a true medical emergency. If not managed adequately and promptly, the patient in status asthmaticus may die as a result of the respiratory changes that develop secondary to respiratory distress. These changes include hypotension and respiratory acidosis.

Pharmacotherapy

The goal of asthma therapy for the patient is to have well-controlled asthma and normal lung function. The common asthma medications prescribed for maintenance or acute relief therapy are listed in **Table 46.1**.

Antiinflammatory drugs

The role of maintenance asthma therapy is either to reduce inflammation or control symptoms. Suppressing inflammation is crucial in decreasing the severity and gaining control of asthma. Therefore the potent antiinflammatory actions of inhaled corticosteroids (ICSs) make these medications the therapy of choice for all types of asthma. When the correct dose is given, the patient's symptoms improve within 2 weeks, but it may take up to several months for full benefits. Steroid inhalers are only available with a prescription. Common types include beclomethasone dipropionate, budesonide, fluticasone propionate, mometasone furoate, and triamcinolone acetonide. Relatively newer inhaled steroid molecules include ciclesonide and flunisolide.

Pharmacokinetics

Significant differences exist in the pharmacokinetic properties of ICSs. All are rapidly cleared from the body, but they show varying levels of oral bioavailability and, more importantly, variation in the absorption rate after inhalation. Oral bioavailability is lowest for fluticasone propionate due to presystemic metabolism, indicating a low potential for unwanted systemic corticosteroid effects. Mathematical modeling has shown pulmonary residence times to be the longest for fluticasone propionate and triamcinolone acetonide but the shortest for budesonide and flunisolide. These properties relate to pulmonary solubility, which appears to be the rate-limiting step in the absorption process.

Mechanism of action

ICSs have potent glucocorticoid activity and work directly at the cellular level by reversing capillary permeability and lysosomal stabilization to reduce inflammation. The onset of action is gradual and may take anywhere from several days to several weeks for maximal benefit with consistent use.

TABLE 46.1 Common asthma medications

Maintenance therapy (to control symptoms)	Acute therapy (for quick relief)
Bronchodilators	
LABAs	
formoterol (Foradil, Symbicort, or Dulera in combination)	
salmeterol (Serevent, Advair in combination)	
vilanterol (Breo in combination)	
theophylline	
Antiinflammatories	SABAs
ICSs	albuterol (ProAir, Proventil, Ventolin)
beclomethasone (QVAR)	levalbuterol (Xopenex)
budesonide (Pulmicort, Symbicort in combination)	Systemic corticosteroids
ciclesonide (Alvesco)	Anticholinergic agents
flunisolide (Aerobid)	ipratropium (Atrovent)
Annuity (Flovent, Armon Air, Advair in combination)	tiotropium (Spiriva)
mometasone (Asmanex)	umeclidinium (Trelegy in combination)
triamcinolone (Azmacort)	
Leukotriene modifiers	
montelukast (Singulair)	
zafirlukast (Accolate)	
zileuton (Zyflo CE)	
Mast cell stabilizers	
Cromolyn (Intal)	
Immunomodulators	
benralizumab (Fasenra)	
dupilumab (Dupixent)	
mepolizumab (Nucala)	
omalizumab (Xolair)	
reslizumab (Cinqair)	
tezepelumab-ekko (Tezspire)	

ICSs, Inhaled corticosteroids; *LABAs,* long-acting beta$_2$-agonists; *SABAs,* short-acting beta$_2$-agonists.

Clinical indications

Inhalation corticosteroids help prevent asthma symptoms. They decrease the number and severity of asthma attacks when used regularly daily. However, they will not relieve an asthma attack that has already started. Most asthma patients can be treated and controlled with inhaled steroids, but some remain uncontrolled despite adequate asthma therapy. In the United States, approximately one-half of asthma patients are uncontrolled.

Contraindications

ICSs should be used cautiously in patients with active or quiescent tuberculosis infection of the respiratory tract; untreated systemic fungal, bacterial, viral, or parasitic infections; or ocular herpes simplex.

Adverse effects

ICSs are now utilized at larger doses and for more extended periods than ever before. Oropharyngeal candidiasis and **dysphonia** are the most commonly recognized adverse effects of therapy, but these topical phenomena cause no significant morbidity and are easily managed. By contrast, there is increasing concern about the potential systemic effects of ICSs. These assumed effects may include adrenal cortex suppression, bone loss, skin thinning, increased cataract formation, decreased linear growth in children, metabolic changes, and behavioral abnormalities. Changes in adrenal function have been noted in patients using medications such as beclomethasone dipropionate and budesonide in doses exceeding 1500 mcg/day.

Toxicities

The systemic effects and toxicity of oral corticosteroids are well known and established. Inhaled steroids have been known to cause relatively minor and localized adverse effects such as oral **candidiasis**. However, less attention has been paid to their systemic effects.

Bronchodilators

Bronchodilators are medications that make breathing easier by relaxing the smooth muscles in the bronchi and widening the airways. Obstruction of the airways, which causes asthma symptoms, may be reversed by short- or long-acting beta$_2$-agonists. These agents work by relaxing smooth muscle around the airway to cause bronchodilation. The three most widely used bronchodilators include:

- Beta$_2$-agonists: such as albuterol, salmeterol, formoterol, and vilanterol
- Anticholinergics: such as ipratropium, tiotropium, umeclidinium, aclidinium, and glycopyrronium
- Theophylline

Beta$_2$-agonists and anticholinergics are available in both short-acting and long-acting forms. Theophylline is only available as an oral tablet in a long-acting form. Albuterol, also known as salbutamol, is approved by the FDA for treating and preventing acute or severe bronchospasm in patients with reversible obstructive airway disease, including exercise-induced bronchospasm.

Pharmacokinetics

Albuterol directly affects the bronchial smooth muscle upon inhalation without initially entering the bloodstream. Trace amounts appear in the blood approximately 2–3 hours after inhalation. Notably, albuterol levels in the body remain low when taken at recommended inhalation doses. The oral form has a half-life of 6 hours. It is metabolized within the liver and primarily excreted through the kidneys.

Mechanism of action

Albuterol acts on beta$_2$-adrenergic receptors, inducing bronchial smooth muscle relaxation and inhibiting immediate hypersensitivity mediator release, particularly from mast cells. Although albuterol also affects beta$_1$-adrenergic receptors, the impact is minimal, exerting little effect on the heart rate. Anticholinergic agents are competitive antagonists of the neurotransmitter acetylcholine at receptor sites within the cholinergic system.

Clinical indications

Albuterol and other bronchodilators treat or prevent acute or severe bronchospasm in patients with asthma, bronchitis, emphysema, and other lung diseases. It is also used to avoid bronchospasm caused by exercise. Theophylline is used with other medicines to treat the symptoms of asthma, bronchitis, emphysema, and other lung diseases. Anticholinergic drugs help treat respiratory disorders such as asthma and COPD. Theophylline is a bronchodilator that relaxes the muscles in the bronchial tubes.

Contraindications

Albuterol is contraindicated in patients with a history of hypersensitivity to it. Rare cases of hypersensitivity reactions, including **urticaria**, rash, and **angioedema**, have been reported after the use of albuterol sulfate. The use of anticholinergics requires caution, particularly with older adults.

Adverse effects

The adverse effects of albuterol include paradoxical bronchospasm, hypokalemia, dysrhythmia, and immediate hypersensitivity reactions. They are associated with anticholinergic agents, which include bronchitis, sinusitis, upper respiratory tract infection, headache, dizziness, and dry mouth. Paradoxical bronchospasm may occur with use as well.

Toxicities

Toxicities of bronchodilators include nervousness, headache, throat or nasal irritation, and muscle aches. More severe signs of toxicity, which are less common, include tachycardia, a feeling of fluttering, or palpitations.

Anticholinergic toxicity includes anhidrosis, mydriasis flushing, mydriasis, urinary retention, delirium, agitation, and hallucinations.

Mast cell stabilizers

Cromolyn sodium is a **mast cell stabilizer** and an alternative therapy for mild persistent asthma. It may also be beneficial in patients with allergic rhinitis. Mast cell stabilizers are not often prescribed due to their dosing frequency and the adverse effects of coughing and wheezing, which may be confused with asthma symptoms. Theophylline relaxes smooth muscle to cause dilation of the airway.

Pharmacokinetics

Cromolyn sodium is administered orally, via nebulization, and intranasally. Very little of the drug is absorbed systemically by any route of administration. It is poorly absorbed from the GI tract. Humans absorb no more than 1% of an administered dose after oral administration, the remainder being excreted in the feces. After administration by inhalation, approximately 8% of the total cromolyn sodium dose administered is absorbed and rapidly excreted unchanged, approximately equally divided between urine and bile.

Mechanism of action

Cromolyn sodium inhibits the release of inflammatory mediators such as histamine and leukotrienes from the sensitized mast cells, causing allergies. It works at the surface, blocking the **degranulation** and further expanding allergies. It is different from antihistamine medications in reducing the action of histamines released from the mast cells.

Clinical indications

Cromolyn oral inhalation is used to prevent mild to moderate bronchial asthma and bronchospasm and for adjunctive treatment of allergic rhinitis and systemic **mastocytosis** in pediatric patients and adults.

Contraindications

Hypersensitivity to cromolyn products or components of the formulation is the absolute contraindication for using cromolyn sodium.

Adverse effects

The most common adverse effects of cromolyn sodium include headache, nausea, abdominal pain, diarrhea, and muscle aches. Serious adverse effects of cromolyn sodium include flushing, **hypoesthesia**, palpitation, premature ventricular contractions, photosensitivity, and behavior changes.

You should remember

Cromolyn sodium may be used cautiously during pregnancy due to low systemic absorption from the various administration routes. It is considered an alternative therapy to ICSs for mild persistent asthma during pregnancy.

Leukotriene modifiers

Leukotriene modifiers, called leukotriene receptor antagonists, can help prevent breathing problems associated with allergies, asthma, and COPD. Examples include montelukast, zafirlukast, and zileuton. Leukotriene modifiers either block or inhibit **leukotrienes** released in response to an allergen and cause constriction of the airways. Patients with allergic rhinitis, aspirin sensitivity, or who smoke cigarettes may be exceptionally responsive to treatment with a leukotriene modifier.

Pharmacokinetics

Montelukast is quickly absorbed following oral administration. It is approximately 99% bound to plasma proteins and metabolized by the liver, and metabolites are excreted mainly via the feces.

Mechanism of action

Montelukast acts by blocking the action of leukotriene in the lungs, resulting in decreased inflammation and relaxation of smooth muscle. Leukotrienes are excreted by various cells, such as mast cells, and are involved in the inflammatory process that may cause asthma and allergic rhinitis signs and symptoms. Leukotriene receptors are found in airway cells, such as macrophages and smooth muscle cells. When bound to leukotriene receptors, montelukast inhibits leukotriene physiologic effects (such as airway edema, smooth muscle contraction, and impairment of regular cellular activity) without exhibiting any agonist activity.

Clinical indications

Montelukast is used to treat chronic asthma and prophylaxis and prevent exercise-induced bronchoconstriction. It is also approved for relieving seasonal and perennial allergic rhinitis symptoms. Montelukast is an orally dosed drug (available as a film-coated tablet, chewable tablet, or oral granules). It is indicated for asthma prophylaxis and chronic treatment in adults and pediatric patients 12 months and older.

Contraindications

Montelukast is contraindicated in patients with a history of hypersensitivity to the drug or its components or patients with phenylketonuria because the chewable tablet contains phenylalanine.

Adverse effects

The adverse effects of montelukast include depression, agitation, anxiety, aggressiveness, memory impairment, insomnia, somnambulism, seizures, paresthesia, hypoesthesia, and suicidal thoughts. Some patients with asthma may develop **systemic eosinophilia** or be associated with vasculitis. Other adverse effects of montelukast include headaches, fever, fatigue, **rhinorrhea**, pharyngitis, laryngitis, sinusitis, **epistaxis**, conjunctivitis, myalgia, arthralgia, and hepatotoxicity.

Toxicities

Acute overdosage with montelukast has been reported with doses as high as 1000 mg in adults and children. However, clinical and biological signs in such cases were relatively benign, including headaches, thirst, sleepiness or hyperactivity, vomiting, and abdominal pain. In case of overdose with montelukast, classical supportive therapies such as gastric lavage, adsorption with activated carbon, clinical monitoring, and, if necessary, supportive treatment may be used. Unfortunately, there is no known antidote for montelukast overdosage. In addition, no data exist concerning the efficiency of hemodialysis and peritoneal dialysis for removing montelukast from the body.

Immunomodulators

Immunomodulators are drugs that change the body's immune response. They mainly target pathways that treat various cancers. Immunomodulators are divided into two categories: immunostimulants and immunosuppressants. Immunostimulants are drugs designed to improve the body's resilience to infections by boosting the immune system's baseline response, which is particularly important in deficient immune systems.

Omalizumab (Xolair) is the first available immunomodulator therapy for children over 6 years with severe allergic asthma. Nucala (mepolizumab) has been approved for treating severe eosinophilic asthma in the pediatric population 6 years old and above. There are a variety of other products, including bevacizumab (Fasenra), sarilumab (Dupixent), reslizumab (Cinqair), and tezepelumab-ekko (Tezspire).

Pharmacokinetics

Omalizumab is administered via subcutaneous injection every 2–4 weeks based on serum IgE levels and body weight. Absorption is slow after subcutaneous injection, with peak serum concentrations achieved at 7–8 days with 62% bioavailability. It is metabolized in the liver, and the clearance relies on the clearance of IgG. Omalizumab is excreted through bile, and the half-life is about 24–26 days.

Mechanism of action

Omalizumab inhibits the binding of IgE to the high-affinity IgE receptor on the surface of both mast cells and basophils. The reduction in surface-bound IgE on cells limits the degree of release of mediators of the typical allergic response. Unlike in asthma, where a 95% reduction in serum IgE levels is required to modify allergen response, the mechanism for chronic urticaria is not as well understood. Chronic urticaria does not involve a classic allergen-driven response.

Clinical indications

Omalizumab treats moderate-to-severe persistent asthma in adults and pediatric patients 6 years or older when a patient's asthma has not been controlled sufficiently on other asthma medicines. This medicine will not relieve an asthma attack that has already started. Omalizumab injection is also used to treat chronic rhinosinusitis with nasal polyps in patients who have tried nasal corticosteroids but need additional relief.

Contraindications

Contraindications include a severe hypersensitivity reaction to omalizumab, and there have been reported cases of anaphylaxis. Due to the risk of anaphylaxis, patients must be closely observed for an appropriate period after omalizumab administration.

Adverse effects

The most common adverse effects associated with omalizumab are localized injection site reactions and headache. Although omalizumab is generally considered to have an excellent safety profile, there are some significant concerns regarding the potential adverse effects of the drug. The significant adverse effects of omalizumab can be categorized into four groups: systemic reactions, likely effects on malignancy, risk of parasitic disease, and immunological effects (**serum sickness**). Anaphylaxis is a possible adverse effect of omalizumab and requires extra monitoring by the provider. Patients should have access to prefilled epinephrine-containing autoinjectors for self-administration. These are called *EpiPen autoinjectors*.

You should remember

Asthma worsens in pregnant females and is associated with obstetrical complications such as fetal growth restriction, preterm delivery, and preeclampsia. Omalizumab is a recombinant humanized monoclonal antibody approved for treating severe persistent asthma.

Inhalation drugs

Inhalers are small, handheld devices that allow the patient to breathe medicine in through the mouth and into the lungs. Types include metered doses, dry powder, and soft mist inhalers. They usually treat asthma and COPD. Bronchodilators and corticosteroids are common inhaled medications.

Metered-dose inhaler

Metered-dose inhalers (MDIs) are the mainstay of asthma and COPD therapy worldwide. They are pocket-size handheld drug delivery devices that utilize the energy of compressed propellant for aerosol generation (see **Fig. 46.1**). An MDI is a specified dose that provides a specific dose of the active agent in each puff.

Dry powder inhaler

A dry powder inhaler (DPI) is an asthma treatment option for older kids and teens. Using a DPI allows medicine to get deep into the lungs. Unlike other inhalers, which deliver a puff of medicine, these inhalers hold the drug as a dry powder. The advantages of using a DPI over an MDI are that it is less time consuming. It is important to advise

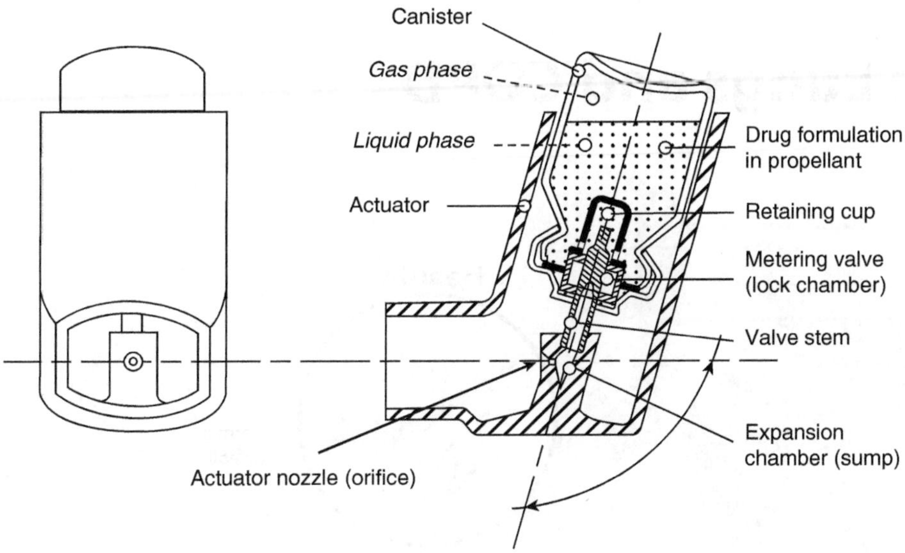

FIG. 46.1 Various metered-dose inhalers.

patients not to shake the inhaler before use. Also, keep the inhaler dry and only clean it with a dry cloth, as contact with moisture may affect the powder.

Nebulizer

A nebulizer is a small machine that turns liquid medicine into an easily inhaled mist.

The MDI or DPI devices are as effective and less time consuming than administering the medicine with a nebulizer. The time to give a medication with a nebulizer depends on the volume of the drug. Nebulization treatments usually take at least 5 minutes but may last over 20 minutes. The nebulizer is bulky, more expensive, and requires more maintenance. Nebulizers are commonly used to treat asthma, CF, COPD, and other respiratory diseases or disorders. Medications such as corticosteroids or bronchodilators may be administered via nebulizers. Corticosteroids can decrease inflammation in the airways, and bronchodilators open the airways to relieve congestion. A *small-volume nebulizer* mixes the desired medication into a fine mist that can be inhaled into the lungs. This allows the medication to work quickly.

Chronic obstructive pulmonary disorder

COPD is a group of disorders that permanently impair lung function. These disorders include **emphysema** and chronic **bronchitis**. According to the WHO, COPD is the third leading cause of death worldwide, with 65 million people suffering from it and over 3 million people dying each year globally. It is also estimated that approximately 90% of the mortality rate occurs in low- to middle-income countries. COPD prevalence and mortality are predicted to increase even more in the coming decades. Continuous exposure to ruinous molecules can lead to abnormal inflammatory responses, permanent tissue damage to the respiratory system, and irreversible pathological changes. Other factors that can lead to the development of COPD include genetics and aging.

Smoking and air pollution are the most common causes of COPD. People with COPD are at higher risk of other health problems. The most common COPD conditions are emphysema, chronic bronchitis, and chronic asthma that is not fully reversible. COPD is often referred to as a "smoker's disease." However, although smoking is one of the main risk factors for developing COPD, people who never smoke may also develop COPD.

The clinical manifestations of COPD are dyspnea on exertion, cough, wheezing, fatigue, weight loss, and progressive disability. With COPD, there is *air trapping* in which mucus plugs and narrowed airways are causative. There is also hyperinflation on expiration. The airways are pulled open during inspiration, and gases can flow past the obstruction. However, during expiration, decreased elastic recoil of the bronchial walls results in airway collapse, and normal expiratory airflow is prevented (see **Fig. 46.2**).

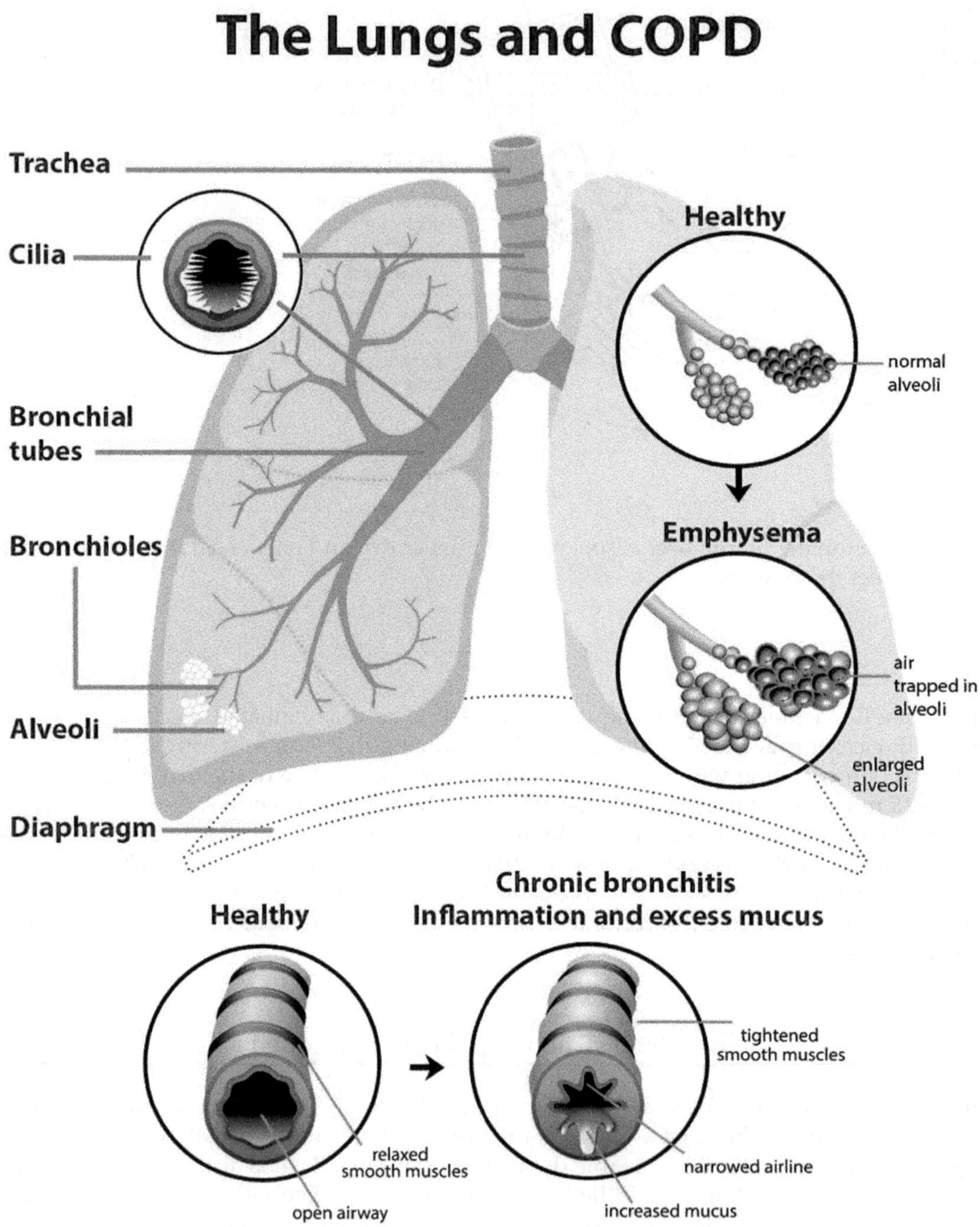

FIG. 46.2 The mechanisms of air trapping in chronic obstructive pulmonary disease.

Mostly, treatment methods are palliative and designed to prevent further impairment due to infection, including quitting smoking, supplemental oxygen, and medications. Many patients with COPD have mild forms of the disease for which little therapy is needed other than smoking cessation. Even for more advanced stages of the disease, effective treatment can control symptoms and slow progression, reduce the risk of complications and exacerbations, and improve patients' ability to lead an active life. Various therapeutic medications are used for

COPD, including bronchodilators, corticosteroids, and antibiotics, which could be administered alone or in combination.

Cystic fibrosis

CF is a progressive genetic disease that causes sticky, thick mucus to build up in organs, including the lungs and pancreas. There are about 40,000 children and adults living with CF in the United States (and an estimated 105,000 people have been diagnosed with CF across 94 countries), and CF can affect people of every racial and ethnic group. The mucus builds up the airways in the lungs and traps bacteria, causing infections, inflammation, and respiratory failure. Patients with CF may have various signs and symptoms, including wheezing, dyspnea, frequent pneumonia or bronchitis, persistent coughing, poor growth or weight gain, salty-tasting skin, difficulty with bowel movements, and **clubbing of fingers** (see **Fig. 46.3**). In most cases, CF is diagnosed during childhood by newborn screening, sweat test, genetic test, chest X-ray, lung function test, and sputum culture. There is no cure for CF, but treatment can ease symptoms, reduce complications, and improve quality of life. Close monitoring

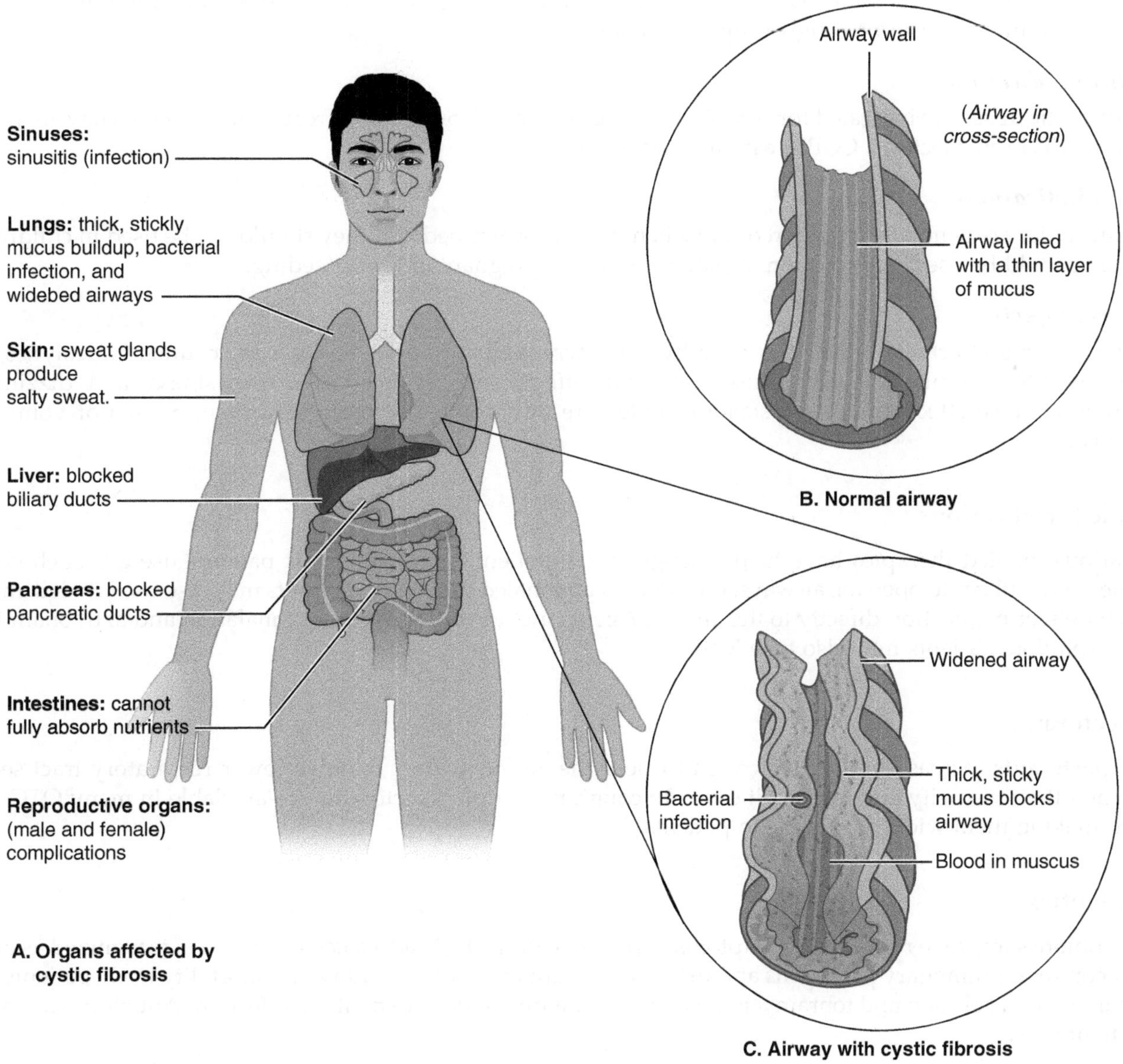

FIG. 46.3 (A) The organs affected by cystic fibrosis. (B) A cross-section of a normal airway. (C) A cross-section of an airway with cystic fibrosis.

and early, aggressive intervention are recommended to slow the progression of CF, which can lead to a longer life. Managing CF is complex, including mucolytics, expectorants, inhaled medications (bronchodilators), and antibiotics.

Mucolytic drugs

Mucolytic drugs break up mucus to clear it out of the lungs more easily. They can be given in oral, intravenous, and nebulizer forms. Mucolytics are part of a more general group of medications called mucoactive agents. Examples of mucolytics include *N*-acetylcysteine (Mucomyst), bromhexine (Mucolyte), guaifenesin (Mucinex), and dornase alfa (Pulmozyme). Acetylcysteine also has antiinflammatory and antioxidant properties.

Pharmacokinetics

Oral acetylcysteine is rapidly absorbed and slowly excreted and is available in the lung in an active form for at least 5 hours at high concentrations.

Mechanism of action

Mucolytic drugs reduce mucus viscosity in the airways. Dissolving the chemical bonds within the secretions makes them thin and can be coughed up more readily.

Clinical indications

Mucolytic drugs are indicated for chronic lung or breathing disorders that create thick mucus. They are frequently used for CF, bronchiectasis, COPD, asthma, and emphysema.

Contraindications

Mucolytics are generally considered safe when used as prescribed, but they should not be used in children under 6. They should be used with caution in patients who are pregnant or breastfeeding.

Adverse effects

The adverse effects of mucolytics vary by drug type and formulation. Over-the-counter mucolytics such as guaifenesin or bromhexine may cause mild side effects such as headache, drowsiness, and dizziness. The common adverse effects of acetylcysteine include sore throat, loss of voice, chest pain, nausea or vomiting, and diarrhea.

Inhaled medications

Various inhaled therapies have helped lengthen CF patients' survival. Most patients use a bronchodilator by inhaler or nebulizer to open the airways, followed by an inhaled mucolytic. Patients may also use inhaled antibiotics, which deliver medication directly to the airway. Agents include tobramycin for inhalation and aztreonam for inhalation solution. Patients may also take ICSs.

Expectorants

Expectorants increase productive cough to clear the airways. They dissolve lower respiratory tract secretions, reducing their viscosity and making it easier to cough them up. Expectorants are available in many OTC preparations, making them widely available to patients.

Antibiotics

Antibiotics improve respiratory symptoms in patients with CF. *Pseudomonas aeruginosa* is recognized as one of the most common pulmonary pathogens and the predominant cause of morbidity and mortality in CF patients. Aztreonam inhalation solution and tobramycin inhalation solution are used to treat the infection. Antibiotics are discussed in **Chapter 49**.

You should remember

There is no cure for CF, but treatment can ease symptoms, reduce complications, and improve quality of life. Close monitoring should begin early, and aggressive intervention is recommended to slow the progression of CF, which can lead to a longer life.

You should remember

P. aeruginosa is an opportunistic pathogen that is a leading cause of morbidity and mortality in CF patients and immunocompromised individuals. Due to its remarkable ability to resist antibiotics, eradicating *P. aeruginosa* has become increasingly challenging.

Key Terms

Allergic rhinitis
Angioedema
Bronchitis
Clubbing fingers
Conjunctivitis
Degranulation
Dysphonia
Emphysema
Epistaxis
Expectorants
Hypoesthesia
Hypoxia
Leukotrienes
Mast cell stabilizer
Rhinorrhea
Serum sickness
Systemic eosinophilia
Urticaria
Wheezing

Clinical Case Studies

Clinical Case Study 1

A 31-year-old female with a history of bronchial asthma presented to the emergency department with a 3-day history of progressive dyspnea after cold exposure. She was on a regular MDI of albuterol, one puff four times daily, at home. She described having a cough and wheezing with no fever, rhinorrhea, or upper respiratory tract symptoms.

Critical Thinking Questions

1. What are the most critical factors for developing asthma?
2. What is the mechanism of action for albuterol?
3. What are the contraindications of albuterol?

Clinical Case Study 2

An 85-year-old male patient stopped smoking 2 years ago. He was a chronic smoker who consumed two packs of cigarettes per day for 55 years. The patient came to the emergency department with complaints of dyspnea, cough with expectoration, and palpitations. The patient had a history of hypertension for 12 years and had cataract surgery. The patient was given nebulized bronchodilators, furosemide 40 mg, and an injection of methylprednisolone. Based on examination findings and the patient's history of smoking, a provisional diagnosis of COPD was made.

Critical Thinking Questions

1. What are the causes of COPD?
2. What are the clinical manifestations of COPD?
3. What are the various therapeutic medications used for COPD?

Clinical Case Study 3

A 17-year-old patient with no family history of CF was brought to the emergency department with a chronic cough, wheezing, dyspnea, and very salty-tasting skin and was previously treated unsuccessfully for asthmatic bronchitis. She suffered from three episodes of pneumonia in the previous 4 years. Head and chest CT after the last pulmonary infection revealed bilateral bronchiectasis and sinusitis.

Critical Thinking Questions

1. What are the causes of CF?
2. What are the signs and symptoms of CF?
3. How is CF diagnosed?

Further Reading

[1] T. Des Jardins, G.G. Burton, Clinical Manifestations and Assessment of Respiratory Disease, eighth ed., Mosby, 2019.
[2] S. Duggins Davis, M. Rosenfeld, J. Chmiel, Cystic Fibrosis – A Multi-Organ System Approach (Respiratory Medicine), Humana Press, 2020.
[3] F. Earlstein, Asthma Explained – Asthma Facts, Diagnosis, Symptoms, Treatment, Causes, Effects, Alternative Medicines, Therapeutic Methods, History, Myths, and More! Facts and Information, , LLC, Pack & Post Plus, 2017.
[4] Global Initiative for Chronic Obstructive Lung Disease, Pocket Guide to COPD Diagnosis, Management and Prevention – A Guide for Health Care Professionals, GICOLD, 2022.
[5] S. Karpel, Linz's Comprehensive Respiratory Diseases, Jones & Bartlett Learning, 2019.
[6] A. Melan, Cystic Fibrosis (CF) – A Manual for Those Who Suffer from Cystic Fibrosis and the Search for a Health Medication Really the Most Effective, Melan, 2022.
[7] J. Middleton, Asthma – Pathophysiology, Diagnosis and Treatment, American Medical Publishers, 2023.
[8] H. Nakamura, K. Aoshiba, Chronic Obstructive Pulmonary Disease – A Systemic Inflammatory Disease (Respiratory Disease Series – Diagnostic Tools and Disease Managements), Springer, 2017.
[9] L. Nici, R. ZuWallack, Chronic Obstructive Pulmonary Disease – Co-Morbidities and Systemic Consequences (Respiratory Medicine), Humana Press, 2012.
[10] V. Nikam, S. Sawarkar, G. Mahajan, S. Jagtap, Natural Immunomodulators – Promising Therapy for Disease Management, Bentham Books, 2023.
[11] D.M. Orenstein, J.E. Spahr, D.J. Weinger, Cystic Fibrosis – A Guide for Patient and Family, fourth ed., Wolters Kluwer / Lippincott, Williams, and Wilkins, 2011.
[12] M. Pokorski, Respiratory Regulation – Clinical Advances (in Experimental Medicine and Biology, Book 755), Springer, 2013.
[13] G. Swanson, The Complete Asthma Guide – an Asthma Book for Adults and Children that Teaches How to be Asthma Free Naturally, Z Media, 2022.
[14] WAO, R.F. Lockey, D.K. Ledford, Asthma – Comorbidities, Coexisting Conditions, and Differential Diagnosis, Oxford University Press, 2017.

CHAPTER

47

Allergic rhinitis and common cold drugs

OUTLINE

LEARNING OUTCOMES

After studying the chapter, readers should be able to:

1. Describe the pathophysiology of allergic rhinitis.
2. List the four OTC antihistamines.
3. Explain the contraindications of antihistamines.
4. Describe the function of mast cell stabilizers.
5. Describe the direct local effect of fluticasone.
6. Explain the adverse effects of fluticasone.
7. Discuss the mechanism of action of pseudoephedrine.
8. Describe the adverse effects of pseudoephedrine.

The Science of Pharmacology
https://doi.org/10.1016/B978-0-443-29038-1.00047-6

9. Explain the pharmacotherapy for the common cold.
10. Describe the toxicity of dextromethorphan.

Overview

Allergic rhinitis is an inflammatory disorder of the nasal mucosa triggered by allergen exposure, which triggers immunoglobulin E–mediated inflammation. It causes symptoms of nasal congestion, rhinorrhea, sneezing, and nasal itching. Other symptoms include sleep disturbance, fatigue, altered mood, and cognitive function compromise that impairs quality of life and productivity. Allergic rhinitis can also be associated with comorbid conditions such as nasal polyps, asthma, and atopic dermatitis. The common cold is a mild upper respiratory tract infection. Colds are the most common illness. Adults have an average of two to three colds yearly, and children have even more. Colds are more common in the winter and spring. More than 200 viruses can cause a cold, but rhinoviruses are the most common type. The viruses that cause colds are very contagious. They can spread from person to person through the air and close personal contact. People can also get infected when they touch something with the virus and then touch their eyes, mouth, or nose.

Treatments with proven effectiveness for cold symptoms in adults include over-the-counter analgesics, zinc, nasal decongestants with or without antihistamines, and ipratropium for cough. The only established safe and effective treatments for children are acetylcysteine, honey (for children 1 year and older), and nasal saline irrigation.

Physiology of the upper respiratory tract

The respiratory tract consists of the upper and lower airways. The upper airways begin from the nares and mouth and end at the larynx. Being extrathoracic, these airways are impacted by barometric pressure impinging on their external surface. The lower airways include the extrathoracic and intrathoracic portions of the trachea, the extrapulmonary and intrapulmonary bronchi, and the bronchioles, alveolar ducts, and alveoli, which are intrathoracic and intrapulmonary. The nose and mouth represent two parallel pathways by which air enters and leaves the system. The nasal cavity and nasopharynx have a large surface area and tortuous airflow path conducive to filtering, warming, and humidifying ambient air. For more discussion, see **Chapter 45**.

Pathophysiology of allergic rhinitis

Allergic rhinitis, commonly known as *hay fever,* is an allergic reaction that causes congestion, nasal itching, sneezing, and eye watering. Triggers can include insects, mold, pet dander, and pollen. The condition can sometimes be severe, but relief can be provided through allergy medications, **allergy shots**, and lifestyle changes.

The pathophysiology of allergic rhinitis involves early and late allergic responses. It is triggered by exposure to **allergens** recognized by antigen-specific **immunoglobulin E** on **mast cells** and basophil receptors in presensitized individuals. The early-phase reaction is signified by mast cell degranulation. This phase is linked to a rapid onset of acute nasal symptoms over minutes, plus ocular symptoms. The symptoms are caused by histamine release, mostly from mast cells in the nasal mucosa. This early-phase histamine release, along with the effects of other proinflammatory solid cytokines such as leukotrienes and **eicosanoids**, also increases vascular permeability. This leads to the development of edema.

The late-phase reaction develops over hours following allergen exposure. It involves the cellular recruitment of basophils, neutrophils, monocytes, eosinophils, and T lymphocytes and the release of mediators that influence the inflammatory response. The late-phase inflammatory reaction involves tissue remodeling, additional tissue edema, and nasal congestion. Because of mucosal inflammation, the tissues react more intensely to allergen exposure. Late-phase reactions and modifications of tissue responsiveness contribute to bronchial hyperresponsiveness.

Pharmacotherapy

Most patients with allergic rhinitis need pharmacotherapy to control their symptoms. Management of allergic rhinitis is affected by the frequency and severity of symptoms, the patient's age, and any concurrent conditions. Antihistamines, intranasal corticosteroids, and mast cell stabilizers commonly treat allergic rhinitis.

Antihistamines

Antihistamines are a class of drugs commonly used to treat symptoms of allergies. They help treat conditions caused by the body's immune system producing too much histamine. People with allergic reactions to pollen and other allergens most commonly use antihistamines. **Table 47.1** summarizes the selective antihistamines.

Fexofenadine is a nondrowsy second-generation antihistamine that helps with "allergic" symptoms. It is an over-the-counter medication that has been approved for use in both children and adults. Children should be 6 months old or older, depending on the indication for use.

Pharmacokinetics

Fexofenadine is rapidly absorbed, reaching peak plasma concentrations 1 hour after oral administration and 1 hour after the oral suspension. Maximum histamine inhibition is achieved approximately 1–2 hours after administration. It is a long-acting antihistamine that can be administered once a day. Fexofenadine has approximately 60%–70% plasma protein binding. Fexofenadine undergoes minimal hepatic metabolism. The mean elimination half-life is approximately 14 hours after administering. Fexofenadine is excreted in feces via biliary excretion (80%) and urine (12%). The half-life may be significantly prolonged in patients with renal disease.

Mechanism of action

The mechanism of action of fexofenadine is to selectively antagonize H1 receptors on the surface of cells in different organ systems. It is a second-generation H1 receptor blocker. Fexofenadine also affects inflammatory

TABLE 47.1 OTC antihistamine combinations.

Generic name	Trade name	Route of administration
brompheniramine	Dimetapp Children's Cold and Allergy	PO
cetirizine	Zyrtec-D, Allertec	PO
chlorpheniramine	Actifed Cold and Allergy Tablets, Chlor-Trimeton Allergy/Decongestant Tablets, Sudafed PE Sinus and Allergy Tablets, Triaminic Cold/Allergy, Tylenol Allergy Multi-Symptoms Gels	PO
clemastine	Tavist Allergy Tablets	PO
diphenhydramine	Benadryl Allergy/Cold Caplets, Sudafed PE Nighttime Cold, Tylenol PM Gelcaps	PO
doxylamine	Unisom, Advil PM, NyQuil	PO
fexofenadine	Allegra-D	PO
loratadine	Claritin-D, Alavert	PO
triprolidine	Actifed Plus	PO

mediators. Compared to other first-generation antihistamines, fexofenadine crosses the blood-brain barrier to a minimal extent and thus does not cause drowsiness like other H1 blockers. Second-generation antihistamines such as fexofenadine, cetirizine, and loratadine have less affinity for cholinergic and alpha-adrenergic receptors and display minimal anticholinergic effects.

Clinical indications

Fexofenadine prevents and treats allergy symptoms such as red and itchy eyes, sneezing, a runny or stuffy nose, and hives. It is also used to treat seasonal allergic rhinitis and chronic idiopathic urticaria. Fexofenadine is approved for use in both children and adults. Children should be 6 months old or older, depending upon the indication for use.

Contraindications

Fexofenadine is contraindicated in patients who have hypersensitivity. It should be used with caution in people with renal impairment, severe hypertension, severe coronary artery disease, and dysrhythmia.

Adverse effects

Side effects of fexofenadine include allergic reactions, headaches, **aphonia**, coughing, epistaxis, vomiting, diarrhea, sleepiness, dry mouth, dizziness, **leukopenia**, back pain, chills, and rashes. The most common adverse effects are vomiting, drowsiness, fatigue, and dry mouth, which may occur in larger doses.

Toxicities

Fexofenadine may have cardiotoxic effects and blocked cardiac potassium channels, which, when taken in large doses, cause prolonged QT intervals, which can lead to fatal arrhythmias. According to FDA guidelines, fexofenadine has replaced terfenadine in the United States because it does not block potassium channels.

You should remember

Histamine is an important chemical that plays a role in several bodily processes. It stimulates gastric acid secretion, plays a role in inflammation, dilates blood vessels, affects muscle contractions in the intestines and lungs, and affects heart rate. It is also released if the body encounters a threat from an allergen. Histamine causes vessels to swell and dilate, leading to allergy symptoms.

Intranasal corticosteroids

Steroid sprays (prescription or OTC) include beclomethasone, budesonide, ciclesonide, flunisolide, fluticasone furoate, fluticasone propionate, mometasone, and triamcinolone.

Intranasal corticosteroids are the first-line treatment for allergic rhinitis and greatly relieve symptoms for most patients. They are more effective than oral antihistamines for symptom relief; they differ regarding dosage frequency, the spray device, and cost. For patients with severe symptoms, a nasal decongestant may be needed for a few days before starting a nasal steroid to reduce nasal swelling, allowing the spray to reach more areas inside the nasal passages. Symptom relief from a steroid spray is often within the first day, but the full effect can take days to weeks; nasal steroids are most effective when used regularly and daily. Table 47.2 summarizes intranasal corticosteroids. Fluticasone is an example of these drugs that are discussed in detail here.

Fluticasone is a corticosteroid given via the nasal, oral inhalation, or topical routes. The route of administration depends on the patient's diagnosis. Nasal fluticasone can treat allergic and nonallergic rhinitis, nasal polyps, and allergies. Inhaled fluticasone is used for treating asthma. Inhaled steroids slightly improve lung function and improve COPD symptoms.

Pharmacokinetics

Fluticasone propionate is cleared from hepatic metabolism by cytochrome P450. It is eliminated more than 90% in the feces and about 2% in the urine. Fluticasone has a longer plasma elimination half-life when given by the inhaled route, approximately 15 hours, compared to 8 intranasally. It is 99% protein bound.

TABLE 47.2 Corticosteroids and miscellaneous drugs for allergic rhinitis.

Generic name	Trade name	Route of administration
Corticosteroids		
beclomethasone	Beconase AQ, Qnasl, Qvar	Intranasal
budesonide	Rhinocort Aqua	Intranasal
ciclesonide	Omnaris, Zetonna	Intranasal
flunisolide	Nasalide, Nasarel	Intranasal
fluticasone	Flonase, Veramyst	Intranasal
mometasone	Nasonex, Sinuva	Intranasal
triamcinolone	Nasacort AQ	Intranasal
Miscellaneous drugs		
cromolyn	NasalCrom	Intranasal
ipratropium	Atrovent	Intranasal
montelukast	Singulair	PO

Mechanism of action

Fluticasone has a direct local effect of vasoconstriction and antiinflammatory activity. Glucocorticoids inhibit the initial inflammatory events such as vasodilation, vascular permeability, and leukocyte emigration. Fluticasone directly decreases inflammatory cells such as eosinophils, monocytes, mast cells, macrophages, and **dendritic cells**. It reduces the number of these cells and the number of cytokines they produce. This medication also directly increases beta$_2$ receptors on airway smooth muscle and decreases mucus gland secretions.

Clinical indications

Fluticasone is indicated for congestion, runny nose, sneezing, nasal itching, nasal swelling, asthma, and nasal polyps. Fluticasone nasal spray controls hay fever symptoms, allergies, nonallergic rhinitis, or nasal polyps but does not cure these conditions. Inhaled fluticasone is used to treat asthma and COPD.

Contraindications

Fluticasone is contraindicated in patients with hypersensitivity to the medication. It should not be used as a primary treatment for acute bronchospasm.

Adverse effects

The adverse effects of intranasal fluticasone include a bloody nose, cough, fever, sore throat, fatigue, dyspnea, headache, muscle pain, and stuffy nose. Less common adverse effects include blurred vision, change in vision, and blindness.

Toxicities

The toxicity with several fluticasone propionate products, including the nasal spray and the inhaler, is possible. However, it is scarce. An overdose may cause metabolic acidosis and **hyperlactatemia**.

You should remember

Fluticasone nasal sprays may cause eye conditions such as cataracts and glaucoma. Patients who use this medication should have a yearly eye exam to check for these conditions. They should be checked sooner if they experience eye problems such as cloudy or reduced vision.

Mast cell stabilizers

The mast cell releases the inflammatory mediators involved in type I allergic reactions (histamine, leukotrienes, prostaglandins, and cytokines). Cromolyn sodium and nedocromil sodium, mast cell–stabilizing agents, comprise an essential group of mild to moderate antiinflammatory drugs.

They prevent histamine release by stabilizing the mast cell membrane. These agents are most effective when used before antigen exposure. Cromolyn sodium is available in an intranasal form OTC. Cromolyn is available as a first-line drug for managing mild allergic reactions. It also manages bronchial asthma, allergic rhinitis, and certain allergic eye conditions such as **vernal conjunctivitis, keratitis**, and keratoconjunctivitis. Generally, cromolyn sodium is relatively safe and has fewer side effects. Nedocromil is much more potent than cromolyn sodium. It is FDA approved in the United States as an inhaled preparation for asthma and relieves nasal symptoms of hay fever and other nasal allergies. It is also available as an ophthalmic formulation for allergic conjunctivitis.

Decongestants

Decongestants are medicines that can provide short-term relief for nasal congestion. They reduce the swelling of the blood vessels in the nose, which helps open the airways. They are available in various formulations over the counter. Most people can use decongestants safely, but they are not suitable for everyone. **Table 47.3** summarizes nasal decongestants.

Pseudoephedrine relieves nasal congestion caused by allergies, hay fever, and colds. It is also used to relieve sinus congestion and pressure temporarily. Pseudoephedrine is in a class of medications called nasal decongestants. It works by causing constriction of the capillaries in the nasal passages.

Pharmacokinetics

Pseudoephedrine is active after oral administration and is easily absorbed from the GI tract. The onset of action occurs after 30 minutes, and after 1–3 hours, the drug reaches its maximum concentration in the serum. The duration of effect of the immediate-release tablet is 3–8 hours. When using the extended-release formulation, this time is twice as long. Pseudoephedrine is mainly excreted unchanged in the urine. Only a small amount is metabolized in the liver to the active metabolite. The half-life decreases when the urine is acidic and increases when the urine is alkaline but ranges between 3–16 hours.

Mechanism of action

Pseudoephedrine is a sympathomimetic with a mixed direct and indirect mechanism of action. It directly stimulates beta-adrenergic receptors and indirectly stimulates alpha-adrenergic receptors, causing the release of endogenous norepinephrine from the granularity of neurons.

TABLE 47.3 Nasal decongestants.

Generic name	Trade name	Route of administration
naphazoline	Privine	Intranasal
oxymetazoline	Afrin 12 Hour, Neo-Synephrine 12 Hour, others	Intranasal
phenylephrine	Afrin 4–6 Hour, Neo-Synephrine 4–6 Hour, others	Intranasal
pseudoephedrine	Sudafed	PO
tetrahydrozoline	Tyzine	Intranasal
xylometazoline	generic only	Intranasal

Clinical indications

Pseudoephedrine relieves nasal or sinus congestion caused by the common cold, **sinusitis**, hay fever, and other respiratory allergies. It is also used to relieve ear congestion caused by otitis media. Some of these preparations are available only with a prescription.

Contraindications

Contraindication of pseudoephedrine includes hypersensitivity to the drug and treatment with monoamine oxidase inhibitors currently or in the last 2 weeks. It should be used with caution in patients with hypertension, coronary artery disease, liver or renal impairment, benign prostatic hyperplasia, diabetes mellitus, hyperthyroidism, **narrow-angle glaucoma**, and mental agitation. Pseudoephedrine should not be used during pregnancy, lactation, and age under 2 years. The extended-release form of the drug should not be used until the age of 12 years.

Adverse effects

The adverse effects of pseudoephedrine include headache, nausea or vomiting, dysuria, fatigue, anxiety, dyspnea, insomnia, tremors, hypertension, tachycardia, and **xerostomia**.

Toxicities

The symptoms of an overdose include seizures, hallucinations, tachycardia, hypertension, dyspnea, coma, and circulatory collapse. In extreme cases, death may occur. Symptoms of overdose also include headache, dizziness, anxiety, **tinnitus**, blurred vision, **euphoria**, ataxia, chest pain, tachycardia, palpitations, increased or decreased blood pressure, increased thirst, sweating, difficulty urinating, nausea, and vomiting. More frequently observed symptoms in children are dry mouth, wide and rigid pupils, hot flashes, fever, and digestive tract dysfunctions.

You should remember

Do not give any over-the-counter cough and cold medicine to children under 4. Using these medicines might cause severe or possibly life-threatening side effects.

You should remember

The law bans over-the-counter sales of cold medicines that contain pseudoephedrine, which is commonly used to make methamphetamine. Cold medicine containing pseudoephedrine is limited to behind-the-counter sales. The amount of pseudoephedrine an individual can purchase each month is limited, and individuals must present photo identification to purchase products containing pseudoephedrine. In addition, pharmacies are required to keep personal information about purchasers for at least 2 years.

Drugs for the common cold

The "common cold" is a benign, self-limited syndrome caused by over 200 viruses. It is the most frequently occurring acute illness in the United States and affects patients of all ages. The common cold is easily spread to others. However, the most common causative viruses are the *rhinoviruses*. It is spread through airborne droplets that are coughed or sneezed into the air and then inhaled by another individual. For unknown reasons, more colds occur during the cold season, from early fall through late winter. This may be due to schools being in session, people staying indoors near each other, and low humidity drying out the nasal passages. The common cold is associated with a substantial economic burden, including the cost of treatment and the loss of productivity.

Everyone is at risk for the common cold. Children and older adults suffer more from common colds yearly than adults because their immune systems are weak. The average child has 6–10 colds per year, while the average adult has only two to four colds per year.

Patients with underlying lung disease, smokers, and those who are immunocompromised (cancer patients or AIDS) typically have more severe symptoms than those not suffering from these conditions.

Symptoms include a stuffy, runny nose, a scratchy, tickly throat, sneezing, eye watering, a low-grade fever, a sore throat, a mild hacking cough, muscle and bone aches, headache, mild fatigue, chills, and a watery discharge from the nose that eventually thickens and becomes yellow or green.

Pharmacotherapy for cold symptoms in adults includes over-the-counter analgesics, zinc, nasal decongestants with or without antihistamines, and ipratropium for cough. Acetylcysteine, nasal saline irrigation, and intranasal ipratropium are the only established safe and effective treatments for children. Over-the-counter cold medications should not be used in children younger than 4.

Antitussives

Antitussives are medicines that suppress coughing. Antitussive therapy can be either specific or nonspecific. Definitive or specific antitussive therapy depends on determining the etiology or operant pathophysiological mechanism and initiating a particular treatment. Because the cause of chronic cough can almost always be determined, it is possible to prescribe specific therapy that can be almost uniformly successful. Nonspecific antitussive therapy is directed at the symptom; it is indicated when definitive treatment cannot be given. For adults, the most common antitussives include products containing dextromethorphan or codeine. Codeine requires a prescription, but a person can find OTC products containing dextromethorphan (see **Table 47.4**). Dextromethorphan is one of the most common compounds found in most over-the-counter antitussives.

Pharmacokinetics

Dextromethorphan is rapidly absorbed from the GI tract, enters the bloodstream, and crosses the blood-brain barrier. Upon initial absorption, it undergoes rapid metabolism via cytochrome P450. It takes about 2 hours to reach peak concentrations. Due to its extensive first-pass metabolism, dextromethorphan has low oral bioavailability. The plasma half-life of dextromethorphan is about 2–4 hours after therapeutic dosing and is primarily excreted in the urine.

Mechanism of action

The primary mechanism of action for dextromethorphan as a cough suppressant is unknown. However, it may act on the central nervous system's pulmonary vagal afferent fibers synapse—this site in the brainstem functions as a gate for the cough reflex. It decreases the sensitivity of these cough receptors and interrupts cough impulse transmission.

Clinical indications

Dextromethorphan temporarily relieves coughs caused by the flu, the common cold, or other conditions. It does not cure the cause of the cough or speed recovery. It is indicated in chronic dry cough or unproductive cough. It is also used for acute dry cough that interferes with normal function or sleep.

TABLE 47.4 Antitussives and expectorants.

Generic name	Trade name	Route of administration
Opioid antitussives codeine hydrocodone/homatropine	Hycodan, Hydromet	PO
Nonopioid antitussives benzonatate dextromethorphan	Tessalon Delsym, Robitussin DM, others	PO PO
Expectorant guaifenesin	Mucinex, Robitussin, others	PO
Mucolytics acetylcysteine dornase alfa	Mucomyst Pulmozyme	Inhalation Inhalation

Contraindications

Dextromethorphan should be avoided in patients with known hypersensitivity. It should not be used with monoamine oxidase inhibitors (MAOI) or for 2 weeks after stopping the MAOI drugs.

Adverse effects

Adverse effects of dextromethorphan are rare. However, the most common symptoms include nausea, vomiting, GI discomfort, drowsiness, **nystagmus**, and dizziness.

Toxicity

Dextromethorphan toxicity may occur due to its OTC misuse. One life-threatening toxicity associated with this drug abuse is **serotonin syndrome**. Due to its action on serotonin reuptake inhibition, if patients are already on typical SSRI or MAOI antidepressants, drug toxicity potentiates excess serotonin in the body, potentially leading to serotonin syndrome. The symptoms include headache, agitation, confusion, tachycardia, hypotension, high fevers, seizures, irregular heartbeat, and **mydriases** and can lead to unconsciousness.

Expectorants and mucolytics

Expectorants are agents that discharge or expel mucus from the respiratory tract. They are used to treat the symptoms of respiratory tract infections, including the common cold, bronchitis, cystic fibrosis, and pneumonia. This condition may cause a buildup of mucus in the lungs. Two expectorant ingredients are available in the United States, including guaifenesin and potassium iodide. Guaifenesin is the most commonly used expectorant in many cold, cough, and flu medications. Examples of guaifenesin include Mucinex and Robitussin.

Potassium iodide is widely used in breathing treatments for people with asthma, chronic bronchitis, or emphysema. Guaifenesin is typically safe to use if taken as directed. Potential side effects of guaifenesin can include headache, dizziness, fatigue, nausea, vomiting, and constipation.

Key Terms

Allergens
Allergy shots
Antitussives
Aphonia
Benign prostatic hyperplasia
Dendritic cells
Eicosanoids
Epistaxis
Euphoria
Immunoglobulin E
Keratitis
Leukopenia
Mast cells
Mydriases
Narrow-angle glaucoma
Nystagmus
Serotonin syndrome
Sinusitis
Tinnitus
Vernal conjunctivitis

Clinical case studies

Clinical case study 1

A 36-year-old female has had a history of nasal congestion that worsened over time, plus recurrent sinus infections. She eventually developed rhinorrhea, sneezing, and chronic nasal blockage. The rhinorrhea temporarily improved during a Caribbean vacation. The patient is diagnosed with allergic rhinitis and is given fexofenadine.

Critical thinking questions

1. What does the pathophysiology of allergic rhinitis involve?
2. What is fexofenadine?
3. How does histamine affect the symptoms of allergic rhinitis?

Clinical case study 2

A 44-year-old male with a history of heavy smoking and chronic bronchitis went to an urgent care clinic because he had a common cold for several days with a runny nose, coughing, low fever, and dyspnea. The patient had also a history of asthma in the past. He coughed up sputum in the morning. Treatment included pseudoephedrine, dextromethorphan, and acetaminophen.

Critical thinking questions

1. What is the indication for pseudoephedrine?
2. What are the contraindications for pseudoephedrine?
3. What is the clinical indication for dextromethorphan?

Further reading

[1] S.H. Evans, The Sinus Solution – the Ultimate Guide to Getting Permanent Relief from Chronic Sinusitis, Evans, 2020.
[2] C. Juan, Allergic Rhinitis – A Comprehensive Guide to the Understanding, Treatment, and Recovery from Allergic Rhinitis, Juan, 2024.
[3] R.F. Lockey, D.K. Ledford, Allergens and Allergen Immunotherapy – Subcutaneous, Sublingual, and Oral, sixth ed., CRC Press, 2020.
[4] D. Louis, Allergic Rhinitis – the Complete Guide on Everything You Need to Know About Allergic Rhinitis, Causes, Cure, Prevention and Management, Louis, 2020.
[5] Medwiz Healthcare Communications, Allergic Rhinitis – Comprehensive Management and Emerging Innovations, Medwiz Healthcare Communications, 2023.
[6] C. Pereira, Corticosteroids – A Paradigmatic Drug Class, IntechOpen, 2021.
[7] N. Popov, Common Cold – A Complete Guide on Treatment of the Common Cold and 10 Tips to Prevent it, Popov, 2022.
[8] F. Ryan, Virusphere – from Common Colds to Ebola Epidemics – Why we Need the Viruses that Plague Us, Prometheus, 2020.
[9] L.D. Thomson-Smith, Allergic Rhinitis – the Causes and Consequences, Facebook Publishing, 2013.
[10] A. Zanasi, G.A. Fontana, D. Mutolo, Cough – Pathophysiology, Diagnosis and Treatment, Springer, 2020.
[11] V. Zinserling, Infectious Pathology of the Respiratory Tract, Springer, 2021.

UNIT IX

Chemotherapeutic drugs

CHAPTER

48

Antiviral drugs

OUTLINE

The Science of Pharmacology
https://doi.org/10.1016/B978-0-443-29038-1.00048-8

LEARNING OUTCOMES

After study of the chapter, readers should be able to:

1. Identify the characteristics of viruses.
2. Explain the effect of viruses on the host.
3. Identify the drugs for influenza infections.
4. Explain the indications for acyclovir.
5. Discuss the HPV immunizations.
6. Describe the drugs used for hepatitis C.
7. Explain the classifications of drugs for viral hepatitis.
8. Describe the adverse effects of tenofovir alafenamide.
9. Explain the preexposure prophylaxis therapy for HIV.
10. Describe the types of COVID-19 therapies used in the United States.

Overview

Viruses are microscopic organisms that can infect hosts such as humans, plants, or animals. They are small genetic information (deoxyribonucleic acid [DNA] or ribonucleic acid [RNA]) inside a protective shell (capsid). Some viruses also have an envelope. Viruses can't reproduce without a host. Some common diseases caused by viruses include the flu, the cold, human herpesviruses (HHVs), enteroviruses, human papillomaviruses (HPVs), and coronavirus disease 2019 (COVID-19). They are obligate intracellular organisms that must reside within a living host cell to survive and reproduce. Viruses enter healthy cells, live and replicate within living cells, and use their DNA and RNA to generate more viruses. The growth cycle of viruses depends on host cell enzymes and cell substrates for viral replication. Except for human immunodeficiency virus (HIV) and certain kinds of viral hepatitis, viruses are self-limiting illnesses that usually do not require treatment with a specific antiviral. Current antivirals target influenza, herpes, and hepatitis. Viruses are particles that infect and replicate inside cells.

Characteristics of viruses

Viruses are microscopic organisms that can infect hosts such as humans, plants, or animals. They can replicate only inside the cells of their host. Viruses have a relatively simple structure comprising the genome, the capsid, and the envelope. The **genome** is the virion's inner core, composed of single- or double-stranded DNA or RNA

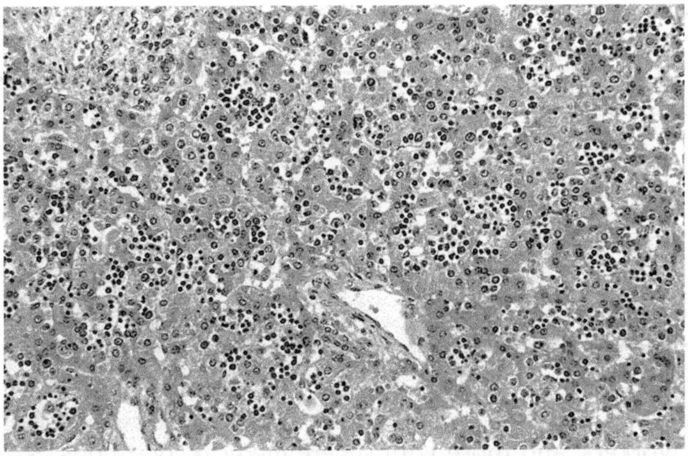

FIG. 48.1 The structure of the human immunodeficiency virus.

molecules, but not both. The viral **capsid** is a protein coat that surrounds and protects the genome. It also plays a role in the **virion** and host cell fusion process. Fusion occurs when virions attach themselves to host cells in preparation for infecting the cells. The envelope is the outermost layer of the virion and is present in some, but not all, viruses. A depiction of HIV is shown in **Fig. 48.1**. The HIV-1 virion consists of a core of identical strands of viral RNA molecules of viral enzymes in a core capsid structure primarily composed of structural viral protein p24.

At least six classes of DNA viruses and 14 classes of RNA viruses are known to infect humans. Some of the more prominent viral illnesses include smallpox (poxviruses), sore throat and conjunctivitis (adenoviruses), warts (papovaviruses), influenza (orthomyxoviruses), respiratory infections (coronaviruses, rhinoviruses), gastroenteritis (rotaviruses, Norwalk-like viruses), HIV, herpes, and hepatitis viruses.

Viruses are divided into categories such as family and genus, based on similar features such as size, shape, and the type of genetic material they carry. Some common viruses include influenza viruses, HHV, enteroviruses, HPVs, hepatitis viruses, orthopoxviruses, and coronaviruses. Some viruses have unique qualities, such as retroviruses and oncoviruses.

Effective drug therapy is currently available for only a few active viral infections. HIV belongs to the retroviruses. Many viral infections, such as chickenpox, are survivable. Some viral illnesses have been reduced by developing effective vaccines, such as for polio, smallpox, measles, chickenpox, hepatitis B (HepB), and COVID-19. However, many other viral infections are either fatal or have much more severe long-term outcomes, such as hepatitis and HIV infection.

The effect of viruses on the host

Viruses are widespread in the environment, and most viral infections may not even be symptomatic before the host's immune system eliminates them. Host immune responses to viral infections are classified as either nonspecific or specific. Nonspecific immune responses include phagocytosis of viral particles by leukocytes such as neutrophils, macrophages, monocytes, and T lymphocytes (T cells). Another nonspecific immune response is the release of cytokines from these leukocytes. Cytokines are biochemical substances such as histamine and tumor necrosis factor that stimulate other protective immune functions. In addition, these activated immune system cells may also phagocytize infected host cells to curb the growth and spread of infection. These immune responses are collectively called cell-mediated immunity, which is nonspecific in that it does not involve antibodies specific to a given antigen.

Influenza viruses

Influenza viruses are the Orthomyxoviridae family of viruses, including influenza A and B, which cause the flu—strains of influenza A also cause avian flu (bird flu) and swine flu (H1N1). Seasonal influenza is an acute respiratory infection caused by influenza viruses that occur worldwide. It causes illnesses that range in severity and sometimes lead to hospitalization and death. Most patients recover from fever and other symptoms within a week without

TABLE 48.1 Drugs for influenza infections

Generic names	Trade names	Route of administration
amantadine	Symmetrel	PO
baloxavir	Xofluza	PO
rimantadine	Flumadine	PO
oseltamivir	Tamiflu	PO
peramivir	Rapivab	IV
zanamivir	Relenza	Inhalation

medical attention. However, influenza can cause severe illness or death, particularly among high-risk groups, including infants, older adults, pregnant females, health workers, and those with severe medical conditions. Seasonal epidemics occur mainly during winter, while in tropical regions, influenza may occur throughout the year, causing outbreaks to be more irregular. **Table 48.1** summarizes drugs for influenza infections. Amantadine and rimantadine are no longer recommended for the prevention or treatment of influenza A due to the increasing resistance of the recent circulating strains of the virus.

Oseltamivir

Oseltamivir is an antiviral agent primarily used to treat and prevent influenza A and B viruses. The recommended dosage for treatment is 75 mg orally twice daily for five days in adults and adolescents aged 13 years and older. For prevention, the recommended dose is 75 mg orally once daily for at least 10 days. Oseltamivir can be initiated within 48 hours of symptom onset for treatment and within 48 hours of exposure for prophylaxis.

Pharmacokinetics

Oseltamivir is well absorbed orally and undergoes extensive conversion to its active metabolite, oseltamivir carboxylate, primarily in the liver. The onset of action is typically within 48 hours of initiation. The drug is excreted mainly unchanged in the urine, with a half-life of approximately 6–10 hours in adults with normal renal function. Renal impairment may increase the half-life and require dosage adjustment.

Mechanism of action

Oseltamivir works by inhibiting the neuraminidase enzyme, essential for releasing progeny virus from infected cells. By inhibiting this enzyme, oseltamivir prevents the spread of influenza virus within the respiratory tract.

Clinical indications

Oseltamivir is indicated for treating uncomplicated acute illness due to influenza A or B infection in patients aged 2 weeks and older who have been symptomatic for no more than 48 hours. It is also indicated for preventing influenza in 1-year-old and older patients. The CDC recommends an annual flu shot to help protect people each year from new influenza virus strains.

Contraindications

Oseltamivir is contraindicated in patients with known hypersensitivity to the drug or any component of the formulation. Caution should be exercised in patients with renal impairment.

Adverse effects

Common adverse effects of oseltamivir include nausea, vomiting, and headache. Rare but serious adverse effects may consist of neuropsychiatric events such as delirium, hallucinations, and abnormal behavior, particularly in pediatric patients. These events may occur primarily in the setting of influenza, but some reports have occurred in patients without known influenza infection.

Toxicity

Oseltamivir toxicity is rare but may manifest as neuropsychiatric symptoms or allergic reactions. In case of overdose, supportive care should be provided and symptomatic treatment initiated as necessary. There is no specific antidote for oseltamivir overdose.

Herpes simplex virus

Herpesviridae is a large family of viruses. There are several types, including herpes simplex virus type 1 (HSV-1), HSV-2, varicella-zoster virus, cytomegalovirus, and Epstein-Barr virus. Although there can be anatomic overlap between the two types of HSV, HSV-1, commonly known as oral herpes, affects the mouth and face.

In contrast, HSV-2 infection is most commonly associated with blisters on both male and female genitalia and is referred to as **genital herpes**. HSV-2 infection is most commonly associated with perioral blisters. HSV is highly transmissible through close physical contact. Although antiviral medications are not curative, they can speed up remission and reduce the duration of painful symptoms. This is especially true if the medications are started early in an outbreak. Patients may be prescribed an ongoing lower dose of antiviral drugs to prevent epidemics. HSV infections can become severe, even life-threatening when the patient is immunocompromised or is a newborn infant. Neurological complications of HSV-2 infection in infants include encephalitis, myelitis, and polyradiculopathy. The best strategy to prevent transmission to the newborn infant is usually delivery by **cesarean section** for any mother with active genital herpes lesions.

Varicella-zoster virus is a type of HHV (HHV-3) that commonly causes chickenpox (**varicella**) in childhood, remains **dormant** for many years, and can then reemerge in later adulthood as painful herpes zoster lesions known as **shingles**. The lesions often occur in similar patterns on the body (see **Fig. 48.2**). Chickenpox is usually a self-limiting disease of childhood. It is highly contagious and easily spread by direct contact with broken-down lesions. The most common clinical manifestation is skin lesions that follow nerve tracts, known as **dermatomes**, along the skin surface. Zoster lesions are often quite painful, and some patients require opioids for pain control. In addition, postherpetic **neuralgia** remains following shingles outbreaks in up to 50% of older adult patients. Early administration of antiviral drugs such as acyclovir may speed recovery, but this effect is usually mild. **Table 48.2** summarizes drugs for HHV infections. The varicella virus vaccine is now routinely recommended for healthy children older than 1 year of age who have not had chickenpox. Two vaccines are available to prevent herpes shingles in patients 50 or older.

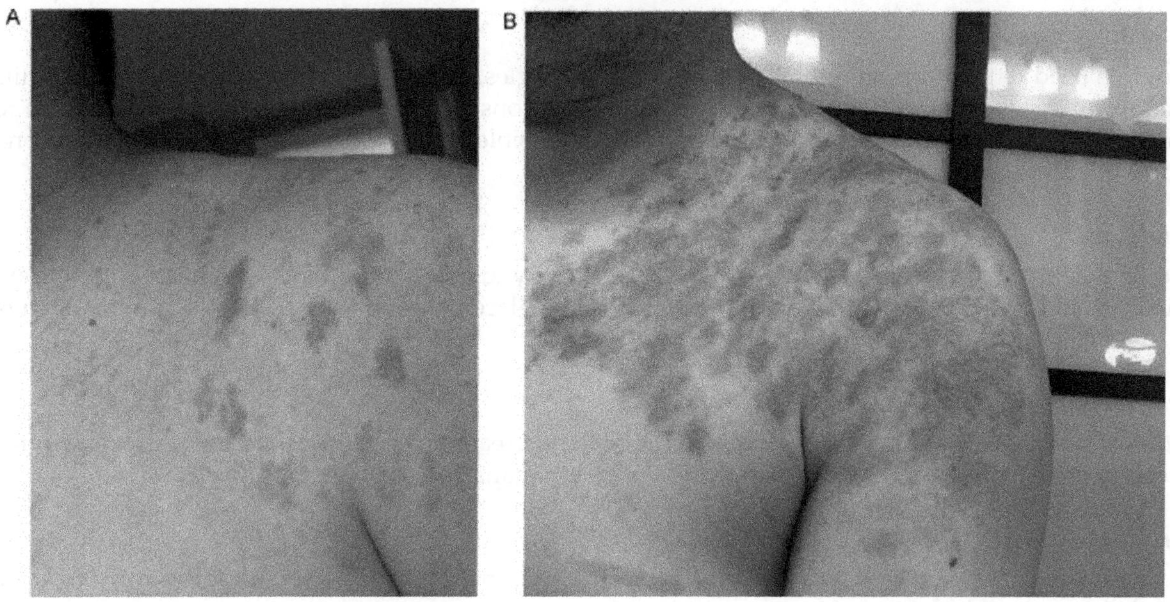

FIG. 48.2 Distribution of shingles on the skin (A) after 1 day and (B) after 6 days.

TABLE 48.2 Drugs for herpesvirus infections

Generic name	Trade name	Route of administration
acyclovir	Zovirax	PO, IV, topical
brincidofovir	Tembexa	PO
cidofovir	Vistide	IV
famciclovir	Famvir	PO
foscarnet	Foscavir	IV
ganciclovir	Cytovene	PO, IV
valacyclovir	Valtrex	PO
valganciclovir	Valcyte	PO
docosanol	Abreva	Topical
penciclovir	Denavir	Topical
trifluridine	Viroptic	Ophthalmic

Acyclovir

Acyclovir is an effective antiviral agent widely used to treat HHV infections. Although generally safe, it can cause acute renal impairment from intratubular crystal deposition when administered intravenously, particularly at high doses. Acyclovir is a drug for treating rare human infections caused by cercopithecine HHV-1 (B virus).

Pharmacokinetics

Acyclovir is slowly and poorly absorbed from the GI tract, and bioavailability decreases with increasing doses. It is widely distributed into tissues, the brain, and body fluids. Plasma protein binding is relatively low at 9%–33%. Acyclovir is eliminated primarily by glomerular filtration with a small addition from tubular secretion.

Mechanism of action

Acyclovir is an antiviral drug that acts as a specific inhibitor of HHV DNA polymerase by acting as an analog to deoxyguanosine triphosphate. Incorporating acyclovir triphosphate into DNA results in chain termination because the absence of a 3′ hydroxyl group prevents the attachment of additional nucleosides.

Clinical indications

Acyclovir is used to treat the symptoms of chickenpox, shingles, and herpes virus infections of the genitals, lips, mouth, skin, and nervous system, as well as herpes virus infections in newborns. It is also used to prevent recurrent genital herpes infections. Acyclovir is best used as soon as possible after the symptoms of herpes infection or shingles occur. This drug cannot cure herpes.

Contraindications

Acyclovir is contraindicated in patients with hypersensitivity to it. It should be used with caution intravenously in patients with kidney disease. It has been shown to cross the placenta but may still be used cautiously in pregnant people.

Adverse effects

The adverse effects of acyclovir taken orally include allergic reactions, headaches, dizziness, confusion, hallucinations, seizures, sensitivity to sunlight, itchy, dry, flaky skin, nausea, vomiting, and diarrhea.

Toxicity

The toxicity of acyclovir may be neurotoxicity, including tremors, myoclonus seizures, **dysarthria**, ataxia, hallucinations, delirium, or coma.

Human papillomaviruses

HPVs are part of the *Papillomaviridae* family of viruses. HPV is a small double-stranded DNA virus that commonly infects humans. The infection is typical in young adults. Viral load and viral type are the primary cofactors, progressing from sickness to cervical intraepithelial lesions and cancer. Smoking, hormonal exposure, and HIV are additional exposures that increase the risk of progression to cancer. They cause *genital warts* (see **Fig. 48.3**). Some types of HPV can lead to cancers. HPV is the most common sexually transmitted infection in the United States. There were about 43 million HPV infections in the United States in 2018, mostly in people in their late teenage years and early 20s. There are many different types of HPV. About 85% of people will get an HPV infection in their lifetime. Vaccinating all 11- to 12-year-old adolescents can protect them long before exposure. The CDC recommends two doses of HPV vaccine for all adolescents at age 11 or 12 years. A two-dose schedule is recommended for people who get the first dose before their 15th birthday. The second dose should be given 6–12 months after the first dose.

A three-dose schedule is recommended for people who get the first dose after their 15th birthday. In a three-dose series, the second dose should be given 1–2 months after the first dose, and the third should be given 6 months after the first dose. The minimum intervals are 4 weeks between the first and second doses, 12 weeks between the second and third doses, and 5 months between the first and third doses. If a vaccine dose is administered after a shorter interval, it should be readministered after another minimum interval has elapsed since the most recent amount. If the vaccination schedule is interrupted, vaccine doses do not need to be repeated (no maximum interval).

HPV immunizations are generally safe in individuals with HIV because they are not live virus vaccines. In those individuals with HIV who have advanced immunosuppression with low CD4 counts, live vaccines can cause a potentially life-threatening disseminated infection because of the live pathogen in the vaccine.

You should remember

The CDC recommends three doses of HPV vaccine (at 0, 1–2, and 6 months apart) for people ages 9 to 26 years if they have certain immunocompromising conditions. People with lower immune responses, such as HIV infection, cancer, transplantation, or autoimmune disease, or taking immunosuppressant medications, should receive three doses to ensure maximum benefit. However, children with asthma, diabetes, and other conditions that do not suppress the immune response to vaccination can receive a two-dose schedule.

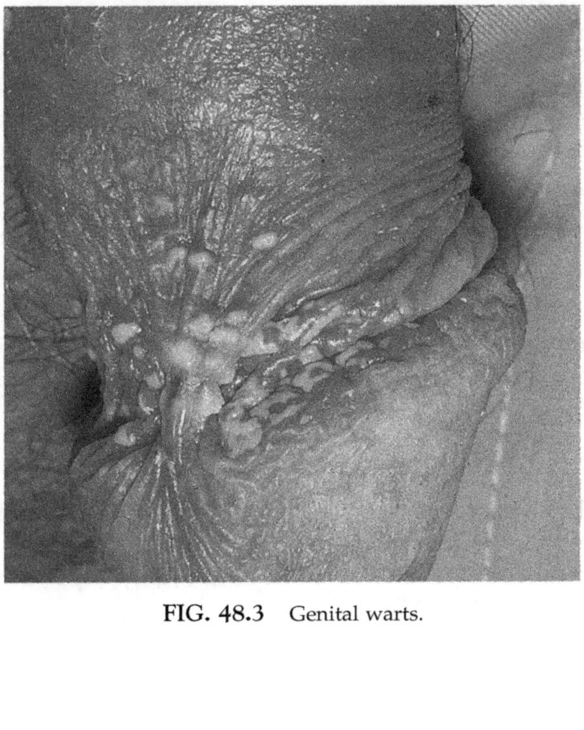

FIG. 48.3 Genital warts.

Viral hepatitis

Hepatitis is liver inflammation that can result in cell damage and liver dysfunction. Several factors, including alcohol abuse, medications, and viruses, can cause hepatitis. Hepatitis can be further characterized as acute or chronic. Acute hepatitis is generally treatable, whereas chronic hepatitis can lead to liver failure. Viral hepatitis includes HepA, HepB, HepC, HepD, and HepE. HepA, HepB, and HepC are the most common types, and we focus on these types in this chapter.

- HepA is caused by a virus that enters the mouth and replicates in the liver. Symptoms occur more often in older children and adults. It is transmitted through the fecal-oral route from contact with an infected person or from ingestion of food or water that has been contaminated. Some affected people have no symptoms and are unaware that they are infected. The incubation periods are between 2 weeks and 6 months after exposure. There may be fatigue, fever, loss of appetite, nausea, vomiting, abdominal pain, light-colored stools, dark urine, jaundice, and joint pain. Symptoms of chronic viral hepatitis may require decades to develop. The HepA vaccine is an inactivated whole-virus vaccine. It is recommended as part of routine immunizations for all children starting at 1 year of age. The series is two doses, with the second given at least 6 months after the first. HepA vaccine is to be administered by intramuscular injection. There are different doses and formulations for children and adults. Two brands are licensed in the United States for children and adults: VAQTA (Merck) and HAVRIX (GlaxoSmithKline). Pediatric formulations are approved for children 12 months to 18 years. The pediatric formulations are 0.5 mL per dose; adult formulations are 1 mL per dose. Contraindications include severe allergic reactions to vaccine components (including neomycin). Individuals with moderate to severe illness should wait until they recover before getting vaccinated. Another vaccine is available as a combination of HepA and HepB called TWINRIX (GlaxoSmithKline). This is a three-dose series given intramuscularly at 0, 1, and 6 months. HepA was routinely recommended as part of childhood immunization in 2006.
- HepB is a viral infection of the liver. The condition can be acute or chronic. Chronic disease can result in cirrhosis, liver failure, and liver cancer. Most adults with HepB recover fully, even with severe symptoms. This is known as a chronic infection. The signs and symptoms of HepB may include fatigue, icterus, abdominal pain, loss of appetite, nausea, vomiting, dark urine, and joint pain. Blood tests, liver ultrasound, and biopsy evaluations confirm chronic HepB. The virus can be found in blood, bodily fluids, semen, and serous fluids. **Papillomaviridae** transmission may include perinatal, sexual contact, and exposure to contaminated needles. In infants infected via perinatal transmission, 90% will become chronically infected with Hep B without postexposure prophylaxis. HepB vaccine is the only vaccine given to babies at birth. It is a recombinant vaccine that is administered via IM injection. Hep B causes about 14,000 new infections annually. Still, about 880,000 adults in the United States are estimated to have chronic HepB. About 66% of infected people are unaware of their condition. In 2020 the rate of new cases was about 12 times higher in Asian Pacific Islanders than in non-Hispanic Caucasians. HepB is one of the leading causes of liver cancer.
- HepC infection has caused an epidemic, with approximately 170 million people infected worldwide and 3–4 million people newly infected each year. An increasing number of patients with cirrhosis will develop **hepatocellular carcinoma**. Unfortunately, there is no vaccine available for HepC. The current standard therapy for HepC consists of pegylated interferon-α, administered once weekly, plus daily oral ribavirin for 24–48 weeks. **Table 48.3** summarizes medicines that are used for viral hepatitis.

Tenofovir

Tenofovir alafenamide (TAF) is an antiviral approved by the FDA for the treatment of chronic HBV in adults and children 12 years of age and certain older patients. There is an older version called tenofovir disoproxil; TAF was reformulated to absorb more quickly, meaning that lower drug levels are in the blood, resulting in fewer kidney- and bone-related side effects.

Pharmacokinetics

TAF has a very low bioavailability when orally administered. Its bioavailability increases by 65% with a high-fat meal. It is eliminated predominantly in the feces (37%) and <1% in the urine by tubular secretion and glomerular filtration. TAF's half-life is 30 minutes. The clearance of tenofovir is highly dependent on the patient's renal function.

TABLE 48.3 Drugs for viral hepatitis

Generic name	Trade name	Route of administration	Indication
adefovir dipivoxil	Hepsera	PO	HBV
elbasvir/grazoprevir	Zepatier	PO	HCV
entecavir	Baraclude	PO	HBV
glecaprevir/pibrentasvir	Mavyret	PO	HCV
lamivudine	Epivir	PO	HBV
sofosbuvir	Sovaldi	PO	HCV
sofosbuvir/velpatasvir	Epclusa	PO	HCV
telbivudine	Tyzeka	PO	HBV
tenofovir alafenamide	Vemlidy	PO	HBV
Peg IFN-α-2a	Pegasys	SC	HCV, HBV

INF-α, Interferon-α.

Mechanism of action

TAF inhibits HBV polymerase, which in turn inhibits DNA synthesis and viral replication of HBV.

Clinical indications

TAF is used to treat chronic HBV infection in patients with compensated liver disease. It is also used against HIV and HSV-2.

Contraindications

TAF has no listed contraindications but should be used cautiously in patients with liver disease other than HepB and kidney disease. In patients with HIV and HBV coinfection, TAF should not be used as a single agent of HIV treatment due to the risk of resistance development.

Adverse effects

Tenofovir's adverse effects include headache, decreased bone mineral density, dizziness, tachycardia, back pain, muscle stiffness, dyspnea, cough, fever, chest pain, chills, skin redness, loss of appetite, and diarrhea.

Toxicity

Administration of high doses of tenofovir has been reported to produce bone toxicity reported as osteomalacia and reduced bone mineral density and to produce some degree of renal toxicity.

Retroviruses

Retroviruses are RNA viruses that use particular proteins to make DNA. Rotavirus infection is a very contagious virus that causes severe diarrhea. Before the development of a vaccine, most children had been infected with the virus at least once by age 5. Since the introduction of routine rotavirus immunization, rotavirus incidence has decreased by about 80% in the United States. Rotavirus gastroenteritis is common in infants and young children. Those under 5 years old are most vulnerable. Early signs and symptoms include fever, abdominal pain, vomiting, and 3–7 days of watery diarrhea.

HIV infection and AIDS

HIV infection is a common and devastating viral infection. There are 39 million people worldwide with HIV infection and over 1.2 million people in the United States. In 2023 there were 34,800 new people who were diagnosed with

HIV in the United States. The rate of infection has decreased since 2016. The most common routes of transmission of HIV are sexual activity, intravenous drug use, and perinatal transfer from mother to child. African Americans have a rate of HIV infection seven times higher than that seen in White Americans. No solid evidence to date confirms transmission of HIV by casual contact, including hugging, kissing, coughing, sneezing, swimming in pools, and sharing of food, water, eating utensils, or toilet facilities. HIV is also not transmitted by insect bites, unlike some other viral illnesses. The risk for transmission to healthcare workers by percutaneous (needlestick) injuries is approximately 0.3%. Performing hand hygiene and maintaining standard precautions to avoid contact with all body fluids during patient care can dramatically reduce the risk of caregiver infection. In accidental exposure, the healthcare professional should receive prophylactic therapy.

Preexposure prophylaxis (PrEP) is an exciting therapy that is given when people are at very high risk for HIV. A combination of tenofovir disoproxil and emtricitabine (Truvada) is FDA approved for daily use as PrEP to help prevent an HIV-negative person from getting HIV from a positive sexual partner or a positive partner who uses injection drugs. Two other FDA-approved PrEP medications are Descovy (TAF and emtricitabine) and a long-acting injection called Apretude (cabotegravir). PrEP is highly effective (up to 90%) in preventing HIV if it is used as prescribed. This is an area in which patient education and adherence are vital. PrEP is much less effective when it is not taken consistently.

HIV is a member of the retrovirus family and RNA viruses and is unique in its use of the enzyme reverse transcriptase during its replication process. This enzyme promotes the synthesis of complementary DNA molecules from the viral RNA genome. A second enzyme, integrase, encourages the integration of this viral DNA into the host cell DNA. This hybrid DNA complex is known as a provirus. It produces new mature HIV virions that infect other host cells. Another important enzyme is protease, which chemically separates the new viral RNA from viral protein molecules. These components are initially synthesized into one significant macromolecular strand, and the protease enzyme carefully breaks up this strand into its essential elements (see **Fig. 48.4**).

HIV infection that is untreated or treatment resistant eventually leads to severe immune system failure, with death occurring secondary to opportunistic infections. Acquired immunodeficiency syndrome (AIDS) often progresses over several years. Various health organizations, including the CDC and the WHO, have published classification systems describing the different "stages" of this infection. The most recent WHO model lists four stages as follows:

- Stage 1: asymptomatic infection
- Stage 2: mild symptoms: early, general symptoms of the disease
- Stage 3: advanced symptoms
- Stage 4: severe symptoms, often leading to death

Patients who are effectively treated with drug therapy usually do not progress through all of these stages, or at least such progression is slowed considerably (by years). Advances in antiretroviral drug therapy have given rise to increasingly more significant numbers of long-term survivors of HIV infection. Highly active antiretroviral therapy (ART) refers to combinations of antiretroviral drugs ("cocktails") that are now standard for treating HIV-infected patients. This combination therapy (highly active ART) is started immediately upon confirmation of HIV infection. Opportunistic infections are treated with infection-specific antimicrobial drugs as they arise. Prophylactic treatment for opportunistic infections is also standard and is most frequently given when a patient's

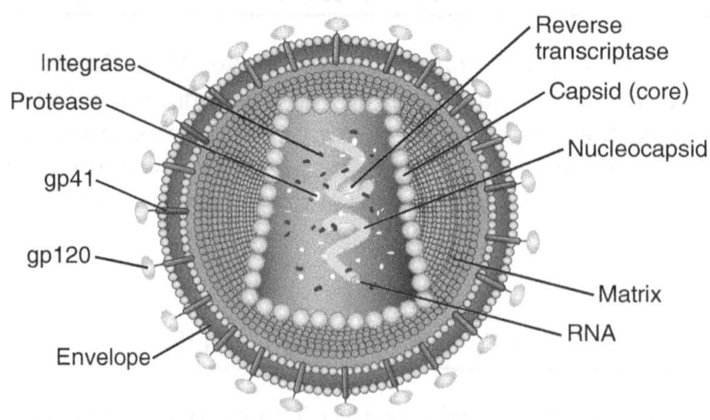

FIG. 48.4 Human immunodeficiency virus.

CD4 count falls below 200 cells/mm^3. Opportunistic malignancies such as **Kaposi sarcoma** and lymphomas are also treated with specific antineoplastic medications and with radiation and surgery as indicated. Long-term survival is defined as living with HIV infection for at least 15 years after infection. **Table 48.1** summarizes antiretroviral drugs used to treat HIV.

TABLE 48.1 Antiretroviral drugs used to treat HIV

Generic name	Trade name	Route of administration
Nucleoside reverse transcriptase inhibitors	Ziagen	PO
abacavir	Epzicom	PO
abacavir/lamivudine	Trizivir	PO
abacavir/zidovudine/lamivudine	Videx EC	PO
didanosine (enteric coated)	Videx	PO
didanosine (dideoxyinosine)	Emtriva	PO
emtricitabine	Epivir	PO
lamivudine	Zerit	PO
stavudine	Viread	PO
tenofovir disoproxil	Descovy	PO
tenofovir alafenamide	Truvada	PO
tenofovir/emtricitabine	Retrovir	PO, IV
zidovudine		
Nonnucleoside reverse transcriptase inhibitors		
delaviridine		
efavirenz	Rescriptor	PO
etravirine	Sustiva	PO
nevirapine	Intelence	PO
	Viramune	PO
Protease inhibitors		
atazanavir	Reyataz	PO
darunavir	Prezista	PO
fosamprenavir	Lexiva	PO
indinavir	Crixivan	PO
lopinavir/ritonavir	Kaletra	PO
nelfinavir	Viracept	PO
ritonavir	Norvir	PO
saquinavir mesylate	Invirase	PO
tipranavir	Aptivus	PO
Fusion inhibitor		
enfuvirtide	Fuzeon	SC
Entry inhibitor		
maraviroc	Selzentry	PO
Capsid inhibitor	Sunlenca	PO, SC
Lenacapavir		
Integrase inhibitors		
Cabotegravir	Apretude	IM
Dolutegravir	Tivicay	PO
Elvitegravir	Vitekta	PO
Raltegravir	Isentress	PO
Combination therapies		
Tenofovir alafenamide/emtricitabine/	Genvoya	PO
elvitegravir/cobicistat	Biktarvy	PO
Tenofovir alafenamide/emtricitabine/bictegravir		

SC, Subcutaneous.

Abacavir

Abacavir is a nucleoside reverse transcriptase inhibitor (NRTI) that is not recommended for use as monotherapy. It can be taken by mouth as a tablet or solution, and it is an approved treatment option for children older than 3 months.

Pharmacokinetics

Abacavir is rapidly and well absorbed following oral administration (83%). About 50% of the drug binds with plasma protein. It is metabolized in the liver, and the half-life is about 2 hours. Abacavir is eliminated from the kidneys and the feces.

Mechanism of action

The effect of abacavir is due to its intracellular anabolite, carbovir triphosphate, which interferes with HIV viral RNA-dependent DNA polymerase, inhibiting viral replication.

Clinical indications

Abacavir is used to treat HIV-1 infection in combination with other antiretroviral drugs. It is commonly used with abacavir/lamivudine/zidovudine, abacavir/dolutegravir/lamivudine, and abacavir/lamivudine.

Contraindications

Abacavir is contraindicated in patients with hypersensitivity to it, people carrying the HLA-B*5701 allele, and those with severe hepatic damage. It should be used with caution in patients with coronary artery disease and patients at increased risk of myocardial infarction due to hyperlipidemia and cardiovascular events.

Adverse effects

Abacavir's adverse effects include fever, cough, headache, rash, tachypnea, abdominal pain, nausea, vomiting, diarrhea, hematuria, and arthralgia.

Toxicities

The primary toxicity associated with abacavir treatment is a potentially life-threatening hypersensitivity reaction.

Didanosine

Didanosine is in the NRTI class and is used in combination with other medicines for the treatment of HIV infection. It cannot cure or prevent HIV infection or AIDS. But it slows down the destruction of the immune system from HIV. This may help delay the development of problems usually related to AIDS or HIV disease. Didanosine inhibits HIV replication by competing with naturally occurring adenosine for incorporation into the growing viral DNA chain, causing inhibition of the viral polymerase and chain termination. Didanosine is an effective and generally well-tolerated drug in previously untreated and ART-experienced patients with HIV infection. Given once or twice daily, it has a vital role as a component of triple-combination regimens for the treatment of patients with symptomatic or asymptomatic HIV infection. Common adverse effects of didanosine include rash, fever, headache, diarrhea, nausea, vomiting, abdominal pain, and **asthenia**. Other adverse effects include severe hypersensitivity reactions, hepatotoxicity, severe metabolic acidosis, peripheral neuropathy, **lipodystrophy,** and pancreatitis.

Emtricitabine

Emtricitabine is in the NRTI class used for the treatment of HIV infection in adults, children, and infants. It is always used in combination with other HIV medicines. Emtricitabine is also used in combination therapy for preexposure prophylaxis to prevent HIV infection. The drug works by inhibiting HIV reverse transcriptase, preventing transcription of HIV RNA to DNA. The adverse effects of emtricitabine are similar to those of other NRTIs and include headache, muscle weakness, arthralgia, fatigue, fever, abdominal pain, nausea, vomiting, diarrhea, depression, anxiety, insomnia, rhinitis, cough, and pharyngitis. One of the specific adverse effects of emtricitabine is hyperpigmentation of the palms and soles, especially in African American patients.

Stavudine

Stavudine is in the NRTI class with activity against type 1 HIV. It is used in combination with other agents in the treatment of HIV infection. Stavudine slows the progression of HIV in those who have advanced symptoms, early symptoms, or no symptoms at all. It helps to decrease the amount of HIV in the body, inhibits the HIV reverse transcriptase enzyme competitively, and acts as a chain terminator of DNA synthesis. Common adverse effects include diarrhea, headache, nausea, vomiting, and rash. Less common but potentially severe adverse reactions include an allergic reaction, pancreatitis hepatotoxicity, tingling in the hands or feet, and peripheral neuropathy.

Tenofovir

Tenofovir is an NRTI used in combination with other drugs to treat HIV. It works for both HIV infection and chronic HepB virus infections. Tenofovir blocks the effectiveness of reverse transcriptase, an enzyme required for each virus to make copies of itself. Blocking reverse transcriptase can reduce the amount of the virus in the blood. The more common adverse effects of tenofovir include headache, nausea, vomiting, rash, back pain, and depression.

Zidovudine

Zidovudine is used for treating HIV-1. It is in the NRTI class of drugs. It was the first medication to be approved by the FDA for the treatment of HIV. The adverse effects of zidovudine include headaches, myalgias, insomnia, nausea, vomiting, diarrhea, lactic acidosis, peripheral myopathy, hepatotoxicity, and bone marrow suppression. Zidovudine is contraindicated for patients with severe life-threatening hypersensitivity reactions to the drug, including anaphylaxis and Stevens-Johnson syndrome. Anaphylaxis may present with dyspnea, diffuse rash, and hypotension. Stevens-Johnson syndrome is an excruciating blistering skin condition. Prompt discontinuation of zidovudine therapy is critical if any of these symptoms arise.

Nevirapine

Nevirapine is a drug used in the management and treatment of HIV. It is in the non-NRTI class of medications and is utilized in conjunction with other ART agents. This medication often is used as part of newborn antiretroviral regimens to prevent perinatal transmission of HIV. Nevirapine can cause severe, life-threatening liver impairment and allergic reactions. The adverse effects include fever, sore throat, chills, rash, fatigue, nausea, loss of appetite, vomiting, hematuria, pale stools, jaundice, stomach pain, arthralgia, edema of the face, dysphasia, hoarseness, and dyspnea.

Darunavir

Darunavir is in the class of protease inhibitors (PIs). It is used in combination with ritonavir and other drugs for the treatment of HIV. As a second-generation PI, darunavir is designed to combat resistance to standard HIV therapy. The adverse effects of darunavir include loss of appetite, nausea, myalgia, arthralgia, and dark urine. Body fat redistribution may occur. Hypersensitivity reactions may also occur with use; darunavir must be discontinued in these cases. This medication should be used with caution in patients with severe liver disease, hypokalemia, and hypomagnesemia.

Fosamprenavir

Fosamprenavir is in the class of PIs. It is an antiretroviral agent used for the treatment and postexposure prophylaxis of HIV-1 infection. It may slow down the destruction of the immune system caused by HIV or delay the complications of AIDS. However, this medicine cannot cure or prevent HIV infection. The adverse effects of fosamprenavir include chills, fever, white spots in the mouth, sore throat, skin rash, bruising, itching, sweating, fatigue, chest pain, cough, nausea, vomiting, diarrhea, back pain, and hematuria.

Indinavir

Indinavir is an antiretroviral PI used for the treatment and prevention of HIV infection and AIDS. The FDA approved indinavir in 1996, as it was among the first HIV PIs authorized in the United States. Indinavir has decreased the likelihood of death due to AIDS progression. It is no longer available in the United States or Europe, as it has many adverse effects, and there are better drugs.

Lopinavir/ritonavir

Lopinavir/ritonavir is a PI structurally related to ritonavir. The FDA approved it as a coformulation with ritonavir under the brand name Kaletra.

Pharmacokinetics

Lopinavir is poorly absorbed orally due to its high first-pass metabolism. It is administered with ritonavir to increase its plasma concentration and prolong its half-life. Both medications are highly protein bound (>98%) and primarily metabolized by the liver via CYP3A4 enzymes. Both components are mainly eliminated in the feces, with some excretion in the urine.

Mechanism of action

Lopinavir/ritonavir works by the lopinavir component binding to the catalytic site of the HIV protease, thereby preventing the cleavage of viral polyprotein precursors into mature, functional proteins necessary for viral replication. The result is the formation of immature, noninfectious viral particles. The ritonavir component inhibits the CYP3A metabolism of lopinavir, allowing increased plasma levels of lopinavir.

Clinical indications

Lopinavir/ritonavir is specifically used for the treatment of HIV-1 infection in adults and children 2 weeks and older. It is no longer recommended as a component of initial therapy for the treatment of HIV due to the release of integrase inhibitor combination products.

Contraindications

Lopinavir/ritonavir is contraindicated in patients with hypersensitivity, dysrhythmia, **porphyria**, pancreatitis, diabetes mellitus, heart disease, and **hemophilia**. Other adverse effects include diarrhea, dyslipidemia, and hepatic disorders.

Adverse effects

It can cause severe, life-threatening adverse effects, which include allergic reactions such as toxic epidermal necrolysis, Stevens-Johnson syndrome, liver impairment, pancreatitis, hyperglycemia, hypertriglyceridemia, uremia, hyperbilirubinemia, dysrhythmia, and skin rash. Other possible adverse effects include headache, fatigue, abdominal pain, nausea, and diarrhea. Coadministration with drugs that are CYP3A inducers may decrease lopinavir plasma concentrations, resulting in the potential loss of virologic response and possible development of resistance.

Toxicities

The toxicity of lopinavir/ritonavir includes liver impairment, pancreatitis, dysrhythmia, severe skin rash, allergic reactions, and drug interactions.

Ritonavir

Ritonavir is a PI used together with other medicines for the treatment of HIV infection and AIDS in adults and children. It may delay the complications of AIDS or HIV infection from occurring. Ritonavir cannot prevent HIV from spreading to other people. Ritonavir binds to the protease active site and inhibits the enzyme's activity. This inhibition prevents cleavage of the viral polyproteins. The adverse effects of ritonavir include nausea, vomiting, abdominal pain, diarrhea, rhabdomyolysis, malaise, dizziness, hyperlipidemia, hypertriglyceridemia, and insomnia. Ritonavir contraindications include patients with a known allergic reaction to the medication. Hypersensitivity reactions may result in toxic epidermal necrolysis and Stevens-Johnson syndrome.

Tipranavir

Tipranavir is a PI that is used to treat HIV-1 when it is resistant to more than one PI. It is a sulfonamide-containing dihydropyran and a nonpeptidic PI that targets the HIV protease. It is administered along with ritonavir to treat HIV.

Pharmacokinetics

CYP3A metabolizes tipranavir. When combined with ritonavir in vitro, it inhibits CYP1A2, CYP2C9, CYP2C19, CYP2D6, and CYP3A in addition to inducing glucuronidase and the drug transporter P-glycoprotein.

Mechanism of action

Tipranavir inhibits the processing of the viral Gag and Gag-Pol polyproteins in HIV-1-infected cells, preventing the formation of mature virions. It binds to the active site of the protease enzyme with fewer hydrogen bonds than peptidic PIs, resulting in increased flexibility and better adjustment to amino acid substitutions at the active site. The drug's strong hydrogen-bonding interaction with the amide backbone of the protease active site Asp30 may lead to its activity against resistant viruses.

Clinical indications

Tipranavir is indicated for combination antiretroviral treatment of HIV-1-infected adult patients with evidence of viral replication who are highly treatment experienced or have HIV-1 strains resistant to multiple PIs.

Contraindications

Tipranavir is contraindicated in patients with modern or severe hepatic impairment. Extreme caution should be utilized in patients with chronic HepB or HepC coinfection with HIV. It is also contraindicated for use with drugs that are highly dependent on CYP3A for clearance or are potent CYP3A inducers.

Adverse effects

The most common adverse effects in adults are abdominal pain, diarrhea, nausea, vomiting, **pyrexia**, fatigue, and headache. It may also lead to high triglyceride or cholesterol levels or increased liver transaminases. The most frequent adverse effects in children are similar to those seen in adults, but the rash is more common than in adults.

Toxicities

Tipranavir toxicities may cause thirst, hunger, unexplained weight loss, increased urination, fatigue, and itchy and dry skin.

Enfuvirtide

Enfuvirtide is a medication administered subcutaneously for the treatment of HIV infection in adults and children 6 years of age or older, weighing at least 24 lb, whose infection is not well controlled by ongoing treatment with other HIV medicines.

Pharmacokinetics

Enfuvirtide reaches peak serum concentration 8 hours after subcutaneous administration. Its half-life is approximately 4 hours. As a peptide, it undergoes catabolism to its component amino acids.

Mechanism of action

Enfuvirtide is a fusion inhibitor that interferes with the penetration of HIV-1 in body cells. It has potent, selective inhibition of the membranes of viruses and cells, explicitly inhibiting the function of the gp41 transmembrane glycoprotein of HIV-1.

Clinical indications

Enfuvirtide injection is indicated for use to treat HIV-1 infection in combination with other antiviral agents in patients previously treated with other HIV medications but with evidence of HIV-1 replication despite being on ART.

Contraindications

Enfuvirtide is contraindicated in patients with known hypersensitivity reactions. It should be used with caution in patients with coagulation disorders or those who have rash, hypotension, and elevated serum liver transaminases, as those symptoms may represent a hypersensitivity reaction to the medication.

Adverse effects

Enfuvirtide may cause itching, swelling, pain, tingling, discomfort, tenderness, redness, bruising, or pain at the injection site. It may also cause tiredness, myalgia, nausea, loss of appetite, weight loss, stomach pain, nausea, diarrhea, arm or leg pain, flulike symptoms, nasal congestion, cold sores, dry mouth, eye pain, itching, redness, or tearing.

Toxicities

Local injection site reactions, including pain and discomfort, induration, erythema, nodules, cysts, pruritus, and ecchymosis, signify enfuvirtide toxicity. Reactions are usually mild to moderate but can be more severe and may represent hypersensitivity to the drug.

Entry Inhibitors and Integrase Inhibitors

Entry inhibitors are a relatively new class of antiretroviral medications for treating HIV-1 infections. They are also known as fusion inhibitors and are used in combination therapy. Patients with HIV who have become resistant to NRTIs, non-NRTIs, and PIs will likely benefit from entry inhibitors because they are a different class of drugs. Currently, there are several entry inhibitors that the FDA has approved for HIV treatment. An example is maraviroc, where adverse effects include fever, chills, cough, rash, fatigue, dizziness, nausea, and diarrhea.

Integrase inhibitors are therapeutic medications active against both HIV-1 and HIV-2. They are now a preferred drug class for HIV treatment. They were discovered in 2007. The HIV-1 integrase is the main enzyme in the replication mechanism of retroviruses. It transfers virally encoded DNA into the host chromosome, a necessary event in retroviral replication. These drugs destroy the virus over time, especially newer integrase inhibitors such as dolutegravir, bictegravir, and cabotegravir. Older integrase inhibitors, including raltegravir and elvitegravir, have shown some resistance to HIV. The adverse effects of integrase inhibitors include mouth lesions, fatigue, fever, nausea, loss of appetite, and hematuria.

Dolutegravir

Dolutegravir is a medication approved for the treatment of HIV infection in adults and children weighing at least 30 kg who are at least 12 years old, either as a stand-alone therapy or in combination with other antiretroviral agents.

Pharmacokinetics

Dolutegravir exhibits rapid absorption, with peak plasma concentrations reaching approximately 2–3 hours after oral administration. Its half-life ranges from 12–14 hours, allowing for once-daily dosing. UDP-glucuronosyltransferase 1A1 primarily metabolizes dolutegravir and is consequently eliminated through feces and urine.

Mechanism of action

Dolutegravir is an integrase inhibitor that interferes with the integration of viral DNA into the host genome, thereby inhibiting HIV replication. It selectively inhibits the catalytic activity of the HIV-1 integrase enzyme, preventing the incorporation of viral genetic material into human chromosomal DNA.

Clinical indications

Dolutegravir is indicated for the treatment of type 1 HIV infection in treatment-naive individuals and those who have previously received ART. It is also used for PrEP to reduce the risk of sexually acquired HIV-1 infection in high-risk adults.

Contraindications

Dolutegravir is contraindicated in individuals with known hypersensitivity reactions to the drug. It should be used with caution in patients with severe hepatic impairment.

Adverse effects

Common adverse effects associated with dolutegravir include headache, insomnia, fatigue, nausea, diarrhea, and abnormal dreams. Additionally, it may cause hypersensitivity reactions, hepatotoxicity, and immune reconstitution syndrome. Rare but serious side effects include severe skin reactions, liver problems, and psychiatric symptoms.

Toxicities

Dolutegravir toxicity primarily manifests as neuropsychiatric adverse effects such as insomnia, abnormal dreams, and mood changes. Additionally, there have been reports of hypersensitivity reactions, hepatic toxicities, and metabolic abnormalities in some patients.

Coronavirus

Coronaviruses are a subfamily of viruses. Severe acute respiratory syndrome coronavirus 2 (SARS-CoV-2), the virus that causes COVID-19, is the most well-known coronavirus. But other types of coronaviruses cause mild illnesses, like a cold. Coronaviruses usually cause mild to moderate upper respiratory symptoms like the common cold. However, three new coronaviruses have emerged from animal reservoirs over the past 20 years and have caused severe and widespread illness and death throughout the world. COVID-19 was first reported as manifesting late in 2019 in Wuhan, China. Since then, it has spread across the globe. Today, COVID-19 has 702,779,668 global cases and 6,979,269 deaths. In the United States alone, there are 103,436,829 cases and over 1 million deaths. While there have been rare cases of COVID-19 spreading between animals and humans, more often, the spread is via close person-to-person contact, primarily via respiratory droplets. The virus can also spread via contact with contaminated surfaces. The highest level of contagion is several days before and after symptom onset because the viral load is most significant in respiratory secretions. High risks of transmission are within nursing homes, long-term care facilities, jails and prisons, ships, churches, gymnasiums, drinking and eating establishments, and meatpacking facilities.

The new version of coronavirus called SARS-CoV-2 causes COVID-19. The virus spreads quickly within 6 feet by respiratory droplets that can be inhaled or enter another person's mouth, nose, or eyes. Sometimes the virus spreads from exposure to droplets or aerosols in the air that remain there for minutes to hours—known as airborne transmission. Most patients with COVID-19 may have a few symptoms or none. However, severe illnesses and deaths have occurred—primarily in older adults, those who smoke, and those with concurrent cancer, diabetes mellitus, obesity, immunocompromise, sickle cell disease, and diseases of the heart, kidneys, liver, or lungs. Serious complications may include acute respiratory distress syndrome, arrhythmias, cardiomyopathy, acute myocarditis, thromboembolism, pulmonary emboli, disseminated intravascular coagulation, and sepsis. The duration and effectiveness of immunity after having contracted COVID-19 are unknown. Most patients develop neutralizing antibodies that appear to wane over time.

Treatment of COVID-19 is supportive primarily for mild to moderate cases, and treatment is based on disease severity. The severity levels are mild, moderate, severe, and critical. Supportive treatment includes vital care management, mechanical ventilation, corticosteroids, immunomodulators, and vasopressors. Two medications, remdesivir and nirmatrelvir/ritonavir, are FDA approved for treating COVID-19. Molnupiravir is authorized to treat COVID-19 under emergency use authorization.

Remdesivir

Remdesivir is a prescription medication approved for the treatment of COVID-19 in adults and pediatric patients (12 years of age and older, weighing at least 40 kg) who require hospitalization for the management of severe COVID-19 illness or in nonhospitalized patients who are at high risk of progression to severe disease.

Pharmacokinetics

Remdesivir is administered intravenously and rapidly distributed throughout the body. Following administration, it is metabolized into its active form, GS-441524, which exhibits antiviral activity against RNA viruses. The half-life of remdesivir is approximately 1 hour, while the half-life of GS-441524 is around 24 hours. Remdesivir and its metabolites are primarily eliminated from the kidney.

Mechanism of action

Remdesivir acts as a nucleotide analog prodrug that inhibits viral RNA polymerases, preventing the replication of RNA viruses such as SARS-CoV-2. By incorporating into viral RNA chains, remdesivir disrupts viral RNA synthesis, ultimately inhibiting viral replication and reducing viral load in infected individuals.

Clinical indications

Remdesivir is indicated for treating COVID-19 in hospitalized patients who require supplemental oxygen, mechanical ventilation, or extracorporeal membrane oxygenation. It is used to shorten the time to recovery in these individuals and is not recommended for patients with mild illness who do not require hospitalization. It may be administered outside of the hospital to people who are at high risk for progression to severe COVID-19 disease.

Contraindications

Remdesivir is contraindicated in individuals with known hypersensitivity to the drug or any of its components. It should be used with caution in patients with severe renal or hepatic impairment.

Adverse effects

Common adverse effects include nausea, vomiting, diarrhea, and elevated liver enzymes. Additionally, remdesivir may cause an infusion-related reaction characterized by low blood pressure, nausea, vomiting, sweating, and shivering.

Toxicities

The most significant toxicity associated with remdesivir is hepatic dysfunction, which may manifest as elevated liver enzymes and hepatotoxicity. Patients should be monitored regularly for signs of liver injury, and treatment should be discontinued if significant liver function abnormalities occur.

Nirmatrelvir/ritonavir

Nirmatrelvir/ritonavir (Paxlovid) is a medication indicated for the treatment of mild to moderate COVID-19 in individuals who are at high risk for progression to severe disease, including those aged 12 years and older and weighing at least 40 kg (approximately 88 lb).

Pharmacokinetics

Nirmatrelvir/ritonavir is an oral medication comprising two active ingredients. Nirmatrelvir is a SARS-CoV-2 PI, while ritonavir is a pharmacokinetic enhancer that inhibits CYP3A-mediated metabolism to increase nirmatrelvir's plasma concentration. Following oral administration, peak plasma concentrations of nirmatrelvir are reached within approximately 2–4 hours. Both nirmatrelvir and ritonavir undergo hepatic metabolism primarily by CYP3A enzymes.

Mechanism of action

Nirmatrelvir/ritonavir inhibits the activity of the SARS-CoV-2 main protease (3CL protease), which is essential for viral replication. Blocking this enzyme interferes with the virus's ability to replicate and spread within the body, reducing viral load and mitigating disease progression.

Clinical indications

Nirmatrelvir/ritonavir is indicated for the treatment of mild to moderate COVID-19 in individuals aged 12 years and older who are at high risk for progression to severe disease. This includes individuals with certain underlying medical conditions or those who are immunocompromised.

Contraindications

Nirmatrelvir/ritonavir is contraindicated in patients with known hypersensitivity to nirmatrelvir, ritonavir, or any excipients in the formulation. It is also contraindicated in patients with severe hepatic impairment or those who are taking medications that are potent CYP3A inhibitors or inducers.

Adverse effects

Common adverse effects associated with nirmatrelvir/ritonavir include diarrhea, nausea, and vomiting. Ritonavir may cause GI upset, headache, fatigue, and elevated liver enzymes.

Toxicities

The most notable toxicity associated with nirmatrelvir/ritonavir is hepatotoxicity, characterized by elevated liver enzymes. Patients should be monitored for signs of liver injury, and treatment should be discontinued if significant liver function abnormalities occur. Additionally, it may interact with other medications, particularly those metabolized by CYP3A enzymes, requiring dose adjustments or avoidance of concomitant use.

Molnupiravir

Molnupiravir is an oral antiviral medication developed for the treatment of COVID-19 in adults who have tested positive for the virus and are at high risk for severe illness.

Pharmacokinetics

Molnupiravir is rapidly absorbed after oral administration, reaching peak plasma concentrations within 2–4 hours. Its half-life is approximately 20 hours. Molnupiravir is metabolized in the liver primarily by hydrolysis and is excreted mainly through urine and feces.

Mechanism of action

Molnupiravir is a prodrug metabolized in the body to the active form, NHC (β-D-N4-hydroxycytidine). NHC works by causing errors in viral RNA replication during the virus's life cycle, ultimately leading to viral mutagenesis and inhibition of viral replication.

Clinical indications

Molnupiravir is indicated for the treatment of mild to moderate COVID-19 in adults who have tested positive for the virus and are at high risk for progression to severe illness. It is not recommended for use in individuals with severe renal or hepatic impairment.

Contraindications

Molnupiravir is contraindicated in pregnant individuals due to potential fetal harm based on animal studies. It is also contraindicated in individuals with a history of hypersensitivity to molnupiravir.

Adverse effects

Common adverse effects associated with molnupiravir include nausea, diarrhea, headache, and fatigue. It may also cause increases in liver enzymes, although severe hepatotoxicity is rare.

Toxicities

Molnupiravir toxicity may manifest as gastrointestinal symptoms, including nausea, vomiting, and diarrhea. Patients should be monitored for signs of liver dysfunction, and treatment should be discontinued if significant liver enzyme elevations occur. Additionally, the potential for teratogenicity in pregnant individuals underscores the importance of contraception during and after treatment with molnupiravir.

You should remember

There are three antiviral therapies indicated for the treatment of COVID-19 infection. Nirmatrelvir/ritonavir and molnupiravir are oral antiviral medications used to treat mild to moderate COVID-19 infection in high-risk individuals. Remdesivir is indicated for hospitalized or nonhospitalized COVID-19 patients with a high risk of progression to severe disease.

Key Terms

Capsid
Cesarean section
Dormant
Ecchymosis
Genital herpes
Genome
Hepatocellular carcinoma
Human papillomaviruses
Induration
Neuralgia
Pyrexia
Shingles
Varicella
Virion
Warts

Clinical Case Studies

Clinical Case Study 1

A 41-year-old male with no significant medical history presented with altered mental status, fever, and general fatigue. There was considerable neck stiffness. Laboratory tests revealed highly elevated CRP and leukocytosis. Bacterial meningitis was initially suspected, and medications were administered. The patient was admitted to the ICU and intubated. Additional tests revealed the patient to have a severe HSV-2 infection, which had caused myelitis. Treatment with acyclovir and prednisolone was successful.

Critical Thinking Questions

1. What are the clinical indications of acyclovir?
2. What are the contraindications of acyclovir?
3. What are the adverse effects of acyclovir?

Clinical Case Study 2

A 38-year-old female was complaining of constant fatigue, nausea, muscle aches, and mild pain in the right upper quadrant. Blood tests, liver ultrasound, and biopsy evaluations confirm chronic HepB. There is no history of vaccination for HepB. The patient admitted to being an alcoholic for many years. Treatment begins with TAF.

Critical Thinking Questions

1. What are the differences between TAF and tenofovir disoproxil?
2. What are the pharmacokinetics of tenofovir?
3. What are the adverse effects of tenofovir?

Clinical Case Study 3

A 37-year-old male with HIV infection and AIDS on zidovudine for 7 months and didanosine for 4 months developed abdominal pain, nausea, vomiting, diarrhea, and dyspnea. Blood testing showed severe metabolic acidosis. Serum bilirubin and enzymes were only modestly elevated. The patient had no history of liver or biliary tract disease or alcohol abuse. Tests for viral hepatitis were negative. Despite intensive support, mechanical ventilation, bicarbonate therapy, and dialysis, he developed progressive hepatic and multiorgan failure and died 1 week after admission.

Critical Thinking Questions

1. What is the mechanism of action for didanosine?
2. What are the common adverse effects of didanosine?
3. What are the contraindications of zidovudine?

Further Reading

[1] J. Adams, V.J. Merluzzi, The Search for Antiviral Drugs – Case Histories from Concept to Clinic, Birkhauser, 2013.
[2] American Academy of HIV Medicine, W.D. Hardy, Fundamentals of HIV Medicine 2023, Oxford University Press, 2023.
[3] E. De Clercq, R.T. Walker, Antiviral Drug Development – A Multidisciplinary Approach (NATO Science Series A: 143), Springer, 2012.
[4] A. Gholamrezanezhad, M.P. Dube, Coronavirus Disease 2019 (Covid-19) – A Clinical Guide, Wiley-Blackwell, 2023.
[5] L. Jefferson, Human Papillomavirus (HPV) 1 – Unlocking the Secrets of HPV – your Roadmap to Health and Empowerment, Jefferson, 2023.
[6] W.M. Kazmierski, Antiviral Drugs – from Basic Discovery Through Clinical Trials, Wiley, 2012.
[7] K. Lee, The History of HIV/AIDS – Discovery and Early Cases – from Patient Zero to Millions – HIV/AIDS Awareness, Lee, 2023.
[8] J.J. Li, Conquest of Invisible Enemies – A Human History of Antiviral Drugs, Oxford University Press, 2022.
[9] X. Liu, P. Zhan, L. Menendez-Arias, V. Poongavanam, Antiviral Drug Discovery and Development (Advances in Experimental Medicine and Biology, Book 1322), Springer, 2021.
[10] B.T. Rouse, C.W. Dence, Herpes simplex Virus – Pathogenesis, Immunobiology and Control (Current Topics in Microbiology and Immunology, 179), Springer, 2011.
[11] E. Sandler, Antiviral Drugs – from Basic Discovery Through Clinical Trials, Hayle Medical, 2023.
[12] A.M. Skalka, Discovering Retroviruses – Beacons in the Biosphere, Harvard University Press, 2018.
[13] H.C. Thomas, A.S. Lok, S.A. Locarnini, A.J. Zuckerman, Viral Hepatitis, fourth ed., Pearson/Wiley-Blackwell, 2013.
[14] V.G. Wilson, Viruses – Intimate Invaders, Springer, 2022.

CHAPTER

49

Antibacterial drugs

OUTLINE

The Science of Pharmacology
https://doi.org/10.1016/B978-0-443-29038-1.00049-X

LEARNING OUTCOMES

After study of the chapter, readers should be able to:

1. Identify the classifications of penicillins.
2. Explain the contraindications of penicillins.
3. Identify the broad-spectrum and extended-spectrum penicillins.
4. Explain the categories of cephalosporins.
5. Discuss the adverse effects of vancomycin.
6. Describe the contraindications of tetracyclines.
7. Explain the adverse effects of fluoroquinolones.
8. Describe the clinical indications of fluoroquinolones.
9. Explain the categories of macrolides.
10. Describe the adverse effects of macrolides.

Overview

Antibiotics can treat or prevent most bacterial infections. They are not effective against viral infections or other infections. They work by killing bacteria or stopping them from spreading. However, many mild bacterial infections get better on their own without using antibiotics. Each antibiotic is effective only against certain types of bacteria. When selecting an antibiotic to treat a patient with an infection, the cause must be detected. For example, some infections are caused only by certain types of bacteria. Because of the widespread use and misuse of antibiotics, bacteria may survive and develop resistance to the effects of the antibiotic. For example, 50 years ago, *Staphylococcus aureus* was susceptible to penicillin. However, over time, strains of this bacteria developed an enzyme able to break down penicillin, making the drug ineffective. Researchers responded by creating a form of penicillin that the enzyme could not break down, but after a few years, the bacteria adapted and became resistant to this modified penicillin. Other bacteria have also developed resistance to various antibiotics.

Penicillins

Penicillins are some of the most commonly prescribed antibiotics. This group includes many individual medications such as penicillin G, penicillin V, amoxicillin, ampicillin, nafcillin, oxacillin, dicloxacillin, carbenicillin, cloxacillin, ticarcillin, and piperacillin/tazobactam (see **Table 49.1**).

Some bacteria produce enzymes that can inactivate **s** antibiotics. Therefore beta-lactamase inhibitors such as clavulanate or sulbactam, along with specific penicillins to inhibit these enzymes, are given. Typical combinations of penicillin for these purposes include the following:

- Ampicillin/sulbactam
- Amoxicillin/clavulanate
- Piperacillin/tazobactam

Pharmacokinetics

The liver does not metabolize most penicillin derivatives. Oral or injection have different bioavailabilities. Penicillin is rapidly excreted in the urine as water soluble; some are in bile. Penicillin has a relatively short half-life of about 2 hours.

TABLE 49.1 Various penicillins.

Generic names	Brand names	Route of administration
penicillin G	Pen G	IM, IV
penicillin V	Veetids	PO
amoxicillin	Amoxil	PO, IV[a]
ampicillin	Omnipen	PO, IM, IV
nafcillin	Unipen, Nallpen	IM, IV
oxacillin	Bactocill	IM, IV
dicloxacillin	Dycill, Dynapen	PO
carbenicillin[a]	Geocillin	PO
cloxacillin[a]	Cloxapen, Orbenin	PO, IM, IV
piperacillin/ tazobactam	Zosyn	IV

[a]*Not available in the United States.*

Mechanism of action

Penicillins inhibit bacterial transpeptidase enzymes involved in synthesizing the bacterial cell wall. These enzymes are called penicillin-binding proteins. Penicillins prevent these enzymes from creating cross-links between peptide chains in the cell wall. Subsequently, penicillins activate the bacteria's endogenous autolytic system, leading to cell lysis and death. Beta-lactamase inhibitors prevent the degradation of the beta-lactam ring in penicillin, which can occur when certain species of bacteria express the enzyme beta-lactamase.

Penicillin V and penicillin VK are orally administered as a solution for reconstitution and tablets, respectively. Penicillin V has a bioavailability of around 65% after passing stomach acid. It is excreted in urine by tubular secretion. Approximately 20%–65% of an oral dose is excreted in urine as unchanged drug and metabolites within 6–8 hours; small amounts are removed in feces and bile.

Clinical indications

Penicillin is one of the most commonly used antibiotics globally; it has a wide range of clinical indications. It is effective against infections involving gram-positive cocci, gram-positive rods, most anaerobes, and gram-negative cocci such as *Neisseria*. Certain bacterial species have obtained penicillin resistance, including enterococci. Enterococci infections now receive treatment with a combination of penicillin and either ceftriaxone or gentamicin. Specific gram-negative bacteria are also resistant to penicillin. However, later generations of broad-spectrum penicillins are effective against gram-negative bacteria. Second-generation penicillins (ampicillin and amoxicillin) are effective against *Proteus mirabilis, Shigella, Haemophilus influenzae, Salmonella,* and *Escherichia coli.* Third-generation penicillins such as carbenicillin are used for gram-negative bacteria. Fourth-generation penicillins such as piperacillin are effective against the same bacterial strains as third-generation penicillins and *Klebsiella*, enterococci, *Pseudomonas aeruginosa,* and *Bacteroides fragilis*. Penicillin has a limited crossing of the **blood-brain barrier** and can only treat a few bacterial meningitis infections. The most common indications for penicillin G include pneumonia, strep throat, staph infection, diphtheria, meningitis, gonorrhea, and syphilis.

Contraindications

Contraindications of penicillin include a previous history of severe allergic reactions to penicillin. It should be avoided in patients with **Stevens-Johnson syndrome**. The penicillins are safe to use during pregnancy and nursing. Penicillin has an antagonistic effect with tetracycline, and there is a greater risk for mortality when treating pneumococcal meningitis than using penicillin alone.

Adverse effects

The adverse effects of penicillins G and V include rash, urticaria, nausea, vomiting, diarrhea, and abdominal pain. In addition, penicillin G can have other adverse reactions, including fever, chills, headache, tachypnea, tachycardia, hypotension, flushing, and muscle spasms. Hypersensitivity reactions with penicillin often occur. The reaction happens within 20 minutes postadministration. It is manifested by laryngospasm, urticaria, bronchospasm, edema, pruritis, hypotension, vascular collapse, and death. Penicillin injection reactions are treated with corticosteroids, epinephrine injection (EpiPen), antihistamines, bronchodilators, and immunotherapy (desensitization).

Toxicities

Penicillin toxicity is rare compared to other antibiotics. It can be administered at high doses without harming patients. However, penicillin can cause local toxicity due to high-dose injections at sensitive sites such as the eye's anterior chamber or the **subarachnoid space**.

You should remember

Penicillin G can be administered either intravenously or intramuscularly. It is available in 1 million units, 5 million units, and 20 million units per vial. Because stomach acid degrades penicillin G more quickly and has less than 30% bioavailability, it is a parenterally administered drug. Because of the short half-life, penicillin G is usually administered in divided doses 4–6 hours apart.

Aminopenicillins

The aminopenicillins are semisynthetic modifications of natural penicillin with a broader spectrum of activity effective against gram-positive and gram-negative bacteria. Natural penicillin is effective chiefly against gram-positive organisms. Aminopenicillins are also effective against certain **rickettsiae**, giant viruses, and **protozoa**. These antibiotics include amoxicillin, amoxicillin/clavulanic acid, ampicillin, and ampicillin/sulbactam. Adding a beta-lactamase inhibitor results in much greater efficacy against gram-negative organisms and some β-lactamase-producing gram-positive and anaerobic organisms.

Extended-spectrum penicillins

The extended-spectrum penicillins are less active against gram-positive and anaerobic organisms than penicillin G, but they have much greater efficacy against gram-negative species, including *P. aeruginosa*. Extended-spectrum penicillins include piperacillin/tazobactam and ticarcillin/clavulanate.

Penicillinase-resistant penicillins

Penicillinase-resistant penicillins, also known as antistaphylococcal penicillins, are antibiotics that are not inactivated by the penicillinase enzyme. Some bacteria produce the enzyme penicillinase that destroys the beta-lactam ring of the antibiotic, making penicillin ineffective. Penicillinase-resistant penicillins are used to treat resistant strains of staphylococci and other infections. Specific conditions, which include **endocarditis**, bacteremia, meningitis, pneumonia, osteomyelitis, cystitis, and pharyngitis, can be treated with penicillinase-resistant penicillins. Penicillinase-resistant penicillins include nafcillin, cloxacillin, oxacillin, and dicloxacillin.

Cephalosporins

Cephalosporins are beta-lactam antimicrobials used to treat infections from gram-positive and gram-negative bacteria. The five generations of cephalosporins are helpful against meningitis, skin infection, resistant bacteria, and other infections. First-generation cephalosporins are used against most gram-positive cocci and some gram-negative bacteria, including *E. coli, Klebsiella pneumoniae,* and *P. mirabilis*. Second-generation cephalosporins are helpful against *H. influenzae, Moraxella catarrhalis,* and *Bacteroides* species. Third-generation cephalosporins have less activity against most gram-positive organisms but have increased coverage against *Neisseria species*, enterobacteriaceae, and *H. influenzae*. Fourth-generation cephalosporins have a similar scope to third-generation cephalosporins but with additional coverage against gram-negative bacteria with antimicrobial resistance, for example, those with beta-lactamases. Fifth-generation cephalosporins have coverage against methicillin-resistant staphylococci and penicillin-resistant pneumococci.

First-generation cephalosporins include cefazolin, cephalothin, cephapirin, cephradine, cefadroxil, and cephalexin. First-generation cephalosporins have active coverage against most gram-positive cocci such as *Staphylococcus* spp. and *Streptococcus* spp. while having minimal coverage against gram-negative bacteria. Gram-negative bacteria that are more susceptible to first-generation cephalosporins are *P. mirabilis, E. coli,* and *K. pneumoniae.* Oral first-generation cephalosporins are commonly prescribed against uncomplicated skin and soft tissue infections such as cellulitis and abscesses due to *Staphylococcus* or *Streptococcus* species.

Additionally, clinicians can use them for bone, respiratory tract, genitourinary tract, biliary tract, and bloodstream infections, otitis media, and surgical prophylaxis. Cefazolin is the cephalosporin of choice for surgical prophylaxis. One non–FDA-approved indication is using first-generation cephalosporins for endocarditis prophylaxis for those susceptible to and undergoing dental or respiratory procedures.

Second-generation cephalosporins are divided into the second-generation and the cephamycin subgroups. Some of the second-generation subgroups include cefuroxime and cefprozil. The cephamycin subgroup includes cefmetazole, cefotetan, and cefoxitin. Within the first subgroup, cefuroxime has increased coverage against *H. influenzae.* Indications for cefuroxime also include Lyme disease in pregnant females and children. The cephamycin subgroup has increased coverage against anaerobes, including *Bacteroides* species. Second-generation cephalosporins have less activity against gram-positive cocci than first-generation cephalosporins but have increased activity against gram-negative bacilli. They are often prescribed to treat respiratory infections such as bronchiolitis or pneumonia. Other indications for second-generation cephalosporins are similar to first-generation indications (bone, respiratory tract, genitourinary tract, biliary tract, bloodstream infection, otitis media, and surgical prophylaxis). In addition to the gram-negative bacteria covered by first-generation cephalosporins, second-generation cephalosporins also have coverage against *H. influenzae* and *M. catarrhalis.*

Third-generation cephalosporins include cefotaxime, ceftazidime, cefdinir, ceftriaxone, cefpodoxime, cefoperazone, and cefixime. This generation has extended gram-negative bacteria coverage, often used to treat gram-negative infections resistant to first- and second-generation or other beta-lactam antimicrobials. The gram-negative spectrum of activity includes *Enterobacter* spp. and *Klebsiella aerogenes*. When given IV, third-generation cephalosporins can penetrate the blood-brain barrier and cover bacteria in the cerebrospinal fluid, especially ceftriaxone and cefotaxime. Ceftriaxone can be given to treat meningitis caused by *H. influenzae, Neisseria meningitidis,* or *Streptococcus pneumoniae.* Ceftriaxone is also used to treat gonorrhea and **Lyme disease**. Ceftazidime, very importantly, has *P. aeruginosa* coverage.

The fourth-generation cephalosporin includes cefepime. Cefepime is a broad-spectrum antimicrobial that can penetrate the cerebrospinal fluid. Cefepime has an additional quaternary ammonium group, allowing it to better penetrate the outer membrane of gram-negative bacteria. Similar to the activity of cefotaxime and ceftriaxone, cefepime can cover *S. pneumoniae* and methicillin-sensitive *S. aureus* (MSSA). Similar to ceftazidime, cefepime, very importantly, can cover for *P. aeruginosa.* In addition to the gram-negative bacteria that the third generation covers (*Neisseria* spp., *H. influenzae,* and *Enterobacteriaceae*), cefepime can provide coverage against beta-lactamase–producing gram-negative bacilli. Although effective against gram-positive and gram-negative bacteria, cefepime is reserved for severe systemic infections.

The fifth-generation cephalosporin includes ceftaroline. Ceftaroline is also a broad-spectrum antimicrobial and thus can cover susceptible gram-positive and gram-negative organisms. However, what makes it unique from the rest of the cephalosporins is its coverage against methicillin-resistant *S. aureus* (MRSA). Ceftaroline can also cover *Listeria monocytogenes* and *Enterococcus faecalis*. However, ceftaroline does not cover *P. aeruginosa*.

Pharmacokinetics

Cephalosporins comprise about half of the available beta-lactam antibiotics. Some pharmacokinetic properties of oral cephalosporins, such as absorption or plasma profile, are variable. In contrast, metabolism is minimal, and they are eliminated by the kidney, except cefixime, which is excreted primarily in bile. Tissue distribution is good and, for some compounds, elevated.

Most cephalosporins can only be administered parenterally. Among agents that are absorbed from the GI tract, those with bioavailabilities of 85%–90% include cefroxadine, cefadroxil, cefsumide, cephalexin, cephradine, cefacetrile, and cefazaflur.

Mechanism of action

The mechanism of action of cephalosporins is similar to that of penicillin. Like the penicillins, cephalosporins bind to penicillin-binding proteins, interfering with cell wall enzymes and causing bacterial death.

Clinical indications

Cephalosporins treat various bacterial infections, especially for people allergic to penicillin. They indicate the treatment of sinusitis, strep throat, otitis media, pneumonia, meningitis, urinary tract infections, and gonorrhea.

Contraindications

One of the contraindications of cephalosporins is if patients are allergic to them. Caution should be utilized in patients who have had an anaphylactic reaction to penicillin or other beta-lactam antimicrobials. The cross-reactivity is thought to be due to similar side chains between some cephalosporins and some penicillin products, but it is not due to the beta-lactam ring.

Ceftriaxone is contraindicated in neonates with hyperbilirubinemia because of reports that ceftriaxone displaces bilirubin from albumin, increasing the free bilirubin concentrations and increasing the risk of jaundice in neonates. Ceftriaxone reacts to a calcium-containing solution, and it can precipitate in the lungs and kidneys of infants less than 28 days old, which could be life-threatening. Therefore ceftriaxone is also contraindicated in infants under 28 days old if they are expected to receive calcium-containing products.

Adverse effects

Cephalosporins are generally safe and have low toxicity. Adverse effects include lack of appetite, nausea, vomiting, diarrhea, and abdominal pain. Less common adverse reactions include hypersensitivity, vitamin K deficiency, **pseudomembranous colitis**, and hemolytic anemia.

Toxicities

After testing the effects of high-dose cephalosporins in rabbits, there is new evidence of nephrotoxicity due to its impact on the mitochondrial system of the kidneys. Cefepime overdose can result in seizures and encephalopathy. Studies show it to potentially result from cefepime crossing the blood-brain barrier and displaying concentration-dependent gamma-aminobutyric acid (GABA) antagonism, which can also occur with toxic doses of penicillin G. Other studies show altered mental status and a triphasic wave discharge on electroencephalogram. Discontinuation of cefepime demonstrates normalization of cognitive status.

Carbapenems

Carbapenems are a class of beta-lactam antibiotics active against many aerobic and anaerobic gram-positive and gram-negative organisms. Thienamycin was the first carbapenem to be discovered in 1976. Carbapenems possess the broadest spectrum of activity and the greatest potency against bacteria of all the beta-lactam antibiotics. Because of this characteristic, they are often reserved for more severe infections or used as "last-line" agents. Carbapenems include imipenem, meropenem, doripenem, and ertapenem (see **Table 49.2**). Carbapenems are usually reserved for known or suspected multidrug-resistant bacterial infections.

TABLE 49.2 Various carbapenems.

Generic names	Trade names	Route of administration
biapenem	Omegacin	IM, IV
doripenem	Doribax	IV
ertapenem	Invanz	IM, IV
imipenem/cilastatin	Primaxin	IM, IV
meropenem	Merrem	IV
panipenem/betamipron	Carbenin	IV

Pharmacokinetics

Carbapenems are poorly absorbed orally, so they can only be used by injection. They generally have low bioavailability. The development of oral carbapenems is currently underway. Ertapenem and imipenem-cilastatin can also be administered intramuscularly. They are mainly eliminated via the kidneys, and dose adjustment is necessary in patients with renal impairment. Both imipenem and meropenem can penetrate the cerebrospinal fluid in patients with meningitis because these carbapenems have large volumes of distribution and penetrate well into infected tissues or organs. The elimination half-life of most carbapenems is around 1 hour, except for ertapenem, which has a 3.8-hour half-life, which allows its once-daily use.

Mechanism of action

Carbapenems can inhibit cell wall synthesis by binding to penicillin-binding proteins. Therefore they cause bacterial cell wall defects and swelling, leading to bacterial death.

Clinical indications

Carbapenems are indicated mainly as **empiric monotherapy** in severe conditions such as **endometritis**, osteomyelitis, bacteremia, meningitis, **peritonitis**, bronchitis, pneumonia, **febrile neutropenia**, nephritis, and pelvic infections. They are also helpful in treating mixed bacterial infections and aerobic gram-negative bacterial infections that are not susceptible to other beta-lactam antibiotics.

Contraindications

The carbapenems are contraindicated in patients who are hypersensitive to these drugs because of an increased risk of seizures in children with central nervous system infections. Patients with kidney disease must be closely monitored when they are treated with a carbapenem.

Adverse effects

Carbapenems are generally well tolerated, and the incidence of hypersensitivity to them is low. However, the typical clinical adverse effects include local injection soreness, nausea, abdominal pain, and skin reactions. Seizures are the most severe side effect, especially with imipenem.

Toxicities

Like other beta-lactam antibacterials, carbapenems have a neurotoxic potential higher than penicillins and cephalosporins. Seizures can occur with imipenem/cilastatin. The liver damage due to the meropenem is usually mild and self-limited.

Vancomycin

Vancomycin (Vancocin) is a tricyclic glycopeptide antibiotic that destroys bacteria in the intestines. It is the drug of choice for treating MRSA infections and is typically utilized as empiric therapy for hospitalized patients with suspected MRSA infections.

Pharmacokinetics

Vancomycin is poorly absorbed via the GI tract and is only given orally to treat *Clostridioides difficile* infections. It is most commonly administered intravenously. However, systemic absorption (up to 60%) may occur following intraperitoneal administration. Approximately 50% of serum vancomycin is protein bound. Because almost 75%–80% of the drug is excreted unchanged in the urine after the first 24 hours following administration, there is seemingly no apparent metabolism of the drug. About 75%–80% of vancomycin is excreted from the kidneys. The half-life is approximately 6 hours.

Mechanism of action

Vancomycin is bactericidal by inhibiting the polymerization of peptidoglycans in the bacterial cell wall. Therefore it prevents the synthesis and polymerization within the peptidoglycan layer. This inhibition weakens bacterial cell walls and ultimately causes leakage of intracellular components, resulting in bacterial cell death.

Clinical indications

Vancomycin treats and prevents various bacterial infections caused by gram-positive bacteria, including MRSA. It is also effective for streptococci, enterococci, and methicillin-susceptible *S. aureus* infections. Vancomycin is also used to treat *C. difficile*-associated diarrhea, pseudomembranous colitis, *Staphylococcus enterocolitis,* osteomyelitis, and endocarditis.

Contraindications

Vancomycin is contraindicated in patients with known hypersensitivity. Rapid bolus administration may cause hypotension, shock, and, rarely, cardiac arrest. It should be used with caution in patients with inflammatory bowel disease such as ulcerative colitis, Crohn disease, kidney disease, or hearing loss.

Adverse effects

Common adverse effects of intravenous vancomycin injection include nephrotoxicity, hypotension, and hypersensitivity reactions. Anaphylaxis is a type of hypersensitivity reaction that can occur with vancomycin. Vancomycin infusion is an infusion-related reaction associated with rapid IV infusion of vancomycin. Symptoms include flushing, pruritus, and an erythematous rash on the face, neck, and upper torso. If an infusion reaction occurs with vancomycin administration, the IV infusion rate may be slowed down to prevent the response from recurring. Less common adverse effects include local phlebitis, chills, drug fever, skin rash, eosinophilia, and reversible neutropenia.

Toxicities

Vancomycin is associated with nephrotoxicity. Generally this toxicity is presented as proximal tubular cell injury with or without necrosis and as acute interstitial nephritis. Ototoxicity is rare with vancomycin monotherapy. However, it is common in patients receiving excessive vancomycin doses and concurrent ototoxic medications such as aminoglycosides, loop diuretics, and antineoplastic agents.

You should remember

Oral vancomycin is categorized as a category B drug for use in pregnancy. In contrast, intravenous vancomycin injection is category C. Vancomycin should not be used during pregnancy unless the benefits outweigh the risks of the medication. When vancomycin is needed, maternal blood levels of vancomycin should be monitored to decrease the risk of nephrotoxicity and ototoxicity in the fetus.

Tetracyclines

The tetracyclines, discovered in the 1940s, are broad-spectrum antibiotics with activity against many gram-positive and gram-negative bacteria and atypical organisms such as **chlamydiae**, mycoplasmas, rickettsiae, and protozoan parasites. The advantages of these agents are the lack of significant adverse side effects, which has led to their extensive use in treating human infections. They are also used prophylactically against malaria. Although tetracyclines have essential roles in human medicine, the emergence of microbial resistance has limited their effectiveness. In clinical practice, tetracyclines have been responsible for selecting resistant organisms. Various tetracyclines are listed in **Table 49.3**.

Pharmacokinetics

First-generation tetracyclines feature low lipophilia and are usually available in oral form only. Their absorption ranges from 25% to 60%. Most first-generation tetracyclines are not metabolized. Instead, they are eliminated by renal excretion. Second-generation tetracyclines are three to five times more lipophilic, enhancing tissue penetration. Doxycycline, the most common member of this group, has a bioavailability of more than 80%. The bile concentration of doxycycline is 10–25 times higher than its serum concentration. High concentrations of doxycycline are also found in the liver and kidneys. Primarily, doxycycline is excreted in bile to feces. Part of doxycycline is inactivated in the

TABLE 49.3 Various tetracyclines.

Generic name	Trade name	Route of administration
chlortetracycline	Aureomycin	PO, IV, Topical
oxytetracycline	Terramycin	IM, IV
tetracycline	Achromycin	PO
demeclocycline	Declomycin	PO
rolitetracycline	Reverin	PO
lymecycline	Tetralysal	PO
clomocycline	Megaclor	PO
methacycline	Rodomycin	PO
doxycycline	Vibramycin	PO
minocycline	Minocin	PO, IV
tigecycline	Tygacil	IV
eravacycline	Xerava	IV
omadacycline	Nuzyra	PO, IV

liver, and the kidneys excrete 40%. Extended-spectrum tetracycline derivatives include tigecycline, eravacycline, and omadacycline

Mechanism of action

Tetracyclines inhibit protein synthesis by preventing aminoacyl-tRNA attachment to the ribosomal acceptor A site. They specifically inhibit the 30S ribosomal subunit. Once the binding process stops, a cell cannot maintain proper function and will be unable to grow or further replicate.

Clinical indications

Tetracyclines are used to treat infections caused by bacteria, including respiratory tract infections and certain infections of the skin, eye, intestinal, lymphatic, genital, and urinary systems. They are also indicated for other diseases spread by ticks, lice, mites, and infected animals. The medication should be taken 2–3 hours before or after using any magnesium, aluminum, or calcium product. The extended-spectrum tetracycline derivatives have activity against pathogens that resist other tetracyclines, such as extended-spectrum beta-lactamase infections.

Contraindications

Tetracyclines are contraindicated in patients who have shown hypersensitivity to them or in children younger than 8 years. In Canada, minocycline and tetracycline are recommended to be avoided in complete renal failure and those with hepatic dysfunction. Tetracyclines are not recommended for use during pregnancy because of the risk of hepatotoxicity in the mother, the potential for permanent discoloration of teeth in the fetus, as well as impairment of fetal long bone growth. Tetracycline usage is also associated with teeth discoloration in children under 8. Thus they generally should be avoided in pediatric patients under age 8. If necessary, doxycycline is the preferred agent.

Adverse effects

The most common adverse effects of tetracyclines include GI tract such as abdominal pain, nausea, vomiting, diarrhea, and loss of appetite. Some patients may have **photosensitivity** when taking the medication. Rare adverse effects of tetracyclines include hepatotoxicity, intracranial hypertension, worsening renal failure, and esophageal strictures.

Toxicities

When patients overdose with tetracyclines, the medication must be discontinued immediately. High doses of tetracyclines can result in liver failure and death.

You should remember

Tetracyclines are dosed differently in adults and children. Adults may receive 1 g of tetracyclines daily, divided into 500 mg twice or 250 mg four times daily. Higher doses, such as 500 mg four times daily, may be given for more severe infections. Pediatric patients above 8 can receive a daily dose of 25 mg/kg up to 50 mg/kg, divided into four equal doses.

Fluoroquinolones

Fluoroquinolones are broad-spectrum antibiotics used to treat bacterial infections. There are three classes of fluoroquinolones: the first, second, and third generations.

The first generation includes cinoxacin and nalidixic acid. These drugs are less commonly used today due to minimal serum levels and increased risk of bacterial resistance. They are only recommended for uncomplicated urinary tract infections and not for patients with poor renal function.

Second-generation drugs have increased gram-negative activity and broad clinical applications for complicated urinary tract infections, sexually transmitted diseases, pneumonia, and skin infections. These drugs include ciprofloxacin, enoxacin, lomefloxacin, norfloxacin, and ofloxacin. Ciprofloxacin is particularly effective against *P. aeruginosa* and can treat osteomyelitis caused by susceptible organisms. Ofloxacin has excellent activity against *Chlamydia trachomatis*.

The third generation, including levofloxacin, gatifloxacin, moxifloxacin, and sparfloxacin, have expanded activity against gram-positive organisms, particularly penicillin-sensitive and penicillin-resistant *S. pneumoniae*, and atypical pathogens such as ***Mycoplasma pneumoniae*** and *Chlamydia pneumoniae*. They are helpful in the treatment of community-acquired pneumonia, acute sinusitis, acute exacerbations of chronic bronchitis, urinary tract infections, and gonorrhea. **Table 49.4** summarizes various fluoroquinolones.

Pharmacokinetics

Fluoroquinolones are broad-spectrum antibiotics with good oral bioavailability. The pharmacokinetics of levofloxacin and moxifloxacin are excellent. Oral bioavailability is 90%–99%, and there is extensive penetration into tissues and body fluids, and it has an elimination half-life of 6–12 hours. Most fluoroquinolones are metabolized in the liver and excreted in urine. Moxifloxacin is eliminated primarily in bile.

TABLE 49.4 Various fluoroquinolones.

Generic name	Trade name	Route of administration
ciprofloxacin	Cipro	PO, IV
delafloxacin	Baxdela	PO, IV
gatifloxacin	Zymaxid	Ophthalmic
gemifloxacin	Factive	PO
levofloxacin	Levaquin	PO, IV
moxifloxacin	Avelox	PO, IV
ofloxacin	Floxin	PO, otic, ophthalmic

Mechanism of action

Fluoroquinolones block DNA replication and inhibit bacterial cell synthesis and cell division, ultimately leading to the bacteria's death. They act by inhibiting two enzymes involved in bacterial DNA synthesis. These DNA topoisomerases are not present in human cells but are essential for bacterial DNA replication, enabling these agents to be both specific and bactericidal.

Clinical indications

The fluoroquinolones are used for the treatment of several bacterial infections, including sinusitis, bacterial bronchitis, pneumonia, urinary tract infections, septicemia and intraabdominal infections, joint and bone infections, skin infections, typhoid fever, anthrax, and bacterial gastroenteritis. In 2016 the FDA released warnings regarding fluoroquinolones leading to serious adverse effects. Because the risk of severe side effects outweighed the benefits for patients with acute bacterial sinusitis, acute bacterial exacerbation of chronic bronchitis, and uncomplicated urinary tract infections, the FDA determined that fluoroquinolones should be reserved for use in patients with these conditions who have no alternative treatment options. Fluoroquinolones are no longer recommended for the empiric treatment of gonorrhea because of increasing resistance worldwide.

Contraindications

Fluoroquinolones are contraindicated in patients who experience hypersensitivity. They are not routinely recommended in children younger than 18 because they may cause cartilage damage; however, they may be considered an alternative option for patients with no other treatment options. They must be used with caution in older adults, those with renal impairment, and patients who are on systemic corticosteroids.

Adverse effects

The adverse effects of fluoroquinolones are generally safe. The most frequent side effects are nausea, dyspepsia, and vomiting. However, severe side effects include tendonitis, tendon rupture (**Achilles tendon**), peripheral neuropathy, myalgia, fatigue, **arthralgia**, exacerbation of myasthenia gravis, difficulty walking, burning pain, depression, loss of memory, insomnia, vision, hearing, taste, and smell alterations.

Toxicities

Fluoroquinolone toxicity ranges from tendon rupture and muscle pain to depression and psychosis.

Macrolides

Macrolides are drugs used to treat various bacterial infections. Azithromycin, clarithromycin, and erythromycin are commonly employed to treat diseases such as pharyngitis, sinusitis, and pneumonia. They are also used in uncomplicated skin infections and otitis media in children. **Table 49.5** summarizes various macrolides.

Pharmacokinetics

The pharmacokinetic properties of macrolide antibiotics differ based on their chemical structure. In low-pH environments such as in the stomach, erythromycin is degraded.

Macrolide absorption in the intestine is thought to be limited by P-glycoprotein. They are lipophilic and widely distributed in blood and tissues. Erythromycin is metabolized in the liver by the cytochrome P450 and eliminated

TABLE 49.5 Various macrolides.

Generic names	Trade names	Route of administration
azithromycin	Zithromax	PO, IV
clarithromycin	Biaxin	PO
erythromycin	Emicin, ATS	PO, IV, topical, ophthalmic
fidaxomicin	Dificid	PO

primarily via feces. Eighty percent is inactivated through demethylation before they are excreted in the bile and urine.

Mechanism of action

Macrolides bind to the 50S subunit of the bacterial ribosome and block the initiation of protein synthesis. They all consist of a large lactone ring, so they prevent the growth of bacteria.

Clinical indications

Macrolides are effective in treating atypical community-acquired pneumonia, ***Helicobacter pylori*** (as part of triple therapy), chlamydia, and acute nonspecific urethritis. They are also used to treat ***Legionella* species** and *Corynebacterium diphtheriae*. When penicillin is contraindicated, macrolides are the drug of choice for group A streptococcal and pneumococcal infections.

Contraindications

Macrolides are contraindicated with known hypersensitivity to macrolides and a history of cholestatic jaundice or hepatic dysfunction associated with prior macrolide use. They should be used with caution during pregnancy and breastfeeding in patients with myasthenia gravis, as well as in elderly clients and those with cardiovascular disease.

Adverse effects

The most common adverse effects of macrolides in adults are headache, dyspepsia, diarrhea, nausea, abnormal taste, and abdominal pain. Like other kinds of antibiotics, pseudomembranous colitis can occur with macrolide use, ranging in severity from mild to life-threatening. The other adverse effects include seizures, confusion, hallucinations, and vertigo.

Toxicities

Toxicities of macrolides include hepatotoxicity. In patients with hemodialysis-dependent kidney failure, treatment with azithromycin is associated with an increased risk of sudden cardiac death.

Aminoglycosides

Aminoglycosides are broad-spectrum bactericidal antibiotics frequently prescribed for children, primarily for infections caused by gram-negative pathogens. The aminoglycoside class includes gentamicin, amikacin, tobramycin, neomycin, plazomicin, paromomycin, and streptomycin.

Pharmacokinetics

Aminoglycosides are poorly absorbed orally but are well absorbed from the pleural cavity, peritoneum, joints, and topically (skin and conjunctiva of the eyes). They are administered IV but may be given IM if IV access is unavailable. Aminoglycosides are excreted by glomerular filtration and have a serum half-life of 2–3 hours; the half-life increases exponentially as the glomerular filtration rate falls, such as in renal insufficiency in older patients.

TABLE 49.6 Various aminoglycosides.

Generic names	Trade names	Route of administration
gentamicin	Cidomycin, garamycin	IM, IV, topical, ophthalmic
amikacin	Amikin	IM, IV, inhalation
tobramycin	Nebcin	IM, IV, inhalation, ophthalmic
neomycin	(generic only)	PO, topical
plazomicin	Zemdri	IV
paromomycin	Humatin	PO
streptomycin	Rimosidin	IM

Mechanism of action

Aminoglycosides are bactericidal agents that bind to the bacteria's ribosomal 30S subunit. This binding misreads the genetic code and disrupts translation, making the bacteria unable to synthesize protein.

Clinical indications

Aminoglycosides are used for empiric therapy in combination with other antibiotics for patients with severe illness; this includes empiric treatment for patients with infective endocarditis, sepsis, complicated intraabdominal infections, and complicated genitourinary infections. Typically, aminoglycosides should not be used for more than 48 hours due to the risk of toxicity associated with prolonged use. It is recommended that adequate dosing and clearance be ensured in addition to audiometric and vestibular testing to monitor for ototoxicity. They are part of directed combination treatment for **brucellosis**, **listeriosis**, and CNS **nocardiosis**. Aminoglycoside monotherapy is indicated for tularemia in children and multidrug-resistant gram-negative pathogens.

Contraindications

Aminoglycosides are contraindicated in patients who have hypersensitivity to aminoglycoside therapy and should be avoided in patients with myasthenia gravis because of the risk of prolonged neuromuscular blockade.

Adverse effects

The main adverse effects of aminoglycosides include ototoxicity, neuromuscular blockade, and nephrotoxicity. Liver damage from aminoglycosides is rare, perhaps because the other adverse effects limit the amount that can be given. Gentamicin, tobramycin, and streptomycin more frequently result in vestibular damage, while kanamycin and amikacin cause more cochlear damage. Aminoglycoside serum levels are typically obtained to monitor patients and prevent supratherapeutic drug concentrations that may lead to toxicity. Kanamycin has been discontinued in the United States.

Toxicities

There is no antidote for the toxicities of aminoglycosides. However, agents with protective effects on the ear and kidney may help prevent aminoglycoside-induced toxicity. In particular, *N*-acetylcysteine demonstrates promising protective effects on patients using aminoglycosides.

You should remember

Neomycin can cause irreversible deafness, so it is no longer used parenterally. It is considerably more ototoxic than kanamycin, which has also been discontinued in the United States. Sufficient absorption may occur after prolonged oral administration to cause ototoxicity, especially in the presence of renal impairment.

Sulfonamides

Sulfonamides are one of the oldest recognized groups of antibacterial agents. They are synthetic **bacteriostatic** antimicrobials with a broad spectrum against gram-positive and gram-negative organisms. However, many strains of an individual species may be resistant. Bacterial sensitivity is the same for the various sulfonamides, and resistance to one sulfonamide indicates resistance to all. Sulfonamides include mafenide, sulfacetamide, sulfadiazine, sulfamethizole, sulfamethoxazole, sulfanilamide, and sulfasalazine (see **Table 49.7**).

Pharmacokinetics

Most sulfonamides are readily absorbed orally, and they are also absorbed through the vaginal mucosa. The sulfonamides are widely distributed throughout all tissues. High levels are achieved in synovial, pleural, peritoneal, and ocular fluids. Sulfonamides are bound to plasma proteins from 15%–90%. There are differences between species in binding. They are metabolized mainly by the liver and excreted by the kidneys.

TABLE 49.7 Various sulfonamides.

Generic names	Trade names	Route of administration
mafenide	Sulfamylon	Topical
sulfacetamide	Klaron, Ovace	Topical
sulfadiazine	Lantrisul, Neotrizine	Topical
sulfamethizole, sulfamethoxazole	Bactrim, Septra	PO, IV[a]
sulfanilamide	Azulfidine, Diamox, Gantrisin	PO
sulfasalazine	Azulfidine, Delzicol, Dipentum	PO
sulfisoxazole	Gantrisin Pediatric, Truxazole	PO

[a]*Sulfamethoxazole/trimethoprim is available as IV.*

Mechanism of action

Sulfonamides act as competitive inhibitors of the bacterial enzyme dihydropteroate synthetase. This enzyme typically uses para-aminobenzoic acid (PABA) to synthesize the necessary folic acid. The inhibited reaction is usually required in these organisms to synthesize folic acid. Without it, bacteria cannot replicate and survive.

Clinical indications

Sulfa drugs are still commonly used to treat a variety of bacterial infections. They treat urinary tract infections, otitis media, acute exacerbations of chronic bronchitis, and **traveler's diarrhea**. Topical sulfonamides can treat burns, vaginitis, and ocular diseases. They are also employed to treat **vulvovaginal candidiasis** caused by *Candida albicans*. Trimethoprim/sulfamethoxazole effectively treats community-acquired soft tissue infections and urinary tract infections.

Contraindications

Sulfa drugs are contraindicated in patients who have had an allergic reaction to them, have a history of drug-induced immune thrombocytopenia with the use of sulfonamides, or have porphyria. The use of sulfonamides in the first trimester and throughout pregnancy might be associated with congenital malformations. They should not be given to infants less than 2 months old.

Adverse effects

Adverse effects of sulfa drugs can result from oral and often topical use. They can cause increased skin sensitivity to sunlight, headache, nausea, diarrhea, abnormal skin blistering, fatigue, and dizziness. Hyperkalemia and hypoglycemia may also occur with use.

Toxicities

Though rare, adverse effects due to sulfa drug toxicity can include severe allergic skin rashes, drug fever, Stevens-Johnson syndrome, agranulocytosis, serum sickness, aplastic anemia, nephritis, confusion, pancreatitis, ataxia, and seizures. These adverse effects can co-occur with hepatotoxicity.

Key Terms

Achilles tendon
Arthralgia
Bactericidal
Bacteriostatic
Blood-brain barrier
Brucellosis
Chlamydiae
Empiric monotherapy
Endocarditis
Endometritis
Febrile neutropenia

Helicobacter pylori
***Legionella* species**
Listeriosis
Lyme disease
Mycoplasma pneumoniae
Nocardiosis
Peritonitis
Photosensitivity
Porphyria
Protozoa
Pseudomembranous colitis
Rickettsiae
Stevens-Johnson syndrome
Subarachnoid space
Traveler's diarrhea
Vulvovaginal candidiasis

Clinical case studies

Clinical case study 1

A 27-year-old female is in her first trimester of pregnancy. Serologic testing for syphilis reveals the presence of late latent syphilis. Standard treatment for this stage of syphilis in pregnancy consists of three weekly intramuscular injections of penicillin G benzathine. The patient has no known allergic reaction to penicillin. However, her mother previously had an allergic reaction to penicillin. A medical assistant administers the intramuscular injection. The patient is asked to stay in the office for 20 minutes. After 10 minutes, she develops severe allergic reactions.

Critical thinking questions

1. What are the indications for penicillin G?
2. What are the signs and symptoms of allergic reactions to penicillin G?
3. What are the treatments for allergic reactions to penicillin G?

Clinical case study 2

A 70-year-old male was brought to the emergency department because of fever, altered mental status, and hiccups. The patient was started on vancomycin, ceftriaxone, and metronidazole as empiric treatment for bacteremia. His condition declined, and the ceftriaxone was replaced with cefepime. Blood cultures were positive for *S. aureus*, and all three sets of cultures grew the methicillin-resistant form of the bacterium known as MRSA. The patient rebounded from his condition.

Critical thinking questions

1. How is vancomycin bactericidal?
2. What are the indications for vancomycin?
3. What are the toxicities associated with vancomycin?

Clinical case study 3

A 24-year-old female was diagnosed with Rocky Mountain spotted fever and treated with doxycycline. Her condition continued to improve gradually, but on a checkup several weeks later, she reported that she was pregnant.

Critical thinking questions

1. Which organisms are affected by tetracyclines?
2. What are the risks associated with tetracycline use during pregnancy?
3. What are the most common adverse effects of tetracyclines?

Further reading

[1] J. Alton, A. Alton, Alton's Antibiotics and Infectious Disease – the Layman's Guide to Available Antibacterials in Austere Settings, Alton First Aid LLC, 2018.
[2] R. Alves, Aminoglycosides – Pharmacology, Clinical Uses and Health Effects, Nova Science Publishers Inc, 2016.
[3] B. Arsic, P. Novak, G. Kragol, J. Barber, M. Grazia Rimoli, F. Sodano, Macrolides – Properties, Synthesis, and Applications, De Gruyter, 2018.
[4] D. Bagchi, A. Das, B.W. Downs, Viral, Parasitic, Bacterial, and Fungal Infections – Antimicrobial, Host Defense, and Therapeutic Strategies, Academic Press, 2022.

[5] A. Gafar Hossion, Vancomycin – Biosynthesis, Clinical Uses and Adverse Effects (Pharmacology Research Safety Testing and Regulation), Nova Science Publishers Inc, 2014.
[6] J.C. Gallagher, C. MacDougall, Antibiotics Simplified, fifth ed., Jones & Bartlett Learning, 2022.
[7] T.P. Gauthier, Learn Antibiotics – A Collection of Resources for Antimicrobial Drugs, Gauthier, 2022.
[8] A.R. Hauser, Antibiotic Basics for Clinicians, third ed., Wolters Kluwer, 2022.
[9] B. Levine, EMRA Antibiotic Guide, twentieth ed., Emergency Medicine Residents' Association, 2022.
[10] J. Lopez, Tetracycline Handbook – A Clinician's Guide to Antifungal and Bacterial Infection Mastery, Lopez, 2023.
[11] R. Mahmud, Y. Ai Lian Lim, A. Amir, Medical Parasitology – A Textbook, Springer, 2017.
[12] A. Rusu, V. Uivarosi, C. Tanase, Focus on Antibiotics – New Challenges and Steps Forward in Discovery and Development, MDPI, 2023.
[13] D. Sarkar, Sulfonamides – an Overview, Nova Science Publishers Inc, 2020.
[14] C. Walsh, T. Wencewicz, Antibiotics – Challenges, Mechanisms, Opportunities, ASM Press, 2016.

CHAPTER

50

Antituberculosis drugs

OUTLINE

LEARNING OUTCOMES

After study of this chapter, readers should be able to

1. Describe the classifications of mycobacterium infections.
2. Explain the two critical types of pathophysiologic of tuberculosis.
3. List the first-line drugs for treating tuberculosis.
4. Explain the importance of the pharmacokinetics of isoniazid.

https://doi.org/10.1016/B978-0-443-29038-1.00050-6

5. Discuss the contraindications of pyrazinamide.
6. Describe the adverse effects of rifampin.
7. Discuss the mechanism of action of ethambutol.
8. Describe leprosy and the drug of choice for treatment.
9. Explain the *Mycobacterium avium* complex and its treatment.

Overview

Mycobacterial infection is a heterogeneous group of infectious diseases caused by obligate aerobic bacteria, most often *Mycobacterium tuberculosis*. Tuberculosis (TB) is a chronic, severe pulmonary and systemic disease. It is spread through the air when people with lung TB cough, sneeze, or spit. Even though it is more common in developing countries, it is increasing in developed countries, probably due to the rise in AIDS cases and the increasing number of drug-resistant strains of *M. tuberculosis*. In addition to immunocompromised people, other population groups who are at increased risk include minorities, people of lower socioeconomic status, people who consume alcohol, prisoners, and older patients. Oropharyngeal and intestinal TB is contracted by drinking milk contaminated with *Mycobacterium bovis*. This is rare in countries where milk is routinely pasteurized. However, it is still seen in countries with tuberculous dairy cows and unpasteurized milk. In the United States, TB is primarily a disease of older adults, immigrants from high-burden countries, racial and ethnic minorities, and people with AIDS. Certain illnesses may also increase the risk of TB, which includes malnutrition, alcoholism, diabetes mellitus, silicosis, Hodgkin lymphoma, kidney failure, and immunosuppression.

Classifications of *Mycobacterium* infections

Mycobacterial infections have three types: TB, nontuberculous mycobacteriosis, and leprosy. TB is a systemic infectious disease involving the respiratory, genitourinary, and lymphatic systems caused by *M. tuberculosis*. Extrapulmonary TB remains a significant clinical problem because symptoms and signs may be difficult to recognize due to TB. **Miliary TB** is responsible for up to 10% of predominantly extrapulmonary cases. HIV-related miliary TB is rapidly progressive and almost always fatal without treatment. Nontuberculous mycobacteria (NTM) have been commonly implicated as opportunistic pathogens in patients with underlying disease or immunosuppression, including AIDS. *Mycobacterium avium* complex (MAC) multiplies a type of NTM and is the most common cause of NTM disease in humans. *Mycobacterium leprae* is the causative pathogen for **leprosy**. It is an infection of the skin, mucous membranes, and peripheral nerves. Leprosy is rare in some parts of the world. However, it remains a significant problem in other parts such as Brazil, India, and Indonesia.

The mycobacteria that most commonly cause TB and leprosy are found in the soil and indoor and outdoor water sources and are recognized to colonize poorly sanitized medical equipment. **Atypical mycobacteria** most commonly infect immunocompromised individuals and young children.

Pathogenesis of tuberculosis

TB is separated into two critical pathophysiologic types: "primary" TB, which occurs in the nonimmune host, and "secondary" TB, which occurs in the host immune to *M. tuberculosis*. The many clinical-pathologic patterns of TB are shown in **Fig. 50.1**.

Primary TB is a disease that develops in a previously unexposed and therefore unsensitized person. Clinically significant disease develops in about 5% of newly infected people. With primary TB, the source of the organism is exogenous. In most people, the primary infection is contained, but in others, primary TB is progressive. Progressive primary TB more often resembles acute bacterial pneumonia with lobe consolidation, **hilar adenopathy**, and **pleural effusion**.

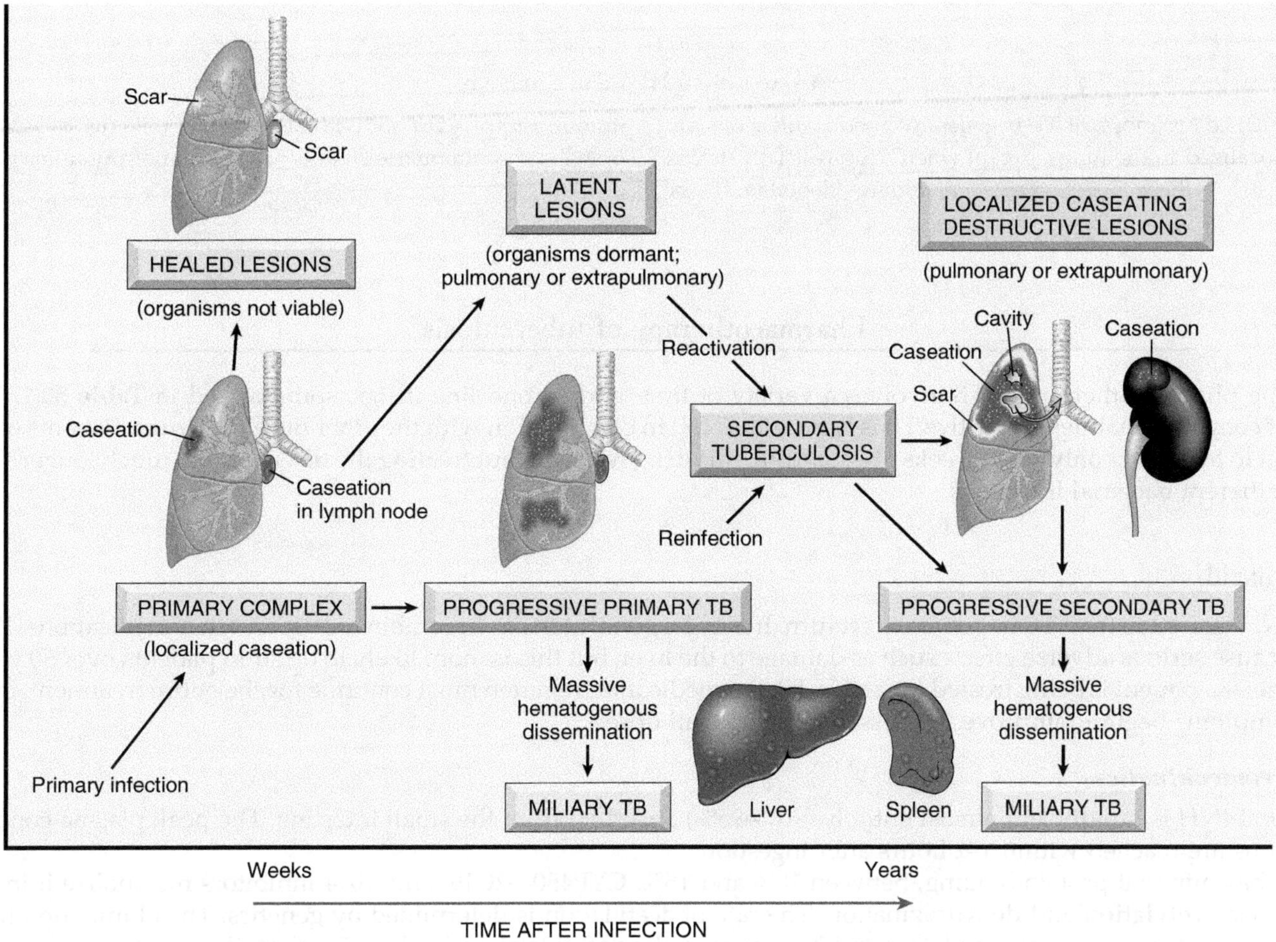

FIG. 50.1 The clinical-pathologic patterns of tuberculosis.

Secondary TB arises in a previously sensitized host and is a reactivation of a dormant TB infection. It may follow shortly after primary TB, but more commonly, it appears many years after the initial infection, usually when host resistance is weakened. Secondary pulmonary TB classically involves the apex of the upper lobes of one or both lungs. As a result, the regional lymph nodes are less prominently involved early in secondary disease than in primary TB. On the other hand, cavitation occurs readily in the secondary form.

Diagnosis of tuberculosis

Diagnosis of pulmonary TB includes the patient's history of potential exposure to the disease, skin TB test, blood test, chest X-ray, and sputum culture. In contrast to secondary TB, progressive primary TB in adults can be challenging to diagnose. Pulmonary disease diagnosis is based in part on the history and physical and radiographic findings of consolidation or cavitation in the apices of the lungs. Ultimately, however, tubercle bacilli must be identified. Acid-fast smears and cultures of the sputum of patients suspected of having TB should be performed. Culture in solid agar media shows growth at 3–6 weeks, but culture in liquid media can provide an answer within 2 weeks.

Polymerase chain reaction (PCR) amplification of *M. tuberculosis* DNA allows for a more rapid diagnosis. A PCR test identifies the presence of *M. tuberculosis* genetic material and, if the organism is detected, whether it is resistant to rifampin. This PCR assay is as sensitive as culture in acid-fast smear-positive samples, but it is slightly less sensitive in smear-negative TB and substantially less sensitive in children. Thus culture remains the gold standard because it allows for drug susceptibility testing. Multidrug resistance is now seen more commonly than in previous years; hence, most newly diagnosed cases in the United States are treated with at least four drugs unless the bacterium's susceptibility from the source case is known.

You should remember

The prognosis of TB is generally good if infections are localized to the lungs, except when drug-resistant strains cause them or occur in older, debilitated, or immunosuppressed individuals at high risk for developing extrapulmonary TB and progression of pulmonary disease.

Pharmacotherapy of tuberculosis

The pharmacotherapy of TB involves a variety of first- and second-line drugs, summarized in **Table 50.1**. The most common treatment for active TB is isoniazid (INH) in combination with the other first-line drugs. Patients often begin to feel better only a few weeks after starting this drug regimen, but treating the disease takes much longer than for different bacterial infections.

Isoniazid

INH is used to treat TB or prevent its return. It may be given alone or in combination with other medications. INH can cause serious adverse effects such as damage to the liver, but this is more likely to occur in patients over 50 years of age. If a patient is being treated for active TB, the medication regimen must continue for the entire treatment, even if symptoms begin to improve. It is essential to take all doses.

Pharmacokinetics

Oral INH is rapidly and almost entirely (90%–95%) absorbed from the small intestine. The peak plasma concentrations are reached within 1–2 hours after ingestion.

It has minimal protein binding, between 10% and 15%. CYP450, -2C19, and -3A4 inhibitors metabolize it in the liver via **acetylation** and dehydrazination. The rate of acetylation is determined by genetics. The elimination half-life is 0.5–1.6 hours in fast acetylators and 2–5 hours in slow acetylators. The drug is primarily excreted in the urine but also the feces.

TABLE 50.1 First- and second-line drugs for treating tuberculosis.

Generic name	Trade name	Route of administration
First-line drugs	Myambutol	Oral
EMB	Hydra, Hyzyd, Isovit	Oral, IM
INH	Rifater, Tebrazid	Oral
PZA	Mycobutin	Oral
rifabutin	Rifadin, Rimactane	Oral, IV
RIF	Priftin	Oral
rifapentine		
Second-line drugs	Amikin	IV/IM
amikacin	Sirturo	Oral
bedaquiline	Capastat Sulfate	IM, IV
capreomycin	Seromycin	Oral
cycloserine	Deltyba	Oral
delamanid	Trecator	Oral
ethionamide	Kantrex	IM, IV
kanamycin	Levaquin	Oral, IV
levofloxacin	Avelox	Oral
moxifloxacin	Floxin	Oral
ofloxacin	Paser	Oral
PAS	Dovprela	Oral
pretomanid		

EMB, Ethambutol; *INH*, isoniazid; *PAS*, para-aminosalicylic acid; *PZA*, pyrazinamide; *RIF*, rifampin.

Mechanism of action

INH is a prodrug that inhibits the formation of the mycobacterial cell wall. It must be activated by a bacterial catalase-peroxidase enzyme in *M. tuberculosis* known as KatG. The antimicrobial activity of INH is selective for mycobacteria, probably due to its inhibition of mycolic acid synthesis. The drug inhibits an **enoyl reductase** called InhA by forming a **covalent adduct** with the nicotinamide adenine dinucleotide **cofactor**.

Clinical indications

INH is an antibiotic indicated in the first-line treatment of active *M. tuberculosis* infection. Active TB infection can present as chills, fever, night sweats, cough, **hemoptysis**, and weight loss.

Contraindications

INH is contraindicated with severe hypersensitivity reactions that include drug-induced hepatitis; previous INH-associated liver damage; severe adverse reactions, including drug fever, chills, and arthritis; and acute liver disease of any cause.

Adverse effects

The two primary adverse effects of INH are nausea and diarrhea. Increases in hepatic serum transaminases, jaundice, and hepatitis may occur with use. INH is also associated with peripheral neuropathy, paresthesia, and sensory impairment, which may require discontinuation. Rare adverse effects include blurred vision or vision loss with or without eye pain, convulsions, fever, sore throat, joint pain, mental depression, mood or other mental changes, skin rash, and unusual bleeding or bruising.

Toxicities

Acute ingestion of 1.5 g of INH or more can lead to mild toxicity, but acute ingestion of over 20 mg/kg can cause convulsions. Signs of liver toxicity include fatigue, anorexia, nausea, myalgia, **arthralgia**, jaundice, and liver failure.

Pyrazinamide

Pyrazinamide (PZA) is an antimicrobial agent most commonly used to treat active TB during the initial phase of therapy, which is usually in the first 2 months of treatment. It is combined with other antibiotic agents. This drug has a relatively narrow spectrum of action. It has clinically significant antibacterial activity against *M. tuberculosis* and *Mycobacterium africanum*.

Pharmacokinetics

PZA is well absorbed orally and crosses inflamed meninges. It is a crucial part of the treatment of tuberculous meningitis. PZA bioavailability is over 90%. The liver metabolizes the drug, and the metabolic products are excreted in the urine and eliminated in 9–10 hours.

Mechanism of action

The mechanism of action of PZA has yet to be fully understood. It is converted to pyrazinoic acid in susceptible strains of *Mycobacterium*, which lowers the environment's pH. It does not have the same actions as most antibiotics, having little to no activity against growing tubercle bacilli. PZA is primarily active against nongrowing microorganisms. Unlike other drugs for TB, its activity increases with decreasing metabolic activity.

Clinical indications

PZA is indicated for the initial treatment of active TB in adults and children when combined with other anti-TB agents. It is never used independently and has no other indicated medical uses. *M. bovis* and *M. leprae* are innately resistant to this drug.

Contraindications

PZA is contraindicated in known hypersensitivity, severe liver damage, and acute **gout**. Liver transaminases and uric acid must be monitored before and during treatment.

Adverse effects

The most common adverse effect is arthralgia, which is not usually severe and only affects about 1% of patients. PZA can precipitate gout flares because it decreases renal excretion of uric acid. The most dangerous adverse effect is dose-related hepatotoxicity. Less common adverse effects include nausea, vomiting, anorexia, **sideroblastic anemia**, skin rash, pruritus, urticaria, dysuria, **interstitial nephritis**, malaise, fever, and porphyria.

Toxicities

PZA toxicities may result in the previously listed adverse effects, plus adverse effects on blood clotting mechanisms or vascular integrity.

Rifampin

Rifampin, or rifampicin, is an antimicrobial used to manage and treat diverse mycobacterial and gram-positive bacterial infections. It is used alone or with other antimicrobials to treat TB and asymptomatic carriers of *Neisseria meningitidis.*

Pharmacokinetics

Approximately 80% of rifampin is transported in blood, bound to plasma proteins (albumin). It is well distributed in various tissues and likely undergoes **deacetylation** in hepatocytes. Its oral bioavailability is 90%–95%, and protein binding is 80%. The drug is metabolized in the liver and intestinal walls. The elimination half-life is 3–4 hours. Rifampin is excreted via the feces (60% to 65%) and urine (about 30%).

Mechanism of action

Rifampin is believed to inhibit bacterial DNA-dependent RNA polymerase. This occurs because the drug binds to the polymerase subunit within the DNA/RNA channel, directly blocking RNA transcription. This effect is believed to be dose related.

Clinical indications

Rifampin is used along with other medications to treat TB in different areas of the body. It is also used for patients in close contact with a person who has meningococcal disease but does not have infectious symptoms; it helps prevent the bacteria from spreading to other people. It may also be an adjunctive agent for various infections, including endocarditis or bone and joint diseases.

Contraindications

Rifampin should be avoided in patients with a history of allergy to the drug or preexisting liver diseases. It is contraindicated in patients receiving atazanavir, darunavir, fosamprenavir, saquinavir, or tipranavir. This is because rifampin has the potential to significantly decrease plasma concentrations of these antiviral drugs, which may cause a loss of antiviral efficacy, the development of viral resistance, or both.

Adverse effects

Rifampin has many adverse effects, including blurred vision, diarrhea, psychomotor agitation, **petechia**, chest pain, dizziness, fever, headache, heartburn, nausea, hives, difficulty concentrating, fainting, tachycardia, fatigue, menstrual changes, jaundice, behavior changes, loss of appetite, muscle weakness, paresthesias, and abdominal distention. Discoloration of the teeth, urine, feces, saliva, sweat, and tears may also occur.

Toxicities

Rifampin can cause toxicity that is either related to dosage (affecting the liver) or treatment duration. Dose-related toxic effects become apparent after 9–15 g of the drug are taken. Various symptoms of overdose can manifest, including **metabolic acidosis** and **thrombocytopenia**. Additional toxicity includes convulsions, oliguric renal failure, cholestatic jaundice, and hypersensitivity reactions, including rifampin-induced flulike syndrome. There is no specific antidote available for rifampin toxicity.

Ethambutol

Ethambutol is a bacteriostatic drug that inhibits cell wall synthesis. It is used in the management and treatment of TB. In most cases, ethambutol is used along with other anti-TB drugs. It is also used as a component of a combination regimen to treat NTM infections.

Pharmacokinetics

Ethambutol is rapidly and well absorbed (over 80% of the dose) in the small intestine. The protein binding of ethambutol is 20%–30%, and it is metabolized in the liver. Ethambutol is 50% eliminated in the urine as the unmetabolized parent compound and 8% to 15% as inactive metabolites. Also, 20%–22% of each dose is eliminated unchanged in the feces. Ethambutol has a half-life of 3.3 hours in patients with normal kidney function and up to 7–15 hours in end-stage renal disease.

Mechanism of action

The mechanism of action of ethambutol has yet to be fully understood. It is believed to exert its bacteriostatic activity by inhibiting arabinosyl transferase, an enzyme that polymerizes arabinose into arabinan and then arabinogalactan, a constituent of bacterial cell walls. This results in impaired mycobacterial cell wall synthesis.

Clinical indications

Ethambutol is combined with other anti-TB drugs to treat pulmonary TB. When administered daily, it has a long duration of action and a moderate therapeutic window. The drug is also used to treat MAC and *Mycobacterium kansasii*.

Contraindications

Ethambutol is contraindicated in patients known to be hypersensitive to the drug, with known **optic neuritis**, and in those unable to understand or report visual side effects or vision changes (such as young children or unconscious patients).

Adverse effects

The adverse effects of ethambutol include optic neuropathy, optic neuritis, retrobulbar neuritis, peripheral neuropathy, hepatotoxicity, mental confusion, disorientation, hallucinations, and psychosis. The other adverse effects include decreased visual activity, **scotoma**, color blindness, visual field defects, and blurred vision.

Toxicities

One of the most well-known signs and symptoms of toxicity is optic neuritis, which is dose related. More than 40% of adults develop toxicity at doses higher than 50 mg/kg. Up to 3% of adults develop toxicity at 15 mg/kg/day.

Drugs for leprosy

Leprosy, or **Hansen disease**, is a slowly progressive infection caused by *M. leprae* that mainly affects the skin and peripheral nerves. Despite its low communicability, leprosy remains endemic among people living in several developing tropical nations.

The source of infection and transmission route is unknown; however, human respiratory secretions or soil are likely origins. *M. leprae* is taken up by macrophages and disseminates in the blood, but it replicates primarily in relatively soft tissues of the skin and extremities. It proliferates best at 32°–34°C, the temperature of the human skin. Like *M. tuberculosis*, *M. leprae* secretes no toxins, and its virulence is based on the properties of its cell wall. It is similar to *M. tuberculosis* in that immunization with Bacille Calmette-Guérin (BCG) vaccine confers some protection against *M. leprae* infection. Cell-mediated immunity is manifested by delayed-type hypersensitivity reactions to dermal injections of a bacterial extract called lepromin.

Lepromatous leprosy involves the skin, peripheral nerves, anterior eye chamber, upper airways, hands, testes, and feet. The vital organs and CNS are rarely affected, presumably because the core temperature is too high for the growth of *M. leprae*. Macular, papular, or nodular lesions form on the face, ears, wrists, elbows, and knees. With progression, the nodular lesions **coalesce** to yield distinctive leonine facies, a facial appearance that can resemble a lion's face. Most skin lesions are hypoesthetic or anesthetic. Lesions in the nose may cause persistent inflammation and bacilli-laden discharge. Dapsone belongs to a class of drugs known as **sulfones**, and it is used to treat leprosy.

Dapsone

Dapsone is an antibiotic used in multidrug regimens to treat leprosy and **dermatitis herpetiformis**. Initially investigated as an antibiotic agent in 1937, it was first used for leprosy treatment in 1945.

Pharmacokinetics

Dapsone is rapidly and nearly completely absorbed orally—the peak concentration occurs in 4–8 hours. The plasma half-life varies between individuals from 10–50 hours, with an average of 28 hours. Dapsone is metabolized in the liver via acetylation and hydroxylation by the CYP450 enzyme system, specifically CYP2E1, a CYP2C9 and CYP3A substrate. About 85% of dapsone is eliminated in the urine.

Mechanism of action

Dapsone is **bacteriostatic** in action. It inhibits the synthesis of dihydrofolic acid by competing with para-aminobenzoic acid for the active site of dihydropteroate synthetase, thereby inhibiting folic acid synthesis.

Clinical indications

Dapsone treats leprosy and helps control dermatitis herpetiformis. It is combined with one or more other medicines to treat leprosy. It may also be used to treat *Toxoplasma gondii* encephalitis or *pneumocystis* pneumonia in patients with HIV. Dapsone is available as a tablet.

Contraindications

The contraindications of dapsone include hypersensitivity to dapsone. It should be used with caution in patients with severe anemia and **agranulocytosis**. Deaths from agranulocytosis, **aplastic anemia**, and other blood dyscrasias are reported with dapsone administration. Dapsone should be avoided in patients with allergy to sulfonamide, glucose-6-phosphate dehydrogenase deficiency, liver or renal impairment, cardiopulmonary disease, peripheral neuropathy, and pregnancy.

Adverse effects

The adverse effects of dapsone include nausea, vomiting, abdominal pain, anorexia, pancreatitis, decreased hemoglobin, neutropenia, tachycardia, cholestatic jaundice, and albuminuria.

Toxicities

The toxicity of dapsone includes fatigue, headache, dizziness, tachycardia, weakness, dyspnea, seizures, and coma. Hepatoxicity or delayed hypersensitivity reactions such as drug rash with eosinophilia and systemic symptoms or Stevens-Johnson syndrome/toxic epidermal necrolysis may occur.

You should remember

Dapsone syndrome may develop after 2–6 weeks after therapy. The symptoms include fever, rash, and hepatitis. This clinical symptom can resemble infectious mononucleosis. Blood work will show peripheral eosinophilia and elevated liver enzymes. It is life-threatening if untreated.

Drugs for *Mycobacterium avium* complex

Mycobacterium avium and *M. intracellulare* are separate species, but the infections they cause are so similar that they are referred to as *M. avium* complex, or MAC. MAC is standard in soil, water, dust, and domestic animals. Clinically significant infection with MAC is uncommon except among people with T-cell immunodeficiency due to AIDS and immunosuppression resulting from treatment for transplant rejection or autoimmune diseases. In patients with marked T-cell immunodeficiency, MAC causes widely disseminated infections, and organisms proliferate abundantly in many organs, including the lungs and gastrointestinal system. Patients are feverish with drenching night sweats and weight loss. In the rare case of MAC in a person without HIV, the organisms primarily infect the lung, causing a productive cough and sometimes fever and weight loss.

MAC is resistant to many antibiotics and anti-TB drugs. However, it is somewhat susceptible to macrolides (clarithromycin or azithromycin), rifamycins (rifampin, rifabutin), ethambutol, clofazimine, fluoroquinolones (ciprofloxacin, levofloxacin, moxifloxacin), aminoglycosides (amikacin), and inhaled amikacin liposomal suspension. Generally, MAC is treated with daily doses of three antimicrobials for at least 12 months after sputum culture conversion. First-line drugs often include azithromycin or clarithromycin, ethambutol, and either rifampin or rifabutin. Additional agents, especially in patients with cavitary or advanced bronchiectatic lung diseases, include amikacin or fluoroquinolones.

Key Terms

Acetylation
Aplastic anemia
Arthralgia
Atypical mycobacteria
Cofactor
Covalent adduct
Deacetylation
Dermatitis herpetiformis
Enoyl reductase
Hansen disease
Hemoptysis
Hilar adenopathy
Interstitial nephritis
Lepromatous leprosy
Leprosy
Miliary tuberculosis
Optic neuritis
Petechia
Pleural effusion
Sideroblastic anemia
Sulfones
Thrombocytopenia

Clinical Case Studies

Clinical Case Study 1

A 45-year-old male was assessed for progressive shortness of breath, cough, and green-colored sputum production. Sputum test results revealed MAC infection, an atypical type of TB. The patient had previously been diagnosed with active typical TB and was treated successfully with TB drugs. However, for the new atypical infection, the patient was prescribed combination therapy over a year, but his compliance was poor. His intermittent use of the medications resulted in progressive deterioration of his lungs.

Critical Thinking Questions

1. What is the difference between primary and secondary TB?
2. What is the most common treatment regimen for active TB?
3. How is MAC generally treated?

Clinical Case Study 2

A 33-year-old female presented with hypopigmented skin lesions on both hands. PCR testing revealed the lesions to be positive for *M. leprae*. An initial TB workup was positive, and chest radiography revealed subtle infiltrates in the right middle lung lobe. The patient's sputum was culture positive for drug-susceptible TB. Minocycline and dapsone therapy was started for 2 months but then changed to rifampin, INH, PZA, and ethambutol with the addition of dapsone once sputum cultures were reported. After 1 month, repeated sputum cultures were negative for TB.

Critical Thinking Questions

1. What are the clinical manifestations of leprosy?
2. What is the mechanism of action of dapsone?
3. What are the causative pathogens for leprosy and TB?

Further Reading

[1] I.O. Andrade, Tuberculosis Volume I, Andrade, 2024.
[2] I.O. Andrade, Tuberculosis Volume II, Andrade, 2024.
[3] C.M. Anuradha, Anti-Tuberculosis Drug Design, Lap Lambert Academic Publishing, 2023.
[4] G. Battista Migliori, Essential Tuberculosis, Springer, 2021.
[5] J. Brodston, Multiple Drug Resistant Tuberculosis – An Analysis of the Standard Protocol Used in the Detection and Treatment of Multiple Drug Resistant Tuberculosis, 2015.
[6] M.V.N. De Souza, Tuberculosis Treatment – The Search for New Drugs, Bentham Books, 2018.
[7] L.N. Friedman, M. Dedicoat, P.D.O. Davies, Clinical Tuberculosis, sixth ed., CRC Press, 2020.
[8] D.E. Griffith, Nontuberculous Mycobacterial Disease – A Comprehensive Approach to Diagnosis and Management (Respiratory Medicine Series), Humana Press, 2019.
[9] D. Heemskerk, M. Caws, B. Marais, J. Farrar, Tuberculosis in Adults and Children (Briefs in Public Health Book 2), Springer, 2015.
[10] R. Laniado Laborin, Drug Resistant Tuberculosis – Practical Guide for Clinical Management, Bentham Books, 2015.
[11] P.X. Lu, H.Z. Lu, Y.X. Yi, Diagnostic Imaging of Drug Resistance Pulmonary Tuberculosis, Springer, 2024.
[12] G. Riccardi, C. Sala, Tuberculosis Drug Discovery and Development, MDPI, 2019.
[13] K. Sardana, A. Khurana, Jopling's Handbook of Leprosy, 6th Edition, sixth ed., CPS Publishers and Distributors Pvt Ltd, 2022.
[14] D.L. Schlossberg, Tuberculosis and Nontuberculous Mycobacterial Infections, seventh ed., ASM Books, 2017 (Book 36).
[15] C. Teixeira Soares, Histopathological Diagnosis of Leprosy, Bentham Books, 2021.

CHAPTER

51

Antifungal drugs

OUTLINE

LEARNING OUTCOMES

After study of the chapter, readers should be able to:

1. Explain the characteristics of fungi.
2. Identify the most common cause of pulmonary fungal infections.
3. Explain dermatophyte infections and various types.
4. Describe the mechanism of action of nystatin.
5. Explain the systemic fungal infections and their treatments.
6. Describe the clinical indications of amphotericin B.
7. Discuss the clinical indications of nystatin.

The Science of Pharmacology
https://doi.org/10.1016/B978-0-443-29038-1.00051-8

8. Explain the adverse effects of amphotericin B.
9. List drugs for both superficial fungal infections
10. Describe the clinical indications of fluconazole.

Overview

Fungal infections (mycosis) are any disease or condition caused by a fungus (yeast or mold). They usually affect the skin, hair, nails, mouth, throat, lungs, urinary tract, or other body parts. Patients with a weakened immune system are at higher risk for fungal infections. Yeasts and molds now rank among the 10 most commonly isolated pathogens in febrile patients with an impaired immune system. Fungi are mainly opportunistic pathogens that only invade the body if a severely weakened natural defense permits them. Most factors facilitating an invasive fungal infection are unavoidable because they are directly connected to the underlying diseases and their treatment. Fungi are living organisms that are classified separately from plants or animals. They move around by spreading out or sending spores into the air. Only a few of the fungi pathogenic for humans are sufficiently virulent to infect a healthy host. Most are relatively harmless unless they encounter an immunocompromised patient with a weakened defense system that permits them to invade the body.

Characteristics of fungi and fungal infections

Fungi are one-celled or multicellular organisms. They help decompose dead animals and plants to recycle their structures and components in soil. Fungi include **molds**, mushrooms, and **yeasts**. Only about 50 species are implicated in human disease. A few species survive in the normal host flora of the mouth, skin, and urogenital tract.

Some fungi grow slowly, meaning that fungal infections can be present for months before symptoms appear. These infections are generally not transmitted via casual contact. Fungal antigens may cause infections or trigger hypersensitivity responses that cause mold or mildew allergies. Some fungi, such as *Aspergillus flavus*, secrete toxins that cause illness by ingesting contaminated foods such as grains. Patients with immunosuppression can develop frequent fungal infections, and aggressive pharmacotherapy is required. Systemic fungal infections in these patients can be fatal very quickly. Fungal pathogens are described in **Table 51.1**.

Drugs for superficial fungal infections

Superficial fungal infections are common. **Dermatophyte infections** are familiar at all ages and in both sexes, and they have a worldwide distribution. Superficial fungal infections affect the nails, skin, and mucous membranes such as mouth, throat, or vagina. Superficial fungal infections include tinea capitis (scalp), tinea cruris (the groin and inner thighs), tinea pedis (athlete's foot), tinea corporis, tinea manuum (hands), and tinea barbae (face and facial hair). Candidal infections affect skin and mucous membranes, which are also common. They can cause oral thrush, diaper rash, and vaginal yeast.

Treatment modalities include oral and topical agents (see **Table 51.2**). Oral therapies include griseofulvin, terbinafine, fluconazole, ketoconazole, and itraconazole. Topical treatments include nystatin, selenium sulfide, tolnaftate, haloprogin, miconazole, clotrimazole, and sodium thiosulfate. Compliance with what is sometimes a long course of treatment is essential to successful treatment and good personal hygiene.

The efficacy of topical agents in superficial mycoses depends not only on the type of lesion and the actual mechanism of action of the drug but also on the viscosity, hydrophobicity, and acidity of the formulation. Regardless of the type of formulation, topical drug penetration in hyperkeratotic lesions is often precarious. Products used for cutaneous application tend to be manufactured in creams or solutions. Ointments are cumbersome and overly occlusive for macerated or fissured intertriginous lesions. The use of powders applied either in sprays or aerosol form is primarily limited to the foot area and lesions in moist intertriginous areas. Cutaneous formulations are not suitable for oral, vaginal, or ocular use.

TABLE 51.1 Fungal pathogens

Fungus	Type of infection	Description
Systemic		
Aspergillus fumigatus, other species	Aspergillosis	Opportunistic; usually affects the lungs but also can spread to other organs
Blastomyces dermatitidis	Blastomycosis	Starts in the lungs, then spreads to other organs
Candida albicans, other species	Candidiasis	The most common opportunistic fungal infection; it can affect almost all organs
Coccidioides species	Coccidioidomycosis	Starts in the lungs, then spreads to other organs
Cryptococcus neoformans	Cryptococcosis	Starts in the lungs; it is the most common cause of meningitis in AIDS patients
Histoplasma capsulatum	Histoplasmosis	Starts in the lungs, then spreads to other organs
Mucorales species, most commonly *Rhizopus*	Mucormycosis	Opportunistic; affects the blood vessels; causes disorders such as sinus infections and stomach ulcers
Pneumocystis jirovecii	Pneumocystis pneumonia	Opportunistic; usually is pneumonia of the lung but can spread to other organs
Superficial		
Candida albicans, other species	Candidiasis	Affects the nails, oral cavity (thrush), skin, vagina
Epidermophyton floccosum	Various skin infections	Athlete's foot (tinea pedis), jock itch (tinea cruris), etc.
Microsporum species	Tinea capitis	Ringworm of the scalp
Trichophyton species	Various infections	Affects the nails, scalp, and skin
Subcutaneous and cutaneous		
Sporothrix schenckii	Sporotrichosis	Mostly affects the skin and superficial lymph nodes
Mixed species	Chromoblastomycosis	Chronic skin mycosis occurring in subtropical and tropical climates

Nystatin

Nystatin is a polyene-class antifungal medication. It is a topical and oral drug that fights against many yeast and *Candida* species. It is mainly used to treat skin and oropharyngeal candidiasis.

TABLE 51.2 Drugs for superficial fungal infections

Generic name	Trade name	Route of administration
butenafine	Mentax	Topical
ciclopirox (cream, gel, shampoo, or nail lacquer)	Loprox, Penlac	Topical
griseofulvin	Gris-PEG	PO
naftifine	Naftin	Topical
nystatin (topical powder, oral suspension, capsule, cream, ointment)	Nystop, Mycostatin	PO, topical, vaginal suppository
tavaborole	Kerydin	Topical
terbinafine	Lamisil	Topical, PO
tolnaftate	Aftate, Tinactin	Topical
undecylenic acid	Fungi-Nail, Gordochom	Topical
Azoles		
butoconazole	Femstat, Bynazole	Intravaginal cream
clotrimazole cream, intravaginal, troche	Lotrimin AF, Gyne-Lotrimin, Mycelex	Topical cream, intravaginal suppository, PO (troche)
econazole	Spectazole	Topical cream
efinaconazole	Jublia	Topical solution
fluconazole	Diflucan	PO
itraconazole	Sporanox	PO
ketoconazole	Nizoral	Topical cream or shampoo
luliconazole	Luzu	Topical cream
miconazole	Micatin, Monistat-3, Oravig	Topical cream, intravaginal suppository, buccal tablet
oxiconazole	Oxistat	Topical cream
sulconazole	Exelderm	Topical cream
terconazole	Terazol	Intravaginal cream/suppository
tioconazole	Monistat-1, Vagistat-1	Intravaginal ointment

Pharmacokinetics

Systemic absorption of nystatin is minimal following oral administration, and no detectable plasma concentrations are attained following topical or vaginal administration. Because nystatin cannot be systemically absorbed, it is not metabolized in the liver. The majority of orally administered nystatin is eliminated unchanged in the feces.

Mechanism of action

Nystatin exerts its therapeutic effect by forming a membrane-spanning pore in the fungal plasma membrane. The formation of this pore can cause a change in membrane permeability that allows for leakage of intracellular contents and the subsequent disruption of electrochemical gradients required for proper cell function.

Clinical indications

Nystatin is a **polyene ionophore** antifungal used to treat cutaneous, mucocutaneous, and gastrointestinal mycotic infections, particularly those caused by *Candida* species.

Nystatin is ineffective in **dermatophytosis**. It is available as a cream, ointment, oral suspension (100,000 units/mL), and coated pills (500,000 units). It can also be combined with antimicrobials or corticosteroids.

Contraindications

Nystatin tablets are contraindicated in patients with a history of hypersensitivity to any of their components. They are generally not to be used for the treatment of systemic mycoses.

Adverse effects

The adverse effects of nystatin include allergic reactions, irritation inside the mouth, nausea, vomiting, diarrhea, and stomach upset.

Toxicities

There have been no reports of severe toxic effects following overdosage of nystatin—doses over 5 million units daily have resulted in nausea and gastrointestinal upset with no other associated effects.

Griseofulvin

Griseofulvin is an antifungal medication that treats specific yeast and fungal skin, hair, and nail infections. It can be taken by mouth in capsule or tablet form.

Pharmacokinetics

Griseofulvin is an oral medication in 125-, 250-, and 500-mg tablets and is also available as a suspension. It is better absorbed in lower doses. This agent has poor water solubility and is considered lipophilic. It is best taken with a high-fat meal to increase absorption from the GI tract. Therapy for **tinea capitis** lasts 6–12 weeks. Griseofulvin is quickly eliminated from the body and thus must be taken over an extended period to be efficacious.

Mechanism of action

Griseofulvin interacts with microtubules to affect the formation of the mitotic spindle. This interference ultimately inhibits mitosis in dermatophytes. It is a fungistatic agent against *Trichophyton*, *Microsporum*, and *Epidermophyton* species. Notably, it is ineffective in treating dimorphic fungi, yeast (*Malassezia*, *Candida*), and chromomycosis.

Clinical indications

Griseofulvin is an antifungal medication that treats fungal and yeast infections in the skin, hair, and nails. It is the drug of choice in treating tinea capitis and **onychomycosis**. It can be used for superficial fungal infections resistant to treatment with topical antifungal medications.

Contraindications

Griseofulvin is contraindicated in patients with hypersensitivity, hepatic failure, porphyria, and pregnancy (category C). Females who are pregnant should avoid it during their first trimester due to the possibility of causing fetal abnormalities. Patients should wait at least a month after completion of treatment with griseofulvin before becoming pregnant.

Adverse effects

Overall, griseofulvin has few adverse effects. It causes loss of appetite, nausea, vomiting, diarrhea, headaches, fatigue, dizziness, confusion, insomnia, fever, dyspnea, hematuria, and allergic reactions. Other adverse effects include photosensitivity, fixed drug eruption, **petechiae**, pruritus, and **urticaria**. It may also worsen lupus or porphyria.

Toxicities

The toxicities of griseofulvin include chest pain, liver damage, and renal impairments.

Drugs for systemic fungal infections

Systemic fungal infections include coccidioidomycosis, blastomycosis, histoplasmosis, cryptococcosis, mucormycosis, aspergillosis, pneumocystis pneumonia, and systemic candidiasis. Systemic mycoses caused by primary pathogens usually originate in the lungs and may spread to other organ systems. Opportunistic fungal pathogens in

TABLE 51.3 Drugs for systemic fungal infections

Generic name	Trade name	Route of administration
amphotericin B	Abelcet, AmBisome, Amphotec, Fungizone	IV
flucytosine	Ancobon	PO
Echinocandins		
anidulafungin	Eraxis	IV
caspofungin	Cancidas	IV
micafungin	Mycamine	IV
Azoles		
fluconazole	Diflucan	PO, IV
isavuconazonium	Cresemba	PO, IV
itraconazole	Sporanox	PO, IV
ketoconazole	Nizoral	PO, topical
posaconazole	Noxafil	PO (delayed release tablet, suspension)
voriconazole	Vfend	PO, IV

immunocompromised hosts cause most systemic fungal infections. They typically originate either in the lungs (*Aspergillus*, *Cryptococcus*, *Mucorales* spp., as a result of inhalation) or from endogenous flora (*Candida* spp., as a result of infected lines or leakage from the GI tract). They may spread to other organs and cause systemic infections. **Table 51.3** includes systemic fungal medications. Systemic fungal infections are medical emergencies and have high mortality rates, which are significant if appropriate therapy is delayed.

Amphotericin B

Despite its well-known adverse effects and toxicity, amphotericin B is crucial in managing severe systemic fungal infections. However, despite a life-threatening illness, therapy sometimes requires discontinuation. Newer lipid formulations that are less nephrotoxic than conventional amphotericin B are available. They are available as amphotericin B liposomal and an amphotericin B lipid complex. The lipid formulations permit a higher daily dose; provide better delivery to organs within the **reticular endothelial system** such as the lungs, liver, and spleen; have similar efficacy to conventional amphotericin B; and are less nephrotoxic.

Pharmacokinetics

Amphotericin B is administered parenterally due to poor oral absorption. The pharmacokinetics of amphotericin B lipid complex and amphotericin B liposomal are nonlinear, characterized by a dose-dependent increase in the volume of distribution and clearance. Amphotericin B demonstrates concentration-dependent fungicidal activity and postantifungal effect.

Amphotericin B reaches high concentrations in the lungs, kidneys, liver, spleen, and bone marrow. The amphotericin B lipid complex has a higher volume of distribution than liposomal amphotericin B due to its uptake by the reticuloendothelial system. Amphotericin B is not metabolized in the liver, and the primary route of elimination is through the kidneys.

Mechanism of action

Amphotericin B acts by binding to ergosterol in the cell membrane of most fungi. After binding with ergosterol, amphotericin B causes the formation of ion channels, leading to the loss of protons and monovalent cations, which results in depolarization and concentration-dependent cell killing.

Clinical indications

Amphotericin B deoxycholate treats aspergillosis, severe blastomycosis, cryptococcosis, coccidioidomycosis, histoplasmosis, and systemic candidiasis.

Contraindications

Absolute contraindications include a history of anaphylactic reaction to amphotericin B. It must be cautiously used to prevent overdosage, which can cause cardiopulmonary arrest. Amphotericin B should not be administered through rapid intravenous infusion due to the possibility of hypotension, hypokalemia, arrhythmias, and shock.

Adverse effects

Amphotericin B may cause headaches, chills, vomiting, stomach pain, fatigue, and dysuria. The most severe adverse effects include anaphylaxis, nephrotoxicity, hypokalemia, hypocalcemia, hyponatremia, and hypomagnesemia.

Toxicities

Amphotericin B may cause dose-related nephrotoxicity. It also produces fever, **phlebitis**, and tremors. Renal toxicity is dose dependent and cumulative. It is more likely when cumulative doses exceed 6 mg/kg daily.

You should remember

Amphotericin B can be used during pregnancy only if indicated. It is the drug of choice for invasive candidiasis in pregnancy. Using ideal body weight instead of total body weight can reduce potential adverse effects on the fetus. Liposomal amphotericin B is preferred due to its minimal risk of teratogenicity during pregnancy.

Drugs for both systemic and superficial fungal infections

Azoles are the antifungals with the largest and most versatile uses. They have broad spectrums and effectively treat most systemic, subcutaneous, and superficial fungal infections. Azoles can be administered PO and are much safer than many older antifungals. Chemical or therapeutic classes may group them. The two unique chemical classes are *imidazoles* and *triazoles*.

The imidazoles include butoconazole, clotrimazole, econazole, ketoconazole, miconazole, oxiconazole, sulconazole, and tioconazole. The triazoles include fluconazole, isavuconazonium, itraconazole, posaconazole, terconazole, and voriconazole. These drugs are more slowly metabolized than the imidazoles but cause fewer adverse effects.

Another way to classify the azoles is via their therapeutic use as either systemic or topical drugs. The azoles prescribed for systemic and topical infections include fluconazole, itraconazole, isavuconazonium, ketoconazole, posaconazole, and voriconazole. The rest of the azoles are only prescribed for superficial infections.

The azoles interfere with the biosynthesis of ergosterol, which is required for fungal cell membrane construction. Depleting the fungal cells of ergosterol impairs fungal growth. The systemic azoles have a spectrum of activity similar to amphotericin B, but they are less toxic and can be administered PO. Therefore some azoles have replaced amphotericin B in treating less systemic severe fungal infections.

Pharmacokinetics

The pharmacokinetic properties of fluconazole are similar after administration by intravenous or oral routes. In normal individuals, the bioavailability of orally administered fluconazole is more than 90% compared with IV administration. Peak plasma concentrations occur between 1 and 2 hours. Fluconazole is metabolized minimally in the liver. It is an inhibitor of CYP2C9, CYP3A4, and CYP2C19. After oral administration, the half-life is about 30 hours (range: 20–50 hours). Fluconazole clearance is primarily via renal excretion, with approximately 80% of the administered dose appearing as the unchanged drug in the urine.

Mechanism of action

Fluconazole is a fluorine-substituted, bis-triazole antifungal agent. Its mechanism of action involves interruption of the conversion of lanosterol to ergosterol via binding to fungal cytochrome P450 and subsequent disruption of fungal membranes.

Clinical indications

Fluconazole is used to treat vaginal candidiasis, oropharyngeal and esophageal candidiasis, urinary tract infections, peritonitis, and systemic *Candida* infections. It is also effective for candidemia, disseminated candidiasis, pneumonia, coccidioidomycosis, and cryptococcal meningitis.

Contraindications

Fluconazole is contraindicated in individuals with hypersensitivity to it. There are no data regarding cross-hypersensitivity between fluconazole and other azole antifungal agents. It should be avoided in patients with liver or kidney impairment. Safety during pregnancy has not been established.

Adverse effects

Common adverse effects of fluconazole include headache, stomach pain, diarrhea, nausea, vomiting, and rash. Serious adverse effects are uncommon but include jaundice, dark urine, pale-colored stool, easy bruising or infections, tachycardia, irregular heartbeat, and anaphylaxis.

Toxicities

Fluconazole can cause a condition that affects the heart rhythm, known as QT prolongation. This can rarely cause serious fast or irregular heartbeats and other symptoms such as severe dizziness or fainting that require immediate medical attention.

Key Terms

Dermatophyte infections
Dermatophytosis
Fungi
Molds
Onychomycosis
Petechiae
Polyene ionophore
Reticular endothelial system
Tinea capitis
Urticaria
Yeasts

Clinical case studies

Clinical case study 1

A 29-year-old female went to a dermatology clinic because of dry, reddened lesions on her face, arms, hands, and chest. She was prescribed itraconazole, but after 8 days, she returned to the clinic because the lesions had spread even further. The patient had no known family history of such lesions. She also complained of generalized weakness. A variety of blood and urine tests were performed. Skin tests revealed cutaneous dermatophytosis and infection with *T. violaceum*. The patient was instructed to continue the itraconazole, to which a few antifungals were added. She also had to apply Lupi-Aqua lotion twice per day. After only slight improvement, two other drugs (clindamycin and levofloxacin) were added for a short time. After 15 days, the patient's lesions started to disappear, and her generalized weakness was resolved.

Critical thinking questions

1. What are examples of superficial fungal infections?
2. What are the clinical indications of nystatin?
3. What are the adverse effects of griseofulvin?

Clinical case study 2

A 56-year-old male had undergone radiation therapy for a nasopharyngeal carcinoma. More recently, a newly diagnosed oropharyngeal carcinoma was excised. Six weeks after the surgery, an enlarging exophytic lesion at the surgical excision site was found. The initial biopsy did not reveal any malignancy or fungal organisms. Another biopsy under anesthesia was performed because CT imaging indicated it was needed. The patient was treated with long-term amphotericin B and fluconazole because the final culture results showed invasive candidiasis. The surgical site showed no additional lesions after 6 months.

Critical thinking questions

1. What are examples of systemic fungal infections?
2. What is the mechanism of action of amphotericin B?
3. What are the adverse effects of amphotericin B?

Further Reading

[1] A. Basak, R. Chakraborty, S.M. Mandal, Recent Trends in Antifungal Agents and Antifungal Therapy, Springer, 2016.
[2] P.B. Fernandes, New Approaches for Antifungal Drugs, Birkhauser, 2013.
[3] M.A. Ghannoum, J.R. Perfect, Antifungal Therapy, second ed., CRC Press, 2019.
[4] M.L. Grayson, Kucers' the Use of Antibiotics – A Clinical Review of Antibacterial, Antifungal, Antiparasitic, and Antiviral Drugs, Three Volume Set, seventh ed., CRC Press, 2017.
[5] D.R. Hospenthal, M.G. Rinaldi, Diagnosis and Treatment of Fungal Infections (Infectious Disease), second ed., Springer, 2015.
[6] M. Imran, M. Asim Farid, M. Adnan Asghar, Antibacterial and Antifungal Drug Discovery – Benzimidazole Derivatives, Lap Lambert Academic Publishing, 2015.
[7] Z. Iqbal, A. Ali Saleh Jaber, M.A. Mirza, Vaginal Drug Delivery Approach for Antifungal Therapy, Lap Lambert Academic Publishing, 2017.
[8] J.H. Kim, L.W. Cheng, K. Land, Advances in Antifungal Development – Discovery of New Drugs and Drug Repurposing, Mdpi Ag, 2022.
[9] D.J. Krysan, W.S. Moye-Rowley, Antifungal Drug Resistance – Methods and Protocols (Methods in Molecular Biology, Book 2658), Humana Press, 2023.
[10] A. Kumar, Phytoconstituents and Antifungals (Developments in Applied Microbiology and Biotechnology), Academic Press, 2022.
[11] N. Manzoor, Advances in Antifungal Drug Development – Natural Products with Antifungal Potential, Springer, 2024.
[12] A. Rasheed, Synthesis of Anti-fungal Drugs, CreateSpace Independent Publishing Platform, 2015.
[13] A. Rasheed, Analysis of Antifungal Drugs, CreateSpace Independent Publishing Platform, 2017.
[14] M. Sokovic, K. Liaras, Antifungal Compounds Discovery – Natural and Synthetic Approaches, Elsevier, 2020.
[15] J.J. Torrado Duran, D.R. Serrano, J. Capilla, Antifungal and Antiparasitic Drug Delivery, Mdpi Ag, 2020.

CHAPTER

52

Antiprotozoal drugs

OUTLINE

The Science of Pharmacology
https://doi.org/10.1016/B978-0-443-29038-1.00052-X

LEARNING OUTCOMES

After study of the chapter, readers should be able to:

1. List eight types of protozoal infections.
2. Describe the adverse effects of chloroquine.
3. Identify agents that are used to treat malaria.
4. Describe the toxicities of chloroquine.
5. Explain the characteristics of *Entamoeba histolytica* and how to treat it.
6. Discuss the characteristics of trichomoniasis and trypanosomiasis.
7. Describe the clinical indications of metronidazole.
8. Explain the contraindications of pyrimethamine.
9. Describe the characteristics of toxoplasmosis and its treatment.

Overview

Parasitic infectious diseases have an enormous health, social, and economic impact in tropical regions of the world. Diseases caused by protozoa, such as malaria and schistosomiasis, are the cause of most parasite-related morbidity, mortality, and deaths annually. They are common pathogens in tropical and subtropical countries and cause some of the most common intestinal infections in the United States. Many protozoal infections are diagnosed by examination of stool samples, but they are also crucial to the surgical pathologist. Common protozoan infectious diseases include malaria, giardia, and toxoplasmosis. Less common diseases include African trypanosomiasis and amoebic dysentery. Each condition affects the body differently. Protozoal infections are severe infectious diseases responsible for significant mortality and morbidity worldwide.

Classification and pathogenesis of protozoal infections

A **protozoan** is a one-celled organism in animal hosts, soil, and water. Only a few protozoans are pathogenic in humans, yet they cause many illnesses and deaths in Africa, Asia, Central America, and South America. Protozoans thrive in areas with poor sanitation and highly dense populations. Travelers often acquire and bring protozoal diseases from other countries into the United States or Canada. Some protozoal infections occur in immunosuppressed patients. **Table 52.1** summarizes various protozoal infections.

Malaria

Malaria is a life-threatening disease caused by parasites transmitted to people through the bites of infected female ***Anopheles*** **mosquitoes**. Symptoms can be mild or life-threatening. Mild symptoms are fever, chills, and headache. Severe symptoms include fatigue, confusion, seizures, and **dyspnea**. According to the World Health Organization (WHO), globally in 2022 there were an estimated 249 million malaria cases and 608,000 malaria deaths in 85 countries. The WHO African region carries a disproportionately high share of the global malaria burden. Nigeria, with the highest malaria burden of any country, accounted for 50% of the children treated for malaria. Children under 5 accounted for about 80% of all malaria deaths in the region. Roughly 2000 cases of malaria are diagnosed annually in the United States, which are usually connected to international travel.

TABLE 52.1 Various protozoal infections.

Disease (and species)	Description	Infection source
Amebiasis (*Entamoeba histolytica*)	Mostly infects the large intestine to cause severe diarrhea; often travels to the liver and forms abscesses; less often travels to the brain, kidneys, or lungs	Fecal-contaminated water
Cryptosporidiosis (*Cryptosporidium* species)	Infects the intestines to cause diarrhea; common in immunocompromised patients	Fecal-contaminated water
Giardiasis (*Giardia lamblia*)	Infects the intestines to cause abdominal pain, fatigue, and malabsorption	Fecal-contaminated water
Leishmaniasis (various *Leishmania* species)	Affects the blood, liver, skin, spleen, and other body systems	Bite of an infected sand fly
Malaria (various *Plasmodium* species)	Infects red blood cells, causing chills, fatigue, and fever; some species invade the liver and other tissues	Bite of the female *Anopheles* mosquito
Toxoplasmosis (*Toxoplasma gondii*)	Can invade any organ, causing a fatal encephalitis in immunocompromised patients or birth defects in people who are pregnant	Ingestion of contaminated food, water, or soil; congenital transmission; or via infected cat feces
Trichomoniasis (*Trichomonas vaginalis*)	A common sexually transmitted infection causing vaginitis in females and urethritis in males	Via sexual contact with infected fluids or genital areas
Trypanosomiasis (*Trypanosoma cruzi* in America, *Trypanosoma brucei* in Africa)	The American form is Chagas disease, invading cardiac tissue and the autonomic ganglia; the African form is sleeping sickness, causing fatigue and central nervous system depression	The bite of the kissing bug in America or the tsetse fly in Africa

Drugs for malaria

Malaria is a severe infection and always requires treatment with medicine. Multiple drugs must be used to prevent and treat malaria. The most common medications for malaria include artemisinins, chloroquine, and primaquine (see **Table 52.2**).

Chloroquine

Chloroquine targets the erythrocytic stage, which causes symptomatic illness. It has been used as an antimalarial drug since World War II. Resistance to chloroquine has developed in several parts of the world, including Africa, Southeast Asia, and South America. Resistant *P. falciparum* strains have reduced chloroquine's effectiveness in these areas.

TABLE 52.2 Drugs for malaria.

Generic name	Trade name	Route of administration
artemether-lumefantrine	Coartem	PO
artesunate	(generic only)	IV
atovaquone-proguanil	Malarone	PO
chloroquine	Aralen	PO, IM, subcutaneous
doxycycline	Vibramycin, Doryx	PO, IV
hydroxychloroquine	Plaquenil	PO
mefloquine	(generic only)	PO
primaquine	(generic only)	PO
quinine	Qualaquin	PO
tafenoquine	Arakoda	PO

Pharmacokinetics

Chloroquine is extensively distributed and has a terminal elimination half-life of 1–2 months. It is 60% bound to plasma proteins and partially metabolized by the liver, giving rise to its primary metabolite, desethylchloroquine. It is excreted about 50% as an unchanged drug in urine, where urine acidification increases its elimination.

Mechanism of action

Chloroquine prevents heme's polymerization into hemozoin, a toxic byproduct of hemoglobin breakdown. It forms a drug-hemozoin complex and caps the polymerizing chain, thereby preventing additional polymerization. This inhibition causes poisonous heme levels to accumulate, ultimately killing the parasite.

Clinical indications

For malaria prevention, 500 mg once weekly is typically given orally 2 weeks before, during, and up to 4 weeks after exposure to an endemic area. When used as a treatment for extraintestinal amebiasis, chloroquine dosing is 1000 mg daily for 2 days, followed by 500 mg daily for at least 2–3 weeks. For severe or emergent cases of malaria, chloroquine should be administered parenterally.

Contraindications

Chloroquine is contraindicated in patients with sensitivity to any components. It should be avoided in patients with retinal or vision changes unless treating acute malaria. Chloroquine has been proven safe to use during pregnancy and in children.

Adverse effects

The adverse effects of chloroquine include pruritus, abdominal cramps, nausea, vomiting, agranulocytosis, photosensitivity, retinopathy, hearing loss, seizures, paranoia, and hallucinations. Intramuscular injections can cause severe hypotension and hemolytic anemia.

Toxicities

High doses of chloroquine toxicities include retinal damage, long and subtle symptoms of reduced visual acuity, **diplopia**, and bilateral loss of vision. Cardiomyopathy, QT prolongation, and ventricular arrhythmias may also occur with long-term use at high doses. High doses can also cause severe psychiatric conditions such as paranoia, hallucinations, and suicidal ideations.

You should remember

Chloroquine and hydroxychloroquine are often coadministered with other drugs in treating malaria and chronic inflammatory diseases.

You should remember

Preventive chemotherapy includes perennial malaria chemoprevention, seasonal malaria chemoprevention, intermittent preventive treatment of malaria in pregnancy and school-aged children, postdischarge malaria chemoprevention, and mass drug administration. These safe and cost-effective strategies complement ongoing malaria control activities, including vector control measures, prompt diagnosis of suspected malaria, and treatment of confirmed cases with antimalarial medicines.

You should remember

Since October 2021 the WHO has recommended broad use of the RTS, S/AS01 malaria vaccine among children living in regions with moderate to high *P. falciparum* malaria transmission. The vaccine has been shown to reduce malaria and deadly severe malaria among young children significantly. In October 2023, the WHO recommended a second safe and effective malaria vaccine, R21/Matrix-M. The availability of two malaria vaccines is expected to make broad-scale deployment across Africa possible.

Classification of nonmalaria protozoal infections

Several other protozoan infections include amebiasis, giardiasis, cryptosporidiosis, African Trypanosoma, trichomoniasis, and toxoplasmosis. We will discuss only amebiasis, giardiasis, and cryptosporidiosis.

Amebiasis

Amebiasis is an intestinal infection caused by a parasite called *Entamoeba histolytica*, which is spread via human feces. It causes intestinal amebiasis and extraintestinal manifestations. Although 90% of *Entamoeba histolytica* infections are asymptomatic, nearly 50 million people become symptomatic; symptoms include fever, loss of appetite, bloody diarrhea, nausea, cramping, and weight loss may occur with about 100,000 deaths yearly. Amebic infections are more prevalent in countries with lower socioeconomic conditions. **Fig. 52.1** illustrates the lifecycle of *Entamoeba histolytica*.

Entamoeba histolytica can have two forms: the cyst form, which can survive in the environment for a prolonged period, and the trophozoite stage, which is the active and invasive form. After ingesting the cyst, trophozoites can form, invading and penetrating intestinal mucosa and destroying epithelial and inflammatory cells. Amoebic liver abscess formation is the most common extraintestinal complication. Symptoms include fever, jaundice, right upper quadrant pain, and hepatomegaly.

Metronidazole is the first-line treatment for intestinal amebiasis and amebic liver abscesses, followed by a luminal agent. In adults, the typical dose is 500 to 750 mg orally three times daily for 7–10 days. Broad-spectrum antibiotics should be started in patients with fulminant amoebic colitis or signs of **peritonitis**. Surgical intervention may be required with bowel perforation or toxic megacolon (see **Table 52.3**).

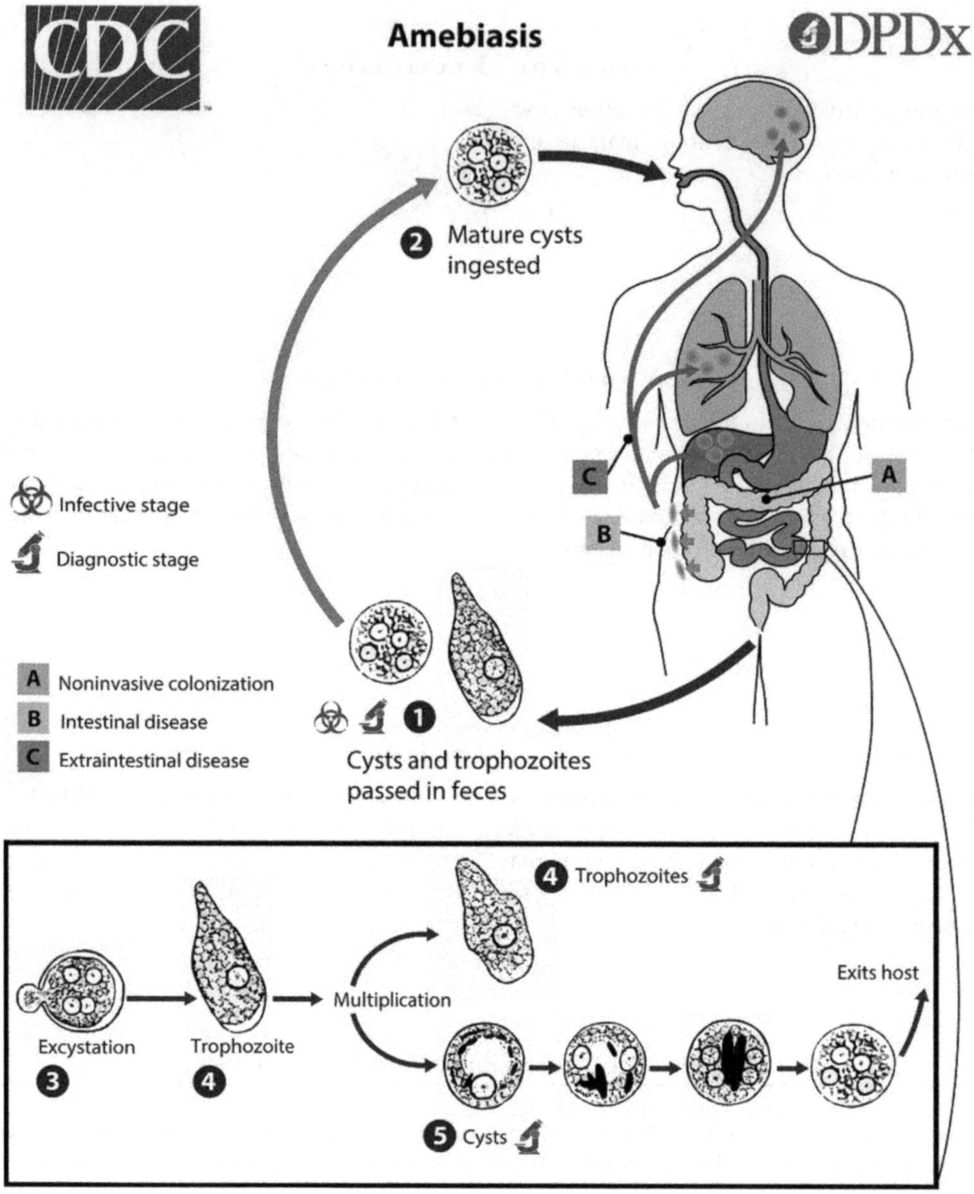

FIG. 52.1 The life cycle of *Entamoeba histolytica.*

Giardiasis

Giardia is an intestinal infection marked by abdominal cramps, bloating, nausea, and watery diarrhea. It is caused by a microscopic parasite found worldwide, especially in areas with poor sanitation and unclean water. Giardiasis is among the most common causes of waterborne disease in the United States. The parasites are found in backcountry streams, lakes, public water supplies, swimming pools, and whirlpool spas and wells. Giardia infection can be spread through food and person-to-person contact. The life cycle of *Giardia duodenalis* consists of two stages: the trophozoite and the cyst. The trophozoite is the vegetative form and replicates in the host's small intestine (see **Fig. 52.2**). Some patients are asymptomatic, but they still carry the parasite and can spread it to others through their stool. For those who do get sick, signs and symptoms usually appear 1–3 weeks after exposure. They may include nausea; watery, sometimes foul-smelling diarrhea that may alternate with soft, greasy stools; abdominal pain; fatigue; and weight loss. Signs and symptoms of giardia infection may last 2–6 weeks, but in some people, they last longer or recur.

Giardiasis usually clears up within a few weeks. However, the patient may have intestinal problems long after the parasites are gone. Several drugs are generally effective against giardia parasites, but only some respond to them.

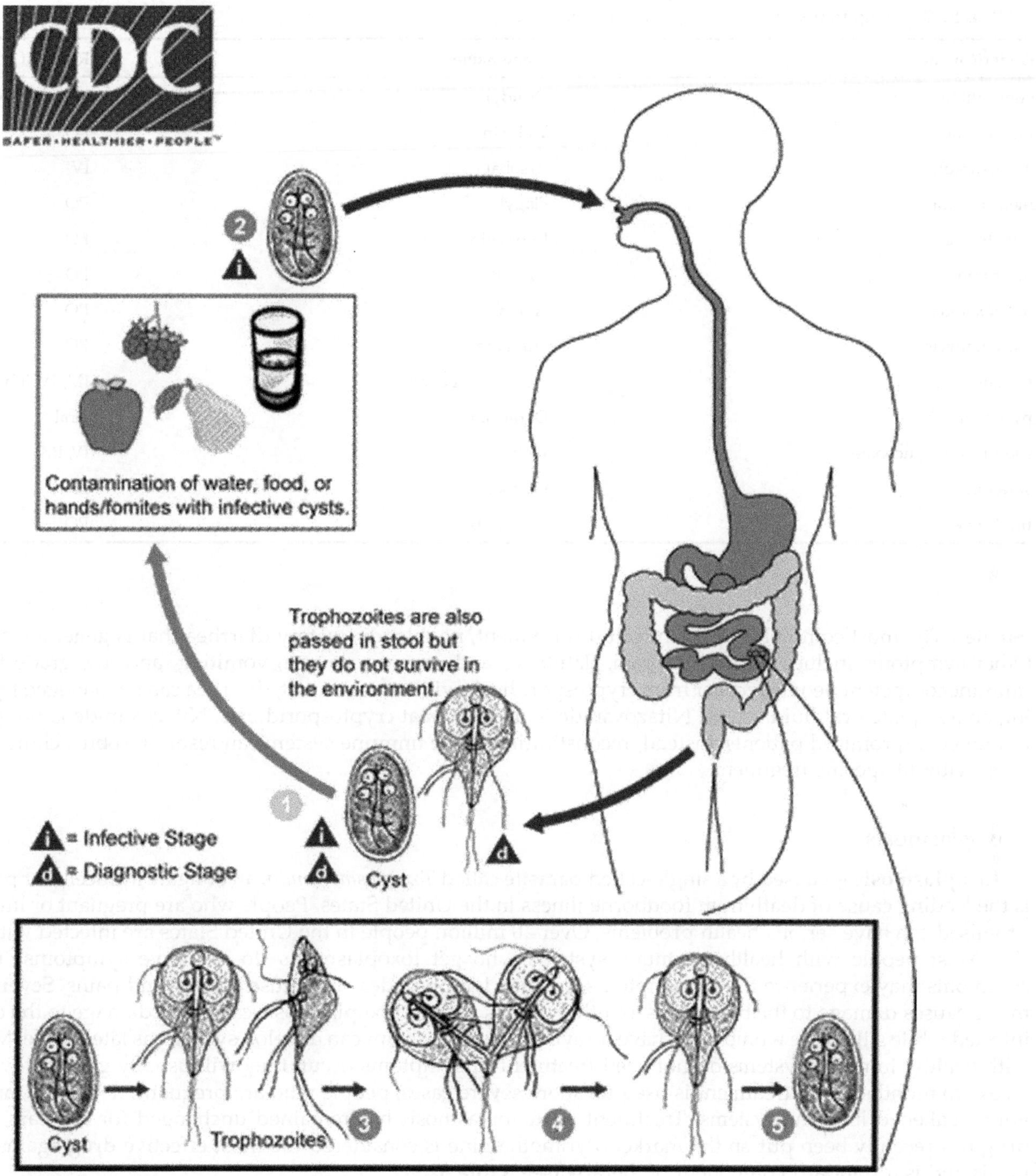

FIG. 52.2 The life cycle of giardiasis.

Prevention is the best defense. Giardiasis can be treated with antibiotic therapy. An intense treatment is with metronidazole 250 mg three times daily or 500 mg twice daily in adults for 5–7 days.

Cryptosporidiosis

Cryptosporidiosis is endemic worldwide; the highest rates are found in low- and middle-income countries. The highest US rates of reported cryptosporidiosis are in young children aged 1–4 and in people aged 15–44, particularly

TABLE 52.3 Drugs to treat nonmalaria protozoal infections.

Generic name	Trade name	Route of administration
eflornithine	Ornidyl	IV
iodoquinol	Yodoxin	PO
melarsoprol	Arsobal	IV
metronidazole	Flagyl	PO
miltefosine	Impavido	PO
nifurtimox	Lampit	PO
nitazoxanide	Alinia	PO
paromomycin	Humatin	PO
pentamidine	NebuPent, Pentam	IM, IV, inhalation
pyrimethamine	Daraprim	Oral
sodium stibogluconate	Pentostam	IV, IM
suramin	Germanin	IV
tinidazole	Tindamax	PO

females. The most common symptom includes frequent, nonbloody, watery diarrhea that is generally self-limited. Other symptoms include abdominal pain, flatulence and urgency, nausea, vomiting, and low-grade fever. Most immunocompetent people recover from cryptosporidiosis without treatment; diarrhea can be managed by maintaining an adequate oral fluid intake. Nitazoxanide is used to treat cryptosporidiosis. Nitazoxanide is not practical in immunocompromised patients. Instead, reconstitution of the immune system can result in robust clinical improvement without specific treatment.

Toxoplasmosis

Toxoplasmosis is caused by a single-celled parasite called *Toxoplasma gondii,* an obligate intracellular protozoan. It is the leading cause of death from foodborne illness in the United States. People who are pregnant or immunocompromised can have serious health problems. Over 40 million people in the United States are infected with the parasite. Most people with healthy immune systems who get toxoplasmosis do not have symptoms. Those with symptoms may experience flulike symptoms, swollen lymph nodes, and muscle aches and pains. Severe toxoplasmosis causes damage to the brain, eyes, or other organs. Ocular toxoplasmosis can cause damage to the eye. Infants infected while still in the womb often have no symptoms at birth but can develop symptoms later in life. Most people with healthy immune systems do not need treatment. If symptoms occur, they will usually go away within a few weeks to months. Drug treatment is used for more severe cases, people who are pregnant, newborns, and patients with weakened immune systems. Treatment for toxoplasmosis has remained unchanged for 20 years, as no new drug has recently been put on the market. Pyrimethamine is considered the most effective drug against toxoplasmosis and is a standard component of therapy (see **Table 52.3**).

You should remember

During pregnancy, toxoplasmosis can pass through the placenta to the fetus. This increases the risk of miscarriage, stillbirth, or severe health problems for the future child. Complications of being born with toxoplasmosis include vision problems, blindness, developmental delays, and learning disabilities.

Trichomoniasis

Trichomoniasis is a sexually transmitted infection caused by the protozoan *Trichomonas vaginalis*. It is the most common nonviral sexually transmitted infection, with more than 156 million new estimated annual cases globally in people between 15 and 49 years of age. About 33% of new infections in this age group occur in Africa, followed by the Americas.

It is treatable and curable. The disease infects the urogenital tract. While most infections are asymptomatic, over 50% of females with the infection have vaginal discharge. Approximately 10% of infected males have urethritis. The parasite is transmitted during sex (oral, vaginal, or anal) and sometimes during delivery of an infant. Proper, consistent use of condoms can prevent the disease transmission. Treatment usually involves metronidazole, though oral tinidazole can also be used.

Trypanosomiasis

Trypanosomiasis, also known as sleeping sickness, is a vector-borne parasitic disease caused by protozoans of the genus *Trypanosoma*. It is transmitted to humans by the bites of **tsetse flies** that have acquired the parasites from infected humans or animals. Tsetse flies are found in sub-Saharan Africa; only some species transmit trypanosomiasis. People involved in agriculture, fishing, animal husbandry, or hunting are the most exposed to the disease. It has a focal distribution that ranges from single villages to entire regions. Incidence can vary between locations.

There are two forms of human African trypanosomiasis (African sleeping sickness) based on the actual parasite. *Trypanosoma brucei gambiense* is found in West and Central Africa and makes up 92% of reported cases. It causes chronic illness, with infections lasting for months or years with no significant signs or symptoms.

American trypanosomiasis, known as **Chagas disease**, occurs mainly in Latin America. It is caused by a different subgenus of *Trypanosoma* and is transmitted differently with very different disease characteristics. The disease can also be transmitted from mother to child by crossing the placenta, via other blood-sucking insects, via accidental infection in laboratories from contact with contaminated needles, and by transmission through sexual contact (though this has only been reported once).

There are three drugs used for *T. brucei gambiense*:

- Pentamidine (IM) during the first stage
- Eflornithine (IV), which is usually administered along with nifurtimox (oral) during the second stage
- Fexinidazole (oral) during the first stage and nonsevere second stage

There are two drugs used for *T. brucei rhodesiense:*

- Suramin (IV) or fexinidazole (oral) during the first stage
- Melarsoprol (IV) during the second stage—but this drug has many adverse effects, including reactive encephalopathy, which is fatal in up to 10% of patients (see **Table 52.3**)

Leishmaniasis

Leishmaniasis is caused by a protozoa parasite from more than 20 species of *Leishmania*. More than 90 species of sandflies transmit the parasites. Patients with HIV who contract leishmaniasis have increased risks of developing full-blown HIV, with high relapse and mortality rates. Antiretroviral treatments are indicated for these patients. Major risk factors for leishmaniasis include poor socioeconomic conditions, malnutrition, deforestation, humans moving into forested areas, increased temperature, increased rainfall, drought, famine, and flooding.

Miltefosine is the drug of choice to treat leishmaniasis. Other medications include amphotericin B, paromomycin, antimonials, azoles (fluconazole, ketoconazole, or itraconazole), pentamidine, and sodium stibogluconate. Prevention and control are based on early diagnosis; effective, prompt treatment; vector control; effective disease surveillance; control of animal reservoir hosts; social mobilization; and strengthening healthcare partnerships.

Drugs for nonmalaria protozoal infections

Amebiasis, giardiasis, and cryptosporidiosis are caused by intestinal parasites, usually acquired through contaminated food or water. These infections affect many people in endemic areas. Amebiasis, giardiasis, and cryptosporidiosis are protozoal intestinal infections mainly spread via poor sanitation. The primary medication used for nonmalaria protozoal infections is metronidazole. Other drugs include eflornithine, iodoquinol, melarsoprol, miltefosine, nifurtimox, nitazoxanide, paromomycin, pentamidine, pyrimethamine, sodium stibogluconate, suramin, and tinidazole (see **Table 52.3**).

Metronidazole

Metronidazole is an antibiotic and antiprotozoal medication that is the mainstay for treating protozoal and anaerobic bacterial infections. It belongs to the nitroimidazole class of antibiotics. However, the antiinfective activity of metronidazole is limited to anaerobic bacteria and protozoa but not fungi.

Pharmacokinetics

Metronidazole is well absorbed after oral administration, reaching peak concentrations in 1–2 hours. Although it starts to work quickly, symptoms may take a few days to resolve. Its half-life is about 8 hours, and it is metabolized in the liver. It is mainly excreted in the urine.

Mechanism of action

Metronidazole inhibits protein synthesis by interacting with DNA. It causes a loss of helical DNA structure and strand breakage, which causes cell death in susceptible organisms.

Clinical indications

Metronidazole treats protozoal infections such as *Trichomoniasis vaginalis, Entamoeba histolytica, Giardia lamblia,* **blastocysts**, and ***Balantidium coli***. It is also used to treat intestinal amebiases, liver amebiasis, bacterial septicemia, bone and joint infections, endocarditis, lower respiratory tract infections, meningitis, brain abscess, endometritis, bacterial vaginosis, and surgical prophylaxis colorectal surgeries. The extended-release tablets are used to treat females with vaginal infections. It is available for oral use, injection, and topical use. The oral medication comes as a tablet, capsule, or suspension. Metronidazole can also be used intravenously or as a topical gel.

Contraindications

Metronidazole is contraindicated in patients with a history of hypersensitivity to the agent. It should be avoided during the first trimester of pregnancy. Patients should not drink alcohol while taking metronidazole tablets, liquid, suppositories, or vaginal gel or for 3 days after finishing treatment. Alcohol can cause side effects such as feeling and being sick, stomach pain, hot flashes, difficulty breathing, a pounding heartbeat (palpitations), and headaches.

Adverse effects

The adverse effects of metronidazole include headache, nausea, vomiting, diarrhea, a slightly metallic taste, vaginitis, confusion, dizziness, genital pruritus, abdominal pain, **xerostomia**, **dysmenorrhea**, urinary tract infection, bacterial infection, flulike symptoms, **pharyngitis**, and sinusitis. Alcohol can cause stomach pain, hot flashes, dyspnea, palpitations, and headaches.

Toxicities

Peripheral neuropathy, dizziness, vertigo, and headache are common symptoms of metronidazole toxicity. Cerebellar toxicity is a rare but severe side effect of metronidazole toxicity, with classic findings on MRI.

You should remember

Prolonged use of metronidazole can cause severe neurological disturbances due to the risk of cumulative neurotoxicity. Monitor for neurologic sequela and discontinue therapy if any abnormal neurologic symptoms occur. Prolonged use of this agent may also result in fungal or bacterial superinfections.

Tinidazole

Tinidazole is an oral broad-spectrum antimicrobial agent used to treat bacterial, protozoal, and parasitic infections and female bacterial vaginosis. It is usually well tolerated. However, it may cause a bitter taste, headache, fatigue, dizziness, and diarrhea. It is also capable of causing anaphylactic and allergic reactions, including bronchospasm, angioedema, and **urticaria**.

Eflornithine

Eflornithine is effective against the protozoans that cause sleeping sickness when administered intravenously. The IV formulation is only available via CDC and WHO distribution programs. Topical eflornithine hydrochloride helps slow the rate of excessive hair growth.

Pharmacokinetics

Eflornithine is not metabolized; its elimination half-life is 1.5–5 hours. Excretion is via the kidneys.

Mechanism of action

Eflornithine is a *suicide inhibitor* that irreversibly binds to ornithine decarboxylase, preventing the natural substrate ornithine from accessing the active site. Its decarboxylation mechanism is analogous to that of ornithine in the active site, where transamination occurs with pyridoxal 5'-phosphate, followed by decarboxylation.

Clinical indications

Eflornithine treats trypanosomiasis in the second phase of the disease, often along with nifurtimox. It is also indicated to treat excess facial hair in females and to reduce the risk of relapse in people with high-risk neuroblastoma.

Contraindications

Contraindications of eflornithine include known hypersensitivity, severe renal or hepatic impairment, preexisting hematologic abnormalities, and eighth cranial nerve impairment. The drug should only be used during pregnancy if the potential benefit outweighs the potential risk to the fetus.

Adverse effects

Adverse effects of eflornithine include **acne**, skin reactions from ingrown hair, hair loss, burning, stinging, tingling, dry skin, itching, redness, rash, hematologic abnormalities, thrombocytopenia, seizures, and reversible hearing loss.

Toxicities

Though rare, toxicities from eflornithine may cause rash, itching, swelling, severe dizziness, and trouble breathing.

Iodoquinol

Iodoquinol is an antiprotozoal medication used to treat the intestinal infection amebiasis. It is described as a halogenated 8-hydroxyquinoline and a direct-acting amebicide. It is active against cysts and **trophozoites** in the intestine.

Pharmacokinetics

Iodoquinol is poorly absorbed from the gastrointestinal tract after oral administration. It is metabolized in the liver and excreted in the feces.

Mechanism of action

Although the mechanism of action of iodoquinol is not fully understood, it appears to act by chelating ferrous ions essential for metabolism.

Clinical indications

Iodoquinol is used to treat *Entamoeba histolytica*. It is active against cysts and trophozoites in the intestinal lumen and is the drug of choice for asymptomatic or moderate amebiasis.

Contraindications

Iodoquinol is contraindicated in patients with a history of hypersensitivity and people with thyroid disorders like hyperthyroidism or goiter. It should be used with caution in patients with renal or hepatic impairment, people with preexisting gastrointestinal issues, and those with preexisting optic neuropathy.

Adverse effects

Iodoquinol is generally safe to use. However, it may cause fever, chills, headache, dizziness, vomiting, abdominal cramps, diarrhea, skin itchiness, and an enlarged thyroid.

Toxicities

Long-term use of high drug doses can lead to blurred vision, eye pain, clumsiness, unsteadiness, increased weakness, muscle pain, numbness, tingling, pain, or weakness in the hands or feet.

Melarsoprol

Melarsoprol is a trivalent arsenical compound first introduced in 1949. It is used to treat late-stage African trypanosomiasis. It is only available as an intravenous injection via the CDC's investigational drug protocol.

Pharmacokinetics

Melarsoprol's maximum plasma levels are about 15 minutes after injection. It is metabolized to its active metabolite, melarsen oxide. Its half-life is less than 1 hour, though bioassays indicate a 35-hour half-life. This is often associated with pharmacologic agents with active metabolites in the liver.

Mechanism of action

Melarsoprol interacts with thiol groups of critical proteins, depriving the parasite of its primary sulfhydryl antioxidant and inhibiting trypanothione reductase. The drug also deprives the parasite of the essential enzyme system that reduces trypanothione.

Clinical indications

Melarsoprol is an arsenic-containing medication used to treat African sleeping sickness, especially in the second stage of the disease caused by *T. brucei rhodesiense* when the CNS is involved. It is typically used in combination with corticosteroids to reduce the risk of drug-induced encephalopathy.

Contraindications

The contraindications of melarsoprol are glucose-6-phosphate dehydrogenase deficiency; pregnancy, depending on the mother's condition; and known hypersensitivity.

Adverse effects

The adverse effects of melarsoprol include hypertension, heart damage, encephalopathy, numbness and tingling of the extremities, vomiting, and albuminuria. This systemic febrile reaction is accompanied by headache, myalgia, tachycardia, and **hyperventilation**.

Toxicities

The toxicities of melarsoprol may result in reactive encephalopathy, which can be fatal in up to 50% of cases.

Pyrimethamine

Pyrimethamine is an inhibitor of dihydrofolate reductase and causes tetrahydrofolate deficiency. It is an antiparasitic prescription medication approved for toxoplasmosis.

Pharmacokinetics

Pyrimethamine is well-absorbed after oral administration, reaching peak serum concentrations 2–6 hours after the dose. It is eliminated in the urine (16%–32%) over approximately 3 days and is often used as a single dose.

Mechanism of action

Pyrimethamine interferes with the regeneration of tetrahydrofolic acid from dihydrofolate by competitively inhibiting the enzyme dihydrofolate reductase. Tetrahydrofolic acid is essential for DNA and RNA synthesis in many protozoa.

Clinical indications

Pyrimethamine is a folic acid antagonist used as an antimalarial or combined with a sulfonamide to treat toxoplasmosis.

Contraindications

Pyrimethamine is contraindicated in patients with known hypersensitivity and patients with documented **megaloblastic anemia** due to folate deficiency.

Adverse effects

Pyrimethamine has a variety of adverse effects, including hematuria, tongue irritation or soreness, **dysuria**, insomnia, anemia, xerostomia, sore throat, dizziness, pinpoint red spots on the skin, chills, pale skin, joint or muscle pain, bleeding gums, loss of appetite, unusual tiredness, fainting, arrhythmias, cough, hives, vomiting, dysphagia, lower back or side pain, diarrhea, fever, and pancytopenia.

Toxicities

The most notable toxicity of pyrimethamine is dose-related bone marrow suppression. This may result in thrombocytopenia, **granulocytopenia**, or megaloblastic anemia. In high doses, hematologic abnormalities should be anticipated, though they may be difficult to distinguish from those related to HIV infection.

Suramin

Suramin is an antiparasitic that exerts its effects by causing parasites to lose energy and die. It is used to treat trypanosomiasis and river blindness (**onchocerciasis**). It is also only available as an IV injection via the CDC's investigational drug protocol.

Pharmacokinetics

Suramin binds extensively to plasma proteins (>99%), accumulates during treatment, and is not significantly metabolized. It is slowly excreted in the urine, resulting in its persistence in plasma for several weeks after treatment ends. It does not penetrate the CNS.

Mechanism of action

Suramin's mechanism of action is believed to involve the parasite's ability to selectively uptake the drug via receptor-mediated **endocytosis** when the drug is bound to low-density lipoproteins and, to a lesser extent, other serum proteins.

Clinical indications

Suramin is used to treat African trypanosomiasis caused by *T. brucei rhodesiense* and *onchocerciasis*.

Contraindications

The contraindication of suramin is known as hypersensitivity. It should be used with caution in patients with optic atrophy and renal or liver damage.

Adverse effects

The adverse effects of suramin include dizziness, shock, fatigue, exfoliative dermatitis, headache, diarrhea, **polydipsia**, nausea, nephrotoxicity, optic atrophy, pancytopenia, immediate hypersensitivity reactions, fever, and renal impairment.

Toxicities

Suramin can be life-threatening because of toxic effects such as vomiting, acute hypersensitivity-like reactions, and, later on, neurologic, ocular, renal, and hepatic abnormalities.

Key Terms

Acne
Amebiasis
Anopheles mosquitoes
Balantidium coli
Blastocysts
Chagas disease
Cryptosporidiosis
Diplopia
Dysmenorrhea
Dyspnea
Dysuria
Entamoeba histolytica
Giardia
Heme
Hemozoin
Leishmaniasis
Malaria
Megaloblastic anemia
Onchocerciasis
Peritonitis
Pharyngitis
Polydipsia
Protozoan
Toxoplasmosis
Trichomoniasis
Trophozoites
Trypanosomiasis
Tsetse flies
Urticaria
Xerostomia

Clinical Case Studies

Clinical Case Study 1

A 56-year-old female returned from a visit to Africa and soon developed a cyclic fever that lasted for 7 days. Her family also reported she had mental status changes. On arrival at the emergency department, the patient was lethargic and soon was in respiratory distress. She was intubated and mechanically ventilated. A malaria smear was positive, and she was diagnosed with severe malaria accompanied by multiorgan failure. Intravenous chloroquine and primaquine were given. The patient began improving by the third day.

Critical Thinking Questions

1. What is the description of malaria infection, and how must it be treated?
2. How does chloroquine work in the treatment of malaria?
3. How is chloroquine used to prevent malaria?

Clinical Case Study 2

A 62-year-old male presented with colicky abdominal pain and watery diarrhea. He was a farmer who regularly used cow manure for crop fertilization. Physical examination revealed abdominal tenderness. Laboratory tests showed low total protein and albumin. An abdominal CT scan revealed a slight intestinal wall thickening. A *G. duodenalis* trophozoite was found in a fecal smear, and giardiasis was diagnosed. Metronidazole was given for 10 days, and the patient's symptoms resolved entirely.

Critical Thinking Questions

1. What is the mechanism of action for metronidazole?
2. What are the clinical indications for metronidazole?
3. What are the adverse effects of metronidazole?

Further Reading

[1] E. Ali, Anti-Malaria Drugs and P. falciparum Gametocytes Prevalence – and Drug Resistance Following Treatment of Uncomplicated P. falciparum Malaria, Lap Lambert Academic Publishing, 2013.

[2] A. Al-Mamun, T. Ahmed, S. Kumar Kundu, Metronidazole Extended Release Solid Dosage Form – Development of Extended Release Formulation and in Vitro Bioequivalence Study of Metronidazole Solid Dosage Form, Lap Lambert Academic Publishing, 2013.

[3] F. Ariey, F. Gay, R. Menard, Malaria Control and Elimination (Methods in Molecular Biology), Human Press, 2019.

[4] R.B. Becker, The Role of Antimalarial Medications in Combating Malaria, Becker, 2022.

[5] G.J. Blokdijk, Chloroquine Phosphate, second ed., CreateSpace Independent Publishing Platform, 2018.

[6] S. Eugenia, Comprehensive Guide to Giardiasis – Understanding, Management, and Holistic Health, Eugenia, 2024.

[7] A. Farid, Cryptosporidiosis – A Problem to be Solved, Lap Lambert Academic Publishing, 2021.

[8] K. Frank, Metronidazole – Guide to Treat Bacterial, Pneumonia and Other Respiratory Tract Infections; Certain Infections of Skin, Eye, Lymphatic, Intestinal, Genital and Urinary Systems, Frank, 2022.

[9] K. Hurst, Amebiasis – Diagnosis, Prevention and Treatment, American Medical Publishers, 2023.

[10] P. Kendrekar, Drug Development for Malaria – Novel Approaches for Prevention and Treatment, Wiley-VCH, 2022.

[11] S. Kumar, S. Pal, Structure-Based Drug Design for Malaria, Lap Lambert Academic Publishing, 2019.

[12] H.M. Staines, S. Krishna, Treatment and Prevention of Malaria – Antimalarial Drug Chemistry, Action and Use (Milestones in Drug Therapy), Springer, 2012.

CHAPTER

53

Cancer chemotherapy

OUTLINE

LEARNING OUTCOMES

After study of the chapter, readers should be able to:

1. Describe the classifications of chemotherapy.
2. Explain the biological and monoclonal therapies.
3. Discuss the clinical indication of alkylating and antimetabolite agents.
4. Describe the adverse effects of antimicrotubule agents.
5. List the trade names of fluorouracil, teniposide, bleomycin, and doxorubicin.

The Science of Pharmacology
https://doi.org/10.1016/B978-0-443-29038-1.00053-1

6. Explain the anticancer antibiotics and their indications.
7. Discuss the contraindications of alkylating agents.
8. Describe the adverse effects of antimicrotubule agents.
9. Explain the contraindications of doxorubicin.
10. Discuss neutropenic fever and tumor lysis syndrome.

Overview

Cancer occurs when a single type of cell grows out of control. It can happen in the blood or as a solid tumor mass. The entire mechanism leading to cancer development is not entirely understood. Genetic and environmental factors, age, and gender play a role in the development of cancer or carcinogenesis. Today, treatments to fight cancers include surgery, chemotherapy, radiotherapy, immunotherapy, and targeted therapy. Chemotherapy is one of the most effective ways to treat cancer, along with surgery and radiotherapy. Chemotherapy inhibits cell proliferation and tumor multiplication, thus avoiding invasion and metastasis. However, this results in the toxic effects of chemotherapy due to the impact on normal cells. Inhibition of tumor growth can occur at several levels within the cell and its environment. Chemotherapy can be administered in neoadjuvant, adjuvant, combined, and metastatic settings. Neoadjuvant therapy is a treatment given before the primary treatment. Adjuvant therapy is the treatment given in addition to the initial therapy, which can suppress or eliminate the growth of occult cancer cells. Adjuvant therapy is now the standard for breast, lung, colorectal, and ovarian cancers. Combined modalities such as chemotherapy and radiation are used to shrink the tumor before the surgery or for curative intent in cancers such as head and neck, lung, and colon.

Types of chemotherapy

Three main groups of medications fall under today's modern anticancer therapy umbrella: traditional chemotherapy, hormonal therapy, and biological therapy. Conventional (traditional) chemotherapy, such as doxorubicin and etoposide, will cause cell death of cancerous and healthy cells. This leads to many of the general toxicities and adverse effects seen with traditional chemotherapy, such as **myelosuppression**, nausea, and vomiting. Hormonal therapies control the endocrine system in cancers such as breast and prostate cancer. Biologic therapies have a more focused target, leading to a different spectrum of toxicities depending on the treatment targets.

Traditional therapy

Traditional chemotherapy has been around since 1941, when nitrogen mustard was administered to patients with **lymphoma**. This agent causes cell death by attacking specified points during cell division and typically has more impact on rapidly dividing cells. However, these rapidly dividing cells are not always just cancer cells. Gastrointestinal cells, hair follicles, and **bone marrow** are normal cells that have rapid growth and therefore are more affected by traditional chemotherapy. This is why many give traditional chemotherapy the nickname of "poison," as it kills whatever active cells it encounters. Conventional chemotherapy can be cell cycle phase specific or nonspecific (see **Fig. 53.1**). The cell cycle comprises four phases: G1, S, G2, and M. The G1 phase is when the cell prepares DNA for synthesis and occurs in the S phase. The G2 phase is where the cell prepares for **mitosis** by producing RNA and proteins, and then the M phase is mitosis, where the cellular division into two cells occurs. Depending on the mechanism of action of chemotherapy agents, they can affect different points of the cell cycle, and some affect all phases.

Hormonal therapy

Hormonal therapies typically decrease or remove a hormone related to the growth of a specific tumor from the system. This class of anticancer drugs tends to have less significant organ damage compared to the other groups;

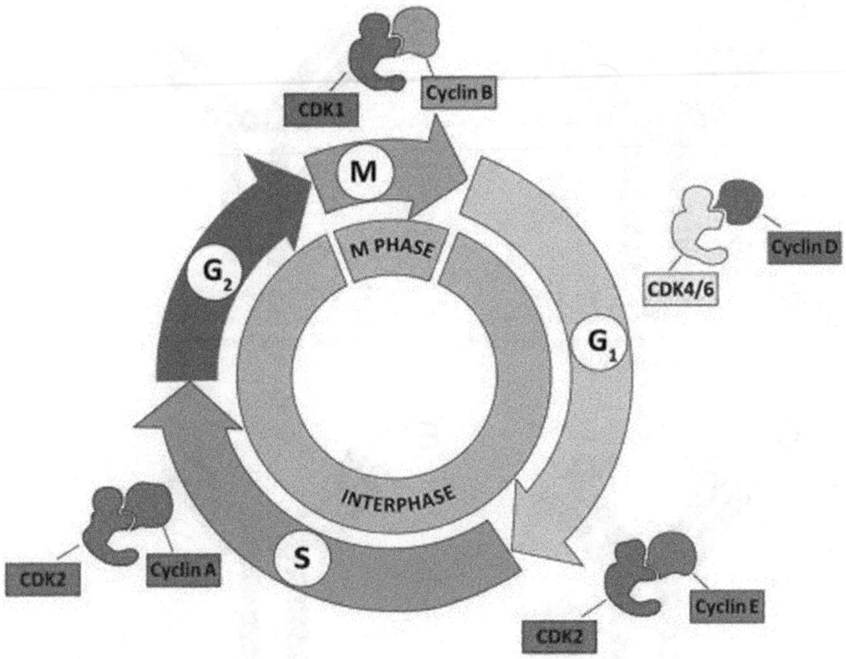

FIG. 53.1 Cell cycle phases.

however, they are not without adverse effects. Corticosteroids can also be used for their killing effects on cancer DNA against a variety of cancers, such as lymphoma and **multiple myeloma**.

Biologic therapy

Biologic therapies consist of targeted therapies, such as monoclonal antibodies (mAbs) and tyrosine kinase inhibitors, and immune-mediated therapies, which can use the patient's immune system to begin an attack on the cancerous cells. Several therapeutic mAbs are now available. Rituximab and trastuzumab were approved in the late 1990s to treat lymphoma and breast cancer, which is a new approach to cancer treatment.

Biologic therapies tend to have adverse effects related to their expected target. For example, bevacizumab is a monoclonal antibody targeting vascular endothelial growth factor (VEGF), while pazopanib is a tyrosine kinase inhibitor targeting VEGF. These drugs have overlapping toxicities, even though they have different mechanisms of action, because they have the same target. Drugs that target VEGF are associated with hypertension and **proteinuria**.

Monoclonal therapy

Monoclonal antibodies are specific antibodies to a single antigen, or target, on the cell surface (see **Fig. 53.2**). They are made by cloning a particular cell for a specific target. There are different ways to manipulate mAbs to change their mechanism of action. Most mAbs directly kill when the antibody interacts with the antigen. However, some mAbs do not cause cell death when they bind with their target, so to achieve cell kill, they have a toxin attached to the mAb, and when the mAb interacts with its target, the mAb and the toxin are internalized by the cell, which then leads to **apoptosis**. An mAb with a toxin attached is called a conjugated monoclonal antibody. The third mechanism of action is when the mAb interacts with a target and prevents signaling cascades that would have led to cell growth and proliferation. An example is bevacizumab, as it targets VEGF, and therefore VEGF cannot bind with its target. This leads to blocking blood vessel growth, which prevents tumor growth by cutting off the nutrient supply to the cancerous cells.

Immune-mediated therapy treats cancer by targeting the immune system and enhancing or inducing a response. Many of these agents are mAbs whose targets are still extracellular (outside the cell). One component of the immune system is the T cell. T cells commonly identify foreign cells in the body and label them for destruction. These drugs can be compared to pressing the gas pedal on a car. The anticancer agents Paratek Pharmaceuticals strengthen the

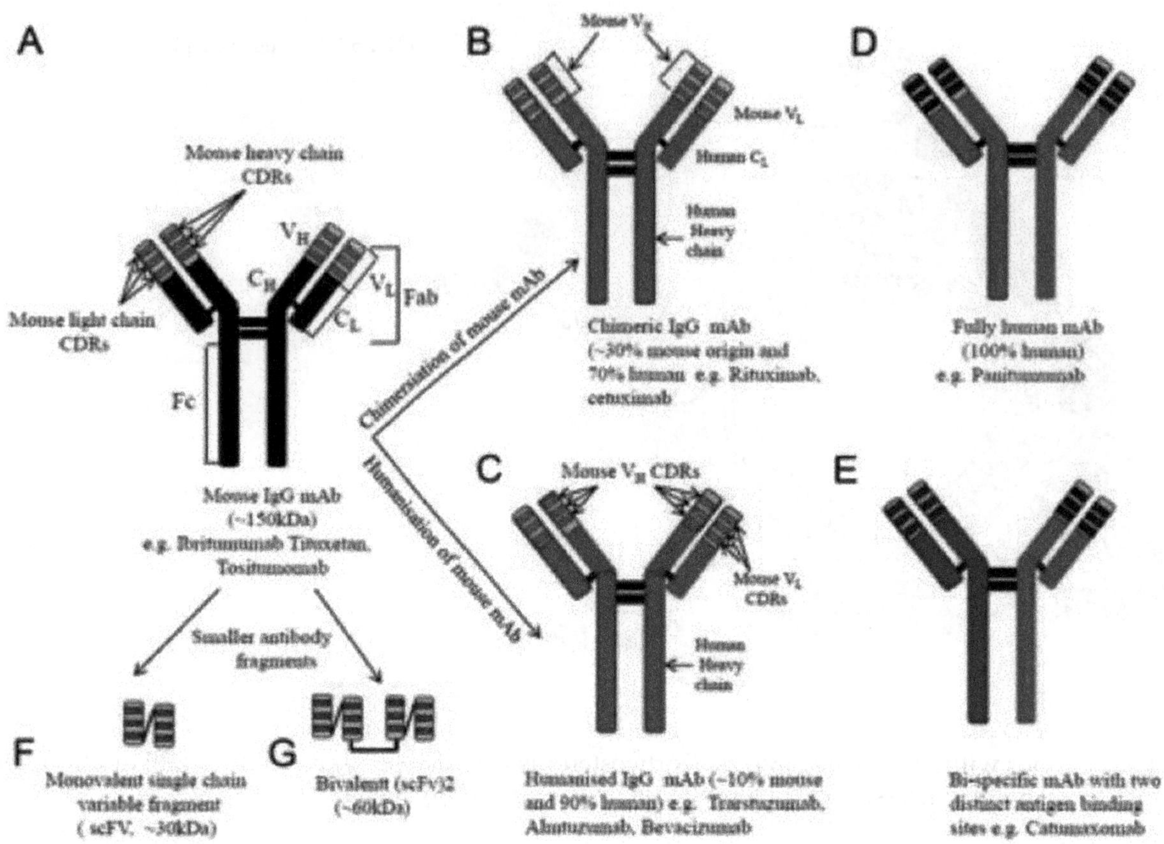

FIG. 53.2 Monoclonal antibody.

immune system (press the gas pedal) and enhance T-cell signaling, thereby increasing the number and duration that T cells can attack foreign cells such as cancer cells.

You should remember

Immunotherapy is intended to improve the immunogenicity of cancer by giving the body a sufficient number of functioning immune cells and related molecules to inspire and strengthen the body's immune response. It is also resistant to cancer, thereby improving the cancer's sensitivity to the anticancer immunity effect.

Chemotherapeutic drug classifications

Chemotherapeutic agents can be classified according to their action mechanism, including alkylating agents, antimetabolites, antimicrotubular agents, and antibiotics.

Table 53.1 summarizes common agents used in the treatment of cancer.

Alkylating agents

Alkylating agents are widely used and significant components of combination chemotherapy. They were among the first anticancer drugs discovered after their effects were seen during their use as chemical weapons during the First World War. They are still the most commonly used pharmacological compounds in chemotherapy. The alkylating agents are the largest anticancer agents, comprising five subgroups: nitrogen mustards, alkyl sulfonates, nitrosoureas, ethylenimines, and triazenes. **Table 53.2** summarizes the various alkylating agents.

TABLE 53.1 Common agents used in the treatment of cancer.

Type of agent	Description
Alkylating agents	Cause replacement of hydrogen by an alkyl group, primarily one that inhibits cell division and growth; five major types: nitrogen mustards, ethylenimines, alkyl sulfonates, nitrosoureas, triazines
Ethyleneimines	Amine compounds containing ethylene linkages between amine groups
Alkyl sulfonates	Direct-acting bacterial mutagens that alkylate DNA, leading to disruption of cancer cell replication
Miscellaneous	Carboplatin, cisplatin, and procarbazine; they stop or slow the growth of cancer cells
Antimetabolites	Prevent cancer cell growth by affecting DNA production; only effective against cells actively participating in cell metabolism; they include purine antagonists, adenosine antagonists, pyrimidine antagonists, and folic acid antagonists
Mitotic inhibitors (plant alkaloids)	Usually are physiologically active organic bases containing nitrogen and usually oxygen, occurring in seed plants; they prevent meiosis (cell division); main examples are vincristine and vinblastine
Antitumor antibiotics	Disrupt protein synthesis in target cells and bind to DNA, causing its fragmentation
Hormone therapy	May selectively suppress growth of certain tissues without causing a cytotoxic action

Pharmacokinetics

The pharmacokinetics of all the alkylating agents have yet to be fully understood. However, chlorambucil is extensively metabolized in the liver, primarily to phenylacetic acid mustard. Oral chlorambucil undergoes rapid GI absorption and plasma clearance. It is almost completely metabolized and has extremely low urinary excretion. Cyclophosphamide is eliminated mainly in the form of metabolites. After intravenous (IV) administration, 10%–20% is excreted in the urine, and 4% is excreted in the bile. Mechlorethamine undergoes rapid spontaneous hydrolysis after IV injection, disappearing from the blood in about 10 minutes. The oral bioavailability of melphalan is variable and is greatly affected by dosing with food (85% when fasting as compared to below 58% with food). The half-life is about 90 minutes. Only 10%–15% of the drug is excreted unchanged in the urine, with the liver metabolizing the rest. The drug requires no hepatic activation and is highly protein bound, especially to albumin.

TABLE 53.2 Alkylating agents.

Generic name	Trade name	Route of administration
chlorambucil (nitrogen mustard)	Leukeran	PO
cyclophosphamide	Cytoxan	PO, IV
ifosfamide	Ifex	IV
mechlorethamine (nitrogen	Mustargen	IV or intracavitary
mustard)	Alkeran	PO, IV
melphalan		
Alkyl sulfonates	Busulfex	PO, IV
Busulfan		
Nitrosoureas	BCNU	PO, intraperitoneal injection
Carmustine	CCNU	PO
Lomustine	Mustophoran	IV
Fotemustine		
Ethyleneimines	Hexalen	PO
altretamine	Thiotepa	IV, intravesicular (directly into the bladder)
thiotepa (injection)		
Triazenes	DTIC-Dome	IV
dacarbazine	Berenil	IM
diaminazene aceturate	Temodar	PO, IV
temozolomide		

Mechanism of action

Alkylating agents are a class of antineoplastic or anticancer drugs that inhibit the transcription of DNA into RNA, thereby stopping protein synthesis. Alkylating agents substitute alkyl groups for hydrogen atoms on DNA, forming cross-links within the DNA chain and thereby cytotoxic, mutagenic, and carcinogenic effects. This action occurs in all cells, but alkylating agents primarily affect rapidly dividing cells, which do not have time for DNA repair.

Clinical indications

Alkylating agents are indicated for treating brain, lung, breast, ovary, and testicular cancer, leukemia, lymphoma, Hodgkin disease, melanoma, multiple myeloma, and sarcoma.

Contraindications

Alkylating agents are contraindicated in patients with known allergies to drugs, bone marrow suppression, renal failure, liver dysfunctions, pregnancy, and lactation.

Adverse effects

Adverse effects seen with alkylating agents include myelosuppression, hemorrhagic cystitis, and GI toxicity. In experimental models, cyclophosphamide can cause neutropenia.

Toxicities

All the alkylating agents have significant toxicities, but the predominant toxicities are to the bone marrow and gastrointestinal tract. Most agents have been shown to cause transient serum aminotransferase elevations in a proportion of patients.

You should remember

Nitrogen mustards are a necessary antineoplastic therapy known as DNA-alkylating agents. They are highly reactive and produce several adverse effects. To minimize these undesirable effects, combining nitrogen mustards with a steroidal hormone with affinity for its receptor can lead to highly selective and less toxic antineoplastic therapeutics. Nitrogen mustard is a highly toxic alkylating agent that causes severe skin injury and neutrophilic inflammation.

Antimetabolites

Antimetabolites are among the most important agents used in cancer chemotherapy. They are the next class of substances that may compete, replace, or inhibit some specific metabolites. They represent a relatively large group of anticancer drugs that structurally resemble natural substrates but differ enough to interfere with their metabolism. There are three types of antimetabolites. They are also called antimetabolite antagonists. Purine antagonists, pyrimidine antagonists, and folic acid antagonists are examples of antimetabolites. **Table 53.3** summarizes the various antimetabolites.

Pharmacokinetics

Antimetabolites are readily absorbed from the small intestine. After IV injection, the plasma half-life is approximately 90 minutes. The drug is metabolized by methylation in the liver and by the hepatic enzyme xanthine oxidase. They are primarily excreted in the urine.

Mechanism of action

The mechanism of action is based on their ability to enter into competitive relationships with structurally similar metabolites of the living, which causes a lack of the corresponding metabolite. Therefore it decreases the activity of vital biochemical processes in the cell. To interfere with the synthesis of DNA constituents, the most common antimetabolites should be structural analogs of purine and pyrimidine bases or folate cofactors.

TABLE 53.3 Antimetabolites.

Generic name	Trade name	Route of administration
capecitabine	Xeloda	PO
fluorouracil	Adrucil	IV
mercaptopurine	Purinethol	PO
methotrexate	Rheumatrex, Trexall	PO, IM, IV

Clinical indications

Antimetabolites are used to treat various cancers, including some forms of leukemia and lymphoma, lung cancer, and breast cancer.

Contraindications

Antimetabolites are contraindicated in patients with known allergies to the drug, peptic ulcer, bone marrow suppression, pregnancy, lactation, liver dysfunction, and renal impairment.

Adverse effects

The adverse effects of antimetabolites include myelosuppression, hair loss, nausea, vomiting, loss of appetite, fatigue, skin rash, elevation of liver enzymes, and diarrhea. These symptoms depend on the specific drug and the patient's dosage.

Toxicities

Antimetabolite toxicity primarily stems from their mechanism of disrupting DNA and RNA synthesis. Because these chemotherapy drugs target rapidly dividing cells, they inadvertently damage healthy, fast-growing tissues, resulting in side effects like bone marrow suppression, gastrointestinal distress, and liver enzyme elevation.[1–4]

Antimicrotubular agents

Antimicrotubular agents, also known as mitotic inhibitors or plant alkaloids, block cell growth by stopping mitosis. These drugs interfere with cellular structures that help move chromosomes during mitosis, so they are used to treat cancer. Microtubules are an essential part of the intracellular cytoskeleton structure and have unique polymerization dynamics critical for many cellular functions, including cell division and control. Antimicrotubule agents include polymerizing agents (paclitaxel and docetaxel) and depolymerizing drugs (vincristine and vinorelbine). **Table 53.4** summarizes the various antimicrotubular agents.

Pharmacokinetics

The antimicrotubular agents exert their cytotoxic effects by binding to tubulin, causing metaphase arrest. The bioavailability of etoposide varies between 25% and 75%, with 97% protein binding. It is metabolized in the liver via CYP3A4. The oral elimination half-life is 6 hours. For the IV form, this is 6–12 hours in adults and 3 hours in children. Etoposide is excreted via the kidneys and feces. For teniposide, protein binding is nearly 100%, with metabolism via the liver mediated by CYP2C12. The elimination half-life is 5 hours, and the drug is excreted via the kidneys and feces. Vinblastine sulfate is metabolized via the liver, mediated by CYP3A4. The elimination half-life is 24.8 hours, and it is excreted via the kidneys and bile ducts. Vincristine has a protein binding of about 44%. It is metabolized by the liver mainly via CYP3A4 and CYP3A5. The elimination half-life averages 85 hours, within a range of 19–155 hours. It is excreted via the feces (70%–80%) and urine (10%–20%). Vinorelbine has a 29%–57% bioavailability ±14%. Protein binding is 79%–91%. It is metabolized via the liver and mediated by CYP3A4. The elimination half-life is 27.7–43.6 hours. The drug is excreted in the feces (46%) and urine (18%).

Mechanism of action

Antimicrotubular agents promote apoptosis in cancer cells. They affect mitosis by acting on tubulin to prevent microtubule polymerization.

TABLE 53.4 Antimicrotubular agents.

Generic name	Trade name	Route of administration
etoposide	VePesid, Etopophos	PO, IV
teniposide	Vumon	IV
vinblastine sulfate (injection)	Vinblastine sulfate	IV
vincristine	Vincasar PFS	IV
vinorelbine	Navelbine	IV

Clinical indications

Antimicrotubule agents are widely used alone or in combination with other anticancer drugs. They are indicated to treat lung, breast, ovarian, bladder, prostate, melanoma, and esophageal cancers. Although there has been a rapid expansion of the number of classes of compounds with antineoplastic activity, few have played a more vital role in the curative and palliative treatment of cancers than the antimicrotubule agents. While the vinca alkaloids have been the only subclass of antimicrotubule agents that have had broad clinical applications in oncologic therapeutics over the last several decades, the taxanes, led by the prototypic agent taxol, are emerging as another very active class of antimicrotubule agents.

Contraindications

Contraindications of antimicrotubule agents include known hypersensitivity, pregnancy, solid tumors with baseline polymorphonuclear neutrophils of less than 1500 cells per cubic meter, and AIDS-related **Kaposi sarcoma** with baseline polymorphonuclear neutrophils of less than 1000 cells per cubic meter.

Adverse effects

The adverse effects of antimicrotubule agents include mouth ulcers, chest pain, arrhythmia, arthralgia, nausea, vomiting, and diarrhea. A significant limitation of using microtubule-targeted agents is the high rate of neuropathy induced by these compounds. Neutropenia is often the most frequent and severe adverse effect in combination regimens.

Toxicities

Antimicrotubules can cause cardiotoxicity by reducing coronary flow via vasoconstriction and conduction abnormalities. They also induce histamine release, which causes bradycardia and AV conduction delays.

Antibiotics

Anticancer antibiotics are chemicals microorganisms produce with anticancer activity. The classification of anticancer antibiotics mainly includes mitomycin, bleomycin, actinomycin, anthracyclines, guanorycin, enediyne, and anthracyclines. In addition, their anticancer effects are also very complex and compelling. Anthracyclines are anticancer antibiotics that mainly include daunorubicin, doxorubicin, epirubicin, and mitoxantrone. Doxorubicin is used here as the primary antibiotic example. **Table 53.5** summarizes the antitumor antibiotics.

Pharmacokinetics

The distribution half-life of doxorubicin is about 5 minutes. The binding of this drug and its major metabolite (doxorubicinol) to plasma proteins is 75% independent of plasma concentration of doxorubicin up to 1.1 mcg/mL.

Mechanism of action

Anticancer antibiotics inhibit uncontrolled proliferation, aggressive growth, and metastasis. Doxorubicin has two proposed mechanisms of action: it acts in the cancer cell via intercalation into DNA and disruption of topoisomerase II–mediated DNA repair. It generates free radicals that damage cellular membranes, DNA, and proteins.

TABLE 53.5 Antitumor antibiotics.

Generic name	Trade name	Route of administration
bleomycin	Blenoxane	IM, IV, subcutaneous
daunorubicin	Cerubidine	IV
doxorubicin	Adriamycin PFS	IV
epirubicin	Ellence	IV
idarubicin	Idamycin	IV
mitomycin	Mutamycin	IV
plicamycin	Mithracin	IV
valrubicin	Valstar	Instilled into the urinary bladder

Clinical indications

Doxorubicin has a broad clinical anticancer spectrum. It is generally used for solid cancers and is effective against malignant lymphoma, breast, lung, liver, gastric, and soft tissue sarcoma. It can also have a good effect on acute leukemia. Adriamycin is used to treat many childhood cancer patients. It is one of the most commonly used anthracyclines in adults and children. Mitomycin is an anticancer drug isolated from *Actinomycin* culture, which is effective in multiple solid cancers. Plicamycin is mainly used in the treatment of testicular embryonal cancer and various malignant cancers caused by hypercalcemia. It is also used for glioma and lymphoma.

Contraindications

Contraindications of doxorubicin include hypersensitivity, recent myocardial infarction or congestive heart failure, acute infections, and severe liver impairment.

Adverse effects

Doxorubicin's adverse effects include soreness, redness, and peeling of the hands and feet. The **hand-foot syndrome** involves tingling, numbness, pain, and dryness. Less often, doxorubicin can cause a rash, itching, or areas of skin darkening.

Toxicities

Acute cardiac toxicity of doxorubicin occurs within days of administration and occurs in about 11% of patients. This manifests as reversible myopericarditis, left ventricular dysfunction, or arrhythmias.

Chemotherapy-induced adverse effects

The adverse effects and long-term sequelae of chemotherapy remain a significant source of concern. Chemotherapy-induced adverse effects are often incompletely effective, frequently do not address potential longer-term sequelae, or may even induce other adverse effects. This chapter discusses myelosuppression and neutropenic fever in detail.

Myelosuppression

Myelosuppression is the most common dose-limiting adverse effect of traditional chemotherapy, although it is not seen with all agents. To understand myelosuppression, first, look at how the bone marrow works to make new cells. The average bone marrow makes various cells with three main groups of cells: white blood cells (WBCs), red blood cells, and platelets. WBCs can be neutrophils, eosinophils, basophils, monocytes, or lymphocytes. With myelosuppression, some or all of these cells are decreased.

Regarding myelosuppression, neutrophils are typically the most impacted WBCs. This is likely due to its short lifespan of about 6–12 hours and its rapid turnover into new cells. Following chemotherapy, a low point in the neutrophil count is typically seen around 10–14 days. The neutrophil count typically recovers by 3–4 weeks after chemotherapy. Neutrophils are needed in the body to help fight off infections. When the absolute neutrophil count falls below 500, the risk of infection increases; this is called neutropenia.

Neutropenic fever

In a person with neutropenia, the signs and symptoms of infection may not be easily seen. This is because one needs neutrophils to yield a response such as redness, swelling, or development of pus. Without these signs, the remaining symptom is a fever. **Neutropenic fever** is defined as a single temperature taken orally of 101°F (38.3°C) or an oral temperature of 100.4°F (38°C) sustained for 1 hour. These fevers are in a patient with neutropenia, defined as less than 500 neutrophils/mcL or less than 1000 neutrophils/mcL, with the expectation to decline to less than 500 neutrophils/mcL over the next 48 hours.

When a person has neutropenic fever, it is considered an oncologic emergency. Depending on an initial risk assessment, a patient can be treated with oral antibiotics as an outpatient or must be admitted to the hospital for IV antibiotics. The primary qualities of the antibiotics selected for neutropenic fever are broad coverage of infectious bacteria, including a specific organism called *Pseudomonas*. Selection of antibiotics can be based on multiple factors, including recent antibiotic exposure, drug allergies, infection history, possible sources of infection/likely pathogens, insurance coverage, side effects, drug-drug interactions, and antibiotic sensitivities at the institution.

Tumor lysis syndrome

Certain types of cancer, such as **acute lymphoblastic leukemia**, **acute myeloid leukemia**, and highly aggressive non-Hodgkin lymphoma, have an increased risk for the development of **tumor lysis syndrome** (TLS). In general, a cancer with a high proliferation rate and high response rate to chemotherapy carries an increased risk of TLS. Other risk factors include renal dysfunction, dehydration, hypotension, and acidic urine. TLS is an oncologic emergency that occurs when cancer cells are destroyed spontaneously or due to anticancer therapy. When lysed, these cells release uric acid from the breakdown of DNA, potassium, phosphorus, and electrolytes within the intracellular ions. This leads to hyperuricemia, hyperkalemia, and hyperphosphatemia, which can cause damage to the kidneys, heart, and brain. Hyperphosphatemia can lead to hypocalcemia due to the binding of phosphorus and calcium to form crystals.

Key Terms

Acute lymphoblastic leukemia
Acute myeloid leukemia
Apoptosis
Kaposi sarcoma
Lymphoma
Mitosis
Multiple myeloma
Myelosuppression
Neutropenic fever
Proteinuria
Tumor lysis syndrome

Clinical Case Studies

Clinical Case Study 1

A 45-year-old female was diagnosed with cancer of the left breast. Tests revealed it to be an aggressive carcinoma. The patient underwent surgery and received traditional chemotherapy, followed by radiotherapy and endocrine therapy. Unfortunately, the cancer metastasized to the lymph nodes and bones. The patient was a good candidate for biologic therapy and was given atezolizumab monotherapy followed by paclitaxel. After 2 years of follow-up, the cancer was still in remission.

Critical Thinking Questions

1. How does traditional chemotherapy work?
2. What do biological therapies consist of?
3. What is paclitaxel classified as?

Clinical Case Study 2

A 47-year-old male was hospitalized with advanced colon cancer that had metastasized to his liver. Surgery was performed, and nearly 90% of the colon had to be removed. Three chemotherapy treatments were given, combining fluorouracil, oxaliplatin, and leucovorin. Follow-up CT scans showed that these treatments had shrunk multiple liver tumors. Portal vein embolization was performed to increase the size of the liver in preparation for primary liver resection. An extended right hepatectomy was then performed, and nearly 70% of the liver was removed. The pathology report revealed that the chemotherapy had killed all of the liver cancer cells. Additional CT scans showed no signs of cancer. Four months of adjuvant chemotherapy with oral capecitabine were given, lowering the chances of recurrence. The patient has survived for three years after the treatments.

Critical Thinking Questions

1. What is the trade name of capecitabine, and how is it administered?
2. What are antimetabolites and their classification?
3. How do antimetabolites work?

Further Reading

[1] B.A. Chabner, D.L. Longo, Cancer Chemotherapy, Immunotherapy and Biotherapy, sixth ed., Wolters Kluwer, 2018.
[2] E. Chu, V.T. DeVita Jr., Physicians' Cancer Chemotherapy Drug Manual, twenty-fourth ed., Jones & Bartlett Learning, 2024.
[3] G.S. Goldberg, R. Airley, Cancer Chemotherapy – Basic Science to the Clinic, second ed., Wiley Blackwell, 2020.
[4] M. Javle, M. Jivraj Borad, Handbook of Targeted Cancer Therapy and Immunotherapy – Gastrointestinal Cancer, Lippincott, Williams, and Wilkins, 2023.
[5] R.J. Jones, T.M. McCormick, Rogue Cells – A Conversation on the Myths and Mysteries of Cancer, Johns Hopkins University Press, 2024.
[6] P.E. Marik, Cancer Care – the Role of Repurposed Drugs and Metabolic Interventions in Treating Cancer, Front Line Covid-19 Critical Care Alliance, 2023.
[7] J. McKay, T. Schacher, The Chemotherapy Survival Guide – Everything you Need to Know to Get Through Treatment, third ed., New Harbinger Publications, 2010.
[8] National Cancer Institute, Chemotherapy and you, NCI, 2019.
[9] M. Olsen, K. LeFebvre, S. Walker, E. Prechtel Dunphy, Chemotherapy and Immunotherapy Guidelines and Recommendations for Practice, second ed., Oncology Nursing Society, 2023.
[10] T.J. Priestman, Cancer Chemotherapy – an Introduction, third ed., Springer, 2012.
[11] S. Reich, The Ultimate Cancer Therapy Survival Guide – Navigating the Cancer Treatment Labyrinth with Success, Reich, 2023.
[12] G. Rodgers, N.S. Young, The Bethesda Handbook of Clinical Hematology, fifth ed., Wolters Kluwer, 2024.
[13] R.T. Skeel, S.N. Khleif, Handbook of Cancer Chemotherapy, Wolters Kluwer / Lippincott, Williams, and Wilkins, 2011.
[14] J. Stegall, Cancer Secrets – an Integrative Oncologist Reveals How to Fight Cancer Using the Best of Modern Medicine and Natural Therapies, second ed., Cancer Secrets, 2023.

UNIT X

Special topics

CHAPTER

54

Immunizations

OUTLINE

LEARNING OUTCOMES

After study of the chapter, readers should be able to:

1. Describe the role of B and T lymphocytes.
2. Explain the necescity of booster vaccines.
3. Compare the classifications of vaccines.
4. Discuss some examples of inactivated vaccines.
5. Identify some examples of live attenuated vaccines.
6. Explain the polysaccharide vaccines.

The Science of Pharmacology
https://doi.org/10.1016/B978-0-443-29038-1.00054-3

7. Describe the hepatitis A and B vaccinations.
8. Explain the COVID-19 pandemic.
9. Describe Japanese encephalitis and the effectiveness of its vaccine.
10. Describe yellow fever and how it is transmitted to humans.

Overview

The development of vaccines is one of the most significant milestones in medicine. The studies and concepts of modern immunization date back to the 1790s with Edward Jenner's work on preventing smallpox disease through vaccination with the cowpox virus. In the late 1800s Louis Pasteur created the first live attenuated, or weakened, bacterial vaccine and later developed the first rabies vaccine. Since then, vaccines for at least 26 diseases have been developed. Vaccines have saved a multitude of lives and prevented pain, suffering, and complications from diseases that were previously untreatable. The WHO estimates immunization prevents 2–3 million deaths annually. With expanded immunization globally, an additional 1.5 million deaths could be prevented. Failure to immunize can cause serious illness from vaccine-preventable diseases. High levels of vaccination are required for the immunity of the community. Although an estimated 91% of children were immunized against measles in the United States in 2019, measles outbreaks have been reported in multiple states due partly to underimmunization.

The immune system

The immune system is a complex network of cells, organs, and proteins. It defends the body against infection and "remembers" each microorganism that has intruded into the body before and has been defeated. Therefore it can recognize and destroy the microbe quickly if it enters the body again. Immune system abnormalities can lead to infections, allergic diseases, immunodeficiencies, and autoimmune disorders. An autoimmune disorder can develop when there is a malfunction of the immune system. The immune system cells include neutrophils, basophils, eosinophils, monocytes, and lymphocytes. The lymphoid cells contain the immune system and supporting cells, forming a scaffold-like tissue structure. T lymphocytes (T cells) and B lymphocytes (B cells) protect against **antigens**. Activated T cells coordinate the immune response. **Macrophages** are vital because they phagocytize foreign substances and help activate T cells. They are assisted by the **dendritic cells**, which capture antigens and return them to the **lymph nodes**. The **reticular cells** are similar to fibroblasts and produce the reticular fiber stroma, a network that supports other cells in the lymphoid organs and tissues.

The two main types of lymphocytes are B lymphocytes and T lymphocytes. B lymphocytes make **antibodies**, and T lymphocytes help control immune responses and kill tumor cells. They are found in blood circulation, lymphoid tissues, and various organs. Most lymphocytes are short lived, with an average lifespan of a week to a few months, but a few live for years. Some lymphocytes migrate to the **thymus**, where they mature into T cells. Others remain in the bone marrow, where they develop into B cells.

For the most robust immune response, T cells and B cells work together and cause the increased production of a series of particular B cells that can evolve into **plasma cells**, which generate antibodies to the vaccine antigen. These antibodies can bind to the antigen and help the body eliminate the threat. After the threat is subdued, some evolved B cells will remain in the body as *memory* B cells. These cells can be activated later when the same antigen is detected. When the B cells are activated, they can multiply rapidly and produce many antibodies to target the antigen or disease.

The immune system's initial response to a vaccine that causes the production of antibodies and memory B cells is called priming. Vaccines are given as a priming series followed by a booster. The booster vaccine causes the memory B cells to be activated, resulting in a more robust and longer-lasting response to the antigen than the reaction after only a priming series.

Classification of vaccines

Vaccines are classified as live attenuated and inactive. Live attenuated vaccines are prepared from a virus or bacteria—attenuated means "to weaken." Modifications are made to the virus or bacteria, allowing it to replicate and stimulate immunity without causing the disease. Live attenuated vaccines include measles/mumps/rubella (MMR), varicella, rotavirus (RV), yellow fever, oral typhoid, and intranasal live attenuated influenza vaccine (LAIV).

Inactivated vaccines are prepared by growing the bacteria or virus in the laboratory and then inactivating it by treating it with chemicals or heat. Some vaccines are made from the inactivated whole virus (such as polio, hepatitis A [HepA], and rabies). Other vaccines are made from subunits of the bacteria or virus (such as acellular pertussis, influenza, hepatitis B [HepB], and human papillomavirus [HPV]). Different vaccines are still made from the **bacteria's toxoids** (such as diphtheria and tetanus). For vaccines made from fractions of the virus or bacteria, the inactivated product is then further modified or purified to obtain the desired component. These products do not replicate in the body and cannot cause disease.

Vaccine antigens

Antigens are substances that mobilize the body's adaptive defenses and are the ultimate targets of all adaptive immune responses. The term "antigen" means "antibody generating." Most of them are large and complex, natural or synthetic molecules that are foreign to the body. Therefore they are considered to be intruders and referred to as "nonself." Antigens may be complete or incomplete. Whole antigens have both immunogenicity and reactivity. **Immunogenicity** is the ability to stimulate specific lymphocytes (B cells) to multiply. Reactivity is the ability to react with activated lymphocytes and antibodies released by immunogenic reactions.

A vaccine antigen is a live or inactivated substance foreign to the body that causes an immune response. The antigen is the part of the vaccine that the body responds to, leading to disease immunity. There are two main categories of vaccine antigens: protein antigens and polysaccharide antigens. The type of antigen the vaccine is made from is essential in causing an immune response. Different antigen types can give more robust and longer-lasting immune responses compared to others. This response is a factor in why different vaccines (protein antigens) are provided at certain ages.

Protein antigens provide a robust response and perfect immune memory. They cause T cells to interact with B cells to produce particular antibody-producing plasma cells and memory cells. Live, attenuated, killed, and conjugated vaccines are all protein antigens. A conjugated vaccine is formed when a polysaccharide is chemically attached to a protein. This attachment places the conjugate vaccine in the protein antigen group.

Polysaccharide antigens are made from a carbohydrate piece of the bacterial cell wall. This type of antigen triggers B cells directly, without the help of T cells in the germinal center of the lymph nodes. Antibody-producing plasma cells result from this response. However, they are relatively short lived and have poor memory induction. Pure polysaccharide vaccines cause poor immune responses in children under 2 years old.

Route of vaccine administration

Administration of vaccines involves a series of actions, which include assessing patient vaccination status, screening for contraindications, preparing and administering vaccines properly, and documenting the vaccines administered. Professional standards for medication administration, manufacturer instructions, and organizational policies and procedures should always be followed when applicable. The route of administration varies depending on the types of vaccines, the patient's age, and the manufacturing guidelines.

Intranasal

The LAIV is the only vaccine administered intranasally. Follow manufacturer guidance for administration. The syringe has a clip that separates the dose into two 0.1-mL sprays. One spray (0.1 mL) will be given in each nostril while the patient sits and breathes normally. Do not repeat the dose if the patient sneezes or expels the dose.

Oral

Oral vaccines are safe, easy to administer, and convenient for all ages. They have been successfully developed to protect from many infectious diseases acquired through oral transmission. Oral delivery of vaccines represents the most attractive mode of administration over other delivery routes because oral vaccination is noninvasive, safe, and straightforward to execute, showing good patient compliance and clinical practicality. RV, adenovirus, cholera vaccine, and oral typhoid vaccines are the only vaccines administered orally in the United States. Administer oral vaccines first if multiple vaccines are required. Administer slowly to the inside of the mouth on one side, between the cheek and the gum in an infant. If the baby spits the dose out, it is not recommended to give another dose. The oral polio vaccine is administered in other countries.

Intramuscular

The preferred site for IM injection in infants 12 months old and younger is the **vastus lateralis muscle**. A 22- to 25-gauge, 5/8-inch needle can be used for neonates and preterm infants if the skin is stretched flat between the finger and thumb during administration. For babies 1 month and older, use a 1-inch needle.

In children 1–2 years old, the vastus lateralis muscle is still the preferred site, but the **deltoid muscle** may also be used if muscle mass is large enough. Use a 22- to 25-gauge needle. For the thigh, a 1-inch needle should be used; for the deltoid, a 5/8-inch needle can be used if the skin is stretched flat between the thumb and forefinger during administration.

The deltoid muscle is the preferred injection site in children 3–18 years old. A 22- to 25-gauge needle that is 5/8 to 1 inch long should be used. For most older children, a 1-inch needle length is preferred. If the 5/8-inch needle is used, the skin should be stretched flat between the thumb and forefinger during administration.

Subcutaneous

The preferred subcutaneous (SC) site for infants under 12 months old is the fatty tissue on the thigh. If necessary, the upper outer triceps may also be used. The upper outer triceps should be used for children 1 year and older. A 5/8-inch, 23- to 25-gauge needle should be used. The needle should be inserted at a 45-degree angle into the SC tissue.

Multiple vaccine administration

If multiple vaccines must be administered, separate anatomical sites are used. If the same muscle group must be used, the injection sites must be separated by at least 1 inch. It is important to remember that oral vaccines are given first before any other types of vaccines. One reason for this is that, for example, infants will likely be less upset before injections and more likely to ingest the oral liquid. The more painful vaccines, such as MMR, pneumococcal conjugate (PCV15 or PCV20), and HPV, should be administered last. Examples of combination vaccines include diphtheria, tetanus, and pertussis (DTaP), trivalent IPV (three strains of the inactivated polio vaccine), MMR, MMR-varicella, DTaP-*Haemophilus influenzae* type B (Hib), and Hib-HepB.

Vaccination schedules

Vaccination schedules are updated regularly and posted on the Centers for Disease Control and Prevention (CDC) immunization schedules webpage. Factors that must be considered include immune system development in children, maternal antibodies in infants, and the immunogenicity of vaccine antigens at different stages of development. Research on the time between doses and the timing of catch-up schedule doses has also been considered.

Children from birth through 6 years

Pediatric formulations for children 6 weeks through 6 years of age include DT (the generic formulation only, which does not include pertussis) and DTaP, which has various trade names from different manufacturers. Combination products that contain additional vaccine antigens are often used for infants. These include DTaP-IPV and DTaP-IPV-Hib. Other products containing DTaP-IPV are approved for 4- to 6-year-old children for the fourth IPV dose and the fifth DTaP dose only. The CDC vaccination schedules for children 6 weeks through 6 years are shown in **Fig. 54.1**.

Children 7 Years Through 17 years

Children 7 or older and adults can receive the Td vaccine. Once again, this product does not include pertussis. Tdap is FDA approved for individuals 10 years of age and older. The primary vaccination series consists of five doses at 2, 4, 6, and 15 to 18 months and between 4 and 6 years of age. Booster doses are recommended at 11 to 12 years of age with Tdap and then every 10 years after that with Td. If the infant series was not given or was started late, the

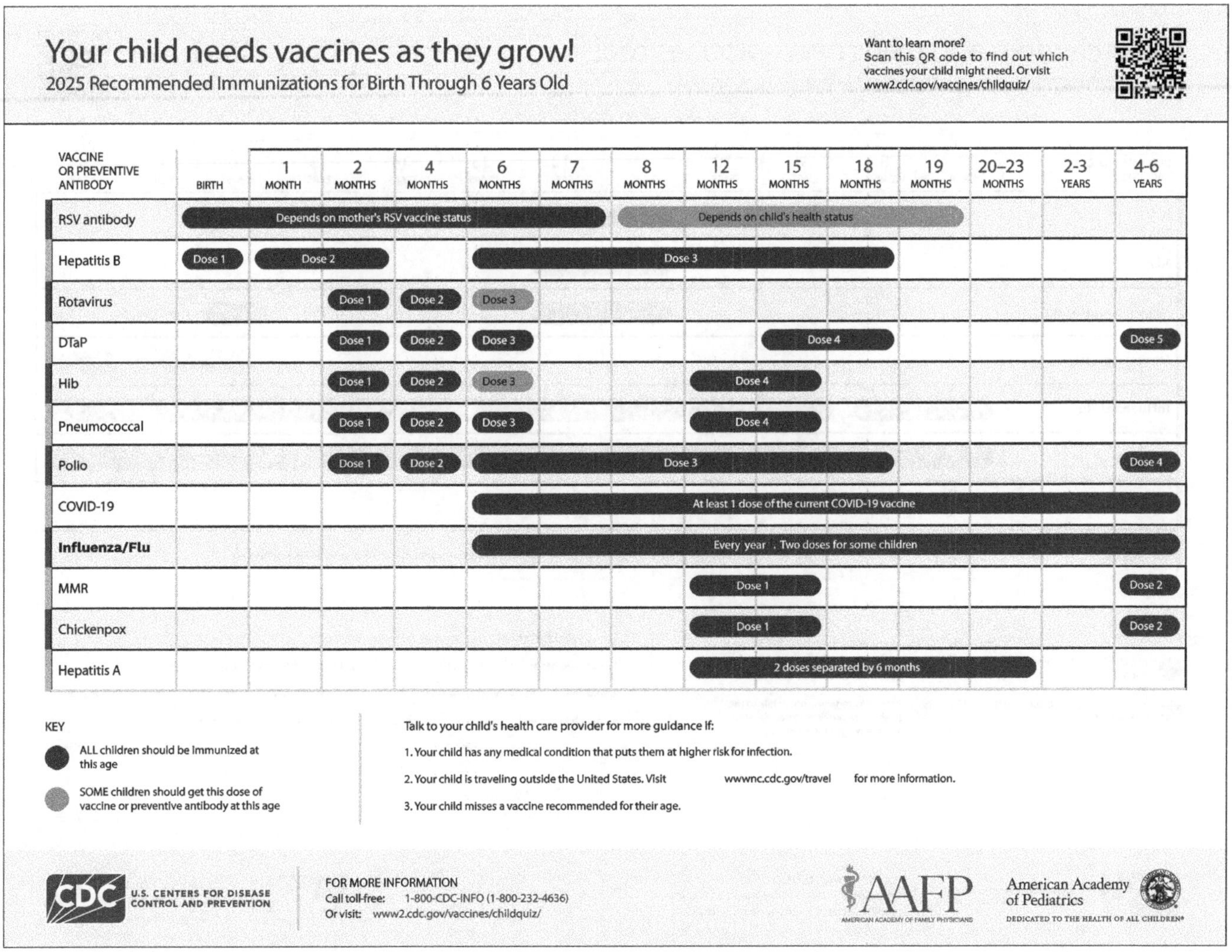

FIG. 54.1 CDC vaccination schedules for children 6 weeks through 6 years.

catch-up schedule specifies the dose timing and formulations to be used. Each of these vaccines is a 0.5-mL IM injection. The CDC vaccination schedules for children 7 years through 18 years are shown in **Fig. 54.2.**

Adult immunizations

Vaccination is recommended throughout life to prevent vaccine-preventable diseases and their sequelae. The primary focus of vaccination programs has historically been directed to childhood immunizations. For adults, chronic diseases have been the primary focus of preventive and medical healthcare, though there has been increased emphasis on preventing infectious diseases. However, adult vaccination coverage remains low for most routinely recommended vaccines. Though adults are less susceptible to falling prey to traditional contagious agents, the probability of exposure to infectious agents has increased due to globalization and growing travel opportunities within and across countries. Thus there is an urgent need to address the problem of adult immunization.

The adult immunization enterprise is more complex, encompassing various vaccines and a diverse target population. There needs to be a coordinated public health infrastructure to support an adult immunization program as there is for children. Moreover, there is little coordination among adult healthcare providers regarding vaccine provision. Substantial improvement in adult vaccination is needed to reduce the health consequences of vaccine-preventable diseases among adults. Routine assessment of adult patient vaccination needs, recommendations, and offers of vaccines required for adults should be incorporated into the regular clinical care of adults. Despite the availability of vaccines, many adults remain unvaccinated because they are unaware of the need for adult

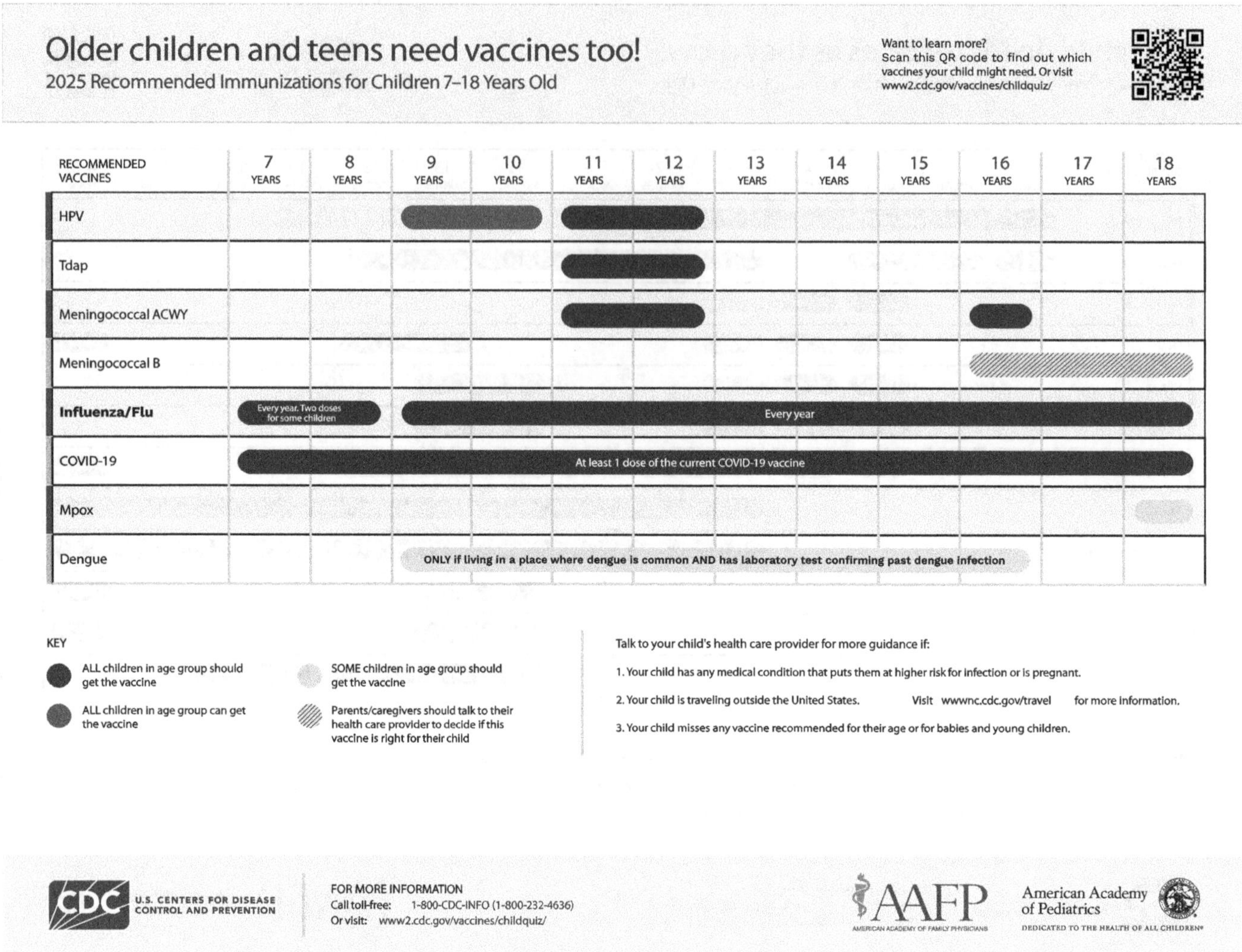

FIG. 54.2 CDC vaccination schedules for children 7 years through 18 years.

vaccines or are misinformed about vaccines and the diseases that vaccines are designed to prevent. Thus there is an urgent need to address the problem of adult immunization.

Contraindications and precautions

Any vaccine may be contraindicated in persons with proven anaphylactic hypersensitivity to any vaccine component. A precaution is a condition that may increase the risk of an adverse reaction following immunization or compromise the vaccine's ability to produce immunity. Generally vaccines are deferred when a precaution is present. However, there may be circumstances when the benefits of giving the vaccine outweigh potential risks or when reduced vaccine immunogenicity may significantly benefit an immunocompromised individual. Some precautions and contraindications depend on whether a vaccine is a live attenuated product or a nonlive product.

Mild illnesses, with or without fever (such as an upper respiratory tract infection or **otitis media**), do not increase the risk of adverse events after immunization or interfere with the response to vaccines. There are no associated contraindications or precautions, so these should not be used as a reason to withhold or delay immunization. The only exception is when nasal congestion is present, which could impede the delivery of LAIV to the nasopharyngeal mucosa. In these cases, the nonlive influenza vaccine can be offered.

A vaccine is contraindicated in a person with a documented history of confirmed anaphylaxis after the previous administration of the same vaccine. However, exceptions may apply (such as the Imvamune and mRNA

COVID-19 vaccines). There are no contraindications or precautions associated with a history of a febrile seizure after a previous immunization. Children with a history of febrile seizures have no increased risk of developing any seizure disorder. Vaccines are generally safe for people with skin disorders. Vaccines should be administered to a nonaffected area of the skin for comfort. Some smallpox vaccines and Bacille Calmette-Guérin (BCG) are exceptions to this. Imvamune vaccine can be safely administered in people with eczema (atopic dermatitis). The BCG vaccine is contraindicated when there is extensive skin disease or burns. Live vaccines such as MMR and varicella are contraindicated in people with known severe immunodeficiencies such as congenital immunodeficiencies, hematologic or solid tumors, or receipt of chemotherapy or in people with human immunodeficiency virus (HIV) who are severely immunocompromised.

You should remember

There are no contraindications or precautions associated with a history of fainting after a previous immunization. The likelihood of fainting can be reduced by lowering stress for patients awaiting immunization. These measures include short waiting times, a comfortable room temperature, preparation of vaccines out of view of recipients, and privacy during administration. People should be immunized while seated or lying down.

Prevention of infectious diseases by vaccines

Vaccines have significantly contributed to global reductions in morbidity and mortality by reducing the incidence of serious infectious diseases. Today, people worldwide experience the benefits of immunizations, beginning in infancy. Vaccines have saved many lives while preventing pain, suffering, and complications from previously untreatable diseases. Today, many vaccines that should be given are available, which will be discussed in this chapter.

Diphtheria, tetanus, and pertussis

Diphtheria is a severe infection caused by *Corynebacterium diphtheriae* strains that make toxins. It can lead to difficulty breathing, dysrhythmia, and even death. Other symptoms include fever, malaise, sore throat, and decreased appetite. Severe disease can cause swelling of the lymph nodes and swelling in the neck. The CDC recommends vaccines for infants, children, teens, and adults to prevent diphtheria.

Tetanus is a disease caused by a toxin produced by *Clostridium tetani*. **Spores** of the organism are found in soil and typically enter the body through a cut or wound. The spores grow and form toxins that cause muscle spasms and convulsions. The disease often starts with muscle spasms in the jaw, causing lockjaw, and then spreads to other muscles. The neonatal form of tetanus is usually caused by infection of the infant's umbilical stump, which rarely occurs in the United States.

Pertussis, also called **whooping cough**, is a disease caused by a bacterium called *Bordetella pertussis*. The toxin is produced by bacteria contributing to symptoms such as runny nose, sneezing, fever, and rapid-fire coughing, followed by a whooping noise as the patient inhales. Complications include bacterial pneumonia, seizures, **encephalopathy** from reduced oxygen supply to the brain, and death. Pertussis is contagious and transmitted through contact with respiratory droplets.

A combination of diphtheria toxoid, tetanus toxoid, and pertussis antigens are used in vaccine formulations. A variety of products containing combinations of these antigens are available. The child's age will dictate which products can be used. The abbreviations are for diphtheria (d or D), tetanus (T), and acellular pertussis (ap).

The primary vaccination series consists of five doses at 2, 4, 6, and 15–18 months and 4–6 years of age for DTaP. Booster doses are recommended at 11–12 years of age with Tdap and then every 10 years after that with Td. If the infant series was not given or started late, the catch-up schedule specifies dose timing and formulations to be used. Each vaccine is a 0.5-mL IM injection, regardless of the product. People should receive a vaccine every 10 years for diphtheria and tetanus; additional emergency booster doses should not be given for tetanus.

You should remember

Pertussis vaccines should be delayed if a child has an evolving neurologic condition. Examples include uncontrolled epilepsy, infantile spasms, and progressive encephalopathy. Once treatment has been initiated and the conditions have stabilized or resolved, the recommendation is to reconsider the benefits and risks of vaccinating.

Poliomyelitis

Poliomyelitis is a highly infectious disease caused by a virus. It invades the nervous system and can cause total **paralysis** in a matter of hours. The virus is transmitted person to person and spreads mainly through the fecal-oral route or, less frequently, by contaminated water or food and multiplies in the intestine. Initial symptoms are fever, fatigue, headache, vomiting, stiffness of the neck, and pain in the limbs. One in 200 infections leads to irreversible paralysis (usually in the legs). Among those paralyzed, 5%–10% die when their breathing muscles become immobilized.

The disease is considered eradicated in the United States but may occur in other countries. There are three serotypes of poliovirus: P1, P2, and P3. Inactivated poliovirus vaccine (IPV) is available as an individual vaccine, but several combination products containing IPV are also known as DTaP-IPV combinations.

IPV combination vaccines are 0.5-mL doses given by IM injection as part of routine infant immunization. The primary series is started in infants at 2, 4, 6, and 18 months, followed by a final dose at 4–6 years of age. The IPV individual vaccine can also be given through SC injection. Oral polio vaccines are used in other countries.

Haemophilus influenzae type B

Hib is a bacteria that can cause severe infections, especially in infants. The bacteria have six serotypes with a polysaccharide capsule (types A–F). The polysaccharide is the primary factor associated with virulence. Of the six capsular types of *H. influenzae*, Hib is responsible for more than 90% of systemic infections. This organism primarily causes **pneumonia** and **meningitis** in young children, and it is a significant public health concern in many parts of the world, with as many as 3 million cases of severe disease occurring every year. The increasing resistance of Hib to antibiotic agents has been reported from many parts of the world, and vaccination is the only public health tool that can rapidly reduce the incidence of Hib disease globally.

Vaccination against Hib for infants begins at 2 months of age. Three doses are required for Hib vaccines at 2, 4, and 6 months, with a booster at 12–18 months of age. All Hib-containing products are to be given through IM injection. The dose for all products is 0.5 mL.

Rotavirus

RV is a diarrheal illness caused by a virus in the Reoviridae family. It enters through the mouth and replicates in the cells of the small intestine. Infections can cause vomiting, fever, and severe diarrhea, leading to dehydration. The virus is transmitted through the fecal-oral route. The highest disease rates are in children 3–35 months of age. RV vaccination is recommended for all infants who do not have a contraindication and should be given before they turn 8 months old. Two live oral RV vaccine formulations are available: RV1 (ROTARIX, GSK) and RV5 (ROTATEQ, Merck).

Contraindications include severe allergic reactions to components or reactions following the prior dose, latex allergy (for RV1 only), and a history of intussusception (a condition where a segment of the intestine slides inside the next segment, like a telescope). Infants with **severe combined immunodeficiency** (SCID) should not receive the vaccine. Consult an immunologist or infectious diseases specialist before administering to infants with known or suspected altered immunocompetence (compromised immune system); acute, moderate, or severe **gastroenteritis**; or other critical illnesses.

Influenza

Influenza is a very contagious viral illness that affects people of all ages. The most common forms are influenza A and B. The classic symptoms of influenza are rapid-onset fever, muscle aches, sore throat, cough, and headache. Other symptoms may also occur. Complications of the illness include pneumonia, heart inflammation, and worsening of preexisting lung diseases.

Influenza vaccine should be administered yearly before and during flu season (October–March). It is recommended that you vaccinate by the end of October. There are two types of influenza vaccine: LAIV and inactivated influenza vaccine. The inactivated influenza vaccine is an IM injection. In children 6 months old through 8 years old, two doses of flu vaccine are required as a priming series during the first immunization season. These doses should be separated by 4 weeks. Children 8 years old and under who have not received two doses in previous years will require two doses in the current season. After the child has received the initial priming doses, only one dose will be needed in the following years.

LAIV is administered intranasally, with 0.1 mL in each nostril while the patient is upright. Children must be at least 2 years old to receive this live vaccine. It is approved for healthy people between the ages of 2 and 49 who are not pregnant.

Measles/mumps/rubella

Measles is a disease caused by a virus and is highly contagious through contact with respiratory and aerosolized droplets. It causes a high fever, cough, runny nose, eye redness, and a rash that develops 3–5 days after the first symptoms. Complications from the disease include diarrhea, ear infection, pneumonia, encephalitis, seizures, and death.

Mumps is a viral infection that usually affects **parotid glands**. Swollen glands may be tender or painful. It may also cause headaches, muscle aches, fever, decreased appetite, and malaise. Mumps can also cause **orchitis**, meningitis, and encephalitis. The virus is transmitted through airborne transmission and direct contact with droplets or saliva.

Rubella, also known as German measles, is caused by a virus. It causes low-grade fever, malaise, swelling of lymph nodes, joint pain, and rash. It can cause congenital rubella syndrome in neonates from infection during pregnancy. Deafness is the most common effect, but other congenital defects can also occur, including eye defects, heart defects, and neurological abnormalities. Rubella is spread through airborne and respiratory droplet transmission.

The MMR vaccine is a live attenuated virus vaccine. A second live attenuated virus vaccine includes MMR and varicella antigens (MMRV). All children 12 months of age and older should receive the MMR vaccine. A second dose should be given at 4–6 years of age. About 5% of people will respond only partially to one dose. The MMR vaccine is contraindicated in a severe allergic reaction, history of anaphylaxis to neomycin, congenital immunodeficiency, HIV infection, leukemia, lymphoma, and malignancy.

The contraindications and precautions for MMRV and MMR are the same, with one exception: MMRV contraindications include a personal or family history of seizures. In these cases, separate MMR and varicella vaccines should be used.

You should remember

Tuberculin skin testing can be done at the same time as MMR or 4 weeks after MMR. However, it is recommended that it be avoided until 4 weeks after MMR vaccination due to the risk of false-negative results due to the suppression of response by the MMR vaccine.

Hepatitis A

HepA is caused by a virus that enters the mouth and replicates in the liver, causing abdominal pain, nausea, malaise, fever, and jaundice. The incubation period is about 4 weeks. Symptoms occur more often in older children and adults. It is transmitted through the fecal-oral route from contact with an infected person or from ingestion of food or water that has been contaminated. The HepA vaccine is an inactivated whole-virus vaccine. The HepA vaccine is recommended for all children between 12 months and 18 years of age living in the United States. It is also recommended for others who are at increased risk of infection. The series is two doses, with the second given at least 6 months after the first. HepA vaccine is to be administered by IM injection.

Hepatitis B

HepB is the world's most common severe liver infection. It is caused by the HepB virus that attacks and injures the liver. Two billion people have been infected, and about 300 million people are living with a chronic HepB infection. Each year, up to 1 million people die from HepB, even though it is preventable and treatable. The condition can be acute or chronic. Chronic disease can result in cirrhosis, liver failure, and liver cancer. HepB is transmitted through contact with infected blood or certain bodily fluids. The virus is most commonly transmitted from an infected person who is pregnant to their baby during childbirth due to the blood exchange that happens between mother and baby. It is also transmitted through unsterile medical or dental equipment, unprotected sex, or unsterile needles or by sharing personal items such as razors, toothbrushes, nail clippers, and body jewelry.

The HepB vaccine is the only vaccine given to babies at birth. It is administered via IM injection. HepB products are available in single-dose vials and prefilled syringes. The HepB vaccine is recommended within 24 hours of birth for all medically stable infants with a birthweight of at least 2 kg if the mother is HepB surface antigen negative. If the baby's birthweight is less than 2 kg, the dose can be given at 1 month of age on discharge from the hospital. If the mother is HepB surface antigen positive or unknown, the vaccine should be offered without regard to birthweight and within 12 hours of birth. In the routine series of three doses of the HepB vaccine, the first dose is typically given within 24 hours after birth, the second dose is given 1–2 months after the first dose, and the third dose is shared between 6 and 18 months. Four doses are permitted if a combination product is used for subsequent doses. Contraindications and precautions include severe allergic reactions to components (yeast protein, latex in prefilled syringes packaging) and moderate to severe illness.

The routine series is three doses of the HepB vaccine, typically given at 0 months, 1–2 months, and 6–18 months of age. Four doses are permitted if a combination product is used for subsequent doses. Catch-up schedules for specific age groups allow for two doses of certain products. Contraindications and precautions include severe allergic reactions to components (yeast protein, latex in prefilled syringes packaging) and moderate to severe illness.

You should remember

The HepB vaccine is recommended for all infants, children, or adolescents younger than 19 who have not been vaccinated, all adults aged 19 through 59, and adults aged 60 years or older with risk factors for HepB infection.

Varicella

Varicella (chickenpox) is an acute infectious disease caused by the varicella-zoster virus, a DNA virus from the herpesvirus group. After the primary infection, varicella-zoster virus stays in the body (in the sensory nerve ganglia) as a latent infection. The disease has two manifestations: the primary infection causes chickenpox, and the recurrent infection causes herpes zoster or **shingles**. Chickenpox is characterized by a rash that begins on the face and progresses to the trunk and extremities.

The varicella vaccine protects against chickenpox (varicella), a common and contagious viral childhood illness. It also protects against shingles. Varicella vaccine is a live attenuated vaccine. **Children under age 13 should get two doses**. The first is at ages 12 through 15 months, and the second is at ages 4 through 6 years. **People 13 years and older** who have never had chickenpox or received the vaccine should get two doses at least 28 days apart. People who have cancers or have HIV/AIDS or another disease that affects the immune system should not get the varicella vaccine.

Human papillomavirus

HPV is a sexually transmitted infection that can cause genital warts, cervical cancer, and anogenital cancer. There are many different serotypes, but types 16 and 18 are high-risk types that cause 70% of cervical cancers. HPV vaccine can protect against exposure. If HPV vaccination is initiated at ages 9–14 years, a two-dose series is recommended with 6–12 months between doses. If HPV vaccination is started at age 15 or older, a three-dose series is required with doses at 0, 1–2 months, and 6 months from the first dose. Immunocompromising conditions require a three-dose series as well. Children with a history of sexual abuse or assault can be vaccinated beginning at 9 years of age. Each dose is a 0.5-mL IM injection.

Meningococcal disease

The bacterium *Neisseria meningitidis* causes meningococcal disease. Several types cause illness worldwide: types A, B, C, W, and Y. Infection with the bacteria can cause sepsis and meningitis. Transmission occurs through aerosolized respiratory droplets or direct contact. Symptoms of the disease include nausea and vomiting, a fever, headache, stiff neck, sensitivity to light, and changes in mental status. Infection can progress rapidly and can be fatal in up to 40% of people who have **meningococcemia**.

Routine vaccination begins with one dose of MenACWY at 11–12, followed by a booster at 16–18. MenACWY is required at a younger age for patients with certain medical conditions or high-risk situations such as HIV infection or persistent complement component deficiency. Two vaccines are available that protect against serogroups A, C, W, and Y:

- MenACWY-D contains polysaccharide components conjugated to diphtheria toxoid. It can be given in persistent complement component deficiency, a specific type of immune system disorder, and for travel to particular regions to children as young as 9 months. However, patients 9–23 months with specific conditions such as **asplenia**, **sickle cell disease**, or HIV infection should not receive this vaccine until 2 years of age. MenACWY-D is available in single-dose vials that do not require reconstitution.
- MenACWY-CRM contains polysaccharide components conjugated to a protein called CRM197. Following the appropriate immunization schedule, children with certain high-risk conditions (including HIV) should be vaccinated as early as 2 months old.

People aged 16–23 at high risk for meningitis (i.e., complement component deficiency, functional or anatomic asplenia, or those taking complement inhibitor medications) should also receive a serogroup B meningococcal vaccine (MenB). They also need to obtain a booster dose of MenB 1 year after the first dose and every 2–3 years after. Individuals in that age group who do not have these high-risk conditions **may** receive a MenB vaccine, especially if they are at risk of meningococcal disease due to living in on-campus college housing.

Contraindications for meningococcal vaccines include severe allergic reactions to components of the vaccine and moderate or severe illness.

Pneumococcal disease

Pneumococcal disease is caused by the bacterium *Streptococcus pneumoniae*. The bacteria have many serotypes, but those with a polysaccharide capsule are the most pathogenic. In children, pneumococcal disease can cause ear infections, pneumonia, **bacteremia**, and meningitis.

Three pneumococcal vaccines are available: 23-valent polysaccharide PPSV23 (Pneumovax23, Merck), the 15-valent PCV15 (Vaxneuvance, Pfizer), and the 20-valent PCV20 (Prevnar 20, Pfizer).

PCV15 and PCV20 are pneumococcal conjugate vaccines, including capsular polysaccharide conjugates for 15 and 20 serotypes. These vaccines are available as a prefilled 0.5-mL syringe administered IM. The PCV15 or the PCV20 vaccine should be administered as a four-dose series for all infants at 2, 4, 6, and 12–15 months old. For adults 65 and older and people 19–64 with specific high-risk medical conditions who have never received a PCV vaccine, PCV15 or PCV20 may be given. If PCV15 is used, this should be followed by a dose of PPSV23 1 year later. If PCV20 is administered, a dose of PPSV23 is NOT indicated. Refer to the CDC vaccine schedule for the most up-to-date recommendations.

The PPSV23 contains polysaccharide capsule components of 23 different serotypes of the bacteria. Because it is a polysaccharide vaccine, it is less effective in young children. PPSV23 is a 0.5-mL dose given primarily through IM injection and should only be given to children 2 years of age and older with certain medical conditions.

Contraindications for pneumococcal vaccines include severe allergic reactions to a pneumococcal vaccine or any vaccine containing diphtheria toxoid.

You should remember

Patients without a spleen or a functioning spleen, with sickle cell disease, or who are immunocompromised, have HIV, have a cochlear implant, or have a cerebrospinal fluid leak are at increased risk for pneumococcal disease.

Respiratory syncytial virus vaccines

Respiratory syncytial virus (RSV) causes infections of the lungs and respiratory tract. It's so common that most children have been infected with the virus by age 2. RSV can also infect adults. The virus is generally spread through direct contact such as via droplets from another person's cough or sneeze that then contact another person's eyes, nose, or mouth. It can also be spread by touching a surface upon which the virus is present, such as a doorknob, and then touching the face before washing the hands. In adults and older, healthy children, RSV symptoms are mild and typically mimic the common cold. It can cause severe infection in some people, including infants, especially premature infants, older adults, people with heart and lung disease, or anyone with a weak immune system (immunocompromised).

Older adults in nursing homes or long-term care facilities have the most severe illnesses and complications. Symptoms include a runny nose, decreased appetite, coughing, sneezing, fever, and wheezing. While most people recover in 1–2 weeks, the condition can become severe and cause shortness of breath and low oxygen levels. RSV may lead to worsening medical conditions such as asthma, chronic obstructive pulmonary disease, or congestive heart failure. Older adults and infants who become very ill with RSV may need to be hospitalized, which can be fatal.

The RSV vaccines can prevent lower respiratory tract disease caused by RSV. There are currently two RSV vaccines approved in the United States: RSVPreF3 (Arexvy, GlaxoSmithKline) and RSVpreF (Abrysvo, Pfizer). These vaccines contain a recombinant RSV F protein antigen stabilized in the prefusion conformation (preF). RSVpreF3 is monovalent, meaning it only includes the F protein of RSV subgroup A, whereas RSVpreF is bivalent, meaning it consists of the F proteins for RSV subgroups A and B. A single vaccine dose of 0.5 mL is administered IM.

The CDC recommends that adults 60 years or older receive one dose of the RSV vaccine, based on discussions between the patient and healthcare provider. Studies are ongoing as to whether revaccination may be needed for some patients. The RSV vaccine can be given at the same time as other vaccines. People who are pregnant are recommended to receive a single dose of RSVpreF (Abrysvo) during weeks 32 through 36 of pregnancy from September through January to prevent severe RSV disease in infants.

The vaccine provider must be told if the patient has had an allergic reaction after a previous dose of the vaccine or if any severe, life-threatening allergies are present. People with a cold or another minor illness can still receive the vaccine. Those who are moderately or severely ill should wait until they recover before getting the RSV vaccine.

COVID-19 vaccines

COVID-19 was a global coronavirus outbreak in 2019. It is an infectious disease caused by the severe acute respiratory syndrome coronavirus 2 virus. The first cases of novel coronavirus were detected in China in December 2019, with the virus spreading rapidly to other countries worldwide. The scientists focused on one "prototype" coronavirus and created a vaccine. That vaccine could then be customized to fight different coronaviruses.

The four approved vaccines in the United States are Pfizer-BioNTech, Moderna mRNA COVID-19, Novavax subunit COVID-19, and Johnson & Johnson's vector COVID-19 vaccines. All of these vaccines are injected IM in the deltoid muscle. The advantages of getting COVID-19 vaccines include a lower risk of severe illness, hospitalization, and death from COVID-19 than unvaccinated people. Updated COVID-19 vaccines can help restore the decreased protection from the previous vaccinations. The updated vaccine formulations provide added protection against the recent Omicron subvariants that are more contagious than the previous ones.

The vaccine's adverse effects include severe allergic reactions, **myocarditis**, and **pericarditis** associated with mRNA COVID-19 vaccination, mostly among males ages 12–39. These rare risks may be further reduced with a longer interval between the first and second doses. Cases of myocarditis and pericarditis have also been reported in people who received the Novavax COVID-19 vaccine. There is a potential cause-and-effect relationship between the J&J/Janssen COVID-19 vaccine and a rare and severe adverse event: blood clots with low platelets (thrombocytopenia syndrome).

You should remember

The two mRNA vaccines, Pfizer and Moderna, authorized by the FDA and recommended by the CDC, are very safe and very good at preventing severe or fatal cases of COVID-19. The risk of serious side effects associated with these vaccines is minimal.

Tuberculosis vaccine

Tuberculosis (TB) is an infectious disease that most often affects the lungs and is caused by bacteria. It spreads through the air when infected people cough, sneeze, or spit. About a quarter of the global population is estimated to have been infected with TB bacteria. About 5%–10% of people infected with TB will eventually get symptoms and develop TB. Those who are infected but not (yet) ill with the disease cannot transmit it. TB is usually treated with antibiotics and can be fatal without treatment. In certain countries, the BCG vaccine is given to babies or small children to prevent TB. The vaccine prevents TB outside of the lungs but not in the lungs.

TB mainly affects adults in their most productive years. However, all age groups are at risk. Over 80% of cases and deaths are in low- and middle-income countries. TB occurs in every part of the world. In 2021 the most significant number of new TB cases occurred in WHO's South-East Asian Region (46%), followed by the African Region (23%) and the Western Pacific (18%). Around 87% of new TB cases occurred in the 30 high–TB-burden countries, with more than two-thirds of the global total in Bangladesh, China, the Democratic Republic of the Congo, India, Indonesia, Nigeria, Pakistan, and the Philippines.

The BCG vaccine is not given as part of the routine vaccination schedule and is provided only when a child or adult is thought to have an increased risk of contracting TB. The BCG vaccine should only be given once in a lifetime. The vaccine is most effective in infants and children aged under 16. BCG vaccination is rarely given to anyone over 16 because there is little evidence that it works well in adults. However, it is given to adults aged 16–35 who are at risk of TB through their work, such as some healthcare workers, veterinary staff, and abattoir workers.

Ebola vaccine

Ebola is a severe and often deadly disease caused by a virus. Symptoms include fever, diarrhea, vomiting, bleeding, and usually death. Ebola can occur in humans and other primates (gorillas, monkeys, and chimpanzees). The Ebola outbreak in West Africa began in March 2014 and was the largest hemorrhagic viral epidemic in history. Almost 40% of the people who developed Ebola in this outbreak died. There is no known cure for Ebola. Experimental treatments have been used, but none have been thoroughly tested to see if they work well and are safe.

The Ebola vaccine is a live virus vaccine administered IM. The vaccine contains a weakened strain of the vesicular stomatitis virus that has been altered to include a gene from the Ebola virus (EBOV). There are currently two approved Ebola vaccines: a single-dose Ad5-EBOV vaccine in China and a two-dose recombinant vesicular stomatitis virus/human adenovirus serotype 5 (rVSV/Ad5) vaccine approved in the Russian Federation "for emergency use." In addition, there are two investigational vaccines, the rVSV-ZEBOV vaccine made by Merck and the Ad26 ZEBOV/MVA-BN-Filo vaccine. Ervebo (Ebola Zaire vaccine) is approved by the FDA for preventing disease caused by the EBOV (species *Zaire ebolavirus*) in individuals 18 years of age and older as a single-dose administration. Ervebo is a replication-competent, live attenuated rVSV vaccine manufactured by Merck.

Becoming infected with EBOV from the vaccine is impossible because it only contains a gene from the EBOV, not the whole virus. Specifically, it includes a gene for the EBOV glycoprotein that replaces the gene for the native VSV glycoprotein.

The vaccine is given as a single-dose vaccine. It is safe and protective against the EBOV (species *Z. ebolavirus*) only, which has caused the most significant and deadly Ebola outbreaks to date. This is the first FDA-approved vaccine for an ebolavirus. Side effects of the Ebola vaccine include headache, fever, muscle pain, fatigue, nausea, skin rash (including blisters), and abnormal sweating. The Ebola vaccine is contraindicated in people with weakened immune systems, females who are pregnant or breastfeeding, and children younger than 1 year old.

Anthrax

Anthrax is a severe infectious disease. It is caused by gram-positive, rod-shaped bacteria known as *Bacillus anthracis,* which occurs naturally in soil and often affects animals worldwide. There are four types of anthrax: cutaneous (involving the skin), inhalation (affecting the lungs), gastrointestinal (affecting the digestive system), and injection anthrax (affecting the skin or other body parts).

Anthrax can cause illness if humans come into contact with infected animals or contaminated animal products, resulting in severe disease. However, anthrax is not contagious among humans. Infection occurs when anthrax spores enter the body and are activated. The bacteria can then multiply and spread, producing toxins. This may happen if humans breathe in the spores or consume contaminated food or water or if the spores enter a wound. Anthrax is less common in the United States than in Central and South America, sub-Saharan Africa, central and southwestern Asia, southern and eastern Europe, and the Caribbean. It can cause blisters or bumps, inflammation, ulcerations, fever, chills, chest discomfort, shortness of breath, confusion, dizziness, coughing, nausea, vomiting, stomach pain, headache, extreme sweating, fatigue, body aches, sore throat, painful swallowing, hoarseness, diarrhea, flushing of the face, red eyes, fainting, and abscesses.

The anthrax vaccine is not currently recommended for the general population anywhere globally. However, because anthrax spores were sent via the mail with criminal intent in the United States following September 11, 2001, any presumed incidents related to bioterrorism in the future would almost immediately cause a reevaluation of the current recommendations. In all likelihood, revised recommendations for receipt of the anthrax vaccine would only target groups at high risk of exposure based on the situation. The risk for exposure to anthrax in the United States is low. Currently, the anthrax vaccine is only recommended in the United States for military personnel, lab personnel, and handlers of animals or animal products who are at the highest risk for exposure to anthrax spores. The vaccine is given as a series of five shots. After the first shot, the vaccine is given 3 weeks, 6 months, 12 months, and 18 months later, annually or every 3 years after that, depending on risk.

The anthrax vaccine is approved by the FDA and recommended for adults 18 through 65 years of age who are at risk of exposure to anthrax bacteria, including certain laboratory workers who work with *B. anthracis*, people who handle potentially infected animals or their carcasses, some military personnel (determined by the Department of Defense), and some emergency and other responders whose response activities might lead to exposure.

The CDC recommends five IM doses for preexposure vaccination at 0, 1, 6, 12, and 18 months, followed by annual boosters. For postexposure immunization, the CDC recommends three SC doses at 0, 2, and 4 weeks in conjunction with a 60-day course of appropriate antimicrobial agents—the preferred injection site for muscle in the upper arm. The selected site for SC injections is the fatty tissue over the deltoid muscle. Use a needle length appropriate for the age and size of the recipient. The vaccine is made by taking a strain of the bacterium and growing it in the laboratory. The bacteria release several harmful toxins into the surrounding broth. These toxins are responsible for disease in those infected with the anthrax bacteria. The toxins are then inactivated with formaldehyde so they can no longer cause disease. The anthrax bacteria are filtered out of the vaccine. Therefore the anthrax vaccine is similar to the "acellular" pertussis vaccine.

You should remember

The safety and efficacy of administering the anthrax vaccine during the same visit as other licensed vaccines have not been evaluated. If an anthrax vaccine is to be given during the same visit as another injectable vaccine, the vaccines should be administered at different injection sites, if possible. Each vaccine should be issued with a separate syringe.

Mpox (formerly monkeypox)

The monkeypox virus is an orthopoxvirus that causes **mpox** (formerly known as monkeypox), a disease with symptoms similar to smallpox, although less severe. While smallpox was eradicated in 1980, mpox continues to occur in countries of Central and West Africa. Since May 2022 cases have been reported from countries without previously documented mpox transmission outside the African region. Two distinct clades of the monkeypox virus have been identified: clade I (formerly known as the Congo Basin [Central African]) clade and clade II (the former West African clade).

Mpox is a zoonosis, a disease transmitted from animals to humans, with cases often found close to tropical rainforests where some animals carry the virus. Evidence of monkeypox virus infection has been found in animals, including squirrels, Gambian pouched rats, dormice, different species of monkeys, and others. The disease can also spread from humans to humans. It can be transmitted through contact with bodily fluids, skin lesions, or internal mucosal surfaces, such as in the mouth or throat, respiratory droplets, and contaminated objects. People with mpox often get a rash that may be located on the head, hands, feet, chest, face, or mouth or near the genitals, including the penis, testicles, labia, vagina, and anus. The incubation period is 3–17 days. During this time, a person does not have symptoms and may feel fine.

JYNNEOS is the only vaccine that is FDA approved to prevent mpox disease. It has also been approved for the prevention of smallpox disease. It is a live virus vaccine that contains Modified Vaccinia Ankara-Bavarian Nordic (MVA-BN), a weakened, nonreplicating *Orthopoxvirus*. JYNNEOS may be safely used in significantly immunocompromised individuals who may not be indicated or recommended to receive certain live vaccines. This vaccine is approved for use in individuals 18 years of age and older who are determined to be at high risk for smallpox or mpox infection. JYNNEOS is approved for intradermal or SC administration as a two-dose series, 4 weeks apart.

The vaccination is given in the forearm. It can also be given SC under the skin on the back of the upper arm or intradermally on the upper back below the scapula. If you ever have keloid scars or are under age 18, the vaccine should be given SC. Getting the vaccine intradermally or SC appears to be equally effective against mpox. The second dose should be given 28 days after the first dose.

Immunizations during pregnancy

Certain vaccines are safe and recommended for people before, during, and after pregnancy to help keep them and their babies healthy. The antibodies mothers develop in response to these vaccines protect them, cross the placenta, and help protect their babies from serious diseases early in life. Vaccinating during pregnancy also helps protect a mother from transmitting certain conditions to the newborn. The CDC recommends that people who are pregnant get up to three vaccines **during** every pregnancy: the inactivated flu vaccine (the injection, not the live nasal flu vaccine), the Tdap vaccine, and, depending on the timing of pregnancy, the RSVpreF vaccine. People who are pregnant should get the Tdap vaccine between 27 and 36 weeks of each pregnancy. This vaccine is recommended during every pregnancy, regardless of how long it has been since the mother previously received the Tdap vaccine. The RSVpreF vaccine (Abrysvo) is recommended during weeks 32 through 36 of pregnancy during September through January to prevent severe RSV disease in infants. It is safe to receive most vaccines right **after** giving birth, even while breastfeeding. People who are pregnant should not get HPV, MMR, live flu (nasal), varicella, yellow fever, typhoid fever, and Japanese encephalitis (JE) vaccines.

Travel-related diseases

Vaccines protect travelers from serious diseases. Based on the location of travel and the prevalence of disease in that area, vaccination against one or more of the following diseases may be recommended before travel. Some countries require proof of immunization for certain diseases such as HepA or yellow fever. Traveling in developing countries and rural areas may require more vaccines for tourists. If a traveler is pregnant or people have an ongoing illness or weakened immune system, they may need additional vaccines. It is essential to be up to date on routine vaccinations. While measles is rare in the United States, it is more common in parts of Asia and Africa. Depending on the travel location and the disease's prevalence in that area, vaccination against one or more of the following diseases may be recommended before the trip.

Typhoid fever

Typhoid fever and paratyphoid fever are life-threatening, systemic illnesses collectively known as enteric fever. Symptoms include fever, headache, abdominal pain, diarrhea or constipation, decreased appetite, and fatigue.

Vomiting and diarrhea are more common in children. It is transmitted primarily through the consumption of contaminated water or food. There are two different vaccines available for typhoid fever that are different. Typhoid vaccine live oral Ty21a (Vivotif, Emergent BioSolutions) is an oral live attenuated vaccine for persons 6 years and older. The dose is one capsule by mouth every other day for four doses. Doses should be administered with cool water 1 hour before and 2 hours after a meal. The doses should be completed at least 1 week before travel. A booster is needed every 5 years if there is continued exposure. One dose of the injectable inactivated typhoid vaccine (Typhim Vi, Sanofi Pasteur) is given at least 2 weeks before travel for people 2 years old and older. A booster is required every 2 years if indicated.

Contraindications for Ty21a include pregnancy and a history of allergy to any vaccine component. Avoid use in immunocompromised persons, during acute febrile illness, and therapies, malignant neoplasms, and transplants.

Japanese encephalitis

JE is caused by a virus transmitted to humans through mosquito bites. It is most common in rural areas in Southeast Asia, the Pacific Islands, and the Far East. The virus is found in pigs and birds and is passed to mosquitoes when they bite infected animals. It cannot be spread from person to person. Most people infected by the JE virus have either no or mild, short-lived symptoms, often mistaken for flu. Around 1 in every 250 people infected with JE develop more severe symptoms as the infection spreads to the brain. This usually happens 5–15 days after infection. Up to one in every three people who develop these more severe symptoms will die due to the disease. In those who survive, these symptoms tend to improve slowly.

The JE vaccine is more than 90% effective. The duration of protection with the vaccine is unclear, but its effectiveness decreases over time. Doses are given either IM or SC. Several inactivated vaccines and one type of live attenuated vaccine are currently used worldwide: inactivated mouse brain–derived vaccines, inactivated Vero cell–derived vaccines, primary hamster kidney cell–derived vaccines, purified vaccines, and live attenuated vaccines.

The inactivated vaccine (manufactured as IXIARO) is the only JE vaccine licensed and available in the United States. This vaccine was approved in March 2009 for use in people aged 17 years and older and in May 2013 for use in children 2 months through 16 years of age. Other JE vaccines are manufactured and used in other countries but are not licensed in the United States. IXIARO is given as a two-dose series, with the doses spaced 28 days apart. Adults aged 18–65 can get the second dose as early as 7 days after the first dose. The last amount should be given at least 1 week before travel. A booster dose (third dose) should be given if a person has received the two-dose primary vaccination series one year or more previously and there is a continued risk for JE virus infection or potential for reexposure. For adults and children aged 3 years or older, each dose of IXIARO is 0.5 mL. For children aged 2 months through 2 years, each amount is 0.25 mL.

There is currently no cure for JE. Treatment involves supporting the body's functions to fight off the infection. An infected person must usually be admitted to the hospital for fluids, oxygen, and medication to treat symptoms. A severe allergic reaction after a previous dose of IXIARO, any other JE vaccine, or any component of IXIARO is a contraindication to further doses. The vaccine contains protamine sulfate, a compound known to cause allergic reactions in some people. The administration of IXIARO to females who are pregnant should usually be deferred. However, females who are pregnant who must travel to an area with high infection risk should be vaccinated.

Cholera

Cholera is a diarrheal illness caused by the toxins produced by *Vibrio cholerae*. The cholera vaccine available in the United States, Vaxchora, by PaxVax, is an oral dosage form that should be taken at least 10 days before travel. This vaccine is not approved for children. The CDC recommends vaccination for people traveling to or living in areas of active cholera transmission.

Vaxchora (lyophilized CVD 103-HgR) is a single-dose, oral vaccine FDA approved in the United States for use in people aged 2–64 who are traveling to an area of active cholera transmission. Vaxchora should be taken at least 10 days before travel to a place of active cholera transmission. The vaccine manufacturer reports that Vaxchora reduces the chance of moderate and severe diarrhea in people by 90% at 10 days and 80% 3 months after. How long protection lasts beyond 3–6 months after vaccination is unknown.

The cholera vaccine should be postponed in the presence of any acute illness. A history of severe systemic reaction or allergic response following a prior dose of cholera vaccine is a contraindication to use further. Females who are pregnant are vulnerable to complications of cholera. Killed oral cholera vaccines are not recommended for females who are pregnant, though there is no evidence of harmful effects during pregnancy.

Yellow fever

Yellow fever is caused by a virus that is transmitted by mosquitos. It can cause fevers, flulike symptoms, achiness, jaundice, and severe liver disease, leading to death. No treatment exists. Yellow fever vaccine is a live virus vaccine made from the 17D strain of the virus. It is recommended for persons 9 months and older traveling to or living in high-risk areas. Only one dose is needed for most travelers. Certain groups, such as persons who have received a bone marrow transplant after the original vaccination, females who were pregnant during immunization, and HIV-infected persons, may require additional doses due to decreased response. The vaccine is 0.5 mL administered through SC injection (or IM injection).

Yellow fever vaccine is contraindicated in persons with an allergy to the vaccine component, persons less than 6 months of age, symptomatic HIV infection, thymus disorder, and immunocompromising conditions.

Rabies

Rabies is a fatal disease that mandates proper prophylaxis after rabies virus exposure to prevent death. It is caused by lyssavirus, a disease that affects the nervous system. The virus is typically transmitted to humans through the bite of an infected animal. The condition causes pain and numbness, fever, weakness, and headache. These symptoms may last for days. Symptoms then progress to cerebral dysfunction, anxiety, confusion, agitation, **hydrophobia**, spasms, coma, and death. The rabies vaccine is recommended before travel to certain countries as preexposure prophylaxis. It is also recommended as postexposure prophylaxis (PEP) after contact with or a bite from certain animals.

There are two rabies vaccines available. The first is a human diploid cell culture vaccine manufactured by Sanofi. The second is the purified chick embryo cell vaccine (RabAvert, Bavarian Nordic) produced in chick embryo cell culture. These vaccines protect against human rabies and are nerve tissue and cell culture vaccines. WHO recommends replacing nerve tissue vaccines with more efficacious, safer vaccines developed through cell culture as soon as possible.

A two-dose preexposure prophylaxis schedule has replaced the three-dose program to watch for up to 3 years. Doses are administered on days 0 and 7. High-risk groups that require preexposure prophylaxis are veterinarians and their staff, animal handlers, rabies researchers, certain laboratory workers, and people who may be in regular contact with rabies virus or animals that may carry the virus. Certain travelers whose activities may lead them to places near potentially rabies-infected animals and where medical treatment is not readily available should also have preexposure prophylaxis.

The vaccination series for PEP in persons previously vaccinated is two doses at 0 and 3 days. In previously unimmunized persons, human rabies immunoglobulin (HRIG) and four doses of rabies vaccine are required at days 0, 3, 7, and 14 for persons not immunosuppressed. Five doses are required for patients who are immunosuppressed at days 0, 3, 7, 14, and 28. HRIG is infiltrated around the bite site and provides rapid passive immune protection with a half-life of approximately 21 days. It is administered only once, on the first day of the PEP regimen. A maximum of the recommended dosage of HRIG should be given because excessive HRIG can partially suppress the active production of antibodies. If the HRIG was not administered on day 0, it may be administered up to and including day 7 of the PEP regimen. Beyond day 7, HRIG is not indicated, as the patient's antibody response to the vaccine occurs in that time frame. The recommended dosage of HRIG is 20 IU/kg body weight for all ages, including children. Infiltrate as much of the HRIG as possible into and around the bite wound. Administer the remaining HRIG IM at a site distant from the first vaccination site, generally in the quadriceps or deltoids. If there is no wound, such as following a bat-in-the-bedroom exposure, administer the entire HRIG dose IM in the deltoid or quadriceps muscles.

Contraindications for preexposure prophylaxis include a history of life-threatening systemic hypersensitivity reaction to any vaccine component. However, due to the fatality of rabies, there are no contraindications to PEP. Human diploid cell culture vaccine (IMOVAX) contains albumin, phenol red indicator, and neomycin. Pregnancy and concurrent immunosuppressive therapy are precautions.

Wrong vaccine

Confusion often occurs due to misunderstanding vaccine names, abbreviations, and components of combination products. For example, Tdap is mistaken for DTaP, and MMRV (which contains varicella vaccine) is mistaken for

MMR. Pneumococcal vaccine errors have occurred from administering the incorrect PPSV23 product when PCV15 or PCV20 was intended.

You should remember

Vaccine errors often do not cause direct patient harm. However, vaccination with subtherapeutic doses, incorrect products, or expired vaccines can leave patients susceptible to disease. To prevent medication errors with vaccines, it is essential to understand and learn from the mistakes that have been reported.

Vaccine storage

From the time a vaccine is manufactured until it is administered, it must be stored at the correct temperature to ensure its effectiveness. Keeping a product refrigerated throughout the supply chain is called the cold chain. The cold chain must remain unbroken. All vaccines must be stored at cold temperatures. Vaccines that require storage in the freezer (−50°C to 15°C) are MMRV and VAR. (ZOSTAVAX, not a pediatric vaccine, is stored in the freezer.) The MMR vaccine can be stored in the refrigerator or freezer (−50°C to +8°C). The MMR and MMRV vaccine diluent should be stored in the refrigerator or at room temperature. The mRNA COVID-19 vaccines should be stored at frozen temperatures until the expiration date or at refrigerator temperatures for up to 10 weeks for the Pfizer BioNTech vaccine or up to 30 days for the Moderna vaccine. All other vaccines must be stored in the refrigerator (2°C to 8°C) and not frozen. Always follow manufacturer instructions for storage.

Key Terms

Anthrax
Antibodies
Antigens
Asplenia
Bacteremia
Cholera
Conjugated vaccine
Deltoid muscle
Dendritic cells
Diphtheria
Ebola
Encephalopathy
Human papillomavirus
Hydrophobia
Immunogenicity
Japanese encephalitis
Lymph nodes
Mpox
Macrophages
Measles
Meningitis
Meningococcemia
Mumps
Orchitis
Otitis media
Paralysis
Parotid glands
Plasma cells
Pneumococcal disease
Pneumonia
Poliomyelitis
Rabies
Reticular cells

Rubella
Severe combined immunodeficiency
Shingles
Sickle cell disease
Spores
Tetanus
Thymus
Tuberculosis
Typhoid fever
Varicella
Vastus lateralis muscle
Whooping cough
Yellow fever

Clinical Case Studies

Case Study 1

A 1-year-old infant accidentally received a double dose of the same vaccine because an error was made in double checking the generic components of two trade-name drugs: MMRII and Priorix. These trade name drugs contain the live MMR vaccines. The error was correctly reported, and the family received an apology.

Critical Thinking Questions

1. How are the MMRII and Priorix vaccines given?
2. What resources must be checked to determine which vaccines are needed for infants and when?
3. What is the correct way to report vaccine administration errors and adverse events?

Case Study 2

A 28-year-old female was diagnosed with cervical cancer, which caused chronic pelvic pain and bleeding after intercourse. She had never received the HPV vaccine. Her treatment included weekly chemotherapy sessions, daily radiation, and internal radiation-placement treatments. Though she survived the cancer, her procedures resulted in her being infertile. The patient now does much work advocating for the importance of early HPV vaccination.

Critical Thinking Questions

1. What factors make it more likely that HPV infection will progress to cancer?
2. What is the vaccination schedule for HPV?
3. What precautions are taken regarding HPV vaccination if a person has HIV?

Case Study 3

A 45-year-old male vacationed in Japan and returned home to the United States, where he developed a headache that worsened until he became confused, had slurred speech, and could not walk without assistance. In the local emergency department, he started hallucinating. He also had a high fever, neck stiffness, ataxia, and increased muscle tone. A brain MRI revealed hyperintensities in the deep gray nuclei and possible subacute infarcts in the right thalamus and midbrain. Tests showed him to be positive for JE. The patient was treated with broad-spectrum antibacterial agents and acyclovir. He slowly improved and was discharged within 2 weeks, recovering completely.

Critical Thinking Questions

1. How is JE spread from animals to humans?
2. What are the available types of JE vaccines?
3. How is the JE vaccine administered?

Further Reading

[1] A.K. Abbas, A.H. Lichtman, S. Pillai, Cellular and Molecular Immunology, tenth ed., Elsevier, 2021.
[2] J. Alter, Vaccines (21St Century Skills Innovation Library), Cherry Lake Publishing, 2010.
[3] R. Bansal, Antibodies and their Role in Therapeutics (Biotechnology), Bansal, 2021.
[4] M. Blaxill, D. Olmsted, Vaccines 2.0: The Careful Parent's Guide to Making Safe Vaccination Choices for your Family, Skyhorse, 2015.
[5] W. Cook, K. Klaas, Mayo Clinic Guide to your Baby's First Years, second ed., Mayo Clinic Press, 2020.
[6] T. Cowan, S. Fallon Morell, Vaccines, Autoimmunity, and the Changing Nature of Childhood Illness, Chelsea Green Publishing, 2018.

[7] T. Doan, F. Lievano, M. Swanson-Mungerson, S.M. Viselli, Lippincott Illustrated Reviews: Immunology (Illustrated Reviews Series), third ed., Wolters Kluwer Health, 2021.
[8] L. Feder, L. Hoang, The Parents' Concise Guide to Childhood Vaccinations – Revised and Updated (2^{Nd}) Edition – Practical Medical and Natural Ways to Protect your Child, Hatherleigh Press, 2017.
[9] S. Humphries, R. Bystrianyk, Dissolving Illusions – Disease, Vaccines, and the Forgotten History, CreateSpace Independent Publishing Platform, 2013.
[10] D.A. Lenox, Pneumococcal Vaccine: How to Protect yourself from Pneumococcal Disease, Leddnox, 2022.
[11] R. Rappuoli, L. Vozza, Vaccines in the Global Era: How to Deal Safely and Effectively with the Pandemics of our Time, WSPC, 2022.
[12] A.R. Rees, A New History of Vaccines for Infectious Diseases: Immunization – Chance and Necessity, Academic Press, 2022.
[13] S. Schama, Foreign Bodie: Pandemics, Vaccines, and the Health of Nations, Ecco, 2023.
[14] P. Thomas, J. Margulis, The Vaccine-Friendly Plan: Dr. Paul's Safe and Effective Approach to Immunity and Health-from Pregnancy Through your Child's Teen Years, Ballantine Books, 2016.
[15] USAF Counterproliferation Center, and Penny Hill Press Inc, The Anthrax Vaccine Debate: A Medical Review for Commanders, CreateSpace Independent Publishing Platform, 2016.
[16] C.E. Davis, The International Traveler's Guide to Avoiding Infections, Book 1, Johns Hopkins University Press, 2012.
[17] H.C.J. Ertl, Rabies and Rabies Vaccines, Springer, 2020.
[18] R.M. Gullberg, Health Advice & Immunizations for Travelers – Intended for International Travelers & Travel Clinics, Gullberg, 2021.
[19] U. Ikidde, Essential Family and Travellers' Health – Health Advice everyone should Know, WriterMotive, 2017.
[20] J.S. Mackenzie, A.D.T. Barrett, V. Deubel, Japanese Encephalitis and West Nile Viruses (Current Topics in Microbiology and Immunology, Book 267), Springer, 2012.

CHAPTER

55

NSAIDs and acetaminophen

OUTLINE

LEARNING OUTCOMES

After study of the chapter, readers should be able to:

1. Describe nonopioid analgesics.
2. Explain the indications of acetaminophen.
3. Compare the mechanism of action of acetaminophen with NSAIDs.
4. Discuss the nonselective COX inhibitors.
5. Identify the common adverse effects of NSAIDs.
6. Explain the contraindications of acetaminophen.
7. Describe the pharmacokinetics of NSAIDs.
8. Explain the contraindications of NSAIDs.

Overview

Nonopioid analgesics are commonly used to treat mild and moderate acute and chronic pain. They can be used as monotherapy but have greater efficacy with weak and strong opioids. Unlike opioids, long-term use of nonsteroidal antiinflammatory drugs (NSAIDs) does not lead to physical dependence. One of the main disadvantages of the NSAIDs is the risk of gastrointestinal side effects, especially bleeding into the digestive tract. This is increased significantly in ulcerative disease, higher doses, and the elderly (over 65 years) with concomitant administration of corticosteroids, anticoagulants, or other NSAIDs. Acetaminophen and NSAIDs are the preferred analgesics for mild to moderate pain and are usually used before prescribing opioid analgesics.

The Science of Pharmacology
https://doi.org/10.1016/B978-0-443-29038-1.00055-5

Acetaminophen

Acetaminophen is an antipyretic analgesic used to treat mild to moderate pain (from headaches, **menstrual periods**, toothaches, backaches, **osteoarthritis**, or cold/flu aches and pains) and to reduce fever. Acetaminophen is the first-line treatment for most mild to moderate acute pain. The injectable form of acetaminophen is indicated for mild to moderate pain in patients 2 years of age or older.

Although acetaminophen is available over the counter, it has caused severe liver damage when taken at higher doses. Acetaminophen can cause sudden liver failure, sometimes resulting in the need for **liver transplantation**, and it can also cause death. Most cases of liver injury are associated with using acetaminophen at doses exceeding recommended maximum daily limits and often involve more than one acetaminophen-containing product. Be cautious when prescribing, preparing, and administering acetaminophen to avoid **dosing errors** that could result in accidental overdose and death. **Table 55.1** summarizes the dosing of different forms of acetaminophen.

Mechanism of action

The mechanism of action of acetaminophen is believed to be due to the activation of descending serotonergic inhibitory pathways in the CNS and other nociceptive systems.

Pharmacokinetics

Acetaminophen is rapidly absorbed from the GI tract and quickly distributed throughout the body. Peak plasma concentrations are achieved within 30–60 minutes. Food may delay time to peak concentration, but the extent of absorption is not affected. It is usually metabolized in the liver and kidneys by P450 enzymes. No toxicity is observed with therapeutic doses under 4 g per day.

Clinical indications

It relieves pain and fever. Acetaminophen can also be combined with other active ingredients in medicines that treat allergies, coughs, colds, flu, and sleeplessness. In prescription medicines, acetaminophen is found with different active ingredients to treat moderate to severe pain. Acetaminophen injection (Ofirmev) is indicated for managing mild to moderate pain in patients 2 years of age or older and managing moderate to severe pain when combined with opioid analgesia in patients 2 years and older. Oral and rectal acetaminophen is indicated to relieve minor aches, pains, and headaches temporarily.

Contraindications

Contraindications to using acetaminophen include hypersensitivity to acetaminophen, severe hepatic impairment, or severe active hepatic disease. Unfortunately, acetaminophen can harm children even if it is appropriately given. A study conducted in more than 30 countries shows that acetaminophen increases the chances of developing asthma, eczema, and allergic runny nose later in childhood if used in a child's first year of life. It is never safe to use

TABLE 55.1 Acetaminophen dosing.

Generic name	Trade name	Average dosage range (mg/day)	Dosage form (in mg)
Para-aminophenol			
acetaminophen (oral)	Tylenol, many others	325–1000	80, 160, 325, 500, 650
acetaminophen (injection)	Ofirmev	100–4000	10 mg/mL, 80 mg/0.8 mL, 80 mg/mL, 80 mg/5 mL, 120 mg/5 mL, 160/5 mL, 325 mg/10.15 mL, 500 mg/5 mL, 500 mg/15 mL, 650 mg/20.3 mL, 650 mg/25 mL

acetaminophen while alcohol is consumed because it can collectively irritate the stomach and lead to ulcers, internal bleeding, and liver damage.

Adverse effects

Although acetaminophen is available over the counter, it has been known to cause severe liver damage when taken at higher doses. Acetaminophen can cause sudden liver failure, sometimes resulting in liver transplant or death. Most cases of liver injury are associated with using acetaminophen at amounts that exceed the recommended maximum daily limits and often involve more than one acetaminophen-containing product. Be cautious when prescribing, preparing, and administering acetaminophen to avoid dosing errors that could result in accidental overdose and death. The ADRs associated with acetaminophen include nausea, vomiting, and headache. Dosing depends on the formulation and route of administration.

Toxicities

In adults, an acute ingestion of more than 150 mg/kg or 12 g of acetaminophen is considered a toxic dose and poses a high risk of liver damage. Acute ingestion of 250 mg/kg or more in children poses a significant risk for acetaminophen-induced hepatotoxicity. Acetaminophen can lead to acute liver failure, which may only be treated with an emergent liver transplant. Acetaminophen toxicity is the second most common cause of liver transplantation worldwide and the most common cause in the United States. It is responsible for 56,000 emergency department visits, 2600 hospitalizations, and 500 deaths annually in the United States.

You should remember

Chronic liver failure occurs over many years and may cause fatigue, loss of appetite, vomiting blood, jaundice, disorientation, edema, and ascites. Acetaminophen has direct hepatotoxic potential when taken as an overdose and can cause acute liver injury and death from acute liver failure. Taking acetaminophen for a long time with alcohol causes liver failure.

Nonsteroidal antiinflammatory drugs

NSAIDs promote pain relief by decreasing acute and subacute tissue damage and inflammatory processes. They are among the most widely used therapeutics. Their antiinflammatory, antipyretic, and analgesic activities represent a choice treatment for various inflammatory diseases such as arthritis and rheumatism and relieve the pains of everyday life. From a historical viewpoint, the first NSAID with therapeutic benefits was aspirin, which has now been used for more than 100 years as an NSAID. The cyclooxygenase (COX) enzyme was first identified as the therapeutic target of NSAIDs in 1971, showing that these antiinflammatory substances block the biosynthesis of prostaglandins that contribute to various physiological and pathophysiological functions. They are also referred to as **COX** inhibitors because they block the action of COX. This enzyme promotes the synthesis of inflammatory **prostaglandins** at the site of tissue damage. Most NSAIDs are considered *nonselective* COX inhibitors because they inhibit COX-1 and COX-2. However, inhibition of the COX enzyme subtype for each NSAID is more concerning COX-blocking activity. Some NSAIDs are more likely to impede COX-1 (ibuprofen, naproxen, ketorolac), and others are more likely to inhibit COX-2 (meloxicam, diclofenac, celecoxib). This difference in inhibition is clinically relevant because of unintended adverse drug reactions caused by blocking these enzymes.

For example, COX-1 enzymes generate prostaglandins that improve blood flow to the gastric mucosa and kidneys and decrease **platelet aggregation**, which can help reduce bleeding. When NSAIDs block COX-1, they can lead to harmful reactions such as GI bleeding, ulceration, and kidney damage. However, COX-2 enzymes generate prostaglandins that activate nociceptors and produce inflammation. When NSAIDs block COX-2, beneficial pain relief occurs. Selective COX-2 inhibition can also result in unintended reactions, including ischemic cardiovascular events such as myocardial infarction and stroke. Therefore two of the three COX-2 particular medications initially approved in the United States—rofecoxib (Vioxx) and valdecoxib (Bextra)—have now been withdrawn from the market. Table 55.2 summarizes the NSAID dosing.

TABLE 55.2 NSAID dosing

Generic name	Trade name	Average dosage range (mg/day)	Dosage form (in mg)
aspirin	Bayer Aspirin, many others	500–4000	81, 325, 500, 650
celecoxib	Celebrex	200–400	50, 100, 200, 400
diclofenac	Cambia, Voltaren	18–150	25, 50, 75, 100
ibuprofen	Advil, many others	200–1200	100, 200, 400, 600, 800
indomethacin	Indocin	20–200	20, 25, 50, 75
ketorolac	Toradol	20–120	10, 15, 60
naproxen	Aleve, many others	200–1000	250, 375, 500

Mechanism of action

NSAIDs block the COX enzyme, which the body uses to manufacture prostaglandins—hormone-like chemicals that contribute to pain, inflammation, and fever. The COX-1 enzyme is present in most body tissues, while the COX-2 enzyme is responsible for inflammation. Therefore the COX-2 inhibitors selectively block COX-2 to reduce pain and inflammation without losing the protection of COX-1 in the GI tract, reducing adverse effects there.

Pharmacokinetics

The NSAIDs are well absorbed from the GI tract, except aspirin. The bioavailability of aspirin is 70% or less due to hydrolysis in the GI tract or during the first pass through the liver. However, the remainder is absorbed as its pharmacologically active metabolite, salicylate. The NSAIDs are extensively bound to plasma proteins, but the clinical significance of interactions between NSAIDs due to displacement from plasma proteins is not known.

Clinical indications

Most NSAIDs are used to relieve mild to moderate pain. They may be beneficial for cancer-related bone pain and chronic low back pain. Topical NSAIDs have similar efficacy as oral NSAIDs, with improved safety when treating small or superficial joint arthritis due to limited absorption. Ketorolac is only indicated for short-term (5 days or less) management of moderate to severe acute pain because of an increased risk of bleeding and cardiovascular disease. NSAIDs are available OTC and as prescription medications. Prescription NSAIDs are indicated for patients with arthritis, gout, menstrual cramps, severe headaches, and generalized body aches.

Contraindications

NSAIDs are contraindicated in people with hypersensitivity or salicylate hypersensitivity and in patients who have experienced an allergic reaction (urticaria, asthma, etc.) after taking NSAIDs. They are generally not recommended for people with kidney disease, heart failure, or cirrhosis or for people who take diuretics, active gastrointestinal bleeding, or peptic ulceration. Ketorolac has several boxed warnings due to its contraindications, which include use in the setting of coronary artery bypass graft surgery, active peptic ulcer disease, recent GI bleed or perforation, advanced renal impairment, suspected or confirmed cerebrovascular bleeding, those with high bleeding risk, use of other NSAIDs, use during labor and delivery, and use as a prophylactic analgesic before major surgery.

Adverse effects

NSAIDs can cause an increased risk of serious (and potentially fatal) adverse cardiovascular thrombotic (blood clot) events, including heart attack and stroke. This can even occur early during treatment and may increase with duration of use. Additionally, NSAIDs can cause an increased risk of severe gastrointestinal inflammation, ulceration, bleeding, and perforation (which may be fatal).

Toxicities

Typical signs and symptoms of NSAID overdose include nausea, vomiting, headache, drowsiness, blurred vision, and dizziness. Seizures are rarely documented across all NSAID classes, except for mefenamic acid (where seizures occur in over one-third of cases) or following massive ingestion of other agents. Ingestions of over 400 mg/kg of ibuprofen are associated with seizures, **apnea**, hypotension, bradycardia, **metabolic acidosis**, and renal and hepatic dysfunction. Occasionally, these NSAIDs can cause dizziness, blurred vision, seizures, and coma.

You should remember

NSAIDs are the competitive inhibitors of COX, the enzyme that mediates the bioconversion of arachidonic acid to inflammatory prostaglandins. Their use is associated with side effects such as gastrointestinal and renal toxicity. The inhibition of COX-2 produces the therapeutic antiinflammatory action of NSAIDs, while the undesired side effects arise from the inhibition of COX-1 activity. Thus more selective COX-2 inhibitors were thought to have reduced side effects.

You should remember

Recent studies have shown that the relation between the two COX inhibitors is more complex. Indeed, COX-1 may contribute to inflammation, whereas COX-2 is constitutively expressed in several tissues and organs, such as the brain, kidneys, and reproductive tract.

Key Terms

Apnea
Cyclooxygenase
Dosing errors
Gout
Liver transplantation
Menstrual periods
Metabolic acidosis
Osteoarthritis
Platelet aggregation
Prostaglandins

Clinical Case Studies

Clinical Case Study 1

A 66-year-old female who abuses alcohol had taken acetaminophen for several years to buffer her musculoskeletal pain. She was hospitalized with signs and symptoms of impending liver failure. Her signs and symptoms included jaundice of the eyes and skin, upper right abdominal pain, ascites, nausea, vomiting, and confusion. Liver function tests were performed, which indicated severe liver damage, and a CT scan provided visual proof. The patient was put on the list for liver transplantation.

Critical Thinking Questions

1. How is the overuse of acetaminophen linked to the need for a liver transplantation procedure?
2. How often does excessive use of acetaminophen result in a liver transplant?
3. What are the concerns of taking acetaminophen while drinking alcohol?

Clinical Case Study 2

A 71-year-old male visits his primary care physician. He is slightly overweight and has dyslipidemia, hypertension, and osteoarthritis in both knees. His history includes a recent stroke. His current prescriptions include an oral anticoagulant and an NSAID. The patient has been primarily sedentary since retiring 6 years previously and admits to hardly ever being physically active. He is scheduled to begin outpatient physical therapy.

Critical Thinking Questions

1. Why are topical NSAIDs safer to use than oral NSAIDs in treating arthritis?
2. What are prescription NSAIDs indicated for?
3. How do NSAIDs promote pain relief?

Further Reading

[1] L. Arpilor, Signs of liver damage – understand the signs of liver damage, from jaundice to abdominal pain, Learn About Potential Indicators and the Implications for Liver Health (2023). Arpilor.

[2] S.S. Ayoub, R.J. Flower, M.P. Seed, Cyclooxygenases – Methods and Protocols (Methods in Molecular Biology, 644), Humana Press, 2010.

[3] K. Beom Kim, R. Movahed, R.K. Malhotra, J.L. Stanley, Management of Obstructive Sleep Apnea – an Evidence-Based, Multidisciplinary Textbook, Springer, 2021.

[4] P. Burra, Textbook of Liver Transplantation – A Multidisciplinary Approach, Springer, 2022.

[5] A. Javaherian, P. Latifpour, Acetaminophen – Properties, Clinical Uses and Adverse Effects (Pharmacology – Research, Safety Testing and Regulation – Public Health in the 21st Century), Nova Biomedical, 2012.

[6] S. Kaplan, A Comprehensive Guide to Non-steroidal Anti-inflammatory Drugs, Nova Science Publishers Inc, 2021.

[7] A. Lanas, NSAIDs and Aspirin – Recent Advances and Implications for Clinical Management, Springer, 2016.

[8] Y. Oluynin, Osteoarthritis – Current Issues of Treatment, Our Knowledge Publishing, 2022.

[9] L.S. Peterson, Mayo Clinic Guide to Arthritis – Managing Joint Pain for an Active Life, Mayo Clinic Press, 2020.

[10] R. Rajendram, V.R. Preedy, V.B. Patel, C.R. Martin, Treatments, Mechanisms, and Adverse Reactions of Anesthetics and Analgesics, Academic Press, 2021.

[11] R. Rice, Tylenol for Pain and Fever Management – Acetaminophen for Rapid Relief of Pain and Fever Reducer, Rice, 2022.

[12] M. Riley, The Essential Guide to Acetaminophen – Usage, Precautions, Interactions and Side Effects, Interactive Media Licensing, 2021.

[13] S. Saraf, NSAIDs (Nonsteroidal Anti-Inflammatory Drugs) – an Overview, BSP Books, 2019.

[14] R.S. Sinatra, J.S. Jahr, J.M. Watkins-Pitchford, The Essence of Analgesia and Analgesics, Cambridge University Press, 2010.

[15] R. Terkeltaub, N.L. Edwards, Gout – Diagnosis and Management of Gouty Arthritis and Hyperuricemia, fourth ed., Professional Communications, Inc, 2016.

[16] M.G. Tsagareli, N. Tisklauri, Behavioral Study of 'Non-Opioid Tolerance' (Pain and Its Origins, Diagnosis and Treatments – Pain Management Research and Technology), Nova Biomedical, 2012.

[17] D.E. Wesson, Metabolic Acidosis – A Guide to Clinical Assessment and Management, Springer, 2016.

CHAPTER

56

Drugs used in osteoarthritis, rheumatoid arthritis, and gout

OUTLINE

LEARNING OUTCOMES

After study of the chapter, readers should be able to:

1. Explain the pathophysiology of osteoarthritis and gout.
2. Describe the systemic damage of rheumatoid arthritis.
3. List drugs for relieving the pain of osteoarthritis and gout.
4. Describe the disease-modifying antirheumatic drugs.

The Science of Pharmacology
https://doi.org/10.1016/B978-0-443-29038-1.00056-7

5. Explain the clinical indications for adalimumab.
6. Describe the adverse effects of adalimumab.
7. Explain the first-line agents for treating gout.
8. Describe the clinical indications of allopurinol.
9. Discuss the mechanism of action for colchicine.
10. Explain the adverse effects of allopurinol.

Overview

Some common joint diseases include osteoarthritis (OA), gout, rheumatoid arthritis (RA), and ankylosing spondylitis. These diseases affect the joints, bones, tendons, ligaments, cartilage, and surrounding muscles and may cause pain, swelling, and reduced range of motion. OA is a degenerative joint disease in which the tissues in the joint break down over time. It is the most common type of arthritis and is more common in older people. People with OA usually have joint pain and stiffness briefly after rest or inactivity. Certain factors may make it more likely to develop the disease, such as obesity, aging, history of injury or surgery to a joint, and family history of OA. RA is a chronic autoimmune disease that primarily affects joints, causing inflammation and joint pain. Females are two to three times more likely than males to get RA and do so about 10 years of age earlier on average. The disease is also often more severe in females than in males. In some patients, RA causes more general symptoms at first, such as fatigue, loss of appetite, and low fever. It can be treated with medication, physical therapy, and occupational therapy. Gout is a metabolic disorder that causes inflammation of the joints. The inflammation is triggered by tiny needle-shaped crystals of uric acid that mainly build up in the joints. Unfortunately, there is no cure for gout. However, it can be treated with medication and self-management strategies.

Osteoarthritis

OA is the most common form of arthritis, affecting millions worldwide. It occurs when the protective cartilage cushions at the ends of bones wear down over time. Annual costs from lost productivity and treatment of OA in the United States are estimated to be more than 65 billion dollars. However, OA implies an inflammatory disease. It is considered an intrinsic disease of **cartilage** in which **chondrocytes** respond to biochemical and mechanical stresses, resulting in the breakdown of the **matrix** via increases in the production of inflammatory cytokines and cartilage-degrading enzymes. OA appears quietly, without an apparent initiating cause, as an aging phenomenon. The disease usually affects a few joints but can be generalized. In about 5% of cases, OA appears in younger individuals with some predisposing factors such as joint deformity, a previous joint injury, or an underlying systemic disease such as **hemochromatosis**, diabetes mellitus, **ochronosis**, and significant obesity that places joints at risk. Therefore it is called secondary OA. Biological sex has some influence on the distribution of joint pain. The knees and hands are more commonly affected in females and the hips in males. OA symptoms often develop slowly and worsen over time. Signs and symptoms of OA include pain, stiffness, tenderness, bone spurs, loss of flexibility, and joint swelling. Pain worsens with joint use and is relieved by rest.

There is no single test for diagnosing OA. The condition may be diagnosed through a physical exam, X-rays, MRI, and blood tests. In some cases, joint fluid samples are taken to look for other causes of joint pain.

Pathophysiology of osteoarthritis

OA primarily involves only one or a few joints. The joints commonly involved include the hips, knees, lower lumbar and cervical vertebrae, proximal and distal **interphalangeal joints** of the fingers, first **carpometacarpal joints**, and first **tarsometatarsal joints**. **Heberden nodes**, prominent osteophytes at the distal interphalangeal joints, are common in females. The wrists, elbows, and shoulders are usually spared. In chronic cases, joint deformity can occur, but this differs from joint deformities resulting from RA. However, the severity of the disease can be diagnosed by X-ray. Although OA can damage any joint, the disorder most commonly affects the joints in the hands, knees, hips, and spine.

Pharmacotherapy of osteoarthritis

There is no cure for OA, but the condition does not necessarily get worse over time. Many treatments are available to help relieve the symptoms, focusing on managing pain and improving joint function. Patients may benefit from medication for mild symptoms that come and go. More severe symptoms may require regular use of drugs. Topical treatments include nonsteroidal antiinflammatory drug (NSAID) creams and capsaicin creams. Systemic NSAIDs such as celecoxib, ibuprofen, naproxen, and diclofenac are the most used medications to treat OA. Acetaminophen has fallen out of favor for the treatment of OA due to safety concerns with its potential effects on the liver and non–clinically significant effects on pain. Corticosteroid injections may be used for severe cases. However, they are only sometimes utilized due to the short duration of relief and evidence that they may accelerate OA progression. Opioids such as codeine may also help relieve severe pain but should only be used when all other treatment options have failed. Duloxetine may be utilized for patients with pain in multiple joints. Nonpharmacologic measures to treat OA include weight management, aerobic and strengthening exercises, assistive devices, braces, and foot orthotics.

You should remember

Exercise is one of the most important treatments for OA, regardless of age or fitness level. Physical activity should include exercises to strengthen the muscles and improve general fitness. Being overweight often makes OA worse, as it places extra strain on the knee joints.

Rheumatoid arthritis

RA is a chronic inflammatory disorder of autoimmune origin that may affect many tissues and organs. However, it primarily attacks the joints, producing nonsuppurative proliferative and inflammatory **synovitis**. RA often progresses to destruction of the articular cartilage and **ankylosis** of the joints (see **Fig. 56.1**). Systemic damage may

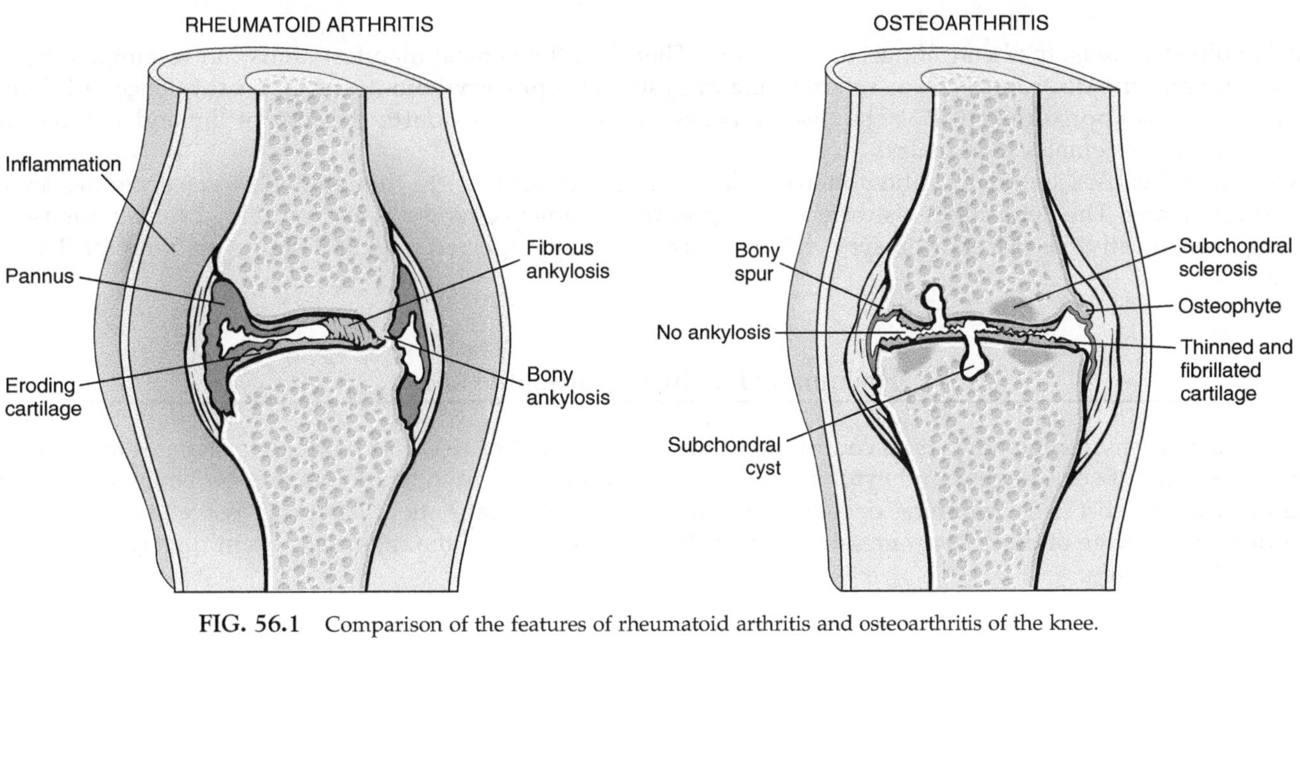

FIG. 56.1 Comparison of the features of rheumatoid arthritis and osteoarthritis of the knee.

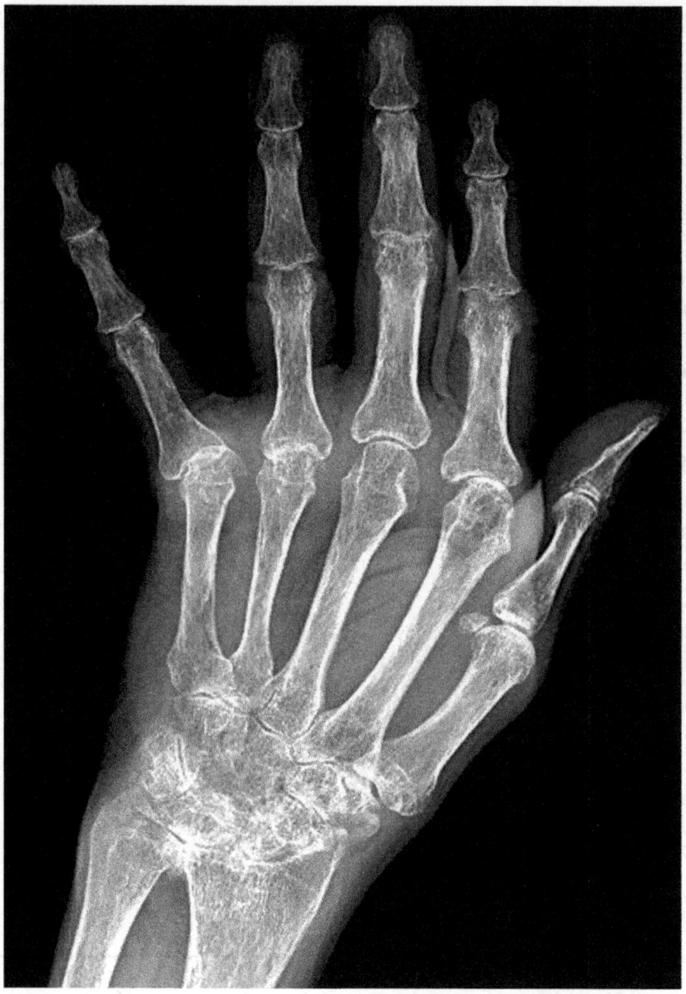

FIG. 56.2 X-ray of a hand affected by rheumatoid arthritis.

involve blood vessels, the heart, lungs, and the skin. Therefore the clinical manifestations can resemble other systemic autoimmune disorders such as **scleroderma** or **systemic lupus erythematosus**. The prevalence of RA in the United States is approximately 1%. The disease peaks in the second to fourth decades of life and is three times more common in females than males.

Chronic RA causes joint deformities, often starting at the hands and wrists, though the lower extremities are usually affected later. The deformities also affect the supporting ligaments, tendons, and muscles, causing intense pain during normal activities. Most or all synovial joints are eventually affected. **Fig. 56.1** shows an X-ray of RA of the hand.

Rheumatoid arthritis pathophysiology

Genetic and environmental factors contribute to the development of RA. The pathologic changes are caused by antibodies against self-antigens and cytokine-mediated inflammation. Involved joints are swollen, warm, painful, and particularly stiff in the morning or following inactivity. The typical patient has progressive joint enlargement and decreased range of motion, progressing to complete ankylosis, with the most significant damage occurring in the first 4 or 5 years.

Pharmacotherapy of rheumatoid arthritis

Nonpharmacologic therapies are essential in the management of RA. **Range of motion** and joint- and muscle-strengthening exercises help patients continue to perform normal daily activities. Psychological counseling may help deal with the possible debilitation that can develop. **Ambulation** may require braces, canes, splints, or walkers. Losing weight helps reduce stress on inflamed joints, and adequate rest helps reduce pain.

The main goals of pharmacotherapy are to reduce pain, manage inflammation, and increase physical abilities. Therapy is started with NSAIDs because they relieve pain and inflammation. Doses are usually higher than those given to patients with OA. However, aspirin is not recommended for long-term therapy due to adverse effects related to **platelet aggregation** and GI bleeding. Acetaminophen can relieve pain and fever but not inflammation. Analgesics can relieve symptomatic pain but only slightly aid in slowing disease progression.

For moderate to severe RA, corticosteroids may be used to relieve symptoms associated with flare-ups. They are only used short term, and severe rebound symptoms can occur if discontinued abruptly. Corticosteroids therefore are given in the lowest possible daily doses. To slow or modify tissue damage from RA, *disease-modifying antirheumatic drugs (DMARDs)* are used. They modify immune and inflammatory responses, reduce mortality rates, improve symptoms, and enhance quality of life. The DMARDs are classified as *nonbiologic, biologic (tumor necrosis factor [TNF] or anti-TNF),* and *biologic (non–anti-TNF)*. **Table 56.1** summarizes the DMARDs used for RA.

Methotrexate is often considered the first-line therapy for RA. Other nonbiologic DMARDs used for initial therapy include hydroxychloroquine and sulfasalazine. Nonbiologic DMARDS such as azathioprine and leflunomide

TABLE 56.1 Disease-modifying antirheumatic drugs used for rheumatoid arthritis.

Generic name	Trade name	Route of administration
Nonbiologic DMARDs		
azathioprine	Azasan, Imuran	PO
cyclosporine A	Neoral, Sandimmune	PO
hydroxychloroquine	Plaquenil	PO
leflunomide	Arava	PO
methotrexate	Otrexup, Rheumatrex, Trexall	PO, subcutaneous
sulfasalazine	Azulfidine	PO
Biologic DMARDs (anti-TNF drugs)		
adalimumab	Humira	Subcutaneous
certolizumab pegol	Cimzia	Subcutaneous
etancercept	Enbrel	Subcutaneous
golimumab	Simponi	Subcutaneous
infliximab	Remicade	IV
Biologic DMARDs (non–anti-TNF drugs)		
abatacept	Orencia	IV
anakinra	Kineret	Subcutaneous
rituximab	Rituxan	IV
sarilumab	Kevzara	Subcutaneous
tocilizumab	Actemra	IV, subcutaneous
tofacitinib	Xeljanz	PO

DMARDS, Disease-modifying antirheumatic drugs; *TNF*, tumor necrosis factor.

have more adverse effects than the other DMARDs but can be combined with biologic therapies. These therapies are newer types of DMARDs that block steps in the inflammatory response. They also reduce joint inflammation and slow joint damage.

TNF is a natural **cytokine** produced by **macrophages** that activates T cells that mediate inflammation and modulate cellular immune responses. Elevated levels of TNF are found in the synovial fluid of patients with RA. Biologics are effective and relatively nontoxic but extremely expensive. Therefore they are usually only prescribed once conventional therapy has failed. Combinations of biological and nonbiologic drugs are sometimes effective for patients who do not respond to monotherapy.

Methotrexate

Methotrexate is used to treat RA. It is a folate antagonist that inhibits cellular metabolism and reduces inflammation, slowing disease progression. Methotrexate is often prescribed as a first-line treatment for RA, either alone or in combination with other medications.

Pharmacokinetics

Methotrexate is administered orally or via subcutaneous injection and is absorbed from the gastrointestinal tract, reaching peak plasma levels within 1–2 hours when taken orally. Its therapeutic effects in RA typically manifest over 6–12 weeks. The drug's action can persist for several days due to its impact on cellular metabolism. Methotrexate is widely distributed in body tissues, including the liver, kidneys, and bone marrow. It is primarily metabolized in the liver to both active and inactive metabolites and is predominantly excreted through the kidneys, with a smaller fraction eliminated in bile.

Mechanism of action

Methotrexate inhibits dihydrofolate reductase, an enzyme essential for folate metabolism and nucleic acid synthesis. This inhibition disrupts the proliferation of inflammatory cells, thereby reducing inflammation and slowing disease progression in RA.

Clinical indications

Methotrexate is primarily indicated for the treatment of moderate to severe active RA in adults, either as a standalone therapy or in combination with other DMARDs or biologics. It is often used as a first-line treatment because it reduces inflammation and slows disease progression. Additionally, methotrexate is employed off-label for various cancers and autoimmune disorders, although these uses are secondary to its primary role in RA management.

Contraindications

Methotrexate is contraindicated in individuals who are pregnant or breastfeeding due to its teratogenic effects, and it should be avoided in patients with severe liver disease, chronic liver conditions, severe renal impairment, active infections, or significant blood disorders. It has black box warnings for potentially causing severe liver toxicity, bone marrow suppression, pulmonary toxicity, and gastrointestinal toxicity. It can also lead to an increased risk of infections and bleeding.

Adverse effects

Common adverse effects of methotrexate include nausea, vomiting, mouth ulcers, liver enzyme elevations, hair loss, and fatigue.

Toxicities

More serious toxicities of methotrexate include hepatotoxicity, which requires regular monitoring of liver function; renal toxicity, particularly in high doses or in patients with preexisting renal issues; and rare pulmonary toxicity, such as interstitial lung disease or pneumonitis. Methotrexate's potential to cause severe side effects necessitates careful monitoring throughout treatment.

Adalimumab

Adalimumab is a biologic (*biological*) therapy used to treat RA. It is an anti-TNF drug that blocks TNF to reduce inflammation, with effects lasting over 2–12 weeks. The drug is also prescribed for **psoriatic arthritis**, **ankylosing spondylitis**, and **juvenile idiopathic arthritis**. It is not prescribed if arthritis is not active, the patient has an infection, or other treatments have not been tried first. Blood tests and a chest X-ray are required before treatment with adalimumab. The drug is sometimes not prescribed if the patient has had repeated or severe infections, multiple sclerosis, a serious heart condition, lung fibrosis, tuberculosis, or hepatitis B. Adalimumab was the first fully human monoclonal antibody approved by the FDA.

Pharmacokinetics

Administered subcutaneously, adalimumab shows peak levels of absorption in approximately 5 days. Its onset of action is 4–5 weeks, and its duration of action is 10–20 days. However, the distribution, primary metabolism, and primary excretion of adalimumab are unknown.

Mechanism of action

Adalimumab blocks TNF's inflammatory activity, inhibiting the inflammatory cascade. High levels of TNF are often found in patients with RA and other inflammatory disorders. By blocking TNF, adalimumab helps reduce inflammation and symptoms associated with these conditions.

Clinical indications

Adalimumab is indicated for moderate to severe active RA in adults as monotherapy or in combination with methotrexate or other nonbiologic DMARDs. It is also used for mild to severe active polyarticular juvenile idiopathic arthritis in patients 2 years of age and older as monotherapy or in combination with methotrexate. Adalimumab is also used for adult psoriatic arthritis and ankylosing spondylitis. Other indications include moderate to severe active Crohn's disease in adults and children over age 6, mild to severe active ulcerative colitis in adults, moderate to severe chronic plaque psoriasis in specific adults, and noninfectious intermediate, posterior, and **panuveitis** in adults and children over age 2.

Contraindications

Adalimumab has no known contraindications. However, due to its immunosuppressive effects, patients must be monitored for infections or malignancies.

Adverse effects

Adalimumab's adverse effects usually include injection site pain, increased **creatine phosphate**, upper respiratory infection, headache, and rash. This drug has a black box warning because it can suppress the immune system and lead to infections. Latent infections such as hepatitis B and tuberculosis can become reactivated. TNF blockers have been linked to malignancies such as leukemias and lymphomas. Rarely have fatal cases of hepatosplenic T-cell lymphoma occurred.

Toxicities

Adalimumab has been linked to a low rate of serum aminotransferase elevations, but these have been transient, mild, and asymptomatic.

Gout

Gout is an inflammatory condition caused by elevated serum uric acid concentrations. It is a painful form of arthritis. When the body accumulates extra uric acid, sharp crystals can form in the joints (usually the big toe). Sudden outbreaks of symptoms such as pain and swelling occur in periods called gout attacks. Treatment is typically a combination of symptom management and changing one's diet. Most primary gout is caused by increased uric acid biosynthesis for unknown reasons. Some patients may overproduce uric acid due to an enzyme deficiency called secondary gout. Secondary gout can also be caused by decreased uric acid excretion.

Gout usually appears after 20–30 years of **hyperuricemia**. It is more common in males than in females. Gout usually develops in middle age. Females typically do not develop gout before menopause, so they tend to develop the

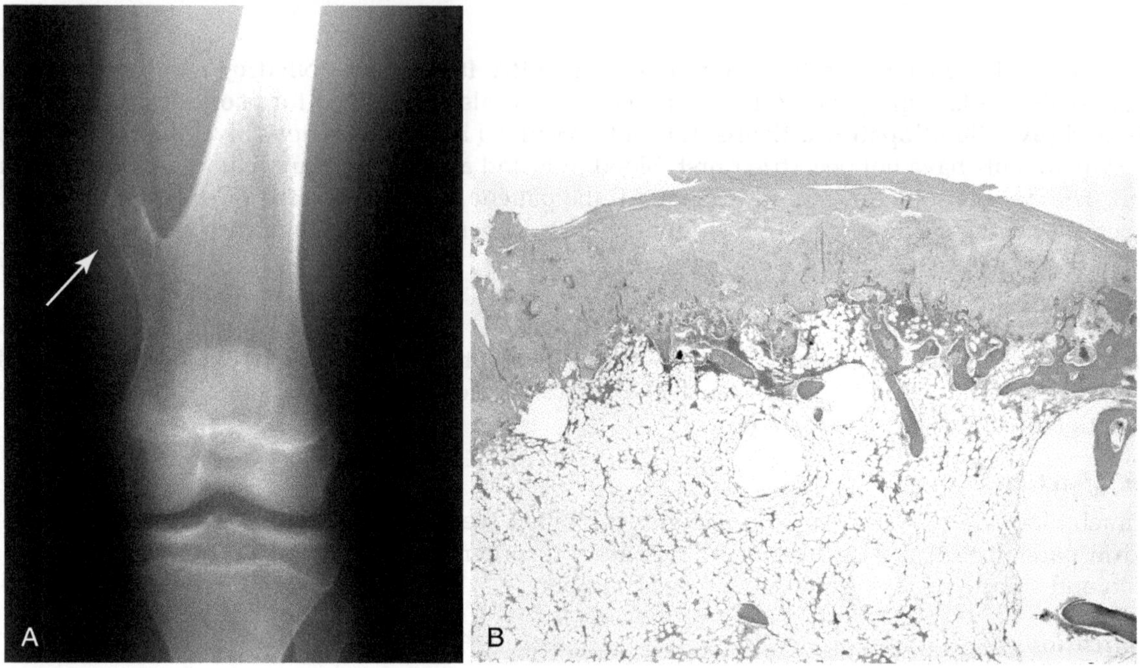

FIG. 56.3 The development of gout.

disease later than males. Less frequently, younger people develop the disease; however, if they do, it tends to be primary gout, which is inherited and runs in families. Heavy alcohol consumption, obesity, drugs such as thiazides that reduce the excretion of urate, and lead toxicity can cause gout.

Gout pathophysiology

Gout pathophysiology involves many factors, but hyperuricemia is the critical risk factor (see **Fig. 56.3**). It is a prerequisite for monosodium urate crystal formation. In most patients, urate underexcretion via renal and GI mechanisms influences the development of hyperuricemia. Many environmental, genetic, and metabolic factors are related to serum urate and alter the synthesis or transport of urate. The most crucial factor for monosodium urate crystal formation is urate supersaturation. Other factors include connective tissue components, pH, and temperature. **Tophus** formation is the primary feature of advanced gout.

Pharmacotherapy of gout

Acute gouty arthritis is treated with NSAIDs, colchicine, or corticosteroids. Preventing gout attacks and treating chronic gout requires using a xanthine oxidase inhibitor, a uricosuric agent, or a combination of these agents, along with lifestyle modifications. Allopurinol is a first-line agent for gout prevention in patients requiring urate-lowering therapy who have no contraindications. Pegloticase, a specialty drug, should be reserved for patients whose treatment has failed. **Table 56.2** summarizes the various pharmacotherapies used for gout.

Colchicine

Colchicine is an alkaloid used to treat acute gout flares because it has potent effects against inflammation and pain. It is also a natural product for **Behçet disease** and **Mediterranean fever**. Due to its narrow therapeutic index and links to deaths in the United States, injectable colchicine was removed from the market, and now only the safe oral form is available.

TABLE 56.2 Pharmacotherapies used for gout.

Generic name	Trade name	Route of administration
allopurinol	Aloprim, Zyloprim	PO, IV
colchicine	Colcrys	PO
febuxostat	Uloric	PO
lesinurad	Zurampic	PO
pegloticase	Krystexxa	IV
probenecid	Probalan	PO

Pharmacokinetics

Oral colchicine is rapidly absorbed in the GI tract. It is widely distributed but concentrated in the kidneys, leukocytes, liver, intestinal tract, and spleen. The onset of action is 12 hours, with a variable half-life of 1.7 to 20.9 hours. The drug is metabolized in the liver and mostly excreted via the feces.

Mechanism of action

Colchicine inhibits neutrophil migration into areas of inflammation, reducing inflammation related to acute gouty arthritis by inhibiting microtubule synthesis.

Clinical indications

Colchicine is indicated for the prevention and treatment of gout flares and familial Mediterranean fever and to reduce risks for myocardial infarction, stroke, coronary revascularization, and cardiovascular death in adults with atherosclerotic disease or multiple cardiovascular risk factors. Off-label uses include Behçet disease, pericarditis, and postpericardiotomy syndrome.

Contraindications

Colchicine is contraindicated in patients with a known hypersensitivity to the drug and in patients with kidney or hepatic impairment. It should be used with caution in people who are pregnant and those with GI, hepatic, or cardiac impairment. Patients with blood dyscrasias must not receive colchicine due to the risk of myelosuppression, leukopenia, thrombocytopenia, and aplastic anemia. The drug should also be used with caution in older adults, debilitated patients, and those with early signs of GI, kidney, liver, or cardiac disease.

Adverse effects

The most significant adverse effects are GI related, occurring in as many as 80% of patients. These effects include nausea, vomiting, abdominal pain, anorexia, and diarrhea. The drug can cause aplastic anemia, bone marrow toxicity, leukopenia, agranulocytosis, or thrombocytopenia. Other adverse effects include hepatotoxicity, **azotemia**, mental confusion, hematuria, proteinuria, and oliguria.

Toxicities

Toxicities from colchicine may cause severe GI distress, paralysis, shock, delirium, respiratory failure, and death (though this is linked to the IV formulation that was discontinued in the United States). Treatment of toxicity may include gastric lavage and hemodialysis.

Allopurinol

Allopurinol is a xanthine oxidase inhibitor used to prevent or lower high uric acid levels in the blood. It works by decreasing uric acid production. The xanthine oxidase inhibitors are classified as purines (such as allopurinol) and "others" (which include febuxostat, topiroxostat, and inositols).

Pharmacokinetics

Allopurinol is given orally or via IV injection. It is 80%–90% absorbed in the GI tract and is widely distributed. Its onset to decreasing serum and urine uric acid occurs at 2–3 days. The drug is secreted in breast milk; less than 1% is bound to plasma proteins. Primary metabolism is via the liver to the active metabolite called **oxypurinol**. The drug is mainly excreted via the kidneys (76%), with 20% excreted in the feces. Its duration of action is 1–3 weeks after being discontinued.

Mechanism of action

Allopurinol reduces uric acid formation via selective inhibition of the action of xanthine oxidase (the enzyme required for uric acid formation). By lowering the formation of uric acid, hyperuricemia is prevented. Allopurinol does not increase the renal excretion of uric acid.

Clinical indications

Allopurinol prevents or lowers high uric acid levels in the blood, regardless of the cause. It is also used to treat gout or gouty arthritis.

Contraindications

Allopurinol is contraindicated with known hypersensitivity or **idiopathic hemochromatosis**. It must be used cautiously in patients with kidney disease, impaired liver function, history of peptic ulcers, lower GI tract disease, bone marrow depression, and during pregnancy.

Adverse effects

The most common and severe adverse effect is a maculopapular rash. Nearly as common are delayed hypertensive reactions, including **Stevens-Johnson syndrome**, fatal **toxic epidermal necrolysis**, and drug reactions with eosinophilia and systemic symptoms. Symptoms of hypersensitivity reactions include a fever, skin rash, hepatitis, eosinophilia, leukocytosis, and progressive kidney failure. Other adverse effects include drowsiness, headache, nausea, vomiting, vertigo, diarrhea, malaise, cataracts, retinopathy, and thrombocytopenia.

Toxicities

Toxicities from allopurinol are rare and have no specific treatment. The patient is treated symptomatically.

Key Terms

Ambulation
Ankylosing spondylitis
Ankylosis
Azotemia
Behçet disease
Carpometacarpal joints
Cartilage
Chondrocytes
Creatine phosphate
Cytokine
Epidermal necrolysis
Gout
Heberden nodes
Hemochromatosis
Hyperuricemia
Idiopathic hemochromatosis
Interphalangeal joints
Juvenile idiopathic arthritis
Macrophages
Matrix
Mediterranean fever
Osteoarthritis
Panuveitis
Platelet aggregation
Psoriatic arthritis
Range of motion

Rheumatoid arthritis
Scleroderma
Stevens-Johnson syndrome
Synovitis
Systemic lupus erythematosus
Tophus

Clinical Case Studies

Clinical Case Study 1

A 63-year-old male presents with pain and stiffness in his right knee that has worsened over the previous 2 years. The knee becomes stiff after standing for about 30 minutes and causes him pain when he climbs the stairs in his house. His mother was diagnosed with OA. An X-ray of his knee shows narrowing of the joint space, mild effusion, and osteophytic projections. The patient was diagnosed with OA and started on oral and topical NSAIDs.

Critical Thinking Questions

1. What is the pathophysiology of OA?
2. How is OA diagnosed?
3. What are some pharmacologic and nonpharmacologic treatments for severe cases of OA?

Clinical Case Study 2

A 61-year-old female has had RA for the past 2 years. She complains of increased joint pain and inflammation, which has begun limiting her daily activities. The patient has been taking naproxen for symptomatic relief and is currently on methotrexate. She was evaluated for her worsening RA and started on adalimumab.

Critical Thinking Questions

1. What are the clinical indications of adalimumab?
2. What are the contraindications of adalimumab?
3. What are the adverse effects of adalimumab?

Clinical Case Study 3

A 56-year-old male has a history of episodic pain and swelling in his big toe. He was recently started on allopurinol. Physical examination reveals a hard lump near his left big toe, plus hot and tender bluish swelling of the right knee and metatarsal. His serum uric acid concentration is 8.2 mg per dL, which is high. Synovial fluid aspirate contains intracellular needle-shaped crystals. The patient is diagnosed with acute gout and is treated with colchicine.

Critical Thinking Questions

1. What are the clinical indications of colchicine?
2. What are the contraindications of colchicine?
3. What are the adverse effects of colchicine?

Further Reading

[1] K. Atkinson, Rheumatoid Arthritis, Juvenile Idiopathic Arthritis, Ankylosing Spondylitis, Psoriatic Arthritis, and Gout – Targeted Biological Treatments, Book 3, Atkinson, 2020.
[2] A. Baring Garrod, A Treatise on Gout and Rheumatic Gout (Rheumatoid Arthritis), Legare Street Press, 2023.
[3] W. Bozeman, Stem Cells for Osteoarthritis, RELATED Media, 2024.
[4] M. Hook, Rheumatoid Arthritis Handbook – A Complete Guide Providing Insights into Understanding, Preventing, Managing, and Treating RA, Hook, 2024.
[5] J. Jenkins, Rheumatoid Arthritis, third ed., How To Books, 2011.
[6] R.C. Koonce, Non-Surgical Treatment Options for Hip Osteoarthritis – an Informative Guide for Patients, OrthoSkool, 2019.
[7] D.S. Newcombe, D.R. Robinson, Gout – Basic Science and Clinical Practice. Springer, 2013.
[8] K. O'Neill Young, Rheumatoid Arthritis Unmasked – 10 Dangers of RA, RA Patient Insights, LLC, 2017.
[9] L.S. Peterson, Mayo Clinic Guide to Arthritis – Managing Joint Pain for an Active Life, Mayo Clinic Press, 2020.
[10] G.M. Pizzo, Rheumatoid Arthritis – A Comprehensive Guide to Understanding, Preventing, Managing, and Treating RA, Pizzo, 2023.
[11] E.K. Poole, A. Guide on Osteoarthritis – How to Regain your Life, what you Need to Know About the Treatment and Management of Osteoarthritis, Poole, 2022.
[12] T.L. Shlotzhauer, Living with Rheumatoid Arthritis, Johns Hopkins Press, 2014.

[13] R. Terkeltaub, N.L. Edwards, Gout – Diagnosis and Management of Gouty Arthritis and Hyperuricemia, fourth ed., Professional Communications, Inc, 2016.
[14] S. Westlake, Hip Osteoarthritis CAN be Cured – Treating OA with Physical Therapy – A Self Help Guide, CreateSpace Independent Publishing Platform, 2016.
[15] P. Wilde, The Physiology of Gout, Rheumatism and Arthritis as a Guide to Accurate Diagnosis and Efficient Treatment, Scholar Select, 2016.

CHAPTER

57

Toxicology

OUTLINE

LEARNING OUTCOMES

After study of the chapter, readers should be able to:

1. Describe symptoms of acute acetaminophen poisoning.
2. Explain the signs and symptoms of an aspirin overdose.
3. Discuss the opiate toxicity and the treatment.
4. List atypical agents of sedative-hypnotics.
5. Describe the common symptoms of atypical antipsychotic poisoning.
6. Explain the signs and symptoms of digitalis poisoning.
7. Describe the complications of lithium poisoning.
8. Explain the symptoms of lead poisoning.
9. Describe the treatments for cyanide poisoning.
10. List the antidotes for carbon monoxide, cyanide, and opiates.

The Science of Pharmacology
https://doi.org/10.1016/B978-0-443-29038-1.00057-9

Overview

A poison is any substance that has the potential to cause harm, and the degree of damage a poison can cause is determined by its dose. Poisons may be substances such as cyanide, arsenic, or strychnine (pesticide), which are considered to be dangerous in small amounts. However, lifesaving drugs and medications are poisons if they are taken in an overdose. Even life-sustaining substances such as water and oxygen can harm the human body if taken excessively. Coming into contact with a potentially harmful substance is known as exposure. Exposures can occur through inhalation, ingestion, dermal, ocular, or parenteral. Accidental poisonings arise far more often at home than through industrial exposure, and the effects are usually acute. Industrial intoxication is more often the result of chronic exposure. Accidental poisoning usually results from the unintentional ingestion of toxic substances, with most occurrences involving children. In most instances, accidental poisonings should be preventable, especially for poisonings of young children via drugs and chemicals found in the home.

Epidemiology

Poisoning is the leading cause of injury-related death in the United States. According to the CDC, there were an estimated 107,543 drug overdose deaths in the United States during 2023—a decrease of 3% from the 111,029 deaths estimated in 2022. Deaths from poisoning exceed deaths from motor vehicle crashes, and drug overdose deaths have tripled since 1990. More than 90% of poisoning deaths reported to the CDC are due to drugs (including illegal drugs). An increase in opioid-related deaths is attributable to the abuse and misuse of these medications. More than 75% of people who abuse opioids report getting them from a friend or family member versus obtaining a legitimate prescription.

About half of all opioid-related deaths involve at least one other drug, such as benzodiazepines or alcohol. Another alarming trend in poisoning is the number of unintentional deaths. Unintentional deaths accounted for 85% of all poisoning deaths in 2023. Specifically, estimated deaths in 2023 from fentanyl were 74,702 in the United States alone.

You should remember

Pediatric exposures occur because naturally curious children learn about their environment by touch and taste. Exposures are unintentional and usually involve small ingestions of substances in their homes, primarily analgesics, due to their ubiquity.

You should remember

The most common poisonings seen today involve nonprescription drugs, household products, solvents, pesticides, and poisonous plants.

Analgesics

Analgesics are responsible for more total exposures and deaths reported to poison centers than any other substance. Several different classes of medications fall into this category, and they all have different mechanisms of toxic action, expected symptoms, and treatments.

Acetaminophen

Acetaminophen (APAP) is found in more than 600 different OTC and prescription medications, and more than 50 million Americans use APAP each week. This drug is used to treat pain and fever. APAP toxicity can occur with acute overdose or with chronic ingestion. Excessive APAP intake can cause liver damage.

Even with a large overdose, symptoms of acute APAP poisoning may be minimal for the first 24 hours because the metabolism of APAP is slow. However, symptoms of toxicity include confusion, **diaphoresis**, abdominal pain, nausea, vomiting, bleeding, jaundice, renal injury, coma, and death. Hepatic damage is the most important manifestation of APAP toxicity and becomes evident 1–2 days after ingestion.

Treatment for APAP overdose should begin with the induction of emesis or gastric lavage, followed by the administration of activated charcoal. *N*-acetylcysteine (NAC) is an effective **antidote** for both acute and chronic APAP poisoning. NAC detoxifies the APAP metabolite, *N*-acetyl parabenzoquinone imine, before it can damage the liver. NAC is always given in a hospital setting; it can be given orally or intravenously (IV). It is most effective when given early on after an acute overdose before liver damage begins. However, NAC is still beneficial when given after a liver injury has started. A special nomogram or algorithm is used to determine the dose and duration of NAC.

Aspirin

Aspirin (ASA) is used for fever, pain, and inflammation. It also prevents heart attacks and ischemic stroke. Like APAP, ASA poisoning can occur with acute or chronic ingestion. It is a member of the salicylate family. The signs and symptoms include nausea, vomiting, **tachypnea**, fever, **tinnitus,** metabolic acidosis, sweating, confusion, seizures, pulmonary and brain edema, coma, and death. There is no antidote for ASA poisoning. Patients with ASA toxicity are often given intravenous sodium bicarbonate and dialysis of the kidneys.

Opioids and opiates

Opioids are pain-relieving medicines that are derived from the poppy plant—for example, heroin and morphine (Duramorph). Opiates are not direct derivatives of the poppy plant, but they are derived from opioids. These include fentanyl (many formulations and trade names), oxycodone (OxyContin), hydrocodone (Vicodin), and codeine. The use of opioids, either by themselves or in combination with other drugs, is a significant cause of the drug overdose crisis in the United States. The vast majority of overdose deaths today are illegally manufactured fentanyl and other potent, synthetic opioids, which may be added to different drugs and consumed unknowingly.

Opioid or opiate toxicity should be suspected when the clinical signs and symptoms of central nervous system (CNS) depression, respiratory depression, and **pupillary miosis** are present. Toxicity from opioids can cause drowsiness, analgesia, **euphoria**, apnea, and constipation.

Some synthetic opioids can produce additional symptoms of overdose. For example, meperidine can cause seizures, and methadone can cause cardiac arrhythmias.

However, the primary toxicity for all opioids is considered to be respiratory depression.

Naloxone is the antidote for respiratory depression due to opioids. It is a competitive antagonist at the opioid receptors, effectively blocking the receptor so the opioid cannot reach it. Naloxone is available in intramuscular, IV, and nasal spray formulations. IV and nasal administration produce rapid effects, reversing opioid toxicity within seconds to minutes. Because respiratory depression is the primary mode of toxicity, another effective treatment for overdose is intubation and mechanical ventilation of the patient until the opioid has been metabolized.

Nonsteroidal antiinflammatory drugs

Nonsteroidal antiinflammatory drugs (NSAIDs) treat fever, pain, and inflammation. Prescription NSAIDs include ketorolac, nabumetone, diclofenac, and meloxicam. OTC NSAIDs include naproxen and ibuprofen. While they have the potential to cause serious adverse effects, NSAIDs are considered to be much safer in overdose compared to APAP, ASA, and opioids. NSAIDs inhibit cyclooxygenase, an enzyme in the pathway that produces pain and inflammatory mediators.

The symptoms of NSAID poisoning, in most cases acute, result in mild to moderate toxicity with nausea, vomiting, and drowsiness. Massive overdoses can result in seizures, coma, hypotension, bleeding, kidney failure, and acidosis. There is no antidote available for NSAID poisoning. Patients' symptoms are managed with supportive care.

Sedative-hypnotics and atypical antipsychotics

Therapeutic sedatives include benzodiazepines and hypnotics used for sleep, such as zolpidem, eszopiclone, and barbiturates. Atypical agents currently available include clozapine (Clozaril), risperidone (Risperdal), olanzapine (Zyprexa), quetiapine (Seroquel), ziprasidone (Geodon), aripiprazole (Abilify), and paliperidone (Invega). Overdose with these drugs may include supportive care such as ventilation for assisted breathing, blood pressure monitoring, and activated charcoal to adsorb any drugs remaining in the stomach. Depending on the pH of the drug taken, alkalinization or acidification of the urine may be attempted to force the excretion of the overdosed drug.

Benzodiazepines

Benzodiazepines are used therapeutically to treat anxiety, promote sleep, or treat seizures. Examples include alprazolam, diazepam, lorazepam, and clonazepam. Benzodiazepines work by increasing the effect of an inhibitory neurotransmitter called gamma-aminobutyric acid (GABA), resulting in generalized depression of the CNS. The symptoms of benzodiazepine poisoning include drowsiness, **slurred speech**, lack of coordination, and coma. Although respiratory arrest is possible, benzodiazepine overdoses are usually not life-threatening unless combined with another CNS depressant drug such as alcohol or an opioid.

To treat benzodiazepine overdose, flumazenil was once a potential antidote. It is a competitive antagonist at the benzodiazepine receptor. Flumazenil can unmask seizures in patients habituated to benzodiazepines or patients who have taken a coingestion of seizure-causing medications. Therefore the risks of flumazenil usually outweigh its benefits in overdose, and it is rarely indicated.

Atypical antipsychotics

Atypical antipsychotics, or second-generation antipsychotics, include drugs such as olanzapine, quetiapine, clozapine, risperidone, ziprasidone, and aripiprazole. The action of atypical antipsychotics is at dopamine and serotonin receptors and causes a variety of effects on the CNS and cardiovascular system. The common symptoms of atypical antipsychotic poisoning include drowsiness, tachycardia, hypotension, and respiratory depression. The treatment for atypical antipsychotics is symptomatic and managed with supportive care. There is no antidote for atypical antipsychotics, and supportive care is used.

Other drugs or toxic substances

Nearly 70% of Americans take at least one prescription medication, and more than $722 billion was spent on prescription drugs in 2023. Medications are everywhere in American homes and, as mentioned previously, account for a large portion of poisonings. Poison centers nationwide are seeing more poisonings from pharmaceuticals than ever before and in every age group. Approximately 530,000 injury incidents occur yearly in outpatient clinics due to medication errors. The two most common reasons for a mistake were taking a double dose and taking the wrong medication. The best way to prevent medication poisoning and medication error is education.

Antihistamines

There is a wide variation in patient tolerance to antihistamines and in the symptoms of poisoning. When poisoned by antihistamines, patients may experience CNS excitement or depression. In adults, drowsiness, **stupor**, and coma may occur. Treatment is supportive and focused on the removal of the unabsorbed drug and the maintenance of vital functions. Convulsions may be controlled with phenobarbital or diazepam.

Digitalis

Digoxin is a digital cardiac glycoside for treating heart failure and **atrial fibrillation**. Toxicity may result from cumulative effects of the drug or from hypokalemia. Increased digoxin levels may also result from concomitant therapy with such drugs as amiodarone, erythromycin, quinidine, tetracycline, and other medications. Signs and symptoms of digitalis poisoning include **cardiac arrhythmias**, nausea, vomiting, seizures, visual abnormalities, dizziness, altered serum potassium levels, and others. The treatment includes activated charcoal, atropine, antiarrhythmics, electrical cardioversion, fragment antigen-binding therapy, and advanced life support. Digitalis poisoning may result in multiple organ failures and recurrence of toxicity after treatment has ended.

Lithium

Lithium is primarily used for bipolar and unipolar depression. It is absorbed, distributed, and eliminated slowly. Acute toxicity usually causes initial GI symptoms followed by CNS complications. Signs and symptoms include nausea, vomiting, memory impairment, **delirium**, hypertension, tachycardia, tremors, seizures, coma, and hypothermia. The treatment consists of advanced life support, fluid therapy, benzodiazepines, whole-bowel irrigation, hemodialysis, amiloride, and other treatments. Complications of lithium poisoning may include permanent encephalopathy, nystagmus, ataxia, and choreoathetosis (the occurrence of involuntary movements).

You should remember

For many years, inducing vomiting was considered to be a mainstay in the treatment of an ingested poison. Syrup of ipecac was once used for toxic ingestions, as it causes vomiting by direct stomach irritation and stimulation of the chemoreceptor triggers in the brain. It is no longer recommended and is not manufactured in the United States.

Methyl alcohol and ethylene glycol

Ingestion of **methyl alcohol** (wood alcohol) or *methanol* produces *metabolic* acids and causes metabolic acidosis. A dose as small as 30 mL can be fatal. Ingestion of only 15 mL of methanol has caused permanent blindness by producing severe optic nerve and CNS toxicity. Symptoms of methanol poisoning usually do not appear until 12–24 hours after ingestion, when toxic metabolites have accumulated in sufficient quantities. Methanol is converted to **formaldehyde** and **formic acid**. Manifestations include headache, dizziness, nausea, vomiting, CNS depression, and respiratory failure. In the treatment of patients with methyl alcohol intoxication, **emesis** and **gastric lavage** are of use only within the first 2 hours after ingestion. IV administration of large amounts of sodium bicarbonate combats acidosis. IV ethanol therapy should be used.

Ethylene glycol is a solvent found in products ranging from antifreeze and de-icing solutions to carpet and fabric cleaners. It has a sweet taste and is intoxicating—factors that contribute to its abuse potential. A lethal dose is approximately 100 mL, and it is metabolized to **glycolaldehyde** and **glycolic acid**. Glycolic acid is degraded to oxalate, which can form **renal stones**. Gastric lavage with ipecac syrup is ineffective because the intestine rapidly absorbs the syrup. Acidosis occurs as ethylene glycol is converted to oxalic and lactic acid. Toxicity manifests in three stages: neurologic symptoms (ranging from drunkenness to coma), which appear within 12 hours; cardiorespiratory disorders (such as tachycardia and pulmonary edema); and flank pain and renal failure (caused by the plugging of the tubules with oxalate crystals).

The enzymes *alcohol dehydrogenase* and *aldehyde dehydrogenase* sequentially metabolize methanol and ethylene glycol into toxic metabolites. This enzyme is also used for ethanol metabolism because alcohol dehydrogenase has an affinity for ethanol 10 times greater than its affinity for methanol or ethylene glycol. IV or oral ethanol is an antidote for methanol and ethylene glycol poisoning.

Lead

Lead is a solid metal that is used in a variety of industries. Children are especially susceptible to lead poisoning, and they can encounter lead in a variety of ways—lead paint, contaminated soil (from deteriorated lead paint, lead industry pollution, lead gasoline emissions), water from plumbing made with lead materials, and imported items such as pottery, jewelry, or folk medicines. The most common source is ingesting lead-based paint or dust from lead-based paint. Lead paint chips can be eaten, or dust from lead paint can be deposited on the hands, toys, or other items the child places in their mouth. Lead is more commonly a chronic poisoning (e.g., a child ingests dust from lead paint in their home over months) but can be acute (e.g., a child lives in a lead paint-free home but ingests a lead fishing-weight foreign body). Homes built in 1978, as required by law, do not contain lead-based paint. However, homes built before 1978 should be expected to contain lead-based paint. The CDC estimates that 24 million housing units in the United States contain deteriorated lead paint and elevated lead-contaminated house dust. Young children reside in 4 million of these homes.

Lead exerts its effects through various mechanisms, affecting different proteins, receptors, and cellular processes. Lead poisoning has an impact on many organ systems. Lead is well absorbed from children's GI tracts and deposited in tissues all over the body, including the bone.

Lead affects many organ systems, but the CNS is of most concern in developing children. Lead poisoning can result in general nonspecific symptoms such as irritability, fatigue, headache, nausea, **metallic taste**, loss of appetite and weight loss, and muscle aches and weakness. CNS symptoms include inability to concentrate, lack of coordination, and tremors. Chronic lead poisoning can cause stunted growth, hearing impairment, learning disabilities, diminished IQ, and impaired behavioral development. Severe lead poisoning can lead to encephalopathy. Symptoms affecting other organ systems include anemia, hypertension, and kidney impairment.

The initial step in the treatment of lead poisoning is to remove the child from the source of lead. It can be challenging if the source of lead is the child's home. Children with elevated lead in the blood are given medications to remove the lead from the child's body. These drugs are called chelating agents, including calcium disodium edetate, dimercaprol, and succimer. Chelating agents bind to lead to a complex that is then excreted in the urine. Calcium disodium edetate and dimercaprol are parenteral medications, and succimer is given orally. Because lead is stored in the bone, removing all of the lead in a child's body can take a significant time, even with chelation.

Additionally, removing lead from a child's body will not reverse neurological damage that has already been done. Because lead poisoning causes permanent neurologic damage to children, prevention is critical. Lead poisoning prevention tips are described in the poison prevention section below.

Arsenic

Arsenic is a cellular toxin readily absorbed through the GI tract and lungs. It has a metallic taste and garlic-like odor and causes extreme GI irritation. Signs and symptoms of arsenic poisoning include nausea, vomiting, hemorrhagic gastroenteritis, cardiogenic shock, ventricular tachyarrhythmias, pulmonary edema, pancytopenia, hemolytic anemia, convulsions, coma, polyneuropathy, renal dysfunction, skin lesions, and others. Arsenic poisoning is treated with advanced life support, endotracheal intubation, fluid therapy, gastric lavage, **gastrotomy, chelation therapy**, hemodialysis, and blood transfusions. Arsenic poisoning may cause neurotoxic effects and multisystem organ failure.

Arsenic is a natural element in water and soil and is easily absorbed by the roots of rice plants. Organic arsenic is considered harmless and bound to sugars in fruits and vegetables. In contrast, inorganic arsenic is considered hazardous, and it may cause lung, bladder, and skin cancer in adults. Inorganic arsenic-containing pesticides were once sprayed on specific crops such as rice and apples, but this was halted mainly in the 1970s in the United States. Even so, rice and rice-related products may have concerning amounts of arsenic. In children, arsenic toxicity can harm normal development and cause brain damage. Brown rice is considered healthier, but it absorbs more arsenic than white rice due to its shell, which is removed to produce white rice. Washing rice a few times, boiling it in hot water, and then cooking it helps to remove arsenic from the rice. There are no FDA standards for arsenic levels in food other than animal products for animals treated with specific drugs. However, there are arsenic thresholds for tap water.

Cyanide

Cyanide is an exceedingly potent and rapid-acting poison, but one for which specific and effective antidotal therapy is available. Cyanide poisoning may result from the inhalation of hydrocyanic acid or the ingestion of soluble inorganic cyanide salts. Parts of many plants also contain substances such as amygdalin, which release cyanide when they are crushed and digested in the acidic environment of the gut. Cyanide poisoning is characterized by drowsiness, tachycardia, headache, seizures, apnea, and cardiac arrest. It may cause death within 1–15 minutes.

Cyanide poisoning is a true medical emergency; however, treatment is highly effective if given rapidly. Diagnosis is made by the characteristic "bitter almond" odor on the victim's breath, but as many as 40% of adults cannot detect this odor due to gene expression. Chemical antidotes should be immediately available wherever emergency medical care is dispensed. Treatment involves the administration of nitrite, which produces methemoglobin in the body.

Methemoglobin can be slowly reduced to hemoglobin. Supportive measures should be instituted immediately, especially artificial respiration with 100% oxygen.

Carbon monoxide

Carbon monoxide (CO) is a colorless, odorless, tasteless, and nonirritating gas in the exhaust of internal combustion engines in concentrations of 3%–7%. CO is responsible for more than 2500 accidental deaths and suicides every year in the United States. The toxic effects of CO are the result of tissue hypoxia. The most characteristic signs of severe CO poisoning are the cherry color of skin and mucous membranes. Treatment requires adequate ventilation in high oxygen concentrations and the absence of CO. If necessary, ventilation should be supported artificially. Pure oxygen should be administered. Cerebral edema should be treated with diuretics and steroids.

Organophosphates

Organophosphate pesticides are compounds that irreversibly inhibit acetylcholinesterase and are absorbed through the skin, lungs, and GI tract. They are widely distributed throughout the tissues and are slowly eliminated by the liver. Symptoms of organophosphate insecticide poisoning include nausea, vomiting, abdominal cramping, headache, blurred vision, and excessive salivation. Toxicity may be achieved between 30 minutes and 2 hours after absorption. Treating patients with organophosphate poisoning includes removing contaminated clothing, washing the skin with soap and water, and using activated charcoal to decontaminate the GI tract. Additional treatment may involve oxygen administration, ventilatory assistance, and treatment of seizures. Cholinergic drugs such as atropine can reverse the symptoms, and pralidoxime can be administered to cleave the organophosphate from acetylcholinesterase if possible. Each organophosphate has a different trait, called enzyme aging, or the covalent binding of the pesticide with acetylcholinesterase, which is permanent, and the enzyme must be regenerated in the body to reestablish function.

Antidotes

Antidotes are drugs or other substances that oppose the action of a poison. An antidote, such as activated charcoal, may be mechanical, which absorbs poisons in the GI tract and prevents their absorption. It may also be chemical, having actions that neutralize the toxin, as well as physiologic, in which its actions oppose the actions of the poison. Specific antidotal therapy is available for only a few poisons. Some systemic antidotes exert their therapeutic effect by reducing the concentration of the toxic substance. They may combine it with the poison or increase its excretion rate. Other systemic antidotes compete with the poison for its receptor site. Specific antidotes, along with their related poisons, are listed in **Table 57.1**.

TABLE 57.1 Poisons and antidotes.

Poison	Antidotes
Acetaminophen	*N*-Acetylcysteine
Benzodiazepines	Flumazenil (Romazicon, others)
Carbon monoxide	Oxygen
Cyanide	Amyl nitrate
Iron	Deferoxamine
Methanol	Ethanol
Opiates	Naloxone (Narcan, others)
Organophosphates	Atropine (Atropen) or pralidoxime

Key Terms

Antidote
Atrial fibrillation
Cardiac arrhythmias
Chelation therapy
Delirium
Diaphoresis
Emesis
Ethylene glycol
Euphoria
Formaldehyde
Formic acid
Gastric lavage
Gastrotomy
Glycolaldehyde
Glycolic acid
Methyl alcohol
Metallic taste
Pupillary miosis
Slurred speech
Stupor
Tachypnea
Tinnitus

Further Reading

[1] I.B. Anderson, N.L. Benowitz, P.D. Blanc, S.Y. Kim-Katz, J.C. Lewis, A.H.B. Wu, K.R. Olson, C. Smollin, Poisoning and Drug Overdose, eighth ed., McGraw Hill/Medical, 2022.
[2] J. Armstrong, O. Pascu, The Toxicology Handbook, fourth ed., Elsevier, 2022.
[3] S. Gilbert, A. Mohapatra, S. Bobst, A. Hayes, S.T. Humes, Information Resources in Toxicology, Volume 2 – the Global Arena, fifth ed., Academic Press, 2020.
[4] R.S. Hoffman, S. Gosselin, L.S. Nelson, M.A. Howland, N.A. Lewin, S.W. Smith, L.R. Goldfrank, Goldfrank's Clinical Manual of Toxicologic Emergencies, second ed., McGraw Hill/Medical, 2023.
[5] K.D. Katz, EMRA and AMCT Medical Toxicology Guide, second ed., Emergency Medicine Residents' Association, 2022.
[6] C.D. Klaassen, Casarett & Doull's Toxicology – the Basic Science of Poisons, ninth ed., McGraw Hill/Medical, 2018.
[7] B.S. Levine, S. Kerrigan, Principles of Forensic Toxicology, fifth ed., Springer, 2020.
[8] C. McQueen, Comprehensive Toxicology, third ed., Elsevier Science, 2018.
[9] K.S. Narayan Reddy, The Essentials of Forensic Medicine & Toxicology, Thirty-fifth ed., Jaypee Brothers Medical Publishers, 2022.
[10] A. Negrusz, G. Cooper, Clarke's Analytical Forensic Toxicology, second ed., Pharmaceutical Press, 2013.
[11] K.R. Olson, I.B. Anderson, N.L. Benowitz, P.D. Blanc, R.F. Clark, T.E. Kearney, S.Y. Kim-Yatz, A.B.H. Wu, Poisoning and Drug Overdose, seventh ed., McGraw Hill/Medical, 2017.
[12] S.M. Roberts, R.C. James, P.L. Williams, Principles of Toxicology, fourth ed., Wiley, 2022.
[13] J. Timbrell, F.A. Barile, Introduction to Toxicology, fourth ed., CRC Press, 2023.

Appendix A: Dosage calculations

Using ratios and proportions to calculate dosages

1. Ratios may be written as 3:4, which means three parts of the drug to 4 parts of the solution or solvent. *Ratios* are used to express the relationship between two or more quantities. Ratios are usually expressed as fractions in drug calculations, as follows:

$$\frac{\text{3 parts of drug}}{\text{4 parts of a solution}} = \frac{3}{4}$$

Proportions show the relationship between two ratios, as follows:

$$\frac{\text{Dose on hand}}{\text{Quantity on hand}} = \frac{\text{Desired dose}}{\text{Desired quantity (X)}}$$

The same formula can be written as follows by using cross multiplication:

$$\text{Desired quantity (X)} = \frac{\text{Desired dose}}{\text{Dose on hand} \times \text{Quantity on hand}}$$

If the dose on hand is 200 mg, the desired dose is 400 mg, and the quantity on hand is 10 mL, what is the desired amount (X)?

$$\frac{\text{Dose on hand (300 mg)}}{\text{Quantity on hand (5 mL)}} = \frac{\text{Desired dose (600 mg)}}{\text{Desired quantity (X)}}$$

When cross multiplying, we find:

$$300 \times X = 5\ \text{mL} \times 600$$

$$300X = 3,000\ \text{mL}$$

$$X = 10\ \text{mL}$$

The dose to be administered is 10 mL.

2. The same proportion method can solve solid dosage calculations as follows:

If the dose on hand is available as 5 mg tablets, and the desired dose is 25 mg/day, how many tablets should be administered each day?

$$\frac{\text{Dose on hand (50 mg)}}{\text{1 tablet}} = \frac{\text{Desired dose (250 mg)}}{\text{Desired quantity (X)}}$$

By cross-multiplying, it is found that:

$$50\ \text{mg} \times X = 250\ \text{mg} \times 1\ \text{tablet}$$

$$50X = 250\ \text{mg}$$

$$X = 5\ \text{tablets/day}$$

Therefore, five tablets should be given daily.

Dosage calculations by weight

Drug dosages are often expressed as milligrams per unit of body weight (usually kilograms rather than pounds) and are commonly used to depict pediatric doses. An example recommended dose of a drug might be 1 mg/kg / 24 hours. This information can be used to calculate the dose for a specific patient or to check that prescribed doses are correct and not significantly under or over the required doses.

Caution must always be used when converting between pounds and kilograms. The formula that should be understood is as follows:

$$\text{Body weight} \times (\text{dose in mg / kg}) = \text{X mg of drug}$$

Example: Chewable tablets for a 110-pound child will be administered at 20 mg/kg/dose. If 500 mg each is administered, how many tablets should be administered to this patient for each dose?

First, convert the patient's weight to kilograms as follows:

$$1\ \text{kg} = 2.2\ \text{lbs}$$

$$\frac{1\ \text{kg}}{2.2\ \text{lbs}} = \frac{\text{X kg}}{110\ \text{lbs}}$$

$$\text{X} = 50\ \text{kg}$$

Next, calculate the total daily dose as follows. For each kg of body weight, you should give 20 mg of the drug.

$$\frac{20\ \text{mg}}{1\ \text{kg}} = \frac{\text{X mg}}{50\ \text{kg}}$$

$$\text{X} = 1,000\ \text{mg}$$

Finally, calculate the number of tablets needed to supply 1,000 mg per dose.

Remember that the concentration of the tablets on hand is 500 mg per tablet.

$$\frac{500\ \text{mg}}{1\ \text{tablet}} = \frac{1,000\ \text{mg}}{\text{X tablets}}$$

$$\text{X} = 2\ \text{tablets per dose}$$

Calculating dosage by body surface area

Using body surface area to calculate pediatric dosages is a very accurate method. Nomograms are charts that use patient weight and height to determine body surface area in square meters (m^2). This body surface area (BSA) is then placed into a ratio with the average adult's body surface area (1.73 m^2). The following formula is then used:

$$\text{Child's dose} = \frac{\text{Child's BSA in m}^2}{1.73\ \text{m}^2} \times \text{Adult dose}$$

Nomogram scales contain metric and avoirdupois values for height and weight, enabling body surface area to be determined in pounds and inches or kilograms and centimeters without making conversions.

A ruler or straightedge is recommended to determine BSA. After selecting the patient's height and weight, place the ruler or straightedge on the nomogram and connect the two points on the height and weight scales representing the patient's values. Where the ruler or straightedge crosses the center column (BSA), the corresponding reading is the value of the BSA in square meters. Substitute the BSA value in the formula to calculate the dosage for this patient. If this child's BSA is 0.52 m^2, and the adult dosage of the required drug is 500 mg, use the following formula to determine the child's dose:

$$\text{Child's dose} = \frac{0.52\text{m}^2}{1.73\ \text{m}^2} \times \text{Adult dose (500 mg)}$$

$$= 0.3 \times 500 \text{ mg}$$

$$= 150 \text{ mg (child's dose)}$$

Calculating IV infusion rates

To calculate the flow rate using the ratio and proportion method, follow these steps:

1. Determine the number of milliliters the patient will receive per hour
2. Determine the number of milliliters the patient will receive per minute
3. Determine the number of drops per minute equal to the milliliters calculated above. The IV set's drop rate must be considered. This is expressed as a ratio of drops per milliliter (gtt/mL).

Example: The prescriber orders 3,000 mL of dextrose 5% in water (D_5W) IV over 24 hours. If the IV set delivers 15 drops per milliliter, how many drops must be administered per minute?

First, calculate mL/hr.

$$\frac{3,000 \text{ mL}}{24 \text{ hrs}} = \frac{X \text{ mL}}{1 \text{ hr}}$$

$$X = 125 \text{ mL/hr or}$$

$$125 \text{ mL} / 60 \text{ min}$$

Next, calculate mL/min.

$$\frac{125 \text{ mL}}{60 \text{ min}} = \frac{X \text{ mL}}{1 \text{ min}}$$

$$X = 2 \text{ mL/min}$$

Finally, calculate gtt/min using the drop rate per minute of the IV set. (IV set drop rate = 15 drops/mL)

$$\frac{15 \text{ gtt}}{1 \text{ mL}} = \frac{X \text{ gtt}}{2 \text{ mL (amount needed/min)}}$$

$$X = 30 \text{ gtt/min}$$

Appendix B: ISMP list of high-alert medications

Type of medication	Examples
Adrenergic Agonists, IV	Epinephrine, norepinephrine, phenylephrine
Adrenergic Antagonists, IV	Labetalol, metoprolol, propranolol
Anesthetic Agents, General, Inhaled and IV	Ketamine, propofol
Antiarrhythmics, IV	Amiodarone, lidocaine
Antithrombotic Agents, including:	
Anticoagulants	Low molecular weight heparin, unfractionated heparin, warfarin
Direct Oral Anticoagulants and Factor Xa Inhibitors	Apixaban, betrixaban, dabigatran, edoxaban, fondaparinux, rivaroxaban
Direct Thrombin Inhibitors	Argatroban, bivalirudin
Glycoprotein IIb/IIIa Inhibitors	Eptifibatide
Thrombolytics	Alteplase, reteplase, tenecteplase
Cardioplegic Solutions	Calcium chloride, magnesium chloride, potassium chloride, sodium chloride
Chemotherapeutic Agents, Parenteral and Oral	Dactinomycin, etoposide, ifosfamide, mitomycin, toposar
Dextrose, Hypertonic, 20% or greater	
Dialysis Solutions, Peritoneal and Hemodialysis	Dextrose monohydrate, eravacycline, sodium chloride
Epidural and Intrathecal Medications	Morphine sulfate, sufentanil citrate
Inotropic Medications, IV	Digoxin, milrinone
Insulin, Subcutaneous and IV	
Liposomal Forms of Drugs and Conventional Counterparts	Liposomal amphotericin B; counterpart agent amphotericin B desoxycholate
Moderate Sedation Agents, IV	Dexmedetomidine, lorazepam, midazolam
Moderate and Minimal Sedation Agents, Oral, for children	Chloral hydrate, midazolam
Opioids, including: IV, Oral, Transdermal, Neuromuscular Blocking Agents	Oral: liquid concentrates, immediate- and sustained-release formulations; Neuromuscular: rocuronium, succinylcholine, vecuronium
Parenteral Nutrition Preparations	SMOFlipid, Intralipid, Nutrilipid
Sodium Chloride for Injection, Hypertonic, greater than 0.9% concentration	
Sterile Water for Injection, Inhalation and Irrigation (excluding pour bottles) in containers of 100 mL or more	
Sulfonylurea Hypoglycemics, Oral	Chlorpropamide, glimepiride, glipizide, glyburide, tolbutamide

Source: Institute for Safe Medication Practices (ISMP), ***https://www.ismp.org***

Appendix C: Answer key to clinical case studies

Chapter 1: Introduction

There are no Clinical Cases in this chapter.

Chapter 2: Pharmacodynamics

Clinical case study 1

1. Warfarin has a narrow therapeutic window and must be used with great care to achieve the desired anticoagulation without excess risk of bleeding.
2. Disorders that affect pharmacodynamics include genetic mutations, malnutrition, thyrotoxicosis, myasthenia gravis, Parkinson's disease, and insulin-resistant diabetes mellitus.
3. Most drug-drug interactions cause heartburn, nausea, headache, and lightheadedness. The most serious interactions of drugs may cause severe hypotension and arrhythmias. Some drug interactions may cause damage to the heart, liver, kidney, and other organs.

Clinical case ctudy 2

1. A drug's safety is determined by comparing the median lethal dose (LD50) and the median effective dose (ED50). A drug with a therapeutic index of 4 or higher is relatively safe unless vast quantities are taken. The danger is much higher for a fatal outcome for a drug with a low therapeutic index 2.
2. Potency is the strength of a drug at a specific dose or concentration. A more potent drug produces therapeutic effects in lower doses compared to other drugs within the same class. Efficacy is the most fantastic maximal response that is created by a drug. Pharmacotherapeutic experts agree that efficacy is nearly always more important than potency.
3. Diphenhydramine is classified as an inverse agonist. It acts at the H1 receptor, reversing the effects of histamine on capillaries to reduce allergic reaction symptoms.

Chapter 3: Pharmacokinetics

Clinical case study 1

1. Solid acids destroy some enteral medications within the stomach. To avoid this, tablets may be coated with a hard, waxy substance that resists acidity. These tablets are known as enteric-coated and dissolve in the small intestine, which has an alkaline environment. Some enteric-coated drugs are so coated because they would otherwise irritate the stomach mucosa if dissolved there.
2. Extended-release tablets or capsules dissolve slowly to provide a longer duration of action. These drugs are used only once or twice daily.
3. Some drugs are available as liquids for people with trouble swallowing tablets or capsules. Liquid forms include elixirs, suspensions, and syrups. They are usually flavored and sweetened extensively, so their bitter taste is not experienced.

Clinical case study 2

1. Drug excretion removes an intact drug, mainly via the kidneys. Drug clearance that depends on kidney function may be affected by kidney disease or reduced cardiac output. Less commonly, the liver can alter consent.
2. The average drug elimination by the kidneys involves glomerular filtration and distal tubular reabsorption. Glomerular filtration occurs when drugs enter the kidneys via the renal arteries. Distal tubular reabsorption occurs when a drug moves to the distal convoluted tubule, where its concentrations are higher than those of the perivascular space.
3. With aging, renal drug excretion decreases. At age 80, clearance is usually reduced to about half of what it was when the individual was 30.

Chapter 4: Pharmacogenomics and drug toxicity

Clinical case study 1

1. Anaphylactic shock is a distinctive, sudden, and severe allergic reaction that may be life-threatening.
2. Anaphylactic shock can cause an extreme loss of blood pressure, urticaria (hives or wheals), diaphragm paralysis, difficulty breathing, and swelling of the oropharynx. Other symptoms include flushed skin, pallor, a feeling of sudden warmth, a "lump" in the throat, difficulty swallowing, nausea, vomiting, diarrhea, abdominal pain, a weak and rapid pulse, runny nose, sneezing, swollen tongue or lips, and wheezing. The result may be cardiac collapse. Anaphylactic shock is a true medical emergency.
3. Treatment of anaphylactic shock must begin immediately. Epinephrine is injected intradermally. Glucocorticoids and antihistamines are injected intravenously, and oxygen is administered.

Clinical case study 2

1. A pharmacokinetic drug-drug interaction occurs when a drug affects another drug's absorption, distribution, metabolism, or excretion. This changes the concentrations of the active drug in the body.
2. Drug-drug interactions occur when a drug changes how tissues respond, or do not respond, to another drug. These interactions can be toxic when the two drugs activate complementary pathways, increasing the effects of both drugs.
3. Clozapine interacts with oral contraceptives and antifungals, even though they are widely different drugs.

Chapter 5: Medication errors

Clinical case study 1

1. The surgeon made the primary error; he should have never written .4 mg IV on the order. A leading zero should have been added for all orders under one total amount, such as milligrams, so the ordered amount said 0.4 mg IV.
2. Medication errors mainly occur when choosing a medication, its dose, and the dosing schedule or dosage.

Clinical case study 2

1. Polypharmacy uses several drugs simultaneously, significantly increasing the risk of medication errors. It is also described as receiving multiple medications, sometimes for the same condition, with conflicting pharmacologic actions. Polypharmacy is most prevalent in older adults but may occur in patients of all ages.
2. Keeping track of multiple medications and healthcare providers is difficult for many older adults. This is complicated further by poor medication information, documentation, and reporting. Keeping track of a patient's medications as they change healthcare providers is medication reconciliation.
3. Medication reconciliation requires accurately listing all medications a patient takes to reduce duplications, dosing errors, omissions, and drug interactions. For hospitalized patients, nurses document all medications previously taken at home, including the dose, frequency, and route. This list is used whenever the patient is admitted to other facilities or transferred to different hospital units. The list is rechecked when a patient is discharged from a hospital. Many possible medication errors have been revealed during medication reconciliation procedures.

Medications considered part of medication reconciliation include prescription medications, OTC medications, herbal supplements, and vitamins.

Chapter 6: Complementary and alternative dietary therapies

Clinical case study 1

1. The patient should be told that garlic is commonly used to prevent and treat vascular diseases, significantly reducing LDL, elevated triglycerides, and hypertension. Other uses for garlic have included treatment for alopecia, breast disease, and upper respiratory infection. A garlic-rich diet seems to have a lower risk of developing colon, prostate, stomach, and breast cancer.
2. Cinnamon also can lower LDL cholesterol.
3. Since she takes warfarin, this patient should be instructed to avoid the following agents: ginger, saw palmetto, dong quai, ginkgo, kava kava, St. John's wort, and ginseng.

Clinical case study 2

1. With this patient's drug regimen, there are concerns about taking St. John's wort, the coronary artery disease medications (ramipril and amlodipine), and the antidepressant (citalopram).
2. St. John's wort can cause loose stools and restlessness, two symptoms of this patient.
3. A person with depression already on medication for the condition might add St. John's wort as self-treatment by being unaware that it interacts negatively with prescribed antidepressants.

Chapter 7: Adverse drug effects and drug interactions

Clinical case study 1

1. An adverse drug reaction is a significant health problem worldwide, with high morbidity and mortality rates ranging from 0.5% to 16.8% in hospitalized children. It is an unpleasant or harmful reaction caused by an intervention related to the use of a drug product. Adverse effects usually predict hazards from future administration and warrant prevention, specific treatment, or alteration of the dosage regimen.
2. The severity of ADRs varies by patient characteristics such as gender, age, genetics, ethnicity, coexisting disorders, or geographic factors. Drug factors include the type of drug, dosage, administration route, treatment duration, and bioavailability.
3. The adverse drug reactions are classified into five categories, which include type A, B, C, D, and E. Type A reactions are predictable from the known pharmacology of a drug and are associated with high morbidity and low mortality rates. Type B reactions are idiosyncratic, bizarre, or novel responses that cannot be predicted from the known pharmacology of a drug and are associated with low morbidity and high mortality. Type C persists for a relatively long time. Type D reactions, called delayed reactions, become apparent after using a medicine. The timing of these may make them more challenging to detect—type E reactions are called end-of-use. They are associated with the withdrawal of a drug.

Clinical case study 2

1. A drug-drug interaction is a pharmacologic or clinical response to administering a combination of drugs that differs from the anticipated effects of the two drugs when given alone.
2. More than 100,000 types of potential drug interactions have been documented, but most do not lead to adverse effects.
3. In an example of a therapeutic drug-drug interaction, drugs used for numbing a specific area, such as local anesthetics, often contain a combination of lidocaine and epinephrine, thereby prolonging the effect of lidocaine in the area of the injection. Reversing agents, such as naloxone (Narcan), are given after surgery to stop the effects of narcotics. Several drugs are given simultaneously for cancer treatment to provide the impact at multiple sites of cancer cell growth. Beneficial drug interactions can improve treatment.

Clinical case study 3

1. Sometimes, interactions occur when a drug affects a preexisting disease or condition. Some disorders can interact with drugs to increase the risk of adverse effects. For example, aspirin increases bleeding in patients with peptic ulcer disease; people with hypertension may be at greater risk for tachycardia with oral decongestants found in over-the-counter cough, cold, and allergy products.
2. Sometimes, helpful drugs in one disease are harmful in another disorder. For example, some beta-blockers taken for heart disease or hypertension can worsen asthma or make it hard for patients with diabetes to know when their blood sugar is too low.
3. Aging can also increase drug interaction risk. For example, sedatives increase the risk of falls in older adults, and lower doses of narcotics are often effective for pain relief. The anticoagulant warfarin causes more bleeding in elderly patients and usually requires a lower dose.

Chapter 8: Drug approval and drug regulations

Clinical case study

1. Today, e-prescribing (electronic prescribing) means that prescriptions originate from a computer instead of the traditional prescription pad. This development has advantages, including tracking patient fulfillment of prescriptions and enabling better monitoring of controlled substance prescriptions.
2. For most drugs, prescriptions are not highly restricted, except for those with a significant potential for abuse. These scheduled drugs are prescribed with certain limitations based on the schedule in which they are classified. Under the Controlled Substances Act, controlled drugs include opioids, sedative-hypnotics, and stimulants in the most rigidly controlled schedules.
3. Schedule II drugs such as oxycodone have high abuse potential that may lead to severe psychological or physical dependence but with accepted medical uses.

Chapter 9: Antimigraine drugs

Clinical case study 1

1. Migraines are signified by pulsating or throbbing pain, usually unilateral, moderate to severe, lasting 4 to 72 hours. They are triggered by hormonal changes (in women), stress, extreme emotions, bright or flickering lights, changes in weather or altitude, alcohol use, certain foods, caffeine, and aspartame.
2. A migraine with an aura develops, with the aura preceding the actual headache by about 30 minutes. The auras are usually visual, such as flashing lights, wavy lines, or vision loss. There may be loss of the ability to speak, tingling, numbness, and weakness in the extremities. The aura may occur without other symptoms, which usually becomes more familiar with continued aging.
3. Severe migraines are treated with serotonin agonists, parenteral dopamine agonists, and narcotic analgesics if these therapies do not work.

Clinical case study 2

1. Migraine without aura is by far the most common type of migraine, affecting 75% of all migraine sufferers. It involves a pulsating headache on one side of the head, which is of moderate to severe intensity.
2. Preventive treatments such as beta-blockers, tricyclic antidepressants, or anti-epilepsy drugs. These medications can reduce the frequency and severity of attacks.
3. Treatments for migraine without aura include over-the-counter painkillers or triptans.

Clinical case study 3

1. Chronic migraine affects about 2% of all migraine sufferers. It is diagnosed when migraines occur 15 or more days per month over three months or longer.

2. The triptans are selective for the 5-HT_1 receptor subtype and are believed to constrict intracranial vessels, stopping migraines whether auras are present.
3. Sumatriptan is contraindicated with uncontrolled hypertension, hypercholesterolemia, a strong family history of cardiovascular disease, chronic severe kidney disease, or hepatic impairment. It must be used cautiously in people with epilepsy.

Chapter 10: Antiseizure drugs

Clinical case study 1

1. Seizure conditions more likely to occur as nocturnal seizures include awakening tonic-clonic seizures, juvenile myoclonic epilepsy, frontal lobe epilepsy, benign Rolandic seizures, and Landau-Kleffner syndrome.
2. Carbamazepine is indicated for tonic-clonic and partial seizures, along with lamotrigine, phenytoin, and valproic acid.
3. In toxic levels, carbamazepine may cause cognitive dysfunction, diplopia, ataxia, drowsiness, induction of hepatic drug metabolism, teratogenicity, and rarely, severe blood dyscrasias and Stevens-Johnson syndrome.

Clinical case study 2

1. An absence of seizure begins in both sides of the brain simultaneously, causing lapses in awareness. The older term for absence seizures was *petit mal seizures*. They start and end quickly, lasting only for a few seconds.
2. The drugs of choice for generalized tonic-clonic seizures include carbamazepine, lamotrigine, phenytoin, and valproic acid.
3. Levetiracetam is an effective monotherapy for newly diagnosed focal epilepsy in adults and is an adjunct drug for partial, myoclonic, and tonic-clonic seizures.

Chapter 11: General anesthesia

Clinical case study 1

1. In general anesthesia, the combined medications used to achieve balanced anesthesia include neuromuscular blockers, opioids, short-acting benzodiazepines, and general anesthetics. Balanced anesthesia begins with administering IV medications before the available drug is given.
2. The respiratory system effects of IV and inhaled general anesthetics include impaired oxygenation, airway irritation, possible laryngospasm, and depressed airway-protective mechanisms.
3. Propofol is now the most widely used intravenous anesthetic because of its high effectiveness and relative safety. It is indicated for induction and maintenance of general anesthesia.

Clinical case study 2

1. Succinylcholine is classified as an anesthesia adjunct and is sold under the trade name Anectine. It is indicated for short-term muscle relaxation in anesthesia, often for the endotracheal intubation procedure.
2. Succinylcholine is contraindicated with malignant hyperthermia, skeletal muscle myopathies, multiple trauma, upper motor neuron injury, extensive or severe burns, extensive denervation of skeletal muscle due to CNS disease or injury, and known hypersensitivity to the drug or its components.
3. Succinylcholine interacts with atracurium, cisatracurium, beta-blockers, inhalation anesthetics, antiarrhythmics, aminoglycosides, bacitracin, clindamycin, lincomycin, polymyxins, tetracyclines, chloroquine, quinine, cholinesterase inhibitors, oral contraceptives, corticosteroids, cyclophosphamide, lithium, magnesium salts, MAO inhibitors, metoclopramide, neostigmine, oxytocin, phenothiazines, procaine, skeletal muscle relaxants, terbutaline, and thiotepa.

Chapter 12: Local anesthesia

Clinical case study 1

1. A spinal block occurs when the local anesthetic penetrates the subarachnoid space between the pia mater and arachnoid membranes. In an epidural block, the local anesthetic is placed into the epidural space, just posterior to the spinal cord or dura mater. The epidural space lies between the posterior longitudinal ligament on the anterior side and the ligamentum flavum posteriorly.
2. Spinal anesthetics work by initially blocking tiny, unmyelinated sympathetic fibers. After this occurs, the myelinated sensory and motor fibers are blocked.
3. A local anesthetic that spreads too high in the spinal column can affect the respiratory muscles, resulting in respiratory distress or failure. Hypotension can also occur because of the developing sympathetic blockade and predisposing factors such as chronic alcohol intake, history of hypertension, and location of the sensory block.

Clinical case study 2

1. The trade name of Novocain is widely known as procaine.
2. Drugs available for local anesthesia are classified as members of the ester or amide families. Amide local anesthetics are generally more therapeutic than esters but can produce more toxic reactions than ester derivatives.
3. Allergic reactions to procaine are usually not in response to the actual drug but to its metabolite, which is known as para-aminobenzoic acid (PABA).

Clinical case study 3

1. Local anesthetics include chemically similar esters and amides, which block sodium channels of the body's excitable membranes. Examples of esters include tetracaine, procaine, benzocaine, and cocaine. The amides include bupivacaine, ropivacaine, and lidocaine.
2. Like prilocaine, lidocaine's half-life is about 1.5 hours. Its length of action is moderate, about 1 to 3 hours.
3. The potential CNS toxicities of local anesthetics include light-headedness, restlessness, sedation, nystagmus, tonic-clonic convulsions, and coma. Other toxicities include respiratory and cardiovascular depression.

Chapter 13: Skeletal muscle relaxants

Clinical case study 1

1. Multiple, rapidly repeated contractions are known as clonic spasms. The other type of muscle spasm, which occurs once over a prolonged period, is called a tonic spasm.
2. Baclofen is often the drug of first choice out of all the skeletal muscle relaxants because of its comprehensive safety margin. It is mainly used for spastic movement disorders, primarily caused by spinal cord injury, multiple sclerosis, or cerebral palsy.
3. Common adverse effects of centrally acting skeletal muscle relaxants such as baclofen include drowsiness, dizziness, weakness, and fatigue. Baclofen also causes headaches, insomnia, dysrhythmias, nausea, vomiting, constipation, and urinary retention.

Clinical case study 2

1. With multiple sclerosis, spasticity occurs in the advanced stages of the disease as myelin sheaths are destroyed. The main motor pathways from the spinal cord to the muscles become interrupted. The affected person's gait is stiff and unbalanced, and they eventually use a wheelchair.
2. Dantrolene, a direct-acting skeletal muscle relaxant, is also indicated for spasticity, especially for the head and neck areas, after spinal cord injury, stroke, or along with multiple sclerosis or cerebral palsy.
3. Tizanidine is contraindicated with psychosis, bradycardia, hypotension, severe liver disease, and decreased kidney function.

Chapter 14: Drug used in parkinson's and other movement disorders

Clinical case study 1

1. The four primary signs of Parkinson's disease are muscle rigidity, bradykinesia, tremors, and postural instability.
2. The two primary medications for Parkinson's disease are the dopaminergic and the anticholinergics. The medications improve symptoms and quality of life, but long-term use results in effects sometimes being gradually lost near the ends of dosing intervals. This can be reduced by adjusting dosing intervals for more frequent doses.
3. Anticholinergics should be avoided in people older than 70 because these individuals are especially susceptible to confusion and hallucinations.

Clinical case study 2

1. Carbidopa-levodopa is classified as a dopaminergic, while trihexyphenidyl is classified as an anticholinergic.
2. The on-off phenomenon of Parkinson's disease is the alteration of symptom-free ("on") and a quick reappearance of symptoms ("off"). The on-off periods can range from a few minutes to several hours. The off periods can occur sometimes, even if the serum drug level is high, and the overall phenomenon is difficult to control. When taking carbidopa-levodopa, doses can be scheduled closer together, or another adjunct medication can be taken during the off period to handle the phenomenon better.
3. Trihexyphenidyl is contraindicated with known hypersensitivity, glaucoma, tardive dyskinesia, cardiac disease, hypertension, prostatic hypertrophy, and liver or kidney impairment.

Chapter 15: Opioid analgesics and antagonists

Clinical case study 1

1. The chronic pain of osteoarthritis is classified as nociceptive somatic chronic pain.
2. About three out of every four chronic pain patients also report depression, and 86% have difficulty sleeping.
3. There is a warning to avoid combined use of opioids with benzodiazepines or other CNS depressants such as alcohol since these combinations can lead to further sedation, respiratory depression, coma, and death. The warnings also discuss the potential risk of addiction, abuse, and misuse.

Clinical case study 2

1. The most common chronic pain condition is persistent low back pain, followed by myofascial pain syndromes.
2. Due to the potential for addiction and abuse and the current opioid crisis, prescribing recommendations for opioids have become more rigid. The legitimate use of these drugs reduces pain successfully, but they can also cause extreme euphoria or an intense "high," leading to dependence and addiction. Factors that must be considered include addiction, abuse, misuse, diversion, dependence, withdrawal, and tolerance.
3. Buprenorphine is used for opioid detoxification, opioid maintenance, and pain management. It is also used for acute, chronic, and opioid dependence. Buprenorphine is a partial opioid receptor agonist that detoxifies and maintains opioid tolerance. It is combined with naloxone in products such as Suboxone. The naloxone is orally inactive, but if snorted or injected, it acts as an opioid antagonist and reverses the effects of buprenorphine, limiting euphoria and risks of an overdose.

Chapter 16: Substance use disorders

Clinical case study 1

1. For cocaine, most users inhale the drug by "snorting" it, taking it orally, or injecting it. The rock form of cocaine is often called crack or crack cocaine and is smoked.

2. Cocaine produces intense euphoria, analgesia, decreased hunger, increased sensory perception, and illusions of physical strength. Large doses increase these effects and cause rapid heartbeat, pupil dilation, elevated body temperature, and sweating.
3. Overdose of cocaine also causes dysrhythmias, stroke, and death from respiratory arrest.

Clinical Case Study 2

1. Hallucinogens such as MDMA can bring on psychoses and related strange behaviors. Stimulants may also cause the same.
2. MDMA is commonly known by the street names of "Ecstasy" or "Molly."
3. The dangerous adverse effects of MDMA include cardiac arrhythmias, heart failure, hypertension, kidney failure, and seizures.

Chapter 17: Neurotransmitters

Clinical case study 1

1. The nicotinic receptors are located in the somatic system, on the motor end plates of skeletal muscle cells, the adrenal medulla, and all postganglionic neurons.
2. The binding of ACh to the nicotinic receptor results in an excitatory effect. The nicotinic receptors are destroyed as *myasthenia gravis* develops.
3. Myasthenia gravis is a chronic autoimmune, neuromuscular disease that causes weakness in the specific skeletal muscles.

Clinical case study 2

1. Problems with the display or use of glutamate are implicated in autism.
2. Problems with the display or use of glutamate are also linked to schizophrenia, obsessive-compulsive disorder, and depression.
3. Autism is a neurological and developmental disorder affecting individuals' interactions, communication, learning, and behavior.

Chapter 18: Adrenergic agonists

Clinical case study 1

1. $Alpha_2$ adrenergic agonists are used to treat hypertension alone or with diuretic agents. They are also used epidurally as an adjunct therapy for severe pain.
2. *Clonidine* works by crossing the blood-brain barrier, stimulating $alpha_2$ receptors in the brainstem to decrease peripheral vascular resistance and lower blood pressure. It is specific for presynaptic two receptors in the vasomotor center.
3. *Clonidine* is also used to treat ADHD, alcohol, opioids, nicotine withdrawal, menopausal flushing, diarrhea, spasticity, and some pain conditions.

Clinical case study 2

1. The $beta_2$ adrenergic agonists are commonly used for asthma. The miscellaneous adrenergic agonists are also sometimes used.
2. Beta2 adrenoreceptors are distributed in the smooth muscle of the bronchioles, blood vessels supplying the brain, heart, kidneys, and the uterus.
3. *Salmeterol* is indicated for moderate-to-severe persistent asthma after previous treatment with a short-acting two agonist in combination with inhaled corticosteroids. The drug is also used for COPD with or without corticosteroids and can be used as monotherapy for exercise-induced bronchospasm.

Chapter 19: Adrenergic antagonists

Clinical case study 1

1. Like the other alpha-adrenergic antagonists, Phenoxybenzamine selectively inhibits alpha adrenoreceptors' actions, producing vasodilation in arterioles to reduce blood pressure. The selective $alpha_1$-antagonists are much safer and are primarily indicated for hypertension. They directly lower blood pressure by blocking alpha1 receptors on arterial smooth muscle.
2. Applications for alpha-receptor antagonists include controlling hypertension and treating patients with peripheral vascular disease, pheochromocytoma, and urinary retention. *Phenoxybenzamine* is also used for hypertension caused by pheochromocytoma and benign prostatic hyperplasia.
3. A contraindication for alpha-receptor antagonists is known hypersensitivity to any of these drugs. Phenoxybenzamine is also contraindicated with coronary artery disease, hypotension, pneumonia, and decreased kidney function.

Clinical case study 2

1. Labetalol non-selectively antagonizes beta-adrenergic receptors but selectively antagonizes alpha-1 adrenergic receptors. After oral administration, the beta-blocking ability is three times that of the alpha-blocking ability. This increases to 6.9 times after IV administration. Antagonism of alpha-1 adrenergic receptors results in vasodilation and decreased vascular resistance.
2. Common adverse effects of beta-receptor antagonists, including labetalol, are dizziness, lethargy, insomnia, and diarrhea. Patients must be taught to take their heart rate and BP and to report a decrease in either. Because these drugs may cause dizziness, patients are advised to change positions slowly. To determine side effects, patients should avoid driving for at least 12 hours after taking the first dose.
3. Labetalol competes with other catecholamines for binding to alpha and beta receptors and has potent yet reversible actions.

Chapter 20: Cholinergic agonists

Clinical case study 1

1. The muscarinic agonists are direct-acting. They enter the synaptic cleft, bind to acetylcholine receptors, and produce the common rest-and-digest responses. Some of these medications cause more acetylcholine to be released into the synaptic cleft, which enhances the physiologic responses to ACh. These agonists work by using the exact mechanism of action as ACh.
2. Bethanechol was approved in 1948 as an oral tablet to stimulate smooth muscle contraction in the digestive and urinary tracts. It is indicated for nonobstructive urinary retention with bladder atony. Off-label uses include treating adynamic ileus and gastric atony.
3. Bethanechol is used cautiously when any disorder that increases GI tract contractions, including recent GI surgery, suspected bowel obstruction, an active ulcer, or inflammatory bowel disease, could worsen. It is also avoided if there is alleged urinary obstruction or recent bladder surgery. Cystitis is another contraindication since the drug can cause bladder contractions to force urine up to the kidneys should the sphincter not open. The drug is also contraindicated with asthma or COPD. It is additionally contraindicated with recent MI, hypotension or hypertension, bradycardia, hyperthyroidism, epilepsy, Parkinson's disease, and peritonitis.

Clinical case study 2

1. Donepezil binds and reversibly inactivates the cholinesterases to inhibit the hydrolysis of acetylcholine. This increases acetylcholine concentrations at cholinergic synapses. Its precise mechanism of action in Alzheimer's disease is not fully understood. The drug also acts as a potent agonist of the $alpha_1$ receptor.
2. Donepezil treats Alzheimer's disease, Lewy body dementia, traumatic brain injury, vascular dementia, and dementia associated with Parkinson's disease.

3. Signs of muscle paralysis signify a cholinergic crisis, respiratory failure, increased respiratory secretions, seizures, coma, and death. A large overdose may require mechanical ventilation to prevent death.

Chapter 21: Cholinergic antagonists

Clinical case study 1

1. The use of muscarinic antagonists has declined due to newer and safer medications being developed.
2. The pharmacokinetics of the muscarinic antagonists are widely similar to *atropine*, with good absorption by almost all routes of administration. Atropine is distributed, crosses the blood-brain barrier and placenta, and small amounts are secreted in the breast milk. It is primarily metabolized in the liver and mostly excreted in the urine. The onset of action is 15 minutes with subcutaneous or IM administration, 30 minutes with oral administration, and 2 to 4 minutes with IV administration. The half-life is 4 hours.
3. Atropine is contraindicated with hyperthyroidism because dysrhythmias may occur. It is contraindicated in severe GI conditions, including ulcerative colitis and ileus, because it can worsen them. Atropine also worsens gastroesophageal reflux disease (GERD) and hiatal hernia, making esophageal injury and aspiration more likely.

Clinical case study 2

1. Some of these drugs, such as ipratropium, block the receptors to decrease the production of cyclic CMP, leading to reduced contraction of smooth muscles in the lung airways. Antimuscarinic antagonists block muscarinic 3 (M3) receptors to prevent acetylcholine binding, resulting in relaxation.
2. Muscarinic antagonists are used for peptic ulcer, irritable bowel syndrome (IBS), dilation of the pupils during ophthalmic examinations, bradycardia, to decrease salivary and respiratory secretions during anesthesia, for bronchodilation, to reverse poisoning with muscarinic mushrooms or organophosphate insecticides, for incontinence, and Parkinsonian symptoms. The antagonists, such as ipratropium, are indicated primarily for treating COPD and asthma exacerbation.
3. Ipratropium may cause dry mouth, sedation, skin flushing, tachycardia, acute angle-closure glaucoma, nausea, palpitations, headache, throat irritation, and urinary retention.

Chapter 22: Anxiety and insomnia drugs

Clinical case study 1

1. The most common anxiety disorders are generalized anxiety disorder, social anxiety disorder, panic disorder, obsessive-compulsive disorder, and post-traumatic stress disorder.
2. Excessive, irrational worry about events or circumstances characterizes generalized anxiety disorder. It often interferes with daily functioning, causing anxiety about health, money, life and death, family, friends, interpersonal relationships, and work.
3. Social anxiety disorder is also known as social phobia. It is characterized by fear and anxiety in social situations, causing extreme distress and impaired ability to function in daily living.

Clinical case study 2

1. Insomnia, acute or chronic, includes trouble falling or staying asleep. Excessive nighttime sleepiness often results in fatigue throughout the day.
2. Insomnia is signified by difficulty falling asleep or staying asleep, awakening too early, or feeling unrefreshed after sleep. It may involve symptoms related to a primary medical illness, a mental illness, other sleep disorders, stressors, or use or exposure to certain substances.
3. The trade name for zolpidem is Ambien. The average daily dosage range is 1.75 to 12.5 mg. The dosage forms are 1.75, 3.5, 5, or 10 mg per oral spray, and the extended-release dosage form is available as 6.25 and 12.5 mg tablets.

Chapter 23: Antidepressants

Clinical case study 1

1. Major depressive disorder (MDD), also known simply as depression, is a mental disorder characterized by at least two weeks of low mood in most situations. It is often accompanied by low self-esteem, loss of interest or pleasure in previously enjoyed activities, low energy, and pain of no identifiable cause.
2. Major depressive disorder runs in families, and those diagnosed have a three times greater chance of having a first-degree relative with the disease.
3. The most effective psychotherapeutic approach to treating depression is cognitive-behavioral therapy (CBT). In some cases, CBT has been proven more effective than antidepressants for major depression. It is also highly beneficial in preventing relapse. Variants of CBT include rational emotive behavior therapy and mindfulness-based cognitive therapy. In contrast, alternative approaches might consist of acceptance and commitment therapy, which focuses on accepting thoughts and feelings while making changes to improve, and interpersonal psychotherapy, which centers on improving interpersonal functioning and relationships. Psychotherapy treats acute symptoms as well as decreases the likelihood of relapses.

Clinical case study 2

1. *Selective serotonin reuptake inhibitors* (SSRIs) are often prescribed as the initial medications for depressive disorders. They are usually first-line drugs since their safety, efficacy, and tolerability are high.
2. The contraindications with the SSRIs include known hypersensitivity, suicidal thoughts, unusual changes in behavior, bradycardia, hypokalemia, hypomagnesemia, recent acute myocardial infarction, seizure disorders, mania, abnormal bleeding, and heart failure.
3. The exact cause of depressive disorders is not always known. However, it is believed to be related to heredity, abnormal levels of neurotransmitters, changes in neuroendocrine function, psychosocial factors, or combinations of all of these. Low mood or sadness often is due to disappointments. These may come from financial problems, illnesses, natural disasters, or deaths of family members and friends.

Chapter 24: Antipsychotic drugs

Clinical case study 1

1. Risperidone is an atypical antipsychotic.
2. Atypical antipsychotics mostly block receptors in the dopamine pathways of the brain. Risperidone mainly decreases brain dopaminergic and serotonergic pathway activity and has a high binding affinity for serotonergic 5-HT2A receptors.
3. Aside from the common adverse effects of the atypical antipsychotics, risperidone often causes gynecomastia. Its adverse severe effects include agranulocytosis. Rarely, risperidone may cause neuroleptic malignant syndrome, such as in this case study.

Clinical case study 2

1. Bipolar disorder is characterized by one or more manic episodes, with or without mixed or psychotic features. A hypomanic stage occurs before progression to full mania. Generally, acute symptoms happen initially, followed by repeated courses of remission and relapse. The remissions are often complete, but many patients have residual symptoms such as manic, depressive, hypomanic, or mixtures of manic and depressive features. The residual symptoms persist for several weeks to six months, with depressive episodes usually lasting longer than manic episodes.
2. Severe bipolar episodes may include psychotic symptoms such as hallucinations or delusions. These psychotic symptoms can be wrongly diagnosed as schizophrenia.
3. Lithium's most serious adverse effects include vomiting, dizziness, diarrhea, cognitive impairment, sedation, and kidney damage.

Chapter 25: Pharmacology of schizophrenia

Clinical case study 1

1. Schizophrenia progresses through several phases, with varied duration and phasic patterns. It involves psychosis, hallucinations, delusions, disordered behavior and speech, flattened affect, cognitive deficits, and occupational and social dysfunction. The five phases are the prodromal, advanced prodromal, early psychosis, middle, and late phases.
2. It is estimated that over 33% of schizophrenia patients are partially or non-compliant about taking their medications. This is serious and increases the risk of relapse, rehospitalizations, self-harm, and treatment costs and reduces the individual's quality of life.
3. With treatment for schizophrenia, most symptoms significantly improve, and the likelihood of a recurrence can be diminished.

Clinical case study 2

1. Hallucinations are sensory perceptions that the person with schizophrenia experiences. They can be auditory, visual, gustatory, olfactory, or tactile, but auditory hallucinations are the most common that are reported.
2. The patient may "hear" voices that abuse, criticize, or comment on their behaviors. The agents may even "talk to each other."
3. Several risk factors contribute to the risk of developing schizophrenia. They include genetics, environment, and structural or functional brain factors. It is not yet possible to use genetic information to predict who will develop schizophrenia. Environmental factors include poverty, stressful surroundings, and exposure to certain viruses or nutritional problems before birth. Differences in brain connections and circuits may be seen in patients with schizophrenia before birth. Changes to the brain during puberty may trigger psychotic episodes in people who are vulnerable due to environmental exposures.

Chapter 26: Attention-deficit/hyperactivity disorder drugs

Clinical case study 1

1. The relative prevalence of ADHD in children is high, affecting approximately 4% of all children, although estimates range from 3% to 11%. It is ranked as the most common neuropsychiatric disorder of childhood. It affects an estimated 5% to 15% of school-age children, with boys affected two to three times more often than girls.
2. Potential causes of ADHD include behavioral, biochemical, genetic, physiologic, and sensorimotor factors. Risk factors include birth weight less than 1,000 grams, head trauma, lead exposure, and potential exposure to alcohol, cocaine, and tobacco during the prenatal period.
3. The most widely used drugs for ADHD are CNS stimulants such as methylphenidate and dextroamphetamine. The dosage is adjusted until an optimal response is achieved. Stimulants make up 75% of the medications taken for ADHD.

Clinical case study 2

1. In adulthood, ADHD is signified by constantly feeling overwhelmed, being a workaholic, excessive talking, having poor tolerance for frustration, a short temper, chronic boredom, quitting jobs abruptly, continual driving infractions, and relationship problems. Adults with ADHD are likelier to have addictions and habits like smoking tobacco products and using illegal substances.
2. It is believed that about 4.4% of adults in the United States have adult attention-deficit disorder. Many eventually realize that they have had a lifelong problem after learning about the diagnosis of ADHD in their children. Many affected adults are of above-average intelligence and highly successful because they have learned strategies that combat their restlessness and lack of attention.
3. The nonstimulant medications such as atomoxetine, developed as of 2003, offer fewer adverse effects plus a longer duration of action (two to four weeks).

Chapter 27: Antihyperlipidemic drugs

Clinical case study 1

1. Bile acid sequestrants (BAS) are FDA-approved for managing hypercholesterolemia.
2. Statins have been linked to some people's muscle pain, digestive problems, and mental fuzziness. Rarely, they may cause liver damage. Rhabdomyolysis is the most severe adverse effect of statin use.
3. Ezetimibe (Zetia) is the only drug in the class of cholesterol-absorption inhibitors.

Clinical case study 2

1. Atherosclerosis is related to dyslipidemia, diabetes mellitus, cigarette smoking, family history, hypertension, obesity, and a sedentary lifestyle. Once the plaques grow or rupture, blood flow can be reduced or obstructed. Atherosclerosis is the most common form of arteriosclerosis. Atherosclerosis is a severe condition resulting in coronary artery disease (CAD), heart attack, and stroke.
2. Triglycerides: Ideal: Below 150 mg/dL. (Borderline high: 150 to 199 mg/dL and High: 200 to 499 mg/dL.)
3. Pitavastatin (Livalo) has a dose range of 1 to 4 mg, and its percentage of LDL lowering capacity is 31 to 41%.

Clinical case study 3

1. Lifestyle changes are the backbone of treating hyperlipidemia. This includes dietary therapy with low total fat, saturated fat, and cholesterol intake. A registered dietitian may be consulted to help patients change their diet. In addition to making healthy food choices, patients must be encouraged to exercise. A reasonable goal is at least 30 minutes of moderate-intensity exercise at least five days a week. All patients should be encouraged to diet and exercise to maintain a healthy weight, limit alcohol use, and avoid tobacco use.
2. For total cholesterol, desirable levels are less than 200 mg/dL. Borderline high levels are 200 to 239 mg/dL, and high levels are 240 mg/dL or higher.
3. For LDL cholesterol, optimal levels are less than 100 mg/dL. **The above** optimal levels are 100 to 129 mg/dL. Borderline high levels are 130 to 159 mg/dL. High levels are 160 to 189 mg/dL, and very high levels are 190 mg/dL or higher.

Chapter 28: Drug effects on angina pectoris and myocardial infarction

Clinical case study 1

1. The four types of angina pectoris include stable angina, relieved by rest and nitroglycerin; unstable angina, induced more quickly than stable angina. This form indicates a worsening coronary artery disease that may progress to myocardial infarction; Prinzmetal's angina is also called *variant angina*. It may occur spontaneously and is unrelated to physical exercise or emotional stress); and microvascular angina is caused by impaired vasodilator reserve, resulting in angina-like chest pain in a person with normal coronary arteries.
2. The cause is usually insufficient coronary blood flow, resulting in a decreased oxygen supply to meet an increased myocardial demand for oxygen in response to physical exertion or emotional stress.
3. Treatment of angina includes nitrates, such as nitroglycerin, isosorbide, beta-adrenergic blockers, and calcium channel blockers. Antiplatelet drugs minimize platelet aggregation and the risk of coronary occlusion. Antilipemic drugs are also given to reduce serum cholesterol or triglyceride levels.

Clinical case study 2

A 38-year-old woman was hospitalized because of severe chest pain that had awakened her from sleep, which radiated to her right shoulder and arm. She was also nauseous on the way to the hospital. The episode lasted about 50 minutes. Her family had no significant atherosclerotic coronary artery disease history, but her mother had hypertension and diabetes mellitus. The patient admitted smoking up to 5 cigarettes daily for six months but did not drink alcohol. The next night in the hospital, the patient experienced additional retrosternal chest tightness for 15 minutes, with more inversions readable on the electrocardiogram (EKG). After a diagnostic cardiac catheterization, the cause of her unstable angina was found to be the dissection of the left anterior descending coronary artery.

Clinical case study 2

1. With unstable angina, the pain increases in frequency and duration. It is induced more quickly than stable angina. This form indicates a worsening coronary artery disease that may progress to myocardial infarction.
2. Coronary atherosclerosis usually occurs at points of turbulence known as vessel bifurcations.
3. Three major anti-ischemia drugs are currently used in managing angina pectoris: β-blockers, nitrates (short- and long-acting), and calcium channel antagonists. Nitrates or β-blockers are usually preferred for the initial treatment of angina, and calcium channel blockers may be added if needed.

Clinical case study 3

1. Angina is chest pain or discomfort caused by insufficient blood flow to the heart muscle. The discomfort may not always be in the chest; it may feel like pressure in the chest, jaw, or arm.
2. Diagnosis of MI is via serial ECGs, serial cardiac markers, and immediate coronary angiography.
3. Aside from reinfarction, the possible complications of acute myocardial infarction include various types of arrhythmias, heart failure, cardiac arrest, angina, infarct extension, cardiogenic shock, mitral valve dysfunctions, aneurysms, cardiac rupture, sinus or AV node dysfunction, embolization, pericarditis, and death. The most common and severe complication of myocardial infarction is arrhythmia.

Chapter 29: Antihypertensive drugs

Clinical case study 1

1. The two main types of hypertension include primary and secondary hypertension. Primary hypertension is multifactorial high blood pressure and does not have one distinct cause. It is also known as idiopathic or essential hypertension. Another medical condition causes secondary hypertension. It can be caused by conditions that affect the kidneys, arteries, heart, or endocrine system.
2. Ninety percent of hypertensive patients are diagnosed with primary hypertension. The remaining 10% of cases are diagnosed with *secondary hypertension*, with identifiable causes or other conditions triggering the hypertension.
3. The risk of an MI or stroke increases for every 20 mm Hg rise in systolic blood pressure and 10 mm Hg rise in diastolic pressure.

Clinical case study 2

1. Factors associated with resistant hypertension are chronic kidney disease, older age, left ventricular hypertrophy, African-American race, female sex, and residence in the southeastern United States. Chronic kidney disease may be the most significant factor affecting resistant hypertension.
2. Before confirming the diagnosis of resistant hypertension, factors such as inappropriate blood pressure technique and lack of medication adherence need to be ruled out.
3. Patients should be encouraged to achieve desired weight loss, restrict salt intake, and reduce alcohol intake to a moderate level. They should also increase regular physical exercise and ingest a high-fiber, low-fat diet.

Clinical case study 3

1. Blood pressure exceeding 180/120 mm Hg is considered a hypertensive crisis (emergency).
2. *Hypertensive crisis* is a frequent cause of admission to the emergency department and may require subsequent access to the hospital. The hypertensive crisis will develop in about 1% of patients with underlying hypertension.
3. Common causes for crisis are nonadherence to antihypertensive medication, lack of a primary care provider, or administration of illicit drugs, such as cocaine.

Chapter 30: Antiarrhythmic drugs

Clinical case study 1

1. Risk factors for atrial fibrillation include advanced age, hypertension, underlying heart and lung disease, congenital heart disease, rheumatic heart disease, mitral stenosis, infarction of the atrial myocardium, and increased alcohol consumption.
2. Atrial fibrillation can be treated with a beta-blocker (esmolol, atenolol) or a calcium channel blocker (verapamil or diltiazem). Depending on patients' symptoms and general health, this medicine may be offered. Digoxin can also be prescribed if other drugs are not suitable. Sometimes, cardioversion can also be used.
3. The complications of atrial fibrillation include stroke, heart failure, cognitive impairment, hypertension, and syncope.

Clinical case study 2

1. The most common causes of ventricular fibrillation include angina, MI, family history of sudden cardiac death, heart surgery, certain medications, electrical shock, electrolyte imbalances, and other arrhythmias.
2. Complications of ventricular fibrillation include hypoxia of the brain, injuries from CPR, long-term disabilities, post-defibrillation arrhythmias, and death.
3. Ventricular fibrillation can be treated with defibrillation and medications. Drugs commonly used for ventricular fibrillation include amiodarone, lidocaine, sotalol, and mexiletine.

Chapter 31: Anti-anemia drugs

Clinical case study 1

1. Iron deficiency anemia happens when patients do not have enough iron. It is usually due to blood loss but may occasionally result in poor iron absorption.
2. Iron deficiency anemia can be diagnosed by measuring a complete blood count. Additional tests may be ordered to evaluate serum ferritin levels, iron, total iron-binding capacity, and transferrin. For patients with iron deficiency, blood tests may reveal low Hg and Hct, low mean cellular volume (MCV), low ferritin, low serum iron, and low iron saturation.
3. The primary mechanism of action of ferrous sulfate is to combine with porphyrin and globin chains to form hemoglobin, which is needed for oxygen delivery from the lungs to other tissues.

Clinical case study 2

1. Pernicious anemia is a complex disease with a clear autoimmune basis. It is a megaloblastic anemia caused by vitamin B12 deficiency secondary to intrinsic factor deficiency. Parietal cells produce and secrete intrinsic factors that bind B12 and facilitate its transport to the terminal ileum for absorption. Vitamin B12 is essential for erythropoiesis and nerve myelination. Common symptoms include headaches, fatigue, weight loss, pale skin, depression, dementia, and peripheral neuropathy.
2. Cyanocobalamin is a synthetic vitamin B12 compound used to treat pernicious anemia, impairment of B12 absorption, Helicobacter pylori infection, gastric atrophy, total or partial gastrectomy, small bowel bacteria overgrowth, pancreatic insufficiency, bowel or pancreas cancers, and malnutrition.
3. The adverse effects of cyanocobalamin include dyspnea, peripheral vascular thrombosis, weight gain, pulmonary edema, and congestive heart failure. Other adverse effects include leg cramps, irregular heartbeats, tingling/numbness, hypokalemia, fatigue, numbness, and joint pain.

Chapter 32: Drugs used in coagulation disorders

Clinical case study 1

1. DVT is the most common cause of pulmonary embolism. Other less frequent sources include fat embolus, amniotic fluid embolus, air bubbles, and DVT in the upper body. Risk factors for pulmonary embolism include a

family history of blood clotting disorders, surgery or injury (especially to the legs), extended bed rest, flying or riding long distances, paralysis, older age, obesity, cigarette smoking, and cancer therapy.
2. Medical history, physical exam, chest X-ray, CAT scan, electrocardiogram, duplex ultrasound, and pulmonary angiogram are performed to diagnose pulmonary embolism.
3. Treatment for PE includes anticoagulants, fibrinolytic therapy, vena cava filter, pulmonary embolectomy, and percutaneous thrombectomy.

Clinical case study 2

1. Dabigatran, rivaroxaban, and apixaban are the newest anticoagulants approved by the FDA in the U.S. Each drug prevents blood clots by inhibiting one clotting factor. These new agents offer several advantages over warfarin.
2. Direct thrombin inhibitors are used for treatments or prevention of acute coronary syndrome, blood clots in the heart due to atrial fibrillation, heparin-induced thrombocytopenia, and VTE. They are a novel class of drugs that have been developed as an effective alternative mode of anticoagulation, especially in patients who suffer from heparin-induced thrombocytopenia, who require dialysis, cardiopulmonary bypass, and for the management of thromboembolic disorders.
3. Direct thrombin inhibitors are contraindicated in severe renal impairment or hemodialysis, hypersensitivity, impairment of hemostasis, active pathologic bleeding, and mechanical prosthetic heart valves.

Chapter 33: Drugs used in heart failure

Clinical case study 1

1. Unhealthy lifestyle habits, such as an unhealthy diet, smoking, using cocaine or other illegal drugs, heavy alcohol use, and lack of physical activity, increase your risk of heart failure.
2. Heart or blood vessel conditions, severe lung disease, or infections like HIV or SARS-CoV-2 raise the risks. Cardiomyopathy, coronary artery disease, hypertension, MI, arrhythmia, diabetes, kidney disease, obesity, or valve abnormalities are also risk factors.
3. Dyspnea usually occurs during exertion and is relieved by rest. Worsening heart failure causes dyspnea at rest and at night, sometimes with a nocturnal cough. As the condition advances, orthopnea is common.

Clinical case study 2

1. Rales are described as an abnormal rattling sound heard when examining unhealthy lungs with a stethoscope.
2. Jugular vein distention occurs as a later symptom of heart failure.
3. The EF is determined by dividing the amount of blood pumped out during contraction ("ejected" from the left ventricle) by the amount at the beginning of the heartbeat. A typical ejection fraction is more significant than 60% and is considered abnormal when below 40%.

Clinical case study 3

1. The most common symptoms are dyspnea, rales, fatigue, and reflecting pulmonary congestion due to low cardiac output.
2. Pitting edema involves a swollen body part with a pit (dimple) after being pressed for a few seconds.
3. Treatment must be immediate for those with acute or worsening heart failure caused by disorders such as acute MI, atrial fibrillation with a very rapid ventricular rate, acute valvular regurgitation, severe hypertension, or pulmonary edema.

Chapter 34: Diuretics

Clinical case study 1

1. Furosemide (Lasix) is classified as a loop diuretic.
2. Thiazide and thiazide-like diuretics are traditionally known as first-line therapy for hypertension uncomplicated by other disease states.

3. Diuretics combined with another antihypertensive agent are more effective in lowering blood pressure than each agent alone. For this reason, they are commonly combined with other antihypertensive agents.

Clinical case study 2

1. Spironolactone is classified as an aldosterone antagonist as well as a potassium-sparing diuretic.
2. Thiazide and thiazide-like diuretics, loop diuretics, and carbonic anhydrase inhibitors are avoided in patients with hyponatremia.
3. Loop diuretics reduce sodium chloride reabsorption in the thick ascending limb of the loop of Henle. This is achieved by inhibiting the Na-K-2Cl carrier in the luminal membrane in this segment, thereby minimizing the entry of luminal sodium and chloride into the cell.

Clinical case study 3

1. Loop diuretics are usually the first choice for treating pulmonary edema, heart failure, nephrotic syndrome, and hepatic cirrhosis; they are also used for hypertension.
2. Spironolactone is metabolized in the liver to canrenone, which has a much longer half-life and is probably responsible for most of the diuretic effect.
3. Potassium-sparing diuretics are contraindicated in patients with hyperkalemia or at risk of developing hyperkalemia. They are also contraindicated in advanced renal failure or chronic kidney disease because these patients are at risk of hyperkalemia. Spironolactone is pregnancy category C, and along with triamterene, it should be avoided in pregnant patients. Eplerenone is a category B medication.

Chapter 35: Drugs affecting the renin-angiotensin-aldosterone system

Clinical case study 1

1. Lisinopril prevents the conversion of angiotensin I to angiotensin II, a potent vasoconstrictor. A decrease in angiotensin II subsequently causes a reduction in aldosterone secretion.
2. The FDA has approved lisinopril for the management of hypertension in adults and children six years of age and older. It is also used as adjunctive therapy in the treatment of heart failure.
3. Lisinopril should be avoided in patients with a history of angioedema, renal failure, bilateral renal artery stenosis, or hyperkalemia. It is contraindicated in pregnant women, category Class D, due to its teratogenic effects.

Clinical case study 2

1. Losartan inhibits angiotensin II-induced vasopressin and adrenal catecholamine release. It also inhibits angiotensin II-induced vasoconstriction and the effects of aldosterone, thereby lowering blood pressure.
2. Losartan is contraindicated in hypersensitivity to losartan or any of its components. It should be avoided during pregnancy as it causes oligohydramnios, resulting in fetal lung hypoplasia and skeletal deformities. Potential neonatal adverse effects are skull hypoplasia, hypotension, renal failure, anuria, and death. Therefore, therapy with the drug should be discontinued when pregnancy is detected.
3. The primary adverse effects of losartan include angioedema, hypotension, hyperkalemia, and renal damage. Other adverse effects are chest pain, anemia, dizziness, fatigue, hypoglycemia, urinary tract infection, nausea, diarrhea, and cough.

Chapter 37: Pharmacotherapy of thyroid disorders

Clinical case study 1

1. Congenital hypothyroidism is usually diagnosed after a standard heel-prick blood sample is obtained at 1 to 2 days of age, which measures levels of T4 and TSH. If the first result is positive, another example is taken from a vein instead of the heel for confirmation. An ultrasound exam or thyroid scan may be recommended to determine the condition's specific cause.

2. Usually, levothyroxine—a synthetic but identical form of thyroxine—is used daily. This medication is often needed throughout the patient's life.
3. Congenital hypothyroidism has been linked to miscarriage, preeclampsia, anemia, stillbirth, and the offspring of patients developing it themselves. It may also cause infertility.

Clinical case study 2

1. The diagnosis is probably the autoimmune condition known as Hashimoto's thyroiditis.
2. For this condition, it is usually recommended that the TSH level be kept under 3.0 milli-international units per liter.
3. Hashimoto's thyroiditis is related to lupus erythematosus, type 1 diabetes, rheumatoid arthritis, and other autoimmune conditions.

Clinical case study 3

1. The likely cause is a toxic multinodular goiter, resulting in symptoms of hyperthyroidism.
2. A thyroid scan is needed to verify the autonomy of the thyroid nodules.
3. Treatment options include radioactive iodine or surgery with antithyroid drug and iodine pre-treatment.

Chapter 38: Adrenocorticosteroids and aldosterone antagonists

Clinical case study 1

1. Corticosteroids are commonly used to treat rheumatoid arthritis, systemic lupus erythematosus, asthma exacerbation, COPD, angioedema, allergy rhinitis, sarcoidosis, contact dermatitis, adrenal insufficiency, congenital adrenal hyperplasia, and replacement therapy after removing pituitary or adrenal cortex tumors.
2. Corticosteroids should be avoided in patients with hypersensitivity to any component of the formulation, concurrent administration of live or live-attenuated vaccines, diabetes mellitus, systemic fungal infection, uncontrolled hyperglycemia, osteoporosis, glaucoma, uncontrolled hypertension, herpes simplex keratitis, varicella infection, and joint infection. Additional relative contraindications include peptic ulcer disease, congestive heart failure, and viral or bacterial infections not controlled by anti-infectives.
3. The adverse effects of corticosteroids depend on the dose, type of steroid, and length of treatment. Adverse effects are more common at higher dosages and with chronic use, though they are not limited to these cases. These effects are seen in up to 90% of patients who take them for more than sixty days. The common adverse effects include weight gain, increased appetite, fatigue, edema, a "puffy" face, acne, and mood changes. Other adverse effects might be osteoporosis, hypertension, gastritis, insomnia, cataracts, glaucoma, diabetes, and agitation.

Clinical case study 2

1. The clinical manifestations of Addison's disease do not appear until at least 90% of the adrenal cortex has been compromised. Addison's disease symptoms usually occur slowly, often over months, and include extreme fatigue, hypotension, weight loss, salt craving, depression, irritability, skin pigmentations, nausea, diarrhea, or vomiting.
2. The causes of Addison's disease may be autoimmune adrenalitis, genetics, tuberculosis, low cortisol levels, or metastatic cancers.
3. Addison's disease is treated with medication to replace the missing hormones. Treatment usually involves steroid replacement therapy for life. Corticosteroid medicines are used to replace the hormones cortisol and aldosterone.

Clinical case study 3

1. The signs and symptoms associated with Conn's syndrome include hypertension, hypokalemia, headache, fatigue, muscle cramps, and palpitations, anxiety, depression, and memory difficulties.
2. Conn's syndrome (hyperaldosteronism) may be primary or secondary. Primary hyperaldosteronism may be caused by hyperplasia or tumors that result in the overproduction of aldosterone. Secondary hyperaldosteronism may be caused by suppression of the renin-angiotensin system and decreased plasma renin activity.

3. The treatment of hyperaldosteronism depends on the cause. If a tumor causes it, adrenalectomy is needed. However, the main goal is to manage hypertension. The most common medications to treat Conn's syndrome are aldosterone antagonists.

Chapter 39: Gonadal hormones and inhibitors

Clinical case study 1

1. Menopause occurs around age 50. For several years preceding menopause, anovulatory cycles become more common. Accordingly, estrogen secretion gradually declines and eventually ceases. Because of the decreased estrogen level, there is reduced negative feedback on the anterior pituitary and increased secretion and pulsatility of FSH and LH at menopause.
2. The causes of menopause may include naturally declining reproductive hormones and oophorectomy, chemotherapy, and radiotherapy.
3. The signs and symptoms of menopause include the decrease of ovarian estrogen and atrophy of the vaginal epithelium, decreased vaginal secretions, decreased breast mass, bone loss, hot flashes, night sweats, dry skin, weight gain, insomnia, sexual dysfunction, urinary incontinence, and mood changes.

Clinical case study 2

1. The causes of infertility might be problems with semen or sperm, a testicular infection, cancer or surgery, mumps, cryptorchidism, or testosterone deficiency. The causes of infertility in females may include ovulation disorders, hyper- or hypothyroidism, polycystic ovary syndrome, endometriosis, and tubal ligation.
2. Clinical indications of clomiphene include ovulatory dysfunction in women desiring pregnancy and male infertility. It is also used in patients diagnosed with polycystic ovarian syndrome, amenorrhea-galactorrhea syndrome, post-oral-contraceptive amenorrhea, and psychogenic amenorrhea. Patients indicated for clomiphene therapy must not have an ovarian cyst, vaginal bleeding, or hepatic impairment.
3. The use of clomiphene is contraindicated in pregnancy, breastfeeding, hepatic impairment, pituitary tumor, endometrial cancer, uterine bleeding, and risk of hypertriglyceridemia.

Clinical case study 3

1. Testosterone replacement therapy is indicated for the treatment of patients with hypogonadism, sexual dysfunction in men, and hot flashes in women. Potential benefits include increased libido and energy levels, bone density, strength, and muscle and cardioprotective effects. Both men and women use a low dose of testosterone, which various routes of administration can take. Testosterone therapy is often used to treat symptoms of hormone deficiency in pre and postmenopausal women.
2. Testosterone is contraindicated in patients with breast or prostate cancers, myocardial infarction, stroke, and untreated obstructive sleep apnea.
3. The adverse effects of testosterone in men include polycythemia, peripheral edema, and cardiac and hepatic dysfunction. Other adverse effects may include hesitation, erectile dysfunction, depression, chest pain, and breast swelling. However, adverse effects of testosterone in women are uncommon if levels are maintained within the female physiological range. The most common are weight gain, hirsutism, and acne, usually reversible with a reduction in dosage or discontinuation.

Chapter 40: Diabetes mellitus and antidiabetic drugs

Clinical case study 1

1. Autoimmunity is considered the primary factor in the pathophysiology of T1D. In a genetically susceptible individual, viral infection may stimulate the production of antibodies against a viral protein, triggering an autoimmune response against antigenically similar beta-cell molecules.

2. Laboratory tests to diagnose diabetes include a fasting blood sugar test, glucose tolerance test, **hemoglobin** A1C test, random blood sugar test, and urine test. In 90% of type 1 diabetes cases, one of these autoantibodies is positive. However, the longer the time passed since diagnosis, the more likely the present autoantibodies will have diminished.
3. There are three primary types of insulin: long-acting, intermediate-acting, and "rapid, ultra-rapid, and short-acting."

Clinical case study 2

1. T2D is often associated with genetic predispositions, environmental factors, lifestyle choices, and the dynamic interactions between these aspects. This ailment is a disease state that involves the dysfunction of insulin-producing pancreatic beta cells, insulin hormone resistance in body cells, or a combination of both. T2D typically begins with a body cell's resistance to insulin, which worsens over time.
2. The classifications of antidiabetic drugs for type 2 diabetes mellitus include biguanide metformin, thiazolidinediones, sulfonylureas, meglitinides, dipeptidyl peptidase-4 inhibitors, glucagon-like-peptide-1 receptor agonists, sodium-glucose-like transporter-2 inhibitors, the amylin mimetic pramlintide, alpha-glucosidase inhibitors, the dopamine agonist bromocriptine, and the bile acid sequestrant colesevelam.
3. The various sulfonylureas include glimepiride, glipizide, and glyburide. Contraindications to the use of sulfonylureas include hypersensitivity to them or drugs with similar structures. Another contraindication is pregnancy. Caution must be used in cases of reduced renal or hepatic function.

Chapter 42: Drugs used for peptic ulcer disease

Clinical case study 1

1. Peptic ulcer disease usually occurs in the stomach and proximal duodenum but may also involve the lower esophagus **or** distal duodenum.
2. The two most common causes of peptic ulcers are infection with Helicobacter pylori and long-term use of nonsteroidal anti-inflammatory drugs such as Advil, Motrin IB, and naproxen sodium (Aleve).
3. The medications used to treat peptic ulcer disease include proton pump inhibitors, H2-receptor antagonists, and antacids.

Clinical case study 2

1. Helicobacter pylori infections are usually treated with two or more antibiotics simultaneously. This helps prevent the bacteria from developing a resistance to one of them.
2. These medications include proton pump inhibitors, bismuth subsalicylate, and histamine (H-2) blockers.
3. Repeat testing for H. pylori is done at least four weeks after treatment. If the tests reveal the infection is still present, additional treatment with a different combination of antibiotics may be required.

Chapter 43: Drugs used for bowel disease and other GI conditions

Clinical case study 1

1. Crohn's disease is one type of inflammatory bowel disease (IBD), a set of chronic, relapsing conditions of unknown origin. It is also known as granulomatous colitis, ileocolitis, and regional enteritis. It is an idiopathic inflammatory disorder that can affect any part of the GI tract, but it usually affects the distal small intestine and proximal large colon.
2. The inflammatory process of Crohn's disease starts in the intestinal submucosa. It spreads to involve the mucosa and serosa in areas that overlie lymphoid tissue. Progression involves neutrophil infiltration of the crypts, leading to abscesses and crypt destruction. The ileocolon is usually involved, though the large and small intestines can also be affected. The inflammation may affect specific haustral segments, creating skip lesions.
3. Sulfasalazine is taken orally and helps reduce irritation and swelling of the intestinal linings. It usually becomes effective in 2 to 4 weeks. However, sulfasalazine should be combined with daily folic acid.

Clinical case study 2

1. Ulcerative colitis can causes ulceration of the colonic mucosa. It extends proximally from the rectum into the colon. Lesions appear in susceptible people between ages 20 and 40.
2. Sulfasalazine treats and prevents acute attacks of mild to moderate ulcerative colitis by helping reduce inflammation and other disease symptoms. It helps stop the body from producing chemicals that cause GI redness and swelling.
3. Sulfasalazine must be avoided if the patient has a history of allergies, significant kidney or liver disease, porphyria, or a glucose-6-phosphate dehydrogenase deficiency.

Clinical case study 3

1. Common factors include reduced colonic motility, delayed stool transit, impaired rectal sensation, and ineffective coordination of the pelvic floor muscles during defecation.
2. The pharmacotherapy of constipation includes laxatives and cathartics. Laxatives soften hard stools or stimulate the movement of the bowels, while cathartics accelerate defecation.
3. Psyllium mucilloid helps relieve constipation, treat irritable bowel syndrome, hemorrhoids, and other GI problems, and help regulate blood glucose levels in patients with diabetes mellitus.

Chapter 44: Vitamins and minerals

Clinical case study 1

1. Common symptoms include chronic fatigue, muscle weakness, bone pain, and an increased risk of falls and fractures.
2. Older adults are at higher risk due to reduced skin synthesis of vitamin D, less outdoor time, and dietary insufficiencies.
3. Interventions include vitamin D supplementation, increased dietary intake of vitamin D-rich foods, and safe sun exposure.

Clinical case study 2

1. Neurological symptoms of vitamin B12 deficiency can include tingling and numbness in the extremities, difficulty concentrating, memory problems, and, in severe cases, neurological damage.
2. Vegans are at risk because vitamin B12 is primarily found in animal products. Without supplementation or consumption of fortified foods, vegans can become deficient.
3. Prevention can be achieved by regularly consuming vitamin B12 supplements, B12-fortified foods, and periodic blood tests to monitor B12 levels.

Chapter 46: Asthma, COPD, and cystic fibrosis drugs

Clinical case study 1

1. The most critical factors for developing asthma are the history of atopic diseases (allergic rhinitis, viral respiratory infection during early childhood, or dermatitis. Respiratory syncytial virus is the most common cause of bronchiolitis in children under one year of age and is associated with wheezing in later childhood.
2. Albuterol acts on β2-adrenergic receptors, inducing bronchial smooth muscle relaxation and inhibiting immediate hypersensitivity mediator release, particularly from mast cells. Although albuterol also affects β1-adrenergic receptors, the impact is minimal, exerting little effect on the heart rate. Anticholinergic agents are competitive antagonists of the neurotransmitter acetylcholine at receptor sites within the cholinergic system.
3. Albuterol is contraindicated in patients with a history of hypersensitivity to it. Rare cases of hypersensitivity reactions, including urticaria, angioedema, and rash, have been reported after the use of albuterol sulfate. The use of anticholinergics requires caution, particularly with older adults.

Clinical case study 2

1. Smoking and air pollution are the most common causes of COPD. People with COPD are at higher risk of other health problems.
2. The clinical manifestations of COPD are dyspnea on exertion, cough, wheezing, fatigue, weight loss, and progressive disability.
3. Various therapeutic medications are used for COPD, including bronchodilators, corticosteroids, and antibiotics, which could be administrated alone or in combination.

Clinical case study 3

1. Cystic fibrosis is a progressive genetic disease that affects the lungs, pancreas, and other organs.
2. Patients with CF may have various signs and symptoms, including wheezing, dyspnea, frequent pneumonia or bronchitis, persistent coughing, poor growth or weight gain, salty-tasting skin, difficulty with bowel movements, and clubbing of fingers.
3. Cystic fibrosis may be assessed with newborn screening, sweat test, genetic test, chest X-ray, lung function test, and sputum culture.

Chapter 47: Allergic rhinitis and common cold drugs

Clinical case study 1

1. The pathophysiology of allergic rhinitis involves early and late allergic responses. It is triggered by exposure to allergens recognized by antigen-specific immunoglobulin E on mast cells and basophil receptors in presensitized individuals. The early-phase reaction is signified by mast cell degranulation. This phase is linked to a rapid onset of acute nasal symptoms over minutes, plus ocular symptoms.
2. Fexofenadine is a nondrowsy second-generation antihistamine over-the-counter treatment for various allergic symptoms.
3. Histamine is released if the body encounters a threat from an allergen. It causes vessels to swell and dilate, leading to allergy symptoms.

Clinical case study 2

1. Pseudoephedrine relieves nasal or sinus congestion caused by the common cold, sinusitis, hay fever, and other respiratory allergies. It is also used to relieve ear congestion caused by otitis media. Some of these preparations are available only with a prescription.
2. Contraindications to pseudoephedrine use include hypersensitivity to the drug, hypertension, coronary artery disease, liver or renal impairment, benign prostatic hyperplasia, diabetes mellitus, hyperthyroidism, narrow-angle glaucoma, mental agitation, and treatment with monoamine oxidase inhibitors currently or in the last two weeks. Pseudoephedrine is also contraindicated in pregnancy, lactation, and age under two years. The extended-release form of the drug should not be used until the age of 12 years.
3. Dextromethorphan temporarily relieves coughs caused by the flu, the common cold, or other conditions. It does not cure the cause of the cough or speed recovery. It is indicated in chronic dry cough or unproductive cough. It is also used for acute dry cough that interferes with normal function or sleep.

Chapter 48: Antiviral drugs

Clinical case study 1

1. Acyclovir is used to treat the symptoms of chickenpox, shingles, and herpes virus infections of the genitals, lips, mouth, skin, and nerves, as well as herpes virus infections in newborns. It is also used to prevent recurrent genital herpes infections. Acyclovir is best used as soon as possible after the symptoms of herpes infection or shingles occur.

2. Acyclovir is contraindicated in patients with kidney disease, a history of allergy to the medication, pregnancy, and lactation. It has been shown to cross the placenta.
3. The adverse effects of acyclovir taken orally include allergic reactions, headaches, dizziness, confusion, hallucinations, seizures, sensitivity to sunlight, itchy, dry, flaky skin, nausea, vomiting, and diarrhea.

Clinical case study 2

1. Tenofovir alafenamide has a very low bioavailability when orally administered. It is eliminated in the urine by tubular secretion and glomerular filtration. Tenofovir's half-life is 32 hours. The clearance of tenofovir is highly dependent on the patient's renal stage.
2. Tenofovir alafenamide is contraindicated in patients with liver disease other than Hep B, kidney disease, and HIV positive.
3. Tenofovir's adverse effects include dizziness, tachycardia, back pain, muscle stiffness, dyspnea, cough, fever, chest pain, chills, skin redness, loss of appetite, and diarrhea. Other adverse effects include hematuria, icterus, edema, insomnia, seizures, and hostility.

Clinical case study 3

1. Didanosine inhibits HIV replication by competing with naturally occurring adenosine for incorporation into the growing viral DNA chain, inhibiting the viral polymerase and terminating the chain.
2. Common adverse effects of didanosine include rash, fever, headache, diarrhea, nausea, vomiting, abdominal pain, and asthenia. Other adverse effects include severe hypersensitivity reactions, hepatotoxicity, severe metabolic acidosis, peripheral neuropathy, lipodystrophy, and pancreatitis.
3. Zidovudine is contraindicated for patients with severe life-threatening hypersensitivity reactions to the drug, including anaphylaxis and Stevens-Johnson syndrome. Anaphylaxis may present with dyspnea, diffuse rash, and hypotension. Stevens-Johnson syndrome is an excruciating blistering skin condition. If any of these symptoms arise, prompt discontinuation of zidovudine therapy is critical.

Chapter 49: Antibacterial drugs

Clinical case study 1

1. The most common indications for penicillin G include pneumonia, strep throat, staph infection, diphtheria, meningitis, gonorrhea, and syphilis.
2. Allergic reactions to penicillin G manifest as laryngospasm, urticaria, bronchospasm, edema, pruritis, hypotension, vascular collapse, and death.
3. To manage penicillin injection reactions, corticosteroids, epinephrine injection (EpiPen), antihistamines, bronchodilators, and immunotherapy (desensitization).

Clinical case study 2

1. Vancomycin is bactericidal by inhibiting the polymerization of peptidoglycans in the bacterial cell wall. Therefore, it prevents the synthesis and polymerization within the peptidoglycan layer. This inhibition weakens bacterial cell walls and ultimately causes leakage of intracellular components, resulting in bacterial cell death.
2.Vancomycin treats and prevents various bacterial infections caused by gram-positive bacteria, including MRSA. It is also effective for streptococci, enterococci, and methicillin-susceptible *Staphylococcus aureus* (MSSA) infections. Vancomycin is also used to treat *Clostridioides difficile*-associated diarrhea, pseudomembranous colitis, *staphylococcus enterocolitis,* osteomyelitis, *and* endocarditis.
3. Vancomycin is associated with nephrotoxicity. Generally, this toxicity is presented as proximal tubular cell injury with or without necrosis and as acute interstitial nephritis. Ototoxicity is rare with vancomycin monotherapy. However, it is common in patients receiving excessive vancomycin doses and concurrent ototoxic medications such as aminoglycosides, loop diuretics, and antineoplastic agents.

Clinical case study 3

1. Tetracyclines are broad-spectrum antibiotics that work against many gram-positive and gram-negative bacteria and atypical organisms such as chlamydiae, mycoplasmas, rickettsiae, and protozoan parasites.
   2.The tetracyclines are contraindicated in pregnancy because of the risk of hepatotoxicity in the mother, the potential for permanent discoloration of teeth in the fetus, as well as impairment of fetal long bone growth. They should be avoided in children before age eight.
3. The most common adverse effects of tetracyclines include GI tract such as abdominal pain, nausea, vomiting, diarrhea, and loss of appetite.

Chapter 50: Antituberculosis drugs

Clinical case study 1

1. Primary tuberculosis is a disease that develops in a previously unexposed and, therefore, unsensitized person. Clinically significant disease develops in about 5% of newly infected people. With primary tuberculosis, the source of the organism is exogenous. Secondary tuberculosis is the pattern of disease that arises in a previously sensitized host. It may follow shortly after primary tuberculosis, but more commonly, it appears many years after the initial infection, usually when host resistance is weakened. It most commonly stems from the reactivation of a latent infection.
2. The most common treatment for active TB is isoniazid in combination with the other first-line drugs.
3. Generally, MAC is treated with daily doses of three antimicrobials for at least 12 months after sputum culture conversion. First-line drugs often include azithromycin or clarithromycin, ethambutol, and either rifampin or rifabutin. Additional agents, especially in patients with cavitary or advanced bronchiectatic lung diseases, include amikacin and streptomycin.

Clinical case study 2

1. Leprosy, or Hansen disease, is a slowly progressive infection caused by M. leprae that mainly affects the skin and peripheral nerves. Despite its low communicability, leprosy remains endemic among people living in several developing tropical nations.
2. Dapsone is an antibiotic used in multidrug regimens to treat leprosy and dermatitis herpetiformis. Initially investigated as an antibiotic agent in 1937, it was first used for leprosy treatment in 1945.
3. The mycobacteria that most commonly cause TB and leprosy are found in the soil and indoor and outdoor water sources and are recognized to colonize poorly sanitized medical equipment. Atypical mycobacteria most commonly infect immunocompromised individuals and young children.

Chapter 51: Antifungal drugs

Clinical case study 1

1. Superficial fungal infections include tinea capitis (scalp), tinea cruris (the groin and inner thighs), tinea pedis (athlete's foot), tinea corporis, tinea manuum (hands), and tinea barbae (face and facial hair). Candidal infections cause skin and mucous membranes, which are also common. They can cause oral thrush, diaper rash, and vaginal yeast.
2. Nystatin is a polyene ionophore antifungal used to treat cutaneous, mucocutaneous, and gastrointestinal mycotic infections, particularly those caused by candida species.
3. The adverse effects of griseofulvin include loss of appetite, nausea, vomiting, diarrhea, headaches, fatigue, dizziness, confusion, insomnia, fever, dyspnea, hematuria, and allergic reactions. Other adverse effects include photosensitivity, fixed drug eruption, petechiae, pruritus, and urticaria. It may also worsen lupus or porphyria.

Clinical case study 2

1. Systemic fungal infections include coccidioidomycosis, blastomycosis, histoplasmosis, cryptococcosis, mucormycosis, aspergillosis, pneumocystis pneumonia, and systemic candidiasis.
2. Amphotericin B acts by binding to ergosterol in the cell membrane of most fungi. After binding with ergosterol, amphotericin B causes the formation of ion channels, leading to the loss of protons and monovalent cations, which results in depolarization and concentration-dependent cell killing.
3. Amphotericin B may cause headaches, chills, vomiting, stomach pain, fatigue, and dysuria. The most severe adverse effects include anaphylaxis, nephrotoxicity, metabolic academia hypokalemia, and hypomagnesemia.

Chapter 52: Antiprotozoal drugs

Clinical case study 1

1. Malaria is a severe infection and always requires treatment with medicine. Multiple drugs must be used to prevent and treat malaria.
2. Chloroquine targets the erythrocytic stage of malaria, which causes symptomatic illness. It has been used as an antimalarial drug since World War II.
3. For malaria prevention, 500 mg is typically given orally two weeks before, during, and up to 8 weeks after exposure to an endemic area, taken weekly.

Clinical case study 2

1. Metronidazole inhibits protein synthesis by interacting with DNA. It causes a loss of helical DNA structure and strand breakage, which causes cell death in susceptible organisms.
2. Metronidazole treats protozoal infections such as Tr*ichomoniasis vaginalis*, *Entamoeba histolytica*, *Giardia lamblia*, blastocysts, and *Balantidium coli.* It is also used to treat intestinal amebiases, liver amebiasis, bacterial septicemia, bone and joint infections, endocarditis, lower respiratory tract infections, meningitis, brain abscess, endometritis, bacterial vaginosis, and surgical prophylaxis colorectal surgeries. The extended-release tablets are used to treat women with vaginal infections. It is available for oral use, injection, and topical use. The oral medication comes as a tablet, capsule, or suspension. Metronidazole can also be used intravenously or as a topical application gel.
3. The adverse effects of metronidazole include headache, nausea, vomiting, diarrhea, a slightly metallic taste, vaginitis, confusion, dizziness, genital pruritus, abdominal pain, xerostomia, dysmenorrhea, urine, urinary tract infection, bacterial infection, flu-like symptoms, pharyngitis, and sinusitis. Alcohol can cause stomach pain, hot flashes, dyspnea, palpitations, and headaches.

Chapter 53: Cancer chemotherapy

Clinical case study 1

1. Conventional (traditional) chemotherapy, such as doxorubicin and eto-poside, will cause cell death of cancerous and healthy cells. This leads to many of the general toxicities and adverse effects seen with traditional chemotherapy, such as myelosuppression, nausea, and vomiting.
2. Biologic therapies consist of targeted therapies, such as monoclonal antibodies and tyrosine kinase inhibitors, and immune-mediated therapies, which can use the patient's immune system to begin an attack on the cancerous cells. Several therapeutic monoclonal antibodies are now available. Rituximab and trastuzumab were approved in the late 1990s to treat lymphoma and breast cancer, which is a new approach to cancer treatment.
3. Paclitaxel is an antimicrotubule agent that is also classified as a polymerizing agent.

Clinical case study 2

1. The trade name of capecitabine is Xeloda, and it is administered orally.
2. Antimetabolites are among the most important agents used in cancer chemotherapy. They are the next class of substances that may compete, replace, or inhibit some specific metabolites. They represent a relatively large group

of anticancer drugs that structurally resemble natural substrates but differ enough to interfere with their metabolism. There are three types of antimetabolites. They are also called antimetabolite antagonists. Purine antagonists, pyrimidine antagonists, and folic acid antagonists are examples of antimetabolites.
3. Antimetabolites prevent cancer cell growth by affecting DNA production; they are only effective against cells actively participating in cell metabolism.

Chapter 54: Immunizations

Clinical case study 1

1. The MMRII and Priorix vaccines are given subcutaneously.
2. The CDC's vaccination schedule for children between 6 weeks and six years must be checked to determine which vaccines are needed for infants and when they are required.
3. After a vaccine is given, it must be reported to the patient's primary care provider and the state's Immunization Information Systems (IIS), if applicable. Any adverse events after the vaccine was given must also be documented and reported to the patient's primary care provider. Documentation of vaccination should be provided to the patient or guardian.

Clinical case study 2

1. Viral load and viral type are the primary cofactors for progressing from infection to cervical intraepithelial lesions and cancer. Smoking, hormonal exposure, and HIV are additional exposures that increase the risk of progression to cancer.
2. Vaccinating all 11- to 12-year-olds can protect them long before exposure. The CDC recommends two doses of HPV vaccine for all adolescents aged 11 or 12 years. A 2-dose schedule is recommended for people who get the first dose before their 15th birthday. In a 2-dose series, the second dose should be given 6–12 months after the first dose. A 3-dose schedule is recommended for people who get the first dose between 10 and 12 years of age. In a 3-dose series, the second dose should be given 1 to 2 months after the first dose, and the third should be given six months after the first dose. The minimum intervals are four weeks between the first and second doses, 12 weeks between the second and third doses, and five months between the first and third doses.
3. Immunizations are generally safe in individuals with HIV, except for live virus vaccines in people with low CD4 counts. In those individuals with HIV who have advanced immunosuppression, live vaccines can cause a potentially life-threatening disseminated infection because of the live pathogen in the vaccine.

Clinical case study 3

1. The Japanese encephalitis virus is found in pigs and birds and is passed to mosquitoes when they bite infected animals. People get the virus when infected mosquitoes then grind them. It cannot be spread from person to person.
2. Several types of inactivated vaccines and a kind of live attenuated vaccine are currently used worldwide to prevent Japanese encephalitis: inactivated mouse brain-derived vaccines, inactivated Vero-cell-derived vaccines, primary hamster kidney (PHK) cell-derived purified vaccines, and live attenuated vaccines.
3. The inactivated vaccine against Japanese encephalitis, IXIARO, is given as a two-dose series, with the doses spaced 28 days apart. Adults aged 18–65 can get the second dose as early as seven days after the first dose. The last amount should be given at least one week before travel. A booster dose (third dose) should be provided if a person has received the two-dose primary vaccination series one year or more previously and there is a continued risk for JE virus infection or potential for reexposure. For adults and children aged three years or older, each dose of IXIARO is 0.5 mL. For children aged two months through 2 years, each amount is 0.25 mL.

Chapter 55: NSAIDs and acetaminophen

Clinical case study 1

1. Although acetaminophen is available over-the-counter, it has caused severe liver damage when taken at higher doses. Acetaminophen can cause sudden liver failure, sometimes resulting in the need for liver transplantation, and it can also cause death.

2. Acetaminophen toxicity is the second most common cause of liver transplantation worldwide and the most common cause in the US. It is responsible for 56,000 emergency department visits, 2,600 hospitalizations, and 500 deaths annually in the United States.
3. It is never safe to use acetaminophen while alcohol is consumed. It can collectively irritate the stomach, leading to ulcers, internal bleeding, and liver damage.

Clinical case study 2

1. Topical NSAIDs have similar efficacy as oral NSAIDs, with improved safety when treating small or superficial joint arthritis due to limited absorption.
2. Prescription NSAIDs are indicated for patients with arthritis, gout, menstrual cramps, severe headaches, and generalized body aches.
3. NSAIDs promote pain relief by decreasing acute and subacute tissue damage inflammatory processes. They are also referred to as COX inhibitors since they block the action of cyclooxygenase (COX). This enzyme promotes the synthesis of inflammatory prostaglandins at the site of tissue damage.

Chapter 56: Drugs used in rheumatoid arthritis, gout, and osteoporosis

Clinical case study 1

1. Osteoarthritis primarily involves only one or a few joints. The joints commonly involved include the hips, knees, lower lumbar and cervical vertebrae, proximal and distal interphalangeal joints of the fingers, first carpometacarpal joints, and first tarsometatarsal joints. Heberden nodes, prominent osteophytes at the distal interphalangeal joints, are common in women. The pathologic changes are caused by antibodies against self-antigens and cytokine-mediated inflammation.
2. There is no single test for osteoarthritis. Diagnosing the condition may include a physical exam, X-rays, MRI, and blood tests. In some cases, joint fluid samples are taken to look for other causes of joint pain.
3. There is no cure for osteoarthritis, but the condition does not necessarily get worse over time. Many treatments are available to help relieve the symptoms, focusing on managing pain and improving joint function. Patients may benefit from medication for mild symptoms that come and go. More severe symptoms may require regular use of drugs. Topical treatments include non-steroidal anti-inflammatory drugs (NSAID) creams and capsaicin creams. Systemic NSAIDs, such as celecoxib, ibuprofen, naproxen, and diclofenac, are the most used medications to treat OA. Acetaminophen has fallen out of favor for the treatment of OA due to safety concerns with its potential effects on the liver and non-clinically significant effects on pain. Corticosteroid injections may be used for severe cases. However, they are only sometimes utilized due to the short duration of relief and evidence that they may accelerate OA progression. Opioids, such as codeine, may also help relieve severe pain but should only be used when all other treatment options have failed. Duloxetine may be utilized for patients with pain in multiple joints. Nonpharmacologic measures to treat OA include weight management, aerobic and strengthening exercises, assistive devices, braces, and foot orthotics.

Clinical case study 2

1. Adalimumab is indicated for moderate to severe active RA in adults as monotherapy or in combination with methotrexate or other non-biologic DMARDs. It is also used for mild to severe active polyarticular juvenile idiopathic arthritis (JIA) in patients two years of age and older as monotherapy or in combination with methotrexate. Adalimumab is also used for adult psoriatic arthritis and ankylosing spondylitis. Other indications include moderate to severe active Crohn's disease in adults and children over age 6, mild to severe active ulcerative colitis in adults, moderate to severe chronic plaque psoriasis in specific adults, and non-infectious intermediate, posterior, and panuveitis in adults and children over age 2.
2. There are no known contraindications regarding adalimumab. However, patients must be monitored for any infections or malignancies.
3. Adalimumab's adverse effects usually include injection-site pain, increased creatine phosphate, upper respiratory infection, headache, and rash. This drug has a black box warning because it can suppress the immune system and lead to infections. Latent infections such as hepatitis B and tuberculosis can become reactivated. The TNF blockers

have been linked to malignancies such as leukemias and lymphomas. Rarely have fatal cases of hepatosplenic T-cell lymphoma occurred.

Clinical case study 3

1. Colchicine is indicated for the prevention and treatment of gout flares and familial Mediterranean fever and to reduce risks for myocardial infarction, stroke, coronary revascularization, and cardiovascular death in adults with atherosclerotic disease or multiple cardiovascular risk factors. Off-label uses include Bechet's disease, pericarditis, and post-pericardiotomy syndrome.
2. Colchicine is contraindicated with a known hypersensitivity to the drug in patients with kidney disease, pregnant women, and those with GI, hepatic, or cardiac impairment. Patients with blood dyscrasias must not receive colchicine. The drug is used with caution in older adults, debilitated patients, and those with early signs of GI, kidney, liver, or cardiac disease.
3. The most significant adverse effects are GI-related, occurring in as many as 80% of patients. These effects include nausea, vomiting, abdominal pain, anorexia, and diarrhea. The drug can cause aplastic anemia, bone marrow toxicity, leukopenia, agranulocytosis, or thrombocytopenia. Other adverse effects include hepatotoxicity, azotemia, mental confusion, hematuria, proteinuria, and oliguria.

Chapter 57: Toxicology

No case studies

Glossary

Absence seizure: A generalized onset seizure that simultaneously begins on both sides of the brain. It is most common in children and typically does not cause any long-term problems. An older term is petit mal seizures.

***Acetyl coenzyme A** (acetyl-CoA):* A central molecule in cell metabolism that plays a crucial role in many cellular processes.

Acetylation: A chemical reaction that adds an acetyl group (CH3C=O) to a molecule or material.

Acetylcholine: A chemical messenger that acts as a neurotransmitter in the brain and others.

Acetylcholinesterase: An enzyme that breaks down acetylcholine into acetic acid and choline.

Achalasia: A condition in which the muscles of the lower part of the esophagus fail to relax, preventing food from passing into the stomach.

Achilles tendon: The tendon connecting calf muscles to the heel bone.

Achlorhydria: A condition in which the stomach does not produce hydrochloric acid, one of the components of gastric acid.

Acne: A common skin condition that happens when hair follicles under the skin become clogged.

Acromegaly: Abnormal growth of the hands, feet, and face, caused by overproduction of growth hormone by the pituitary gland.

Action potential(s): The change in electrical potential associated with the passage of an impulse along the membrane of a muscle cell or nerve cell.

Active transport: The movement of ions or molecules across a cell membrane into a region of higher concentration, assisted by enzymes and requiring energy.

Active zone: Specialized regions of the presynaptic membrane where neurotransmitters are released.

Acupuncture: The insertion of skinny needles through the skin at strategic points on the body. A key component of traditional Chinese medicine, acupuncture is most commonly used to treat pain.

Acute coronary syndrome: Potentially life-threatening conditions occur when a blockage causes blood flow to the heart to slow or stop suddenly.

Acute lymphoblastic leukemia: A cancer of the lymphoid blood cells involving large numbers of immature lymphocytes.

Acute myeloid leukemia: A cancer of the myeloid blood cells involving rapid growth of abnormal bone marrow and blood.

Adaptogenic: Acting to normalize and regulate the systems of the body.

Addison's disease: A disorder involving disrupted functioning of the part of the adrenal cortex. This results in decreased production of two hormones by the adrenal cortex: cortisol and aldosterone.

Additive effect: The combined effect produced by two or more agents' actions equals the sum of their separate effects.

Adenohypophysis: The anterior lobe of the pituitary gland produces and releases most of the gland's hormones.

Adenyl cyclase: An enzyme that synthesizes cyclic adenosine monophosphate (cAMP), a second messenger that regulates many cellular processes.

Adrenal medulla: The inner part of the adrenal gland, located on top of each kidney. It produces norepinephrine and epinephrine, which help control the body's response to stress and increase blood pressure.

Adrenergic agonists: Drugs that work by mimicking the functioning of the sympathetic nervous system.

Adulteration: Deliberately added to increase bulk, enhance or mimic a pharmacological effect, or facilitate drug delivery.

Adverse drug reaction: A response to a noxious and unintended drug that occurs at doses commonly used for prophylaxis, diagnosis, or therapy of disease or modifying physiologic function.

Adverse effect(s): An undesired effect of a drug. They can range from mild to severe and can be life-threatening.

Adynamic ileus: Also called paralytic ileus, a condition in which foods and drinks do not usually pass through the intestines.

Affinity: The extent or fraction to which a drug binds to receptors at any given drug concentration or the firmness with which the drug binds to the receptor.

Agonist: A substance that acts like another substance and stimulates an action.

Agranulocytosis: A severe condition where the body has a dangerously low number of white blood cells.

Akathisia: A state of agitation, distress, and restlessness that is an occasional side-effect of antipsychotic and antidepressant drugs.

Alanine aminotransferase: An enzyme that is usually present in liver and heart cells. ALT is released into the blood when the liver or heart is damaged.

Albumin: The most abundant circulating protein in the blood. It is a family of globular proteins.

Aldosterone: A corticosteroid hormone that stimulates the absorption of sodium by the kidneys and regulates water and salt balance.

Aliphatic: An organic compound containing hydrogen and carbon atoms that are usually linked in chains via single, double, or triple bonds.

Allergen: A substance that can cause an allergic reaction.

***Allergic reactions:* The immune system reacts** to something that does not affect most other people.

Allergic rhinitis: A condition that causes nose inflammation due to an allergic reaction to inhaled allergens.

Alopecia: The partial or complete absence of hair from areas of the body where it usually grows; baldness.

Alpha-adrenergic antagonists: Medications that relax muscle tissue in blood vessels and the prostate gland, improving urine and blood flow.

Alveolar ducts: Small passageways in the lungs that connect the bronchioles to the alveolar sacs.

Alveoli: Tiny air sacs at the end of the bronchioles.

Alzheimer's disease: A brain disorder that slowly destroys memory and thinking skills and, eventually, the ability to carry out the simplest tasks.

Ambulation: The ability to walk independently, either with or without assistance.

Amebiasis: A common parasitic enteral infection. It is caused by any of the amoeba of the *Entamoeba* group.

Amnesia: A partial or total loss of memory.

Ampulla of Vater: The hepatopancreatic ampulla, or the hepatopancreatic duct, is formed by the union of the pancreatic duct and the common bile duct and is precisely located at the major duodenal papilla.

Amyotrophic lateral sclerosis: A progressive nervous system disease that affects nerve cells in the brain and spinal cord, causing loss of muscle control.

Anaphylaxis: An excessive localized enlargement of an artery caused by weakening of the artery wall.
Androgen receptors: A protein that binds to androgens (testosterone).
Androgen: Male sex hormone that is a steroid and includes testosterone and androsterone.
Angina pectoris: A condition marked by severe pain in the chest, often also spreading to the shoulders, arms, and neck.
Angioedema: Swelling under the skin.
Angiotensinogen: A protein that plays a role in regulating blood pressure, fluid balance, and electrolyte homeostasis. It is a critical component of the renin-angiotensin-aldosterone system.
Anhedonia: Inability to feel pleasure.
Anhidrosis: A rare condition in which the sweat glands make little or no sweat. It can affect the whole body or a small part of the body. Severe burns, radiation, infection, inflammation, or other injuries to the skin may cause anhidrosis.
Ankylosing spondylitis: A type of arthritis that causes inflammation in the spine and other joints, resulting in pain and stiffness>
Ankylosis: A condition where the bones in a joint fuse abnormally, resulting in stiffness and restricted movement.
Anorexia: Loss of appetite.
Anorgasmia: Regular difficulty reaching orgasm.
Anovulatory cycles: A menstrual cycle where an egg is not released from the ovaries.
Antagonist: A substance that acts against and blocks an action.
Antepartum: The period before childbirth.
Anterograde amnesia: Inability to form new memories after the event that caused the amnesia.
Anthrax: A severe disease usually caused by Bacillus anthracis bacteria. It is found naturally in soil worldwide and commonly affects livestock and wild animals. People typically get sick with anthrax if they come in contact with infected animals or contaminated animal products.
Anti-nuclear antibodies: A type of antibody that binds to the nucleus of a cell, attacking the body's healthy cells.
Antidote: A substance that stops the harmful effects of a poison.
Antigens: Any substance that causes the body to make an immune response against that substance. Antigens include toxins, chemicals, bacteria, viruses, or other substances outside the body. Body tissues and cells, including cancer cells, also have antigens on them that can cause an immune response.
Antitussives: Help prevent coughing by working on the part of the brain that controls the action.
Antrum: The lower part of the stomach, where food mixes with gastric juice and is stored until it moves into the small intestine.
Anuria: The lack of urine production. It can happen as a result of shock, severe blood loss, or heart or kidney failure. It can also occur from medications or toxins. Anuria is an emergency and can be life-threatening.
Anxiety disorders: A mental illness that causes excessive and uncontrollable feelings of fear and anxiety that can significantly impair a person's daily life.
Anxiolysis: A level of sedation in which a person is very relaxed and may be awake.
Apathy: Lack of feeling or emotion.
Aphonia: A voice disorder that causes a person to lose their voice or be unable to produce sound.
Aplastic anemia: A rare but severe blood disorder that occurs when the bone marrow is unable to produce enough new blood cells.
Apnea: The temporary cessation of breathing. It can occur in infants, children, and adults and can be caused by some conditions, including sleep apnea.
Apoptosis: The death of cells, which occurs as a normal and controlled part of an organism's growth or development.
Apothecary system: This system, used for measuring and weighing drugs and solutions, was brought to the United States from England during the colonial period; the metric system has now replaced it.
Areflexia: Absence of deep tendon reflexes.
Arginine vasopressin deficiency: A rare disorder characterized by polydipsia and polyuria.
Arrhythmia(s): An irregular heartbeat or a problem with the rate or rhythm of the heart.
Arterioles: A tiny blood vessel that branches from an artery and delivers blood to capillaries.
Arthralgia: Pain in a joint caused by injury, infection, inflammation, and immune disorders, such as rheumatoid arthritis, lupus, Sjogren's syndrome, or systemic lupus erythematosus.
Ascites: An abnormal accumulation of fluid in the abdomen.
Aspartate aminotransferase: An enzyme that promotes the transfer of an amino group from glutamic acid to oxaloacetic acid and, when present in abnormally high levels in the blood is a diagnostic indication of heart attack or liver disease
Asplenia: The absence of a spleen.
Asthenia: Abnormal physical weakness or lack of energy.
Asthma: A chronic lung disease that causes inflammation and tightening of the muscles around the airways, making breathing difficult.
Asystole: The state of total cessation of electrical activity from the heart.
Ataxia: The loss of complete control of bodily movements.
Atrial fibrillation: The most common type of heart arrhythmia, an irregular and often very rapid heart rhythm that can lead to blood clots in the heart.
Atrial natriuretic peptide: A hormone secreted from the right atrium in response to atrial stretch from hypervolemia and hypertension.
Atrioventricular node: A small mass of heart tissue connecting the electrical systems of the atria and ventricles.
Atypical antipsychotics: Agents that block receptors in dopamine pathways, used to treat schizophrenia, bipolar disorder, autistic irritability, and as adjuncts for depression
Atypical cystic fibrosis: A milder form of the disease that can affect one organ or multiple organ systems to varying degrees.
Atypical drugs: A group of new drugs that affect multiple neurotransmitter receptors, including dopamine, serotonin, norepinephrine, and histamine. They differ from typical antipsychotic agents in producing significantly fewer extrapyramidal symptoms and having a lower risk of tardive dyskinesia in vulnerable clinical populations at doses that produce comparable control of psychosis.
Atypical mycobacteria: Also known as non-tuberculous mycobacterial infections, they are caused by bacteria found in soil, water, and animals.
Autism: A broad range of conditions involving poor social skills, repetitive behaviors, speech problems, and nonverbal communication.

Autonomic nervous system: A part of the peripheral nervous system that controls involuntary bodily functions, such as heart rate, blood pressure, and digestion.
Autoreceptors: Receptors on nouns that respond to the neurotransmitters released by the same cell.
Azotemia: An excess of nitrogenous waste products in the blood.
Bacteremia: The presence of bacteria in the blood.
Bactericidal: Having the ability to kill bacteria.
Bacteriostatic: The agent prevents the growth of bacteria.
Balanced anesthesia: Anesthesia produced by smaller doses of two or more agents is considered safer than the usual large dose of a single agent.
Balantidium coli: An intestinal parasite that causes the infection balantidiasis.
Barcoding: An automatic identification technology that allows data to be collected rapidly and accurately from all aspects of a company's operations, including manufacturing, inspection, transportation, and inventory elements.
Baroreceptors: Receptors sensitive to changes in pressure.
Barrett's esophagus: A condition that occurs when the lining of the lower esophagus changes due to damage from stomach acid.
Basal metabolic rate: Refers to the amount of energy the body needs to maintain homeostasis.
Bechets' disease: A rare, chronic inflammatory disorder that affects blood vessels and multiple body parts.
Benign prostatic hyperplasia: A noncancerous condition that causes the prostate gland to enlarge. It is the most common prostate condition in men over 50.
Beta-adrenergic antagonists: These medications, also called beta-blockers, reduce blood pressure by blocking the effects of the hormone epinephrine.
Beta-amyloid: An amyloid derived from a more significant precursor protein and is the primary plaque component in Alzheimer's disease.
Biliary excretion: Active secretion of drug molecules or their metabolites from hepatocytes into the bile. The bile then transports the drugs to the gut, where the drugs are excreted.
Bioavailability: The proportion of a drug or other substance that enters the blood circulation when introduced into the body and can have an active effect.
Biotransformation: The alteration of a drug or a substance within the body.
Bipolar disorder: Also called manic-depression, involving extreme emotional highs and extreme depression.
Black cohosh: A member of the buttercup family, its flowers and roots were commonly used in traditional Native American medicine. Today, it's a famous women's health supplement claimed to help with menopause symptoms, fertility, and hormonal balance.
Blastocysts: Ball of cells that forms early in a pregnancy, about five to six days after a sperm fertilizes an egg.
Bloating: A feeling of fullness or swelling in the abdomen, often caused by gas in the intestines.
Blood dyscrasia: Any disorder of the blood, bone marrow clotting proteins, or lymph tissue. The causes of these issues may include genetic factors, medications, infections, or exposure to toxins.
Blood-brain barrier: A network of blood vessels and tissue that is made up of closely spaced cells and helps keep harmful substances from reaching the brain; it lets some substances, such as water, oxygen, carbon dioxide, and general anesthetics, pass through.
Bone marrow: A soft, highly vascular modified connective tissue that occupies the cavities of most bones and occurs in two forms.
Bowman's capsule: A cup-shaped sac in the kidney surrounding the glomerulus, the first step in filtering blood to create urine.
Bradycardia: A type of arrhythmia, or abnormal heart rhythm, that occurs when the heart beats slower than 60 times per minute.
Brain circuits: Connections of neurons through which electrical activity occurs.
Brainstem: The central trunk of the brain, consisting of the medulla oblongata, pons, and midbrain, and continuing downward to form the spinal cord.
Bronchial tree: The bronchi are the branches of the tree within the lungs.
Bronchioles: A tiny branch of air tubes in the lungs.
Bronchitis: An infection of the bronchi.
Brucellosis: An infectious disease caused by a family of bacteria called *Brucella*. Humans generally acquire the disease through direct contact with infected animals, by eating or drinking contaminated animal products, or by inhaling airborne agents.
Buccal route: Placing a drug between gums and cheek, where it also dissolves and is absorbed into blood circulation.
Bundle of His: A bundle of specialized muscle fibers in the heart that carries electrical signals from the atrioventricular (AV) node to the ventricles.
Calcitonin: A polypeptide hormone secreted by the parafollicular or C cells of the thyroid gland; it is involved in plasma calcium homeostasis and decreases the bone resorption rate.
Candidiasis: A fungal infection caused by an overgrowth of the yeast Candida. It can affect different parts of the body in various ways.
Cannabinoids: The chemical compounds that are the active principles of marijuana.
Capsid: The protein shell that encloses a virus's genetic material, acting as a protective coating around the viral nucleic acid, allowing it to attach to host cells and deliver its genome during infection.
Carboxylesterase: An enzyme catalyzes the hydrolysis of esterified chemicals, including pesticides, drugs, and lipids.
Cardiac cycles: The series of events that occur between the start of one heartbeat and the start of the next.
Cardiac decompensation: Inability of the heart to maintain adequate circulation; it is marked by dyspnea, venous engorgement, cyanosis, and edema.
Cardiac output: The amount of blood the heart pumps in a minute.
Cardiogenic shock: A life-threatening condition in which the heart suddenly cannot pump enough blood to meet the body's needs.
Cardiomyocytes: The cells that make up the myocardium and are responsible for the heart's contraction and relaxation.
Carpometacarpal joints: The joints in the hand that connect the carpal bones to the metacarpal bones.
Cartilage: A tough, flexible tissue that provides structure and support to the body and helps bones move smoothly.
Catabolism: The breakdown of proteins into absorbable monomers for further degradation or reassembly.
Catatonia: A state of immobility and stupor related to a disturbed mental state.
Catecholamine: Sympathomimetic amines, including dopamine, epinephrine, and norepinephrine, are essential for physiological responses to stress.

Cathartics: A substance that accelerates defecation. This is similar to a laxative, which is a substance that eases defecation, usually by softening feces.
Caudal block anesthesia: Produced by injection of a local anesthetic into the caudal canal, the sacral portion of the spinal canal.
Celiac artery: A short, wide artery that supplies blood to the foregut and is the first major branch of the abdominal aorta.
Celiac disease: A damage to the small intestine that interferes with the absorption of nutrients from food; it occurs when the body reacts abnormally to gluten.
Cerebral edema: Swelling of the brain. It is a relatively common phenomenon with numerous causes.
Cesarean section: A surgical procedure performed to deliver a baby through incisions made in the mother's abdomen and uterus.
Chagas disease: A potentially life-threatening disease caused by the parasite Trypanosoma cruzi.
Chamomile: An aromatic European plant of the daisy family with white and yellow flowers.
Chelation therapy: A medical procedure that uses a chemical solution to remove heavy metals and other toxins from the body.
Chemical names: The chemical compound that shows the names of each of its elements or sub-compounds.
Cheyne-Stokes Breathing: Breathing involves alternating periods of rapid breathing and long pauses. This event may develop in heart failure, stroke, brain trauma, or a tumor.
Child-Pugh liver impairment: A system for assessing the prognosis — including the required strength of treatment and necessity of liver transplant — of chronic liver disease, primarily cirrhosis. It forecasts the increasing severity of your liver disease and your expected survival rate.
Chlamydiae: A common sexually transmitted infection caused by the bacterium Chlamydia trachomatis. It can affect people of all ages but is most common in young people, especially women.
Cholecystokinin: A polypeptide hormone secreted in the small intestine; it stimulates gallbladder contraction and secretion of pancreatic enzymes.
Cholera: A bacterial disease that causes severe diarrhea, vomiting, and dehydration. It is caused by the bacterium Vibrio cholerae and is spread through contaminated food or water.
Choline acetyltransferase: An enzyme that produces acetylcholine in the brain.
Cholinergic antagonists: Drugs that bind to but do not activate cholinergic receptors, blocking the actions of acetylcholine or cholinergic agonists.
Cholinergic crisis: Overstimulation at neuromuscular junctions due to excessive acetylcholine because of inactivity of the AChE enzyme.
Cholinergic receptors: Membrane proteins that are activated by the acetylcholine. They are involved in signal transduction in the nervous system and play a role in memory, cognitive, and autonomic functions.
Chondrocytes: The only specialized cell type found in the cartilage tissue.
Choreiform movement: A jerking or writing movement.
Chromaffin cells: Make epinephrine and norepinephrine. They are found in the adrenal glands or ganglia.
Chronic obstructive pulmonary disease (COPD): A chronic lung condition that reduces airflow to and from the lungs. It is caused by lung damage that leads to inflammation and swelling in the airways.
Chronotropy: The effect on the rate or timing of a physiological process, such as the heart rate.
Chyme: The semifluid mass of partly digested food expelled by the stomach into the duodenum.
Ciliary body: A ring-shaped structure in the eye that produces aqueous humor, nourishes the lens and cornea, and helps the eye focus.
Circumflex artery: A coronary artery that supplies oxygenated blood to the left side of the heart.
Cirrhosis: A chronic liver disease that occurs when the liver is damaged over time and healthy liver cells are replaced by scar tissue. This scarring, also known as fibrosis, makes it difficult for the liver to function correctly.
Clearance: The rate at which the active drug is removed from the body; and for most drugs at steady state, clearance remains constant so that drug input equals drug output.
Clonic spasms: A repeated, involuntary muscle twitch or jerking motion.
Clubbing fingers: A physical sign characterized by bulbous enlargement of the ends of one or more fingers or toes.
Cofactor: A non-protein chemical compound bound to a protein and required for the protein's biological activity.
Cognitive-behavioral therapy: One of the most common and best-studied forms of psychotherapy. It is a combination of two therapeutic approaches, known as cognitive therapy and behavioral therapy.
Coiled loops: A series of loops or rings wound together or a single loop within that series.
Collecting tubule: The last part of a long, twisting tube that collects urine from the nephrons (cellular structures in the kidney that filter blood and form urine) and moves it into the renal pelvis and ureters. Also called a collecting duct.
Colonoscopy: A procedure in which a flexible fiber-optic instrument is inserted through the anus to examine the colon.
Combination drugs: Two or more drugs combined into a single dosage form.
Commensal: A relationship between two species in which one benefits from the other without harming or benefiting it.
Comorbidities: The simultaneous presence of two or more diseases or medical conditions in a patient.
Complement fixation: Combining complement with the antigen-antibody complex, rendering the complement inactive or fixed.
Computerized physician order entry: The process of providers entering and sending treatment instructions – including medication, laboratory, and radiology orders – via a computer application rather than paper, fax, or telephone.
Conchae: Three pairs of turbinates are commonly described along the lateral walls of the nasal cavity: the superior, middle, and inferior.
Congestive heart failure: A complex clinical syndrome characterized by inefficient myocardial performance, resulting in compromised blood supply to the body.
Conjugated vaccine: A type of vaccine that combines a weak antigen with a solid antigen to create a more robust immune response.
Conjugation: Chemical combination or linkage of chemical groups to organic molecules, often to produce a water-soluble form and allow more ready excretion.
Conjunctivitis: An inflammation or infection of the conjunctiva, the transparent layer covering the white of the eye and the inner eyelid.
Conn's syndrome: Primary aldosteronism caused by hyperplasia or tumors.
Constitutive activity: Also known as basal activity, it is ligand-independent and produces a second messenger without an agonist.
Coronary sinus: A large vein in the heart that carries deoxygenated blood from the myocardium to the right atrium.
Coronary sulcus: A groove on the heart's surface that separates the atria from the ventricles.

Corpus luteum: A mass of cells that forms in an ovary. It is a temporary organ that appears every menstrual cycle and disappears if fertilization does not occur.

Corticotropin:

Covalent adduct: A complex formed when a covalent bond joins two species

Crash cart: A crash cart or code cart is a set of trays or drawers on wheels used in hospitals for transportation and dispensing of emergency medication or equipment at the site of medical or surgical emergency for life support protocols to save someone's life potentially.

Creatine phosphate: A high-energy molecule stored in muscles, critical in providing chemical energy for cell activity and viability.

Creatinine clearance: The volume of blood plasma cleared of creatinine, a muscle waste, over a specific period.

Creatinine kinase: An enzyme that helps produce energy in muscles and other tissues:

Creatinine: A chemical waste product that results from the breakdown of muscle tissue and protein digestion in food.

Cretinism: A congenital condition caused by a deficiency of thyroid hormone during prenatal development and characterized by small stature, intellectual disability, dystrophy of the bones, and a low basal metabolism.

Crohn's disease: A chronic inflammatory disease of the intestines, especially the colon and ileum, associated with ulcers and fistulae.

Cryptorchidism: A condition in which one or both testicles fail to move from the abdomen, where they develop before birth, into the scrotum. It may increase the risk of the development of testicular cancer. They are also called undescended testicles.

Cryptosporidiosis: A contagious disease that causes watery diarrhea. It is caused by parasites called Cryptosporidium.

Crypts: A sterile invagination composed of goblet, stem, and Paneth cells, which can secrete mucus and antimicrobial peptides such as cryptdins.

Crystalluria: The presence of crystals in the urine.

Cushing's syndrome: Moon-shaped face, fat accumulation around the torso, fat loss from extremities, and easy bruising due to elevated levels of cortisol that are caused either by excess production of the hormone ACTH from an adrenal or pituitary tumor or by high doses of corticosteroid hormones.

Cyanosis: A bluish color of mucous membranes and skin.

Cycloplegia: Paralysis of the eye's ciliary muscle, resulting in a loss of accommodation.

Cyclothymia: A rare mood disorder similar to bipolar disorder but less intense.

Cystitis: A bladder infection that causes inflammation of the lower urinary tract. It is the most common type of urinary tract infection.

Cystoscopy: A thin, tube-like instrument that looks inside the bladder and urethra. It has a light and a lens for viewing and may have a tool to remove tissue.

Cytochrome P450: A group of enzymes metabolizing foreign substances and liver drugs.

Cytokine storm: The uncontrolled, sometimes life-threatening, excessive release of cytokines (such as chemokines, interferons, or interleukins) in the body from an aggressive, pro-inflammatory immune response resulting from an overreaction of the immune system.

Decompensated heart failure: A syndrome in which a structural or functional change in the heart leads to an inability to eject or accommodate enough blood; it requires immediate treatment.

Defibrillation: A procedure that uses an electric shock to restore a normal heartbeat and treat life-threatening heart arrhythmias.

Deglutition: The process of swallowing, which is the movement of food, liquids, or saliva from the mouth to the stomach.

Degranulation: A cellular process that releases molecules from granules, which are secretory vesicles found in some cells.

Delirium tremens: A rapid onset of confusion usually caused by withdrawal from alcohol.

Delirium: An acutely disturbed state of mind that occurs in fever, intoxication, and other disorders and is characterized by restlessness, illusions, and incoherence of thought and speech.

Delusions: Rigid, false beliefs that conflict with reality.

Dementia: A decline in mental ability that interferes with daily life. It is caused by brain damage or disease that destroys nerve cells, leading to a loss of cognitive functioning. Dementia can affect memory, thinking, language, judgment, and behavior.

Dendritic cells: A type of immune cells that play a vital role in the body's immune response.

Depolarization: Reversing the charge across a cell membrane of neurons and causing an action potential.

Dermatitis herpetiformis: A chronic, intensely itchy, blistering skin manifestation of gluten-sensitive enteropathy, commonly known as celiac disease.

Dermatome: An area of skin in which sensory nerves derive from a single spinal nerve root.

Dermatophytosis: A common fungal infection of hair, skin, or nails.

Designer drugs: A structural or functional analog of a controlled substance designed to mimic the pharmacological effects of the original drug while avoiding classification as illegal and detection in standard drug tests.

Detrusor muscles: The smooth muscle component of the urinary bladder facilitates contraction of the bladder wall during micturition.

Diabetic ketoacidosis: A dangerous complication of diabetes mellitus in which the chemical balance of the body becomes dangerously acidic.

Diaphoresis: Sweating, especially to an unusual degree, as a symptom of a disease or a side effect of a drug.

Diaphragm: A condition caused by pressure on the phrenic nerve or damage to the nerve.

Diaphragm: A dome-shaped muscle that separates the chest cavity from the abdominal cavity, primarily functioning as the primary muscle responsible for breathing by contracting and relaxing to facilitate inhalation and exhalation; essentially, it controls the volume of the chest cavity to allow air to move in and out of the lungs.

Diathesis: A tendency to suffer from a particular medical condition.

Diphtheria: A contagious disease caused by a toxin-producing bacteria that can affect the respiratory tract and other body parts.

Diplopia: A pathological condition of vision in which a single object appears double.

Distal convoluted tubule: A short segment of the nephron in the kidney that plays a critical role in regulating electrolytes and fluid volume.

Diuresis: An increase in the amount of urine made by the kidney and passed from the body.

Dong Quai: An aromatic herb of the parsley family, native to China and Japan, the root of which is used to treat premenstrual syndrome, menstrual cramps, menopausal symptoms, and other gynecological complaints.

Dopamine: A neurotransmitter that plays a significant role in reward-motivated behaviors and, therefore, drug or alcohol addiction.

Dormant: Inactive but capable of becoming active.

Dose-response relationship: Increasing levels of exposure are associated with either an increasing or decreasing risk of the outcome.

Dosing errors: An incorrect dosage form occurs when a patient receives a dosage different than prescribed.
Downregulation: A decrease in the number of receptors on the surface of target cells, making the cells less sensitive to a hormone or another agent.
Dromotropy: The conduction speed of electrical impulses in the heart is affected.
Drug interaction: A reaction that occurs when a drug is taken with another drug, food, beverage, supplement, or when taken with certain medical conditions.
Drug monograph: A publication that specifies for a drug (or class of related drugs) the types and amounts of ingredients it may contain, the conditions and limitations for
Drug-drug interactions: When two or more drugs react with each other, either prescription or over-the-counter.
Duchenne muscular dystrophy: A severe form of muscular dystrophy caused by a genetic defect that usually affects boys and is characterized by the progressive loss of muscle.
Dwarfism: Short stature that results from a genetic or medical condition; generally defined as an adult height of 4 feet 10 inches or less.
Dysarthria: Difficult or unclear articulation of speech that is otherwise linguistically normal.
Dyskinesia: An impairment of voluntary movement.
Dyslipidemia: An abnormal amount of lipids and lipoproteins in the blood.
Dysmenorrhea: Painful menstrual cramps or periods.
Dyspareunia: Painful sexual intercourse due to medical or psychological causes.
Dyspepsia: A discomfort or pain in the upper abdomen that can occur during or after eating.
Dysphonia: Having an abnormal voice.
Dyspnea: Difficulty breathing, gasping, and breathlessness.
Dystonia: A state of abnormal muscle tone resulting in muscular spasms and abnormal posture, typically due to neurological disease or a side effect of drug therapy.
Dysuria: A symptom that describes painful or uncomfortable urination, often described as a burning, stinging, or itching sensation in the urethra or urethral meatus.
Ebola: A rare but often deadly infectious disease affecting humans and non-human primates. It is caused by an ortho-ebolavirus primarily found in sub-Saharan Africa.
Ecchymosis: A small bruise caused by blood leaking from broken blood vessels into the tissues of the skin or mucous membranes.
Echinacea: A coneflower of North America. It is used in herbal medicine mainly for its antibiotic and wound-healing properties.
Eclampsia: A form of toxemia of pregnancy characterized by albuminuria, hypertension, and convulsions.
Ectopic heartbeat: Originating in an area of the heart other than the sinoatrial node (pacemaker).
Efficacy: The maximum response that can be achieved with a drug.
Eicosanoids: Lipid-based signaling molecules that play a unique role in innate immune responses, including inflammation, blood pressure regulation, and brain physiology
Ejection fraction: A measurement of the percentage of blood leaving the heart each time it squeezes.
Embolism: Obstructing an artery, usually by a clot of blood or an air bubble.
Emesis: The forceful ejection of some or all of the stomach's contents through the mouth.
Emphysema: A progressive chronic lung condition in which the alveoli are damaged or destroyed. When this happens, it causes the tiny air sacs to rupture and create one big air pocket instead of many tiny ones. Air becomes trapped in the damaged areas and does not move the oxygen correctly through the body.
Empiric monotherapy: A treatment that uses a single antibiotic, or β-lactam agent, before the results of blood cultures and antibiotic susceptibility tests are known.
Endocarditis: An inflammation of the heart chambers and valves' inside lining.
Endocardium: The innermost layer of the heart, lining the chambers and covering the heart's valves, papillary muscles, and chordae tendineae.
Endocytosis: The uptake by a cell of material from the environment by invading the plasma membrane; it includes both phagocytosis and pinocytosis.
Endometriosis: A chronic condition where tissue similar to the lining of the uterus grows outside of the uterus.
Endometritis: An infection and inflammation of the uterus lining (endometrium).
Endometrium: The inner lining, consisting of the functional and basal endometrium.
Endoplasmic reticulum: A network of interconnected membranes within a cell that functions to produce, modify, and transport proteins and lipids, essentially acting as a factory assembly line within the cell; it can be either "rough" with attached ribosomes for protein synthesis or "smooth" for lipid production depending on its structure.
Endothelial cells: The cells that line the inside of blood vessels, lymph vessels, and the heart.
Entamoeba histolytica: A protozoan that causes intestinal amebiasis and extra-intestinal manifestations.
Enteral route: Absorption of a drug via the GI tract, including oral, gastric, or duodenal routes.
Enterocytes: Cells of the intestinal lining.
Enteroendocrine cells: Specialized cells in the gastrointestinal tract that produce and release hormones in response to stimuli.
Epicardium: A tissue layer that covers the heart and the roots of the great arteries.
Epidermal necrolysis: A life-threatening skin disorder characterized by blistering and peeling skin.
Epidural block anesthesia: An epidural nerve block is a procedure to block pain by injecting anesthetic medication into the epidural space. The epidural space is the area between the inner wall of the vertebral column and the outermost of the dura mater that surrounds the spinal cord.
Epilepsy: A neurological disorder marked by sudden recurrent episodes of sensory disturbance, loss of consciousness, or convulsions associated with abnormal electrical activity in the brain.
Epinephrine: A neurotransmitter and a hormone. It plays a vital role in the body's "fight-or-flight" response.
Epistaxis: A nosebleed is a loss of blood from the tissue lining the inside of the nose.
Erythema multiforme: A skin disorder considered an allergic reaction to medicine or an infection.
Erythrocytes: A type of blood cell made in the bone marrow and found in the blood. They contain a protein called hemoglobin, which carries oxygen from the lungs to all body parts.

Erythropoietin: A glycoprotein hormone that acts on stem cells of the bone marrow to stimulate red blood cell production.
Ethmoid bone: One of the eight bones of the cranium. It is situated at the roof of the nasal cavity and between the two orbital cavities.
Ethylene glycol: A synthetic liquid substance that absorbs water. It is odorless but has a sweet taste. It makes antifreeze and de-icing solutions for cars, airplanes, and boats.
Euphoria: A feeling or state of intense excitement and happiness.
Excipient: An inactive substance that serves as the vehicle or medium for a drug or other active substance.
Excitatory postsynaptic potential: A graded depolarization caused by the arrival of a neurotransmitter at the postsynaptic membrane. It develops from chemically gated ion channels that open in the plasma membrane, leading to membrane depolarization.
Excitotoxicity: A process that occurs when neurons are damaged or die due to excessive or prolonged exposure to excitatory amino acids, particularly glutamate.
Exclusivity: The right to have or do something limited to only one person or organization.
Excretion: The removal of drugs and their metabolites from the body.
Exfoliation: The process of removing dead skin cells from the skin's surface to improve its appearance.
Exfoliative dermatitis: A severe skin condition that causes extreme shedding of the top layers of the skin.
Exocytosis: A cellular process that moves large molecules and wastes out of a cell.
Expectorants: Medications that thin mucus in the lungs and throat, making it easier to cough up and remove from the lungs.
Extended-release: This method slowly releases a drug in the body over an extended period, significantly reducing dosing frequency.
Extrapyramidal reactions: Involuntary, uncontrollable movements.
Extrasystoles: A prematurely occurring beat of one of the heart's chambers that leads to momentary arrhythmia but leaves the fundamental rhythm unchanged.
Facet joint: The connections between the bones of the spine. The nerve roots pass through these joints from the spinal cord to the arms, legs, and other body parts.
Facilitated diffusion: The transport of substances across a cell membrane from an area of higher concentration to an area of lower concentration with the help of a transport molecule.
Factor Xa inhibitors: A class of blood thinners that prevent blood clots from forming or treating existing clots.
Fallopian tubes: Bilateral conduits between the female pelvis's ovaries and uterus.
Fasciculations: A brief, spontaneous contraction of a few muscle fibers.
Fat embolus: This occurs when fat globules enter the bloodstream, usually after a bone fracture or other trauma.
Fatty acids: Monoprotic acids, such as those found in animal and vegetable fats and oils, are saturated or unsaturated compounds with even carbon atoms. Examples include palmitic, stearic, and oleic acids.
Febrile neutropenia: A severe condition that occurs when a patient with neutropenia develops a fever.
Fertility: The ability of an organism to reproduce through natural sexual activity.
Fertilization: The process where a male sperm fuses with a female gamete to form a zygote, marking the initiation of development of a new individual organism; essentially, the union of two reproductive cells to create a new life.
Fetal-placental barrier: The tissues between maternal and fetal blood must be crossed to enable exchange.
Fibroblasts: A type of cell that contributes to the formation of connective tissue, a fibrous cellular material that supports and connects other tissues or organs in the body. They secrete collagen proteins that help maintain the structural framework of tissues.
Fibromyalgia: A chronic disorder characterized by widespread musculoskeletal pain, fatigue, and tenderness in localized areas.
Fidgety movements: Accelerated small neck, trunk, and limb movements.
First-order kinetics: A constant proportion of the drug is eliminated per unit time. The elimination rate is proportional to the amount of drug in the body. The higher the concentration, the greater the amount of drug eliminated per unit of time.
First-pass elimination: Presystemic metabolism, also called first-pass metabolism.
First-pass metabolism: The metabolism of drugs or chemicals in the liver or intestine before they reach the systemic circulation.
Flutter: A type of arrhythmia that causes the upper chambers of the heart to beat too quickly:
Formaldehyde: A chemical commonly used to kill germs and to preserve laboratory specimens and tissues. It is also used to make building materials (such as wood), glue, fabric, paint, fertilizers, pesticides, and other substances.
Formic acid: A colorless, corrosive liquid with a strong, pungent odor.
Formulary: An official list giving details of medicines that may be prescribed.
Free radicals: Any molecular species capable of independent existence that contains an unpaired electron in an atomic orbital.
Frequency distribution curves: Graphic depictions showing that in any given population, a range of doses is necessary to achieve a single, given effect in each of the individuals of that population. The dose at which 50% of the individuals show the response has been arbitrarily set to zero.
Full agonist: Having high efficacy, producing a complete response while occupying a relatively low proportion of receptors.
Fundus: The dome-shaped upper left part of the stomach stores gas and food when the stomach is full.
Fungi: A group of eukaryotic microorganisms, some of which are capable of causing superficial, cutaneous, subcutaneous, or systemic disease.
G-proteins: A family of proteins that act as molecular switches within cells, transmitting signals from external stimuli to the cell's interior by binding to and hydrolyzing guanosine triphosphate to regulate cellular processes.
Galactosemia: A rare hereditary disorder causing an inability to convert the simple sugar called galactose into glucose.
Gallstone: Solid cholesterol, bilirubin, and bile deposits in the gallbladder or bile ducts.
Gamma-aminobutyric acid: An amino acid that acts as a neurotransmitter in the central nervous system to reduce neuronal excitability and inhibit nerve transmission.
Ganglionic blockers: Agents that block transmission at the sympathetic and parasympathetic ganglia of the autonomic nervous system.
Gangrene: A severe condition that occurs when body tissue dies due to a lack of blood flow or a bacterial infection.
Gap junctions: Membrane channels that connect adjacent cells and allow the exchange of small molecules, substrates, and metabolites. They are a common form of intercellular communication and are critical for the function of many cells and tissues.
Gastric lavage: A medical procedure that removes the stomach's contents using a tube.
Gastric pits: Indentations in the stomach lining that lead to gastric glands.

Gastrin: A polypeptide hormone secreted by specific cells of the pyloric glands; it strongly stimulates the secretion of gastric acid and pepsin; it also weakly stimulates the secretion of pancreatic enzymes and gallbladder contraction.
Gastrinoma: A gastrin-secreting tumor usually found in the pancreas or duodenum. Duodenal wall tumors are frequently small and multiple.
Gastroesophageal reflux disease (GERD): A chronic digestive disorder that occurs when stomach acid flows back into the esophagus. It is caused by a malfunction of the lower esophageal sphincter, the muscle that usually closes to prevent stomach contents from flowing back up.
Gastroparesis: Paralysis of the stomach, also called gastroparalysis and gastroplegia.
Gastrostomy: An opening into the stomach from the abdominal wall, made surgically for food introduction.
Gastrotomy: The operation of cutting into the stomach.
Gene therapy: The transplantation of normal genes into cells in place of missing or defective ones to correct genetic disorders.
General anesthesia: A state of controlled unconsciousness induced by medication to prevent patients from feeling pain or being aware of their surroundings during surgery or other procedures.
Generalized anxiety disorder: A mental disorder that causes people to experience excessive and uncontrollable worry about everyday events.
Generalized seizures: Those that originate from multiple brain foci, characterized by general rather than localized neurologic symptoms; they may be tonic-clonic and may progress from a focal seizure.
Generic name: The official nonproprietary name of a drug under which it is licensed and identified by the manufacturer.
Genital herpes: A chronic sexually transmitted infection caused by the herpes simplex virus.
Genome expression: The process by which the information encoded in a gene is used to direct the assembly of a protein molecule.
Genome: The complete set of genetic information in an organism. It provides all of the information the organism requires to function.
Genomics: The branch of molecular biology concerned with the structure, function, evolution, and mapping of genomes.
Genotoxicity: Substances that may bind directly to DNA or act indirectly, leading to DNA damage by affecting enzymes involved in DNA replication.
Gestational diabetes: A condition during pregnancy that involves a defect in how the body processes and uses glucose in the diet; the pancreas is not engaged, while the placenta is implicated.
Ghrelin: A hormone secreted by the stomach cells that promotes hunger, decreases after eating, and promotes growth hormone secretion.
Giardia: A microscopic parasite that causes giardiasis, a common intestinal illness in diarrhea.
Gingival hyperplasia: An oral condition that causes your gums to overgrow.
Ginkgo biloba: An extract of ginkgo leaves that is held to enhance mental functioning by increasing blood circulation to the brain.
Ginseng: The root of a plant found in countries such as China, Russia, and America, which some people believe is good for your health.
Glaucoma: A group of eye diseases that cause vision loss by damaging the optic nerve.
Glomerular filtration rate: A measure of how well the kidneys function by estimating how much blood passes through the filters each minute.
Glomerulonephritis: A condition in which the tissues in the kidney become inflamed and have problems filtering waste from the blood.
Glomerulus: A network of vascular tufts encased in the capsule of the kidney.
Glucocorticoids: Involved in the metabolism of carbohydrates, proteins, and fats; they have anti-inflammatory activities.
Gluconeogenesis: The synthesis of glucose from noncarbohydrate sources, such as amino acids and glycerol. It occurs primarily in the liver and kidneys whenever the supply of carbohydrates is insufficient to meet the body's energy needs.
Glutamate: A salt or ester of glutamic acid, especially one that functions as a neurotransmitter that excites central nervous system cells.
Glutamine: An amino acid that plays a role in many bodily functions, such as the brain and immune system.
Glutaminergic receptor: A group of receptors in the central nervous system that mediate excitatory neurotransmission.
Glycine: A building block for making proteins in the body. It also transmits chemical signals in the brain, which are used for schizophrenia and improving memory.
Glycogen: An extensively branched glucose polymer that humans use as an energy reserve.
Glycogenolysis: The process of breaking down glycogen, a stored energy source in the liver and muscles, to produce glucose.
Glycolaldehyde: A simple organic molecule considered the smallest possible sugar molecule. It is often described as a potential precursor to more complex biomolecules, potentially playing a role in the origin of life due to its presence in interstellar space.
Glycolic acid: A chemical compound with various uses, including in skin care products and as a metabolite in ethylene glycol poisoning.
Goldenseal: A North American woodland plant of the buttercup family with a bright yellow root used in herbal medicine.
Gonadotropin-releasing hormone: A hormone that regulates the reproductive system by stimulating the release of other hormones from the pituitary gland.
Gonadotropin: Hormones that regulate the reproductive system, including the development, growth, and function of the ovaries and testes.
Gout: A disease in which defective metabolism of uric acid causes arthritis, especially in the smaller bones of the feet, deposition of chalkstones, and episodes of acute pain.
Grand mal seizures: A form of epilepsy characterized by tonic-clonic seizures in two phases: the tonic phase, in which the body becomes rigid, and the clonic phase, in which there is uncontrolled jerking. Tonic-clonic seizures may or may not be preceded by an aura and are often followed by headache, confusion, and sleep.
Gustatory: Related to the sense of taste.
Gynecomastia: Overdevelopment or enlargement of breast tissue in men or boys.
Half-life: The time required for half of a drug to undergo a process.
Hallucinations: Experiences of perceptions that are not real.
Hansen disease: A chronic infectious disease caused by Mycobacterium leprae. The disease affects the skin, the peripheral nerves, mucosal surfaces of the upper respiratory tract, and the eyes. Leprosy is known to occur at all ages, ranging from early childhood to old age.
Hapten: A small molecule combined with a larger carrier, such as a protein, can elicit antibodies and bind specifically to it.
Heart failure: A severe condition that occurs when the heart is unable to pump enough blood and oxygen to the body's organs.
Heberden nodes: Bony lumps that develop on the distal interphalangeal (DIP) joints of the fingers
Helicobacter pylori: A type of bacteria that causes infection in the stomach. It is the leading cause of peptic ulcers, and it can also cause gastritis and stomach cancer.
Hemarthrosis: A condition of articular bleeding that is into the joint cavity.

Hematopoiesis: The process of creating blood cells and bone marrow cells in the body.

Hematopoietic growth factors: A group of hormone-like proteins that regulate the production and maturation of blood cells.

Hematuria: The presence of blood or blood cells in the urine.

Heme: The part of specific molecules that contains iron. The heme part of hemoglobin is the substance inside red blood cells that binds to oxygen in the lungs and carries it to the tissues.

Hemifacial spasm: A neuromuscular disorder characterized by frequent involuntary contractions of the muscles on one side of the face.

Hemochromatosis: A disorder of iron metabolism characterized by excessive iron accumulation in the liver and other tissues and by the development of severe cirrhosis.

Hemodynamic response: A rapid delivery of blood to active neuronal tissue. Complications in this response arise in acute coronary syndromes and pulmonary arterial hypertension.

Hemolysis: The breakdown of red blood cells. Some diseases, medicines, and toxins may cause red blood cells to break down faster.

Hemolytic anemia: A disorder in which red blood cells are destroyed faster than they can be made.

Hemophilia: A rare, inherited bleeding disorder that prevents blood from clotting properly.

Hemoptysis: Coughing or spitting up blood from the respiratory tract.

Hemorrhagic stroke: A type of stroke that occurs when a blood vessel in or on the brain ruptures, causing bleeding into the brain or between the brain and skull.

Hemosiderosis: The accumulation of excess iron in the body as a direct result of multiple blood transfusions.

Hemozoin: A crystalline, iron-containing pigment produced by malaria parasites as a waste product of hemoglobin digestion

Hepatic congestion: A condition that occurs when blood backs up in the liver due to increased pressure or compromised blood flow.

Hepatic portal circulation: A portal vein carrying blood from the stomach, small intestine, and spleen to the liver, where hepatocytes alter the nutrients carried by the blood before passing into the systemic circulation.

Hepatic portal circulation: A unique circulatory system that connects two systems of capillary beds: one in the sinusoidal area of the liver and the other in the wall of the small intestine and spleen. Its blood flow to the liver is unique because it receives deoxygenated and oxygenated blood.

Hepatocellular carcinoma: Primary liver tumor that is the most common type of liver cancer in adults

Hepatocytes: The primary parenchymal tissue of the liver.

Herbals: Products derived from plants or their oils, roots, seeds, berries, or flowers. They have been used for many centuries. Herbal supplements are believed to have healing properties.

High-alert medications: Drugs that bear a heightened risk of causing significant patient harm when they are used in error. Although mistakes may or may not be more familiar with these drugs, the consequences of a mistake are more devastating to patients.

High-altitude sickness: A group of symptoms that can occur when a person ascends to a higher altitude too quickly.

Hilar adenopathy: Enlargement of the lymph nodes within the lung hilum can be an essential finding for underlying pathology.

Hirsutism: A condition that causes excessive growth of dark or coarse body hair in a male-like pattern, such as on the face, chest, and back. It is the most common endocrine disorder in women.

HMG-CoA reductase inhibitors: Lipid-lowering medications used in the primary and secondary prevention of coronary heart disease.

Homeostatic downregulation: The process by which a cell decreases the quantity of components such as RNA or proteins in response to external stimuli.

Human papillomavirus infection: The most common sexually transmitted infection in the United States. There are more than 200 types of HPV, and most infections cause no symptoms and resolve on their own within two years. However, some types of HPV can cause genital warts, precancerous lesions, and certain types of cancer.

Human papillomaviruses: A group of viruses that can cause warts and some types of cancer:

Humanistic therapies: Focus on free will, human potential, and self-discovery.

Huntington's disease: A rare, inherited, and progressive brain disorder that causes uncontrolled movements, emotional problems, and loss of thinking ability.

Hydramnios: A condition that occurs when too much amniotic fluid builds up during pregnancy.

Hydrolysis: A typical chemical reaction where water is mainly used to break down the chemical bonds between a particular substance.

Hydrophobia: An extreme fear of water, significantly when associated with painful laryngeal spasms caused by rabies.

Hydrostatic pressure: The force a fluid exerts in a confined space due to gravity. In physiology, hydrostatic pressure is essential for blood pressure and fluid movement in and out of blood vessels.

Hydroxylation: A chemical process that adds a hydroxyl group (-OH) to an organic compound.

Hyperaldosteronism: A condition that occurs when the adrenal glands produce too much aldosterone, the hormone responsible for balancing potassium and sodium in the body.

Hyperglycemia: An abnormality in the circulating blood, especially in patients with diabetes mellitus.

Hyperintensities: Features of the white matter in imaging studies that predict an increased risk of stroke, dementia, and death.

Hyperkinetic: Related to hyperactive behaviors.

Hyperplasia: Increased cell production in a normal tissue or organ. It may be a sign of abnormal or precancerous changes.

Hypertensive crisis: A sudden, severe increase in blood pressure 180/120 mm Hg or greater. It is a medical emergency. It can lead to a heart attack, stroke, or other life-threatening health problems.

Hyperthyroidism: A condition in which the thyroid gland produces too much thyroid hormone.

Hyperuricemia: A condition with too much uric acid in the blood.

Hypervigilance: A state of heightened awareness and watchfulness.

Hypnosis: A state of focused attention and deep relaxation where a person is more responsive to suggestions.

Hypoadrenalism: A rare disorder that occurs when the adrenal glands do not produce enough hormones.

Hypoesthesia: A partial or total loss of sensation in the body. It can involve a tingling sensation and make a person less sensitive to touch, temperature, vibration, or pain.

Hypogonadism: A condition that occurs when the body's sex glands, or gonads, produce little to no sex hormones.

Hypomanic stage: A component of bipolar disorder in which there is increased energy, activity, mood, or behaviors before full mania occurs.

Hypopnea: The condition of taking shallow breaths for 10 seconds or longer while asleep, with the airflow being at least 30% lower than usual.
Hypothalamus: A portion of the brain below the thalamus, which links the endocrine system to the nervous system, regulates metabolic processes, and synthesizes and secretes neurohormones.
Hypoxia: A medical condition that occurs when the body's tissues do not have enough oxygen to maintain homeostasis.
Idiopathic hemochromatosis: A rare, chronic disease that causes iron building in the body.
Idiosyncratic responses: Adverse effects that cannot be explained by the known mechanisms of action of the offending agent do not occur at any dose in most patients and develop mostly unpredictably in susceptible individuals only.
Ileocecal valve: A sphincter muscle at the junction of the ileum and colon.
Immunogenicity: The ability of a substance to cause an immune response in an organism.
Immunoglobulin E: An antibody that plays a crucial role in allergic reactions and the body's response to parasites.
Impotence: The inability to have an erection of the penis adequate for sexual intercourse. Also called erectile dysfunction.
Induction: The initial therapy used when treating a disease.
Induration: The thickening and hardening of soft tissues, specifically the skin, results from an inflammatory process caused by various triggering factors.
Infiltration injections: Local anesthesia is produced by injecting the anesthetic solution directly into the area of terminal nerve endings.
Influx: Movement of a substance into the cell.
Infundibulum: A hollow funnel-shaped mass in front of the tube cinereum that extends to the posterior lobe of the pituitary gland.
Ingredients: Any substance intended for incorporation into a finished drug product.
Inhibitory postsynaptic potential: A synaptic response that reduces the likelihood of a neuron firing an action potential. IPSPs occur when transmitter molecules bind to receptors, causing an influx of negatively charged ions that hyperpolarize the postsynaptic membrane.
Inotropic: A substance that increases or decreases the force of muscular contractions.
Inotropy: Refers to the myocardium contractions and changes the force of those contractions.
Insomnia: A sleep disorder involving trouble falling asleep or staying asleep.
Intermittent claudication: Lower extremity skeletal muscle pain that occurs during exercise.
Interphalangeal joints: The hinge-shaped joints that connect the phalanges of the fingers and toes.
Interstitial nephritis: A condition where there is inflammation within the kidneys.
Interstitial nephritis: A kidney condition that causes inflammation in the renal interstitium, the area between the kidney tubules.
Intrinsic activity: The maximal possible effect that a drug can produce. Medicines that bind to a receptor and create an intense action have high intrinsic activity related to efficacy.
Intrinsic factor: A protein the stomach produces that helps the body absorb vitamin B12.
Intrinsic factors: A protein that helps the intestines absorb vitamin B12. It is made by cells in the stomach lining.
Inverse agonists: A drug that binds to the same receptor as an agonist but induces a pharmacological response opposite the agonists.
Ion trapping: The accumulation of a chemical across a cell membrane due to a difference in pH and the chemical's pKa value.
Iris: The colored part of the eye that surrounds the pupil. It regulates the amount of light that enters the eye. Lens: The lens is an explicit part of the eye behind the iris that helps to focus light and images on the retina.
Iritis: An inflammation of the iris.
Irritable bowel syndrome: A common condition characterized by abdominal discomfort associated with altered bowel movements. The main symptom of IBS is abdominal pain or discomfort associated with a change in bowel habits.
Ischemic stroke: A life-threatening condition that occurs when blood flow to the brain is blocked.
Islet of Langerhans: Also called the pancreatic islets, these regions contain the pancreas's endocrine cells. They comprise 2% of the pancreas's volume and are essential in glucose metabolism.
Isoforms: Any of two or more functionally similar proteins with a similar but not an identical amino acid sequence.
IsozymesEach of two or more enzymes with identical functions but different structures.: Each of two or more enzymes with identical functions but different structures.It is a manifestation of peripheral arterial disease, which includes atherosclerotic stenosis of arteries in the extremities.
Japanese encephalitis: A viral infection of the brain that is spread by infected mosquitoes.
Jaundice: Yellow staining of the skin and sclerae of the eyes by abnormally high blood levels of the bile pigment bilirubin.
Juvenile idiopathic arthritis: The most common type of arthritis in kids and teens. It typically causes joint pain and inflammation in the hands, knees, ankles, elbows, and wrists.
Juxtaglomerular apparatus: A specialized structure formed by the distal convoluted tubule and the glomerular afferent arteriole.
Juxtaglomerular cells: Located in the walls of the afferent and efferent arterioles in the kidney. They produce, store, and release renin.
Kaposi's sarcoma: A cancer that causes red or purple patches of abnormal tissue to grow under the skin. A rare cancer that is often linked to HIV infection:
Keratitis: An inflammation of the cornea of the eye.
Keratomalacia: An eye disorder that involves drying and clouding of the cornea in people with undernutrition.
Ketoacidosis: A severe life-threatening condition requiring immediate treatment. Symptoms include nausea, vomiting, abdominal pain, and rapid breathing.
Kinesiophobia: An irrational and debilitating fear of physical movement or activity due to a fear of painful injury or reinjury.
Kwashiorkor: A form of malnutrition caused by protein deficiency in the diet, typically affecting young children in the tropics.
Lacrimal glands: Almond-sized glands located in the upper, outer part of the eye's orbit that produce tears.
Lassitude: A state of physical or mental weariness and lack of energy.
Legionella species: A type of gram-negative bacteria that can cause Legionnaires' disease and Pontiac fever.
Leishmaniasis: A parasitic disease caused by the bite of an infected sandfly and the infection with Leishmania parasites:
Lepromatous leprosy: A type of leprosy that causes widespread skin lesions and affects the nervous system.
Leprosy: A slowly progressing bacterial infection that affects the skin, peripheral nerves in the hands and feet, and mucous membranes of the nose, throat, and eyes. Destruction of the nerve endings causes the affected areas to lose sensation.
Lethargy: A lack of energy and enthusiasm.

Leukocytes: Also known as white blood cells (WBCs), are cells in the blood that are part of the immune system and help the body fight infection and disease

Leukopenia: A decrease in white blood cells in the blood (usually neutrophils).

Leukotrienes: A group of inflammatory mediators produced in leukocytes and involved in allergic and inflammatory responses.

Libido: A person's overall sexual drive or desire for sexual activity. Biological, psychological, and social factors influence libido.

Ligamentum flavum: A ligament that binds adjacent vertebral laminae to each other.

Ligand: A ligand is a substance that forms a complex with a biomolecule to serve a biological purpose.

Lipid profile: A blood test that can measure the amount of cholesterol and triglycerides in the blood.

Lipodystrophy: A group of genetic or acquired disorders in which the body cannot produce and maintain healthy fat tissue.

Lipogenesis: A metabolic process that converts fatty acids and glycerol into fats, or triglycerides, for storage in fat.

Lipolysis: The metabolic process through which triacylglycerols break down via hydrolysis into their constituent molecules.

Listeriosis: A bacterial infection caused by eating food contaminated with Listeria monocytogenes. It can lead to severe illness, including meningitis, encephalitis, and sepsis, and can sometimes be fatal.

Liver transplantation: A surgical procedure that replaces a diseased or damaged liver with a healthy liver from a donor.

Loading dose: A dose of medication, often more significant than subsequent doses, administered to establish a therapeutic level of the medication.

Locus ceruleus: A nucleus in the pons involved in responses to stress and panic.

Loop of Henle: Extended U-shaped tubule portion that conducts urine within each nephron.

Lou Gehrig's disease: A progressive neurodegenerative disease that affects nerve cells in the brain and spinal cord. It is also called amyotrophic lateral sclerosis (ALS).

Lutein hormone: A hormone that plays a vital role in the reproductive system and is produced in the pituitary gland.

Lyme disease: An inflammatory disease caused by a spirochete *(Borrelia burgdorferi)* that is transmitted by ticks and usually characterized by an initial rash followed by flulike symptoms, including fever, joint pain, and headache. If left untreated, the disease can result in chronic arthritis and nerve and heart dysfunction.

Lymph nodes: Small, bean-shaped immune system clusters that filter lymphatic fluid and help the body fight infection and disease.

Lymphoma: A type of blood cancer affecting the lymphatic and immune systems.

Ma huang: An extract of ma huang containing ephedrine and related alkaloids is used as a dietary supplement.

Macrocytic: Red blood cells that are larger than usual.

Macrophages: A type of white blood cell that surrounds and kills microorganisms, removes dead cells, and stimulates the action of other immune system cells.

Macula densa: **A** group of specialized cells in the nephron that monitors sodium levels in the fluid passing through the kidney's convoluted tubule.

Maintenance doses: The maintenance rate [in mg/h] of drug administration equals the rate of elimination at a steady state.

Major depressive disorder: Also called depression, a mood disorder causing a persistent feeling of sadness and loss of interest in life.

Malaria: A life-threatening disease caused by parasites that infect red blood cells and are transmitted by the bite of an infected mosquito. A single-celled parasite of the genus Plasmodium causes it.

Malathion: An insecticide classified as an organophosphate that controls mosquitos and other pests, including lice.

Malignant hyperthermia: A severe reaction to certain anesthetics involving dangerously high body temperature, muscle abnormalities, and tachycardia.

Marasmus: Severe undernourishment causing an infant's or child's weight to be significantly low for their age (e.g., below 60 percent of average).

Mast cells: The cells in the connective tissue that contain many granules rich in histamine and heparin.

Mastalgia: Pain or discomfort in one or both breasts.

Mastication: The process by which the teeth crush and grind food. It is the first step in the process of digestion.

Mastocytosis: A rare disease that happens when your body makes too many mast cells.

Matrix: An extensive network of proteins and other molecules that surround, support, and give structure to cells and tissues in the body.

Measles: A highly contagious viral disease that causes a rash, fever, cough, runny nose, and other symptoms.

Median effective dose: The dose produces a response of 50% of the maximum obtainable.

Median lethal dose: The dose causing mortality in 50% of animals.

Medication administration record: A written record of medications prescribed for and administered to a patient.

Medication cartridges:

Medication error: Mistakes in prescribing, dispensing, and giving medications.

Medication reconciliation: The process of identifying the most accurate list of all medications that the patient is taking.

Mediterranean fever: An inherited autoinflammatory disease characterized by recurrent episodes of fever and acute inflammation of the membranes lining the abdomen, joints, and lungs.

Medulla oblongata: The part of the brain that connects the brainstem to the spinal cord. It's located at the base of the skull and is responsible for several essential functions.

MedWatch program: **This program a**llows healthcare professionals and consumers to report serious problems that they believe may be associated with the medical products they prescribe, dispense, or use.

Megaloblastic anemia: A blood disorder that occurs when the bone marrow produces abnormally large red blood cells. It is a type of macrocytic anemia.

Melanoma: The most invasive skin cancer with the highest risk of death. At the same time, it is a severe skin cancer and highly curable if diagnosed early.

Melatonin: A hormone that helps regulate the body's sleep-wake cycle and circadian rhythm.

Meningitis: A severe infection that causes inflammation of the membranes that cover the brain and spinal cord.

Meningococcemia: A bloodstream infection caused by Neisseria meningitidis.

Menopause: The time in a woman's life when the periods stop.

Menstrual cycle: The monthly hormonal changes from the beginning of one menstrual period to the start of the next.

Menstrual periods: The monthly vaginal bleeding that occurs when the lining of the uterus sheds.

Metabolic acidosis: Characterized by an increase in the hydrogen ion concentration in the systemic circulation, resulting in a serum HCO3 less than 24 mEq/L.

Metabolic encephalopathy: A group of neurological disorders that occur when a chemical imbalance in the blood affects the brain. Some underlying conditions, such as diabetes, liver disease, renal failure, heart failure, drug overdose, and bacterial meningitis, can cause this imbalance.

Metallic taste: A lost or changed sense of smell can cause a metallic taste in the mouth. It may be caused by oral hygiene, nutrient deficiencies, infections, and taking certain supplements.

Methyl alcohol: A colorless, flammable, and highly toxic organic chemical compound. It is used to make antifreeze, pesticides, windshield wiper fluid, paint thinner, certain types of fuel, and other substances. It is also called wood alcohol.

Microcytic: Red blood cells that are smaller than usual.

Micromedex: Easy-to-use online tool to effectively manage and update hospital formulary and communicate the most current information facility-wide.

Microscopic colitis: Swelling and irritation, called inflammation, of the large intestine.

Microsomal enzyme system: A collection of enzymes in the smooth endoplasmic reticulum of liver cells that modify molecules to make them more polar and less lipid-soluble.

Migraine headaches: Moderate to severe headaches, often on one side of the head.

Miliary tuberculosis: A potentially fatal and severe form of tuberculosis that occurs when the bacteria Mycobacterium tuberculosis spreads through the bloodstream and affects multiple organs.

Milk thistle: A flowering herb related to the daisy and ragweed family. It is native to Mediterranean countries.

Mindfulness-based cognitive therapy: A type of psychotherapy that uses cognitive behavioral methods with mindfulness meditative practices.

Mineralocorticoids: A class of steroid hormones regulating the body's water and salt balance.

Minimum effective concentration: The minimum plasma concentration of a drug needed to achieve sufficient drug concentration at the receptors to produce the desired pharmacologic response.

Miosis: Excessive constriction of the pupil of the eye.

Miscarriage: The spontaneous loss of a fetus before the 20th week of pregnancy.

Mitosis: A process in which a cell replicates its chromosomes and then divides into two identical daughter cells:

Mitral valve: One of four valves in the heart that keep blood flowing in the right direction. Each valve has flaps called leaflets that open and close once during each heartbeat.

Modulation: The functional and morphologic fluctuation in response to changing environmental conditions.

Molds: A type of fungi microscopic organism that grows in long filaments called hyphae.

Monitored anesthesia care: A type of anesthesia that involves administering sedatives to a patient while continuously monitoring their vital signs.

Monoaminergic systems: Networks of neurons that use monoamine neurotransmitters, which regulate emotion, arousal, and some forms of memory.

Morbidity: Having a disease or a symptom of disease, or the amount of disease within a population.

Mortality: The number of deaths in a particular group in a certain period.

Motilin: A hormone that regulates the gastrointestinal tract, helping to move food through the digestive system.

Mpox: Previously known as monkeypox, it is a viral illness caused by the monkeypox virus, a species of the genus Orthopoxvirus.

Mucositis: A complication of some cancer therapies in which the lining of the digestive system becomes inflamed. They are often seen as sores in the mouth.

Multiple myeloma: A cancer of plasma cells that is generally incurable.

Multiple sclerosis: A chronic, typically progressive disease involving damage to the sheaths of nerve cells in the brain and spinal cord, whose symptoms may include numbness, impairment of speech and muscular coordination, blurred vision, and severe fatigue.

Multiple sclerosis: A chronic, typically progressive disease involving damage to the sheaths of nerve cells in the brain and spinal cord, whose symptoms may include numbness, impairment of speech and muscular coordination, blurred vision, and severe fatigue.

Mumps: A contagious viral infection that causes painful swelling of the salivary glands, usually in the cheeks and jaw. It is spread by contact with saliva or respiratory droplets from an infected person, and it's as contagious as the flu.

Muscarinic antagonists: Agents that competitively block cholinergic responses.

Muscarinic receptors: G-coupled protein receptors involved in the parasympathetic nervous system. The only exception to these receptors is the sweat glands, which possess muscarinic receptors but are part of the sympathetic nervous system.

Myalgia: A painful sensation evolving from muscle tissue.

Myasthenia gravis: A chronic autoimmune disorder in which antibodies destroy communication between nerves and muscles, resulting in skeletal muscle weakness.

Mycoplasma pneumoniae: A common respiratory pathogen that produces diseases of varied severity ranging from mild upper respiratory tract infection to severe atypical pneumonia. Although rarely fatal, it is a significant cause of acute respiratory tract infections.

Mydriases: An unusual dilation or widening of the pupils. There are various causes of this fixed dilation of the pupils. The condition may be caused by dilating eye drops from an eye exam.

Mydriasis: Prolonged dilatation of the pupil of the eye.

Myelosuppression: A condition that occurs when the bone marrow's activity is reduced, resulting in a decrease in red blood cells, white blood cells, and platelets.

Myocardium: The Middle layer of the heart walls. Which is responsible for the contractile function of the cardiac pump.

Myoclonic seizure: Characterized by brief, jerking muscle or muscle group spasms. They often occur with atonic seizures, which cause sudden muscle limpness.

Myofascial pain syndromes: A chronic condition that causes muscle pain and fascia, the thin connective tissue surrounding muscles (epimysium).

Myometrium: The middle layer of the uterine wall, consisting mainly of uterine smooth muscle cells but also of supporting stromal and vascular tissue.

Myopathy: Any disorder of the skeletal muscles.
Myxedema: Severe hypothyroidism, leading to decreased mental status, hypothermia, and other symptoms related to slowed function in multiple organs; it is a medical emergency with a high mortality rate.
Narrow therapeutic index: Drugs where slight differences in dose or blood concentration may lead to serious therapeutic failures and adverse drug reactions that are life-threatening or result in persistent or significant disability or incapacity.
Narrow-angle glaucoma: Also called closed-angle or angle-closure glaucoma, the eye pressure increases very quickly compared to the more common open-angle glaucoma.
Necrosis: The death of most or all of the cells in an organ or tissue due to disease, injury, or failure of the blood supply.
Necrotizing enterocolitis: The death of tissue in the intestine. It occurs most often in premature or sick babies.
Nephritic syndrome: A clinical syndrome that presents as hematuria, elevated blood pressure, decreased urine output, and edema.
Nephron: A single kidney unit that filters the blood and forms urine from waste products.
Nephrotoxicity: Rapid deterioration in kidney function due to toxic effects of medications and chemicals.
Nerve block anesthesia: A nerve block is an anesthetic and anti-inflammatory injection that treats pain by targeting a specific nerve or group of nerves.
Neural plexuses: Networks of nerves in the body that supply sensory and motor nerves to different regions.
Neuralgia: A sharp, shocking pain that follows the path of a nerve and is due to irritation or damage to the nerve.
Neuroglycopenia: Glycopenia in the brain, usually due to hypoglycemia, affects the function of neurons and alters brain function and behavior; if prolonged or recurrent, it can cause loss of consciousness, brain damage, and death.
Neurohypophysis: the posterior lobe of the pituitary gland.
Neurokinin receptor: A receptor involved in some physiological processes, including pain and stress.
Neuroleptanalgesia: The combination of a potent sedative analgesic agent (an opioid) and a tranquilizer.
Neuroleptic malignant syndrome: A life-threatening neurologic emergency associated with the use of antipsychotic agents and characterized by a distinctive clinical syndrome of mental status change, rigidity, fever, and dysautonomia.
Neuromodulators: Substances that do not directly activate ion-channel receptors but that, acting together with neurotransmitters, enhance the excitatory or inhibitory responses of the receptors.
Neuromuscular blockers: Agents that paralyze skeletal muscles by blocking the transmission of nerve impulses at the myoneural junction.
Neuromuscular junctions: A highly specialized synapse between a motor neuron nerve terminal and its muscle fiber responsible for converting electrical impulses generated by the motor neuron into electrical activity in the muscle fibers.
Neurotoxicity: Damage to the brain or peripheral nervous system from exposure to toxic substances.
Neurotransmitters: The chemical agents released by neurons to stimulate other neurons, muscles, or gland cells, thus allowing impulses to be passed from one cell to the next throughout the nervous system.
Neutral antagonists: Those that bind equally to active and inactive states of G-protein-coupled receptors, blocking actions of agonists and inverse agonists.
Neutropenia: A condition where there are abnormally low levels of neutrophils in the blood.
Nicotinic receptors: Channel proteins that open after binding to acetylcholine to allow cation diffusion.
Nicotinic: Refers to the effects of nicotine on nerve fibers and the nicotinic acetylcholine receptors.
Nocardiosis: An infectious disease caused by *Nocardia*, which is a gram-positive bacillus with a branching hyphae morphology found throughout the environment in soil, decomposing vegetation, and other organic matter.
Nociceptive pain: A receptor in the form of a naked dendrite that responds to a pain stimulus.
Nocturnal cough: a cough that occurs at night.
Nocturnal enuresis: The involuntary release of urine during sleep. It is a common condition that affects children, teenagers, and adults.
Nocturnal seizure: A form of epilepsy that can cause abnormal movement or behavior during sleep.
Norepinephrine: A chemical messenger that functions as a hormone and a neurotransmitter in the body.
Normal flora: Microorganisms are always present on or in a person and usually do not cause disease.
Normocytic: Characterized by red blood cells that are normal in size and usually also in hemoglobin content.
Nystagmus: Rapid involuntary movements of the eyes.
Obsessive-compulsive disorder: A mental disorder that causes people to have unwanted, recurring thoughts and feelings.
Obstructive jaundice: A condition characterized by the obstruction of bile flow from the liver to the small intestine.
Oculogyric crisis: Spasmodic movements of the eyeballs into a fixed position, usually upwards. These episodes generally last minutes but can range from seconds to hours.
Olfaction: The sense of smell, a unique sensory modality that plays a crucial role in mating, survival, and shaping the quality of life in humans.
Oligo-ovulatory: A condition that causes irregular or infrequent ovulation and periods.
Oligohydramnios: Decreased amniotic fluid volume for gestational age. The most common causes are premature rupture of membranes and placental insufficiency.
Oliguria: A reduced amount of urine production.
On-off phenomenon: A state in which an individual exhibits a rapid fluctuation of akinetic and choreoathetotic movements when treated with dopa for Parkinson's disease.
Onchocerciasis: A rare tropical parasitic disease transmitted by a black fly. Infection by the parasite can cause eye and skin problems. In humans, the parasitic worms live under the skin.
Onychomycosis: A fungal infection of the nail that causes discoloration, thickening, and separation from the nail bed.
Oocyte: The female gamete cell.
Open-angle glaucoma: A chronic, irreversible, and progressive optic neuropathy that occurs when the drainage canals of the eye become clogged. This leads to a gradual increase in eye pressure and a loss of peripheral vision. It is the most common type of glaucoma.
Opioid crisis: A devastating consequence of the opioid epidemic that includes increases in opioid misuse and related overdoses.
Optic neuritis: An inflammatory condition that demyelinates the optic nerve and degrades vision in one or both eyes.
Orange Book: A freely accessible list maintained by the FDA describing all pharmaceutical drugs that have been proven safe and effective.

Orchitis: The inflammation of the testicle unilaterally or bilaterally, usually caused by viruses and bacteria.
Orexin: A neuropeptide that regulates arousal, wakefulness, and appetite.
Orgasm: The final part of the sex act, which involves the contraction of sexual organs and a sudden release of endorphins, leading to a feeling of pleasure.
Oromandibular dystonia: A focal dystonia that affects the mouth, jaw, and tongue, making speaking difficult.
Orphan drugs: Drugs that treat rare diseases and conditions are considered both therapeutic and commercial orphans because they have too small a patient population to render their development commercially viable.
Orthostatic hypotension: A condition that occurs when blood pressure drops suddenly after standing up from a sitting or lying down position.
Osmoreceptors: Sensory neurons in the brain that detect changes in the body's osmotic pressure and help maintain fluid balance.
Osmotic pressure: The minimum pressure that needs to be applied to a solution to prevent the inward flow of its pure solvent across a semi-permeable membrane.
Osteoarthritis: Degeneration of joint cartilage and the underlying bone, most common from middle age onward. It causes pain and stiffness, especially in the hip, knee, and thumb joints.
Osteocalcin: A protein found in bone that plays a role in bone formation, calcium homeostasis, and energy metabolism.
Osteomalacia: Softening of the bones, typically through vitamin D or calcium deficiency.
Osteoporosis: A bone disease that causes bones to become weak and more likely to break. It occurs when the amount and thickness of bone tissue decreases or when the structure of bone changes.
Otitis media: An ear infection and middle ear inflammation that occurs when fluid builds up behind the eardrum.
Ototoxicity: Ear poisoning from drug or chemical exposure often impairs hearing and balance.
Ovulation: A phase in the menstrual cycle when the ovary releases an egg (ovum).
Ovum: The female reproductive cell.
Oxidation: A process that occurs when atoms or groups of atoms lose electrons.
Pallidotomy: The surgical inactivation of a part of the basal ganglia in treating involuntary movements (as in Parkinson's disease).
Pancytopenia: A lower-than-normal number of red and white blood cells and platelets in the blood.
Paneth cells: Specialized epithelial cells in the small intestine that play a vital role in maintaining the health of the intestinal tract.
Panic disorder: An anxiety disorder characterized by unexpected and repeated episodes of intense fear accompanied by physical symptoms.
Panuveitis: Inflammation of all layers of the uvea of the eye, which includes the iris, ciliary body, and choroid. These make up the middle layer of the eye.
Paracrine hormones: Local hormones that act on nearby cells without entering the bloodstream.
Paradoxical hyperactivity: The condition in which administration of stimulant drugs to hyperactive children leads to a decrease in their excessive motor activity.
Parafollicular cells: Also known as C-cells, are a type of cell in the thyroid gland that produces calcitonin.
Paralysis idiopathic: Paralysis occurs when the exact cause is unknown.
Paralytic ileus: A condition that occurs when the muscles of the intestines are paralyzed, preventing food from passing through.
Paranasal sinuses: Hollow, air-filled spaces in the skull and facial bones around the nose.
Paranoia: A mental disorder in which a person has an extreme fear and distrust of others. A paranoid person may have delusions that people are trying to harm them.
Parasympathomimetics: A class of drugs that mimic the effects of acetylcholine to activate the parasympathetic nervous system.
Parathyroid hormone: A hormone that regulates calcium levels in the blood and phosphorus and vitamin D levels. Parathyroid glands secrete it.
Parenteral route: Any non-oral means of administration, generally interpreted as injecting directly into the body, bypassing the skin and mucous membranes.
Paresthesia: A feeling of numbness, burning, or tingling, usually in the extremities, such as the hands and feet.
Parietal cells: Cells in the stomach that produce hydrochloric acid and intrinsic factors, which help with digestion and the absorption of vitamin B12.
Parkinson's disease: A progressive disease of the nervous system marked by tremors, muscular rigidity, and slow, imprecise movement, chiefly affecting middle-aged and older adults. It is associated with degeneration of the brain's basal ganglia and a deficiency of the neurotransmitter dopamine.
Parotid glands: The largest of the three primary pairs of salivary glands, on either side of the face, just below and in front of the ears.
Partial agonist: This agonist produces sub-maximal activation even when occupying the total receptor population and, therefore, cannot produce the maximal response.
Partial placenta previa: A condition where the placenta partially covers the cervix.
Partial pressure: The pressure that would be exerted by one of the gases in a mixture if it occupied the same volume on its own.
Partial prothrombin time: Measures how long it takes for a patient's blood to clot and is used to assess the function of clotting factors.
Partial seizure: A partial (focal) seizure occurs when unusual electrical activity affects a small brain area. It is a simple partial seizure when the seizure does not involve awareness.
Passive diffusion: A process by which an ion or molecule passes through a cell wall via a concentration gradient or from an area of high concentration to an area of low concentration.
Pepsin: A stomach enzyme that digests proteins found in ingested food.
Pepsinogen: A protein digestive enzyme produced by the stomach that is converted into pepsin by stomach acid.
Peptic ulcers: A sore in the stomach lining or the duodenum.
Perception: The ability to see, hear, or become aware of something through the senses.
Peristalsis: Series of involuntary muscle contractions that move food and other substances through the body.
Peritoneum: A serous membrane that lines the abdominal cavity, consisting of two layers: the parietal peritoneum, which lines the abdominal wall, and the visceral peritoneum, which covers the abdominal organs.
Peritonitis: A life-threatening condition that involves inflammation of the peritoneum, the tissue that lines the abdominal wall and covers most of the abdominal organs.

Pernicious anemia: A condition in which the body cannot properly absorb vitamin B12, leading to a lower-than-normal number of red blood cells.
Peroxisomes: Specialized for carrying out oxidative reactions using molecular oxygen.
Petechia: Tiny bleeding spots under the skin or in the mucous membranes.
pH: A measure of hydrogen ion concentration, a measure of the acidity or alkalinity of a solution. The pH scale usually ranges from 0 to 14.
Phantom limb pain: The perception of pain or discomfort in a limb that is no longer there. It is most commonly presented as a sequela of amputation.
Pharmacogenetics: The branch of pharmacology concerned with the effect of genetic factors on reactions to drugs.
Pharmacogenomics: The branch of genetics concerned with how an individual's genetic attributes affect the likely response to therapeutic drugs.
Pharmacogenomics: The branch of genetics concerned with how an individual's genetic attributes affect the likely response to therapeutic drugs.
Pharmacokinetics: The branch of pharmacology concerned with the movement of drugs within the body.
Pharmacopeia: A book describing drugs, chemicals, and medicinal preparations especially.
Pharyngitis: The inflammation of the mucous membranes of the oropharynx. In most cases, the cause is an infection, either bacterial or viral.
Phenylketonuria: Also known as PKU, a rare inherited disorder with increased phenylalanine, an amino acid, in the blood; this is toxic to the CNS.
Pheochromocytoma: A tumor of the chromaffin cells, most often found in the medulla of the adrenal gland.
Phlebitis: A condition where a vein becomes inflamed, usually in the legs, and can be caused by infection, injury, or irritation.
Phospholipids: A class of lipids that are the primary components of cell membranes and essential for life.
Photophobia: A painful sensitivity to or extreme intolerance of bright light.
Photosensitivity: Having a chemical, electrical, or other response to light.
Pill rolling motions: A circular movement or tremor of the tips of the thumb and the index finger when brought together, as seen in Parkinson's disease.
Pitting edema: A condition where fluid builds up under the skin, causing swelling and a persistent indentation when pressure is applied.
Pituitary gland: The endocrine gland at the base of the brain that secretes hormones to control metabolism, growth, sexual maturation, reproduction, and blood pressure.
Placebo: A harmless pill, medicine, or procedure prescribed more for the psychological benefit of the patient than for any physiological effect.
Plasma albumin: A significant contributor to maintaining the osmotic pressure of plasma and assists as a carrier protein for steroids, fatty acids, and thyroid hormones in the blood. It also plays a significant role in stabilizing extracellular fluid volume.
Plasma cells: White blood cells (B lymphocytes) that produce antibodies to fight infection:
Plasma osmolarity: The number of particles of solute per liter of solution, whereas the term osmolality refers to the number of solute particles per kilogram of solvent.
Platelet aggregation: The process by which platelets adhere to each other at sites of vascular injury has long been recognized as critical for hemostatic plug formation and thrombosis.
Platelet aggregation: The process by which platelets adhere to each other to form a hemostatic plug. I
Pleural effusion: An abnormal fluid collection between the thin layers of tissue (pleura) lining the lung and the chest cavity wall.
Pneumococcal disease: A severe bacterial infection caused by Streptococcus pneumoniae.
Pneumonia: A lung infection that causes the air sacs to fill with fluid or pus, making breathing difficult.
Poliomyelitis: A viral infection that affects the central nervous system. It is highly contagious and can cause paralysis, but large-scale vaccination programs have helped eliminate it from most parts of the world.
Polycystic kidney disease: A genetic disorder that causes fluid-filled sacs, called cysts, to grow in the kidneys. The cysts can start to develop in the kidneys at any time, from before birth to adulthood. It is a chronic condition that can lead to kidney failure.
Polycystic ovary syndrome: A condition in which a female has little or no menstruation, is infertile, has excessive body hair, and is obese; the ovaries may contain several cysts.
Polycythemia: An increase in the blood's total red blood cell mass.
Polydipsia: Excessive thirst or excess drinking.
Polymorphism: A condition involving one or several variants of a particular DNA sequence, usually a variation at a single base pair.
Polymyalgia rheumatica: A chronic inflammatory disorder that causes pain and stiffness in the neck, shoulders, and hips.
Polymyositis: An uncommon inflammatory disease that causes muscle weakness affecting both sides of the body.
Polypharmacy: The simultaneous use of multiple drugs by a single patient for one or more conditions.
Pons: The most significant part of the brainstem, located above the medulla and below the midbrain.
Porphyria: A rare hereditary disease in which the blood pigment hemoglobin is metabolized abnormally. Porphyrins are excreted in the urine, which becomes dark; other symptoms include mental disturbances and extreme skin sensitivity to light.
Portal hypertension: Elevated pressure in the portal venous system. The portal vein is a central vein that leads to the liver. The most common cause of portal hypertension is cirrhosis of the liver.
Post-traumatic stress disorder: A mental health condition that can develop after experiencing or witnessing a traumatic event.
Postganglionic neurons: Part of the autonomic nervous system and are responsible for regulating the activity of many organs in the body.
Potency: The quantity of drug necessary. Produce a given effect, or it may refer to the maximum response achieved with the drug.
Potentiate: The effect of increasing the power or effectiveness of a drug or other treatment.
Preeclampsia: A disorder of pregnancy characterized by high blood pressure and, often, a significant amount of protein in the urine; it begins after 20 weeks of pregnancy **and**
Premenstrual syndrome: Any of a complex of symptoms (including emotional tension and fluid retention) experienced by some women in the days immediately before menstruation.
Presynaptic opioid receptors: Located in axon terminals and reduce neurotransmission by inhibiting the release of excitatory neurotransmitters.
Primary bronchi: The first and most extensive branches of the respiratory tree, and are the two primary tubes that branch off from the trachea and supply air to each lung.
Primary hypertension: Unknown causes of hypertension.
Prinzmetal's angina: Characterized by chest pain at rest with transient ischemic electrocardiographic changes in the ST segment, with a prompt response to nitrates. Pt is also called vasospastic or variant angina.

Prodrome: An early symptom indicating the onset of a disease or illness.
Prodrugs: A compound with little or no pharmacological activity that metabolizes inside the body and converts into a pharmacologically active drug compound.
Proliferation: A rapid multiplication of parts or the increase in the number of something.
Prostaglandin: A group of lipids made at tissue damage or infection sites involved in dealing with injury and illness. They control inflammation, blood flow, clot formation, and labor induction.
Proteinuria: A condition where there is an excess of protein in the urine:
Proteonomics: The study of proteomes, which are proteins produced in an organism, system, or biological context.
Prototype drug: An individual drug that represents a drug class – a group of medications having similar chemical structures, mechanism of action, and mode of action.
Protozoan: A microscopic, single-celled organism that can invade and live in the cells and tissues of humans.
Proximal convoluted tubule: A renal tubule segment in the kidney that reabsorbs water and solutes from the glomerular filtrate and returns them to the bloodstream.
Pseudocholinesterase: An enzyme in the liver that metabolizes certain drugs, including anesthesia and local anesthetics.
Pseudomembranous colitis: A severe colon inflammation caused by an overgrowth of the bacterium Clostridioides difficile.
Psoriatic arthritis: A chronic inflammatory disease that affects the joints and tendons. It is often associated with the skin condition psoriasis.
Psychodynamic therapies: Those who focus on the psychological roots of emotional suffering use self-reflection and self-examination.
Psychostimulants: Psychotropic substances that can stimulate the CNS.
Pulmonary arteries: Blood vessels that carry deoxygenated blood from the right side of the heart to the lungs.
Pulmonary edema: A life-threatening condition that occurs when too much fluid builds up in the lungs, making it difficult to breathe.
Pulmonary embolectomy: A major surgical procedure that removes a pulmonary embolism.
Pulmonary embolism: A blockage in a lung artery caused by a blood clot that has traveled from elsewhere in the body. It is a life-threatening medical emergency that requires immediate treatment.
Pulmonary hypertension: A severe condition that occurs when the blood pressure in the lungs is abnormally high.
Pulmonary trunk: A short, thick artery that carries deoxygenated blood from the heart to the lungs.
Punctate keratopathy: Corneal inflammation of diverse causes characterized by scattered, acceptable, punctate corneal epithelial loss or damage.
Purkinje fibers: Specialized nerve cells that transmit electrical signals to the heart's ventricles, causing them to contract. This contraction allows blood to flow from the heart to the rest of the body.
Pylorus: The part of the stomach that connects to the duodenum.
Pyrexia: The elevation of core body temperature above normal.
Rabies: A fatal viral disease that attacks the central nervous system and is spread through the bite or scratch of an infected animal.
Radiculopathy: A set of conditions in which one or more nerves are affected and do not work correctly.
Range of motion: The distance and direction a joint can move from fully extended to fully flexed. It is a measure of flexibility that involves the muscles, ligaments, tendons, bones, and joints.
Rational emotive behavior therapy: A psychotherapy that attempts to resolve emotional and behavioral problems and any disturbances of them.
Raynaud's syndrome: A disease characterized by spasms of the arteries in the extremities, especially the fingers (Raynaud's phenomenon). It is typically brought on by constant cold or vibration and leads to pallor, pain, numbness, and, in severe cases, gangrene.
Red man syndrome: An infusion-related reaction to vancomycin. It typically consists of pruritus, an erythematous rash that involves the face, neck, and upper torso.
Reflex tachycardia: An increased heart rate to compensate for decreased blood pressure.
Reflexes: An automatic, involuntary, and nearly instantaneous response to a stimulus. They allow the body to adapt to a changing environment and protect itself from injury or damage.
Refractory periods: Inactivity after a neuron or muscle cell has undergone excitation. As the cell is repolarized, it will not respond to any stimulus during this period.
Regional anesthesia: A type of pain management for surgery that numbs a large part of the body, such as from the waist down.
Regurgitation: The act of bringing swallowed food back into the mouth.
Renal corpuscle: a filtration unit in the kidney that filters blood and forms urine.
Renin: An enzyme secreted by the kidney that is part of a physiological system that regulates blood pressure.
Repolarization: The process by which a cell's membrane potential returns to its normal resting state after a nerve impulse or action potential.
Resistant hypertension: a blood pressure that remains above goal despite concurrent use of three antihypertensive agents of different classes taken at maximally tolerated doses.
Restless legs syndrome: A chronic neurological disorder that causes an uncontrollable urge to move the legs.
Reticular cells: A type of fibroblast that provides structural support and is involved in the immune response.
Reticular endothelial system: A group of cells in the body that remove dead or abnormal cells, tissues, and foreign substances.
Reticular formation: A diffuse network of nerve pathways in the brainstem connecting the spinal cord, cerebrum, and cerebellum and mediating the overall level of consciousness.
Retinoic acid: A nutrient that the body needs in small amounts to function and stay healthy. It is made in the body from vitamin A and helps cells to grow and develop, especially in the embryo.
Retinoids: A class of chemical compounds that are natural derivatives of vitamin A or are chemically related to it.
Rhabdomyolysis: A severe syndrome due to muscle injury; release of contents from muscle fibers into the bloodstream can lead to renal failure.
Rheumatic heart disease: A condition that occurs when the heart valves are permanently damaged by rheumatic fever.
Rheumatoid arthritis: A chronic autoimmune disease that causes joint pain, swelling, stiffness, and loss of function.
Rhinorrhea: A condition where the nasal cavity is filled with a significant amount of mucus fluid.
Rickettsiae: A diverse collection of obligately intracellular Gram-negative bacteria found in ticks, lice, fleas, mites, chiggers, and mammals.
Risk-benefit ratio: The ratio of the risk of an action to its potential benefits.
Rituals: Activities that involve gestures, words, actions, or objects, always performed in a particular order.

Rubella: Also known as German measles, it is a contagious viral infection that is usually mild.
Rugae: A series of folds or wrinkles in the wall of an organ.
Sacral hiatus: The inferior end of the sacral canal at the level of S3-S4 on the dorsal surface, where filum terminale emerges.
Sacroiliac joint: Lies next to the spine and connects the sacrum (the triangular bone at the bottom) with the pelvis (iliac crest). It is a robust, weight-bearing joint that acts as a shock-absorbing structure for all upper body forces.
Saddle block anesthesia: A form of spinal anesthesia that produces loss of sensation in the buttocks, perineum, and inner thighs.
Sarcoidosis: A rare disease that causes the immune system to form inflamed lumps called granulomas in the lungs, skin, and eyes.
Sarin: A chemical nerve agent used in warfare.
Saturation kinetics: The kinetics of a reaction or mediated transport when the velocity increases to a plateau as the concentration of a component is increased.
Saw palmetto: A small palm with fan-shaped leaves with sharply toothed stalks, native to the southeastern US.
Scheduled drugs: Are sorted into their schedules based on their potential for abuse, legal status, and medicinal uses.
Schwannomas: A rare, non-cancerous tumor that grows in the nervous system.
Scleroderma: A chronic autoimmune disease that causes the skin and other body parts to harden and thicken. It occurs when the immune system mistakenly attacks healthy tissue, causing inflammation and the body to produce too much collagen.
Scotoma: A visual field abnormality or a blind spot.
Secondary bronchi: The first subdivision of the main bronchi in the lungs.
Secretin: A hormone released into the blood circulation by the duodenum (especially in response to acidity) to stimulate secretion by the liver and pancreas.
Sentinel events: The patient safety event that results in death, permanent harm, or severe temporary harm.
Sepiapterin reductase: A rare genetic disorder that causes movement problems, intellectual disability, and other symptoms.
Sepsis: A life-threatening medical emergency that occurs when the body's immune system has an extreme response to an infection or injury.
Serotonin syndrome: A severe drug reaction caused by medications that build up high serotonin levels in the body. Serotonin is a chemical that the body produces naturally. It's needed for the nerve cells and brain to function.
Serotonin: A chemical messenger that plays a crucial role in many bodily functions, including mood, sleep, digestion, and wound healing.
Serum sickness: An immune-complex-mediated hypersensitivity reaction that classically presents with fever, rash, polyarthritis, or polyarthralgia.
Severe combined immunodeficiency: A rare, inherited genetic disorder that causes a child to be born with a weakened immune system.
Sexual arousal: A state of physiological arousal elicited by sexual contact or by other erotic stimulation.
Sexual promiscuity: The practice of engaging in sexual activity with different partners or being indiscriminate in choosing sexual partners.
Shingles: Also called herpes zoster or zona. Any person who has had chickenpox can develop shingles. This condition erupts along the course of the affected nerve, producing lesions anywhere on the body and may cause severe nerve pain.
Sialorrhea: A condition that occurs when there is too much saliva in the mouth.
Sickle cell disease: An inherited disease in which the red blood cells have an abnormal crescent shape, block small blood vessels and do not last as long as normal red blood cells. Sickle cell disease is caused by a mutation in one of the genes for hemoglobin. It is most common in people of West and Central African descent. Also called sickle cell anemia.
Side effects: Any effect of a drug, chemical, or other medicine that is in addition to its intended effect, especially an effect that is harmful or unpleasant.
Sideroblastic anemia: A type of anemia that results from abnormal utilization of iron during erythropoiesis.
Sigma receptors: Protein cell surface receptors that bind ligands; when activated, effects include hypertonia, tachycardia, tachypnea, antitussive effects, and mydriasis.
Sinoatrial node: A small mass of tissue made up of nerve fibers embedded in the musculature of the higher right atrium that originates the impulses stimulating the heartbeat.
Sinus dysrhythmia: A condition where the heart rate varies, typically by more than 10 beats per minute.
Sinusitis: An inflammation of the sinuses and mucous membranes that line them.
Sjögren's syndrome: An autoimmune disease that attacks the glands that make tears and saliva.
Skin abrasions: An abrasion is a superficial rub or wearing off of the skin, usually caused by a scrape or a brush burn.
Skull hypoplasia: An underdevelopment of the skull, which can affect specific bones in the skull, such as the frontal bone, zygomatic bone, or maxilla.
Sleep apnea: A sleep disorder that causes people to stop breathing or breathing shallowly while sleeping.
Slit junctions: Intercellular adhesion complexes in epithelia and endothelia that control paracellular permeability.
Slurred speech: Also called dysarthria. Speech impairment may cause several conditions, including brain injury, stroke, multiple sclerosis, Parkinson's disease, and cerebral palsy. Some substances, such as alcohol, opioids, barbiturates, and benzodiazepines
Smart infusion pumps: Medication delivery devices that use a combination of computer technology and drug libraries to limit the potential for dosing errors.
Smith-Magenis syndrome: A developmental disorder involving intellectual disability, delayed speech and language skills, distinctive facial features, sleep disturbances, and behavioral problems.
Social phobia: An anxiety disorder that causes people to experience persistent fear and anxiety in social situations.
Somatic pain: Originates from damage or inflammation to the body's tissues, such as the skin, muscles, bones, joints, ligaments, tendons, and mucous membranes.
Somatic system: A part of the peripheral nervous system that controls voluntary movement and sensory input.
Somatotropin: A hormone synthesized in and secreted by the anterior lobe of the pituitary gland that promotes growth of the long bones in the limbs and increases the synthesis of protein essential for growth.
Spermatogenesis: The process by which sperm cells are produced in the testicles.
Sphenoid bone: One of the seven bones that articulate to form the orbit. Its shape resembles that of a butterfly or bat with its wings extended.
Sphingolipids: A specialized group of lipids essential to the composition of the plasma membrane of many cell types; however, they are primarily localized within the nervous system

Spinal block anesthesia: A procedure in which a pharmaceutical agent is administered into the subarachnoid space, producing a loss of sensation at and below the level of the block.

Spores: A single-celled reproductive unit produced by certain plants, fungi, and bacteria, which is capable of developing into a new individual without fusing with another cell, essentially acting as a means of asexual reproduction and often able to survive harsh conditions due to its thick protective wall.

Squamous stratified epithelium: A tissue that covers and lines parts of the body and comprises multiple layers of flattened cells that are tightly joined together. Its principal function is to protect the body from wear and tear.

St. John's wort: A plant with yellow flowers used in traditional European medicine as far back as the ancient Greeks.

Stable angina: Chest pain of cardiac origin that has not changed in character, frequency, intensity, or duration for 60 days.

Statins: A class of medications that lower cholesterol and reduce the risk of cardiovascular disease.

Status epilepticus: A seizure that lasts longer than 5 minutes, or having more than one seizure within 5 minutes, without returning to an average level of consciousness between episodes, is called status epilepticus. This is a medical emergency that may lead to permanent brain damage or death.

Sterol: Any group of predominantly unsaturated solid alcohols of the steroid group, such as cholesterol and ergosterol, found in animals, plants, and fungi, especially as components of cell membranes.

Stevens-Johnson syndrome: A rare, severe skin reaction that occurs when the immune system overreacts to a trigger, such as a medication or infection.

Stillbirth: The death or loss of a baby before or during delivery.

Strabismus: A condition in which the visual axes of the eyes are not parallel, and the eyes appear to be looking in different directions.

Striatum: The part of the basal ganglia that coordinates motor and action planning, decision-making, motivation, reinforcement, and reward perception.

Stroke volume: The volume of blood discharged from the ventricle with each contraction; in adults, it is usually about 70 ml.

Stroma: The cells and tissues that support and give structure to organs, glands, or other tissues in the body.

Strychnine: A highly toxic, colorless, bitter, crystalline powder that can cause severe health effects, including death.

Stupor: A state of near-unconsciousness or insensibility.

Subarachnoid hemorrhage: A life-threatening medical emergency that occurs when a blood vessel ruptures and bleeds into the space between the brain and the arachnoid membrane.

Subarachnoid space: The cerebrospinal fluid-filled space between the arachnoid and the pia.

Subdural hematoma: A blood collection that forms between the dura mater and the brain.

Sublingual route: Placing a drug under the tongue to dissolve and absorb into the blood circulation.

Submucosal fibroids: A non-cancerous tumor that grows in the muscle layer of the uterus, just beneath the lining

Substance abuse: The harmful or hazardous use of psychoactive substances, including alcohol and illicit drugs. One of the critical impacts of illegal drug use on society is the negative health consequences experienced by its members.

Substance misuse: A serious public health challenge. It includes the use of illegal drugs and the inappropriate use of legal substances, such as alcohol.

Substantia gelatinosa: A gray matter structure in the spinal cord that plays a crucial role in how the body perceives pain, temperature, and touch.

Sudden infant death syndrome: The term used to describe the sudden death of a baby younger than 1 year of age that does not have a known cause, even after a full investigation.

Supraoptic neurons: Large neurosecretory cells in the hypothalamus that produce and release oxytocin and vasopressin.

Sustained-release: Designed to slowly release a drug in the body over an extended period, significantly to sustain therapeutic levels.

Sympathetic nervous system: A network of nerves that controls the body's "fight-or-flight" response. It is part of the autonomic nervous system, which controls many functions without conscious thought.

Syncope: A brief loss of consciousness caused by a temporary drop in blood pressure that results in decreased blood flow to the brain. A quick onset, short duration, and spontaneous recovery characterize syncope.

Synergistic effect: An interaction between two or more drugs that causes the total effect of the drugs to be greater than the sum of the individual effects of each drug.

Synovitis: A medical condition that involves inflammation of the synovial membrane, the connective tissue that lines joints.

Systemic lupus erythematosus: A disease where a person's immune system attacks and injures the body's organs and tissues. Almost every system of the body can be affected by SLE.

Tachycardia: A heart rate of more than 100 beats per minute at rest.

Tachyphylaxis: A decrease in response to a drug due to prior exposure to the agent, which may be countered by increasing the dose.

Tachypnea: Rapid and shallow breathing faster than usual for a person's age and condition.

Tactile: Related to the sense of touch.

Tardive dyskinesia: A neurological disorder characterized by involuntary movements of the face and jaw.

Teratogen: Any agent that causes an abnormality following fetal exposure during pregnancy. They are usually discovered after an increased prevalence of a particular birth defect.

Terpenes: The primary constituents of essential oils and are responsible for the aroma characteristics of cannabis.

Tertiary bronchi: The third level of branching in the bronchial tree, located at the edge of the lungs.

Tetanus: A bacterial infection that causes muscle spasms and lockjaw, also known as trismus.

Tetracyclic antidepressants: Those that contain four rings of atoms; most of them do not inhibit the reuptake of serotonin.

Thalamus: A large mass of gray matter in the diencephalon; it relays sensory signals, including motor signals, to the cerebral cortex and regulates consciousness, sleep, and alertness.

The Joint Commission: An independent, not-for-profit organization that accredits and certifies health care organizations and programs.

The margin of safety: The ratio of the lethal dose to 1% of the population to the effective dose to 99% of the population (LD1/ED99). It is used to measure drug safety in the pharma industry.

Therapeutic drug monitoring: Measuring the amount of certain medicines in the blood.

Therapeutic index: A ratio that compares the blood concentration at which a drug becomes toxic and the concentration at which the drug is effective. The larger the therapeutic index, the safer the drug is.
Therapeutic range: The dosage range in serum concentration expected to achieve the desired therapeutic effect.
Therapeutic window: The dosage range of a drug or its concentration in a bodily system that provides safe and effective therapy.
Thermogenesis: The process by which organisms produce heat is a typical result of metabolic processes.
Thrombocytes: Small, colorless cell fragments in the blood that form clots and stop or prevent bleeding. They are also called platelets.
Thrombocytopenia: An abnormally low amount of platelets.
Thrombolytics: Medications used to dissolve blood clots.
Thrombosis: Local coagulation or clotting of blood in the circulatory system.
Thrombus: A blood clot that forms inside one of the veins or arteries.
Thymus: A gland in the chest that plays a vital role in the immune system by producing and maturing immune cells, particularly T lymphocytes, and secret thymosin.
Thyroglobulin: A protein produced by the thyroid gland that helps store and synthesize thyroid hormones.
Thyroid-stimulating hormone: Thyrotropin, a hormone secreted by the anterior lobe of the pituitary gland that explicitly has an affinity for and stimulates the thyroid gland.
Thyrotoxicosis: A condition resulting from excessive concentrations of thyroid hormones in the body, such as hyperthyroidism.
Thyrotropin-releasing hormone: A hormone that regulates thyroid gland activity by stimulating the production and release of thyroid-stimulating hormone (TSH) in the pituitary gland.
Thyrotropin: A hormone secreted by the anterior lobe of the pituitary gland that has an affinity for and stimulates explicitly the thyroid gland.
Tinea capitis: A contagious fungal infection that affects the scalp, hair, and hair follicles.
Tinnitus: Ringing or buzzing in the ears.
Tocopherols: A group of organic compounds that act as antioxidants and are essential for human health.
Tocotrienols: A group of compounds belonging to the vitamin E family.
Tolerance: A person's diminished response to a drug occurs when the drug is used repeatedly, and the body adapts to its continued presence.
Tonic spasm: A single, prolonged contraction of a muscle or group of muscles that results in abnormal posturing and rigidity.
Tonic-clonic seizure: The classic type of epileptic seizure consists of two phases to a tonic-clonic seizure – the tonic phase and the clonic phase.
Tophus: A deposit of monosodium urate crystals in the blood of people with longstanding high levels of uric acid in the blood.
Topical route: Application to body surfaces such as the skin or mucous membranes to treat ailments via an extensive range of classes, including creams, foams, gels, lotions, and ointments.
Tourette's syndrome: A disorder involving repetitive movements or sounds (tics) that are difficult to suppress.
Toxic megacolon: An acute form of colonic distension. It is characterized by a very dilated colon, accompanied by abdominal distension and sometimes fever, abdominal pain, or shock.
Toxoplasmosis: An infectious disease caused by the one-celled protozoan parasite *Toxoplasma gondii*. Although most individuals do not experience any symptoms, the disease can be severe and even fatal in individuals with weakened immune systems.
Trachea: A long, U-shaped tube that connects the larynx to the lungs.
Trade name: A commercial name granted by a naming authority for marketing a drug/device product in a particular jurisdiction.
Trancelike state: A half-conscious state, seemingly between sleeping and waking.
Transcranial magnetic stimulation: A noninvasive form of brain stimulation in which a changing magnetic field causes electric currents at certain brain areas through electromagnetic induction.
Transdermal patches: The medicated adhesive pad is placed on the skin to deliver a timed-release dose of medication through the skin into the bloodstream.
Transduction: The action or process of transferring genetic material from one microorganism to another by a viral agent.
Traveler's diarrhea: A gastrointestinal infection that affects many travelers to areas with poor sanitation and limited access to safe drinking water. It's caused by consuming food or water contaminated with bacteria, viruses, or parasites.
Trichomoniasis: A sexually transmitted infection caused by a parasite called Trichomonas vaginalis.
Tricyclic antidepressants: Those that contain three rings of atoms; they are second-line drugs following the SSRIs.
Triglycerides: A type of fat that circulates in the blood and is the most common fat in the body.
Trophic hormones: A type of hormone produced by the anterior pituitary gland under the stimulation of hypothalamic-releasing factors.
Trophozoites: The activated feeding stage in certain protozoa's life cycle, such as malaria-causing Plasmodium falciparum.
Truncal obesity: Abdominal central obesity, in which there is excessive visceral fat around the stomach and abdomen.
Trypanosomiasis: A parasitic disease caused by protozoans of the genus Trypanosoma.
Tryptophan: An essential amino acid that the body needs to function correctly but cannot produce independently.
Tsetse flies: Any of several dipteran flies that occur in Africa south of the Sahara and include vectors of human and animal trypanosomes.
Tuberculosis: A contagious bacterial infection that spreads through the air and usually affects the lungs. The bacteria Mycobacterium tuberculosis causes it.
Tubular reabsorption: The kidneys remove water and solutes from the filtrate and return them to the bloodstream. It is the second major step in urine formation.
Tubular secretion: A process in the kidneys that moves waste products and other substances from the blood into the renal tubules.
Tuft cells: Chemosensory cells in the epithelial lining of the intestines. Similar tufted cells are found in the respiratory epithelium or brush cells.
Tumor lysis syndrome: A life-threatening medical condition that occurs when cancer cells break down rapidly, releasing their contents into the bloodstream.
Tumor necrosis factor: A protein made by white blood cells in response to an antigen or infection.
Typhoid fever: A bacterial infection that causes a high fever, abdominal pain, diarrhea, and other symptoms. It is also called enteric fever and is caused by salmonella bacteria.
Tyrosine: An amino acid that helps the body produce neurotransmitters, hormones, and melanin.
Ulcerative colitis: A chronic inflammatory bowel disease that causes inflammation in the colon and rectum.

Unipolar: A person's mood state is abnormal and only on one side. This is in contrast to bipolar depression, which involves both a depressed mood and a manic mood.
Unstable angina: Chest pain of cardiac origin that is variable, usually increasing in frequency and intensity and with irregular timing.
Upregulation: The increase in the number or density of cell surface receptors for a physiologically active substance, causing an increase in sensitivity in response to persistent exposure.
Uremia: A clinical condition associated with declining renal function and is characterized by fluid overload, electrolyte imbalances, metabolic abnormalities, and physiological changes.
Urticaria: A skin rash known as "hives," presenting with itching, redness, or lumps called "wheels."
Urushiol: A toxic, liquid catechol derivative, the active irritant principle in several species of the plant genus Rhus, as in poison ivy.
Vagal nerves: the primary nerves of the parasympathetic nervous system that control specific body functions such as digestion, heart rate, and immune system.
Vagotonic: Related to vagotonia, which is overactivity or irritability of the vagus nerve.
Valerian: A plant that typically bears clusters of small pink or white flowers. Native to Eurasia, several species have been introduced to North America.
Varicella: A highly contagious disease caused by the varicella-zoster virus.
Varicella: A highly contagious disease marked by an itchy, blister-like rash caused by the varicella-zoster virus (a type of herpesvirus). The virus is easily spread from person to person through contact with mucus, saliva, or fluid from the blisters of an infected person or through droplets released when an infected person coughs or sneezes. Also called chickenpox.
Vasoconstrictor: A drug or nerve that causes blood vessels to narrow or constrict.
Vasodilators: Medications that open or dilate blood vessels, allowing blood to flow more easily.
Vastus lateralis muscle: The vastus lateralis is a muscle in the thigh that is part of the quadriceps muscle.
Vena cava filter: A metal device implanted in the inferior vena cava to prevent blood clots from traveling to the lungs.
Ventilation: The air movement between the environment and the lungs via inhalation and exhalation.
Ventricular fibrillation: A life-threatening arrhythmia occurs when the ventricles twitch instead of beating normally.
Vernal conjunctivitis: A chronic, non-contagious allergic inflammation of the eyes that causes seasonal eye irritation.
Vertigo: A symptom that causes a false sensation of motion or spinning, often described as dizziness.
Vestibular system: A network of structures and neural pathways that helps maintain the balance and sense of orientation.
Villi: Small, finger-like projections that increase the surface area of a membrane and help absorb nutrients.
Virilism: A condition in which females develop male traits such as male pattern baldness or excessive facial hair.
Virion: A complete, infectious virus particle consisting of a nucleic acid genome surrounded by capsid.
Visceral pain: Originates in the internal organs, such as the heart, lungs, bladder, reproductive organs, or digestive system, and the tissue that covers them
Volatile liquid: Liquid that evaporates at room temperature or vaporizes quickly.
Volatile liquids: Liquid that evaporates at room temperature or vaporizes quickly.
Von Willebrand disease: A bleeding disorder that occurs when the blood does not clot properly. It is the most common inherited bleeding disorder in the world and affects people of all races and genders.
Vulvovaginal candidiasis: Vaginal infection with *Candida* species, usually *C. albicans*. Symptoms are generally a thick, white vaginal discharge and vulvovaginal pruritus that is often moderate to severe.
Warts: Non-cancerous skin growths caused by the human papillomavirus.
Wheezing: A high-pitched whistling sound that occurs when breathing in or out and can indicate breathing difficulty.
Whooping cough: A highly contagious bacterial infection affecting the lungs and bronchi. It begins like a cold but becomes severe coughing and gasping for air. Long coughing spells may cause vomiting and broken blood vessels in the eyes and skin. Also called pertussis.
Withdrawal: Discontinuation of the use of an addictive substance.
Wolf-Parkinson-White syndrome: A rare heart condition that causes an arrhythmia. Between the atria and ventriculus.
Xerophthalmia: Abnormal dryness of the conjunctiva and cornea of the eyes is caused by a deficiency in vitamin A.
Xerostomia: A papule, nodule, or plaque in the skin due to lipid deposits; it is usually yellow but may be brown, reddish, or cream-colored.
Xerostomia: Dry mouth caused by insufficient production of saliva.
Xerostomia: Dry mouth caused by insufficient production of saliva.
Yeasts: Single-celled, eukaryotic microorganisms classified as fungi, which reproduce by budding and are commonly used in baking and brewing due to their ability to ferment sugars into alcohol and carbon dioxide.
Yellow fever: A viral disease transmitted to humans through the bite of infected mosquitoes.
Zero-order kinetics: A constant amount of drug is eliminated per unit of time, but the rate is independent of the drug's concentration.
Zollinger-Ellison syndrome: A rare condition in which one or more tumors grow in the pancreas or the upper part of the small intestine.
Zona fasciculata: The thick middle layer of the adrenal cortex.
Zona glomerulosa: The outermost layer of the adrenal cortex.
Zona reticularis: The innermost layer of the adrenal cortex.

Index

Page numbers followed by "*f*" indicate figures, "*t*" indicate tables, and "*b*" indicate boxes.

B

C

D

E

H

I